AF616592

GASTROINTESTINAL MUCOSAL BIOPSY

CONTEMPORARY ISSUES IN SURGICAL PATHOLOGY VOLUME 20

SERIES EDITOR

Lawrence M. Roth, M.D.

Professor of Pathology
Director, Division of Surgical Pathology
Indiana University School of Medicine
Indianapolis, Indiana

Previously published

Vol. 6 Tumors and Tumorlike Conditions of the Ovary
Lawrence M. Roth, M.D., and Bernard Czernobilsky, M.D.

Vol. 7 Pathology of the Testis and Its Adnexa
Aleksander Talerman, M.D. , and Lawrence M. Roth, M.D.

Vol. 9 Pathology of the Vulva and Vagina
Edward J. Wilkinson, M.D.

Vol. 12 Pathology of the Heart and Great Vessels
Bruce F. Waller, M.D.

Vol. 13 Pathology of the Urinary Bladder
Robert H. Young, M.D.

Vol. 15 Pathology of the Prostate
David G. Bostwick, M.D.

Vol. 16 Tumors and Tumor–like Conditions of the Kidneys and Ureters
John N. Eble, M.D.

Vol. 17 Pathology of the Colon, Small Intestine, and Anus, 2nd Ed.
H. Thomas Norris, M.D.

Vol. 18 Tumors and Tumorlike Lesions of Soft Tissue
Vito Ninfo, M.D., E.B. Chung, M.D., M.Sc., Ph.D., and
Andrea O. Cavazzana, M.D.

Vol. 19 Tumors and Tumorlike Lesions of the Uterine Corpus and Cervix
Philip B. Clement, M.D., and Robert H. Young, M.D., M.R.C. Path.

GASTROINTESTINAL MUCOSAL BIOPSY

Harvey Goldman, M.D.
Professor of Pathology
Harvard Medical School
Chairman, Department of Pathology
New England Deaconess Hospital
and
New England Baptist Hospital
Boston, Massachusetts

With the collaboration of

Jihad Hayek, M.D.
Senior Pathologist
Department of Pathology
New England Deaconess Hospital
Boston, Massachusetts

Micheline Federman, Ph.D.
Senior Research Scientist
Department of Pathology
New England Deaconess Hospital
Boston, Massachusetts

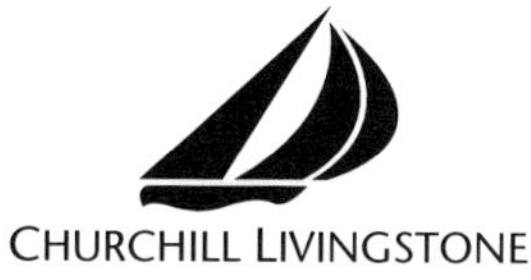

CHURCHILL LIVINGSTONE

New York, Edinburgh, London, Madrid, Melbourne, San Francisco, Tokyo

Library of Congress Cataloging-in-Publication Data

Goldman, Harvey, date
Gastrointestinal mucosal biopsy / Harvey Goldman with the collaboration of Jihad Hayek, Micheline Federman.
p. cm. — (Contemporary issues in surgical pathology ; v. 20)
Includes bibliographical references and index.
ISBN 0-443-08990-6
1. Gastrointestinal system–Biopsy. 2. Gastrointestinal mucosa.
I. Hayek, Jihad. II. Federman, Micheline. III. Title. IV. Series.
[DNLM: 1. Gastrointestinal System—pathology. 2. Gastrointestinal Diseases—pathology. 3. Biopsy. 4. Gastric Mucosa—pathology. 5. Intestinal Mucosa—pathology. WI CO769MS v. 20 1996 / WI 141 G619g 1996]
RC804.B5G65 1996
616.3'307—dc20
DNLM/DLC
for Library of Congress

95-40823
CIP

Distributed in the United Kingdom by Churchill Livingstone, Robert Stevenson House, 1–3 Baxter's Place, Leith Walk, Edinburgh EH1 3AF, and by associated companies, branches, and representatives throughout the world.

Accurate indications, adverse reactions, and dosage schedules for drugs are provided in this book, but it is possible that they may change. The reader is urged to review the package information data of the manufacturers of the medications mentioned.

The Publishers have made every effort to trace the copyright holders for borrowed material. If they have inadvertently overlooked any, they will be pleased to make the necessary arrangements at the first opportunity.

Acquisitions Editor: *Kerry Willis*
Assistant Editor: *Marc Strauss*
Production Editor: *Elizabeth Bowman-Schulman*
Production Supervisor: *Sharon Tuder*

Printed in the United States of America

First published in 1996 7 6 5 4 3 2 1

To the many colleagues, residents, fellows, and students
who have provided the cases and inspiration for this endeavor

and

To Eleonora, with love

Preface

Gastrointestinal Mucosal Biopsy is intended to serve as a guide to the analysis of mucosal biopsies in all portions of the alimentary tract, including the esophagus, stomach, small and large intestines, and anal canal. Presented are the uses, interpretations, and limitations of such biopsies in a wide assortment of inflammatory and tumor conditions, involving both children and adults. Of the inflammatory disorders, there are extensive examples of motor and mechanical diseases, of effects caused by chemical and physical agents, of infectious and ischemic conditions, and of the major idiopathic disorders. Also included are details of mucosal biopsies used to detect and to monitor the assorted tumors, premalignant conditions, and tumor-like lesions that affect each of the gut segments. Major emphasis is placed on the more common disorders, but there is an effort to identify numerous examples of rare conditions as well. The greatest detail is on general concepts and especially on the histologic features and differential diagnosis of the various conditions.

The material is presented in 11 chapters, based on a functional approach with separate material on the esophagus, the stomach, and the duodenum as obtained by upper endoscopy; on the jejunum mainly from aspiration-type biopsy; on the ileum from lower endoscopy or direct evaluation of ileostomy segments; and on the large intestine and anal region from lower endoscopy. The book has 107 tables and 431 illustrations, including 26 in color and 36 electron micrographs. The color photomicrographs contain examples of infectious agents, of cytologic smears, and of special stains. These are presented at the end of Chapter 1 and serve as a reference throughout the book. Many of the specific diagnoses in surgical pathology, particularly those related to types of tumors, depend on immunocytochemical stains. Illustrations of these examples are kept to a minimum, however, because they tend to have a similar appearance in the histologic sections. Rather, representative electron micrographs (listed in the appendix) are provided to help delineate the features.

Gastrointestinal Mucosal Biopsy should serve as a practical handbook for surgical pathologists and other morphologists who examine and interpret mucosal biopsies of the gut. It will also be of use to all physicians and surgeons who participate in endoscopic and other gastrointestinal tract procedures.

Harvey Goldman, M.D.

Acknowledgments

The author is indebted to Dr. Jihad Hayek and Dr. Micheline Federman for their invaluable aid and guidance in the preparation of *Gastrointestinal Mucosal Biopsy*. Dr. Hayek helped to identify the case material and produced all the illustrations of the histologic sections. Dr. Federman contributed the ultrastructural pictures and supervised the overall preparation and quality of the photographs.

We thank the following colleagues who provided microscopic slides or transparencies that were used to prepare the illustrations: Dr. Donald Antonioli for Figs. 4-8A, 9-21, and 9-29; Dr. Karoly Balogh for Figs. 3-1 and 9-32; Dr. Ronald Bardawil for Plates 3A to 3H; Dr. Bertha Garcia and Dr. David Hurlbut for Fig. 8-15; Dr. Harry Kozakewich for Figs. 2-23, 4-31, 6-20, and 9-34; Dr. Cynthia Needham for Plate 2D; Dr. Robert Odze for Figs. 3-2 and 5-1; Dr. Antonio Perez-Atayde for Fig. 7-25; and Dr. Carlos Villamil for Fig. 6-14 and Plate 2A. We are especially grateful to Julie Nuttall Morry, B.S., for producing all the non-color illustrations and to Mrs. Nancy Dalton for transcribing the entire manuscript.

Contents

Color plates appear following page 10.

1

Introduction and Technical Features

This chapter deals with the overall uses, general techniques, and the interpretation of gastrointestinal mucosal biopsy specimens. Chapters 2 through 11 present biopsy findings in the various inflammatory and neoplastic disorders that involve the esophagus, the stomach, the several parts of the small intestine, the colon and rectum, and the anal region.

GENERAL ASPECTS

With the appearance and further development of the flexible fiberoptic endoscopes, there has been a steady increase of their use in the evaluation of many gastrointestinal diseases.[1–3] Instruments are available for the examination of both the upper portion of the gut, including the esophagus, stomach, and most of the duodenum, together with the ampullary region and the connecting bile and pancreatic ducts[4–6]; and of the lower portion, including the rectum, the entire colon, and the distal-most portion of the ileum.[7–9] There currently exist extra-long upper endoscopes that can extend well into the jejunum[10, 11]; additionally, enteroscopes can be applied at the time of surgery.[12, 13]

Types of Endoscopes

The earliest endoscopes were of the rigid type, permitting only a limited examination of the more accessible parts of the distal esophagus and stomach as well as the distal colon. These endoscopes generally permitted only forward views and allowed for a single biopsy, typically of a large mass lesion.

The appearance of flexible forms of endoscopes in the late 1950s revolutionized this field.[14–18] Further developments permitted extensive applications to large portions of the gut, as well as the great ease of obtaining tissue samples and brush specimens from the many regions. Most of the endoscopes used are of the forward-viewing type that allows for direct visualization and obtaining of samples. Side-viewing instruments are employed to examine the region of the ampulla and to cannulate its ducts. The endoscopes for adults have diameters on the order of 3.5 to 4 mm, and scopes used in children are 2 mm in diameter. The latter can be employed in adults in regions of strictures.

The instruments are constructed to permit several channels of flexible fibers, each with a separate function for viewing, biopsy, brushing, photography, and coagulation. As a result, there is a full capacity for detection, biopsy sampling, documentation, and therapy of numerous lesions.

Uses of Endoscopy

The ease of both preparation of the patient and application of an endoscope has led to more examinations of patients for a larger variety of disorders, extending over the course of the lesions.[19–22] Examination and biopsy are now employed not only to render the diagnosis, but also to follow the evolution of the lesions (Table 1-1). Visualization of the gut and biopsies are taken as well to determine the extent of disease, to rate the severity and response to therapy of the disorders, and to detect complications at an early and more treatable stage.

For example, upper endoscopy is frequently used to detect the presence of a gastric peptic ulcer and to follow its course after a specific therapy. Similarly, examination of the colon is extensively used in patients with chronic colitis to identify the disorder, to confirm its chronicity and extent of disease, to evaluate the effects of therapy, and, particularly, to detect early complications such as dysplasia. There is also widespread use of colonoscopy to identify and to remove polyps.[23] This practice was begun in 1969 and is now the primary method for polypectomy, obviating the need for colonic resections in most cases.

Complications

Most endoscopy procedures yield relatively small biopsy samples, and the complication rate is correspondingly very small.[24, 25] Potential difficulties include the appearance of bleeding and, exceptionally, of perforation.[26] Hemorrhage of a noticeable degree occurs in only 1 to 2 percent of cases. It is more commonly associated with a greater amount of blood following the removal of large polyps, particularly in the colon; these involve excision through stalks that may contain larger submucosal arteries.

Perforation of the gut is uncommon, occurring in less than 1 percent of cases. It is seen more often in the colon and usually in cases with extensive colitis. This can be minimized by proper selection of cases and care of examination, avoiding any major trauma during the procedure. Deaths from endoscopy are extremely rare and are related to perforations of the bowel in sick patients.

Table 1-1. General Uses of Endoscopy and Biopsy

Provide specific diagnosis
Determine extent and severity of disease
Follow response to therapy
Detect complications

MUCOSAL BIOPSY SPECIMENS AND TECHNIQUES

Types of Biopsies

A variety of biopsy types can be obtained from the gut (Table 1-2).[17, 18] Tubes can be inserted without the use of endoscopes, leading to suction or aspiration-type biopsies. These are ordinarily obtained from the stomach; the small bowel, particularly areas that are not readily accessed by endoscopes, such as the jejunum; and from the rectum. The suction biopsy samples are big and typically include a portion of the submucosa. The larger size of the sample permits ease of orientation, which is especially helpful in evaluation of the jejunal mucosa where the relation of the height of the villi to the crypts is usually needed.[27, 28] The presence of the

Table 1-2. Types of Mucosal Biopsies

Suction biopsy
Endoscopic biopsy
Pinch
Spike
Grasp (forceps)
Strip
Fine-needle aspiration

submucosa is most important in the study of diseases that tend to involve larger vessels, such as vasculitis and deposition of amyloid.

Biopsies obtained through the endoscope are of several forms and include those taken directly by a bite or pinch of the tissue, a removal following the spike of an area, and the use of forceps to obtain grasp or shave specimens; strip biopsies, taken after injections of glucose solutions into the underlying tissue, allowing for a larger sample; and the insertion of fine needles to obtain cytologic material from areas with large folds or suspected submucosal lesions.[29–31] For polyps, the snare of the underlying area or evident stalk is typically employed together with direct cutting or coagulation of the submucosal tissue.[32] Larger polyps may require removal by multiple pieces.

In obtaining biopsy specimens, it is very important to consider the gross appearance of the lesions, with sampling of any different-appearing areas. The subsequent analysis is helped by obtaining photographs of the gross endoscopy, which can be provided with the specimen submission.

Preparation of Slides

Orientation

For proper orientation of the specimens, it is most helpful for the persons involved in the processing to appreciate the surface topography of the specimens.[33] Many attempts have been made to enhance orientation by applying the specimens to various substances such as filter paper or vegetable matter, presenting the luminal surface for inspection. Exquisite orientation is most needed in the examination of small bowel samples, to permit proper relation of the villous height to crypt depth. For most other specimens, the use of multiple sections often provides ample orientation.

Fixation

Buffered formalin is used in most laboratories and proves to be an adequate fixative, provided one is aware of the tissue shrinkage that occurs. When better cellular appearance is desired, such as in the presence of lymphomas, fixatives that contain heavy metals are available, including Bouin's, B5, and Hollende's solutions. These solutions cause less tissue shrinkage and permit the appearance of larger nuclei with less distortion. Following fixation the tissue samples are passed through a series of solutions, resulting in dehydration and preparation for the paraffin embedding and cutting of the slides.

Sections and Stains

Because many of the lesions are small, it is recommended that at least two to three levels be obtained from each biopsy. As noted above, this also increases the likelihood of obtaining good orientation, and allows for a greater survey to look for tiny areas of organisms, granulomas, and dysplasia. The several sections can even be placed, if needed, on the same glass slide. The hematoxylin and eosin (H & E) stain is routinely employed and is adequate for the great majority of lesions.

Special stains need not be automatically obtained but rather can be selected based on particular needs (Table 1-3). The more commonly used stains include Mallory's or Gomori's trichrome for collagen, Congo Red and metachromatic stains for amyloid, periodic acid–Schiff (PAS) and methenamine silver for fungi, and Gram and acid-fast stains for bacteria and other microorganisms. There are also special stains that can be used to detect and to demonstrate the various types of mucin, including the PAS reaction for neutral glycoproteins, the Alcian Blue stains for the acid mucosubstances, and the high-iron diamine for sulfomucin. In addition, there are many other stains employing

Table 1-3. Common Histochemical Stains

Stain	Substance
Trichrome	Collagen
Congo Red and metachromatic	Amyloid
Methenamine silver	Fungi
Gram and acid-fast	Bacteria and protozoa
PAS	Neutral glycoprotein
Alcian Blue	Acid mucosubstances
High-iron diamine	Sulfomucin
Grimelius'	Endocrine cells

immunocytochemical and other techniques, as described in later sections. Examples of the various special stains are shown in the color plates at the end of this chapter (Plates 1 to 4).

Special Techniques and Procedures

Cytology

For the detection of neoplasms, cytologic examination can be an important adjunct[34] (Plate 3). This is especially helpful in cases with strictures where tissue samples may be difficult to obtain from the interior of the lesion, whereas a brush can access the narrowed area and provide a cytologic smear. As noted above, fine-needle aspiration can be applied to deeper lesions, such as those in the submucosa, to obtain cytologic preparations for study.[30, 31, 35] Even with evident gross lesions on the surface, the cytologic smears can help in the confirmation of tumor. This has been more extensively used in screening for lesions in the esophagus in areas with a high prevalence of squamous cell carcinoma.[36] It also has proven useful in the identification of gastric carcinomas, whereas cytologic examination of the colon and rectum has not been performed as often.[37–39] The smears are typically processed in alcoholic fixative and by Papanicolaou's stain. As with the tissue samples, the smears can also be used for other special stains including immunocytochemical techniques for study of both tumors and infections.[40]

Immunocytochemistry

There are now a great number of immunocytologic stains that can be applied to tissue sections and cytologic smears, to help in the designation of a particular type of tumor (Table 1-4).[41, 42] More commonly used stains are cytokeratins, epithelial membrane antigen, and carcinoembryonic antigen (CEA) for detection of epithelial neoplasms; leukocyte common antigen and many other B-cell and T-cell markers for identifying lymphomas; and vimentin, actin, myosin, and other fibrillar proteins to realize mesenchymal tumors. Furthermore, some tumors are associated with highly individualized markers. Examples include albumin and alpha-fetoprotein for hepatic tumors, cystic fluid protein and both estrogen and progesterone markers that are more commonly seen in breast tumors, and subtypes of cytokeratins that can help to distinguish squamous cell and adenocarcinomas. There are also highly selective markers for the various leukemias and lymphomas, melanomas, and germ cell tumors.

General stains for the endocrine cells include Grimelius' stain, which serves as a histochemical stain for argyrophilic cells, and two immunocytochemical stains for chromogranin and synaptophysin. Of these, the chromogranin stain appears to be the most sensitive, identifying over 90 percent of endocrine cells, and is most widely used. The endocrine lesions are more precisely defined by the use of stains for the specific hormones, including gastrin, somatostatin, glucagon, serotonin, and vasoactive intestinal polypeptide (VIP). These can be present in both

Table 1-4. Examples of Immunocytochemical Stains

Stains	Marker
Cytokeratins, epithelial membrane antigen, and CEA	Epithelia
Leukocyte common antigen, B-cell and T-cell markers	Leukocytes
Vimentin, actin, and myosin	Stromal cells
Chromogranin and synaptophysin	Endocrine cells
Many other specific stains (see text)	

discrete masses and in areas of hyperplasia in various parts of the gut.

Electron Microscopy

Ultrastructural examination of biopsy specimens can be of considerable assistance in defining particular neoplasms, in the detection and distinction of numerous microorganisms, and in the isolation and differentiation of abnormal substances.[43, 44] Examples include the detection of rootlets adjacent to glandular lumens, which help to define an adenocarcinoma as of colonic type; the finding and subtyping of the various microsporidial species in the small bowel of patients with AIDS; and the accurate distinction of amyloid and other fibrillar materials. (See the Appendix for a complete list of electron micrographs presented in this book.)

For this study, samples should be fixed as promptly as possible in either glutaraldehyde or equivalent solutions. If needed, and if the material sought is not destroyed by the prior procedures, samples can be taken from formalin-fixed tissue and even from paraffin-embedded material, which are then reprocessed for the electron microscopic study.

Most of the ordinary examinations involving electron microscopy are of the transmission type. Studies employing scanning electron microscopy can also be helpful in demonstrating the topography and histology of the various parts of the gut.[45] These techniques can further assist in identifying surface microorganisms and in defining features on the surface of the cells that allow for distinction of dysplasia from normal and regenerative epithelia. Such findings have been noted in squamous cell dysplasia of the esophagus and in glandular dysplasia of the colon. The techniques are relatively expensive and time consuming, but may help in especially difficult cases to provide the final diagnosis.

Cell Markers and Flow Cytometry

Special techniques are now routinely used to help in the identification of the particular cell type of leukemias and lymphomas, including those that arise in or extend into the gut.[46] These techniques are employed to define the lymphomas as of the B-cell or T-cell type and to provide the complete immunophenotyping. This information is often needed to rate the biologic behavior of the tumors and the needed therapy.

Flow cytometry has also been extensively investigated in many of the neoplasms of the gut in attempts to determine whether this technique can be used to distinguish malignant from benign tumors, and to assess the behavior of the malignancies.[47, 48] Aneuploidal populations are more commonly seen in malignant lesions but can also be noted in one-half of the benign tumors; when present, it is likely that the lesion represents a neoplasm. Many current investigations are aimed at determining subsets of invasive tumors and of metastases that have more extensive aneuploidy in efforts to better determine the biology and therapy of the lesions.

Other Molecular Techniques

There are current, extensive studies of the gut tumors that employ new molecular techniques, such as in-situ hybridization (ISH) and the detection of altered proteins, DNA, and RNA.[49] Combined with the immunocytochemical stains, there have been many investigations seeking to determine the overexpression of oncogenes, tumor-suppressor gene substances, and other altered growth factors. Examples include the finding of excess p53, c-*myc* and k-*ras* genes, enhanced growth, and altered location of fetal antigens such as sucrase–isomaltase in many neoplasms, both benign and malignant, throughout the gut.[50, 51] At present these are of an experimental nature and are not yet involved in routine diagnoses.

Microbiology and Biochemical Studies

For the many infectious disorders, microbiologic studies may be applied for the detection and fine distinction of organisms that may be otherwise difficult to identify in tissue samples. These are most often used to look for pathogenic viruses but can also aid in detailing the organism in granulomatous disorders. Biochemical studies can be applied to help define the substances present in the various storage disorders.

DISEASE CLASSIFICATION AND TERMINOLOGY

Categories of Diseases

The uses and features of endoscopic evaluation and biopsy are demonstrated in the many inflammatory disorders and tumors that can affect the various portions of the gut (Table 1-5),[33] including developmental, motor and mechanical, and vascular disorders; infections; physical, chemical and drug injuries; the several idiopathic and immunologic disorders; and a variety of miscellaneous conditions in the different parts of the gut.

Table 1-5. Categories of Gastrointestinal Diseases

Developmental
Motor and mechanical
Vascular
Infections
Physical
Chemical and drug
Idiopathic
Immunologic
Depositions
Tumors

Tissue Reactions

Epithelial responses to injury include the acute effects of degeneration and regeneration, the various types of metaplasia, and the development of dysplasia and neoplasia. Both the standard inflammatory reactions and the special features of granulomas can occur, and these are detailed in Chapter 2.

Based on the duration of disease and the characteristic inflammatory reactions, the disorders are separated into acute disease with or without repair, chronic inactive or quiescent disease, and chronic active lesions. There are some differences dependent on location, but, in general, the presence of many mononuclear inflammatory cells together with architectural alterations including glandular atrophy helps to define chronic disease in most parts of the gut.

BIOPSY INTERPRETATION

Artifacts of Preparation

In the evaluation of a biopsy sample, it is necessary to consider and discount any effects that may be due to the preparation of the patient or specimen (Table 1-6), such as the common appearance of mucosal edema of the mucosa due to hypertonic solutions

Table 1-6. Artifacts Due to Preparation

Edema and hemorrhage
Clumping of mononuclear cells
Flattening of epithelium
Loss of epithelial mucus

and a superficial, mild colitis from more caustic enemas.[52] Also, the trauma of the procedure often causes foci of hemorrhage and clumping of mononuclear inflammatory cells, varying degrees of flattening of the surface epithelium, and loss of mucus from the epithelial cells, presumably discharged in response to the irritation.[22] These latter changes can be enhanced by excessive handling of tissue after biopsies are obtained. Support for their nonsignificant nature are the lack of any definite features of degeneration of the epithelial cells and the absence of a neutrophilic reaction. It is best to require the appearance of such degenerative and inflammatory changes before considering any changes to be meaningful.

Microscopic Examination

It is helpful to apply a systematic approach to the examination of the biopsy samples, looking for changes in overall architecture; for alterations in any of the individual components, including the epithelia and elements of the lamina propria; and for the detection of any abnormal substances or agents.

Unlike other tissues of the body, there is a large amount of inflammatory cells in many portions of the gut mucosa, and features of chronic disease are more ordinarily dependent on alterations of the epithelial architecture. The presence of acute or active disease is typically determined by noting definite damage of epithelial cells together with neutrophilic infiltration of the epithelial and lamina propria regions.

Report of Findings

It would be most helpful if all requisition slips were to indicate not only the nature of the specimen, but also the particular reason for performing the endoscopic examination.[53] It would be further useful if this slip and explanation were accompanied by a diagram or photograph indicating the gross endoscopic findings and the sites of biopsy. With the presence of such information, one can proceed with a more intelligent analysis of the biopsy and with the report of its findings.

In the absence of any definite features of disease, including the exclusion of any alterations that might be due to the preparation, biopsies are reported as "within normal limits", "no diagnostic abnormalities", and other variations on the same theme. In many instances, particularly in the evaluation of inflammatory lesions, the report tends to assess the extent of the disease, indicating whether one or all biopsies are involved and whether it is of a focal or diffuse nature. In addition, estimates are made of whether the disease is acute, chronic inactive, or chronic active. Some of the disorders include specific findings, such as the presence of amyloid, the detection of certain microorganisms, and the diagnosis of dysplasia and particular neoplasms. As mentioned previously, it would be best to have a particular question and to provide a specific answer in the final pathology report.

NEW TECHNIQUES

With the enhanced development of the flexible endoscopes over the past three decades, efforts have been directed toward defining the criteria of the many disorders, including those needed for early detection and for the discovery of complications. Lesions that involve the mucosa and, particularly, the superficial portions are easily accessed. There are current attempts to obtain samples from the deeper portions of the mucosa and of the submucosa or other parts of the wall by taking samples after incisions are made into the mucosa, or by fine-needle aspiration of such areas. The precise location of these lesions has been helped by the use of endoscopic ultrasonography and by improvements in the photographic imaging of the lesions.[54–57]

Endoscopes are being developed that will be capable of examining the rest of the small intestine, particularly the jejunum from above and the ileum from the lower part. There are also considerable efforts in improving the treatment of the lesions through endoscopes, since these typically lead to the avoidance of operations and to reduced morbidity. Endoscopes are now widely used for the cauterization of hemorrhagic or ulcerative lesions, the sclerosis of vascular ectasias, the insertion of stents through obstructive areas, and for the potential ablation of small areas of dysplasia or tumor.

In the near future further developments are expected in endoscope optics, in the creation of longer instruments, and in the application of the various therapeutic regimens.

REFERENCES

1. Scott B, Atkinson M: Gastroenterology services: a regional review of changes over a five year period (1981–86). Gut 30:695–700, 1989
2. Goldman H: Era of the mucosal biopsy. pp. 1–10. In Goldman H, Appelman HD, Kaufman N (eds): Gastrointestinal Pathology. Williams & Wilkins, Baltimore, 1990
3. Scott B: Endoscopic demands in the 90's. Gut 31:125–126, 1990
4. Morrissey JF, Reichelderfer M: Gastrointestinal Endoscopy. N Engl J Med 325:1142–1149, 1214–1222, 1991
5. Hunt RH, Cotton PB, Crespi M et al: Role of endoscopy in the diagnosis of cancer. Cancer Res 49:6822–6827, 1989
6. Komorowski RA, Beggs BK, Geenan JE, Venu RP: Assessment of ampula of Vater pathology. An endoscopic approach. Am J Surg Pathol 15:1188–1196, 1991
7. Wolff WI: Colonoscopy: history and development. Am J Gastroenterol 84:1017–1025, 1989
8. Goldin E, Rachmilewitz D: Ileoscopic diagnosis of terminal ileitis. Gastrointest Endosc 30:11–14, 1984
9. Borsch G, Schmidt G: Endoscopy of the terminal ileum. Diagnostic yield in 400 consecutive specimens. Dis Colon Rectum 28: 499–501, 1985
10. Iida M, Yamamoto T, Yao T et al: Jejunal endoscopy using a long duodenofiberscope. Gastrointest Endosc 32:233–236, 1986
11. Chong J, Tagle M, Barkin JS et al: Small bowel push-type fiberoptic enteroscopy for patients with occult gastrointestinal bleeding or suspected small bowel pathology. Am J Gastroenterol 89:2143–2146, 1994
12. Barkin JS, Schonfeld W, Thomsen S et al: Enteroscopy and small bowel biopsy—an improved technique for the diagnosis of small bowel disease. Gastrointest Endosc 31: 215–217, 1985
13. Lewis BS, Kornbluth A, Wayne JD: Small bowel tumors: yield of enteroscopy. Gut 32:763–765, 1991
14. Morrissey JF: The 1982 A/S/G/E Distinguished Lecture: Gastrointestinal endoscopy—20 years of progress. Gastrointest Endosc 29:53–56, 1983
15. Hirschowitz BI: The development and application of fiberoptic endoscopy. Cancer 61: 1925–1941, 1988
16. Hirschowitz BI: Development and application of endoscopy. Gastroenterology 104: 337–342, 1993
17. Haggitt RC, Rubin CE. Endoscopy and endoscopic biopsy. pp. 37–47. In Ming S-C, Goldman H (eds): Pathology of the Gastrointestinal Tract. WB Saunders, Philadelphia, 1992
18. Green PHR: Digestive tract endoscopy and biopsy. pp. 1–6. In Rotterdam H, Sheahan DG, Sommers SC (eds): Biopsy Diagnosis of the Digestive Tract. 2nd Ed. Raven Press, New York, 1993
19. Goldman H, Antonioli DA: Mucosal biopsy of the esophagus, stomach and proximal duodenum. Hum Pathol 13:423–448, 1982
20. Goldman H, Antonioli DA: Mucosal biopsy of the rectum, colon and distal ileum. Hum Pathol 13:981–1012, 1982
21. Haber GB: Role of endoscopy in inflammatory bowel disease. Dig Dis Sci 32:165–255, 1987
22. Goldman H: Interpretation of large intestinal mucosal biopsy specimens. Hum Pathol 25:1150–1159, 1994

23. Wolf WI, Shinya H: Polypectomy via the fiberoptic colonoscope: removal of lesions beyond reach of the sigmoidoscope. N Engl J Med 288:329–332, 1973
24. Shahmir M, Schuman BM: Complications of fiberoptic endoscopy. Gastrointest Endosc 26:86–91, 1980
25. Reiertsen O, Skjoto J, Jacobson CD, Rosseland AR: Complications of fiberoptic gastrointestinal endoscopy—five years' experience in a central hospital. Endoscopy 19:1–6, 1987
26. Pasricha PJ, Fleischer DE, Kalloo AN: Endoscopic perforations of the upper digestive tract: a review of their pathogenesis, prevention, and management. Gastroenterology 106:787–802, 1994
27. Perera DR, Weinstein WM, Rubin CE: Small intestinal biopsy. Hum Pathol 6:157–217, 1975
28. Dobbins WO III: Small bowel biopsy in malabsorptive states. pp. 137–188. In Norris HT (ed): Pathology of the Colon, Small Intestine, and Anus. 2nd Ed. Churchill Livingstone, New York, 1991
29. Levine DS, Reid BJ: Endoscopic biopsy technique for acquiring larger mucosal samples. Gastrointest Endosc 37:332–337, 1991
30. Lange P, Kock K, Laustsen J et al: Endoscopic fine needle aspiration cytology of the stomach. A new diagnostic procedure. Endoscopy 19:72–73, 1987
31. Graham DY, Tabibian N, Michaletz PA et al: Endoscopic needle biopsy: a companion study of forceps biopsy, two different types of needles and salvage cytology in gastrointestinal cancer. Gastrointest Endosc 35:207–209, 1989
32. Tappero G, Gaia E, De Giuli P et al: Cold snare excision of small colorectal polyps. Gastrointest Endosc 38:310–313, 1992
33. Goldman H, Ming S-C: General concepts and methods of examination. pp. 3–13. In Ming S-C, Goldman H (eds): Pathology of the Gastrointestinal Tract. WB Saunders, Philadelphia, 1992
34. Qizilbash AH, Casteli M, Kowalski MA et al: Endoscopic brush cytology and biopsy in the diagnosis of cancer of the upper gastrointestinal tract. Acta Cytol 24:313, 1980
35. Zargar SA, Khuroo MS, Mahajan R et al: Endoscopic fine needle aspiration cytology in the diagnosis of gastro-esophageal and colorectal malignancies. Gut 32:745–748, 1991
36. Tsang TK, Hidvegi D, Horth K, Ostrow JD: Reliability of balloon-mesh cytology in detecting esophageal carcinoma in a population of U.S. veterans. Cancer 59:556–559, 1987
37. Ehya H, O'Hara BJ: Brush cytology in the diagnosis of colonic neoplasms. Cancer 66:1563–1567, 1990
38. Marshall JB, Diaz-arias AA, Barthel JS et al: Prospective evaluation of optimal number of biopsy specimens and brush cytology in the diagnosis of cancer of the colorectum. Am J Gastroenterol 88:1352–1354, 1993
39. Rosman AS, Federman Q, Feinman L: Diagnosis of colon cancer by lavage cytology with an orally administered balanced electrolyte solution. Am J Gastroenterol 89:51–56, 1994
40. Debongnie JC, Mairesse J, Donnay M, Dekonick X: Touch cytology. A quick, simple sensitive screening test in the diagnosis of infections of the gastrointestinal mucosa. Arch Pathol Lab Med 118:1115–1118, 1994
41. Blackman E, Nash SV: Diagnosis of duodenal and ampullary epithelial neoplasms by endoscopic biopsy: a clinicopathologic and immunohistochemical study. Hum Pathol 16: 901–910, 1985
42. Mori M, Ambe K, Adachi Y et al: Prognostic value of immunohistochemically identified CEA, SC, AFP, and S-100 protein-positive cells in gastric carcinoma. Cancer 62: 534–540, 1988
43. Frost AR, Orenstein JM, Abraham AA, Silverberg SG: A comparison of the usefulness of electron microscopy and immunohistochemistry. One laboratory's experience. Arch Pathol Lab Med 118:922–926, 1994
44. Erlandson RA, Rosai J: A realistic approach to the use of electron microscopy and other ancillary diagnostic techniques in surgical pathology. Am J Surg Pathol 19:247–250, 1995
45. Shields HM, Best CJ, Goldman H: Distinction of dysplasia from inflammatory changes in ulcerative colitis: a scanning electron microscopy study with quantitative analyses. Surg Pathol 1:183–192, 1988
46. Grody WW, Weiss LM, Warnke RA et al: Gastrointestinal lymphomas. Immunohistochemical studies on the cell of origin. Am J Surg Pathol 9:328–337, 1985
47. Hood DL, Petras RE, Edinger M et al: Deoxyribonucleic acid ploidy and cell cycle analysis

of colorectal carcinoma by flow cytometry. Am J Clin Pathol 93:615–620, 1990
48. Haggitt RC, Reid BJ, Rabinovitch PS, Rubin CE: Barrett's esophagus. Correlation between mucin histochemistry, flow cytometry, and histologic diagnosis for predicting increased cancer risk. Am J Pathol 131:53–61, 1988
49. Grody WW, Gotti RA, Naeim F. Diagnostic molecular pathology. Modern Pathol 2:553–568, 1990
50. Amin MB, Ma CK, Linden MD et al: Prognostic value of proliferating cell nuclear antigen index in gastric stromal tumors. Correlation with mitotic count and clinical outcome. Am J Clin Pathol 100:428–432, 1993
51. Nikulasson S, Andrews CW Jr, Goldman H et al: Sucrase–isomaltase expression in dysplasia associated with Barrett's esophagus and chronic gastritis and in adenocarcinomas of the gastrointestinal tract. Int J Surg Pathol 2:281–286, 1995
52. Meisel JL, Bergman D, Graney D et al: Human rectal mucosa: proctoscopic and morphological changes caused by laxatives. Gastroenterology 72:1274–1279, 1977
53. Yardley JH, Hamilton SR, Hutcheon DF: How the GI pathologist can interact best with the GI trainee. Gastrointest Endosc 30: 368–371, 1984
54. Mitsunaga A: Diagnosis of submucosal tumors of the upper gastrointestinal tract by endoscopic ultrasonography. Gastrointest Endosc 29:3–15, 1987
55. Nickl NJ, Cotton PB: Clinical application of endoscopic ultrasonography. Am J Gastroenterol 85:675–682, 1990
56. Bladen JS, Anderson AP, Bell GD et al: Nonradiological technique for three-dimensional imaging of endoscopes. Lancet 341:719–722, 1993
57. Williams C, Guy C, Gillies D et al: Electronic three-dimensional imaging of intestinal endoscopy. Lancet 341:724–725, 1993

Color Plates

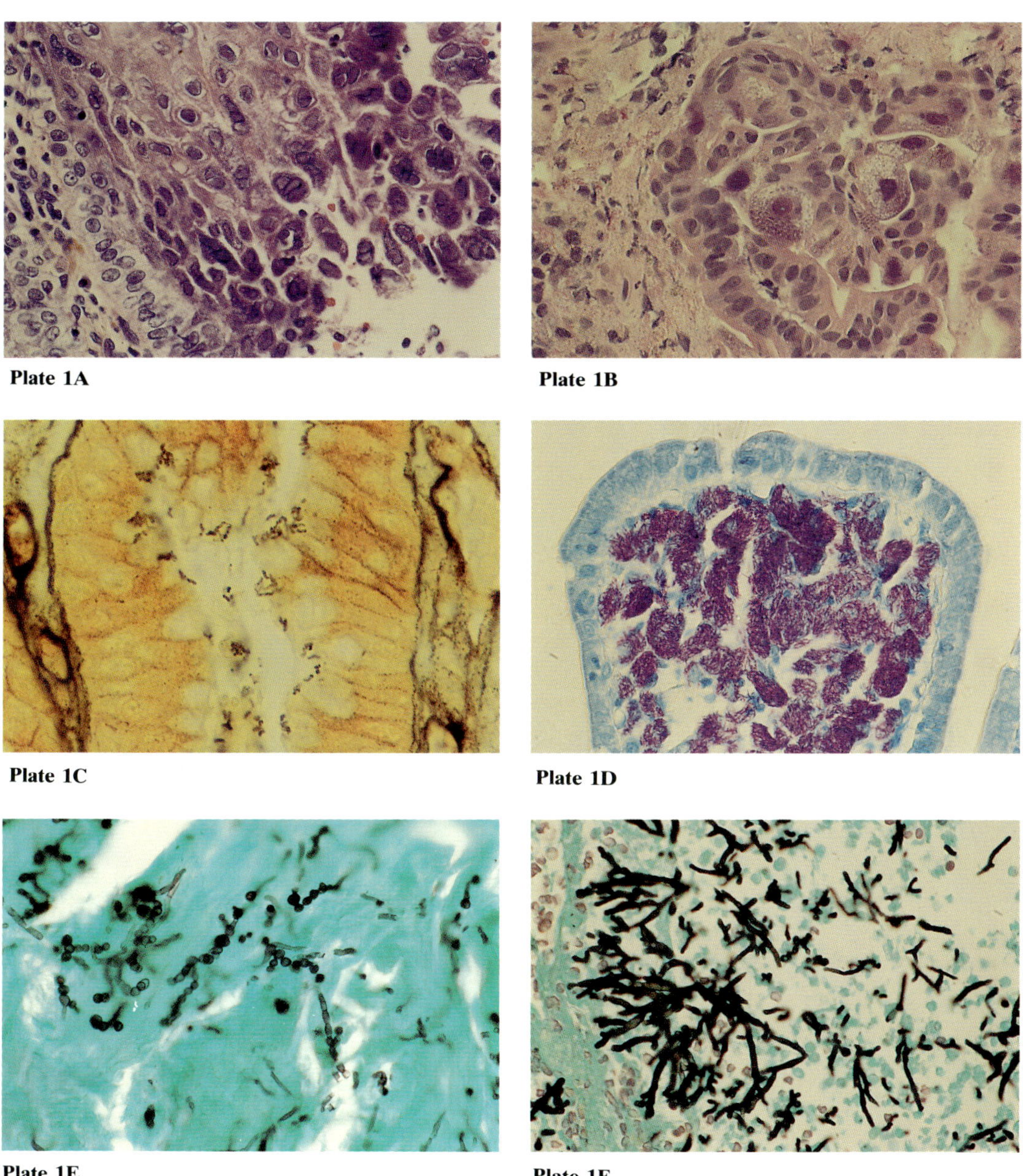

Plate 1A

Plate 1B

Plate 1C

Plate 1D

Plate 1E

Plate 1F

Plate 1. Infectious agents. **(A)** Herpes viral inclusions in squamous epithelial cells (× 285). **(B)** Cytomegalovirus inclusions in glands (× 285). **(C)** *Helicobacter pylori* in lumen of gastric pit. Dieterle silver stain, × 475. **(D)** *Mycobacterium avium intracellulare* in lamina propria macrophages. Acid fast stain, × 285. **(E)** *Candida.* Methenamine silver stain, × 285. **(F)** *Apergillus.* Methenamine silver stain, × 285.

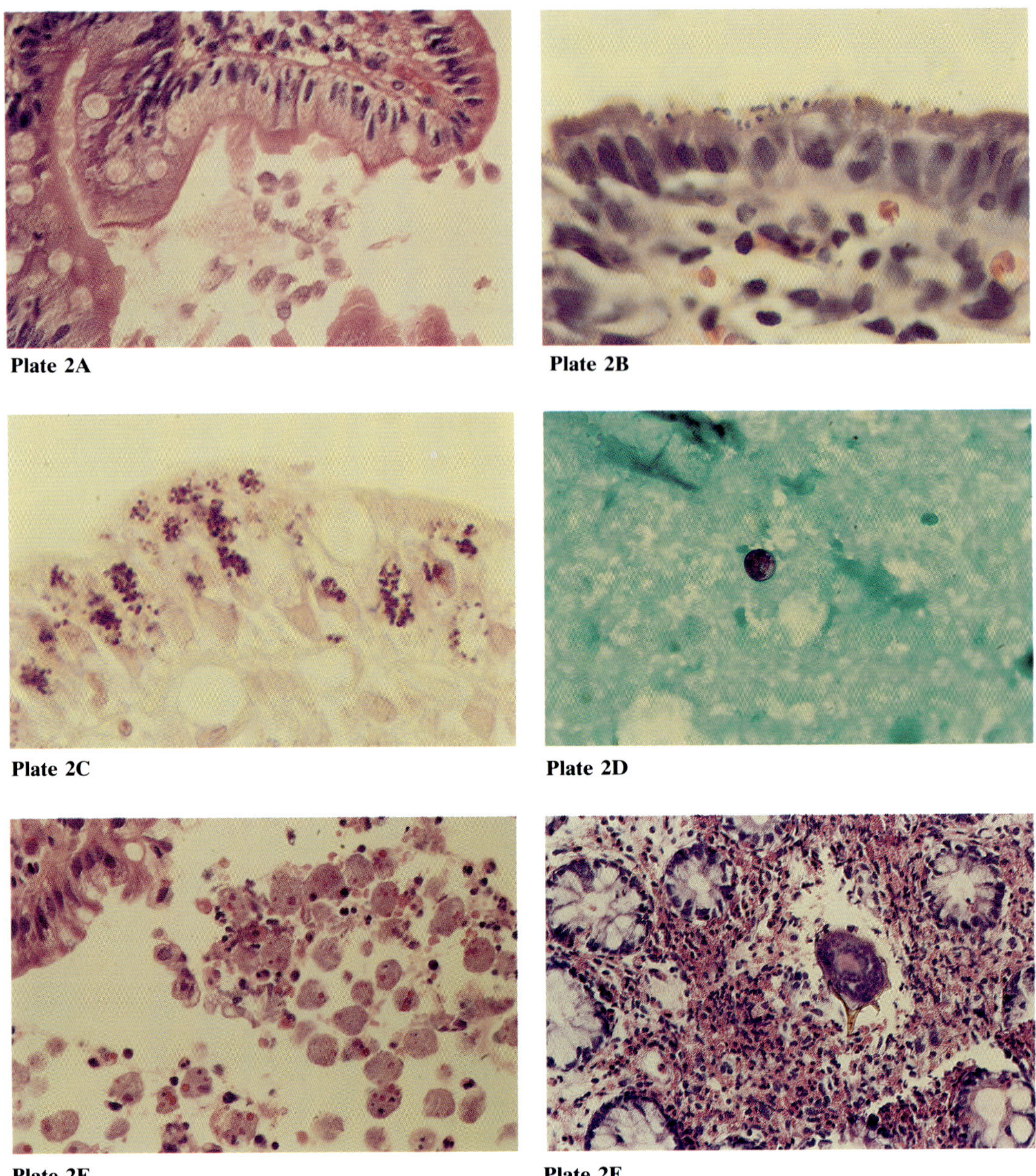

Plate 2A

Plate 2B

Plate 2C

Plate 2D

Plate 2E

Plate 2F

Plate 2. Infectious agents. **(A)** *Giardia lamblia,* in lumen (× 285). **(B)** *Cryptosporidia,* on cell surface (× 475). **(C)** *Microsporidia,* within epithelial cells. Gram stain, × 475. **(D)** *Cyclospora,* in fecal smear. Modified acid fast stain, × 475. **(E)** *Entameba histolyticum* (× 285). **(F)** *Schistosoma* ovum (× 95).

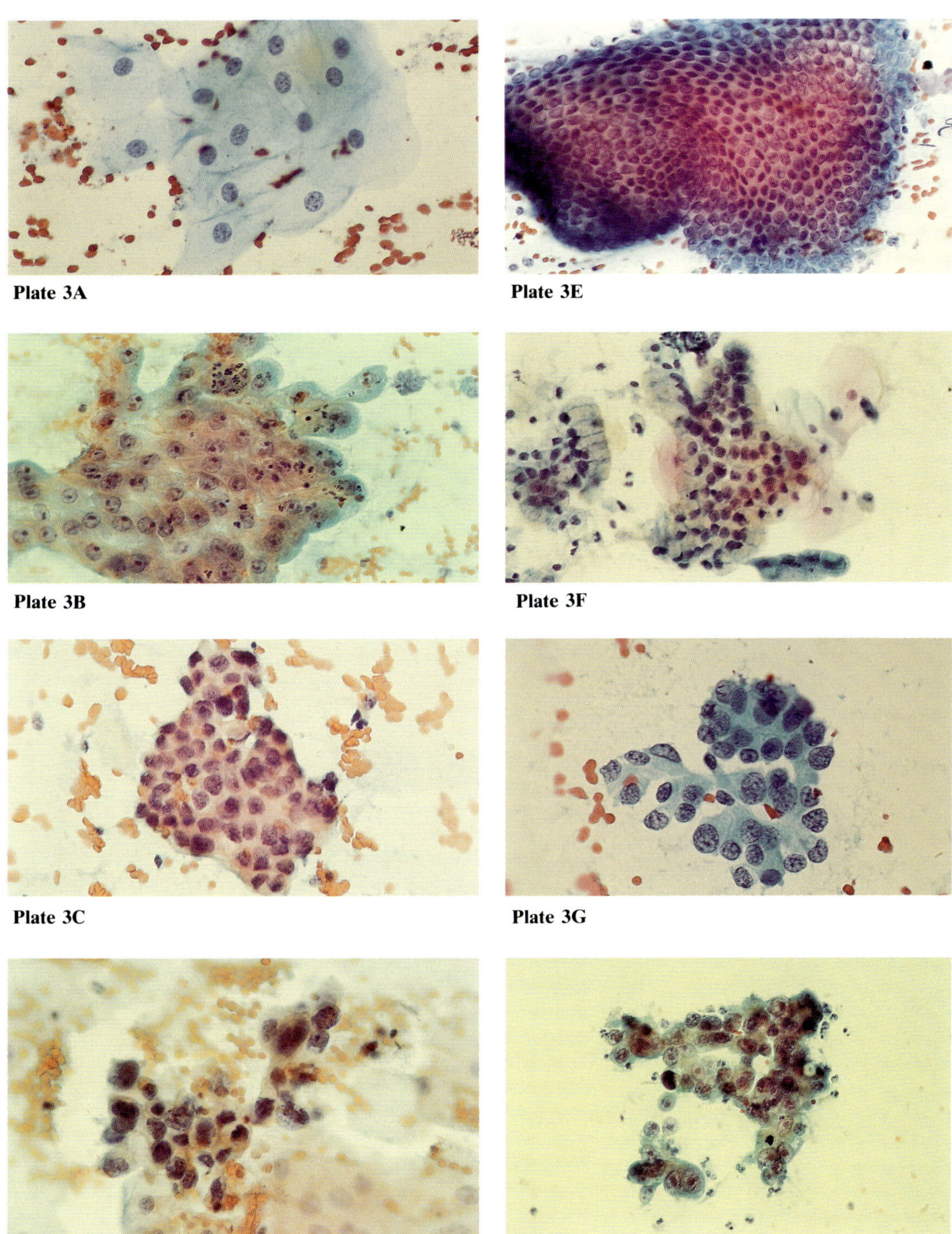

Plate 3. Cytology smears. **(A)** Normal esophageal squamous cells (× 285). **(B)** Inflammatory effect in squamous cells (× 285). **(C)** Squamous cell dysplasia (× 240). **(D)** Squamous cell carcinoma (× 240). **(E)** Normal gastric glandular cells (× 190). **(F)** Inflammatory effect in glandular cells (× 190). **(G)** Glandular dysplasia (× 285). **(H)** Adenocarcinoma (× 190).

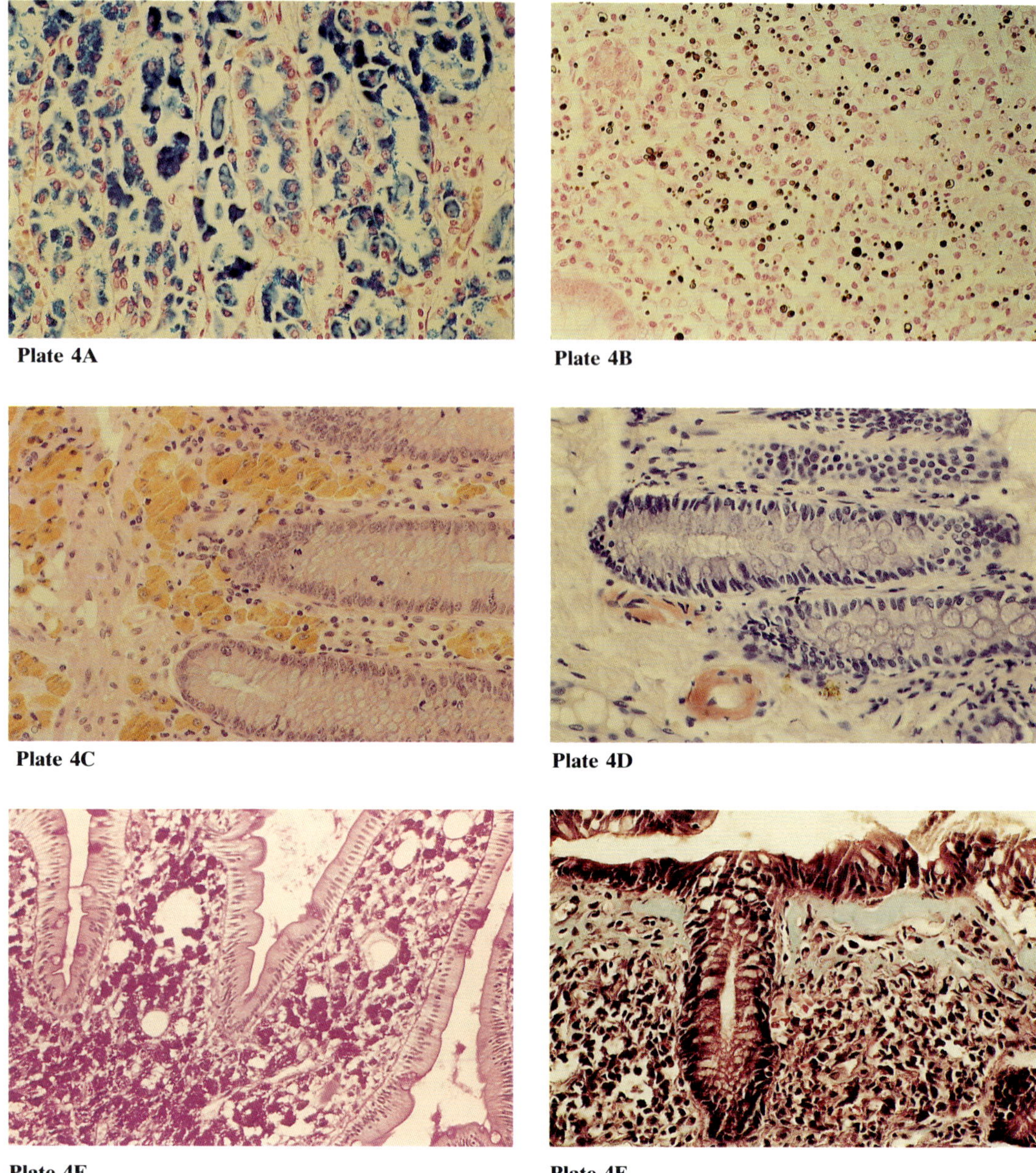

Plate 4. Pigments and special stains. **(A)** Prussian blue reaction for iron in the gastric glands of a patient with hemochromatosis (× 190). **(B)** von Kossa stain for calcium in malakoplakia, located in the macrophages within the colonic mucosa (× 190). **(C)** Deposits of lipofuscin in the brown bowel syndrome, present in the macrophages of the colonic mucosa (× 190). **(D)** Congo red stain for amyloid in the submucosal vessels of the colon (× 190). **(E)** Periodic acid-Schiff (PAS) reaction in Whipple's disease, identifying the bacteria within the macrophages of the lamina propria in the jejunum (× 95). **(F)** Trichrome stain for collagen beneath the surface epithelium in a case of collagenous colitis (× 190).

2

Inflammatory Disorders of the Esophagus

Endoscopy and mucosal biopsy of the esophagus are commonly employed to identify esophagitis, to monitor the course of disease following therapy, and to evaluate mass and stricture lesions (Table 2-1). The inflammatory disorders and their effects are presented in this chapter, and the lesions of dysplasia and general tumors are presented in Chapter 3.

GENERAL ASPECTS

Except for the evaluation of possible tumors, the clinical use of endoscopic examination of the esophagus initially tended to lag behind that of the stomach. As flexible endoscopes became available, there occurred a more frequent inspection of the esophagus to look for evidence of esophagitis, particularly of that due to reflux. It subsequently became evident that many other conditions affect the esophagus, often to a common degree. Examination of this area, to look for a wide variety of inflammatory lesions (either primary or of a secondary nature), for the effects of therapy, and for the development of any complications, is now frequent.[1–3]

Normal Structure

The inner mucosal lining is similar throughout the esophagus[4–7] and consists of a stratified squamous epithelium, a variable quantity of lamina propria, and a thick muscularis mucosae (Table 2-2).

Epithelium

The squamous layer contains basal and prickle cell zones, with the cells showing evident intercellular bridges (Fig. 2-1). There are uncommon keratohyaline granules but no well developed keratin layer in the normal state. The basal zone ordinarily is just a few cells thick and is considered to be normal if it represents 15 percent or less of the entire squamous layer thickness. Portions of the lamina propria, termed *papillae,* extend into the squamous layer, ordinarily up to about

Table 2-1. Uses of Esophageal Mucosal Biopsy

Identify esophagitis
Acute versus chronic disease
Monitor course following therapy
Detect complications
Evaluate mass and stricture lesions

50 percent of the epithelial thickness (Fig. 2-2). Expansion of the basal zone and elongation of the lamina propria papillae represent evidence of repair and are major features of esophagitis, which is described below. These findings have been noted in the distal few centimeters of the normal esophagus, where they may represent evidence of so-called physiologic reflux; whatever the case, their finding in this distal region cannot be considered evidence of clinically significant esophagitis.

Scattered throughout the squamous epithelial layer are a modest number of mononuclear cells, consisting mainly of Langerhans dendritic cells and T lymphocytes,[8] as well as a rare eosinophil, but ordinarily no neutrophils. These intraepithelial inflammatory cells are also increased in cases of esophagitis.

Lamina Propria and Muscularis Mucosae

The lamina propria consists of loose connective tissue in which is a variable amount of inflammatory cells, including mononuclear cell types, eosinophils, occasional lymphoid nodules, and rarely neutrophils. Most of the esophageal glands are contained in the submucosa, but small foci are present in the lamina propria; these glands as well as the ducts are exceptionally detected in biopsies but rarely show any pathologic features. The amount of inflammatory cells is increased in many esophageal disorders, particularly if there is destruction of the squamous epithelium. The muscularis mucosae, consisting of smooth muscle, is relatively thick compared to other portions of the gut; and the novice should not confuse this with the true muscularis propria. Most endoscopic biopsies consist only of the epithelial layer together with a small portion of superficial lamina propria. Larger aspiration type biopsies and material taken from children more often show the full mucosa including the muscular portion.

Structural Variations

Mitoses in the basal zone are rare in the normal state. Their presence together with an expansion of the basal zone represents repair and is commonly noted as a feature of esophagitis. Scattered throughout the basal zone in the normal state are rare endocrine cells and melanocytes[9,10] from which lesions, particularly tumors, can arise. Also rarely seen are other features that are more typical of skin such as the presence of sebaceous glands[11–14] (Fig. 2-3) and of a keratin layer (Fig. 2-4). The sebaceous glands are present in the lower portion of the epithelium and are unassociated with hair development; their appearance is similar to what is encountered in the oral mucosa and known as *Fordyce's lesion.* The finding of a keratin layer on the superficial aspect of the squamous epithelium probably represents an effect of chronic irritation similar to the development of a callus, and it is most often noted following the long-standing presence of some foreign object such as a tube.

Table 2-2. Normal Esophageal Mucosa and Variations

Stratified squamous epithelium
Basal (5–10%) and prickle cell zones
No keratin layer
Intraepithelial mononuclear cells and rare eosinophils
Rare mitoses, endocrine cells and melanocytes at base
Lamina propria (loose connective tissue)
Papillae extend 50% of epithelial thickness
Variable amount of inflammatory cells
Rare glands and ducts
Thick muscularis mucosae (smooth muscle)
Variants
Glycogenic acanthosis
Rare: sebaceous glands, keratosis

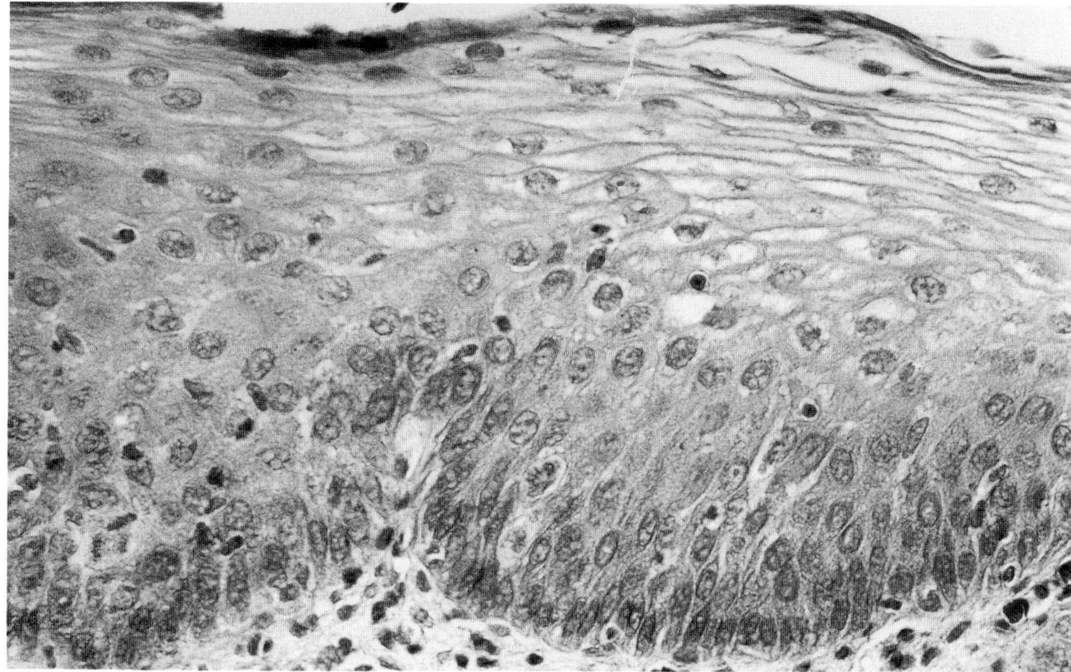

Fig. 2-1. Normal esophagus, showing stratified squamous epithelium with base at the bottom. There are scattered mononuclear cells, consisting of lymphocytes and dendritic cells, within the epithelial layer. The basal zone of squamous cells is limited to a few cells in thickness. There is a small portion of lamina propria at the botom (× 425).

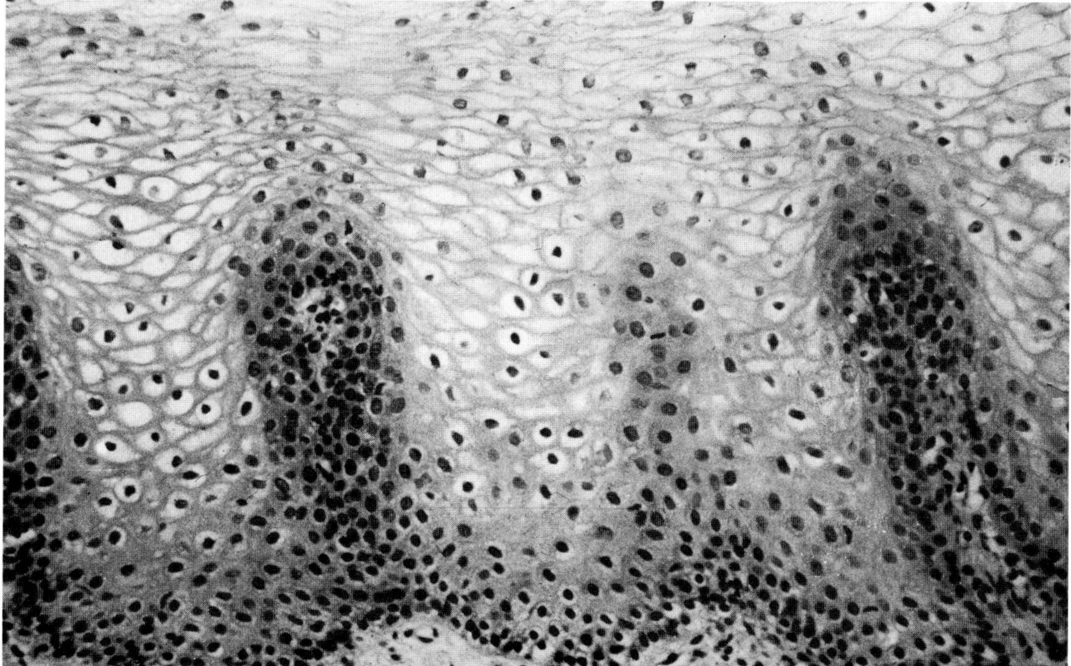

Fig. 2-2. Squamous epithelial layer of the normal esophagus with evident glycogen deposition in the form of vacuolated cytoplasm. The papillae of the lamina propria extend up to about one-half of the epithelial thickness.

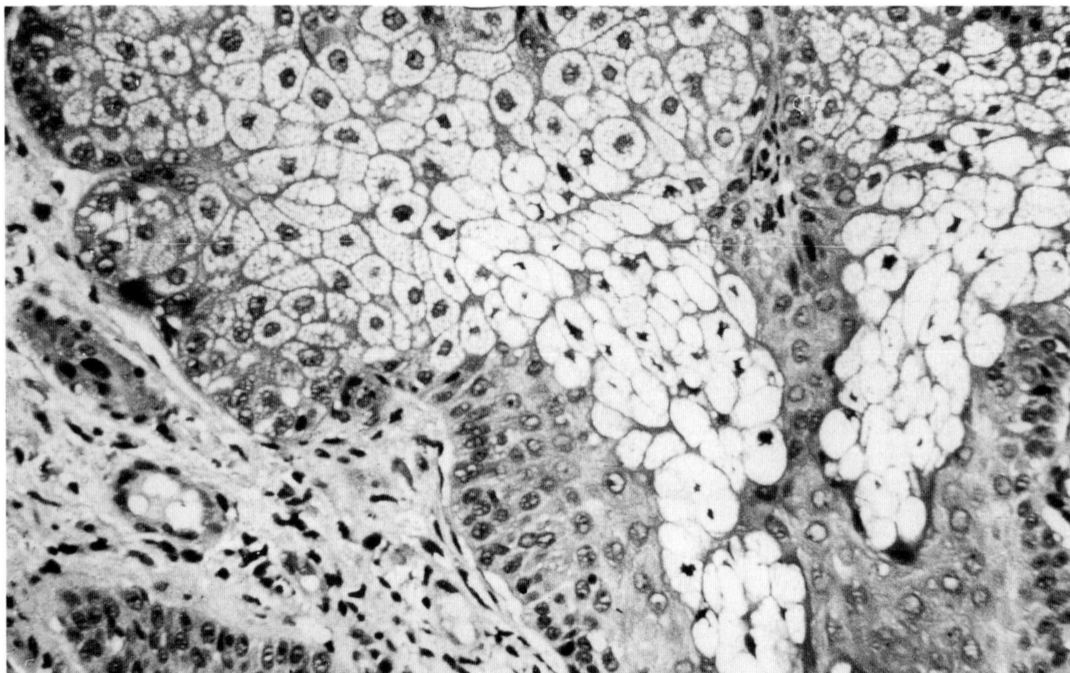

Fig. 2-3. Ectopic sebaceous glands in the esophagus. A portion of the lamina propria appears at the bottom left. Large sheets of sebaceous cells are present, merging with the squamous epithelium. The cells of the sebaceous glands are round, have central nuclei, and finely vacuolated cytoplasm due to the lipid content.

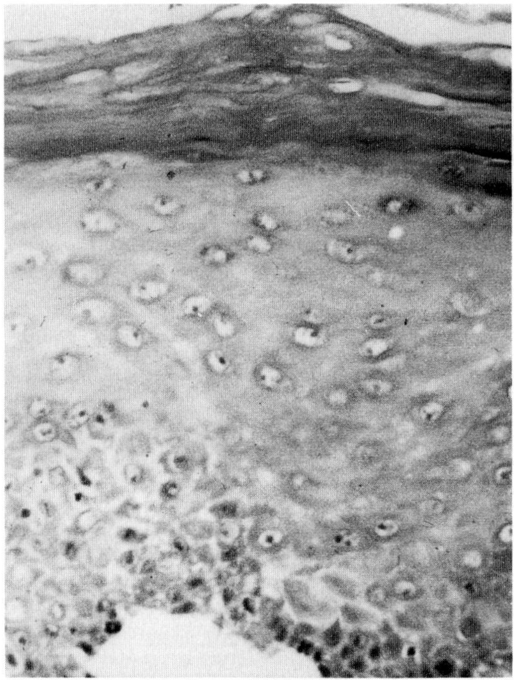

Fig. 2-4. Esophageal squamous epithelium with marked keratosis on the surface. There are no other signs of active inflammation.

Glycogenic Acanthosis

This is a common lesion represented by sharply localized thickenings of the mature squamous prickle cell layer.[15–17] The lesions are typically less than 1 cm in diameter, are multiple, and may be seen in any part of the esophagus.

Biopsies reveal simply a thickening of the mature squamous tissue that is rich in glycogen, and this can be accented by the use of the periodic acid–Schiff (PAS) reaction (Fig. 2-5). There is no associated inflammation or other abnormalities of the squamous cells, there are no mitoses, and the basal zone is not expanded. The lesions are most easily recognized grossly, and superficial biopsies may show only the squamous tissue without other abnormalities. Accordingly, in most instances it is only possible to indicate that there is uninflamed, mature squamous tissue, which is consistent with the entity of glycogenic acanthosis.

The cause of the lesions is not known. Their frequent presence in the distal esophagus, where reflux esophagitis is so common, suggests a localized excess of repair, but this is not established. Biopsies are typically performed to exclude other potential causes of localized thickenings, such as infections and dysplastic areas. The lesion has no clinical significance.

General Pathologic Features

Acute Effects

The majority of the effects seen in esophagitis are of an inflammatory nature and are nonspecific (Table 2-3). Milder lesions lead to lesser damage of the squamous epithe-

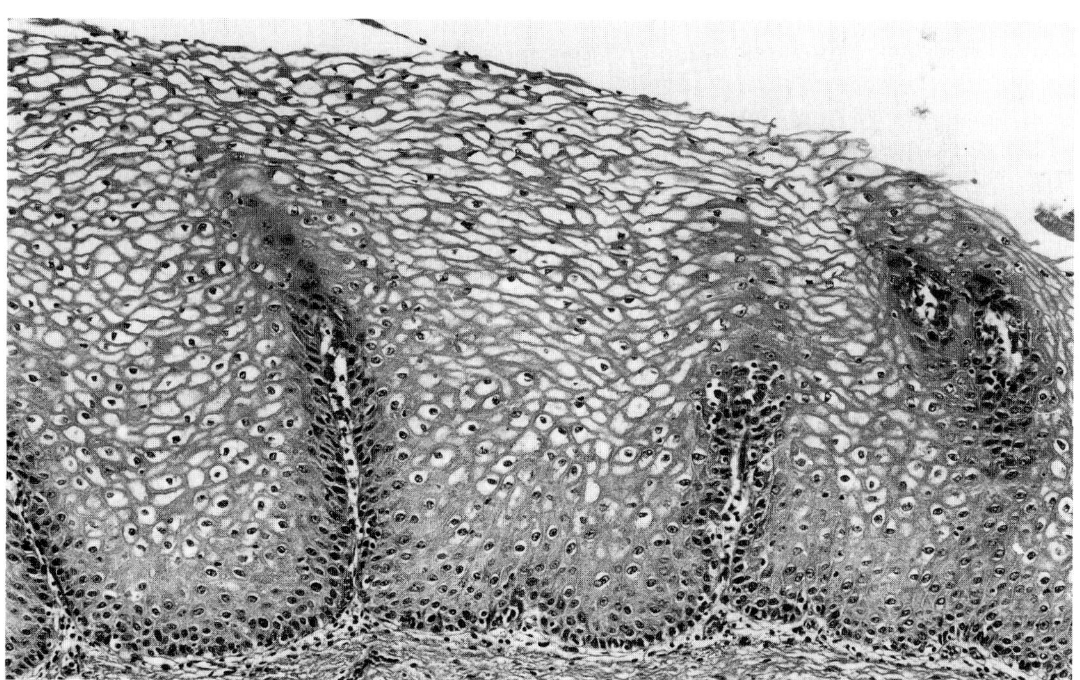

Fig. 2-5. Glycogenic acanthosis of the esophagus. The overall squamous layer is thickened and composed of cells that are vacuolated due to the presence of glycogen. There are no signs of inflammation or repair. The histologic features resemble the normal (Fig. 2-2), and the diagnosis depends on information that the biopsy was taken from a grossly thickened plaque (× 140).

Table 2-3. Histologic Features of Esophagitis

Cellular degeneration and balloon cells
Erosion and ulceration
Granulation tissue
Neutrophils. Increase of eosinophils and mononuclear cells
Basal zone expansion, elongation of papillae, and dilation and rupture of venules
Chronic features
Fibrosis leading to stricture formation
Glandular metaplasia (Barrett's esophagus)
Special features
Granulomas
Inclusions
Microorganisms

lium, with the presence of reversible squamous cell changes and increased inflammatory cells (Fig. 2-6); more marked effects reveal destruction of the innermost lining, represented as superficial erosions that involve part of the squamous layer, or as ulcers that extend into the lamina propria or through to the submucosa. With the milder lesions, the squamous epithelial cells may show swelling due to the increased absorption of water and proteins (termed *balloon cells*)[18]; the presence of increased mononuclear inflammatory cells and of eosinophils within the squamous epithelial layer[19–21] (Fig. 2-7); and the appearance of an expanded basal zone and elongation of the lamina propria papillae together with dilation of the venules.[22–23] In cases with greater destruction, there is granulation tissue formation, and all acute lesions reveal neutrophilic infiltration as well.

Chronic Effects

The chronic lesions reveal persistence of the active effects and the development of complications, which assist in determining this state. In the esophagus, there may be the appearance of increased fibrous tissue leading to stricture formation; but the best marker of chronicity is characterized by a change from the squamous epithelium to a glandular layer.[24] This represents a metaplasia consisting of a mixture of gastric and intestinal-type epithelial cells, known as *Barrett's esophagus,* and is discussed in detail in the section on Reflux Esophagitis.

Biopsy Effects

As in all parts of the gut, the endoscopic examination and biopsy may cause some effects that should be discounted before considering definite injury to this area. These changes tend to be fairly minor in the esophagus and consist mainly of a mild flattening or distortion of the squamous layer, and the uncommon presence of edema or hemorrhage in the lamina propria; the effects of the endoscopic procedure are much more common in the glandular tissues in other parts of the gut. The most significant effect or limitation of the endoscopic biopsy is probably the small nature of the specimens. These often are twisted and less than perfectly embedded. In addition, because of their small nature, they often are over fixed. Accordingly, one must learn to evaluate less-than optimal biopsies in many instances. It would be nice to request larger specimens in all cases, but this proves to be impractical and is probably not necessary for most evaluations.

The various causes of esophageal injury and inflammation, of a primary and secondary nature, are listed in Table 2-4.

DEVELOPMENTAL DISORDERS

Tracheoesophageal Fistula and Esophageal Atresia

Following repair of these lesions, the patients typically show evidence of poor clearance of the esophagus, and this functional state promotes the development of reflux esophagitis.[25,26] Accordingly, children with this disorder are carefully monitored for the appearance of this complication.

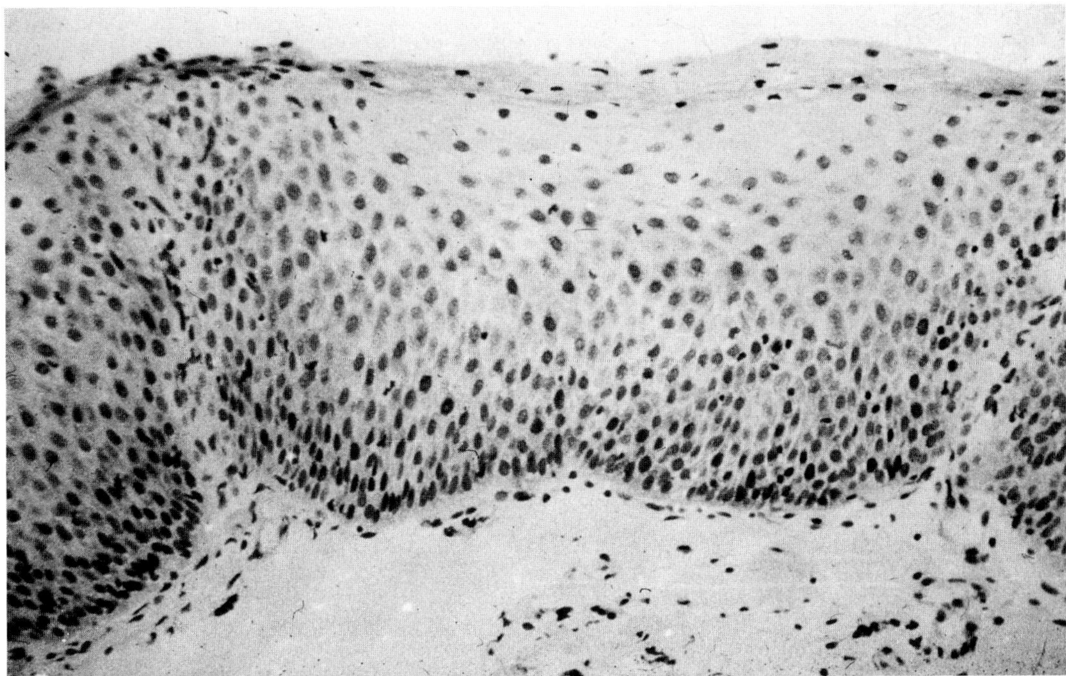

Fig. 2-6. Active esophagitis due to acid reflux. There is both expansion of the basal zone up to one-half of the epithelial thickness and elongated papillae. The lamina propria seen at the bottom is unremarkable.

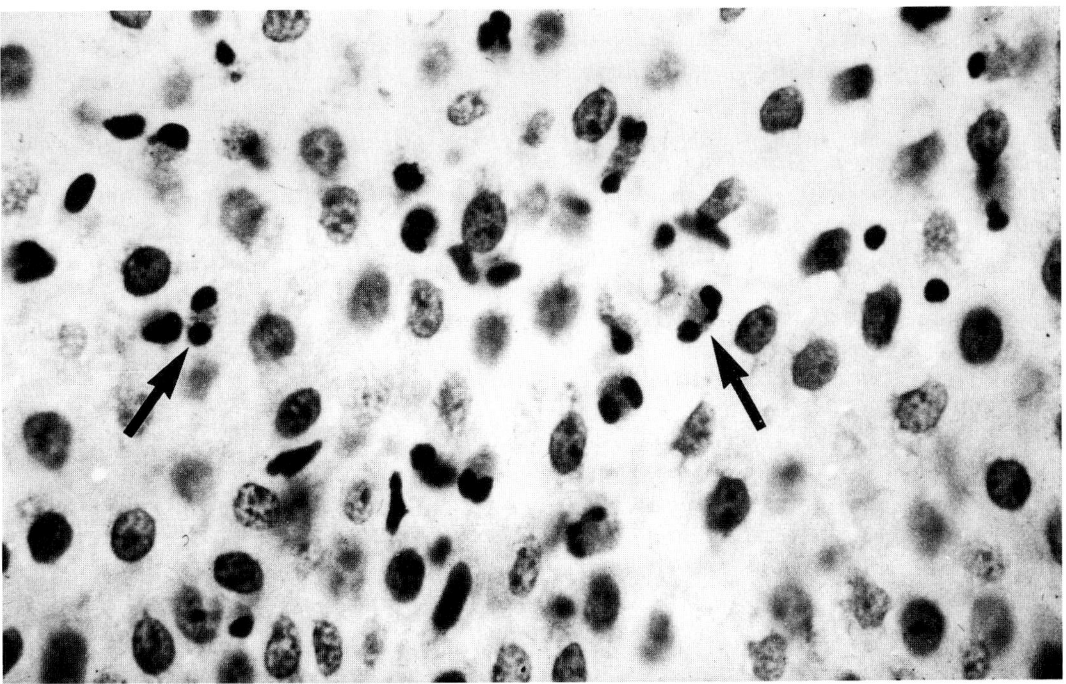

Fig. 2-7. A closer view of the squamous epithelium in active esophagitis, showing a marked infiltration by inflammatory cells. Many are eosinophils, evidenced by the bilobed, dense nuclei and cytoplasmic granules (arrows).

Table 2-4. Causes of Esophagitis

Reflux disease
Acid (peptic), alkaline
Infections
Chemical and drug injury
Radiation and trauma
Allergic and other immune conditions
Neuromuscular disorders
Rare
Behçet's, Crohn's, sarcoidosis
Skin diseases

Cysts and Hamartomas

There are a variety of developmental cysts and hamartomas that can develop in the wall of the esophagus,[27,28] but these do not typically lead to any diagnostic biopsy procedures at the endoscopic level.

Esophageal Webs and Rings

Webs represent redundant mucosal tissue and rings include portions of the esophageal wall, and these may extend into the esophageal lumen and be potential causes of obstruction.[29] They are typically identified by radiographic or gross endoscopic examination, and biopsies are only obtained in the event of overlying inflammatory or ulcer lesions. The biopsies are entirely nonspecific.

The esophageal webs are often multiple,[30,31] and such cases may be associated with the *Plummer-Vinson,* or *Paterson-Kelly syndrome.*[32] The syndromatic cases reveal more webs in the proximal part of the esophagus, reduced gastric acid, and iron deficiency anemia. The epithelium overlying the webs is prone to neoplastic transformation, and biopsies may be employed to detect the dysplastic lesions in the squamous epithelium. Webs can also develop as a complication of cutaneous disorders that can affect the esophagus; this topic is discussed in the section under "Miscellaneous Conditions."

Heterotopic Stomach

Ectopic foci of the normal stomach,[33] typically of the fundic-corpus mucosa, may be found in all parts of the alimentary tract (Table 2-5). They are especially common in the upper esophagus,[34–38] in the duodenum,[39,40] and in *Meckel's diverticula.* The lesions in the esophagus are localized mainly in the proximal quarter and are often referred to as *inlet patch.* The lesions may extend for a few centimeters but are not present in the distal esophagus, helping to differentiate them from the acquired condition of Barrett's esophagus. The heterotopic areas appear as mucoid regions, and biopsies are typically done to confirm the finding and to rule out other inflammatory conditions.

Biopsy Features

The biopsies are diagnostic, revealing mature gastric corpus mucosal tissue that consists of surface and pit-type mucous cells together with the specialized glands containing parietal and chief cells (Fig. 2-8). Bacterial organisms, consistent with *Helicobacter pylori,* may be found adherent to the surface of the mucous cells.[41] The gastric glands are compact, and there is usually no increase of inflammatory cells in the lamina propria. Although the gastric cells are considered to be functional, the rapid transit through the esophagus eliminates in most instances the development of any peptic effects such as ulceration in the adjacent squamous epithelium. This may exceptionally occur and lead to stricture formation.[42] Such ulcers are more commonly seen in areas of the gastrointestinal tract where there may be stasis, such as in Meckel's diverticula and in the rectum.

The main differential diagnosis is with Barrett's esophagus (Table 2-6). The latter is an acquired abnormality that develops in

Table 2-5. Location of Heterotopic Stomach

Common
Upper esophagus (inlet patch)
Duodenum
Meckel's diverticulum
Rare
Other small intestine
Rectum
Duplication cysts

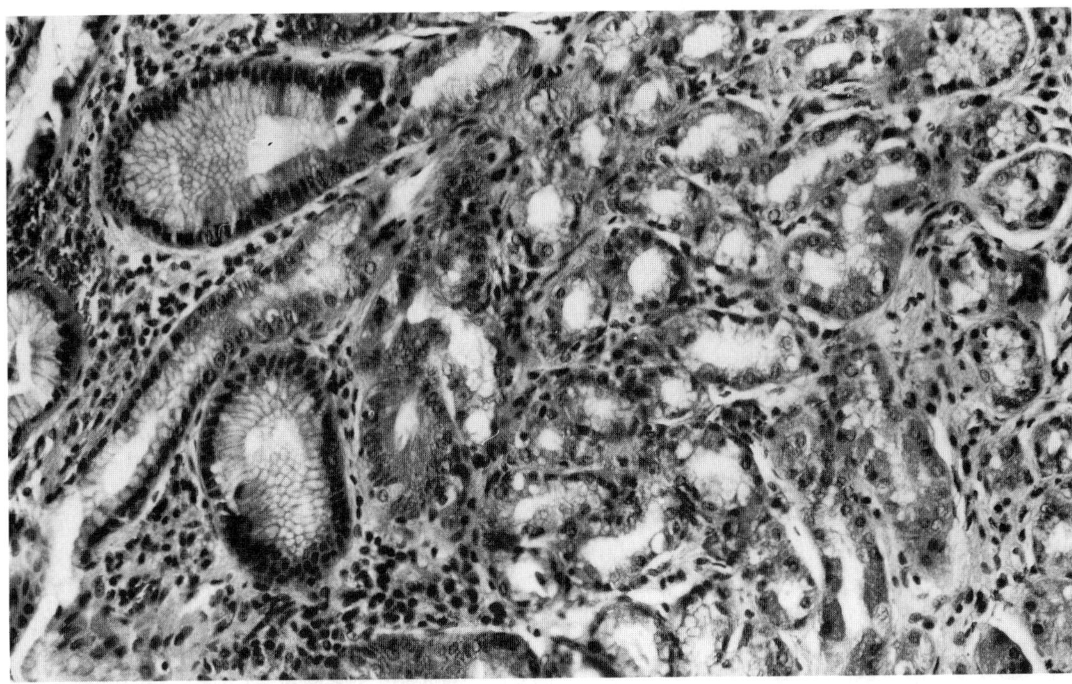

Fig. 2-8. Heterotopic stomach in the esophagus. The biopsy was taken from the proximal esophagus at 15 cm. The surface with gastric-type pits containing mucous cells appears at the left. Most of the lesion is composed of gastric fundic glands, showing a mixture of parietal, chief, and mucous cells (× 210).

chronic inflammatory conditions, usually in peptic esophagitis. The Barrett's lesions are concentrated in the distal portion of the esophagus; if present in the more proximal region, there is continuous involvement of the distal area as well. Microscopic features of Barrett's are entirely different from the heterotopic stomach, revealing a mixture of gastric and intestinal mucous cells and a paucity of the special gastric fundic-type cells. Cases may be seen in which both lesions are present, with the appearance of esophagitis and Barrett's esophagus concentrated in the distal part and the heterotopic stomach largely representing an incidental finding in the proximal portion of the esophagus. There is no evidence to support any relationship between the two lesions. Rarely, tumors can develop from heterotopic stomach, and this should be considered whenever there is an adenocarcinoma in the proximal esophagus.[43]

MOTOR AND MECHANICAL DISORDERS

A variety of motor and mechanical disturbances can affect the transit function of the esophagus and the action of the lower

Table 2-6. Comparison of Heterotopic Stomach and Barrett's Esophagus

Feature	Heterotopia	Barrett's
Surface/pit mucous cells of stomach	Present	Variable
Goblet mucous cells	Absent	Common
Parietal and chief cells	Abundant	Uncommon
Inflammation	Scant	Common

sphincter. These conditions favor stasis and poor acid clearance, leading to the development of inflammatory lesions. Overall, the features are entirely nonspecific, and the diagnosis depends on the full clinical and gross information. Biopsies may be done to evaluate inflammatory lesions that develop.

Achalasia

Included in this category are patients with the idiopathic form and those with *Chagas' disease* where the lesion is due to a chronic infection with *Leishmania.*[44,45] In either case, there is a progressive loss of the ganglia in the distal part of the esophagus and excessive contraction and motility of the esophageal musculature. There results poor opening of the lower sphincter, requiring endoscopic dilation or surgery to open the lumen. This may lead in turn to excessive reflux of gastric contents and poor emptying, and the patient may develop signs of reflux esophagitis. In such instances, biopsies are done to identify the esophagitis, to evaluate the effects of the dilation, and to detect any other complications such as stricture and Barrett's esophagus. An increase in squamous cell carcinoma has also been mentioned in cases with achalasia.

The mucosal biopsies obtained are largely for the evaluation of the esophagitis and are not done to investigate the primary neuromuscular disorder.

Diverticula

Several kinds of esophageal diverticula are encountered, including the pulsion type in the most proximal region, the traction form in the midportion, and those related to healing ulcers that tend to be concentrated in the distal part. These lesions are identified mainly by radiographic and gross endoscopic examinations; biopsies are only exceptionally done to evaluate potential inflammatory lesions in their areas. An exaggeration of ductal structures, referred to as *pseudodiverticula,* has been noted in the distal portion, but this is not typically evaluated by biopsy.[46,47]

Systemic Sclerosis

Chronic connective tissue disorders may affect the esophagus largely by interfering with proper motility. The lesions are most strikingly seen in systemic sclerosis but also may be present to a lesser degree in other conditions such as diabetes mellitus, dermatomyositis, mixed connective tissue disease, *Sjögren syndrome,* and pseudoobstructive disorders.[48–54] Inflammatory lesions leading to stricture development are commonly seen in the more severe examples of systemic sclerosis and were originally thought to be due to the direct connective tissue effects. It is now well established that they are caused instead by damage to the lower esophageal sphincter, favoring excess reflux and the development of reflux esophagitis. Biopsies are done as in all cases of reflux disease to detect the esophagitis and to look for complications such as Barrett's esophagus and stricture formation.

The biopsies are entirely nonspecific and represent those seen in any case of reflux esophagitis. Accordingly, there may be the features of acute or active disease in the squamous epithelium, and the rare development of Barrett's esophagus in these patients. Biopsies are also done to exclude areas of dysplasia and carcinoma.

Mallory–Weiss Syndrome

This syndrome represents small, longitudinally-oriented lacerations that develop at the junction of the esophagus and gastric cardia in patients following episodes of severe retching and vomiting.[55,56] The tears are more commonly seen in alcoholic patients and may lead to severe inflammation and hemorrhage. The diagnosis is ordinarily made by gross inspection, and biopsies are done only if there is suspicion of a tumorous lesion. Histologic examination of the Mallory-Weiss lesion is entirely nonspecific.

VASCULAR DISORDERS

Compared to other portions of the alimentary tract, vascular lesions of the esophagus, other than varices, are rare.

Varices

Marked dilation of the esophageal and gastric veins develop in patients with cirrhosis and other causes of portal hypertension.[57] These are typically manifested by extension into the lumen and have the potential for rupture and significant clinical hemorrhage. The diagnosis is ordinarily established by gross examination.

There is an increasing use of the insertion of sclerotic agents to cause a reduction in these varices. These substances can cause significant inflammation and fibrosis of the adjacent esophageal wall as well as of the variceal lesions. With time, there can develop ulcers and strictures, and biopsies are exceptionally performed to evaluate these and to exclude tumors. Microscopic features are entirely nonspecific (see the section under "Chemical and Drug Disorders" for discussion).

Ischemic Disorders

Ischemic lesions due to poor flow, to obstruction of major vessels, or to vasculitis are rarely seen in the esophagus.[58] Exceptionally, there can develop localized lesions due to either tumors or the effects of radiation that are compromising the blood supply in a small region. Biopsies are rarely evaluated for these conditions.

REFLUX ESOPHAGITIS

Endoscopy and biopsy examination of the esophagus is most often employed to evaluate patients with reflux esophagitis.

Mechanism of Injury

In most instances, injury to the esophagus results from an incompetence of the lower esophageal sphincter, alone or in conjunction with poor clearance of the esophagus.[59–61] Most cases are of unknown etiology, but the lesions also are seen in any patients with equivalent esophageal injuries, such as persons with repair of esophageal atresia, patients with systemic sclerosis and other connective tissue disorders, and those who have had esophageal dilation for achalasia or other strictures.

The most sensitive test to evaluate patients for reflux is esophageal manometry.[62–64] For the best results, this should include a prolonged period, consisting of either an overnight or a full-day examination. Criteria have been established for the number of normal episodes of reflux and for the time of clearance of acid material from the esophagus. A greater number of normal reflux episodes are acceptable in children.[65,66] Other tests that are occasionally employed are simple radiographs to look for reflux, milk technesium scans, and the *Bernstein test* in which acid is inserted into the esophagus to elicit pain. The manometric examination also permits the determination of the esophageal pressures, particularly that of the lower sphincter, to look for any abnormal reduction. Overall, the pressure measurements are the most sensitive but are not routinely employed or continued in most patients. Evaluation of reflux is largely determined clinically by symptoms and by the gross inspection at endoscopy. In this respect, there is a very poor correlation between the macroscopic and biopsy determinations of esophagitis; it is therefore strongly urged that a biopsy be obtained at the time of any endoscopy. Minor gross changes such as erythema may prove to be insignificant and probably due to the procedure itself, whereas patients without major endoscopic features may reveal definite disease on histologic examination.

Hiatal hernias are often seen in patients with reflux esophagitis, but the hernial condition is also very common in the general population. Most studies have shown poor correlations, although operations to correct hernias are still considered in patients with reflux disease. It is important to stress that the simple presence of a hernia does not absolutely signify reflux disease, and biopsy should still be obtained.

Acute Effects

Biopsy Features

Whatever the underlying cause of the reflux, and whether the substance is acid or alkaline,[67,68] the effects on the esophageal epithelium are the same[22,23,69–77] (Table 2-7). The earliest lesion, best represented in experimental studies, consists of degeneration of the superficial squamous cells together with the presence of neutrophils and probably increased eosinophils[20,21] (Figs. 2-6 and 2-7). Also noted are swollen squamous epithelial cells (balloon cells) that are due to the excess absorption of water and protein, probably reflecting damage to the cellular membranes in acute cell injury.[18] These balloon cells can be distinguished from richly glycogenated squamous cells by the use of appropriate stains; the glycogen is accented by the PAS reaction, whereas the balloon cells are positive for immunoperoxidase stains for albumin. There has been debate about the potential utility of eosinophils within the squamous epithelium. These are normally present but at a rare number, probably no more than one to two per biopsy in the distal portion.[78] Any increase of eosinophils should be considered abnormal, and this criterion can be especially helpful in poorly oriented biopsies.

Table 2-7. Stages of Reflux Esophagitis

Acute: necrosis, inflammation, and granulation
Repair: Expansion of basal zone and elongation of papillae
Chronic: Fibrosis and Barrett's
Complications: Dysplasia and adenocarcinoma

Following the reflux injury there are attempts at repair, resulting in several other features: the expansion of the basal zone to more than 15 percent of the epithelial thickness, and best appreciated when more than 25 percent (Fig. 2-9); elongation of the papillae of the lamina propria to more than 75 percent of the relative thickness (Fig. 2-10); and the presence of dilated and ruptured venules within the papillae. All of these features require excellent orientation and proper embedding of the samples and are best accomplished when the biopsies are of a larger aspiration or jumbo type. As mentioned above, it may be difficult to evaluate these features in the usually obtained smaller biopsy samples, and other features such as the number of eosinophils within the epithelial layer may be easier to appreciate.[21,79,80] Also noted is an increase in the amount of mononuclear inflammatory cells, including both dendritic Langerhans cells and lymphocytes, within the epithelium in patients with reflux esophagitis[8,19,74,77]; unless marked, this criterion probably needs a scoring system to be valid.

Several of the features of acute or active esophagitis are present in normal persons in the distal few centimeters of the esophagus, possibly reflecting normal or physiologic reflux.[69] In particular, basal zone expansion and elongation of the papillae have been well documented in this region. In contrast, an increase in the intraepithelial inflammatory cells, including eosinophils, has not been regularly shown in normal persons in this distal area and may continue to be a useful criterion. With more severe disease there is progressive coagulative necrosis of the squa-

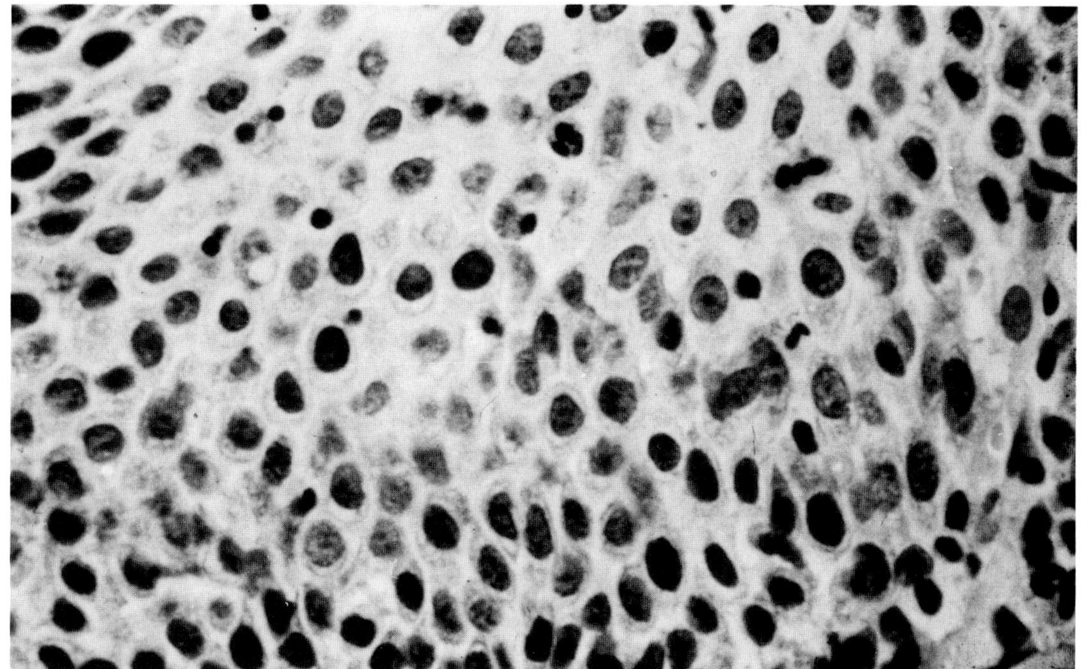

Fig. 2-9. Reflux esophagitis, revealing the marked expansion of the basal zone of squamous cells, which can extend the whole thickness of the epithelial layer. Such cases may be confused with dysplasia (see Ch. 3); the hyperplasia shows a regularity in the size and shape of the cells and of their nuclei.

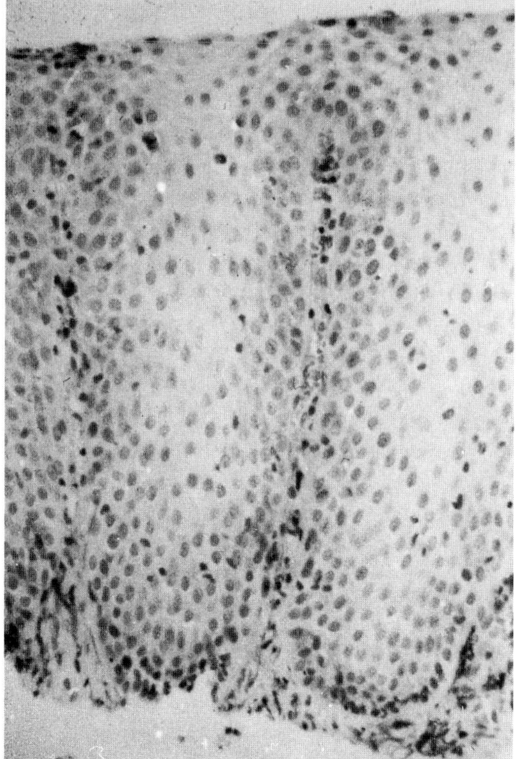

Fig. 2-10. Reflux esophagitis. There is marked elongation of the papillae that extend very close to the epithelial surface appearing at the top. This is often associated with dilated venules, resulting in an erythematous surface.

mous epithelial layer resulting in superficial erosions and in deeper ulcers. Such cases show prominent neutrophils at the base and at the edges of the lesion together with varying amounts of granulation tissue. Biopsy of ulcerated lesions are done not only to confirm the presence of esophagitis but also to rule out other causes such as infections or tumors.

Biopsy Uses

In the evaluation of biopsies of patients with suspected reflux esophagitis, one tries to establish that there is esophagitis, that the disorder is either acute alone or associated with chronic effects, and whether there are other specific lesions noted. In particular, infectious agents or their inclusions and any specialized inflammation such as granulomas are sought. Some disorders are excluded by unusual distribution, such as viral infections and reactions to pills that tend to be focal, and lesions that are more apt to be in the proximal esophagus, such as chronic graft versus host disease and the various cutaneous disorders that can affect the esophagus.

Biopsies are also done to monitor the course of the patient following medical or surgical therapy and to look for complications, particularly the development of chronic disease. With healing of the acute disorder, there is restoration of the normal squamous epithelium. Most patients experience multiple episodes of reflux disease, but well established chronic disease only develops in about 10 to 15 percent of the patients.

Chronic Effects

Although many patients experience multiple attacks of reflux esophagitis, only a small percentage of these progress to chronic disease. The major chronic effects are a fibrosis resulting from deep ulceration and granulation tissue leading to stricture formation,[81] and the appearance of a change in the squamous epithelium to a glandular type, which is called *Barrett's esophagus*[24] (Fig. 2-11). These features serve as markers of chronic esophagitis and predictors of other complications such as the development of epithelial dysplasia and carcinoma.

Barrett's Esophagus

Causes

Although originally described as a congenital abnormality,[82] it has now been firmly established that Barrett's esophagus is a consequence of prolonged injury to the esophagus in both adults and children.[83–87] There results a change or metaplasia from the normal squamous epithelium to a glandular type, consisting of some admixture of gastric- and intestinal-type mucous epithelial cells. The most common cause, simply reflecting the overall greater prevalence, is idiopathic reflux esophagitis. Similar findings can be seen in any other chronic esophagitis including that related to systemic sclerosis, to lye-associated strictures, to the complications of chemotherapy, to the loss of the sphincter following surgery, and to the effects of dilation in patients with achalasia.[88–92]

Biopsy Features

There have been extensive studies of the pathologic features of Barrett's esophagus[24,93–99] (see Fig. 2-11). Grossly, the lesion presents as a mucoid or salmon-colored mucosa replacing parts of the squamous epithelium, which is normally of a pale color and opaque or dull appearance. Three major histologic forms of Barrett's esophagus are regularly noted, including a so-called specialized columnar type, a cardiac form, and an atrophic corpus mucosa (Table 2-8). When all are present, they tend to be arranged in a proximal-to-distal disposition. The most

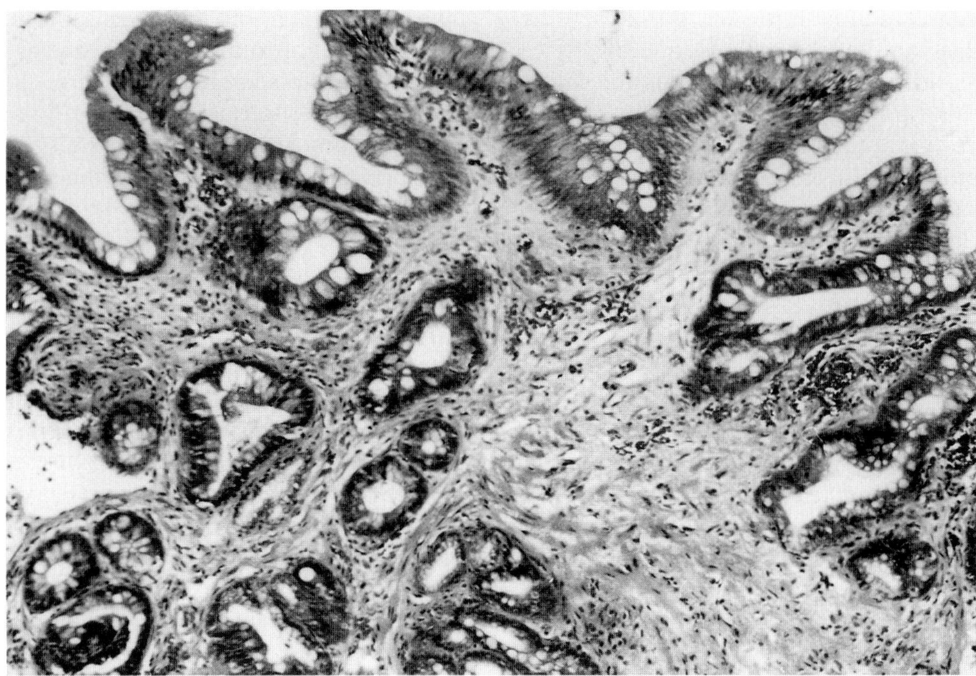

Fig. 2-11. Barrett's esophagus. The squamous layer has been entirely replaced by glandular tissue. The surface and glandular epithelium are composed of columnar cells (× 105).

distinctive is the specialized columnar type, which appears to be an admixture of gastric and intestinal mucous cells (Fig. 2-12). At first glance, this resembles gastric mucosa with areas of intestinal metaplasia in the form of goblet mucous cells. Closer inspection, however, reveals a much greater variety in the forms of mucous cells, including those that resemble normal surface or foveolar gastric mucous cells with the PAS-positive mucin granules confined to the apical portion of the cytoplasm; well formed goblet mucous cells identical to those seen in the normal small and large intestine, with positive reactions for acid mucins; and tall columnar cells with larger amounts of mucus than ordinarily seen in gastric cells and with a more prominent number of surface microvilli that form

Table 2-8. Epithelial Types in Barrett's Esophagus

	Columnar	Cardiac	Fundic
Surface Mucous Cells			
Normal gastric	+	++	++
Columnar	++	±	0
Goblet	++	±	0
Glands			
Cardiac	+	++	0
Parietal/chief	0	±	+
Mucin reactions			
Neutral	+	++	++
Mild acid	++	+	±
Sulfated	++	0	0
Relation to dysplasia	+	0	0

Symbols: 0, none; ±, rare; +, slight; ++, prominent.

an attenuated brush border. Also, these hyperplastic columnar cells frequently reveal both acidic mucins and considerable variation on ultrastructural examination.[95]

The other forms of Barrett's epithelium are more regular in appearance, resembling either cardiac mucosa (Fig. 2-13) or an atrophic fundic type (Fig. 2-14). Both forms exhibit normal surface and gastric pit (foveolar) type mucous cells overlying either well formed cardiac glands or atrophic fundic-corpus glands, showing just vestiges of the specialized glands with a few parietal and chief cells. *Helicobacter pylori* organisms are occasionally found in conjunction with the surface and pit mucous cells[100–102]; when seen, they are usually also present in the gastric antrum in these patients.

Only the appearance of the specialized columnar epithelium is highly distinctive and promptly supportive of the diagnosis of Barrett's esophagus. However, this is not an absolute finding, since the features can also exceptionally be seen in the stomach, representing intestinal metaplasia of the stomach. The appearance of the cardiac- and fundic-types of Barrett's epithelium could just as readily come from the junction of the esophagus and stomach, and the precise localization of the biopsies in such cases is needed to support the diagnosis of Barrett's esophagus. It has recently been established that Barrett's esophagus can exist in a very short version, probably for just a few centimeters above the junction, and it is very important to correlate the gross and microscopic features with reference to the exact localization of the biopsies.[103,104]

Although many of the columnar cells have increased microvilli, most of these are mucous cells. Uncommonly present are well formed intestinal-type absorptive cells with a more complete brush border. Other cellular elements that may be observed are Paneth cells and an increase in the number of endocrine cells of the gastric and intestinal

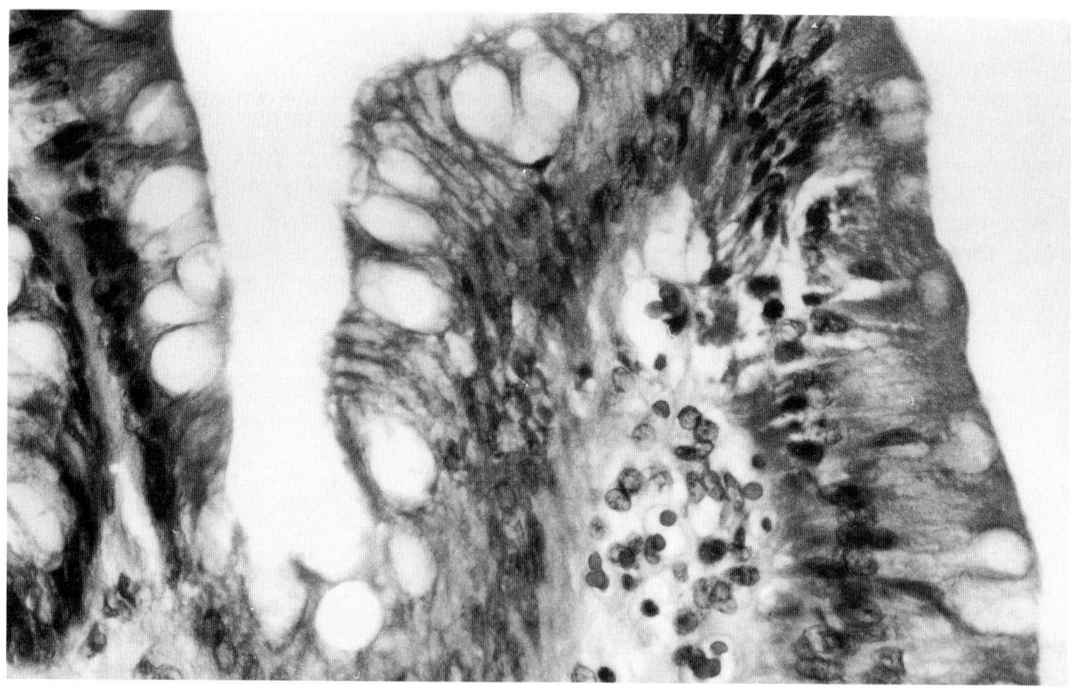

Fig. 2-12. Barrett's esophagus, with surface epithelium of the so-called specialized columnar type. Noted are both goblet and columnar mucous cells (× 425).

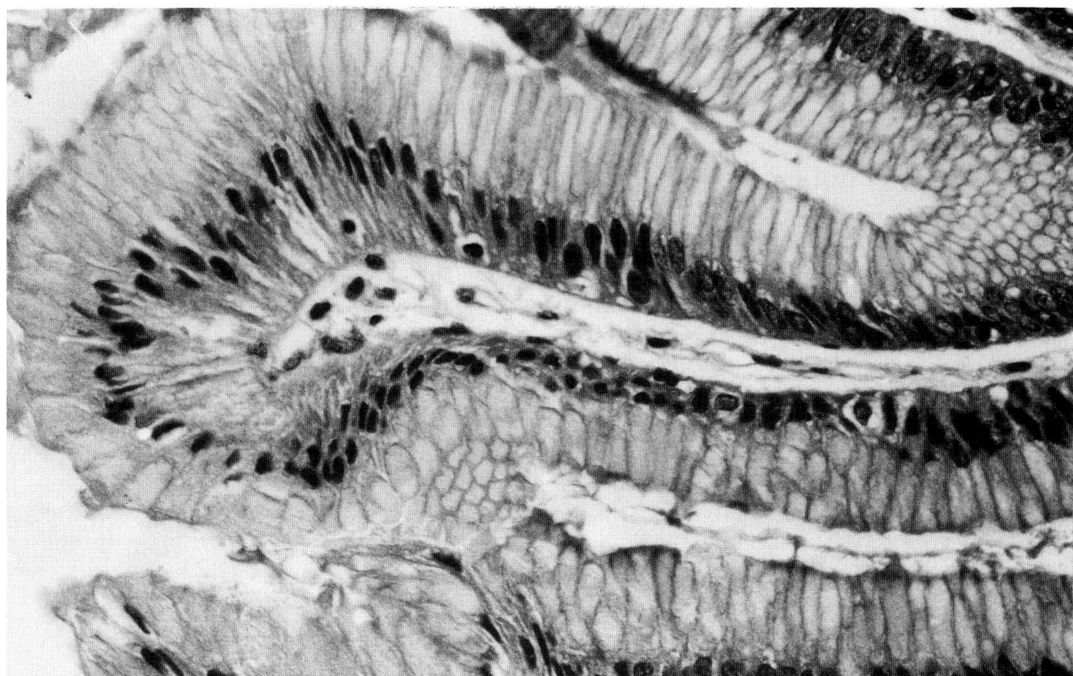

Fig. 2-13. Barrett's esophagus, with surface epithelium of the cardiac type. There is a continuous layer of columnar mucous cells. Compared to the normal cardia, the cells in Barrett's esophagus tend to be taller and to contain the mucin in more than the apical regions (× 425).

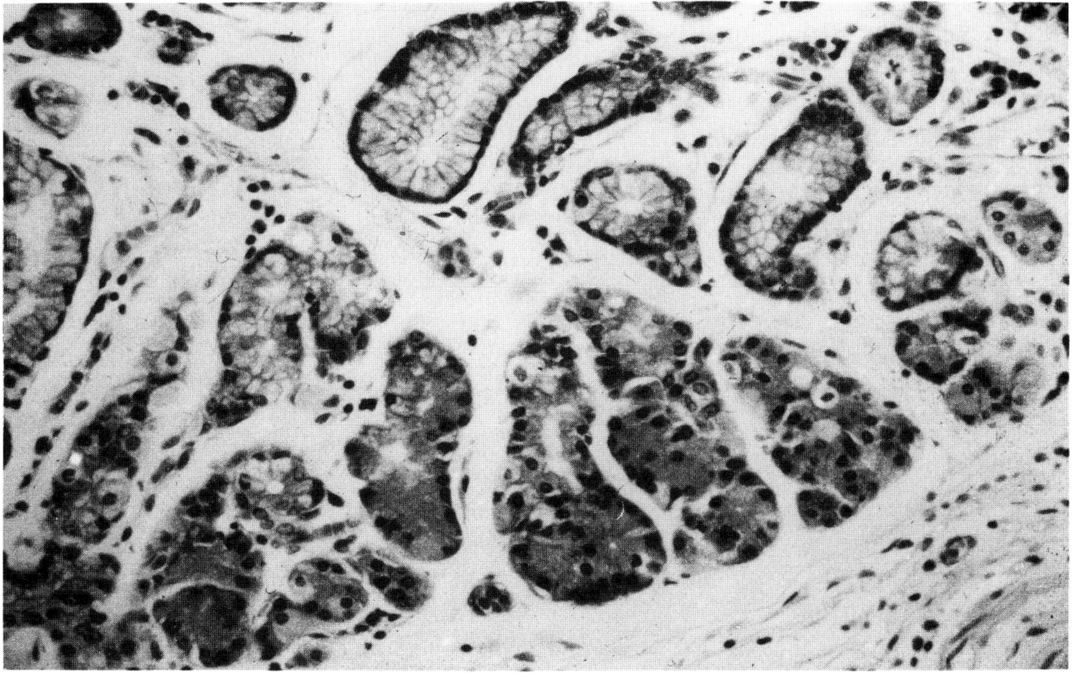

Fig. 2-14. Barrett's esophagus, with epithelium of the atrophic fundic type. There appear shortened gastric pits with mucous cells at the top and markedly atrophic fundic glands at the base. (From Goldman,[1] with permission.)

types.[105,106] Most of the metaplastic areas resemble the incomplete or colonic form, and the complete or small intestinal type of intestinal metaplasia is much less frequent in the areas of Barrett's esophagus.[99] (These types of intestinal metaplasia are described in more detail in Chapter 4.)

With treatment of the chronic esophagitis, there can occur partial resolution of the Barrett's esophagus.[107–109] Biopsy of the epithelial areas reveals a return to squamous epithelium, but complete resolution of Barrett's esophagus is rare.

Biopsy Uses

The notion that Barrett's esophagus can be divided into three distinct forms of epithelium has proven to be an oversimplification. Studies by electron microscopy, both of the transmission and scanning forms, have realized a greater variety and montage of the cells.[95,110,111] This simply reflects the metaplastic process with cells assuming features of both gastric and intestinal differentiation. Nevertheless, at the biopsy level, the separation into the three major forms has practical utility. The development of dysplasia and carcinoma seems to occur preferentially in the specialized columnar form. Overall, endoscopic examination and biopsies of the mucosa are obtained in patients with Barrett's esophagus to render the original diagnosis, to follow the patients after therapy, and for surveillance to identify dysplasia and carcinoma.

Dysplasia and Carcinoma

The major importance of identifying that a patient has chronic esophagitis is the recognition of an increased prevalence of carcinoma in such patients.[111–116] It has been estimated that perhaps 5 to 10 percent of patients with established Barrett's esophagus are at risk for the development of dysplasia or carcinoma, which justifies screening and surveillance programs for their early detection.[117,118] This subject is covered in Chapter 3.

INFECTIONS

Esophageal infections are more commonly seen in debilitated and immunocompromised patients than in immunocompetent patients (Table 2-9). As a result, we are witnessing a considerable increase in the use of biopsy examination for esophageal infections, particularly in patients with the acquired immunodeficiency syndrome (AIDS).[119,120] Special stains are commonly employed, including PAS and methenamine silver for fungi and protozoa, Gram stain for bacteria, and immunocytochemical stains for viral inclusions. It is expected that there will be a more frequent use of in-situ hybridization to improve the sensitivity of infection detection in the esophagus and in other parts of the alimentary tract.[121]

General Features of Infections

The esophageal infections are typically associated with mucosal necrosis leading to erosions and ulcerations, and there is usually a prominent neutrophilic reaction. Granulation tissue is present with the deeper ulcers. All of these features are nonspecific and are seen as well in other types of esophagitis. Specific or diagnostic features include the presence of viral-associated inclusions and of the particular microorganisms, the visualization of which can be facilitated by special stains. Rarely noted in the esophagus are infections associated with a granulomatous inflammation.

Table 2-9. Esophageal Infections

Organism	Pathogenic	Opportunistic
Viruses	Herpes simplex	Cytomegalovirus
	Rare: herpes zoster	HIV, EBV
Bacteria	Gram-negative species	*Actinomyces*
	Helicobacter pylori	*Mycobacterium avium*
	Mycobacterium tuberculosis	
	Treponema pallidum	
Fungi	*Candida*	*Aspergillus*
	Rare	Rare
	Histoplasma	*Phycomycetes*
	Blastomyces	*Paracoccidioides*
	Cryptococcus	*Torulopsis*
Protozoa	*Leishmania* (Chagas')	*Cryptosporidium*
	Rare: *Amoeba*	*Pneumocystis*
Helminths	Rare: flukes	

VIRAL INFECTIONS

Herpes Simplex Infection

Esophageal infection due to herpes simplex, mostly type I, is regularly seen in immunocompetent patients.[122,123] Presumably, these are infections that extend from the lips and oral cavity. An increase in herpes infections is seen in patients who are immunocompromised. These lesions present as focal ulcers, in contrast to the more diffuse effects of reflux esophagitis. Biopsies of the ulcer edges and cytologic smears are distinctive, revealing necrosis and inflammation, neutrophils and mononuclear cells, together with the cytopathic features of the virus[124–127] (see Plate 1A). These include multinucleated squamous cells and purple intranuclear inclusions of the so-called Cowdry types A and B (Figs. 2-15 and 2-16). The type A forms are smaller and surrounded by a clear halo, whereas the type B forms are bigger and tend to fill most of the nuclear space, resulting in a ground glass appearance. Degenerating squamous epithelial cells may show dull-appearing coagulated nuclei that can resemble inclusions; in cases of doubt, immunocytochemical stains for herpes can provide specificity. These stains do not always aid in the detection of the cases; for this, in-situ hybridization holds promise. The inclusions and multinucleated cells are present primarily in the squamous epithelium. Exceptionally, one can encounter these inclusions in glandular epithelial cells, but these are not present in the normal esophageal surface.

Cytomegalovirus Infection

Infection of the esophagus by cytomegalovirus (CMV) is noted almost exclusively in immunocompromised patients[128–131] and can be associated with giant ulcers.[132] Biopsies reveal variably sized intranuclear and very large intracytoplasmic inclusions that tend to stain purple with the H & E stain (Plate 1B). The nuclear inclusions have a prominent halo resembling an owl's eye (Figs. 2-17 and 2-18). They are most prominent in the mesenchymal cells, including fibroblasts, endothelial cells, and probably macrophages. An increasing amount of the inclusions is now noted in epithelial cells, particularly in glandular tissue, but this is not prevalent in the esophagus. The inclusions are readily visualized with H & E stains, and specificity can be provided in doubtful cases by immunocytochemical stains.

Other Viral Infections

Infections of the esophagus with other viral agents are rare and need clinical correlation or special studies for their documenta-

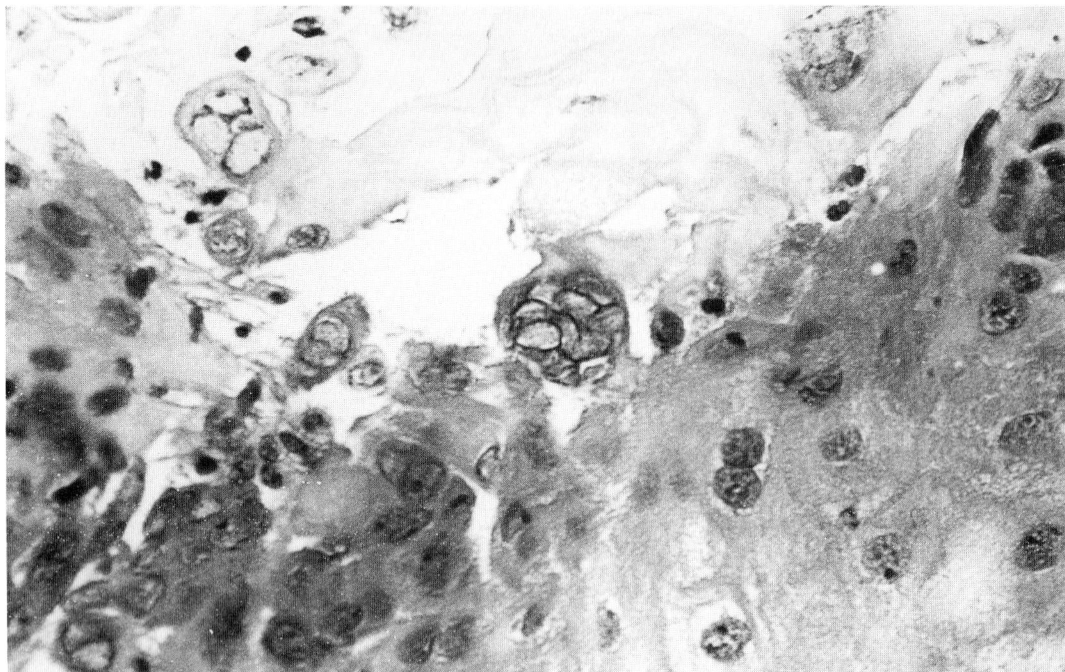

Fig. 2-15. Herpes simplex infection of the esophagus. This is taken from the edge of an ulcer. Noted are multinucleated epithelial cells and numerous intranuclear inclusions (× 640).

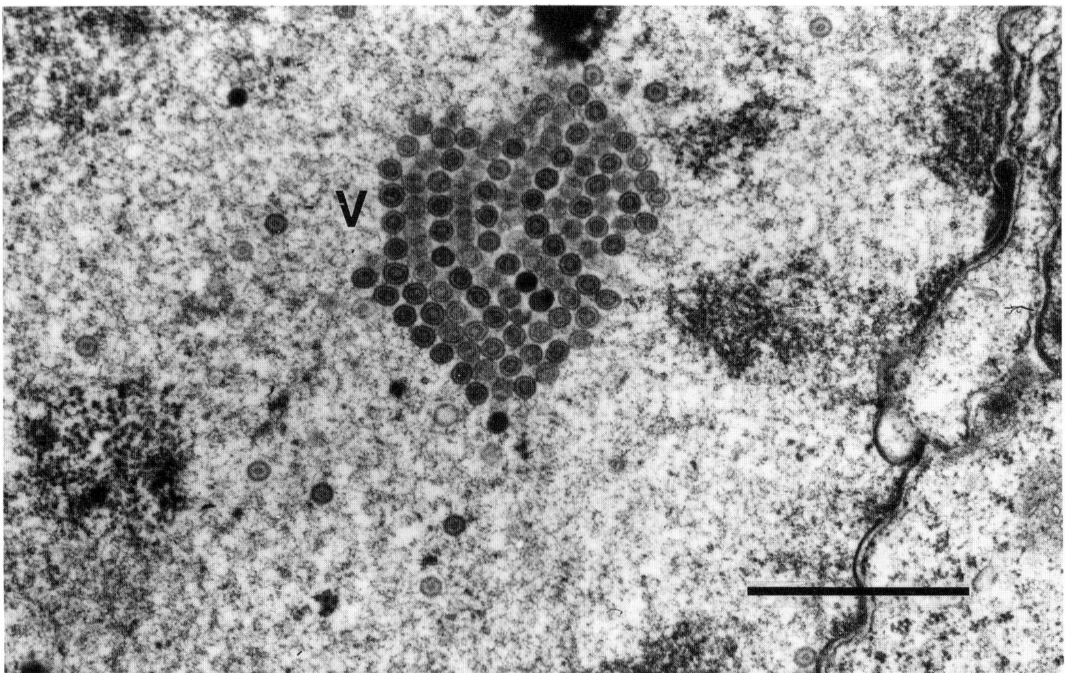

Fig. 2-16. Electron micrograph of herpes simplex virus infected cell (monocytes in culture). Particles (V) seen in the nucleus are naked nucleocapsids with and without cores. The *Herpesviridae,* such as herpes simplex virus, Epstein-Barr virus, and cytomegalovirus, are indistinguishable ultrastructurally (× 28,500; bar = 1 μm).

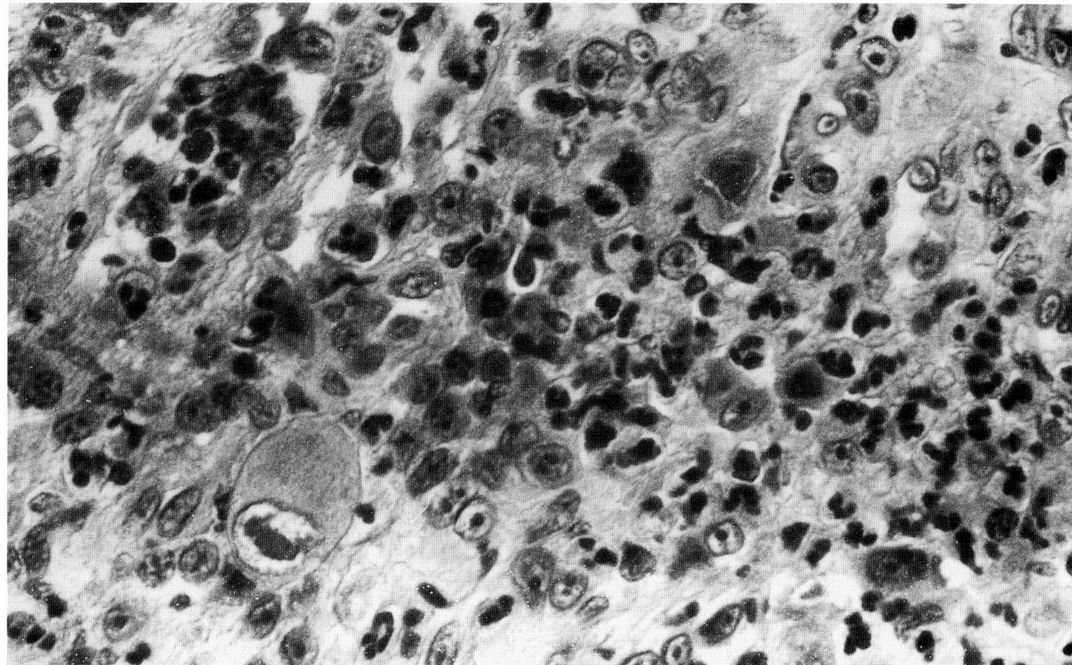

Fig. 2-17. Cytomegalovirus infection of the esophagus: ulceration, marked acute inflammation, and large intranuclear and intracytoplasmic inclusions within the mesenchymal cells. Nuclear inclusions look glassy; cytoplasmic ones appear granular. (× 850).

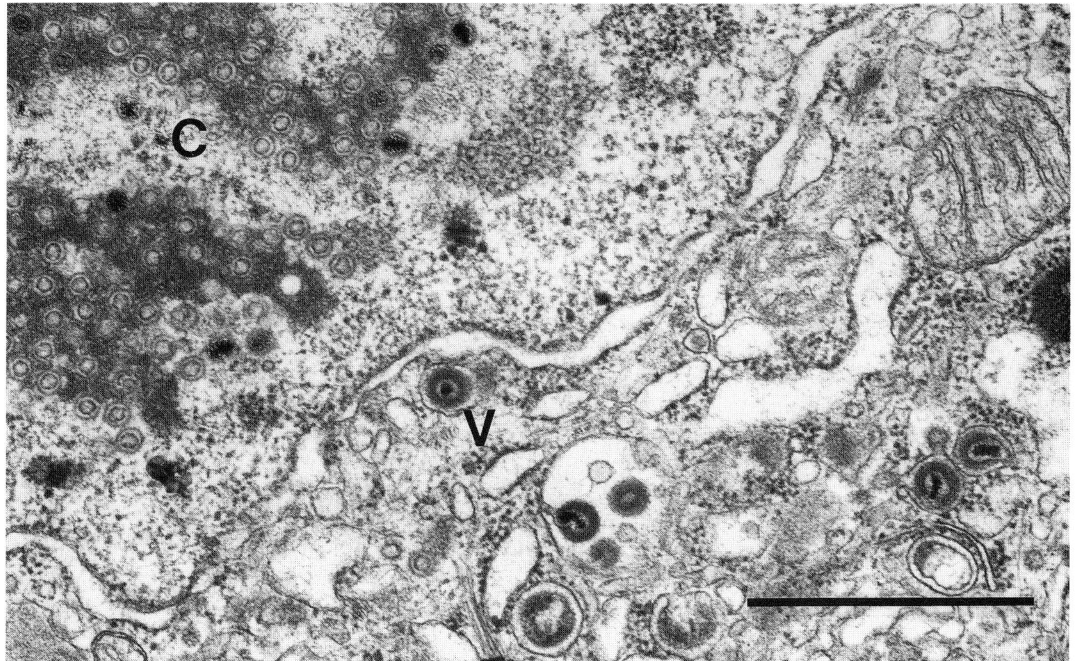

Fig. 2-18. Electron micrograph of CMV-infected cell. Nucleus has numerous particles, some with dense cores, representing nucleocapsid (C) forms. Cytoplasm contains mature viruses (V) with characteristic nucleocapsids and envelopes derived from nuclear membrane (× 37,500; bar = 1 μm).

tion. Included in this category are infections with herpes zoster virus,[133] rubella,[134] HIV,[135–137] and Epstein–Barr virus.[138] Biopsies of such cases are rare, and the features are nonspecific. In recent years, there has been an increasing interest in the association of human papilloma virus (HPV) with the esophagus, analogous to studies of the cervix and the anal canal. The data is conflicting, but there appears to be partial documentation for the presence of HPV in the development of some of the esophageal squamous cell papillomas.[139–141] Although esophageal mucosal biopsies commonly show vacuolization of the cells surrounding the nuclei, resembling koilocytotic changes in the cervical squamous epithelium, there is scant evidence to support HPV in most cases of esophagitis.

Bacterial Infections

Most cases of bacterial infection of the esophagus occur in debilitated patients and those with chronic disorders, and it is probable that the infections reflect a reduced resistance by the patients.[142] In such cases there are seen scattered areas of ulceration and often gram-negative types of bacteria. Both bacteria and fungi may be present in these patients.

Helicobacter pylori

The presence of *H. pylori* is noted in some patients with Barrett's epithelium, particularly adjacent to gastric surface-type mucous cells.[100–102,143] These bacteria are only present in patients who also have the organisms located in the stomach in association with chronic active gastritis. The bacteria probably do not contribute in any way to the development or promotion of the Barrett's esophagus. The organisms can be seen with the H & E stain, and can be accented with either the Giemsa stain or the Dieterle silver stain (Plate 1C).

Other Bacterial Infections

Rare causes of bacterial infections involving the esophagus include syphilis and actinomycosis,[134,144] tuberculosis,[145–146] and *Mycobacterium avium* infection in immunocompromised patients.[147] Syphilis more often affects the stomach, and lesions in the esophagus are exceptional and show no specific abnormality. Infection with *Actinomyces israelii* is more common in the intestines and can be associated with deep ulceration and fistula formation. The diagnosis is afforded by noting the gross sulfur granules composed of the gram-positive filamentous organisms. Tuberculosis is also more frequently noted in the ileocecal region, but cases can appear in the mid-esophagus by a spread from involved hilar lymph nodes. The biopsy features are relatively specific, showing granulomas with prominent caseous necrosis and the bacilli by acid-fast stains. In infection with *Mycobacterium avium,* there is poor granuloma formation but abundant acid-fast positive organisms (Plate 1D). There has also been a rare report of Whipple's disease affecting the esophagus.[134]

Fungal Infections

Fungi that may affect the esophagus include the regular pathogens that uncommonly induce infection in the alimentary tract, and the opportunistic fungi that typically cause disease in immunocompromised hosts.

Candida Infection

The most frequently noted result of fungal pathogens in the esophagus is moniliasis due to various species of *Candida,* including *C. albicans, C. tropicalis,* and *C. krusei.*[148–150] These organisms cause plaques and ulcerations with marked acute inflammation, and can be seen with H & E but may be confused with fibrin strands and nuclear fragments (Fig. 2-19). They are best recognized with the PAS and methenamine silver stains, showing oval spores with small buds and prominent elongation leading to the appearance of non-septate pseudohyphae (Plate 1E). Particularly in immunocompromised patients, there may be coexistent bacterial and viral infections in the same area or in other regions of the esophagus. Simple scraping or brushing of the epithelium can also reveal the organisms,[151] and this detection in an immunocompromised patient is sufficient to lead to therapy. In otherwise normal persons, one would like to see evidence of necrosis of the squamous epithelium to prove that there is an actual infection as opposed to a simple swallowing of the organisms from the throat.

Other Fungal Infections

Other causes of fungal infection in the esophagus are rare. Torulopsosis represents infection due to *Torulopsis glabrata,* which appear as smaller, round organisms without pseudohyphae.[152] In infections due to *Aspergillus* organisms (*A. fumigatus, A. niger,* and *A. flavus*)[153] and to *Phycomycetes* (mucormycosis)[154–155] there is usually more extensive necrosis and deep ulceration. The *Aspergillus* fungi are recognized as relatively slender, septate hyphae that branch at acute angles (Plate 1F), whereas the *Phycomycetes* are broad, nonseptate, and branch at right or obtuse angles (Plate 1G). Both have a propensity to involve vessels, a factor that favors the greater necrosis in these cases.

The pathogenic types of fungi include the agents responsible for histoplasmosis[156,157] and blastomycosis.[158,159] These are usually associated with more generalized involvement of the gastrointestinal tract, and localization to the esophagus is rare. The lesions show variable ulceration and granuloma formation, and the diagnosis depends on the identification of the specific fungi. *Histoplasma capsulatum* appear as tiny organisms that are invariably within macrophages or giant cells and are best visualized with the methenamine silver stain (Plate 1H). *Blastomyces dermatitidis* (the North American form) are larger and show budding. There are also rare reports of esophageal infection due to *Paracoccidioides* (the South American form)[160] and to *Cryptococcus.*[161]

Parasitic Infections

The most important parasitic disease of the esophagus is Chagas' disease due to *Leishmania,* resulting in ganglionic loss and difficulty in opening the lower esophageal sphincter. This is described above in the section on "Motor and Mechanical Disorders."

Protozoan and helminthic infections of the esophagus are otherwise rare and almost exclusively seen in immunocompromised patients. There have been recorded involvement by *Pneumocystis,*[162] *Cryptosporidium,*[163] and infestations with *Amoeba* and flukes.[134] The pathologic features are nonspecific, and the diagnosis requires identification of the organism or its ova.

CHEMICAL AND DRUG INJURY

The specific diagnosis of chemical- and drug-induced disorders of the esophagus is often provided by the clinical history.[164,165] Endoscopy and biopsy are typically done to identify and to localize the extent of the chemical or drug injury, and to rule out infections and tumors that may be present in such patients. There are multiple mechanisms by which chemicals can cause esophageal injury, including simple entrapment of pills in the mucosa, causing a localized ulcer; direct toxicity or an allergic reaction involving the epithelium; and the promotion of vasculitis, infections, or altered motility.[166]

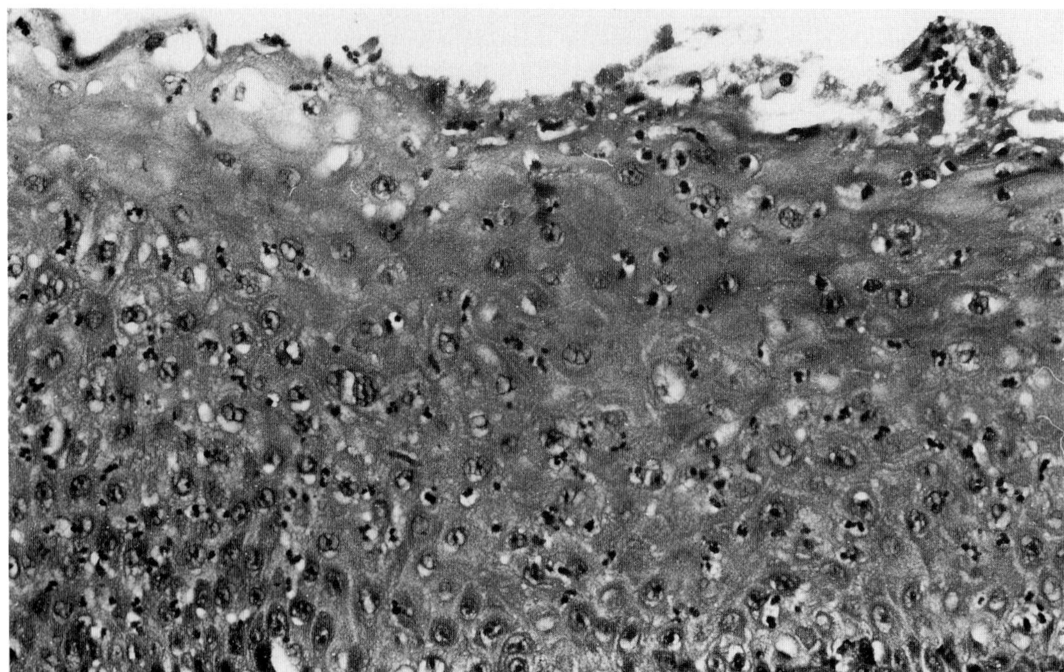

Fig. 2-19. Acute esophagitis due to *Candida albicans* with marked infiltrate of neutrophils within the squamous layer. The fungi can be detected on the surface and in the layer at higher magnification (see Color Plate 1E and Fig. 4-28) (× 210).

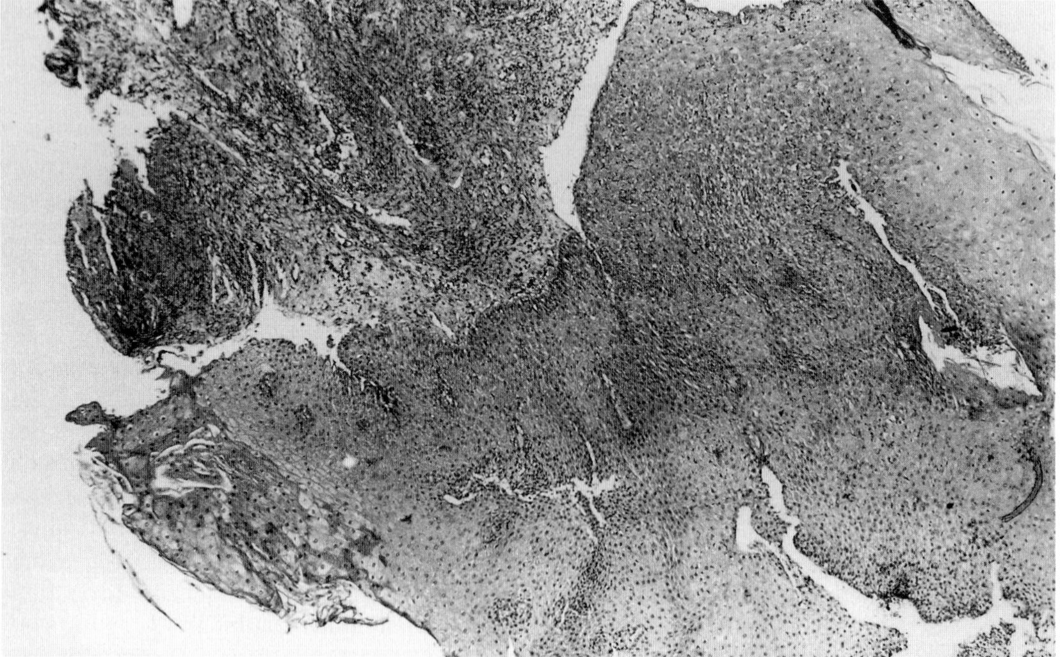

Fig. 2-20. Pill-induced ulcer of the esophagus. There is a sharply localized, focal ulcer of the squamous tissue, appearing at top and left. The ulcerated area is composed of necrotic epithelium, inflammatory cells, and granulation tissue (× 56).

Table 2-10. Example Causes of Pill-Induced Esophagitis

Antibiotics	Anti-Inflammatory Drugs	Miscellaneous Drugs
Clindamycin	Aspirin	Alprenol chloride
Deoxycycline	Indomethacin	Ascorbic acid
Erythromycin	Phenylbutazone	Barbiturates
Lincomycin	Tolmetin	Chloral hydrate
Minocycline	Combinations	Clinitest tablets
Oxytetracycline		Cromolyn sodium
Penicillin		Emepronium bromide
Tetracycline		Estramustine phosphate
Tinidazole		Ferrous salts
		Pantogar
		Potassium chloride
		Quinidine
		Vasopressin

(Modified from Lewis,[165] with permission.)

Corrosive Esophagitis

The ingestion of strong alkali, acids, and other household cleaning products can result in marked spasm and necrosis of either the esophagus or stomach.[167] The lesions in the esophagus tend to be maximal after exposure to alkaline solutions such as lye.[168,169] The diagnosis is readily established by the history, and endoscopy is often performed to determine the extent of injury.[169] Biopsies are not ordinarily obtained. Late effects include the development of fibrosis and stricture[170] and rarely a localized segment of Barrett's esophagus[89]; in which case biopsy may be done for surveillance, looking for the further complications of dysplasia and carcinoma.

Pill-Induced Esophagitis

The most common cause of drug-induced esophagitis is due to the ingestion of tablets that get struck to the mucosal surface and cause a localized burn or chemical injury.[171–175] These are seen with a wide variety of medications and typically occur after inadequate consumption of liquids at the time of taking the pills (Table 2-10). The lesions tend to be sharply localized, and this serves to distinguish them from the more diffuse distribution of reflux esophagitis. Similar focal lesions are seen in many infections.

Biopsies are completely nonspecific, revealing erosion or ulceration together with an acute inflammatory reaction and later with granulation tissue (Fig. 2-20); bullous formation is rarely seen and may relate to a hypersensitivity type of reaction.[176] Biopsies are often done to exclude other lesions, and the diagnosis is established with the aid of the history. The lesions usually heal without sequellae, and complications such as stricture are uncommon; complications are usually due to more caustic substances such as potassium or iron salts.[177–179]

Chemotherapeutic Agents

The esophageal mucosa is commonly injured following the use of chemotherapeutic drugs in the treatment of tumors of the esophagus, lung, and mediastinum.[180–182] These are often employed in conjunction with radiotherapy. There can result ulcerations of the mucosa and the potential for fibrosis and stricture formation.

Biopsies are obtained in cases with persistent ulceration or stricture, largely to exclude opportunistic infection and residual or recurrent tumor. The features of the chemical injury are nonspecific, revealing intact squamous epithelium with enlarged and atypical nuclei in the milder cases (Fig. 2-21); and necrosis, inflammation, and granulation tissue in the severe form.

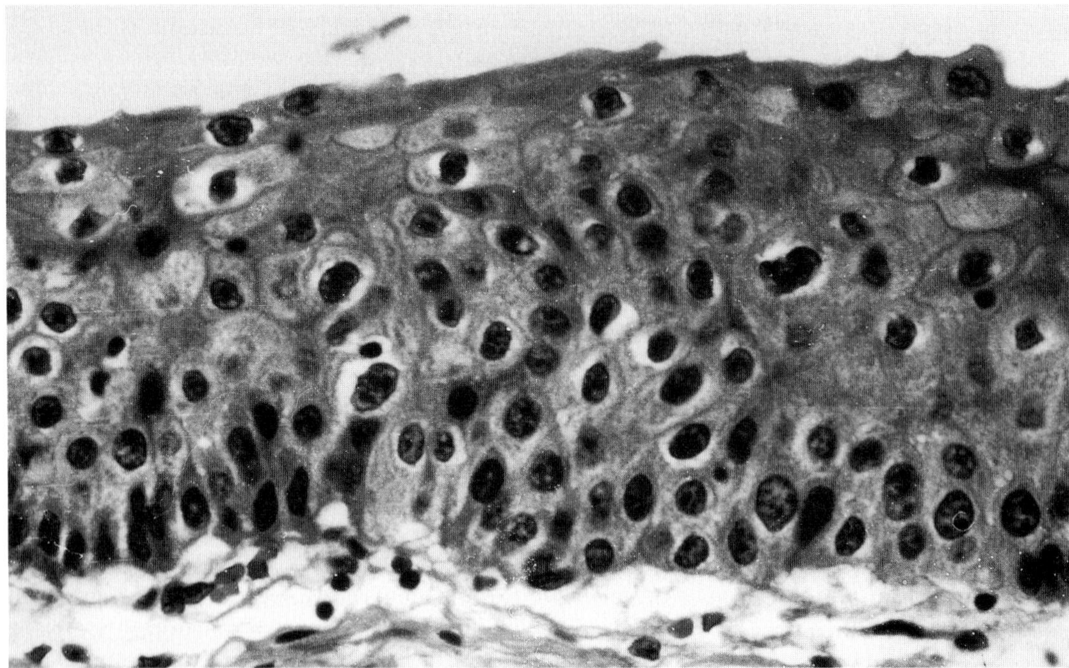

Fig. 2-21. Effect of chemotherapy in the esophagus. The squamous epithelium shows expansion of immature cells with enlarged, slightly irregular and variably hyperchromatic nuclei. The cells have abundant cytoplasm that helps to distinguish this from squamous cell dysplasia (× 640).

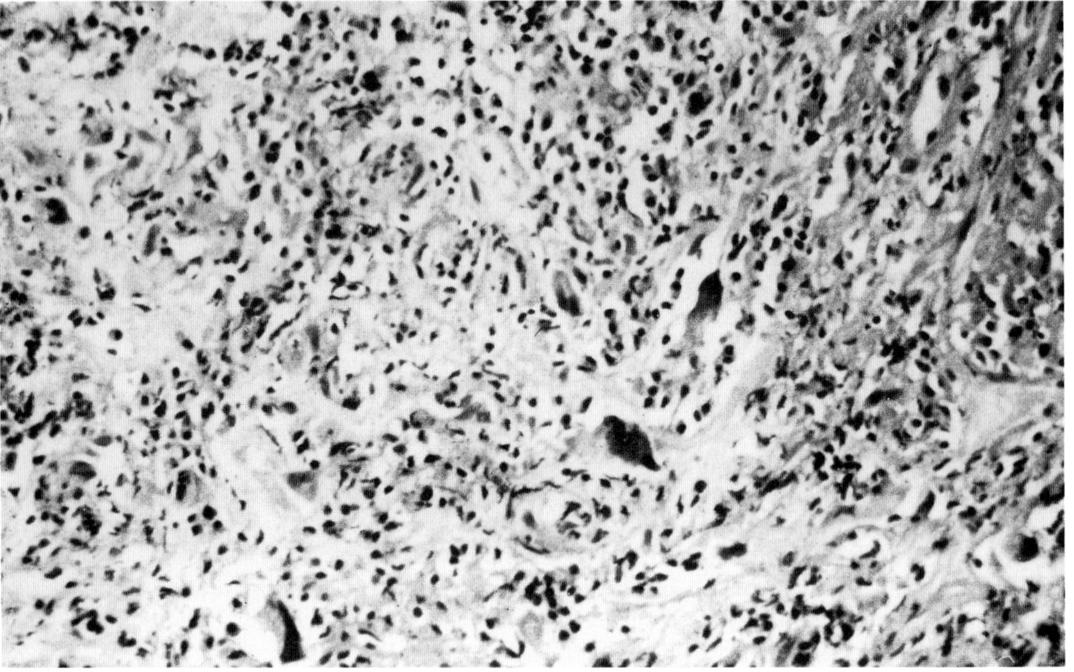

Fig. 2-22. Radiation esophagitis. Photograph is from the base of an ulcer, showing inflammation, fibrosis, and numerous fibroblasts with enlarged and hyperchromatic nuclei.

Sclerotherapy Effects

Sclerosing agents are occasionally instilled into esophageal varices in an effort to control hemorrhage,[183,184] and this may result in more extensive ulceration and fibrosis of the area.[185,186] The diagnosis is readily established by the clinical setting, and biopsies are rarely obtained from such areas.

PHYSICAL DISORDERS

Radiation Injury

Radiation therapy is commonly employed for malignant tumors of the esophagus, the lung, and the mediastinum.[166] Esophageal injury from the radiation is common, with edema and ulceration noted in the early stages, and the potential for stricture as a late event[187–188] (Table 2-11). Biopsies are often obtained in these patients not only to identify radiation injury, but also to exclude recurrent tumor and opportunistic infections.[189–191]

Most of the biopsies are nonspecific, showing only edema, ulceration, or fibrosis. Occasionally noted are prominently dilated vessels and enlarged nuclei within the mesenchymal elements, particularly in the granulation tissue and fibrosis (Fig. 2-22).

Trauma

The appearance of tubes or foreign bodies in the esophagus can cause localized irritation, ulceration, and acute inflammation.[192,193] With the persistent presence of the tube, there can result a keratosis of the squamous epithelium. Biopsies of these cases are rarely obtained and are nonspecific.

Table 2-11. Biopsy Features of Radiation

Nonspecific
Ulceration
Granulation tissue
Fibrosis
Suggestive
Ectatic vessels
Atypical mesenchymal cells
Abnormal glandular proliferation

ALLERGIC AND OTHER IMMUNE DISORDERS

Allergic Esophagitis

Eosinophilic gastroenteritis embraces a group of disorders with prominent infiltrates of eosinophils that can present as mainly mucosal, mural, or serosal disease.[194–195] The mucosal form, also termed *allergic gastroenteritis* because of a probable allergic etiology, is associated with prominent gastric and small-bowel involvement, often leading to iron deficiency anemia and to protein-losing enteropathy.

In the mucosal type of eosinophilic or allergic gastroenteritis, the esophagus is commonly involved. Until recent years, this was not well appreciated because of the lack of sampling of this area. In this disorder the esophagus[196–200] and gastric antrum[201] are most frequently affected; lesser changes are seen in the gastric corpus and they are much more focal in the small intestine and rare in the colon.

Biopsy Features

Biopsies are mainly done to identify the esophagitis and to exclude other causes. The features are relatively nonspecific and resemble those seen in reflux esophagitis.[80,195] The biopsies reveal a prominent basal zone hyperplasia and a marked increase of eosinophils within the squamous epithelial layer, which can be exceptionally pronounced at the luminal aspect (Fig. 2-23). Although the amount and location of the eosinophils may be suggestive of allergic disease, an absolute distinction from reflux esophagitis cannot be made. In such cases, the presence of an ele-

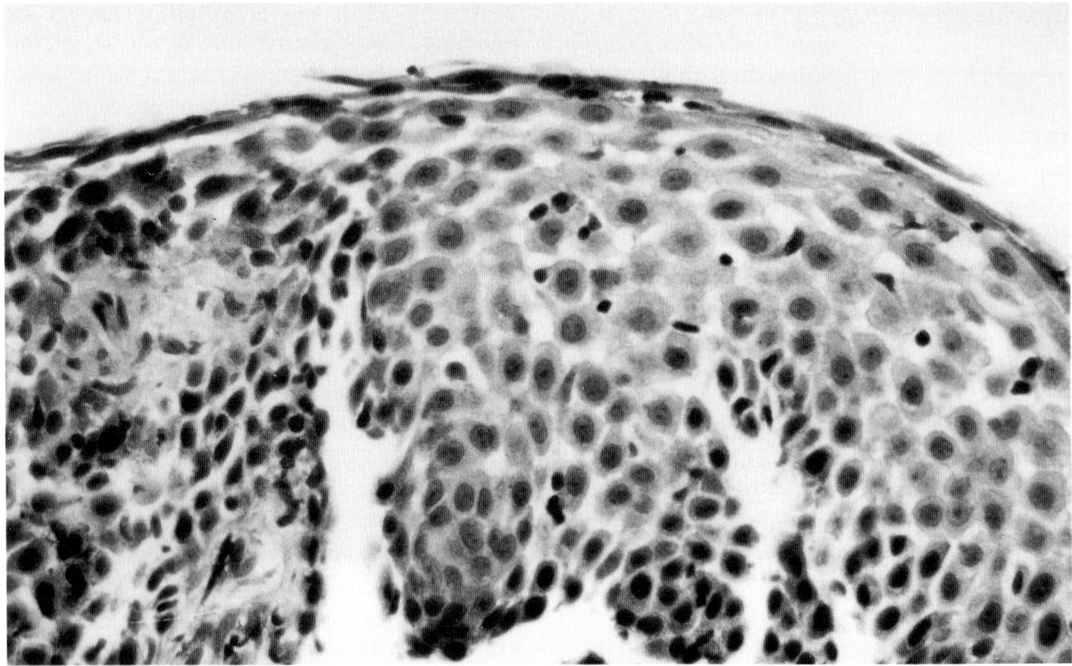

Fig. 2-23. Allergic esophagitis. There is prominent expansion of the basal zone, elongated papillae, and increased inflammatory cells including eosinophils in the squamous layer. The features are often identical to that seen in reflux esophagitis (see Figs. 2-6 and 2-9) (× 425).

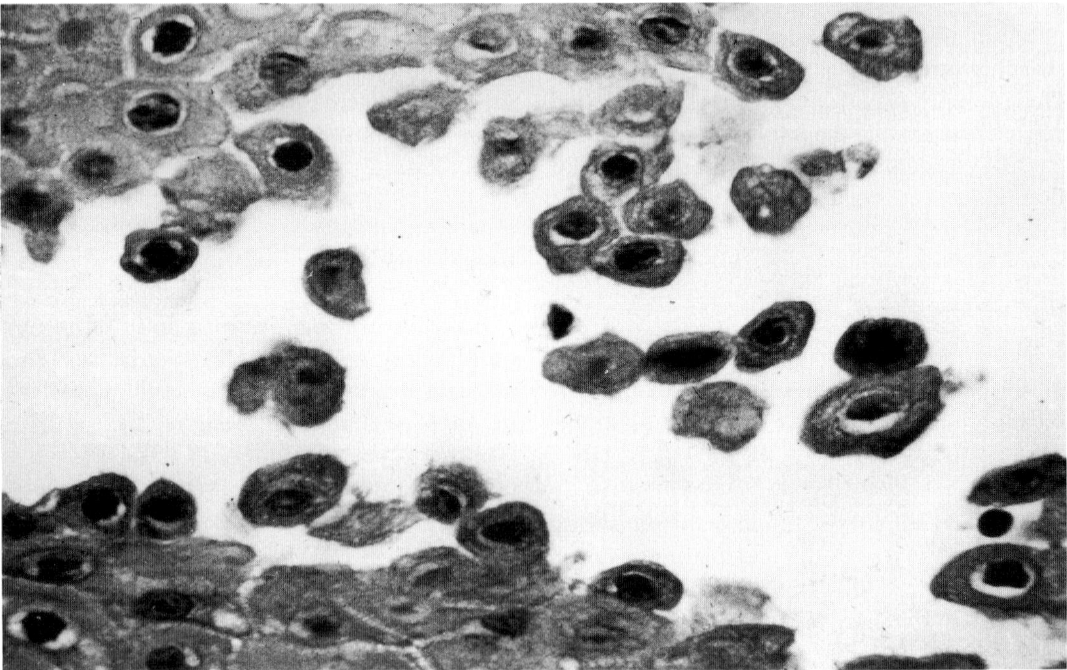

Fig. 2-24. Pemphigus of the esophagus. Noted is a large intraepithelial bulla, due to acantholysis of the squamous cells, and the lack of inflammatory cells.

vated peripheral eosinophil count and of disease affecting the gastric antrum helps to support allergic disease, whereas an abnormal pH probe test would be indicative of a reflux disorder. This differential is more prevalent in children in whom both reflux and allergic disease are more common. The features of allergic disease are discussed further in Chapters 4, 6, and 7.

Other Immunologic Disorders

Acute graft-versus-host disease most often affects the small intestinal mucosa, but esophageal lesions can occur. These present as ulcers, and severe lesions may proceed to strictures.[202]

The upper portion of the esophagus can also be affected in chronic graft-versus-host disease, with features similar to that seen in the skin and consisting of infiltrates of mononuclear inflammatory cells.[203] Biopsies are rarely employed in this area to establish the diagnosis.

Although esophagitis is often seen in patients who take medications, the injury is largely due to a localized physical effect, and damage related to an immunologic mechanism is rare.[176] With any patient who has a immunologic deficiency, opportunistic infections are typically present in the esophagus as well as in other parts of the alimentary tract, and these are discussed in previous sections of this chapter.

MISCELLANEOUS CONDITIONS

Connective Tissue Disorders

As noted above, the esophagus is regularly involved in systemic sclerosis, leading to the promotion of reflux esophagitis.[48,49] There is also exceptional involvement of the esophagus in patients with diabetes mellitus, dermatomyositis and other connective tissue disorders, and with rheumatoid arthritis.[50–53, 204,205] Significant clinical effects in these patients are, however, rare and biopsies are uncommonly employed. These show the nonspecific features of reflux disease.

Depositions

Deposition of amyloid material within the alimentary tract is frequently present in systemic cases of amyloidosis,[206,207] and may be especially prominent in submucosal vessels, in the muscle coats, and in gastric ulcers.[208,209] Its documentation in the esophagus has been rare.[210,211] The substance is recognized as acellular and fractured hyaline material, largely in vessel walls, and confirmed by the observation of green birefringence after staining with Congo Red or by ultrastructural examination (see Fig. 9-46 and Plate 4D).

Localized collections of melanin[10,212] and of lipids[213] have also been rarely noted in the esophagus, mainly concentrated in macrophages within the lamina propria.

Behçet's Disease

Behçet's disease is a rare condition characterized by multiple ulcers of the skin, and genital and oral mucosa. It is thought to be due to a vasculitis, but the exact etiology has never been established. The lesions can involve the ileum and colon, resembling *Crohn's disease,*[214,215] and they may exceptionally affect the esophagus and present as multiple small ulcers.[216–218] Biopsies are entirely nonspecific, revealing the necrosis and inflammation without definite granulomas (see Fig. 8-17). The diagnosis depends on the presence of more characteristic lesions in the genital and intestinal regions.

Granulomatous Disorders

The esophagus is rarely affected in sarcoidosis[219] and in Crohn's disease.[220–224] Noted are focal ulcers and the variable pres-

Table 2-12. Skin Lesions in the Esophagus

Types	Major Features
Pemphigus vulgaris	Intraepithelial bulla Acantholysis IgG and C3 in squamous cells
Familial benign pemphigus (Hailey–Hailey disease)	Suprabasal bulla
Bullous pemphigoid	Subepithelial bulla Minimal inflammation IgG in basement membrane
Epidermolysis bullosa dystrophica and acquisita	Subepithelia bulla Prone to fibrosis, stricture, and web formation
Stevens–Johnson syndrome	Subepithelial bulla Marked inflammation with eosinophils
Lichen planus	Vacuolization of basal zone cells Lymphocytic infiltrate beneath epithelium

ence of granulomas without caseation (see Figs. 4-41 and 4-42). The diagnosis can be suspected on biopsy but ordinarily depends on identifying lesions in more characteristic locations, such as the lungs and liver for sarcoidosis and the intestinal tract for Crohn's disease. Other causes of granulomas include foreign body reactions, tuberculosis, and some fungal infections that are discussed above.

Skin Diseases

Many of the chronic inflammatory conditions of the skin can affect the oral mucosa and the esophagus, and these are summarized in Table 2-12. Most of the diseases are productive of vesicular and bullous lesions, including pemphigus vulgaris,[225–229] familial benign pemphigus,[230] bullous pemphigoid,[231] and epidermolysis bullosa.[232–236] The biopsy features are identical to those seen in the skin. In pemphigus vulgaris, there is prominent acantholysis leading to large bullae within the squamous epithelial layer, and immunofluorescence studies reveal IgG and complement within the squamous cells (Fig. 2-24). The lesion in familial pemphigus, also called *Hailey–Hailey disease,* has less necrosis and smaller lytic areas that are restricted to the superbasal portion of the epithelium.

The other disorders reveal subepithelial bullae, the presence of IgG that is limited to the basement membrane region, and usually only slight inflammation in the acute stage. The cases of epidermolysis bullosa dystrophica[232–234] include many congenital types; blisters appear following minimal trauma, and the lesions are prone to fibrosis leading to web formation and potential strictures in the esophagus. Similar effects have been noted in cases of epidermolysis bullosa aquisita, particularly the link with web production.[235–236] Erythema multiforme, largely due to drug reactions, can also affect the oral mucosa and occasionally the esophagus.[237] This is termed *Stevens–Johnson syndrome* and is characterized by marked inflammation in the lamina propria with many eosinophils and the variable presence of subepithelial bullae. In lichen planus, there are the typical features of vacuolization of the cells in the basal zone and a heavy infiltrate of lymphocytes just beneath the epithelial layer.[238–240]

The patients often present with pain or dysphagia, and most cases also have the characteristic cutaneous lesions that permit a ready diagnosis. Endoscopy and biopsy are done to identify the distinctive bullae, to determine the extent of the disease, and to exclude other blistering disorders such as viral infections. In most cases, the biopsy features are typical, and one should try to obtain fresh frozen material to perform the appropriate immunofluorescent stains for immunoglobulins and complement.

REFERENCES

1. Goldman H, Antonioli DA: Mucosal biopsy of the esophagus, stomach and proximal duodenum. Hum Pathol 13:423–448, 1982
2. Whitehead R: Mucosal Biopsy of the Gastrointestinal Tract. 4th Ed. pp. 3–32. WB Saunders, Philadelphia, 1989
3. Sommers SC: Esophagus. pp. 7–52. In Rotterdam H, Sheahan DG, Sommers SC (eds): Biopsy Diagnosis of the Digestive Tract. 2nd Ed. Raven Press, New York, 1992
4. Geboes K, Desmet K: Histology of the esophagus. Front Gastrointest Res 3:1–17, 1978
5. Fink SM, Barwick KW, Winchenbach CL et al: Reassessment of esophageal histology in normal subjects: a comparison of suction and endoscopic techniques. J Clin Gastroenterol 5:177–183, 1983
6. DeNardi FG, Riddell RH: The normal esophagus. Am J Surg Pathol 15:296–309, 1991
7. Hopwood D, Logan KR, Bouchier IA: The electron microscopy of normal human oesophageal epithelium. Virchows Arch B Cell Pathol 26:345–358, 1978
8. Geboes K, DeWolf-Peeters C, Rutgierts P et al: Lymphocytes and Langerhans cells in the human oesophageal epithelium. Virch Arch A Pathol Anat Histopathol 401:45–55, 1983
9. Tateishi R, Taniguchi H, Wada A et al: Argyrophil cells and melanocytes in esophageal mucosa. Arch Pathol 98:87–89, 1974
10. Ohashi K, Kato Y, Kanno J, Kasuga T: Melanocytes and melanosis of the oesophagus in Japanese subjects: analysis of factors affecting their increase. Virchows Arch A Pathol Anat Histopathol 417:137, 1990
11. Ramkrishnan T, Brinker JE: Ectopic sebaceous glands in the esophagus. Gastrointest Endosc 24:293, 1978
12. Auld RM, Lukash WM, Bordin GM: Heterotopic sebaceous glands in the esophagus. Gastrointest Endosc 33:332–333, 1987
13. Bertoni G, Sassatelli R, Nigrisoli E et al: Ectopic sebaceous glands in the esophagus: report of three new cases and review of the literature. Am J Gastroenterol 89:1884–1887, 1994
14. Marcial MA, Villafana M: Esophageal ectopic sebaceous glands: endoscopic and histologic findings. Gastrointest Endosc 40:630–632, 1994
15. Rywlin AM, Ortega R: Glycogenic acanthosis of the esophagus. Arch Pathol 90:439–443, 1970
16. Bender MD, Allison J, Cuartas F, Montgomery C: Glycogenic acanthosis of the esophagus: a form of benign epithelial hyperplasia. Gastroenterology 65:373–380, 1973
17. Stern Z, Sharon P, Ligumsky M et al: Glycogenic acanthosis of the esophagus. A benign but confusing endoscopic lesion. Am J Gastroenterol 74:261–263, 1980
18. Jesserun J, Yardley JH, Giardiello FM, Hamilton SR: Intracytoplasmic plasma proteins in distended esophageal squamous cells (balloon cells). Modern Pathol 1:175–181, 1988
19. Mangano MM, Antonioli DA, Schnitt SJ, Wang HH: Nature and significance of cells with irregular nuclear contours in esophageal mucosal biopsies. Modern Pathol 5:191–196, 1992
20. Winter HS, Madara JL, Stafford RJ et al: Intraepithelial eosinophils: a new diagnostic criterion for reflux esophagitis. Gastroenterology 83:818–823, 1982
21. Brown LF, Goldman H, Antonioli DA: Intraepithelial eosinophils in endoscopic biopsies of adults with reflux esophagitis. Am J Surg Pathol 8:899–905, 1984
22. Ismail-Beigi F, Horton PF, Pope CE: Histological consequences of gastroesophageal reflux in man. Gastroenterology 58:163–174, 1970
23. Geboes K, Desmet V, VonTrappen G. Vascular changes in the esophageal mucosa: an early histologic sign of esophagitis. Gastrointest Endosc 80:29, 1980
24. Paull A, Trier JS, Dalton MD et al: The histologic spectrum of Barrett's esophagus. N Engl J Med 295:476–480, 1976
25. Winter HS, Madara JL, Stafford RJ et al: Delayed acid clearance and esophagitis after

repair of esophageal atresia. Gastroenterology 80:1317, 1981
26. Werlin SL, Dodds WJ, Hogan WJ et al: Esophageal function in esophageal atresia. Dig Dis Sci 26:796–800, 1981
27. Howes AR, Brady CE, Williams JR et al: Multiple retention cysts of the lower esophagus. J Clin Gastroenterol 4:209–212, 1982
28. Arbona JL, Fazzi JGF, Majoral J: Congenital esophageal cysts: case report and review of literature. Am J Gastroenterol 79:177–182, 1984
29. Goyal RK, Bauer JL, Spiro HM: The nature and location of lower esophageal ring. N Engl J Med 284:1175, 1971
30. Shifleet DW, Gilliam JH, Wu WC et al: Multiple esophageal webs. Gastroenterology 77:556, 1979
31. Janisch HD, Eckardt VF: Histological abnormalities in patients with multiple esophageal webs. Dig Dis Sci 27:503, 1982
32. Entwistle CC, Jacobs A: Histological findings in the Paterson–Kelly syndrome. J Clin Pathol 18:408, 1965
33. Goldman H: Other inflammatory disorders of the intestine. pp. 713–715. In Ming S-C, Goldman H (eds): Pathology of the Gastrointestinal Tract. WB Saunders, Philadelphia, 1992
34. Jabbari M, Goresky CA, Lough J et al: The inlet patch: heterotopic gastric mucosa in the upper esophagus. Gastroenterology 89:352–356, 1985
35. Truong LD, Stroebein JR, McKechnie JC: Gastric heterotopia of the proximal esophagus: a report of four cases detected by endoscopy and review of literature. Am J Gastroenterol 81:1162–1165, 1986
36. Bogomoletz WV, Geboes K, Feydy P et al: Mucin histochemistry of heterotopic gastric mucosa of the upper esophagus in adults: possible pathogenic implications. Hum Pathol 19:1301–1306, 1988
37. Variend S, Howat AJ: Upper oesophageal gastric heterotopia: a prospective necropsy study in children. J Clin Pathol 41:742–745, 1988
38. Borkan-Manesh F, Fornum JB: Incidence of heterotopic gastric mucosa in the upper oesophagus. Gut 32:968–972, 1991
39. Franzin G, Musola R, Negri A et al: Heterotopic gastric (fundic) mucosa in the duodenum. Endoscopy 14:166–167, 1982
40. Spiller RC, Shouska S, Barrison IG: Heterotopic gastric tissue in the duodenum. A report of eight cases. Dig Dis Sci 27:880–883, 1982
41. Flejou JF, Potet F, Molas G et al: Campylobacter-like organisms in heterotopic gastric mucosa of the upper oesophagus. J Clin Pathol 43:961, 1990
42. Steadman C, Kerlin P, Teaque C, Stephenson P: High esophageal stricture: a complication of "inlet patch" mucosa. Gastroenterology 94:521–524, 1988
43. Christensen WN, Sternberg SS: Adenocarcinoma of the upper esophagus arising in ectopic gastric mucosa. Two case reports and review of the literature. Am J Surg Pathol 11:397–402, 1987
44. Adams CWH, Brain RHF, Trounce JR: Ganglion cells in achalasia of the cardia. Virchows Arch A Pathol Anat Histopathol 372:75, 1976
45. Goldblum JR, Whyte RI, Orringer MB, Appelman HD: Achalasia. A morphologic study of 42 resected specimens. Am J Surg Pathol 18:327–337, 1994
46. Bruhlmann WF, Zollikoten CL, Maranta E et al: Intramural pseudodiverticulosis of the esophagus: report of seven cases and literature review. Gastrointest Radiol 6:199, 1981
47. Medeiros JF, Doos WG, Balogh K: Esophageal intramural pseudodiverticulosis: a report of two cases with analysis of similar, less extensive changes in "normal" autopsy esophagi. Hum Pathol 19:928–931, 1988
48. Orringer MB, Dabich L, Zarafonetis CJ et al: Gastroesophageal reflux in esophageal scleroderma: diagnosis and implications. Ann Thorac Surg 22:120, 1976
49. Zamost BJ, Hirschberg J, Ippoliti AF et al: Esophagitis in scleroderma: prevalence and risk factors. Gastroenterology 92:421–428, 1987.
50. Rothstein RD: Gastrointestinal motility disorders in diabetes mellitus. Am J Gastroenterol 85:782–785, 1990
51. Kleckner FS: Dermatomyositis and its manifestations in the gastrointestinal tract. Am J Gastroenterol 53:141, 1970
52. Marshall JB, Kretsihmar JM, Gerhardt DC et al: Gastrointestinal manifestations of mixed connective tissue disease. Gastroenterology 98:1232–1238, 1990

53. Kjellen G, Fransson SG, Lindstrom F et al: Esophageal function, radiography and dysphagia in Sjögren's syndrome. Dig Dis Sci 31:225–229, 1986
54. Schuffler MD, Pope CE: Esophageal motor dysfunction in idiopathic intestinal pseudo-obstruction. Gastroenterology 70:677, 1976
55. Knauer CM: Mallory–Weiss syndrome. Characterization of 75 Mallory–Weiss lacerations in 528 patients with upper gastrointestinal hemorrhage. Gastroenterology 71: 5–8, 1976
56. Graham DY, Schwartz JT: The spectrum of the Mallory–Weiss tear. Medicine (Baltimore) 57:307–318, 1978
57. Spence RAJ, Sloan JM, Johnston GW, Greenfield A: Oesophageal mucosal changes in patients with varices. Gut 24:1024–1029, 1983
58. Patton RB, Sommers SC. The histopathology of infarction and other ulcerative diseases of the esophagus. Am J Clin Pathol 33:516, 1960
59. Dobbs WJ, Hogan WJ, Helm JF et al: Pathogenesis of reflux esophagitis. Gastroenterology 81:376, 1981
60. Bennett JR: Etiology, pathogenesis, and clinical manifestations of gastro-oesophageal reflux disease. Scand J Gastroenterol 23(S146):67, 1988
61. Zaninotto G, DeMeester TR, Schweizer W et al: The lower esophageal sphincter in health and disease. Am J Surg 155:104, 1988
62. Behar J, Bianconi P, Sheahan DG: Evaluation of esophageal tests in the diagnosis of reflux esophagitis. Gastroenterology 71:9, 1976
63. Brand DL, Eastwood IR, Martin D et al: Esophageal symptoms, manometry, and histology before and after anti-reflux surgery: a long-term follow-up study. Gastroenterology 76:1393, 1979
64. Varty K, Evans D, Kapila L: Paediatric gastro-oesophageal reflux: prognostic indicators from pH monitoring. Gut 34: 1478–1481, 1993
65. Winter HS, Madara JL, Stafford RJ et al: Functional and morphological assessment of acid reflux in children. Gastroenterology 78:1293, 1979
66. Black DD, Haggitt RC, Orenstein SR, Whitington PF: Esophagitis in infants. Morphometric histological diagnosis and correlation with measures of gastrointestinal reflux. Gastroenterology 98:1408–1414, 1990
67. Himal HS: Alkaline gastritis and alkaline esophagitis: a review. Can J Surg 20:403, 1977
68. Stoker DL, Williams JG: Alkaline reflux oesophagitis. Gut 32:1090–1092, 1991
69. Weinstein WM, Bogoch ER, Bowes KL: The normal human esophageal mucosa: a histological reappraisal. Gastroenterology 68:40–44, 1975
70. Behar J, Sheahan DC: Histologic abnormalities in reflux esophagitis. Arch Pathol 99:387, 1975
71. Seefeld U, Kregi GJ, Siebenmann RD et al: Esophageal histology in gastroesophageal reflux: morphometric findings in suction biopsies. Am J Dig Dis 22:956, 1977
72. Johnson LF, DeMeester TR, Haggitt RC: Esophageal epithelial response to gastroesophageal reflux: a quantitative study. Am J Dig Dis 23:498, 1978
73. Geboes K, Desmet V, Van Trappen G: Esophageal histology in the early stage of gastroesophageal reflux. Arch Pathol Lab Med 103:205, 1979
74. Bhan I, Leape LL, Ramenofsky ML: Histologic features of esophageal biopsies from children with gastroesophageal reflux. Lab Invest 46:2, 1982
75. Knuff TE, Benjamin SB, Worsham F et al: Histologic evaluation of chronic gastroesophageal reflux. An evaluation of biopsy methods and diagnostic criteria. Dig Dis Sci 29:194, 1984
76. Collins BJ, Elliott H, Sloan JM, McFarland RJ, Love AHG: Oesophageal histology in reflux esophagitis. J Clin Pathol 38: 1265–1272, 1985
77. Wang HH, Mangano MM, Antonioli DA: Evaluation of T-lymphocytes in esophageal mucosal biopsies. Modern Pathol 7:55–58, 1994
78. Tummala V, Barwick KW, Sontag SJ et al: The significance of intraepithelial eosinophils in the histologic diagnosis of gastroesophageal reflux. Am J Clin Pathol 87:43–48, 1987
79. Janisch HD, von Kleist D, Hampel KE: Intraepithelial eosinophils in esophageal reflux. Gastroenterology 85:785, 1983

80. Lee RG: Marked eosinophila in esophageal mucosal biopsies. Am J Surg Pathol 9: 475–479, 1985
81. Marks RD, Richter JE: Peptic strictures of the esophagus. Am J Gastroenterol 88:1160–1173, 1993
82. Barrett NR. The lower esophagus lined by columnar epithelium. Surgery 41:881, 1957
83. Mersian RA, Hermos JA, Robbins AG et al: Barrett's esophagus: clinical review of 26 cases. Am J Gastroenterol 69:458, 1978
84. Herlihy KJ, Orlando RC, Bryson JC et al: Barrett's esophagus: clinical, endoscopic, histologic, manometric and electrical potential difference characteristics. Gastroenterology 86:436–443, 1984
85. Speckler SJ, Goyal RK: Barrett's esophagus. N Engl J Med 315:362–371, 1986
86. Dahms BB, Rothstein FC: Barrett's esophagus in children: a consequence of chronic gastroesophageal reflux. Gastroenterology 86:318–323, 1984
87. Cooper JE, Spitz L, Wilkins BM: Barrett's esophagus in children: a histologic and histochemical study of 11 cases. J Pediatr Surg 22:191, 1987
88. Cameron AJ, Payne WS: Barrett's esophagus occurring as a complication of scleroderma. Mayo Clin Proc 53:612, 1978
89. Spechler SJ, Schimmell EM, Dalton JW et al: Barrett's epithelium complicating lye ingestion with sparing of the distal esophagus. Gastroenterology 81:580–583, 1981
90. Sartori S, Nielson I, Indelli M et al: Barrett's esophagus after chemotherapy with cyclophosphamide, methotrexate, and 5-fluorouracil (CMF): an iatrogenic injury. Ann Intern Med 114:210, 1991
91. Hamilton SR, Yardley JH: Regeneration of cardiac type mucosa and acquisition of Barrett's mucosa after esophagogastrostomy. Gastroenterology 72:669, 1977
92. Jaakkola A, Reinikainen P, Ovaska J et al: Barrett's esophagus after cardiomyotomy for esophageal achalasia. Am J Gastroenterol 89:165–169, 1994
93. Lee RG: Mucins in Barrett's esophagus: a histochemical study. Am J Clin Pathol 81:500–503, 1984
94. Penchmaur M, Potet F, Goldfain D: Mucin histochemistry of the columnar epithelium of the oesophagus (Barrett's oesophagus): a prospective biopsy study. J Clin Pathol 37:607, 1984
95. Zwas F, Schields HM, Doos WG et al: Scanning electron microscopy of Barrett's epithelium and its correlation with light microscopy and mucin stains. Gastroenterology 90: 1932–1941, 1986
96. Rothery GA, Patterson JE, Stoddard DJ, Day DW: Histological and histochemical changes in the columnar lined (Barrett's) oesophagus. Gut 27:1062, 1986
97. Haggitt RC, Reid BJ, Rabinovitch PS, Rubin CE: Barrett's esophagus. Correlation between mucin histochemistry, flow cytometry, and histologic diagnosis for predicting increased cancer risk. Am J Pathol 131:53–61, 1988
98. Jaurequi HO, Davessar K, Hale et al: Mucin histochemistry of intestinal metaplasia in Barrett's esophagus. Modern Pathol 1:188–192, 1988
99. Gottfried MR, McClave SA, Boyce HW: Incomplete intestinal metaplasia in the diagnosis of columnar lined esophagus (Barrett's esophagus). Am J Clin Pathol 92: 741, 1989
100. Paull G, Yardley JH: Gastric and esophageal Campylobacter pylori in patients with Barrett's esophagus. Gastroenterology 95:216–218, 1988
101. Talley NJ, Cameron AJ, Shorter RG et al: Campylobacter pylori and Barrett's esophagus. Mayo Clin Proc 63:1176, 1988
102. Loffeld RJLF, Ten Tije BJ, Arends JW: Prevalence and significance of Helicobacter pylori in patients with Barrett's esophagus. Am J Gastroenterol 87:1598–1600, 1992
103. Ozzello L, Savary M, Roethlisberger B: Columnar mucosa of the distal esophagus in patients with gastroesophageal reflux. Pathol Annu 1:41, 1977
104. Cameron AJ, Lombay CT: Barrett's esophagus: age, prevalence, and extent of columnar epithelium. Gastroenterology 103:1241–1245, 1992
105. Schreiber DS, Apstein M, Hermos JA: Paneth cells in Barrett's esophagus. Gastroenterology 74:1302, 1978
106. Berenson MM, Herbst JJ, Frecton JW: Enzyme and ultrastructural characteristics of esophageal columnar epithelium. Am J Dig Dis 19:895, 1974

107. Brand DL, Ylziasaker JT, Gefand M et al: Regression of columnar esophageal (Barrett's) epithelium after anti-reflux surgery. N Engl J Med 302:844, 1980
108. Hassall E, Weinstein WM: Partial regression of childhood Barrett's esophagus after fundoplication. Am J Gastroenterol 87:1506–1512, 1992
109. Berenson MM, Johnson TD, Markowitz NR et al: Restoration of squamous mucosa after ablation of Barrett's esophageal epithelium. Gastroenterology 104:1686–1691, 1993
110. Levine DS, Rubin CE, Reid BJ, Haggitt RC: Specialized metaplastic columnar epithelium in Barrett's esophagus. A comparative transmission electron microscopic study. Lab Invest 60:418, 1989
111. Thompson JJ, Zinsser KR, Enterline HT: Barrett's metaplasia and adenocarcinoma of the esophagus and gastroesophageal junction. Hum Pathol 14:142–161, 1983
112. Naef AP, Savery M, Ozzello L: Columnar-lined lower esophagus: an acquired lesion with malignant predisposition. Report on 140 cases of Barrett's esophagus with 12 adenocarcinomas. J Thorac Cardiovasc Surg 70:826, 1975
113. Haggitt RC, Tryzellaar J, Ellis FH et al: Adenocarcinoma complicating columnar epithelium-lined (Barrett's) esophagus. Am J Clin Pathol 70:1–5, 1978
114. Hamilton SR, Smith RRL: The relationship between columnar epithelial dysplasia and invasive adenocarcinoma arising in Barrett's esophagus. Am J Clin Pathol 87:301–312, 1987
115. Williamson WA, Ellis FH Jr, Gibb SP et al: Barrett's esophagus. Prevalence and incidence of adenocarcinoma. Arch Intern Med 151:2212–2216, 1991
116. Streitz JM Jr, Ellis FH Jr, Gibb SP et al: Adenocarcinoma in Barrett's esophagus: a clinicopathologic study of 65 cases. Ann Surg 213:122, 1991
117. Reid BJ, Haggitt RC, Rubin CE et al: Observer variation in the diagnosis of dysplasia in Barrett's esophagus. Hum Pathol 19:166–178, 1988
118. Levine DS, Haggitt RC, Blount PL et al: An endoscopic biopsy protocol can differentiate high-grade dysplasia from early adenocarcinoma in Barrett's esophagus. Gastroenterology 105:40–50, 1993
119. Dworkin B, Wormser GP, Rosenthal WS et al: Gastrointestinal manifestations of the acquired immunodeficiency syndrome: a review of 22 cases. Am J Gastroenterol 80:774–778, 1985
120. Rotterdam H, Tsang P. Gastrointestinal disease in the immunocompromised patient. Hum Pathol 25:1123–1140, 1994
121. Wu G-D, Shintaku IP, Chien K, Geller SA: A comparison of routine light microscopy, immunohistochemistry, and in situ hybridization for the detection of cytomegalovirus in gastrointestinal biopsies. Am J Gastroenterol 84:1517–1520, 1989
122. Nash G, Ross J: Herpetic esophagitis: a common cause of esophageal ulceration. Hum Pathol 5:339–345, 1974
123. Owensby LC, Stammer JL, Esophagitis associated with herpes simplex infection in an immunocompetent host. Gastroenterology 74:1305, 1978
124. McKay JS, Day DW: Herpes simplex oesophagitis. Histopathology 7:409–420, 1983
125. Burrig K-F, Borchard F, Feiden W, Pfitzer P: Herpes oesophagitis. II. Electron microscopical findings. Virchows Arch A Pathol Anat Histopathol 404:177–185, 1984
126. Matsumoto J, Sumujoski A: Herpes simplex esophagitis—a study in autopsy series. Am J Clin Pathol 84:96–99, 1985
127. Greenson JK, Beschorner WE, Boitnott JK et al: Prominent mononuclear cell infiltrate is characteristic of herpes esophagitis. Hum Pathol 22:541–549, 1991
128. Hinnant KL, Rotterdam HZ, Bell ET, Tapper ML: Cytomegalovirus infection of the alimentary tract. A clinicopathological correlation. Am J Gastroenterol 81:944–950, 1986
129. Wilcox CM, Diehl DL, Cello JP et al: Cytomegalovirus esophagitis in patients with AIDS: a clinical, endoscopic, and pathologic correlation. Ann Intern Med 113:589, 1990
130. Theise ND, Rotterdam H, Dieterich D: Cytomegalovirus esophagitis in AIDS: diagnosis by endoscopic biopsy. Am J Gastroenterol 86:1123–1126, 1991
131. Chetty R, Roskell DE: Cytomegalovirus infection in the gastrointestinal tract. J Clin Pathol 47:968–972, 1994

132. St. Onge G, Bezahler GH: Giant esophageal ulcer associated with cytomegalovirus. Gastroenterology 83:127, 1982
133. Gill RA, Gebhard RL, Dozeman RL, Sumner HW: Shingles esophagitis: endoscopic diagnosis in two patients. Gastrointest Endosc 30:26–27, 1984
134. Hamilton SR: Esophagitis. pp. 386–401. In Ming S-C, Goldman H (eds): Pathology of the Gastrointestinal Tract. WB Saunders, Philadelphia, 1992
135. Rabeneck L, Boyko WJ, McLean DM et al: Unusual esophageal ulcers containing enveloped virus-like particles in homosexual men. Gastroenterology 90:1882, 1986
136. Bartewlsman JFWM, Lang JMA, van Leeuwen R et al: Acute primary HIV esophagitis. Endoscopy 22:184, 1990
137. Chawla SK, Ramani K, Chawla K et al: Giant esophageal ulcers of AIDS: ultrastructural study. Am J Gastroenterol 89:411–415, 1994
138. Kitchen VS, Helbert M, Francis ND et al: Epstein–Barr virus associated oesophageal ulcers in AIDS. Gut 31:1223–1225, 1990
139. Winkler B, Capo V, Reumann W et al: Human papillomavirus infection of the esophagus. A clinicopathologic study with demonstration of papillomavirus antigen by the immunoperoxidase techniques. Cancer 55:149–155, 1985
140. Poletoske EJ: Squamous papilloma of the esophagus associated with the human papillomavirus. Gastroenterology 102:668–673, 1992
141. Odze R, Antonioli D, Shocket D et al: Esophageal squamous papillomas. A clinicopathologic study of 38 lesions and analysis for human papillomavirus by the polymerase chain reaction. Am J Surg Pathol 17: 803–812, 1993
142. Walsh TJ, Belitsos NJ, Hamilton SR: Bacterial esophagitis in immunocompromised patients. Arch Intern Med 146:1345, 1986
143. Coelho LG, Das SS, Payne A et al: Campylobacter pylori in esophagus, antrum, and duodenum. A histological and microbiological study. Dig Dis Sci 34:445–448, 1989
144. Poles MA, McMeeking AA, Scholes JV et al: Actinomyces infection of a cytomegalovirus esophageal ulcer in two patients with acquired immunodeficiency syndrome. Am J Gastroenterol 89:1569–1572, 1994
145. Gordon AH, Marshall JB: Esophageal tuberculosis: definitive diagnosis by endoscopy. Am J Gastroenterol 85:174–177, 1990
146. Eng J, Sabanathan S: Tuberculosis of the esophagus. Dig Dis Sci 36:536–540, 1991
147. Amberson JB, DiCarlo EF, Metroka CE et al: Diagnostic pathology in the acquired immunodeficiency syndrome. Arch Pathol Lab Med 109:345–351, 1985
148. Knoke M, Bernhardt H: Endoscopic aspects of mycosis in the upper digestive tract. Endoscopy 12:295, 1980
149. Scott BB, Jenkins D: Gastro-oesophageal candidiasis. Gut 23:137–139, 1982
150. Mathieson R, Dutta SK: Candida esophagitis. Dig Dis Sci 28:365–370, 1983
151. Young JA, Elias E: Gastro-oesophageal candidiasis: diagnosis by brush cytology. J Clin Pathol 38:293–296, 1985
152. Tom W, Aaron JS. Esophageal ulcers caused by *Torulopsis glabrata* in a patient with acquired immune deficiency syndrome. Am J Gastroenterol 82:766–768, 1987
153. Young RC, Bennett JE, Vogel CL et al: Aspergillosis: the spectrum of the disease in 98 patients. Medicine 49:147, 1970
154. Lyon DT, Schubert TT, Mantia AG, Kaplan MH: Phycomycosis of the gastrointestinal tract. Am J Gastroenterol 72:379–394, 1979
155. Margolis PS, Epstein A: Mucormycosis esophagitis in a patient with the acquired immunodeficiency syndrome. Am J Gastroenterol 89:1900–1902, 1994
156. Miller DP, Everett ED: Gastrointestinal histoplasmosis. J Clin Gastroenterol 1:233, 1979
157. Cappell MS, Mandell W, Grimes MM, Neu HC: Gastrointestinal histoplasmosis. Dig Dis Sci 33:353–360, 1988
158. Khandekar A, Moser D, Fidler WJ: Blastomycosis of the esophagus. Ann Thorac Surg 30:71, 1979
159. McKenzie R, Khakoo R: Blastomycosis of the esophagus presenting with gastrointestinal bleeding. Gastroenterology 88: 1271–1273, 1985
160. Ziliotta A Jr, Kunzle JE, Takeda FA: Paracoccidioidomycosis of the esophagus: report of a case. Rev Inst Med Trop Sao Paulo 22:261, 1980
161. Jacobs DH, Macher AB, Handler R et al: Esophageal cryptococcosis in a patient with the hyperimmunoglobulin E-recurrent in-

fection (Job's) syndrome. Gastroenterology 87:201–203, 1984

162. Grimes MM, LaPook JD, Bar MH et al: Disseminated Pneumocystis carinii infection in a patient with acquired immunodeficiency syndrome. Hum Pathol 18:307–308, 1987
163. Kazlow PG, Shah K, Benkov KJ et al: Esophageal cryptosporidiosis in a child with acquired immune deficiency syndrome. Gastroenterology 91:1301–1303, 1986
164. Riddell RH, the gastrointestinal tract. pp. 515–606. In Riddell RH (ed): Pathology of Drug-Induced and Toxic Diseases. Churchill Livingstone, New York, 1982
165. Lewis JH: Gastrointestinal injury due to medicinal agents. Am J Gastroenterol 81:819–834, 1986
166. Goldman H, Szabo S: Chemical and physical disorders. pp. 141–170. In Ming S-C, Goldman H (eds): Pathology of the Gastrointestinal Tract. WB Saunders, Philadelphia, 1992
167. Dafoe CS, Ross CA: Acute corrosive esophagitis. Thorax 24:291, 1969
168. Poelman JR, Hausman RH, Holtsma HFW: Endoscopy in lye burns of oesophagus and stomach. Endoscopy 9:172, 1977
169. Oakes DD, Shenck JP, Mark JBD: Lye ingestion. Clinical patterns and therapeutic implications. J Thorac Cardiovasc Surg 83:194, 1982
170. Symbas PN, Vlasis SE, Hatcher CR Jr: Esophagitis secondary to ingestion of caustic material. Ann Thorac Surg 36:73, 1983
171. Collins FJ, Matthews HR, Baker SE, Strakova JM: Drug-induced oesophageal injury. Br Med J 1:1673, 1979
172. Mason SJ, O'Meara TF: Drug-induced esophagitis. J Clin Gastroenterol 3:115, 1981
173. Kikendall JW, Friedman AC, Oyewole MA et al: Pill-induced esophageal injury. Case reports and review of the medical literature. Dig Dis Sci 28:174–182, 1983
174. Bott S, Prakach C, McCallum RW: Medication-induced esophageal injury: survey of the literature. Am J Gastroenterol 82:758–763, 1987
175. Eng J, Sabanathan S: Drug-induced esophagitis. Am J Gastroenterol 86:1127–1133, 1991
176. Heer M, Altorfer J, Burger H-R, Walti M: Bullous esophageal lesions due to cotrimoxazole: an immune-mediated process? Gastroenterology 88:1954–1957, 1985
177. Lambert JR, Newman A: Ulceration and stricture of the esophagus due to oral potassium chloride (slow release tablet) therapy. Am J Gastroenterol 73:508, 1980
178. Bonavina L, DeMeester TR, McChesney L et al: Drug-induced esophageal strictures. Ann Surg 206:173, 1987
179. McCord GS, Clouse RE: Pill-induced esophageal strictures: clinical features and risk factors for development. Am J Med 88:512, 1990
180. Greco FA, Breveton HD, Kent H et al: Adriamycin and enhanced radiation reaction in normal esophagus and skin. Ann Intern Med 85:294, 1976
181. Slavin RE, Dias MP, Saral R: Cytosine arabinoside induced gastrointestinal toxic alterations in sequential chemotherapeutic protocols. Cancer 42:1747, 1978
182. Boal DK, Newburger PE, Teele RL: Esophagitis induced by combined radiation and adriamycin. AJR 132:567–570, 1979
183. Ayres SJ, Goff JS, Warren GH: Endoscopic sclerotherapy for bleeding esophageal varices: effects and complications. Ann Intern Med 98:900, 1983
184. Soehendra N, DeHeer K, Kempeneers I, Frommelt L: Morphological alterations of the esophagus after endoscopic sclerotherapy of varices. Endoscopy 15:291–296, 1983
185. Helpap B, Bollweg L: Morphological changes in the terminal oesophagus with varices, following sclerosis of the wall. Endoscopy 13:229, 1981
186. Evans DMD, Jones DB, Cleary BK, Smith PM: Oesophageal varices treated by sclerotherapy: a histopathologic study. Gut 23:615, 1982
187. Novak JM, Collins JT, Donowitz M et al: Effects of radiation on the human gastrointestinal tract. J Clin Gastroenterol 1:9, 1979
188. Berthrong M, Fajardo LF: Radiation injury in surgical pathology. Part II. Alimentary tract. Am J Surg Pathol 5:153–178, 1981
189. Jennings FL, Arden A: Acute radiation effects in the esophagus. Arch Pathol 69:407, 1960
190. Vanagunas A, Jacob P, Olinger E: Radiation-induced esophageal injury: a spectrum

from esophagitis to cancer. Am J Gastroenterol 85:808–812, 1990

191. Chowhan NM: Injurious effects of radiation on the esophagus. Am J Gastroenterol 85:115–120, 1990
192. Nadi P, Ong GB. Foreign body in the esophagus: a review of 2394 cases. Br J Surg 65:5, 1978
193. Crysdale WS, Sendi KS, Yoo J: Esophageal foreign bodies in children—15 year review of 484 cases. Ann Otol Rhinol Laryngol 100:320, 1991
194. Klein NC, Hargrove RL, Sleisenger MH, Jeffries GH: Eosinophilic gastroenteritis. Medicine 49:299–319, 1970
195. Goldman H, Proujansky R: Allergic proctitis and gastroenteritis in children: clinical and mucosal biopsy features in 53 cases. Am J Surg Pathol 10:75–86, 1986
196. Dobbins JW, Sheahan DG, Behar J: Eosinophilic gastroenteritis with esophageal involvement. Gastroenterology 72:1312, 1977
197. Picus D, Frank PH: Eosinophilic esophagitis. AJR 136:1001–1003, 1981
198. Munch R, Kuhlmann U, Makek M et al: Eosinophilic esophagitis, a rare form of eosinophilic gastroenteritis. Schweiz Med Wochenschr 112:731, 1982
199. Matzenger MA, Daneman A: Esophageal involvement in eosinophilic gastroenteritis. Pediatr Radiol 13:35–38, 1983
200. Katz AJ, Goldman H, Flores AF, Twaroq FJ: Esophageal involvement in allergic (eosinophilic) gastroenteritis. Gastroenterology 88:1438, 1985
201. Katz AJ, Goldman H, Grand RJ: Gastric mucosal biopsy in eosinophilic (allergic) gastroenteritis. Gastroenterology 73:705–709, 1977
202. Ferrara JLM, Deeg HJ: Graft-versus-host disease. N Engl J Med 324:667–674, 1991
203. McDonald GB, Sullivan KM, Schuffler MD et al: Esophageal abnormalities in chronic graft-versus-host disease in humans. Gastroenterology 80:914–921, 1981
204. Nishikai M, Asaba G, Homma M: Rheumatoid esophageal disease. Am J Gastroenterol 67:29, 1977
205. Bretagne JF, Launois B, Ferrand B, Gastard J: Rheumatoid stricture of the esophagus. Gastroenterol Clin Biol 6:709, 1982
206. Kyle RA, Bayrd ED: Amyloidosis: review of 236 cases. Medicine 54:271–299, 1975
207. Gilat T, Spiro HM: Amyloidosis and the gut. Am J Dig Dis 13:619–633, 1968
208. Coughlin GP, Remer RG, Grant AK: Endoscopic diagnosis of amyloidosis. Gastrointest Endosc 26:154, 1980
209. Yamada M, Hatakeyama S, Tsukagoshi H: Gastrointestinal amyloid deposition in A1 (primary or myeloma-associated) and AA (secondary) amyloidosis: diagnostic value of a gastric biopsy. Hum Pathol 16:1206–1211, 1985
210. Heitzman EJ, Heitzman GC, Elliott CF: Primary esophageal amyloidosis: report of a case with bleeding, perforation, and survival following resection. Arch Intern Med 109:595, 1962
211. Busuttil A, More IAR, Jones DG: Amyloid deposits in the trachea and esophagus: ultrastructural confirmation. Laryngoscope 86:850, 1976
212. Sharma SS, Venkateswaran S, Chacko A, Mathan M: Melanosis of the esophagus. An endoscopic, histochemical, and ultrastructural study. Gastroenterology 100:13–16, 1990
213. Remmele W, Engelsing B: Lipid island of the esophagus. Case Report. Endoscopy 16:240–241, 1984
214. Chajek T, Fainaru M: Behçet's disease: Report of 41 cases. Medicine (Baltimore) 54:179, 1975
215. Lakhanpal S, Tani K, Lie JT et al: Pathologic features of Behçet's syndrome: a review of Japanese autopsy registry data. Hum Pathol 16:790–795, 1985
216. Mori S, Yoshihira A, Kawamura H et al: Esophageal involvement in Beçhet's disease. Am J Gastroenterol 78:548–553, 1983
217. Anti M, Marra G, Rapaccini L et al: Esophageal involvement in Behçet's syndrome. J Clin Gastroenterol 8:514–519, 1986
218. Yashiro K, Nagasaho, Hasegawa K et al: Esophageal lesions in intestinal Behçet's disease. Endoscopy 18:57–60, 1986
219. Weisner PJ, Kleinman MS, Coademi JJ: Sarcoidosis of the esophagus. Am J Dig Dis 16:943, 1971
220. LiVolsi VA, Jaretzki A. Granulomatous esophagitis: a case of Crohn's disease limited

to the esophagus. Gastroenterology 64:313, 1973
221. Freedman PG, Dieterich DT, Galthaza EJ: Crohn's disease of the esophagus: case report and review of the literature. Am J Gastroenterol 79:835–838, 1984
222. Freson M, Kottler RE, Wright JP. Crohn's disease of the oesophagus. S Afr Med J 66:417–418, 1984
223. Geboes K, Janssens J, Rutgierts P, Van Trappen G: Crohn's disease of the esophagus. J Clin Gastroenterol 8:31–37, 1986
224. Niv Y: Esophageal involvement in Crohn's disease. Am J Gastroenterol 83:205–206, 1988
225. Wood DR, Patterson JB, Orlando RC: Pemphigus vulgaris of the esophagus. Ann Intern Med 96:189–191, 1982
226. Goldin E, Lijovetsky G: Esophageal involvement by pemphigus vulgaris. Am J Gastroenterol 80:828–830, 1985
227. Barnes IM, Clark ML, Estes SA, Bongiovanni GL: Pemphigus vulgaris involving the esophagus. A case report and review of the literature. Dig Dis Sci 32:655–659, 1987
228. Eliakim R, Goldin E, Livshin R, Okon E: Esophageal involvement in pemphigus vulgaris. Am J Gastroenterol 83:155–157, 1988
229. Trattner A, Lurie R, Leiser A et al: Esophageal involvement in pemphigus vulgaris: a clinical, histologic, and immunopathologic study. J Am Acad Dermatol 24:233, 1991
230. Kahn D, Hutchinson E: Esophageal involvement in familial benign chronic pemphigus. Arch Dermatol 109:718–719, 1974
231. Sharon P, Green ML, Rachmilewitz D: Esophageal involvement in bullous pemphigoid. Gastrointest Endosc 24:122, 1978
232. Johnston DE, Koehler RE, Balfe DM: Clinical manifestations of epidermolysis bullosa dystrophica. Dig Dis Sci 26:1144–1149, 1981
233. Aglia FP, Francis IR, Ellis CN: Esophageal involvement in epidermolysis bullosa dystrophica: clinical and roentgenographic manifestations. Gastrointest Radiol 8:111–117, 1983
234. Ergun GA, Linan AN, Dannenberg AJ, Carter DM: Gastrointestinal manifestations of epidermolysis bullosa. A study of 101 patients. Medicine 71:121–127, 1992
235. Stewart MI, Woodley DT, Briggaman RA: Epidermolysis bullosa acquisita and associated symptomatic esophageal webs. Arch Dermatol 127:373, 1991
236. Weinman D, Stewart MI, Woodley DT, Garcia G: Epidermolysis bullosa acquisita (EBA) and esophageal webs: a new association. Am J Gastroenterol 86:1518–1522, 1991
237. Zweiban B, Cohen H, Chandrasoma P: Gastrointestinal involvement complicating Stevens–Johnson syndrome. Gastroenterology 91:469–474, 1986
238. Lefer LG: Lichen planus of the esophagus. Am J Dermatopathol 4:267–269, 1982
239. Al Shihabi BM, Jackson JM: Dysphagia due to pharyngeal and oesophageal lichen planus. J Laryngol Otol 96:567–571, 1982
240. Dickens CM, Hasteltine D, Walton S, Bennett JR: The oesophagus in lichen planus: an endoscopic study. Br Med J 300:84, 1990

3

Tumors of the Esophagus

The first section of this chapter provides the principal uses of mucosal biopsy, the various specimens that are available, and the potential limitations of these studies. This information applies to tumors throughout other parts of the gut as well. The subsequent sections of the chapter present the specific tumors encountered in the esophagus[1-3] (Table 3-1).

GENERAL ASPECTS

Uses of Mucosal Biopsy

Endoscopic examination and biopsy of the esophageal mucosa are commonly employed to detect tumors and identify their particular type, to determine the extent of the lesions, and to monitor patients following therapy (Table 3-2). Adjunctive therapy, in the form of radiation and chemotherapy, is often added in the malignant cases. Accordingly, a biopsy examination in such patients serves to look not only for recurrent or residual tumor but also for the development of complications of therapy, such as damaging effects from the drugs or radiation and the appearance of opportunistic infections.

Biopsy Material

There have been extensive studies of endoscopy in the evaluation of tumors in the upper gut.[4,5] It is evident that cytologic smears, obtained either independently or, more often, by direct brushing of the mucosa at the time of endoscopy, can be of considerable assistance.[6-9] Studies have demonstrated that about five biopsies are needed to obtain the diagnosis of malignancy in over 95 percent of the cases and that a combination of cytology with histology detects practically all cases.[10,11]

In efforts to improve the yield in tumors that are beneath the mucosa, fine-needle aspiration cytology and intraluminal ultrasound examinations are being tested.[12,13] Also, for lesions showing the earliest neoplastic changes, such as the dysplasias of the squamous or glandular epithelium, modern molecular techniques have been introduced.[14-16] Particularly sought are the overexpression of oncogenes or their products and alterations in the suppressor genes.

Potential Limitations

In many instances the biopsy can demonstrate that there is a tumor or neoplasm, and may be able to differentiate between a be-

Table 3-1. Tumors of the Esophagus

Inflammatory and hyperplastic nodules
Squamous cell papilloma and carcinoma
Adenoma and adenocarcinoma
Endocrine tumors
Lymphoid tumors
Mesenchymal tumors
Melanocytic tumors
Secondary and metastatic tumors

nign and a malignant lesion. However, it is not always possible to identify the specific type of tumor, largely because of the limited sampling, and also due to associated necrosis and inflammation that may distort the cytologic features. Similarly, a biopsy may lead to the determination of a particular cell type, but the limited sampling often does not permit conclusive statements about the differentiation. In many of the benign neoplasms and other non-neoplastic tumors, the biopsy often illustrates several features that are compatible with a particular lesion but may not be completely diagnostic. It is therefore important to correlate the gross appearance with the microscopic findings to secure the best diagnosis.

With the increasing use of endoscopy in tumor assessment, it has become especially important to appreciate the wide range of inflammatory and degenerative effects that can be present as a result of the tumor or its treatment, and that these not be mistaken for malignancy.[17, 18]

BENIGN MUCOSAL TUMORS

Discussed in this section are those lesions that either originate in or dominantly involve the esophageal mucosa (Table 3-3).

Table 3-2. Biopsy Uses in Tumors

Detection of tumor
Identification of specific type
Determination of extent of lesions
Monitor patients following therapy

Table 3-3. Benign Mucosal Tumors of the Esophagus

Cysts, hamartomas, and embryonic rests
Webs and acanthosis
Inflammatory polyp
Fibrovascular polyp
Squamous cell papilloma
Adenoma

Cysts, Hamartomas, and Hyperplastic Lesions

Cysts and Hamartomas

There are a variety of cysts, hamartomas, and embryonic rests that can be present in the esophagus. These may affect any layer and are often more pronounced in the deeper portions, but they exceptionally extend into the mucosal area. Most of the cysts are of the retention type and probably represent dilated ductal structures; these tend to be concentrated in the lower esophagus and are mainly within the submucosa.[19–21] There are several types of duplication cysts that occur both within and outside the esophageal wall, and these have a highly variable epithelium with any combination of esophageal, bronchial, or gastric types.[22] Ectopic foci of thyroid or parathyroid tissues, as well as hamartomas comprised of epithelial and stromal elements including cartilage, have also been rarely noted.[23, 24] In the *Cowden syndrome,* multiple hamartomatous-type lesions are present mainly in the skin and in the gastrointestinal tract[25]; mesenchymal-type nodules are observed in the mucosa, and can exceptionally affect the esophagus.

Hyperplastic Lesions

More commonly noted in the esophageal mucosa are hyperplastic lesions. Glycogenic acanthosis represents localized areas of hyperplasia of the squamous epithelium, particularly of the glycogen-rich prickle cell zone[26–28] (see Fig. 2-5). These are often multiple and more commonly noted in the distal esophagus. Webs are localized excesses of mucosal tissue that may be developmental or occur following injury to the mucosa, particularly in certain skin disorders such as epidermolysis bullosa of both the dystrophica and acquisita types.[29–33] Biopsies of these lesions simply show hyperplasia or acanthosis of the squamous layer without significant inflammation, and the diagnosis requires correlation with the gross findings. Nevertheless, the biopsy does serve to rule out other causes of the epithelial thickening, such as infections or dysplastic lesions. The subjects of glycogenic acanthosis and of esophageal webs are discussed more fully in Chapter 2.

Polyps

Polyps represent a variety of inflammatory and hyperplastic tumors that project into the esophageal lumen and typically have a smooth surface.[34] They more often cause problems when located at a narrow area such as the esophagocardiac junction.[35,36]

Inflammatory Polyps

The inflammatory-type polyps represent areas of excess inflammatory or granulation tissue and typically subside over time. They are usually single and related to some traumatic or inflammatory injury to the esophagus, such as the presence of a tube or the persistence of an ulcer lesion. They are most often composed of well developed granulation tissue, equivalent to the granuloma pyogenicum seen in many other tissues of the body (Fig. 3-1). Biopsies reveal the inflammatory or granulation tissue with variable fibrosis, and also serve to exclude proliferative lesions of the epithelium. Rarely noted in the esophagus is the inflammatory fibroid polyp.[37]

Fibrovascular Polyp

A more striking example of a polypoid tumor in the esophagus is the so-called fibrous or fibrovascular polyp.[38–40] These are typically single and often very large lesions that project into and extend over several centimeters within the esophageal lumen. The surface is smooth and composed in part by mature squamous epithelium and often reveals multiple areas of erosion. Most of the polyp is comprised of relatively mature fibrous, vascular, and occasionally adipose tissue. The lesions are thought to represent an exaggerated hyperplastic response rather than a true neoplasm, and malignant degeneration of such lesions has not been described. Biopsies typically demonstrate just the superficial portion of the lesion, revealing the squamous epithelium that is not dysplastic and the focal erosions. The mucosal biopsies do not usually capture the underlying core of fibrous and vascular tissue. Nevertheless, the combination of the biopsy information together with the striking gross presentation is often sufficient to provide the diagnosis. Other lesions that can present in this fashion are the spindle cell variant of squamous cell carcinoma and mesenchymal tumors, such as leiomyomas, that project from the submucosal compartment. Biopsies of the spindle cell carcinoma would show a mixture of dysplastic squamous epithelium and highly proliferative and atypical spindle cells. The fibrovascular polyps usually require excision because of their large size and potential for obstruction, but follow-up biopsies of the esophagus are not needed.

Squamous Cell Papilloma

Squamous cell papillomas are small wart-like lesions that typically appear in the distal esophagus.[41–44] They usually measure about 5 mm or less in diameter, are most often single, and are mainly observed in adults. At one time they were thought to represent

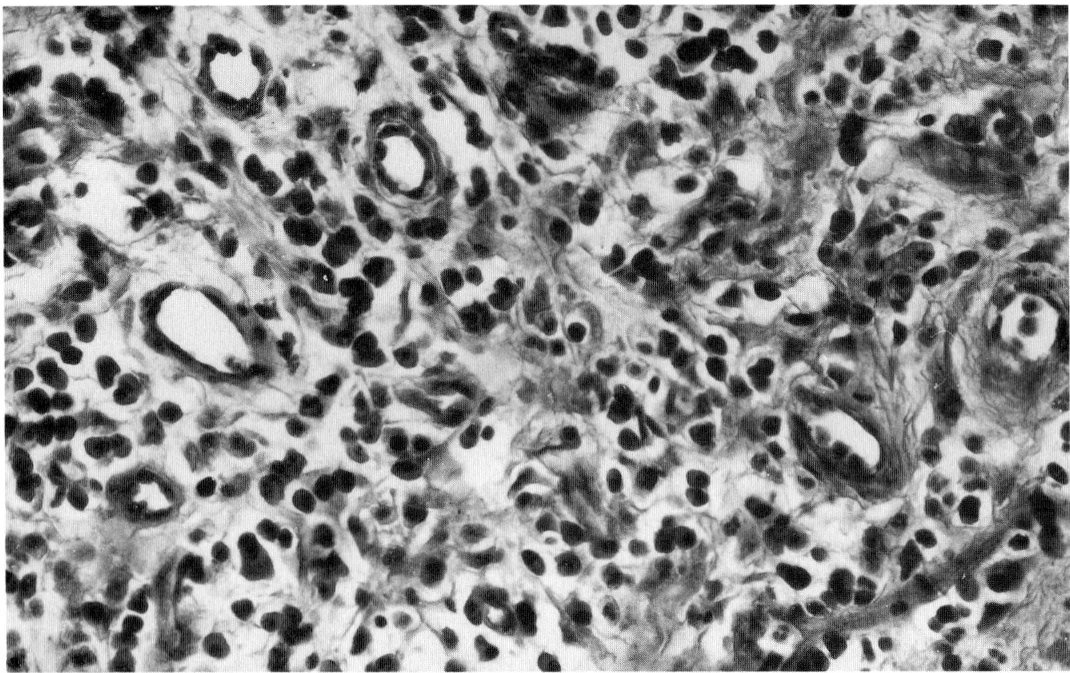

Fig. 3-1. Fibrovascular polyp of the esophagus. Shown is the core of the polyp, consisting of granulation tissue with both acute and chronic inflammatory cells. Other cases show more fibrosis (× 425).

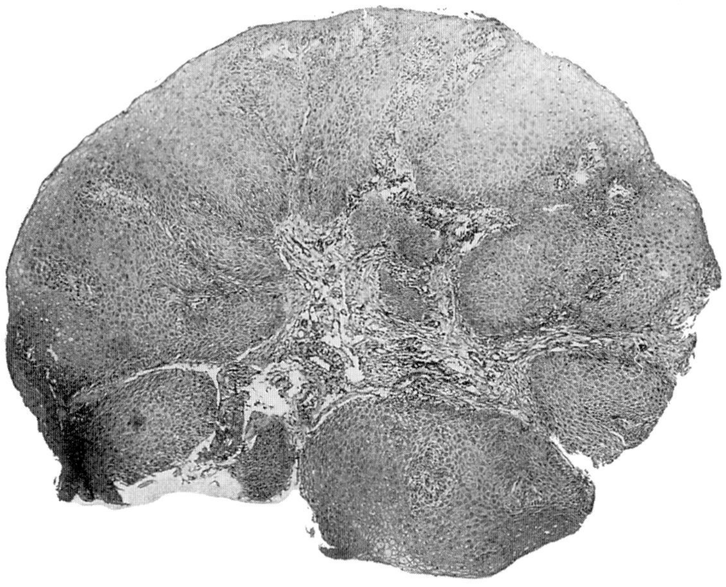

Fig. 3-2. Squamous cell papilloma of the esophagus. There is a prominent papillary hyperplasia of the squamous epithelium overlying a core of inflamed connective tissue. The squamous cells are mature and show no dysplasia (× 43).

excessive repair tissue in cases of reflux esophagitis, with the lesions comparable to fibroepithelial polyps, but this cannot be established in most instances. It has recently been demonstrated that up to one-half of these lesions contain antigens of human papillomavirus, particularly type 16 alone or in combination with type 18.[45–47] Other investigators have not been able to demonstrate this association, however, and the issue is not yet settled.[48]

The lesions are covered by a layer of normal or, more often, thickened squamous epithelium, which overlies a core of mature fibrovascular tissue (Fig. 3-2). Because of the small size of the papillomas, they are frequently encompassed by the biopsy, thus permitting an appreciation of the full architecture of the lesions.[49] Different gross forms have been described, based on the surface contour, and these include an exophytic type with a papillary surface; an endophytic type with a smooth surface; and a spiked type with a marked degree of hyperkeratosis and a strikingly thickened granular zone.[50] With the larger lesions, the mucosal biopsies may reveal only the thickened squamous epithelium. The major differential diagnosis is with other proliferative squamous lesions, particularly squamous cell carcinoma and, especially, the verrucous form. In the carcinomas, there would be some element of dysplasia of the squamous epithelium as well as invasion of the underlying connective tissues. This may prove difficult to see in the very well differentiated or verrucous forms of squamous cell carcinoma, in which the superficial biopsies may show only minimal or no dysplasia and not reveal the invasion in these specimens. Accordingly, it is very important to correlate the biopsy material with the gross appearance. The vast majority of squamous cell papillomas are very small lesions whereas the carcinomas and, particularly, the verrucous type tend to be much larger. Nevertheless, in case of any doubt, further biopsies should be done to be confident that carcinoma has been excluded.

Some cases of multiple squamous cell papillomas also have lesions in the tracheobronchial tree, and there appears to be in these cases some increased association with human papillomavirus.[51] In all patients with multiple squamous cell papillomas, particularly if present in the proximal esophagus or in the associated bronchial tree, the potential for secondary malignancy should be appreciated. In such patients, careful monitoring for the development of dysplasia or early carcinoma is probably indicated.

Adenoma

Benign neoplasms of the glandular epithelium are rarely noted in the esophagus, and practically all are seen in cases of Barrett's esophagus.[52–56] They probably represent localized areas of polypoid dysplasia, and most cases have been described in association with other areas of flat dysplasia. The biopsies are fairly characteristic, revealing prominent palisading and elongation of the nuclei with varying degrees of hyperchromatism. The appearance is usually identical to that of an adenoma in the colon or in other parts of the gastrointestinal tract. Once a diagnosis of an adenoma or glandular dysplasia is made, further examination and biopsy are often needed to confirm the diagnosis and to exclude an associated adenocarcinoma. The finding of these neoplastic lesions also requires consideration of surgery, and this subject is discussed in a later section of this chapter, "Glandular Dysplasia in Barrett's Esophagus".

SQUAMOUS CELL CARCINOMA

Squamous cell carcinoma is the most common form of malignant tumor of the esophagus, reflecting the nature of the esophageal epithelium[57] (Table 3-4). There is, however, an increasing frequency of adenocarcinomas in many of the Western countries.

Table 3-4. Types of Squamous Tumors of the Esophagus

Hyperplastic lesions
Glycogenic acanthosis
Squamous cell papilloma
Squamous cell dysplasia
Squamous cell carcinoma
Variants of squamous carcinoma
Verrucous carcinoma
Spindle cell carcinoma
Basal cell carcinoma

Epidemiology

Squamous cell carcinoma is especially prevalent in large parts of the Orient, particularly in the Hunan Province of China and in Japan, in the Caspian Peninsula of Iran, in Eskimo groups, and in parts of Scandinavia and South Africa.[57–60] The tumors present in adults, and are much more common in men. The earlier lesions of dysplasia and beginning carcinoma are frequently found in the fourth to fifth decades and the cases of more advanced carcinoma about five to ten years later.

The etiology of squamous cell carcinoma is not established. From experimental studies in animals involving squamous epithelium, particularly of the skin, papilloma-inducing viruses and local chemical irritants would seem to be good prospects as risk factors. There are strong associations between the development of these tumors and genetic groups, the types of diets, and the prevalence of alcohol consumption and tobacco smoking[61] (Table 3-5). There has also been a consideration of dietary nitrosamines, since many of the chemical precursors are present in the diets, equivalent to the relationship of these substances to gastric carcinoma. In addition, there is the variable demonstration of human papillomavirus in cases of squamous cell carcinoma, mainly involving types 16 and 18 similar to squamoproliferative lesions in other sites.[62–66] There does not appear to be any direct relationship between the ordinary, single squamous cell papilloma and the development of squamous cell carcinoma.

Table 3-5. Risk Factors in Squamous Carcinoma of the Esophagus

Geographic distribution (genetic groups)
Dietary components
Ethanol and tobacco consumption
Human papillomavirus
Radiation

In the Plummer-Vinson, or Paterson-Kelly syndromes, there are multiple mucosal webs that are concentrated in the proximal esophagus. Some of these cases are associated with iron deficiency anemia and with gastric atrophy. They tend to be more common in the Scandinavian countries, and the patients are prone to the development of squamous cell carcinoma, which typically occurs in the postcricoid region.[67]

Premalignant Conditions and Lesions

Premalignant Conditions

There are many clinical situations and conditions that are associated with an increased frequency of squamous cell carcinoma of the esophagus[68–70] (Table 3-6). Several of these are related to esophageal stasis, and the link with carcinoma may be a prolonged presence of chronic inflammation and excess or irregular growth, similar to the development of tumors in other parts of the gut and body in such situations. The premalignant conditions include cases of esophageal diverticula,[71] stricture,[72] achalasia,[73,74] and possibly prolonged reflux esophagitis.[75,76] Although adenocarcinomas are commonly noted in patients with *Barrett's esophagus,* also occa-

Table 3-6. Predisposing Conditions in Squamous Cell Carcinoma of the Esophagus

Esophageal stricture and diverticula
Achalasia
Celiac disease
Tylosis
Chronic radiation
Plummer–Vinson syndrome
Chronic esophagitis

sionally observed are squamous cell carcinomas, either alone or in conjunction with the glandular tumor in such patients.[77–79] It remains possible that factors underlying the development of chronic esophagitis, whether of innate squamous epithelium or of glandular metaplasia, are operative. Accordingly, biopsy in patients with Barrett's should be considered for both dysplastic squamous and glandular lesions. There is an increased risk of squamous carcinoma in patients who have received prior radiation, which is mainly done for tumors of the esophagus or contiguous structures.[80–82] A possible relationship to human papillomavirus is mentioned above,[62–66] and there is also an increased association of gut carcinomas in patients with tylosis and with celiac disease, including carcinomas of the esophagus.[83,84]

Considering the enhanced prevalence of squamous cell carcinomas in these groups of patients, they probably deserve some element of monitoring or surveillance. This can readily be accomplished by periodic endoscopy with the acquisition of cytologic smears and biopsies to look for squamous cell dysplasia and early carcinoma. Given the relatively low incidence of squamous cell carcinoma in many of the Western countries, however, extensive screening of the general population or even of groups with higher risks in these locations is often not employed.

Premalignant Lesions

Whereas the premalignant conditions identify clinical groups with an increased risk for the development of neoplasia, the term *premalignant lesion* is used to signify an actual transformation into a neoplastic process, typically at the benign level. In turn, patients with these lesions would be at considerable risk for the further development of malignancy. The characteristic lesion in the esophagus is squamous cell dysplasia, which can be readily recognized by cytologic and biopsy examinations. Other candidate lesions have not been clearly shown to be directly predisposed to carcinoma; these include polyps and squamous cell papillomas and are discussed above.

Squamous Cell Dysplasia

In regions where squamous cell carcinoma is highly prevalent, it has been clearly established that the tumor is associated with and probably preceded by squamous cell dysplasia. Of the cases of invasive squamous cell carcinoma, severe or high-grade dysplasia is found in 50 to 60 percent of cases and carcinoma in-situ in 70 percent.[85] The interval between the appearance of dysplasia and carcinoma can range from 2 to 7 years. This association is equivalent to that noted in other portions of the body, principally in the uterine cervix and in the bronchial epithelium. In the Orient, mass surveys of asymptomatic patients by cytologic techniques have been able to detect a substantial number of cases of dysplasia, equivalent to the use of the Pap smear in young women to find cervical lesions.[57,86] Such cytologic information has in turn led to endoscopic examination and biopsy to provide the histologic equivalent for the diagnosis of dysplasia and, in many cases, early squamous cell carcinoma.[87–90] In the Western countries, where the incidence of squamous cell carcinoma is much less, such routine surveys are not done, and we rarely see biopsy material from such asymptomatic patients. More often, smears and biopsies are obtained in patients who are already symptomatic and have tumors beyond the dysplastic or early carcinomatous stage.

Cytologic Features

The cytologic features of squamous cell dysplasia are standard and characteristic (Plates 3A–D), similar to those seen in other parts of the body (Table 3-7). The

Table 3-7. Cytologic Classification for Epithelial Tumors

Negative
Atypical, probably inflammatory
Dysplasia
Mild (low grade)
Moderate and severe (high grade)
Carcinoma

diagnosis is made in part on architectural variation but mainly on the individual cellular features and principally on the characteristics of the nuclei.[6–9,86] In early, mild (low-grade) dysplasia, there is enlargement of the nuclei but still ample cytoplasm; the nuclei show some increase in chromatin that is generally dispersed as well as the lack of a heavy chromatin amount at the edge of the nuclei. There is usually minimal variation either in the size of the nuclei or in their shape. The principal challenge in low-grade dysplasia is to differentiate these cells from those of regenerating or inflamed squamous epithelial cells, and this may not always be possible. Features favoring dysplasia are the absence of inflammatory cells, some degree of variation in nuclear size, and the greater quantity of chromatin material. In regenerating squamous epithelial cells, the nuclei all tend to be almost of equal size, and there is usually very fine chromatin. Nevertheless, there are cases of doubt, and further cytologic or histologic examination may be required to make the distinction between low-grade dysplasia and inflammatory or regenerative epithelium. The cytologic features of moderate to severe (high-grade) dysplasia show even more variation in the size and shape of nuclei, lesser amounts of cytoplasm, and, especially, coarser aggregates of chromatin and their condensation at the nuclear edge. There is usually more confidence in rendering this diagnosis as opposed to inflamed or regenerating squamous epithelium, because of the greater atypicality in the squamous cell nuclei.

Histologic Features

The histologic features of squamous cell dysplasia are similar to those seen in other squamous lesions of the body, such as those that occur in the uterine cervix and bronchial epithelium. In mild (low-grade) dysplasia, there is the presence of immature and atypical squamous cells extending for a portion of the epithelial thickness, whereas in the moderate and severe (high-grade) forms of squamous dysplasia, the cellular alteration extends very close to or involves the complete epithelial thickness (Fig. 3-3). When the latter occurs, the diagnosis of squamous cell carcinoma in-situ is also considered, but this category can just as well be included as the extreme of high-grade dysplasia (Fig. 3-4). There have been large studies conducted in China and Japan correlating the cytologic and biopsy findings in the esophagus, as well as follow-up studies of the patients with established dysplasia. In the Chinese studies, of 150 early esophageal cancers, simple hyperplasia of the adjacent epithelium was present in 95 percent and dysplasia in 68 percent of cases.[91] Most abnormalities were immediately next to the carcinoma, but separate lesions were seen in 20 percent of cases. Carcinoma in-situ was evident in over one-half of the patients. Of 500 cases with severe dysplasia followed for at least 5 years, there was regression to mild dysplasia or benign epithelium in 40 percent, no change in 20 percent, and advancement to carcinoma in 20 percent of cases.[57]

From the above data, it would probably be useful for the cases of squamous cell dysplasia to be divided into low-grade and high-grade categories, similar to what is done in the uterine cervix for squamous lesions and

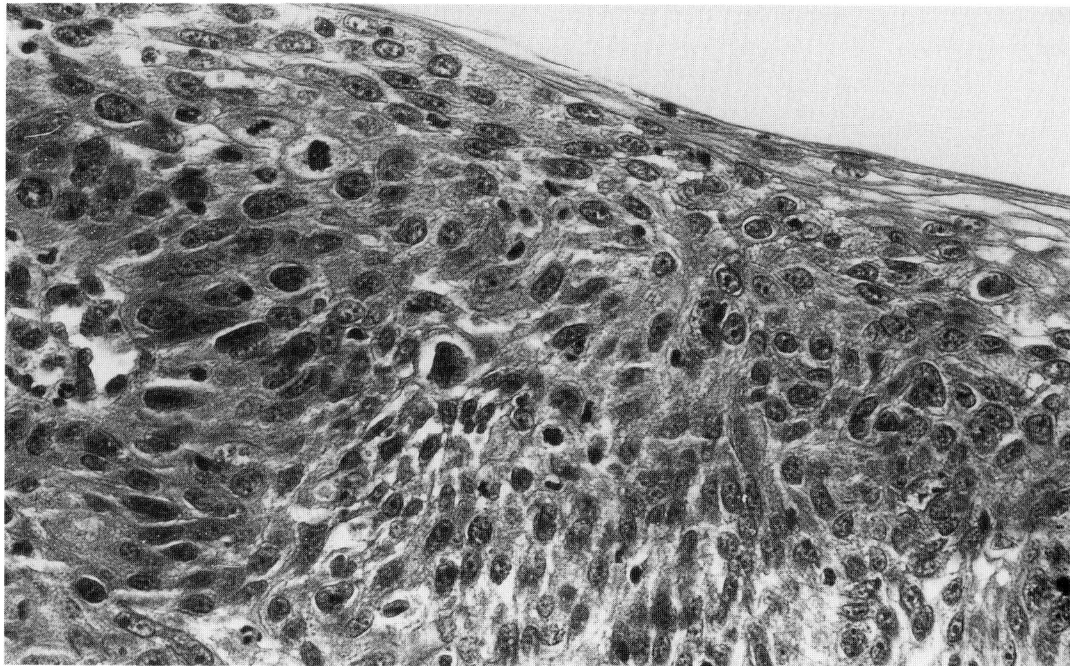

Fig. 3-3. High-grade squamous cell dysplasia of the esophagus. There is marked proliferation of immature and atypical squamous cells extending from the base (at the bottom) to the upper third of the epithelial layer. Maturation is present in the superficial portion, and is best seen in the upper right (× 425).

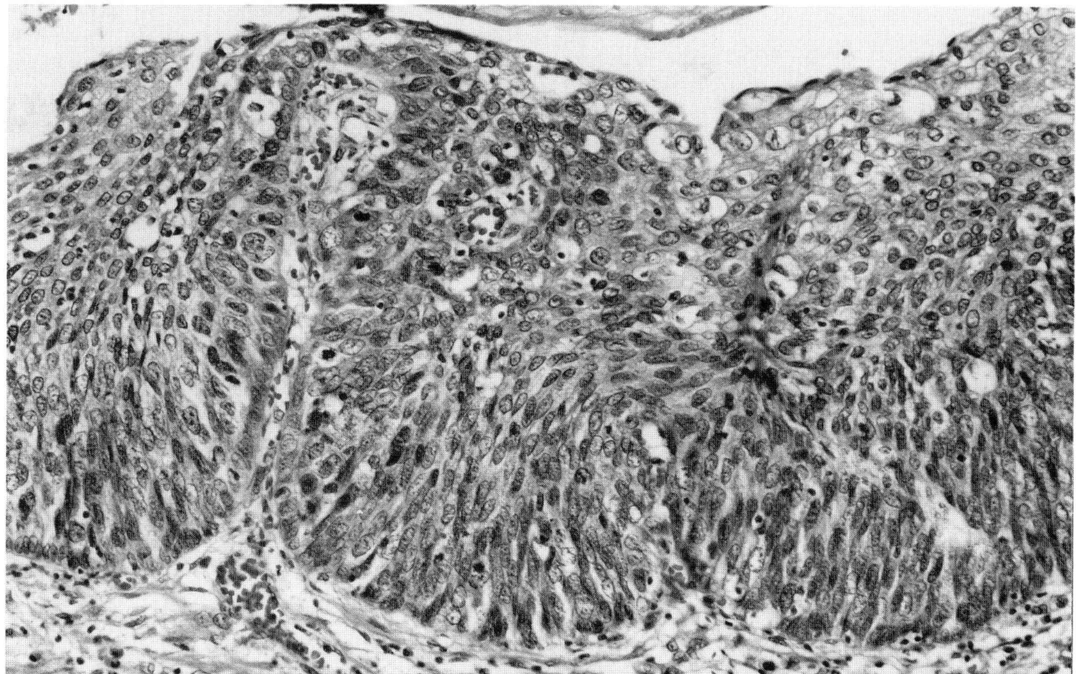

Fig. 3-4. Squamous cell carcinoma in-situ of the esophagus. The immature and abnormal squamous cells extend from the base to the surface of the epithelial thickness. There is no invasion into the lamina propria at the bottom (× 210).

in other parts of the alimentary tract for glandular dysplasia.

Features of Squamous Cell Carcinoma

Unlike the oral mucosa, localized patches of thickened and white epithelium, termed *leukoplakia,* are relatively uncommon in the esophagus.[92] Most of these are due to simple hyperplasia, such as glycogenic acanthosis, or represent inflammatory membranes in fungal or other infections. Their finding as a precursor lesion of squamous carcinoma, such as representative of dysplasia, has not proven helpful in the esophagus.

Early Carcinoma

Early carcinomas represent cases in which the diagnosis is established in patients who are asymptomatic or have minimal problems in countries with a high frequency of the tumor, whereas they are mostly incidental findings in the Western countries.[85,93–97] At a gross level, they have been classified as follows: *occult,* in which there is no gross lesion recognized; *erosive,* showing friability or minimal erosion; *plaque,* with slightly elevated epithelium; and *papilloma,* with a more exaggerated epithelial lesion.[57] At a histologic level, most of these cases represent high-grade dysplasia or carcinoma in-situ.[98] In about one-quarter of the cases, there is extension of tumor into the lamina propria, representing intramucosal carcinoma (Fig. 3-5); about 5 percent of these early cases show further invasion through the muscularis mucosae into the upper part of the submucosa at a histologic but not gross level.

Such minimal gross lesions are sought at endoscopic examination to select for biopsy, and additional random samples are taken in patients with abnormal cytologic smears. The biopsies with carcinoma in-situ are essentially equivalent to high-grade dysplasia, showing the presence of abnormal squamous cells throughout the epithelial thickness or sparing just the most superficial layers (cf. Fig. 3-4). The squamous cells show only modest variation in size and shape of their nuclei but often marked degrees of nuclear irregularity and hyperchromatism. In the endoscopic examination, Lugol's iodine solution is occasionally applied to the surface to try to identify the abnormal areas.[99,100] This solution readily stains the normal and hyperplastic epithelium, which is rich in glycogen, whereas the dysplastic and carcinomatous areas fail to take up the stain because of the loss of glycogen stores in their cytoplasm.

The biopsy diagnosis of early squamous cell carcinoma may at times be difficult, particularly in relatively small and distorted specimens. There is a major need to separate the carcinoma from the much more common finding of basal zone hyperplasia in the reparative phase of the reflux type and other forms of active esophagitis. In the hyperplasia there can be a pronounced proliferation of the immature cells, which extend throughout the entire thickness of the squamous epithelium (cf. Fig. 2-9). The cells, however, show extreme constancy in size, shape, and nuclear features, whereas some variation is evident in the dysplastic and carcinomatous samples. The finding of early invasion must be distinguished from inflammatory changes and reparative epithelium adjacent to ulceration. As in all instances of carcinoma invasion, abnormal cells extending clearly beyond the basement membrane must be documented. These features can be accented by immunoperoxidase stains such as those for keratin, but this does not otherwise permit distinction between benign and malignant cells.[101,102]

Advanced Carcinoma

Most of the cases of squamous cell carcinoma encountered in the Western countries are in the more extensive or advanced stage.

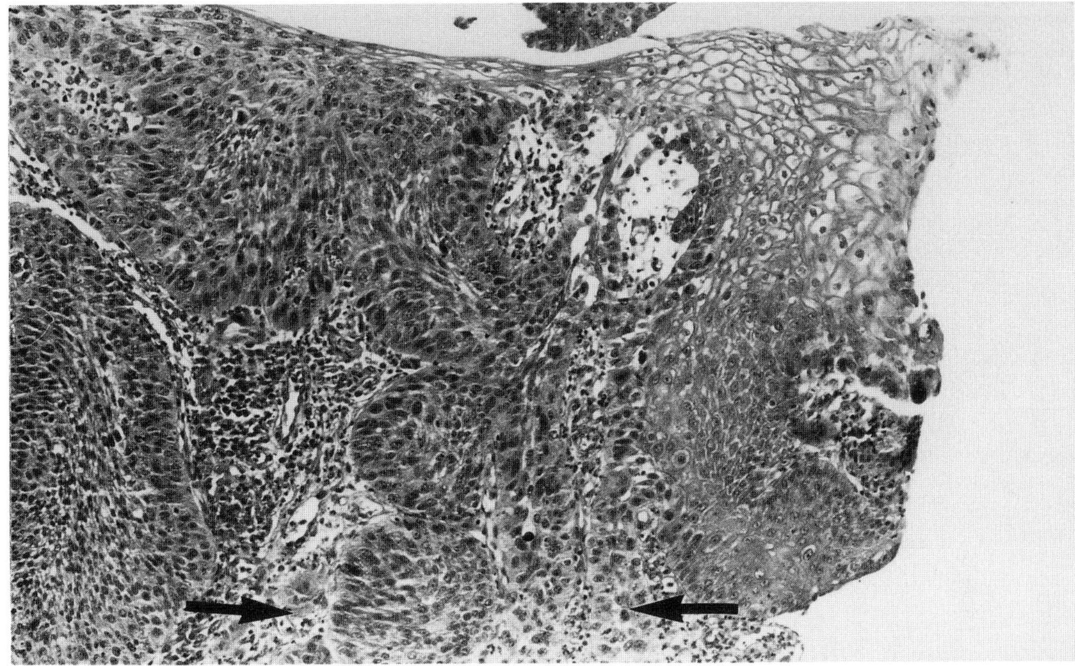

Fig. 3-5. Squamous cell carcinoma of the esophagus, with early invasion. There is a blurring of the squamous nests at the base, and small clusters of carcinoma cells are noted in the lamina propria (arrows). A portion of normal esophagus appears at the right edge (× 140).

These present grossly as polypoid or fungating, as ulcerative, or as infiltrating or stenotic lesions. In these advanced cases, there is gross extension of tumor at least into the submucosa and, in most instances, deep into the wall and to the adventitia. The diagnosis is readily suggested by the radiographic and endoscopic appearance, and biopsies are obtained for confirmation and to determine the specific cell type. A full range of squamous differentiation can be seen in the tumors, extending from those with well formed squamous cells and keratin production to tumors that are composed mainly of broad sheets of undifferentiated cells. Most of the squamous carcinomas in the esophagus are of the well- to moderate-differentiated types (Figs. 3-6 and 3-7). The biopsy samples reflect this but may not be totally accurate in view of their small sample. In any case, the grading of these tumors is not especially helpful in determining their behavior, which is much more dependent on the actual stage of the carcinoma.

There can be problems if there is extensive ulceration, in which case the biopsy samples may fail to reveal viable tumor tissue. In other instances it may be apparent that there is carcinoma, but the samples are too superficial to evaluate for invasion; this is typically not a problem considering the gross features of a big tumor. As in all instances with mucosal biopsies, a sample may only permit a diagnosis of malignancy and may not be able to certify that it is a squamous lesion as opposed to another malignant form. In most instances surgery is indicated and would permit the final diagnosis. However, in those cases where the therapy may vary, additional examination and further biopsies would be needed.

The advanced squamous cell carcinomas of the esophagus commonly extend through the wall and may spread into the mediasti-

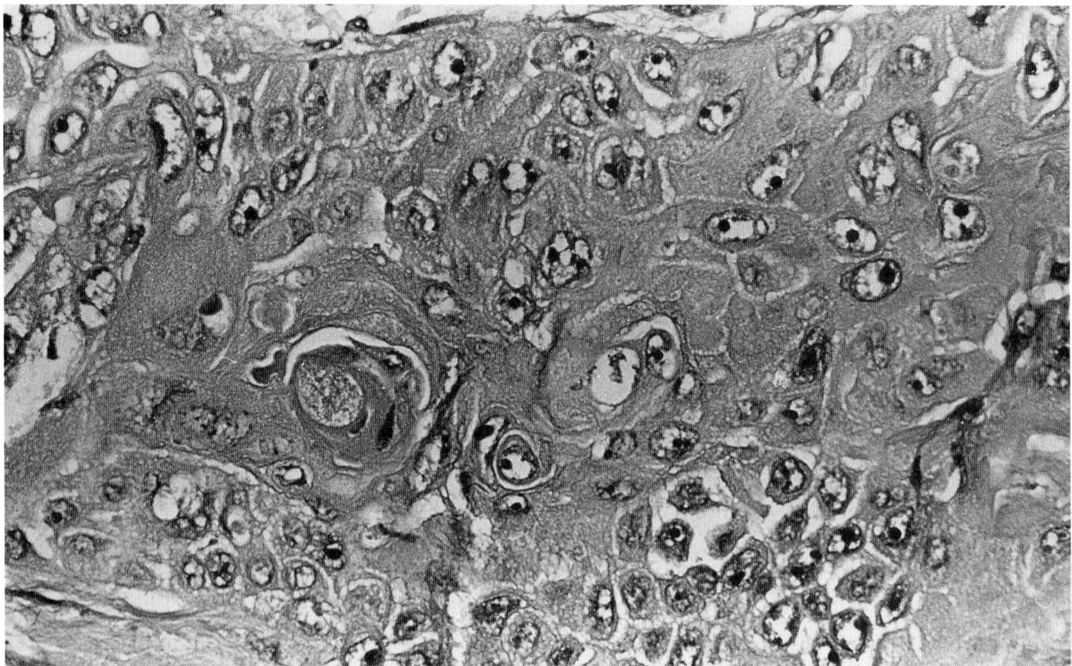

Fig. 3-6. Invasive squamous cell carcinoma of the esophagus. There are large and markedly atypical cells that form sheets. Intercellular bridges between the cells and intracellular keratin production are present (× 425).

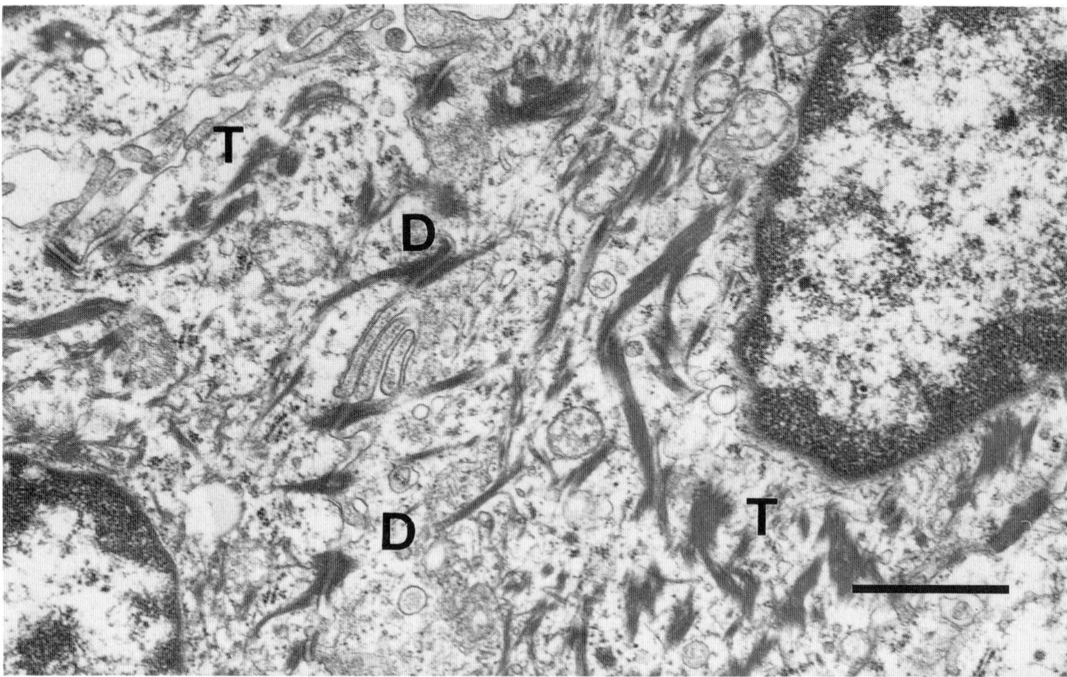

Fig. 3-7. Electron micrograph of squamous cell carcinoma. Variable number of tonofilaments (T) are characteristically present in the cytoplasm, and cells are joined by numerous desmosomes (D) (× 20,000; bar = 1 μm).

num and pericardial sac. Metastases to regional lymph nodes and to lungs are common. The treatment consists of a combination of surgery, radiation, and chemotherapy,[103] and endoscopic examination with biopsy is often done in such patients to check on the results of therapy. At these times, there may be areas of atrophy, ulceration, or stenosis. Biopsies are taken to look for residual or recurrent carcinoma, for the effects of radiation or chemotherapy, and for the development of opportunistic infections, principally those due to herpes virus, cytomegalovirus, and fungal organisms (see Ch. 2). In assessing the mucosa following drug or radiation therapy, it may be particularly difficult to distinguish viable tumor cells from the effects of the therapy.[57] In particular, the radiation and radiomimetic drugs can cause irregularly enlarged and hyperchromatic nuclei in the squamous epithelial cells, including those in the carcinoma.[104–106] Although these may appear highly atypical, they may be arrested cells and not necessarily signs of viable tumor. It is best in such cases to compare the post-therapy samples with the slides of the original tumor in an effort to assess this effect. Also, multiple sections should be obtained to look for less-affected tumor cells.

Special Studies

Scanning electron microscopic examination permits evaluation of the surface contour of cells, which is often abnormal in neoplasms. It has been observed that the microridges on the squamous cells are reduced in cases of esophagitis but markedly increased in areas of squamous cell carcinoma.[107] This would have potential value in cases in which the distinction between esophagitis, dysplasia, or early carcinoma is difficult. However, given the potential effort and expenses involved as opposed to repeating the biopsies, the application of ultrastructural examination has been limited. There have been many studies involving flow cytometry of squamous cell carcinomas that have demonstrated aneuploidy in over three-quarter of the cases.[108–112] Furthermore, there is a strong association between the presence of such atypical growths and advanced tumor, particularly of metastatic lesions. There are also numerous studies demonstrating oncogene products or loss of suppressive genes such as p53 in squamous tumors, but their overall application to diagnosis and to direction of therapy are not yet established.[113–115] As noted above, immunoperoxidase stains can help in showing the epithelial cells and accent their invasion, particularly when in small numbers.

Variant Forms of Squamous Carcinoma

Verrucous Carcinoma

Verrucous carcinoma represents an uncommon form of squamous cell carcinoma that is largely exophytic and associated with marked degrees of keratin production[116,117] (Fig. 3-8). The superficial mucosal biopsies may simply show the excessive keratin and the surface squamous cells without revealing the underlying carcinoma. It is necessary to exclude these lesions from squamous cell papillomas, which is usually easy since the papillomas tend to be very small whereas the verrucous carcinomas are more typically large. Both may show hyperkeratosis, a prominent granular cell layer, and mature squamous cells in the superficial biopsies. Accordingly, deeper samples are needed to establish the dysplastic lesion and the invasion in the verrucous carcinoma.

Spindle Cell (Polypoid) Carcinoma

Spindle cell carcinoma represents squamous cell carcinomas in which a major part of the tumor is in the form of spindle cells.[118–120]

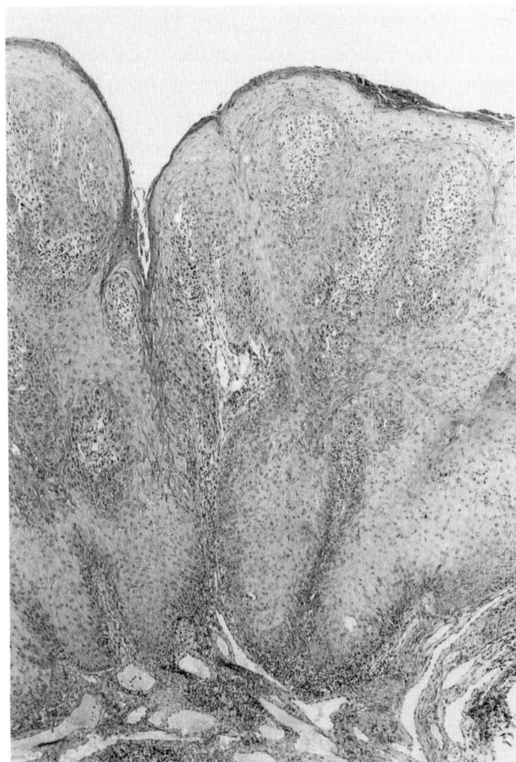

Fig. 3-8. Verrucous carcinoma of the esophagus. There is a large mass of squamous cells, mostly mature, resulting in a papillary growth. The carcinomatous nature is based on the focal atypism of the cells and the demonstration of superficial invasion into the lamina propria, best seen in the lower left (× 48).

They typically present as large polypoid lesions and require distinction from fibrovascular polyps and from mesenchymal tumors that extend into the lumen. Their neoplastic and malignant nature are usually evident on biopsy, revealing the dysplastic cells (Fig. 3-9). If the squamous cell portion is found, the overall entity can be appreciated. If only the spindle cells are seen, the differentiation from mesenchymal type tumors, which are much less common in the esophagus, is needed. Multiple samples are often required to demonstrate the squamous component even in surgical specimens.

These have also been called *carcinosarcomas* in the past, reflecting the presence of both epithelial-type and spindle cells. In addition, there may be areas of metaplastic cartilage and bone formation (Fig. 3-10). However, both ultrastructural and immunocytochemical examinations have illustrated that the spindle cells possess desmosomes and cytochemical markers of epithelial cells.[121,122] These special techniques can be added to the examination of the biopsies to permit the exact diagnosis of the spindle cell variant of squamous cell carcinoma. Given the large polypoid nature of these lesions, they typically require surgery, and

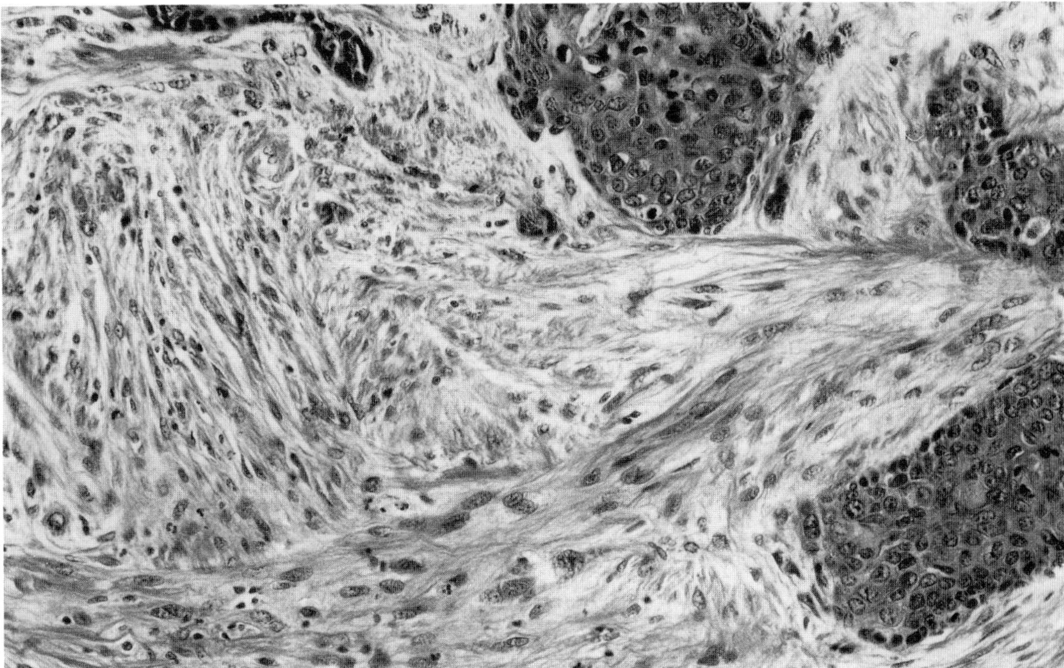

Fig. 3-9. Spindle cell (polypoid) carcinoma of the esophagus. Much of the tumor is in the form of spindle cells. Their squamous nature is based on the association with the mature elements (appearing at the right) and by the demonstration of the same cytokeratins in the spindle cells (× 210).

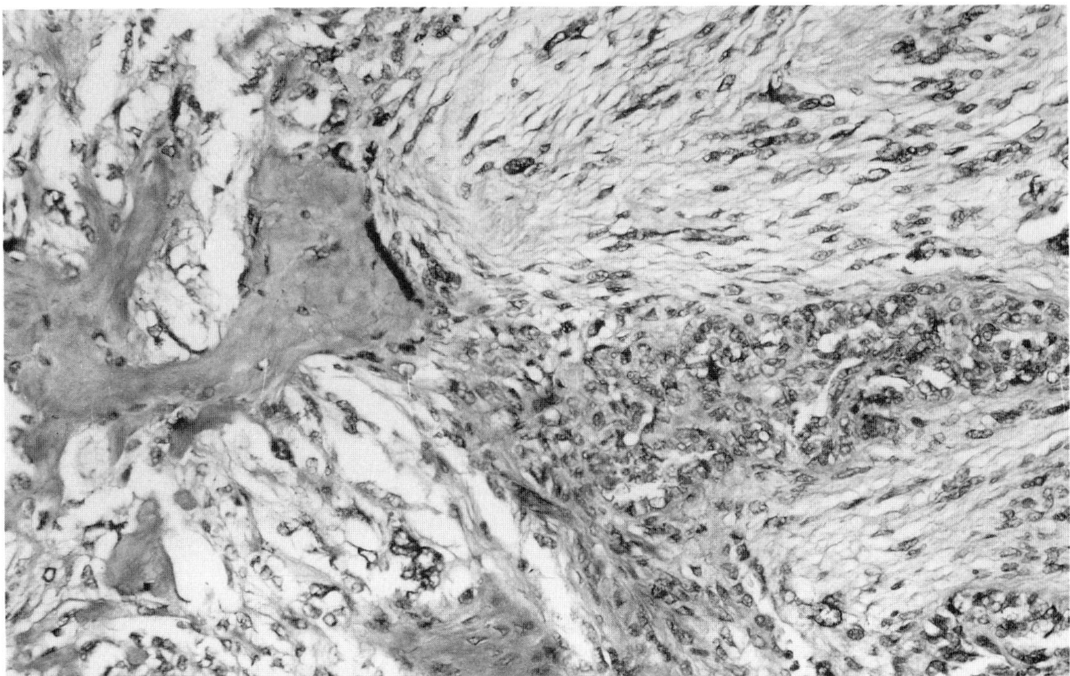

Fig. 3-10. Spindle cell carcinoma of the esophagus, with foci of osseous metaplasia (left). Such tumors have also been called *carcinosarcomas,* but the heterologous tissues seen usually have a benign cellular appearance (× 105).

the final diagnosis may depend on the specimen examination.

Basal Cell Carcinoma

Basal cell carcinomas are equivalent to the common lesions in the skin but are extremely rare in the esophagus.[123]

ADENOCARCINOMA

Epidemiology

There has been a considerable increase in the incidence of adenocarcinoma of the esophagus, principally the distal portion, in many of the Western countries.[124–129] Also noted has been an increase in adenocarcinomas affecting the gastric cardia, and it was thought that some of the esophageal cases may represent extension from those of the stomach. However, it is now established that there is an increase in adenocarcinomas of the entire region involving the distal third of the esophagus, the junction, and the proximal stomach. It is estimated that adenocarcinomas may represent up to 25 to 30 percent of all esophageal carcinomas and over 50 percent of those that present in the distal portion.[125]

Most of the cases of adenocarcinoma of the esophagus appear to be a complication of Barrett's esophagus.[130,131] In contrast to squamous cell carcinoma, the cases are more often seen in the developed and Western countries where reflux esophagitis is so highly prevalent. The tumors are more frequent in men and there is an association with smoking and alcohol consumption, but these relationships are not as large as in cases of squamous cell carcinoma. Clusters of cases are occasionally noted in families,[132] but there are no proven associations with genetic disorders, with general diet, or with other chemical factors. The principle relation appears to be with those conditions that favor the development of chronic esophagitis and, in turn, Barrett's esophagus, which is the dominant precursor for the development of esophageal adenocarcinoma; included are ordinary reflux disease,[133–138] scleroderma[139] and treated achalasia.[140] This is another example of a chronic inflammatory condition that predisposes to the development and growth of malignant tumors. The frequency of carcinoma generally relates to the length of the Barrett's epithelium,[131,141] but tumors in short segments have also been noted.[142]

Sources of Adenocarcinomas

There are several potential sources for adenocarcinomas that involve the esophagus (Table 3-8). They may extend from contiguous structures, particularly from the proximal part of the stomach and rarely from the bronchial tree. Of the adenocarcinomas originating in the esophagus, the great majority arise from Barrett's esophagus, which is a glandular metaplasia that develops in patients with chronic esophagitis.[133–138,143–145] Rarely noted are adenocarcinomas that develop from heterotopic stomach, which typically occurs in the proximal part of the esophagus[146–148]; and from submucosal glands. The latter are more apt to show the variant forms, such as mucoepidermoid carcinoma and adenoid cystic carcinoma.

Whatever the source of the carcinoma, it typically presents as a polypoid or ulcerated mass. Biopsy can reveal the neoplastic glands, and the diagnosis of malignancy is dependent on the finding of markedly dysplastic cells and of invasion into the lamina

Table 3-8. Sources of Adenocarcinoma in the Esophagus

Extension from stomach
Barrett's esophagus
Heterotopic gastric tissue
Submucosal glands
Metastatic tumors

propria or beyond. The source of the adenocarcinoma is determined by demonstrating the associated lesions, such as Barrett's esophagus. In the adenocarcinomas from the other sources, this may not be easily established by biopsy but may depend on full examination of the surgical specimens.[125,149] Nevertheless, the appearance of an adenocarcinoma in the more proximal regions of the esophagus away from the areas of the expected Barrett's would support a different source. Similarly, the finding of adenocarcinoma limited to the most distal region and junction may cause suspicion for extension of a carcinoma of the stomach into the esophagus. It should be stressed that the histologic features of the adenocarcinomas are the same whatever the primary source of the tumor.[124–126] Furthermore, the tumors of the lower esophagus, the junction, and the proximal stomach tend to have not only similar histology but also the same broad epidemiologic features and probable behavior.

Glandular Dysplasia in Barrett's Esophagus

As noted above, the principal cause of adenocarcinoma of the esophagus is chronic esophagitis with glandular metaplasia, and is mainly presented in Chapter 2. The Barrett's glandular epithelium develops whenever there is a chronic irritation. Most cases are due to reflux esophagitis[150–152]; uncommon causes include lye stricture, effects of chemotherapy, systemic sclerosis by virtue of promoting reflux esophagitis, and post-resection or dilation of the esophagus in which the sphincter action is eliminated.[153–157] In all of these situations, there is a replacement of the squamous epithelium by glandular tissue, consisting of a mixture of gastric and intestinal cells.[158] Most of the cells are of a mucinous type and all forms are seen, including those containing neutral glycoproteins and mildly acidic and sulfated mucins.[159–165]

Prevalence and Surveillance

In patients with Barrett's esophagus, it is estimated that 1 to 3 percent may develop carcinoma and that, overall, 5 to 10 percent of the patients will eventually have a carcinoma.[133–138] It has been difficult to establish any specific risk factors in these patients with Barrett's esophagus other than the existence of the metaplastic epithelium. Furthermore, it has been demonstrated that there is the development of abnormal cells, termed *dysplastic epithelium,* which can serve as a marker of existing cancer or increased likelihood of development of carcinoma[136,166–169] (Fig. 3-11). This is analagous to the dysplasia found in the stomach in cases of chronic gastritis[170,171] and that found in the colon in cases of ulcerative colitis.[172] Many assumptions have been made based on the similarity to ulcerative colitis, but it must be remembered that data specific to the esophageal lesions are required. This has been collected over the past several years and more reliable information is now available regarding dysplasia in the esophagus with respect to its incidence and prevalence, cytologic features and degrees of dysplasia, and recommendations regarding therapy.[173–176] As in the colon and stomach, this remains a field in which the information is growing, and the recommendations need constant review.

Given the decided increase in carcinoma development in cases of Barrett's esophagus, it is recommended that such patients have screening and surveillance to look for associated dysplasia.[166–169,173–180] Of all cases of esophageal adenocarcinoma involving the distal esophagus, a great majority reveal dysplasia at their edges or in adjacent regions, supporting the notion that the dysplasia may be a precursor lesion. Furthermore, there have now been sufficient prospective studies to show the appearance and evolution of Barrett's esophagus to dysplasia and to early adenocarcinoma to support this hypothesis. It is not known when to start such endoscopic screening of surveillance, but it is usually

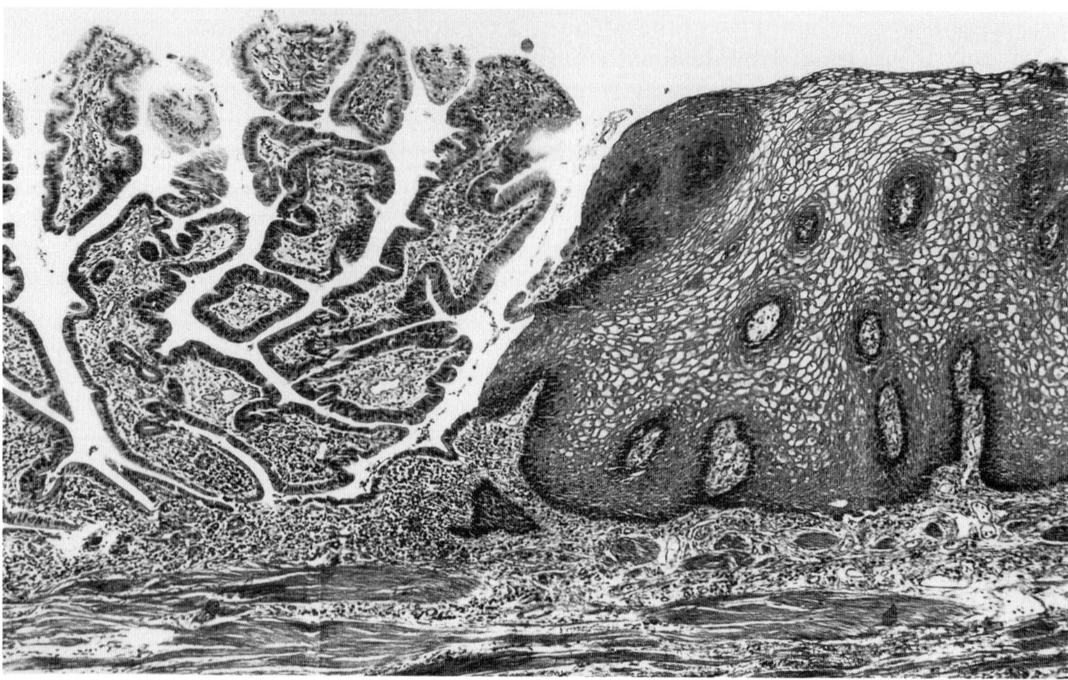

Fig. 3-11. Barrett's esophagus with glandular dysplasia. Photograph is from a resected specimen showing normal squamous epithelium at the right, Barrett's epithelium with a papillary growth of dysplasia at the left, and a part of the muscularis mucosae at the bottom (× 68).

begun at least 10 years after the identification of the Barrett's esophagus.

Gross Features

Sought at endoscopic examination are biopsies of any gross lesions that deviate from the typical mucoid or salmon-colored mucosa. These would include strictures, ulcers, polyps, and plaques. In addition, random samples are obtained from the flat mucosa. There is no rigid protocol indicating the number and location of the biopsies, but the more that can be obtained and the larger the specimens, the greater the likelihood for the detection and easy identification of the dysplasia.[180] In cases with carcinoma, the dysplasia is most often seen in the immediately adjacent mucosa. Additional areas can be found in the uninvolved flat mucosa. Exceptionally, the dysplastic areas occur in a grossly evident polypoid or papillary lesion that is identical to an adenoma. Since the isolated occurrence of an adenoma in the esophagus probably does not occur, in contrast to the colon, the finding of such a lesion should serve as an alert that this represents a polypoid area of dysplasia in Barrett's esophagus.

Cytologic Features

As with squamous tumors, cytologic examination might be of benefit but has been less tested in cases of Barrett's esophagus[181,182] (Plates 3E–H). As we approach days of cost containment, however, the potential use of tubes to obtain cytologic specimens might become the first step in the screening for glandular dysplasia. The benign metaplastic epithelium is appreciated as columnar cells with slightly elongated and eccentric nuclei

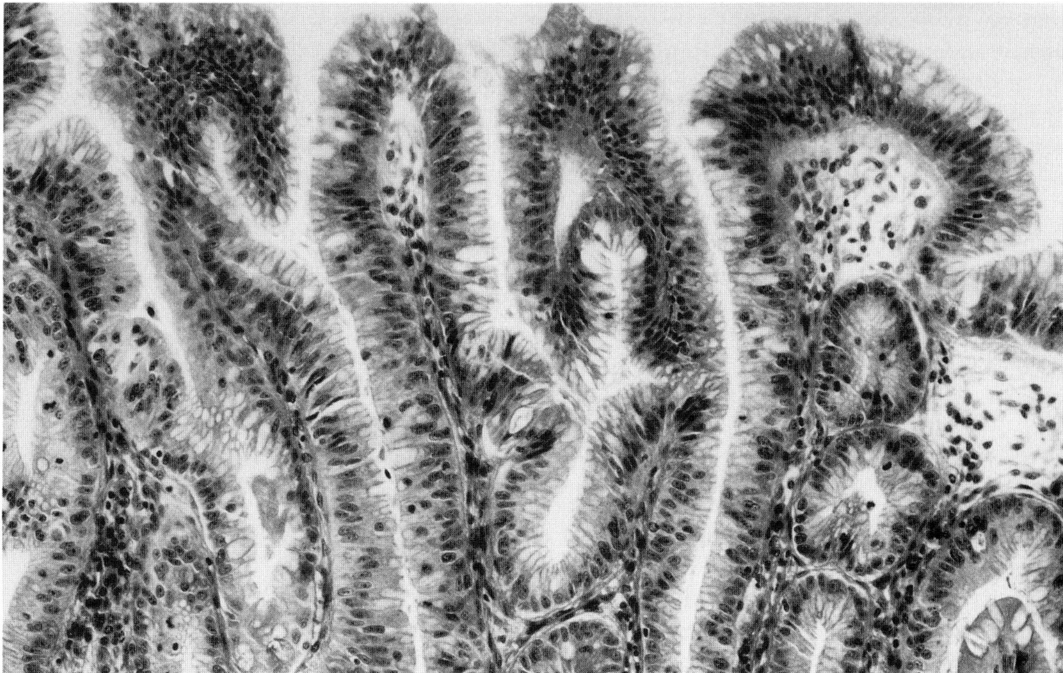

Fig. 3-12. Low-grade glandular dysplasia in Barrett's esophagus. The epithelial cells show elongation of the nuclei but minimal palisading and hyperchromatism. Also noted are ample mucin production and maturation at the surface (× 210).

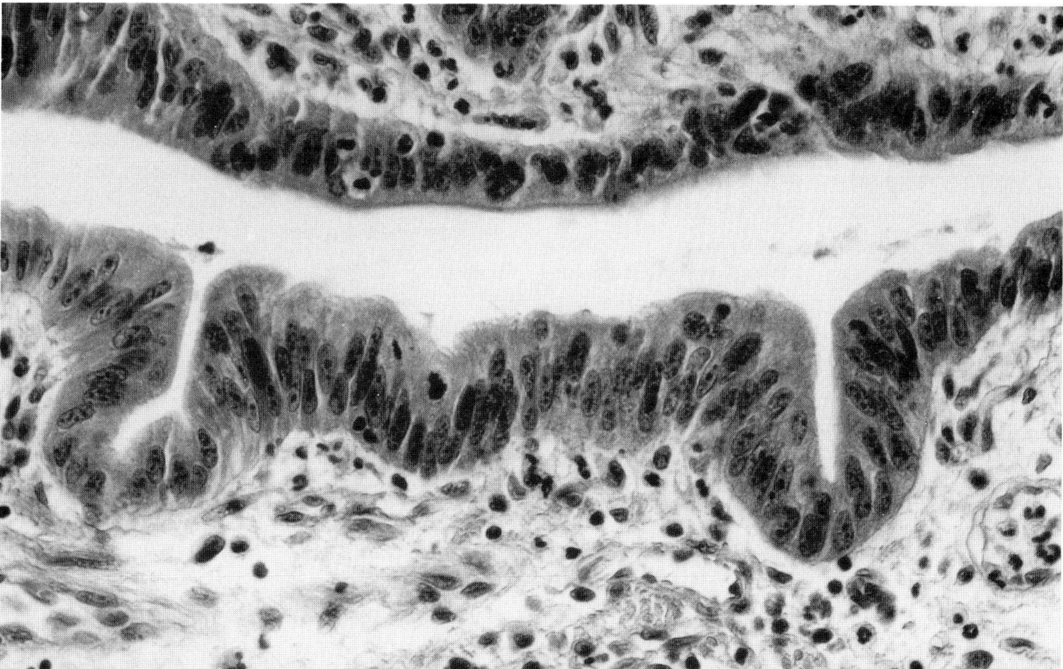

Fig. 3-13. High-grade glandular dysplasia in Barrett's esophagus. The dysplastic gland shows marked variability of nuclei with prominent palisading; irregularity in size, shape, and position; and hyperchromatism. The nuclei are near the surface of the cells, and there is no mucin formation (× 425).

that have fine chromatin; the cells resemble gastric and intestinal mucous cells of a benign nature. The cytologic features of dysplasia are equivalent to those noted in the stomach, revealing enlargement and irregularity of the nuclei with increasing clumps of chromatin. Even greater aberrations in the nuclei with more prominent hyperchromatism and irregularity of the cells are seen in cases that are diagnostic by cytology of adenocarcinoma. In contrast to the squamous tumors, which have nuclei in the center of the cells, the nuclei in adenocarinoma cells are eccentrically placed.

Histologic Features and Classification

The histologic diagnosis of dysplasia on biopsy is principally by the architectural and cytologic features as evidenced on the routine stains (Table 3-9). As in other areas of the gut, there is the need to recognize the full range of inflammatory and regenerative features that can occur in Barrett's esophagus and to exclude these before considering the diagnosis of dysplasia. There may be marked degrees of regeneration, showing many mitoses; the regenerating cells typically contain enlarged nuclei, but they tend to be very regular in position and size and have fine chromatin and central nucleoli. In cases with ulceration or stricture, there is often a great deal of granulation tissue containing enlarged endothelial and fibroblastic cells that must be appreciated and distinguished from dysplasia or invasive carcinoma. This is sometimes difficult in the small, distorted, and potentially overfixed specimens, and caution should be the rule. Following therapy for the reflux disease, there frequently is partial return of the squamous epithelium and this admixture with the glandular tissue should not be confused for an abnormal growth.

Table 3-9. Classification of Dysplasia in Barrett's Esophagus

Negative for dysplasia
Indefinite or suspicious for dysplasia
Positive for dysplasia
Low grade
High grade
Intramucosal carcinoma

In classifying the biopsies, they are rated as negative for dysplasia; indefinite or suspicious for dysplasia; and positive for dysplasia, including low-grade and high-grade degrees (Table 3-9). Low-grade dysplasia is characterized by minimal or no architectural abnormalities, meaning no further irregularity of the glands beyond that expected in Barrett's esophagus, but with the unexplained presence of atypical cells. These cells show an increase in the size and elongation of the nuclei that may palisade and involve any portion of the cell; there is usually no prominent hyperchromatism or loss of polarity of the cells (Fig. 3-12). In high-grade dysplasia, there is even greater abnormality, consisting of occasional elongation and complexity of the glands; of much more prominence of the nuclei with hyperchromatism; and of reductions in the amount of cytoplasm and in the mucin content in the cells (Fig. 3-13). The cases of high-grade dysplasia are more likely to involve a greater area and both the basal and superficial regions of the biopsies, but these are not absolute findings. Increased mitoses are seen but are not a discriminating feature. Similarly, the dysplastic areas may develop a villiform surface, but this can also be seen in metaplastic regions that are negative for dysplasia.

The accuracy in making the histologic diagnosis of dysplasia has been tested, and it was demonstrated that the high-grade cases of dysplasia, which also include in-situ and early invasive carcinoma can be distinguished from the rest of the cases in over 85 percent of the cases.[166] Conversely, the ability to distinguish the negative cases from the rest had a success rate of only 70 percent. This was due in large part to the limited view in the study of the tissue section; in this study, the slides were covered and only a tiny portion of the biopsy sample was inspected, eliminating architectural criteria from the evaluation. It seems to be common practice that the negative biopsies can be sorted out in a much higher percentage of cases.

Special Studies

There were studies to suggest that the finding of metaplasia that is rich in sulfated mucin is more apt to have dysplasia; however, this feature has also been noted in almost one-half of the cases that lack any dysplasia.[159–161] Routine immunohistochemical and ultrastructural examinations have also not yielded any features that help in the diagnosis of dysplasia.[161,183–185] The demonstration of oncogenes, of loss of tumor suppressor genes, and of markers of enhanced growth fraction are more likely to assist in the early diagnosis or in determining specificity for the diagnosis of dysplasia.[186–190] Of interest, it has been noted that sucrase–isomaltase is frequently present in the cytoplasm of dysplastic cells in cases of Barrett's esophagus as well as in those with chronic gastritis and with ulcerative colitis.[191,192] The presence of such markers or their genes holds promise for the improved definition of dysplasia in such patients.

Treatment of Patients with Dysplasia

There are evolving recommendations for actions to be taken based on the biopsy findings.[166,173–176,178–180,193] It is currently suggested that there be routine or repeat examination every 1 to 2 years for cases that are negative for dysplasia; that there be repeat biopsy in cases that are indefinite, with the interval dependent on the degree of suspicion ranging from days to 3 months; and that there probably be repeat biopsy within a few months in cases that are rated as low-grade dysplasia, not only to confirm the diagnosis but also to exclude more severe degrees of dysplasia. In the finding of high-grade dysplasia, it is recommended that this be verified by additional observers or further examinations. The latter also serves to determine the extent of the dysplasia and to uncover any previously unsuspected areas of carcinoma. The biopsy features of carcinoma are sought in the form of cells, either singly or in clusters, that extend into the lamina propria or muscularis mucosae. This finding is made easier with the use of larger, so-called jumbo biopsies that include a more substantial portion of the mucosa.[180] Esophagogastric resection is currently considered for cases that have high-grade dysplasia in association with early carcinoma and also for those cases of high-grade dysplasia that persist. With the improvements in surgical technique and in selection of patients, there is a growing tendency to provide this operation for most patients with confirmed high-grade dysplasia. Examination of the surgical specimen serves to confirm the dysplasia in practically all cases and also realizes the detection of early carcinoma in up to one-quarter of the cases. In most patients detected by surveillance the carcinomas, if present, are at an early stage.[175]

Features of Adenocarcinoma

Early Carcinoma

The earliest cases of adenocarcinoma occurring in Barrett's esophagus are seen in patients who have been part of a surveillance program, and they are almost always associated with the finding of glandular dysplasia. The carcinoma is characterized by the presence of atypical glandular epithelial cells that extend at least into the lamina propria and may research the muscularis mucosae (Fig. 3-14). Such cases are referred to as *intramucosal adenocarcinoma.* When there is more substantial conversion of the mucosa to car-

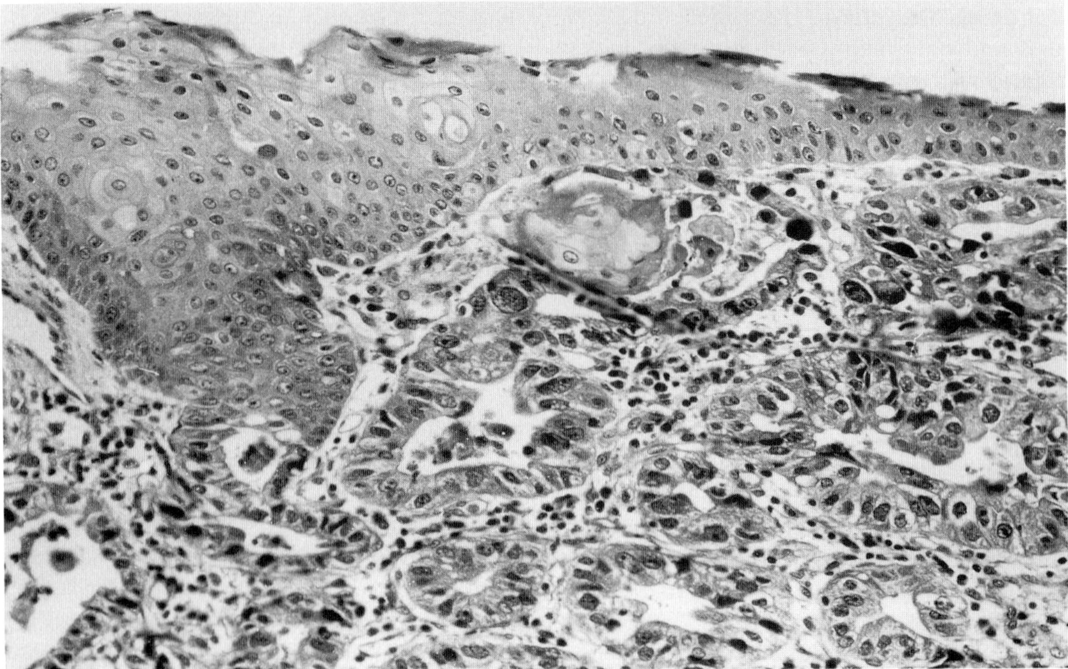

Fig. 3-14. Well differentiated adenocarcinoma in Barrett's esophagus. Present are highly irregular glands with markedly atypical cells in the lamina propria that undermine the normal squamous epithelium (top) (× 210).

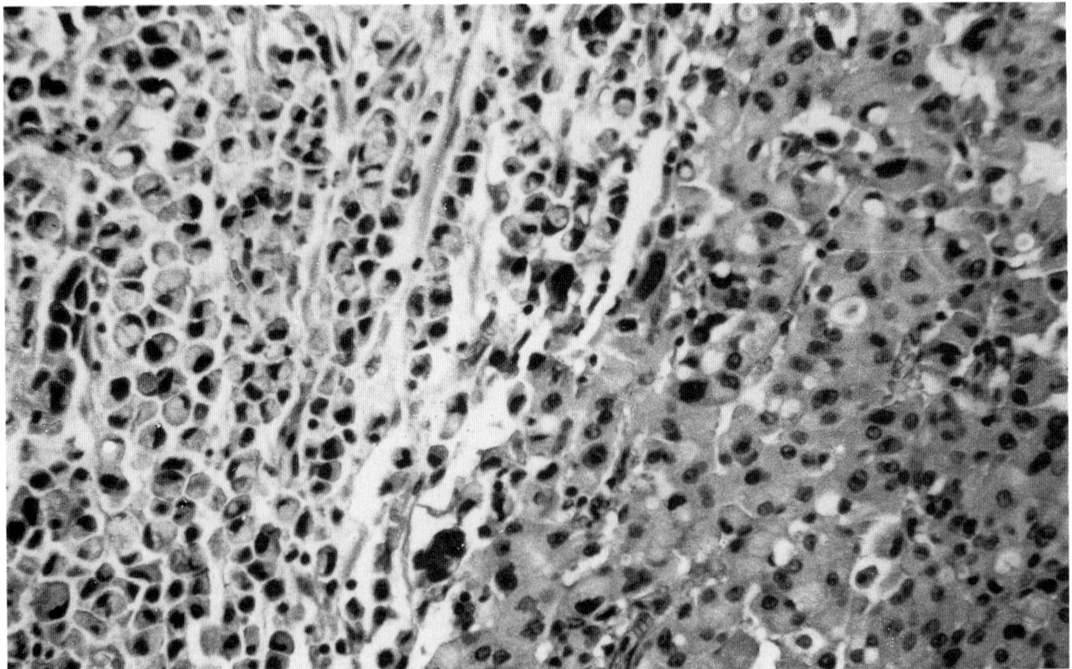

Fig. 3-15. Poorly differentiated adenocarcinoma in Barrett's esophagus. Noted are sheets of tumor cells with many signet ring forms (left).

cinoma, cystic neoplastic glands are frequently seen, similar to what is observed in intramucosal adenocarcinoma of the stomach. The mucosal biopsies usually show some combination of glandular dysplasia and early adenocarcinoma, and complete examination of the surgical specimen is needed to determine the full extent of any invasion.

Advanced Carcinoma

Most cases of esophageal adenocarcinoma that are seen in patients with symptoms are more advanced, with tumor that is grossly invasive into the submucosa or muscularis propria. As with the squamous tumors, these can present as polypoid, ulcerative, or infiltrative masses. They are concentrated in the distal esophagus, a reflection of their development in the areas of Barrett's esophagus. Since the histologic features of the adenocarcinomas complicating Barrett's esophagus and those arising in the stomach (including the proximal part) are identical, their distinction is dependent largely on the actual location of most or all of the tumor.[124–126] In addition, the mucosa adjacent to the tumor may reveal the Barrett's epithelium in the esophageal cases as opposed to chronic gastritis with intestinal metaplasia of the corpus in the gastric cases. The initial distinction may not be totally critical since the same operative procedure is employed for all tumors in this region.

All forms of adenocarcinoma, ranging from those that are well differentiated with evident gland formation to poorly differentiated tumors showing diffuse cells and prominent signet ring cell formation, can be seen[56,125,194] (Fig. 3-15). The prognosis and therapy depend on the stage of the tumor. Unfortunately, most advanced cases present with transmural disease and surgery is often only of a palliative nature. Biopsies of advanced carcinomas typically reveal the irregular gland formation of sheets of cells with prominent necrosis and invasion. Difficulties can arise if the samples are very small, revealing mainly necrosis with scant cellular material or inadequate underlying tissue to evaluate for invasion. Following treatment, biopsies may be obtained to monitor the patients; in such instances, the samples are inspected for recurrent tumor, for effects of therapy, and for the appearance of any infections.

Uncommonly observed in Barrett's cases are other types of tumors, including neuroendocrine carcinoma and adenocarcinoid lesions,[195] adenosquamous types, pure squamous cell carcinomas,[77–79] and choriocarcinoma.[196] There have also been noted carcinomas with a mixture of glandular, squamous, and endocrine differentiation.[197] The development of these other tumors simply reflects the potential for the stem cells to differentiate. Biopsy may recognize any of these subtypes, and their existence in the esophagus in such cases should be accepted rather than requiring spread from other areas.

Special Techniques

Several studies using flow cytometry have demonstrated the presence of aneuploidy, hyperploidy, or expanded G2 fractions in most of the cases with dysplasia and carcinoma.[198–203] It has been suggested that this technique can help the biopsy diagnosis of the dysplasia and early carcinoma cases, but the results have not been uniformly successful.[204] Regular immunocytochemical and ultrastructural examinations have not provided any special assistance in the diagnosis of the adenocarcinomas of the esophagus. More recent attention has been devoted to molecular techniques, with demonstration of increased expression of p53 and c-*erb* in areas of dysplasia and carcinoma.[205–207] In cases that have biopsies that are rated as indefinite or suspicious for dysplasia, the application of flow cytometry or stains for gene abnormalities in subsequent samples might prove useful.

Variant Forms of Adenocarcinoma

The *adenoacanthoma* represents an adenocarcinoma in which there are foci of mature squamous cell metaplasia, whereas the *adenosquamous cell carcinoma* is a tumor in which both the glandular and squamous elements show the cytologic features of malignancy[25,56,208] (Figs. 3-16 and 3-17). They both appear to represent uncommon variants of esophageal adenocarcinoma (Table 3-10) and are most often noted in the distal esophagus. There is no special difference in behavior based on these subtypes. Mucosal biopsy may appreciate these variants but more often shows only the dominant component of adenocarcinoma.

Rarely noted in the esophagus are tumors with salivary gland features such as *mucoepidermoid carcinoma*[209,210] and *adenoid cystic carcinoma.*[211,212] The mucoepidermoid carcinomas are identified by the admixture in the tumor of keratinizing squamous elements and individual columnular or signet ring cells with mucin production (cf. Fig. 11-15). The adenoid cystic carcinoma shows a cribiform pattern of epithelial cells with prominent cyst formation, separated by extensive amounts of collagen (Fig. 3-18). These tumors are probably derived from the submucosal glands in the esophagus, and they tend to be concentrated in the middle portion. The tumors can extend into the mucosa, and biopsies may provide the diagnosis of malignancy but usually not the specific cell type.

Table 3-10. Types of Glandular Tumors in the Esophagus

Glandular dysplasia and adenoma
Adenocarcinoma
Variants of Adenocarcinoma
Adenoacanthoma
Adenosquamous cell carcinoma
Mucoepidermoid carcinoma
Adenoid cystic carcinoma

OTHER TUMORS

As in all parts of the alimentary tract, there is a wide array of additional tumor types that can affect the esophagus (Table 3-11). Most of these are rare. Mucosal biopsy can often assist in the diagnosis of tumor but there may be insufficient material to provide the specific cell type.

Endocrine Tumors

Carcinoid Tumor

Unlike other parts of the gastrointestinal tract, well formed carcinoid tumors are rarely observed in the esophagus.[213,214] They demonstrate nests and ribbons of uniform cells with large round nuclei and fine chromatin. Specificity can be provided by special stains, particularly Grimelius' argyrophil method, and by immunocytochemical stains for endocrine cell markers such as chromogranin and synaptophysin.[215] Ultrastructural examination is also highly specific, revealing the dense core granules that are typical of endocrine differentiation within the cytoplasm of the tumor cells.[216] As in other parts of the gut, clusters of endocrine cells can also be found in cases of adenocarcinoma; when this is especially prominent, the terms *adenocarcinoid tumor* or *composite tumor* are used.[217,218] Such cases have been observed in carcinomas complicating the Barrett's esophagus but are otherwise rare in the esophagus.[195]

Small Cell Carcinoma

Small cell carcinoma of the esophagus is equivalent to the undifferentiated or oat cell type of neuroendocrine carcinoma that is

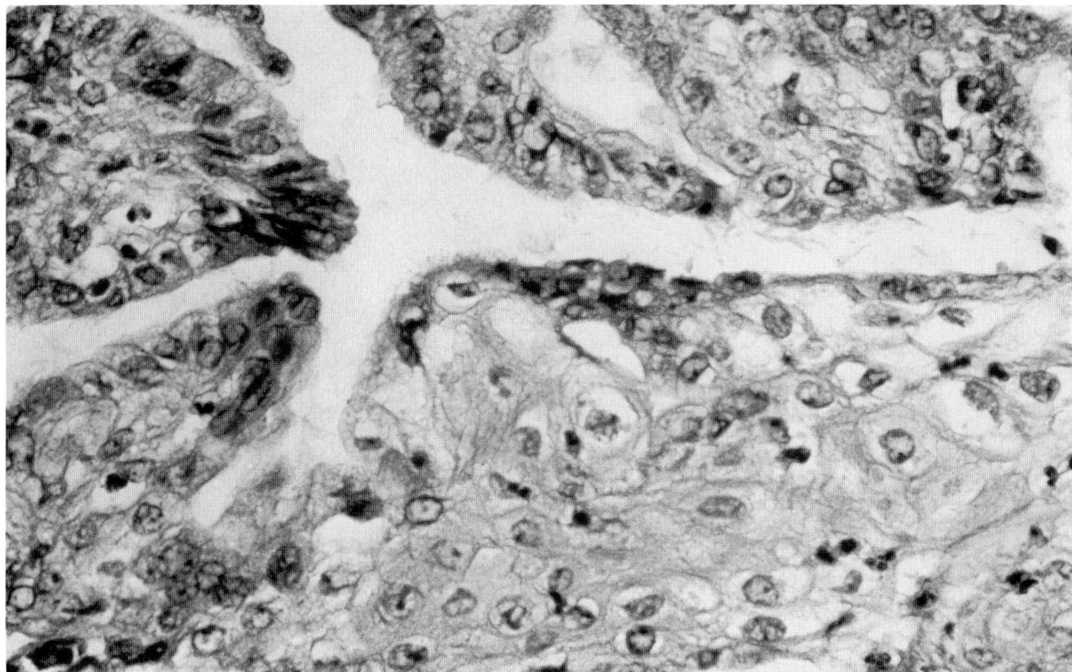

Fig. 3-16. Adenoacanthoma. The tumor is composed mainly of malignant glands, with foci of metaplastic squamous tissue (bottom and right). The squamous cells usually appear benign (× 425).

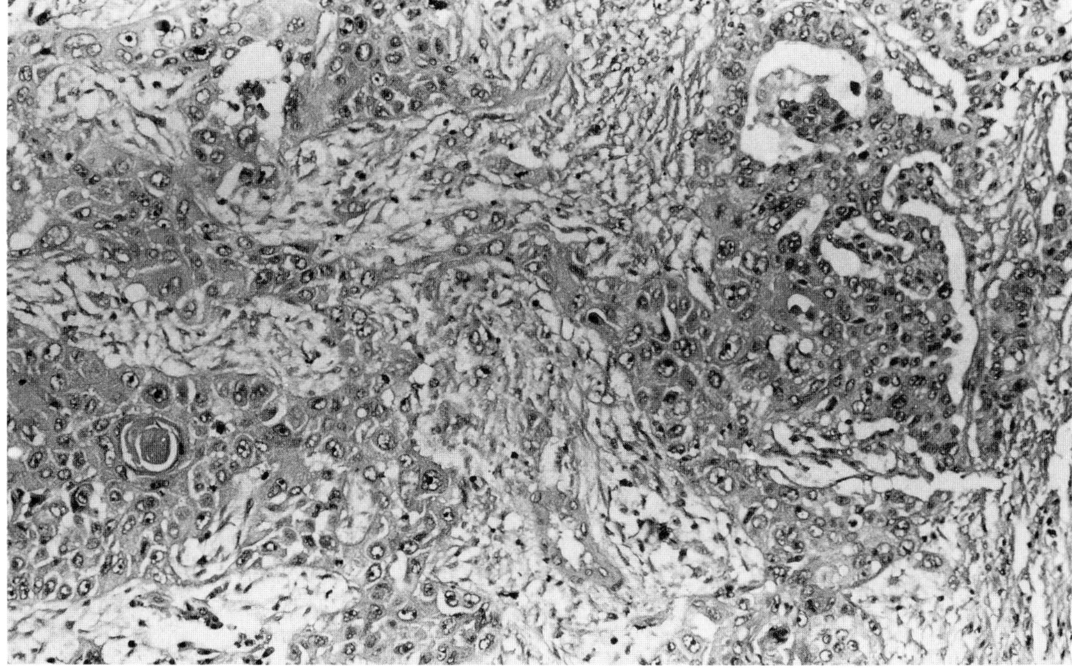

Fig. 3-17. Adenosquamous cell carcinoma of the esophagus. There is a mixture of malignant glandular (upper right) and squamous tumor (× 170).

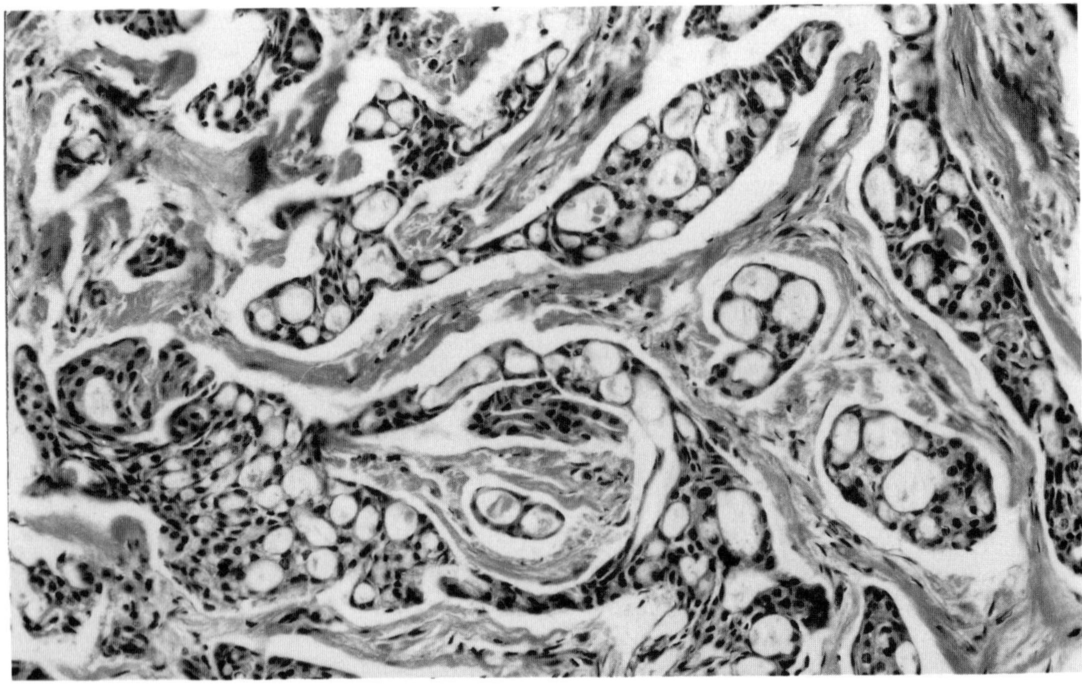

Fig. 3-18. Adenoid cystic carcinoma. There is the characteristic appearance of small nests of tumor cells with prominent microcystic change. The nests are separated by bands of fibrous tissue (× 210).

more typical of the bronchial tree. Rare cases are observed that appear to be primary in the esophagus and can be realized by mucosal biopsy.[219–221] The tumors are composed of solid sheets of cells with oval, dense nuclei, and lack any squamous or glandular differentiation (Fig. 3-19). The main differential is with other small cell tumors, particularly with lymphomas, and these can be sorted out by appropriate immunocytochemical stains (including antibodies to epithelial and endocrine cell markers for the neuroendocrine carcinoma as opposed to leukocyte common antigen for lymphomas), and by electron microscopic examination. Given the much more common prevalence of small cell or oat cell carcinoma in the tracheobronchial tree, it is important to exclude an extension or metastasis from that area in any case that presents in the esophagus.

Table 3-11. Uncommon Tumors of the Esophagus

Endocrine tumors
Carcinoid tumor
Small cell carcinoma
Lymphoid tumors
Benign lymphoid hyperplasia
Malignant lymphoma
Mesenchymal tumors
Leiomyoma
Granular cell tumor
Sarcomas
Other primary tumors
Malignant melanoma
Choriocarcinoma
Secondary and metastatic tumors

Lymphoid Tumors

Benign Lymphoid Hyperplasia

Occasionally seen in esophageal biopsies are small lymphoid nodules, either in the lamina propria or in the upper portion of the submucosa. These are not always associated

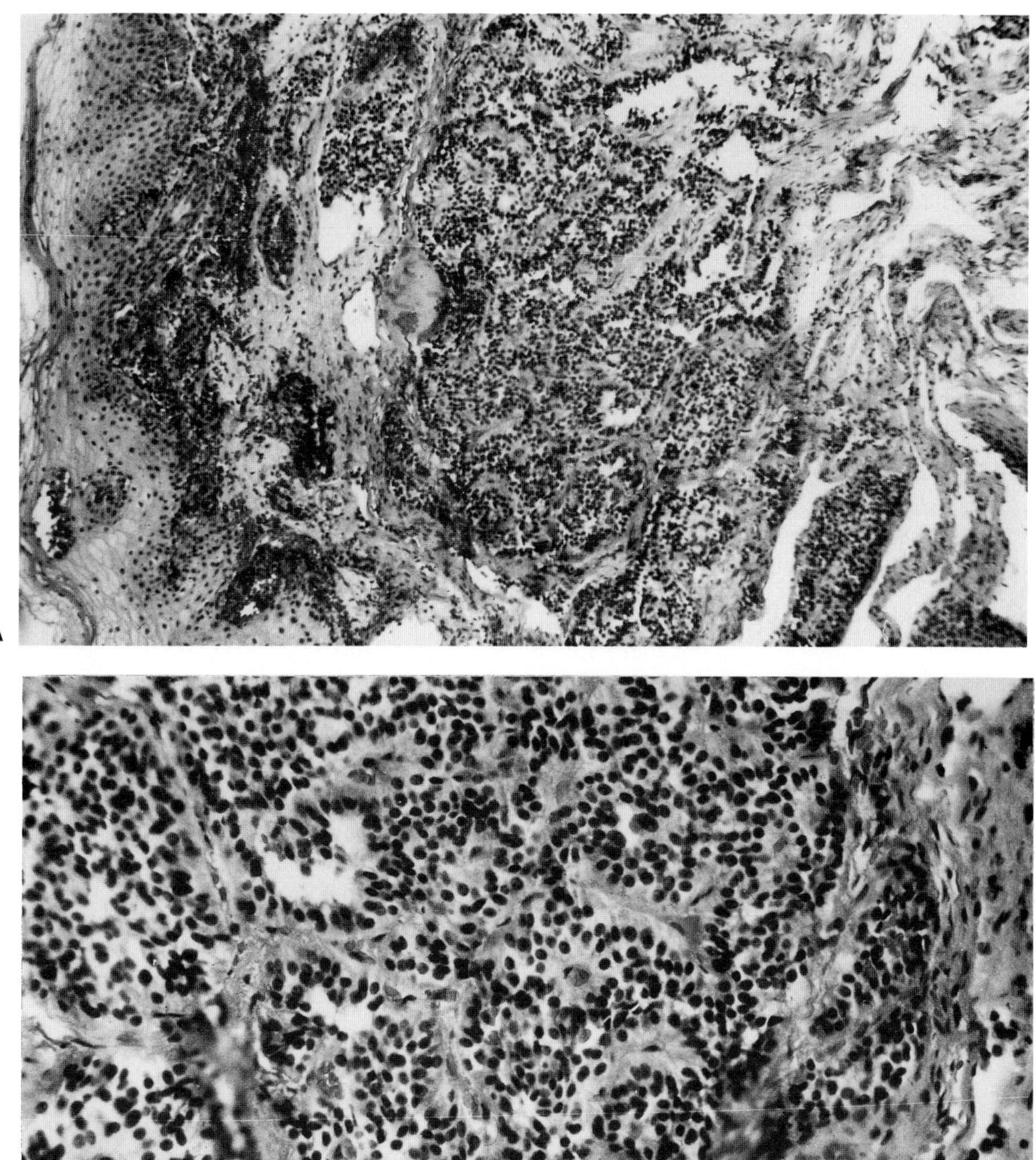

Fig. 3-19. Small cell (neuroendocrine) carcinoma of the esophagus. **(A)** The tumor has irregular edges and is located in the lamina propria; the overlying squamous epithelium appears at left, and a part of the muscularis mucosae appears at right. **(B)** High power of the tumor, showing small cells with dense, slightly elongated nuclei.

with other features of inflammation, and it is possible that these lymphoid nodules are either a normal component or a vestige of a prior injury. Rarely noted is a larger mass or nodule of lymphoid hyperplasia measuring several millimeters and involving both the mucosal and submucosal regions.[222] The benign nature of the infiltrate is appreciated by the presence of well formed follicles. These can be detected by mucosal biopsy, and it is important in such cases to exclude an associated inflammatory condition as well as malignant lymphoma.

Malignant Lymphoma

Compared to other parts of the gastrointestinal tract,[223] the appearance of primary malignant lymphoma in the esophagus is rare.[224–226] The esophagus can also be infiltrated by malignant lymphoma that extends from adjacent areas, such as the mediastinum, or be part of a disseminated process.[227,228] Most of the tumors are of the non-Hodgkin's, B-cell type.[229] (More complete descriptions of lymphoma are provided in Ch. 5 and in Ch. 7.)

Mesenchymal Tumors

Leiomyoma

Both benign and rarely malignant tumors can develop from the mesenchymal elements present throughout the wall of the esophagus.[1,34] Most common are leiomyomas that are frequently seen as incidental findings in surgical and autopsy specimens; they tend to be less than 2 cm in diameter and are usually limited to the wall without extension to the musoca[230] (Fig. 3-20). Rarely noted are an extensive proliferation of such muscle tumors, referred to as *leiomyomatosis*. Symptoms leading to mucosal examination and biopsy occur when the tumors are present in a naturally narrow location, such as the esophagocardiac junction, or when they become larger and develop overlying mucosal ulceration. It is rare, however, for the biopsy to show the mesenchymal elements; rather, only the overlying ulceration or atrophic mucosa is usually seen.

Granular Cell Tumor

Granular cell tumors are benign neoplasms that probably derive from nervous tissue elements. They can be present in many parts of the body including all portions of the alimentary tract.[231] They are occasionally seen in the esophagus as single or multiple nodules, and the diagnosis can be readily made on biopsy.[232–234] The tumors have a characteristic appearance, comprised of large cells with abundant, finely granular cytoplasm and small, benign-appearing nuclei (Figs. 3-21 and 3-22). The granular nature is due to the presence of many lysosomes and can be accented by the PAS reaction. The tumors often have an ill-defined border and may appear to infiltrate the surrounding tissue, but are considered benign lesions. The differential includes nodular collections of macrophages that show more convoluted nuclei, and diffuse or signet ring cell types of carcinomas that reveal malignant-type nuclei as well as larger mucin droplets within the cytoplasm.

Sarcomas

Sarcomas are rare in the esophagus; those that occur include leiomyosarcoma, malignant schwannoma, hemangiopericytoma, synovial sarcoma, and osteosarcoma.[235–240] They present as large masses that may extend into the mucosa. Biopsies in most cases reveal ulceration and malignant tumor without providing specific identification. All of these primary mesenchymal tumors should be distinguished from other lesions that can project into the lumen, including the ordinary carci-

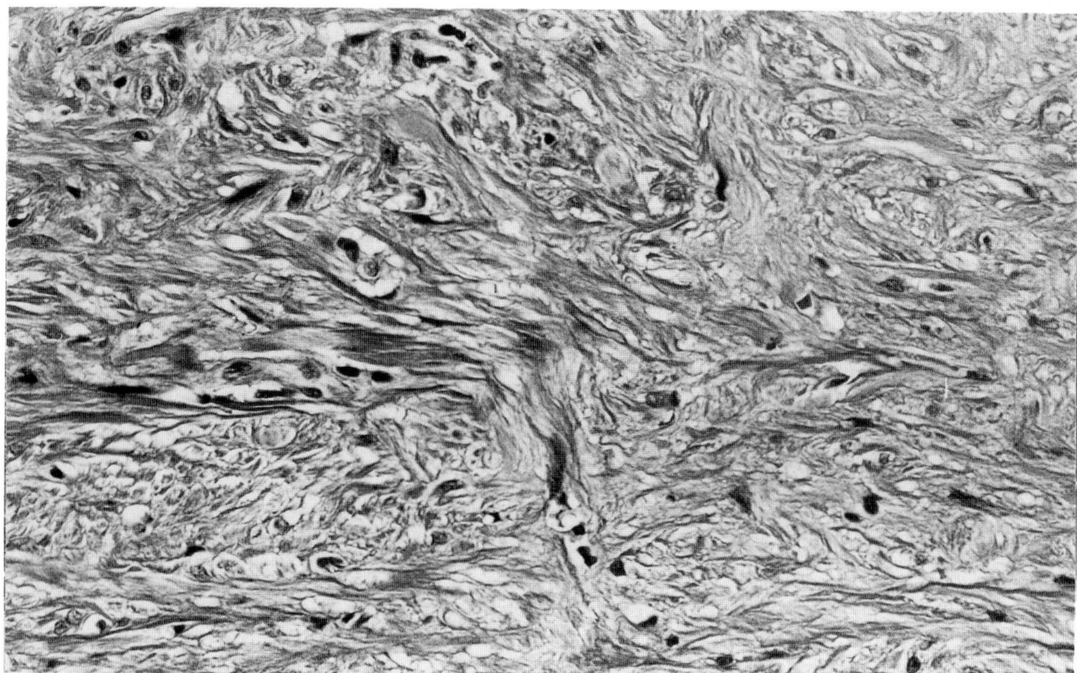

Fig. 3-20. Leiomyoma of the esophagus. The tumor is comprised of slender cells with small nuclei together with abundant fibrous tissue (× 425).

nomas, the large fibrovascular polyps, and the protruding spindle cell type carcinoma. The distinction between sarcoma and the spindle cell variant of squamous cell carcinoma can be particularly difficult. It is important to recognize that the spindle cell variant is more common, and its epithelial nature can be identified by immunocytochemical stain for keratin and also by ultrastructural examination. Given this overall differential, it is useful to obtain material from large, protruding masses for these special studies, which include electron microscopic evaluation.

Other Primary Tumors

Malignant Melanoma

Malignant melanoma can occur in the esophagus as either a primary or metastatic lesion. Melanocytes are normally noted in the esophagus.[241,242] The primary melanomas typically present as polypoid or ulcerated masses that resemble carcinomas, but the biopsy reveals the characteristic large cells with prominent nuclei and nucleoli as well as melanin deposits within the cytoplasm in most cases[243–245] (Fig. 3-23). Immuncytochemical stains for S-100 and melanoma-specific markers can provide assistance,[246] and ultrastructural examination can be particularly helpful in tumors with sparse or no melanin deposits by demonstrating the melanosomes within the cytoplasm[247] (Fig. 3-24). Rarely noted are benign melanocytic proliferations at the edges of the melanoma to support the primary nature[243] (Fig. 3-25). In most cases, the decision that a melanocytic tumor of the esophagus has arisen locally is based on the finding of only a single lesion and the exclusion of its presence in other sites, particularly the skin. Metastatic melanoma can also appear in the esophagus as in other parts of

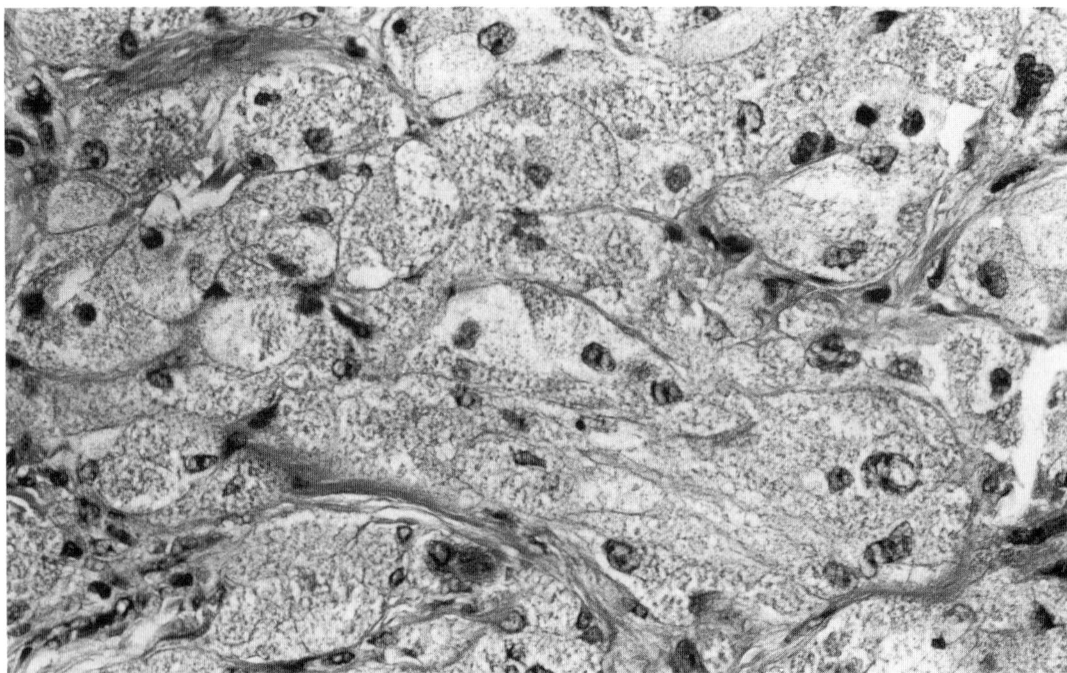

Fig. 3-21. Granular cell tumor of the esophagus. The tumor consists of large cells with abundant, granular cytoplasm and small nuclei. There is no cytologic atypism (× 425).

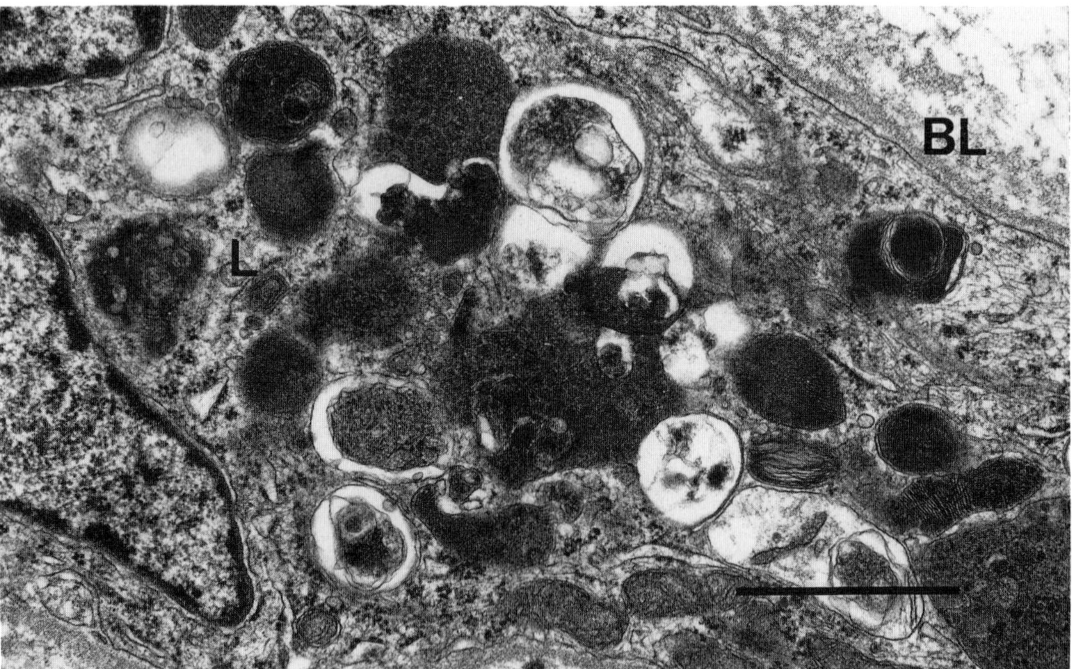

Fig. 3-22. Electron micrograph of granular cell tumor. The cytoplasm contains large numbers of characteristic heterogeneous secondary lysosomes (L), and basal lamina (BL) surround groups of cells (× 28,500; bar = 1 μm).

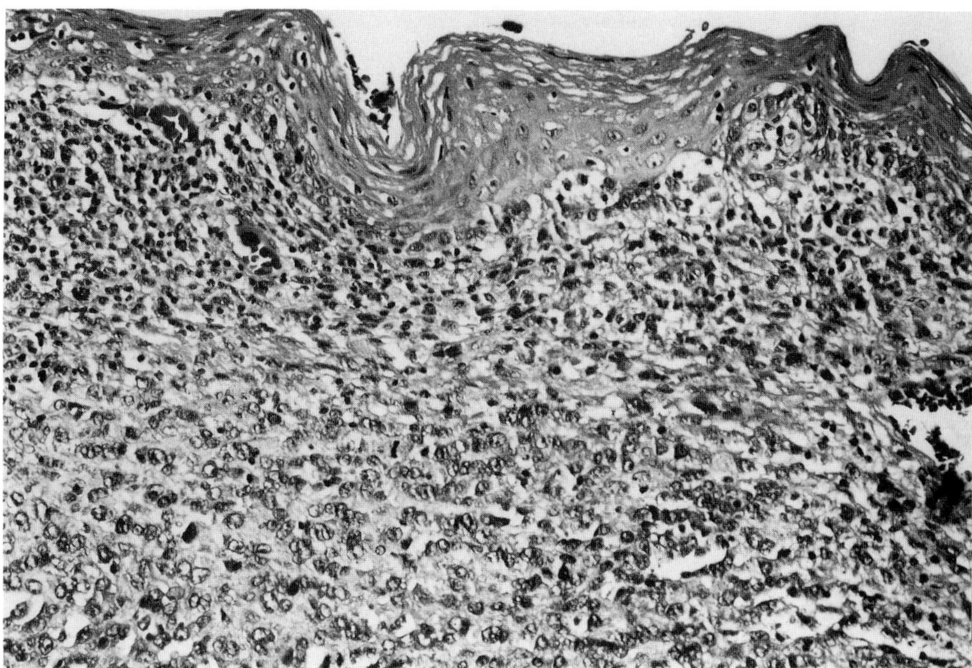

Fig. 3-23. Malignant melanoma of the esophagus. There is a diffuse infiltrate of tumor cells, in the form of sheets and cords, beneath the squamous layer. The primary nature of the melanoma was supported by the finding of junctional activity (see Fig. 3-25) (× 210).

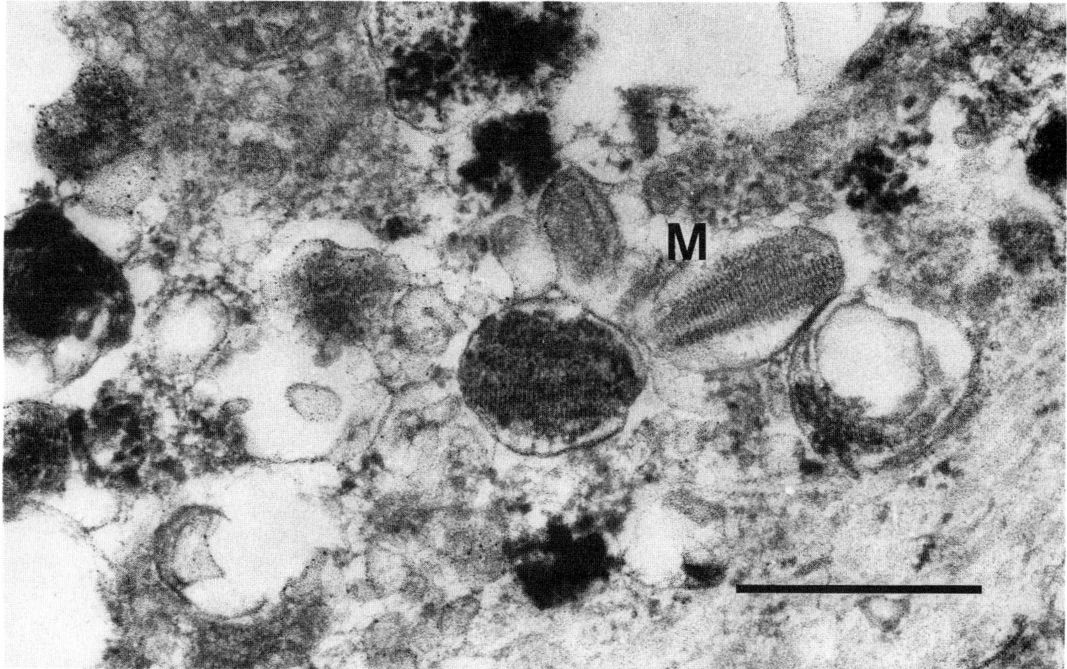

Fig. 3-24. Electron micrograph of malignant melanoma with melanosomes in various stages. Premelanosomes (M) composed of a striated core with and without pigment are diagnostic of the tumor (× 62,500; bar = 0.5 μm).

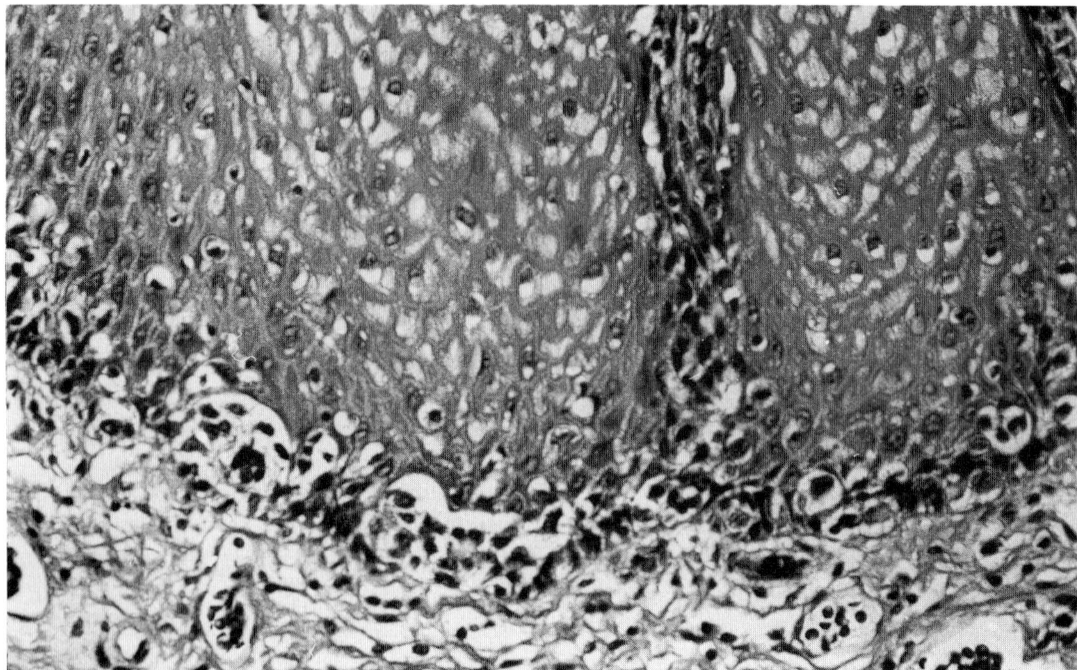

Fig. 3-25. Malignant melanoma of the esophagus. The adjacent squamous epithelium reveals junctional activity at the base. Some of the melanocytic cells are atypical and extend slightly into the squamous layer (× 280).

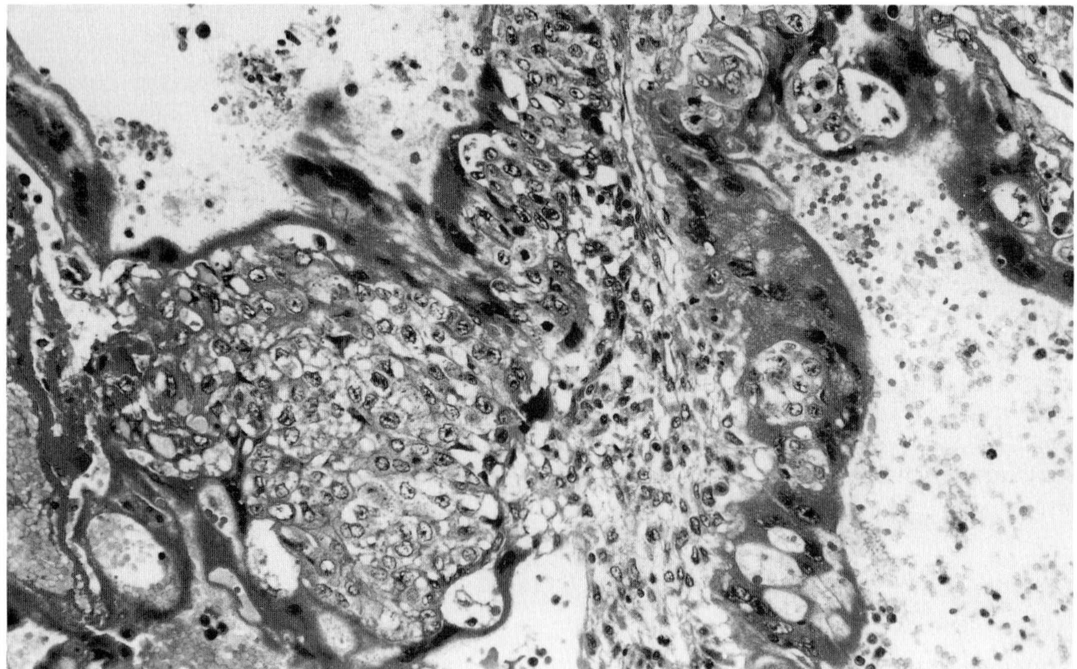

Fig. 3-26. Choriocarcinoma, showing sheets of cytotrophoblastic tumor cells surrounded by the multinucleated syncytial-type cells (× 425).

the alimentary tract[248,249]; lesions in such cases are typically multiple and polypoid.

Choriocarcinoma

Primary choriocarcinomas have been rarely reported in the alimentary tract, particularly in the esophagus and the stomach.[56,196,250] They reveal the characteristic features with large giant cell forms and are thought to be aggressive tumors (Fig. 3-26). It is important to exclude extension of a germ cell tumor from the adjacent mediastinal region.

Secondary and Metastatic Tumors

Many other tumors can appear in the esophagus, as an extension from adjacent organs or as part of a metastatic process.

Secondary Tumors

The most commonly observed secondary tumors are adenocarcinomas of the proximal stomach that extend into the lower part of the esophagus; these must be differentiated from primary esophageal adenocarcinoma. Since the histology of the adenocarcinomas is identical in the two areas, the primary localization is largely dependent on noting where the tumor is grossly present.[125] In addition, the finding of Barrett's esophagus alone or in association with dysplasia provides support for an esophageal origin. Tumors can also extend into the esophagus from the lung and the mediastinum, and these are largely sorted out by radiographic and biopsy studies of the other tissues.

Metastatic Tumors

Metastatic tumors can come to the esophagus from practically any area of the body.[251] More commonly noted are metastases of malignant melanoma,[248,249] and carcinomas of the lungs, breast, kidney, upper airway, skin, and prostate.[252–254] They more often present as multiple tumors in very sick patients, suggesting the likelihood of metastatic disease. Biopsies can help in establishing that there is malignancy and can assess the tumors compared to the original sources. The biopsy also serves to exclude other non-tumor diagnoses, such as ulcers developing from therapy or from secondary infections.

REFERENCES

1. Ming S-C: Tumors of the Esophagus and Stomach. Armed Forces. Institute of Pathology Fascicle 7. 2nd series. Washington D.C., 1973
2. Yang PC, Davis S: Incidence of cancer of the esophagus in the U.S. by histologic type. Cancer 61:612–617, 1988
3. Watanabe H, Jass JR, Sobin LH: WHO Histological Typing of Oesophageal and Gastric Tumors. Springer-Verlag, Berlin, 1990
4. Winawar SJ, Sherlock P, Hajdu SI: The role of upper gastrointestinal endoscopy in patients with cancer. Cancer 37:440, 1976
5. Hunt RH, Cotton PB, Crespi M et al: Role of endoscopy in the diagnosis of cancer. Cancer Res 49:6822–6827, 1989
6. Hanson JT, Thorenson C, Morrissey JF: Brush cytology in the diagnosis of upper gastrointestinal malignancy. Gastrointest Endosc 26:33, 1980
7. Qizilbash AH, Casteli M, Kowalski MA et al: Endoscopic brush cytology and biopsy in the diagnosis of cancer of the upper gastrointestinal tract. Acta Cytol 24:313, 1980
8. Geisinger KR: Endoscopic biopsies and cytologic brushings of the esophagus are diagnostically complementary. Am J Clin Pathol 103: 295–299, 1995
9. Tsang TK, Hidvegi D, Horth K, Ostrow JD: Reliability of balloon-mesh cytology in detecting esophageal carcinoma in a population of U.S. veterans. Cancer 59:556–559, 1987
10. Graham DY, Schwartz JT, Cain GT, Gyorkey F: Prospective evaluation of biopsy number in the diagnosis of esophageal and gastric carcinoma. Gastroenterology 82:228–231, 1982

11. Lal N, Bhasin DK, Malik AK et al: Optimal number of biopsy specimens in the diagnosis of carcinoma of the esophagus. Gut 33:724–726, 1992
12. Zargar SA, Khuroo MS, Mahajan R et al: Endoscopic fine needle aspiration cytology in the diagnosis of gastro-esophageal and colorectal malignancies. Gut 32:745–748, 1991
13. Mitsunaga A: Diagnosis of submucosal tumors of the upper gastrointestinal tract by endoscopic ultrasonography. Gastrointest Endosc 29:3–15, 1987
14. Grody WW, Gatti RA, Naeim F: Diagnostic molecular pathology. Modern Pathol 2: 553–568, 1990
15. Chang F, Syrjanen E, Kurinen K, Syrjanen E: The p53 tumor suppressor gene as a common cellular target in human carcinogenesis. Am J Gastroenterol 88:174–186, 1993
16. Stemmermann G, Heffelfinger SC, Noffsinger A et al: The molecular biology of esophageal and gastric cancer and their precursors. Hum Pathol 25:968–981, 1994
17. Wolf BC, Khettry U, Leonardi HK et al: Benign lesions mimicking malignant tumors of the esophagus. Hum Pathol 19:148–154, 1988
18. Shekitka KM, Helwig EB: Deceptive bizarre stromal cells in polyps and ulcers of the gastrointestinal tract. Cancer 67:2111–2117, 1991
19. Howes AR, Brady CE, Williams JR et al: Multiple retention cysts of the lower esophagus. J Clin Gastroenterol 4:209–212, 1982
20. Arbona JL, Fazzi JGF, Majoral J: Congenital esophageal cysts: case report and review of literature. Am J Gastroenterol 79:177–182, 1984
21. Edgin R, Mekhjian HS: Esophageal retention cyst: unusual cause for dysphagia. J Clin Gastroenterol 3(suppl I):57–59, 1981
22. Qazi FM, Geisinger KR, Nelson JB et al: Symptomatic congenital gastroenteric duplication cyst of the esophagus containing exocrine and endocrine pancreatic tissues. Am J Gastroenterol 85:65–67, 1990
23. Postlethwait RW, Detmer DE: Ectopic thyroid nodule in the esophagus. Ann Thorac Surg 19:98–100, 1975
24. Shah B, Unger L, Heimlich HJ: Hamartomatous polyp of the esophagus. Arch Surg 110:326–328, 1975
25. Sommers SC: Esophagus. pp. 7–52. In Rotterdam H, Sheahan DG, Sommers SC (eds): Biopsy Diagnosis of the Digestive Tract. 2nd Ed. Raven Press, New York, 1992
26. Rywlin AM, Ortega R: Glycogenic acanthosis of the esophagus. Arch Pathol 90: 439–443, 1970
27. Bender MD, Allison J, Cuartas F, Montgomery C: Glycogenic acanthosis of the esophagus: a form of benign epithelial hyperplasia. Gastroenterology 65:373–380, 1973
28. Stern Z, Sharon P, Ligumsky M et al: Glycogenic acanthosis of the esophagus. A benign but confusing endoscopic lesion. Am J Gastroenterol 74:261–263, 1980
29. Shifleet DW, Gilliam JH, Wu WC et al: Multiple esophageal webs. Gastroenterology 77:556, 1979
30. Janisch HD, Eckardt VF: Histological abnormalities in patients with multiple esophageal webs. Dig Dis Sci 27:503, 1982
31. Ergun GA, Linan AN, Dannenberg AJ, Carter DM: Gastrointestinal manifestations of epidermolysis bullosa. A study of 101 patients. Medicine 71:121–127, 1992
32. Stewart MI, Woodley DT, Briggaman RA: Epidermolysis bullosa acquisita and associated symptomatic esophageal webs. Arch Dermatol 127:373, 1991
33. Weinman D, Stewart MI, Woodley DT, Garcia G: Epidermolysis bullosa acquisita (EBA) and esophageal webs: a new association. Am J Gastroenterol 86:1518–1522, 1991
34. Faivre J, Bory R, Moulinier B: Benign tumors of oesophagus: value of endoscopy. Endoscopy 10:264–268, 1978
35. Murney RG, Huston JD: Endoscopic evaluation of the esophagogastric polyp and fold. Gastrointest Endosc 29:294–295, 1983
36. Van der Veer LD, Krama K, Relkin R, Clearfield H: The esophagogastric polypfold complex. Am J Gastroenterol 79: 918–920, 1984
37. LiVolsi VA, Perzin KH: Inflammatory pseudotumors (inflammatory fibrous polyps) of the esophagus. A clinicopathologic study. Am J Dig Dis 20:475–481, 1975
38. Patel J, Kieffer RW, Martin M: Giant fibrovascular polyp of the esophagus. Gastroenterology 87:953–956, 1984

39. Penagini P, Ranzi T, Velio P et al: Giant fibrovascular polyp of the esophagus: report of a case and effects on esophageal function. Gut 30:1624–1629, 1989
40. Avezzano EA, Fleischer DE, Merila MA, Anderson DL: Giant fibrovascular polyps of the esophagus. Am J Gastroenterol 85: 299–302, 1990
41. Parnell SA, Peppercorn MA, Antonioli DA et al: Squamous cell papilloma of the esophagus: report of a case after peptic esophagitis and repeated bougienage with review of the literature. Gastroenterology 74:910, 1978
42. Fernandez-Rodriquez CM, Bodia-Figuerola N, del Arbol R et al: Squamous papilloma of the esophagus: report of six cases with long-term follow-up in four patients. Am J Gastroenterol 81:1059–1068, 1986
43. Sablich R, Benedetti G, Bignucola S, Serraino D: Squamous cell papilloma of the esophagus. Report on 35 endoscopic cases. Endoscopy 20:5–7, 1988
44. Orlowska J, Jarosz D, Gugulski A et al: Squamous cell papillomas of the esophagus: report of 20 cases and literature review. Am J Gastroenterol 89:434–437, 1994
45. Winkler B, Capo V, Reumann W et al: Human papillomavirus infection of the esophagus. A clinicopathologic study with demonstration of papillomavirus antigen by the immunoperoxidase techniques. Cancer 55: 149–155, 1985
46. Poletoske EJ: Squamous papilloma of the esophagus associated with the human papillomavirus. Gastroenterology 102:668–673, 1992
47. Odze R, Antonioli D, Shocket D et al: Esophageal squamous papillomas. A clinicopathologic study of 38 lesions and analysis for human papillomavirus by the polymerase chain reaction. Am J Surg Pathol 17:803–812, 1993
48. Carr NJ, Bratthauer GL, Licky JH et al: Squamous cell papillomas of the esophagus: a study of 23 lesions for human papillomavirus by in-situ hybridization and the polymerase chain reaction. Hum Pathol 25: 536–540, 1994
49. Ravry MJR: Endoscopic resection of squamous papilloma of the esophagus. Am J Gastroenterol 71:398–400, 1979
50. Odze R, Antonioli D, Shocket D et al: Esophageal squamous papillomas. A clinicopathologic study of 38 lesions and analysis for human papillomavirus by the polymerase chain reaction. Am J Surg Pathol 17:803–812, 1993
51. Waterfall WE, Somers S, Desa DJ: Benign oesophageal papillomatosis. J Clin Pathol 31:111–115, 1978
52. Goldman H, Antonioli DA: Mucosal biopsy of the esophagus, stomach and proximal duodenum. Hum Pathol 13:423–448, 1982
53. McDonald GB, Brand DL, Thorning DR: Multiple adenomatous neoplasms arising in columnar-lined (Barrett's) esophagus. Gastroenterology 72:1317–1321, 1977
54. Lee RG: Adenomas arising in Barrett's esophagus. Am J Clin Pathol 85:629–632, 1986
55. Keeffe EB, Hisken EC, Schubert F: Adenomatous polyp arising in Barrett's esophagus. J Clin Gastroenterol 8:271–274, 1986
56. Ming S-C: Adenocarcinoma and other epithelial tumors of the esophagus. pp. 459–477. In Ming S-C, Goldman H (eds): Pathology of the Gastrointestinal Tract. WB Saunders, Philadelphia, 1992
57. Li F-S, Wang Q-L: Squamous cell carcinoma of the esophagus. pp. 439–458. In Ming S-C, Goldman H (eds): Pathology of the Gastrointestinal Tract. WB Saunders, Philadelphia, 1992
58. Huang GL, Wu YK (eds): Carcinoma of the Esophagus and Gastric Cardia. Springer-Verlag, Berlin, 1984
59. Munoz N, Crespi M, Grassi A et al: Precursor lesions of esophageal cancer in high risk populations in Iran and China. Lancet 1:876–879, 1982
60. Dreyer L: The incidence of dysplasia and associated epithelial lesions in the oesophageal mucosa of South African blacks. S Afr Med J 58:406–408, 1980
61. Burch PRJ: Esophageal cancer in relation to cigarette and alcohol consumption. J Chronic Dis 37:793–808, 1984
62. Hille JJ, Markowitz K, Margolius KA, Isaacson C: Human papillomavirus and carcinoma of the esophagus. N Engl J Med 312:1707, 1985
63. Toh Y, Kuwano H, Tanaka S et al: Detection of human papillomavirus DNA in esopha-

geal carcinoma in Japan by polymerase chain reaction. Cancer 70:2234–2238, 1992
64. Chang F, Syrjanen S, Shen Q et al: Screening for human papillomavirus infections in esophageal squamous cell carcinomas by insitu hybridization. Cancer 72:2525–2530, 1993
65. Chen B, Yin H, Dhurandhar N: Detection of human papillomavirus DNA in esophageal squamous cell carcinomas by the polymerase chain reaction using general consensus primers. Hum Pathol 25:920–923, 1994
66. Togawa K, Jaskiewicz K, Takahashi H et al: Human papillomavirus DNA sequences in esophagus squamous cell carcinoma. Gastroenterology 107:128–136, 1994
67. Entwistle CC, Jacobs A: Histological findings in the Paterson–Kelly Syndrome. J Clin Pathol 18:408, 1965
68. Correa P: Precursors of gastric and esophageal cancer. Cancer 50:2554–2565, 1982
69. Ming S-C: Precancerous states of the esophagus and stomach. p. 192. In Carter RL (ed): Precancerous States. Oxford University Press, London, 1984
70. Qiu S, Yang G: Precursor lesions of esophageal cancer in high-risk populations in Hunan Province, China. Cancer 62:551–557, 1988
71. Wychulis AR, Gunnlaugsson GH, Claggett OT: Carcinoma occurring in pharyngoesophageal diverticulum: report of three cases. Surgery 66:976–979, 1969
72. Appelqvist P, Salmo M: Lye corrosion carcinoma of the esophagus: a review of 63 cases. Cancer 45:2655–2658, 1980
73. Peracchia A, Segalin A, Bardini R et al: Esophageal carcinoma and achalasia—prevalence, incidence and results of treatment. Hepato-Gastroenterology 38:514–517, 1991
74. Meijssen NAC, Tilanus HW, van Blankenstein M et al: Achalasia complicated by squamous cell carcinoma: a prospective study in 195 patients. Gut 33:155–159, 1992
75. Kuylenstierna R, Munck-Wikland E: Esophagitis and cancer of the esophagus. Cancer 56:837–839, 1985
76. Oettle GJ, Paterson AC, Leiman G, Segal I: Esophagitis in a population at risk for esophageal carcinoma. Cancer 57:2222–2229, 1986
77. Rosengard AR, Hamilton SR: Squamous carcinoma of the esophagus in patients with Barrett esophagus. Modern Pathol 2:2–7, 1989
78. Rubio CA, Aberg B: Barrett's mucosa in conjunction with squamous carcinoma of the esophagus. Cancer 68:583–586, 1991
79. Parof F, Flejon J-F, Potet F, et al: Esophageal squamous carcinoma in five patients with Barrett's esophagus. Am J Gastroenterol 87:746–750, 1992
80. Goffman TE, McKeen EA, Curtis RE et al: Esophageal carcinoma following irradiation for breast cancer. Cancer 52:1808–1809, 1983
81. Sheril DJ: Radiation-associated malignancies of the esophagus. Cancer 54:726–728, 1984
82. Marchese MJ, Liskow A, Chang CH: Radiation therapy-associated cancer of the esophagus. NY State J Med 86:152–153, 1986
83. Harper PS, Harper RMJ, Howell-Evans AW: Carcinoma of the esophagus with tylosis. Quart J Med 38:317–333, 1970
84. Cooper BT, Holmes GK, Ferguson R, Cooke WT: Celiac disease and malignancy. Medicine (Baltimore) 59:249–261, 1980
85. Anani PA, Gardial D, Savary M et al: An extensive morphologic and comparative study of clinically early and obvious squamous cell carcinoma of the esophagus. Pathol Res Pract 187:214–219, 1991
86. Shen Q: Diagnostic cytology and early detection. p. 157. In Huang CJ, Wu YK (eds): Carcinoma of the Esophagus and Gastric Cardia. Springer-Verlag, Berlin, 1984
87. Crespi M, Grassi A, Munoz N et al: Endoscopic features of suspected precancerous lesions in high-risk areas for esophageal cancer. Endoscopy 16:85–91, 1984
88. Jacob P, Kohrilas PJ, Desai T et al: Natural history and significance of esophageal squamous cell dysplasia. Cancer 65:2731–2739, 1990
89. Dawsey SM, Wang GQ, Weinstein WM et al: Squamous dysplasia and early esophageal cancer in the Linxian region of China: Distinctive endoscopic lesions. Gastroenterology 105:1333–1340, 1993
90. Kuwano H, Baba K, Ikebe M et al: Histopathology of early esophageal carcinoma and squamous epithelial dysplasia. Hepato-Gastroenterology 40:222–226, 1993

91. Mandard AM, Marnay J, Gignoux M et al: Cancer of the esophagus and associated lesions. Hum Pathol 15:660–669, 1984
92. Kaye MD: Esophageal leukoplakia. Gastrointest Endosc 33:254–259, 1987
93. Guanrei Y, He H, Sungliang Q, Yuming C: Endoscopic diagnosis of 115 cases of early esophageal carcinoma. Endoscopy 14:157–161, 1982
94. Schmidt LW, Dean PJ, Wilson RT: Superficially invasive squamous cell carcinoma of the esophagus. A study of seven cases in Memphis, Tennessee. Gastroenterology 91:1456–1461, 1986
95. Rubio CA, Liu F-S, Zhao H-Z: Histological classification of intra-epithelial neoplasms and microinvasive squamous carcinoma of the esophagus. Am J Surg Pathol 13: 685–690, 1989
96. Bogomoletz WV, Molar G, Potet F: Superficial squamous cell carcinoma of the esophagus. A report of 76 cases and review of the literature. Am J Surg Pathol 13:535–546, 1989
97. Yoshinoka H, Shimazu H, Fukumoto T, Baba M: Superficial esophageal carcinoma: a clinicopathological review of 59 cases. Am J Gastroenterol 86:1413–1418, 1991
98. Kuwano H, Matsuda H, Matsuoka H et al: Intra-epithelial carcinoma with esophageal squamous cell carcinoma. Cancer 59:783–787, 1987
99. Mandard AM, Tourneux J, Gignoux M, Blanc L et al: In situ carcinoma of the esophagus: macroscopic study with particular reference to the Lugol test. Endoscopy 12:51–57, 1980
100. Mori M, Adachi Y, Matsushima T et al: Lugol staining pattern and histology of esophageal lesions. Am J Gastroenterol 88:701–705, 1993
101. Burg-Kurland CL, Purnell DM, Combs JW et al: Immunocytochemical evaluation of human esophageal neoplasms and preneoplastic lesions for hCG, HPL, alpha-FP, CEA, and NCA. Cancer Res 46:2936–2943, 1986
102. Hurlimann J, Gardiol D: Immunohistochemistry of dysplasias and carcinomas of the esophageal epithelium. Pathol Res Pract 184:567–576, 1989
103. Huang GJ, Gu XZ, Zhang RG et al: Combined preoperative irradiation and surgery in esophageal carcinoma: report of 408 cases. Chin Med J 94:73–76, 1981
104. Jennings FL, Arden A: Acute radiation effects in the esophagus. Arch Pathol 69:4407, 1960
105. Vanagunas A, Jacob P, Olinger E: Radiation-induced esophageal injury: a spectrum from esophagitis to cancer. Am J Gastroenterol 85:115–120, 1990
106. Chowhan NM: Injurious effects of radiation on the esophagus. Am J Gastroenterol 85:115–120, 1990
107. Goran DA, Shields HM, Bates ML et al: Esophageal dysplasia. Assessment by light microscopy and scanning electron microscopy. Gastroenterology 86:39–50, 1984
108. Kaketani K, Saito T, Koboyashi M: Flow cytometric analysis of nuclear DNA content in esophageal cancer. Aneuploidy as an index for highly malignant potential. Cancer 64:887–891, 1989
109. Rual A, Segalin A, Panozzo M et al: Flow cytometric DNA analysis of squamous cell carcinoma of the esophagus. Cancer 65: 1185–1188, 1990
110. Robasykiewicz M, Reid BJ, Volant A et al: Flow-cytometric DNA content analysis of esophageal squamous cell carcinoma. Gastroenterology 101:1588–1593, 1991
111. Doki Y, Shiozaki H, Tahara H et al: Prognostic value of DNA ploidy in squamous cell carcinoma of esophagus. Analyzed with improved flow cytometric measurement. Cancer 72:1813–1818, 1993
112. Itakura Y, Sasano H, Mori S, Nagura H: DNA ploidy in human esophageal squamous dysplasias and squamous cell carcinomas as determined by image analysis. Modern Pathol 7:867–873, 1994
113. Ozawa S, Ueda M, Ando N et al: Prognostic significance of epidermal growth factor receptor in esophageal squamous cell carcinomas. Cancer 63:2169–2173, 1989
114. Imazeki F, Omata M, Nose H et al: p53 gene mutations in gastric and esophageal cancers. Gastroenterology 103:892–896, 1992
115. Sarbia M, Porschen R, Borchard F et al: p53 protein expression and prognosis in squamous cell carcinoma of the esophagus. Cancer 74:2218–2223, 1994
116. Agha FP, Weatherbee L, Sams JS: Verrucous carcinoma of the esophagus. Am J Gastroenterol 79:844–849, 1984

117. Jasin KA, Bateson MC: Verrucous carcinoma of the oesophagus. A diagnostic problem. Histopathology 17:473, 1990
118. Cho S-R, Henry DA, Schneider V, Turner MA: Polypoid carcinoma of the esophagus: a distinct radiological and histopathological entity. Am J Gastroenterol 78:476–480, 1983
119. Linder J, Stein RB, Roggli VL et al: Polypoid tumor of the esophagus. Hum Pathol 18:692–700, 1987
120. Sasajima K, Takai A, Tamiguchi Y et al: Polypoid squamous cell carcinoma of the esophagus. Cancer 64:94–97, 1989
121. Kuhajda FP, Sun TT, Mendelsohn G: Polypoid squamous carcinoma of the esophagus: a case report with immunostaining for keratin. Am J Surg Pathol 7:495–499, 1983
122. Gal AA, Martin SE, Kernen JA, Patterson MJ: Spindle cell carcinoma of the esophagus. An immunohistochemical study. Cancer 60:2244–2250, 1987
123. Rubio CA, Liu F-S: The histogenesis of the microinvasive basal cell carcinoma of the esophagus. Pathol Res Pract 186:223–227, 1990
124. Kalish RJ, Clancy PE, Orringer MB, Appelman HD: Clinical, epidemiologic, and morphologic comparison between adenocarcinomas arising in Barrett's esophageal mucosa and in the gastric cardia. Gastroenterology 86:461–467, 1984
125. Wang HH, Antonioli DA, Goldman H: Comparative features of esophageal and gastric adenocarcinomas: recent changes in type and frequency. Hum Pathol 17:482–487, 1986
126. MacDonald WC, MacDonald JB: Adenocarcinoma of the esophagus and/or gastric cardia. Cancer 60:1094–1098, 1987
127. Hesketh PJ, Clapp RW, Doos WG et al: The increasing frequency of adenocarcinoma of the esophagus. Cancer 64:526–530, 1989
128. Pera M, Cameron AJ, Trastek VF et al: Increasing incidence of adenocarcinoma of the esophagus and esophagogastric junction. Gastroenterology 104:510–513, 1993
129. Blot WJ, Devesa SS, Fraumeni JF Jr: Continuing climbs in rates of esophageal adenocarcinoma: an update. (letter) JAMA 270: 1320, 1993
130. Levi F, Ollyo J-B, LaVecchia C et al: The consumption of tobacco, alcohol and the risk of adenocarcinoma in Barrett's esophagus. Int J Cancer 45:852, 1990
131. Menke-Pluymers MBE, Hop WCJ, Dees J et al: Risk factors for the development of an adenocarcinoma in columnar-lined (Barrett) esophagus. Cancer 72:1155–1158, 1993
132. Jochem VJ, Fuerst PA, Fromkes JJ: Familial Barrett's esophagus with adenocarcinoma. Gastroenterology 102:1400–1402, 1992
133. Thompson JJ, Zinsser KR, Enterline HT: Barrett's metaplasia and adenocarcinoma of the esophagus and gastroesophageal junction. Hum Pathol 14:142–161, 1983
134. Naef AP, Savery M, Ozzello L: Columnar-lined lower esophagus: an acquired lesion with malignant predisposition. Report on 140 cases of Barrett's esophagus with 12 adenocarcinomas. J Thorac Cardiovasc Surg 70:826, 1975
135. Haggitt RC, Tryzellaar J, Ellis FH et al: Adenocarcinoma complicating columnar epithelium-lined (Barrett's esophagus. Am J Clin Pathol 70:1–5, 1978
136. Hamilton SR, Smith RRL: The relationship between columnar epithelial dysplasia and invasive adenocarcinoma arising in Barrett's esophagus. Am J Clin Pathol 87:301–312, 1987
137. Williamson WA, Ellis FH Jr, Gibb SP et al: Barrett's esophagus. Prevalence and incidence of adenocarcinoma. Arch Intern Med 151:2212–2216, 1991
138. Streitz JM Jr, Ellis FH Jr, Gibb SP et al: Adenocarcinoma in Barrett's esophagus: a clinicopathologic study of 65 cases. Ann Surg 213:122, 1991
139. McKinley M, Sherlock P: Barrett's esophagus with adenocarcinoma in scleroderma. Am J Gastroenterol 79:438–439, 1984
140. Shah AN, Gunby TC: Adenocarcinoma and Barrett's esophagus following surgically treated achalasia. Gastrointest Endosc 30: 294–296, 1984
141. Iftikhar SY, James PD, Steele RJC et al: Length of Barrett's esophagus: an important factor in the development of dysplasia and adenocarcinoma. Gut 33:1155–1158, 1992
142. Schnell TG, Sontag SJ, Chejfec G: Adenocarcinomas arising in tongues or short segments of Barrett's esophagus. Dig Dis Sci 37:137–143, 1992

143. Smith RRL, Hamilton SR, Boitnott JK, Rogers EL: The spectrum of carcinoma arising in Barrett's esophagus. A clinicopathologic study of 26 patients. Am J Surg Pathol 8:563–573, 1984
144. Hassall E, Dimmick JE, Magee JF: Adenocarcinoma in childhood Barrett's esophagus: case documentation and the need for surveillance in children. Am J Gastroenterol 88:282–288, 1993
145. Paraf F, Flejou J-F, Pignon J-P et al: Surgical pathology of adenocarcinoma arising in Barrett's esophagus. Analysis of 67 cases. Am J Surg Pathol 19:183–191, 1995
146. Christensen WN, Sternberg SS: Adenocarcinoma of the upper esophagus arising in ectopic gastric mucosa. Two case reports and review of the literature. Am J Surg Pathol 11:397–402, 1987
147. Jernstrom P, Brewer LA III: Primary adenocarcinoma of the mid-esophagus arising in ectopic gastric mucosa with associated hiatal hernia and reflux esophagitis (Dawson's syndrome). Cancer 26:1343–1348, 1970
148. Sperling RM, Grindell JH: Adenocarcinoma arising in an inlet patch of the esophagus. Am J Gastroenterol 90:150–152, 1995
149. Sarbia M, Borchard F, Hengels KJ: Histogenetical investigations on adenocarcinoma of the esophagogastric junction. An immunohistochemical study. Pathol Res Pract 189:530–536, 1993
150. Herlihy KJ, Orlando RC, Bryson JC et al: Barrett's esophagus: clinical, endoscopic, histologic, manometric and electrical potential difference characteristics. Gastroenterology 86:436–443, 1984
151. Speckler SJ, Goyal RK: Barrett's esophagus. N Engl J Med 315:362–371, 1986
152. Dahms BB, Rothstein FC: Barrett's esophagus in children: a consequence of chronic gastroesophageal reflux. Gastroenterology 86:318–323, 1984
153. Cameron AJ, Payne WS: Barrett's esophagus occurring as a complication of scleroderma. Mayo Clin Proc 53:612, 1978
154. Spechler SJ, Schimmell EM, Dalton JW et al: Barrett's epithelium complicating lye ingestion with sparing of the distal esophagus. Gastroenterology 81:580–583, 1981
155. Sartori S, Nielson I, Indelli M et al: Barrett's esophagus after chemotherapy with cyclophosphamide, methotrexate, and 5-fluorouracil (CMF): an iatrogenic injury. Ann Intern Med 114:210, 1991
156. Hamilton SR, Yardley JH: Regeneration of cardiac type mucosa and acquisition of Barrett's mucosa after esophagogastrostomy. Gastroenterology 72:669, 1977
157. Jaakkola A, Reinikainen P, Ovaska J et al: Barrett's esophagus after cardiomyotomy for esophageal achalasia. Am J Gastroenterol 89:165–169, 1994
158. Paull A, Trier JS, Dalton MD et al: The histologic spectrum of Barrett's esophagus. N Engl J Med 295:476–480, 1976
159. Lee RG: Mucins in Barrett's esophagus: a histochemical study. Am J Clin Pathol 81:500–503, 1984
160. Penchmaur M, Potet F, Goldfain D: Mucin histochemistry of the columnar epithelium of the oesophagus (Barrett's oesphagus): a prospective biopsy study. J Clin Pathol 37:607, 1984
161. Zwas F, Schields HM, Doos WG et al: Scanning electron microscopy of Barrett's epithelium and its correlation with light microscopy and mucin stains. Gastroenterology 90:1932–1941, 1986
162. Rothery GA, Patterson JE, Stoddard DJ, Day DW: Histological and histochemical changes in the columnar lined (Barrett's) oesophagus. Gut 27:1062, 1986
163. Haggitt RC, Reid BJ, Rabinovitch PS, Rubin CE: Barrett's esophagus. Correlation between mucin histochemistry, flow cytometry, and histologic diagnosis for predicting increased cancer risk. Am J Pathol 131: 53–61, 1988
164. Jaurequi HO, Davessar K, Hale JH et al: Mucin histochemistry of intestinal metaplasia in Barrett's esophagus. Modern Pathol 1:188–192, 1988
165. Gottfried MR, McClave SA, Boyce HW: Incomplete intestinal metaplasia in the diagnosis of columnar lined esophagus (Barrett's esophagus). Am J Clin Pathol 92:741, 1989
166. Reid BJ, Haggitt RC, Rubin CE et al: Observer variation in the diagnosis of dysplasia in Barrett's esophagus. Hum Pathol 19: 166–178, 1988
167. Lee RF: Dysplasia in Barrett's esophagus. A clinicopathologic study of six patients. Am J Surg Pathol 9:845–852, 1985

168. Hameeteman W, Tytgat GNJ, Houthoff HJ, Twell JG: Barrett's esophagus: development of dysplasia and adenocarcinoma. Gastroenterology 96:1245–1256, 1989
169. Miros M, Kerlin P, Walker N: Only patients with dysplasia progress to adenocarcinoma in Barrett's oesophagus. Gut 32:1141–1146, 1991
170. Jass JR: A classification of gastric dysplasia. Histopathology 7:181–193, 1983
171. Ming S-C, Bajtai A, Correa P et al: Gastric dysplasia. Significance and pathologic criteria. Cancer 54:1794–1801, 1984
172. Riddell RH, Goldman H, Ransohoff DF et al: Dysplasia in inflammatory bowel disease: standardized classification with provisional clinical applications. Hum Pathol 14:931–968, 1983
173. Skinner DB, Walther BC, Riddell RH et al: Barrett's esophagus. Comparison of benign and malignant cases. Ann Surg 198:554–566, 1983
174. Rice TW, Falk GW, Achkar E, Petras RE: Surgical management of high grade dysplasia in Barrett's esophagus. Am J Gastroenterol 88:1832–1836, 1993
175. Streitz JM, Andrews CW Jr, Ellis FH: Endoscopic surveillance of Barrett's esophagus. Does it help? J Thorac Cardiovasc Surg 105:383–388, 1993
176. Rusch VW, Levine DS, Haggitt R, Reid BJ: The management of high grade dysplasia and early cancer in Barrett's esophagus. Cancer 74:1225–1229, 1994
177. Levine DS, Haggitt RC, Blount PL et al: An endoscopic biopsy protocol can differentiate high-grade dysplasia from early adenocarcinoma in Barrett's esophagus. Gastroenterology 105:40–50, 1993
178. McArdle JE, Lewin KJ, Randall G, Weinstein W: Distribution of dyspasias and early invasive carcinoma in Barrett's esophagus. Hum Pathol 23:479–482, 1992
179. Kruse P, Boesby S, Bernstein IT, Andersen IB: Barrett's esophagus and esophageal adenocarcinoma. Endoscopic and histologic surveillance. Scand J Gastroenterol 28:193–197, 1993
180. Levine DS, Haggitt RC, Blount PL et al: An endoscopic biopsy protocol can differentiate high-grade dysplasia from early adenocarcinoma in Barrett's esophagus. Gastroenterology 105:40–50, 1993
181. Robey SS, Hamilton SR, Gupta PK, Erozan VS: Diagnostic value of cytopathology in Barrett's sophagus and associated carcinoma. Am J Clin Pathol 89:493–498, 1988
182. Geisinger KR, Teot LA, Richter JE: A cooperative cytopathologic and histologic study of atypia, dysplasia, and adenocarcinoma in Barrett's esophagus. Cancer 69:8–16, 1992
183. Levine DS, Rubin CE, Reid BJ, Haggitt RC: Specialized metaplastic columnar epithelium in Barrett's esophagus. A comparative transmission electron microscopic study. Lab Invest 60:418, 1989
184. Levine DS, Reid BJ, Haggitt RC et al: Correlation of ultrastructural alterations with dysplasia and flow cytometric abnormalities in Barrett's epithelium. Gastroenterology 96:355–367, 1989
185. Mills LR, Schuman BM, Assid RT et al: Scanning electron microscopy of dysplastic Barrett's epithelium. Modern Pathol 2:112–116, 1989
186. Abdelatif JMA, Chandler FW, Mills LR et al: Differential expression of C-myc and H-ras oncogenes in Barrett's epithelium. A study using colorimentric in-situ hybridization. Arch Pathol Lab Med 115:880–885, 1991
187. Jankowski J, Coghill G, Hopwood D, Wormsly KG: Oncogenes and oncosuppressor gene in adenocarcinoma of the esophagus. Gut 33:1033–1038, 1992
188. Ramel S, Reid BJ, Sanchez CA et al: Evaluation of p53 protein expression in Barrett's esophagus by two-flow cytometry. Gastroenterology 102:1220–1228, 1992
189. Younes M, Lebovitz RM, Lechago LV, Lechago J: p53 protein accumulation in Barrett's metaplasia, dysplasia, and carcinoma: a follow-up study. Gastroenterology 105:1637–1642, 1993
190. Hong MK, Larkin WB, Herman BE et al: Expansion of the Ki-67 proliferative compartment correlates with degree of dysplasia in Barrett's esophagus. Cancer 75:423–429, 1995
191. Wu GD, Beer DG, Moore JH, Orringer MB et al: Sucrase–isomaltase gene expression in Barrett's esophagus and adenocarcinoma. Gastroenterology 105:837–844, 1993

192. Nikulasson S, Andrews CA Jr, Goldman H et al: Sucrase–isomaltase expression in dysplasia associated with Barrett's esophagus and chronic gastritis and in adenocarcinomas of the gastrointestinal tract. Int J Surg Pathol 2:281–286, 1995
193. Burke AP, Sobin LH, Shekitka KM, Helwig EB: Dysplasia of the stomach and Barrett esophagus: a follow-up study. Modern Pathol 4:336, 1991
194. Pazdur R, Olencki T, Herman GE: Linitis plastica of the esophagus. Am J Gastroenterol 83:1395–1397, 1988
195. Slavin J, Pitson G, Dowling JP: Neuroendocrine carcinoma arising in Barrett's esophagus. Int J Surg Pathol 2:43–46, 1994
196. Wasan HS, Schofield JB, Krausz T et al: Combined choriocarcinoma and yolk sac tumor arising in Barrett's esophagus. Cancer 73:514–517, 1994
197. Banner BF, Memoli VA, Warren WH, Gould VE: Carcinoma with multidirectional differentation arising in Barrett's esophagus. Ultrastruct Pathol 4:205–217, 1983
198. McKinley MJ, Budman DR, Grueneberg D et al: DNA content in Barrett's esophagus and esophageal malignancy. Am J Gastroenterol 82:1012–1015, 1987
199. James PD, Atkinson M: Value of DNA image cytometry in the prediction of malignant change in Barrett's oesophagus. Gut 30: 899–905, 1989
200. Reid BJ, Blount PL, Rubin CE et al: Flow-cytometric and histological progression to malignancy in Barrett's esophagus: prospective endoscopic surveillance of a cohort. Gastroenterology 102:1212–1219, 1992
201. Khan M, Bui HX, del Rosario A et al: Role of DNA content determination by image analysis in confirmation of dysplasia in Barrett's esophagus. Modern Pathol 7:169–174, 1994
202. Menke-Pluymers MBE, Mulder AH, Hop WCJ et al: Dysplasia and aneuploidy as markers of malignant degeneration in Barrett's oesophagus. Gut 35:1348–1351, 1994
203. Haggitt RC: Barrett's esophagus, dysplasia, and adenocarcinoma. Hum Pathol 25:982–993, 1994
204. Fennestry MB, Sampliner RE, Way D et al: Discordance between flow cytometric abnormalities and dysplasia in Barrett's esophagus. Gastroenterology 97:815–820, 1989
205. Hamelin R, Flejou J-F, Muzeau F et al: TP53 gene mutations and p53 protein immunoreactivity in malignant and premalignant Barrett's esophagus. Gastroenterology 107: 1012–1018, 1994
206. Hardwick RH, Shepherd NA, Moorghen M et al: Adenocarcinoma arising in Barrett's oesophagus: evidence for the participation of p53 dysfunction in the dysplasia/carcinoma sequence. Gut 35:764–768, 1994
207. Nakamura T, Nekarda H, Hoelscher AG et al: Prognostic value of DNA ploidy and c-erbB-2 oncoprotein overexpression in adenocarcinoma of Barrett's esophagus. Cancer 73:1785–1794, 1994
208. Bombi JA, Riverola A, Bordas JM et al: Adenosquamous carcinoma of the esophagus. Pathol Res Pract 187:514–519, 1991
209. Pascal RR, Clearfield HR: Mucoepidermoid (adenosquamous) carcinoma arising in Barrett's esophagus. Dig Dis Sci 32:428–432, 1987
210. Sasajima K, Watanabe M, Tabuko K et al: Mucoepidermoid carcinoma of the esophagus. Endoscopy 22:140–143, 1990
211. Sweeney EC, Cooney T: Adenoid cystic carcinoma of the esophagus: a light and electron microscopic study. Cancer 45:1516–1525, 1980
212. Cerar A, Jutersek A, Vidmar S: Adenoid cystic carcinoma of the esophagus. A clinicopathologic study of three cases. Cancer 67:2159–2164, 1991
213. Rankin R, Nirodi NS, Browne MK: Carcinoid tumor of the esophagus. Scott Med J 25:245–249, 1980
214. Siegal A, Swartz A: Malignant carcinoid of oesophagus. Histopathology 10:761–765, 1986
215. Facer P, Bishop AE, Lloyd RV et al: Chromogranin: a newly recognized marker for endocrine cells of the human gastrointestinal tract. Gastroenterology 89:1366–1373, 1985
216. Reyes CV, Wellington J, Gould VE: Neuroendocrine carcinomas of the esophagus. Ultrastruct Pathol 2:367–376, 1980
217. Chong FK, Graham JH, Madoff IM: Mucin-producing carcinoid ("composite tumor") of

upper third of esophagus: a variant of carcinoid tumor. Cancer 44:1853, 1979

218. Klappenbach RS, Kurman RJ, Sinclair CF, James LP: Composite carcinoma–carcinoid tumors of the gastrointestinal tract. A morphologic, histochemical and immunocytochemical study. Am J Clin Pathol 84:137–143, 1985
219. Ignacio AG, Chintapalli K, Choi H: Primary oat cell carcinoma of the esophagus. Am J Gastroenterol 82:78–81, 1987
220. Mori M, Matsukuma A, Adachi Y et al: Small cell carcinoma of the esophagus. Cancer 63:564–573, 1989
221. Law SY-K, Fok M, Lam K-Y et al: Small cell carcinoma of the esophagus. Cancer 73:2894–2899, 1994
222. Sheahan DG, West AB: Focal lymphoid hyperplasia (pseudolymphoma) of the esophagus. Am J Surg Pathol 9:141–147, 1985
223. Appelman HD, Hirsch SD, Schnitzer B, Coon WW: Clinicopathologic overview of gastrointestinal lymphomas. Am J Surg Pathol 9(3):S71–83, 1985
224. Matsaura H, Saito R, Nakajima S et al: Non-Hodgkin's lymphoma of the esophagus. Am J Gastroenterol 80:941–946, 1985
225. Mengoli M, Marchi M, Rota E et al: Primary non-Hodgkin's lymphoma of the esophagus. Am J Gastroenterol 85:737–741, 1990
226. Taal BG, Van Heerde P, Somers R: Isolated primary oesophageal involvement by lymphoma: a rare cause of dyphagia: two case histories and a review of other published data. Gut 34:994–998, 1993
227. Traube M, Waldron JA, McCallum RW. Systemic lymphoma initially presenting as an esophageal mass. Am J Gastroenterol 77:835–837, 1982
228. Agha FP, Schnitzer B: Esophageal involvement in lymphoma. Am J Gastroenterol 80:412–416, 1985
229. Isaacson PG: B-cell lymphomas of the gastrointestinal tract. Am J Surg Pathol 9(3):S117–128, 1985
230. Seremetis MG, Lyons WS, de Guzman V et al: Leiomyomata of the esophagus: an analysis of 838 cases. Cancer 38:2166, 1976
231. Khansur T, Balducci L, Tavassoli M: Granular cell tumor. Cancer 60:220–222, 1987
232. Cornish D, Feinstat T, Schneider P et al: Esophageal granular cell tumor removed by endoscopic polypectomy. Am J Gastroenterol 80:950–953, 1985
233. Brady PG, Nord HJ, Connor RG: Granular cell tumor of the esophagus: natural history, diagnosis, and therapy. Dig Dis Sci 33: 1329–1333, 1988
234. Orlowska J, Pachlewski J, Gugulski A, Butruk E: A conservative approach to granular cell tumors of the esophagus: four case reports and literature review. Am J Gastroenterol 88:311–315, 1993
235. Partyka EK, Sanowski RA, Kozarek RA: Endoscopic diagnosis of a giant esophageal leiomyosarcoma. Am J Gastroenterol 75: 132–134, 1981
236. Patel SR, Anandarao N: Leiomyosarcoma of the esophagus. NY State J Med 90: 371–373, 1990
237. Burke JS, Ranchod M: Hemangiopericytoma of the esophagus. Hum Pathol 12:96–100, 1981
238. Amr SS, Shihabi NK, Hajj H: Synovial sarcoma of the esophagus. Am J Otolaryngol 5:266–269, 1984
239. Bloch MJ, Iozzo RV, Edmunds H Jr, Brooks JJ: Polypoid synovial sarcoma of the esophagus. Gastroenterology 92:229–233, 1987
240. McIntyre M, Webb JN, Browning GCP: Osteosarcoma of the esophagus. Hum Pathol 13:680–682, 1982
241. Tateishi R, Taniguchi H, Wada A et al: Argyrophilic cells and melanocytes in esophageal mucosa. Arch Pathol 98:87–89, 1974
242. Ohashi K, Kato Y, Kanno J, Kasuga T: Melanocytes and melanosis of the oesophagus in Japanese subjects: analysis of factors affecting their increase. Virchows Arch A Pathol Anat Histopathol 417:137, 1990
243. Guzman RP, Wightman R, Ravinsky E, Unruh HW: Primary melanoma of the esophagus with diffuse melanocytic atypia and melanoma in-situ. Am J Clin Pathol 92: 802–804, 1989
244. Sabenathan S, Eng J, Pradhan GN: Primary malignant melanoma of the esophagus. Am J Gastroenterol 84:1475–1481, 1989
245. Stranks GJ, Mathai JT, Rowe-Jones DC: Primary malignant melanoma of the esophagus: case report and review of surgical pathology. Gut 32:828–830, 1991

246. Symmons WF, Grimes MM: Malignant melanoma of the esophagus: histologic variants and immunohistochemical finding in four cases. Surg Pathol 4:222–234, 1991
247. Go ATS, Zirkin RM. Primary malignant melanoma of the esophagus: a case report with endoscopic and electron microscopic studies. Am J Gastroenterol 77:840–843, 1982
248. Butler ML, Van Heertum RL, Teplick SK: Metastatic malignant melanoma of the esophagus: a case report. Gastroenterology 69:1334–1337, 1975
249. Adair C, Ro JY, Sahin AA et al. Malignant melanoma metastatic to gastrointestinal tract. Int J Surg Pathol 2:3–10, 1994
250. Trillo A, Accettullo LM, Yeiter TL: Choriocarcinoma of the esophagus: histologic and cytologic findings. A case report. Acta Cytol 23:69–74, 1979
251. Kadakia S, Parker A, Canales L: Metastatic tumors of the upper gastrointestinal tract: endoscopic experience. Am J Gastroenterol 87:1418–1423, 1992
252. Antler AS, Ough Y, Pitchumoni CS et al: Gastrointestinal metastases from malignant tumors of the lungs. Cancer 49:170–172, 1982
253. Holyokw ED, Nemoto T, Dao TL: Esophageal metastases and dysphagia in patients with carcinoma of the breast. J Surg Oncol 1:97–107, 1979
254. Gore RM, Sparberg M: Metastatic carcinoma of the prostate to the esophagus. Am J Gastroenterol 77:358–359, 1982

4

Inflammatory Disorders of the Stomach

This chapter deals with the inflammatory and ulcerative disorders that affect the stomach. The tumors that affect the stomach are presented in Chapter 5. In instances where the major description of a disorder is found in another chapter, the salient features of the condition affecting the stomach are noted herein.

GENERAL ASPECTS

Endoscopic examination and biopsy of the stomach have been performed for over 40 years; however, the earlier studies were mainly limited to the detection of tumors, and involved rigid instruments and limited biopsy material. Indeed, adequate cytologic study of the stomach only became possible with the introduction of the flexible endoscopes and the potential use of brushings. At present, endoscopy and biopsy of the stomach are extensively employed for the detection and fine evaluation of gastritis; for the localization of ulcers and the determination of whether they are benign or malignant; and for the evaluation and precise identification of mass lesions [1–3] (Table 4-1). Endoscopic study is commonly done for patients with persistent upper abdominal pain, hematemesis, and possible obstructive disorders.

Normal Structure

There are three types of gastric mucosa, represented in the cardia, in the fundus and corpus, and in the antrum (Table 4-2). The differences are principally in the specialized epithelial glands and to a lesser extent in the features of the lamina propria.[4–7] The muscularis mucosae appears to be the same in all regions.

Common Features

All parts of the stomach are covered by a continuous layer of surface mucous cells that extend into the gastric pits, or *foveolae* (Fig. 4-1). This epithelium is composed of columnar mucous cells, with the mucus granules

Table 4-1. Uses of Gastric Mucosal Biopsy

Identify gastritis
Monitor disease following therapy
Detect complications
Distinguish between benign and malignant ulcers
Evaluate mass lesions

concentrated in the luminal quarter of the cell cytoplasm. The mucus is in the form of a neutral glycoprotein, and stains strongly with the periodic acid–Schiff (PAS) reaction, and negatively with Alcian Blue and other stains for acid mucins, under normal circumstances.[8–10] By ultrastructural examination, the granules are relatively dense when compared to other mucous-type cells.

At the base of the gastric pits are the neck mucous cells, which are somewhat shorter than the surface mucous cells and have irregular granules dispersed throughout the cytoplasm. This is the zone for regenerative activity and subsequent differentiation of the cells within the stomach. Biopsies of the normal mucosa, whether from the antrum or the corpus, show only a rare mitosis. When these are easily seen, there is almost certainly considerable regeneration of the gastric pits, correlating with a healing or chronic process.

Neuroendocrine cells are also present throughout the gastric mucosa.[11–13] These are concentrated in the lower portions of the glands, commonly have a relatively clear cytoplasm, and vary considerably in their types and function (Fig. 4-2). Most of the endocrine cells in the antrum are of the gastrin-producing G-cell type (Fig. 4-3), whereas those in the corpus and fundus are mainly of the enterochromaffin-like (ECL) cells. Other endocrine cells scattered throughout the stomach include the D cells, which form somatostatin, and the enterochromaffin (EC) cells, which release serotonin. In most inflammatory disorders of the stomach there occur slight proliferations of these endocrine cells, without any special functional effect. Under special circumstances, mainly in cases of chronic gastritis, they undergo hyperplasia and tumor formation, which is described in a later section.

Table 4-2. Normal Gastric Epithelial Cells

Cell Type	Major Product/ Function
Surface/pit mucous cell	Neutral mucin
Neck mucous cell	Regenerative cell
Fundus/corpus	
Parietal cell	Acid and B_{12} intrinsic factor
Chief cell	Pepsinogens
Antrum/cardia	
Mucous Cell	Neutral mucin
Neuroendocrine cells	Gastrin, somatostatin, serotonin

Cardiac Mucosa

The cardiac mucosa is present for only a few centimeters, extending from the distal end of the squamous-lined esophagus (Fig. 4-4). It is covered by gastric surface-type mucous cells that extend into pits that vary greatly in length; the rest of the mucosa shows irregular glands filled with mucous cells that resemble (and are probably identical to) those found in the antrum. In these mucous cells, the granules tend to fill the complete cytoplasm, are larger in diameter, and are paler by ultrastructural examination than those seen in the surface mucous cells. They are mainly composed of neutral glycoproteins as evidenced by positive PAS reaction, and staining negatively for acid mucin. In the cardiac mucosa, there is a considerable amount of lamina propria due to the invariable presence of a large amount of inflammatory cells, both of the mononuclear cell and granulocytic types. It appears that the cardiac mucosa is normally inflamed, and one should avoid a diagnosis of gastritis in this area unless there is evident necrosis or a considerable increase in neutrophils.

Fundic and Corpus (Body) Mucosa

This mucosa represents the traditional part of the stomach, with the characteristic specialized glands that extend from the gas-

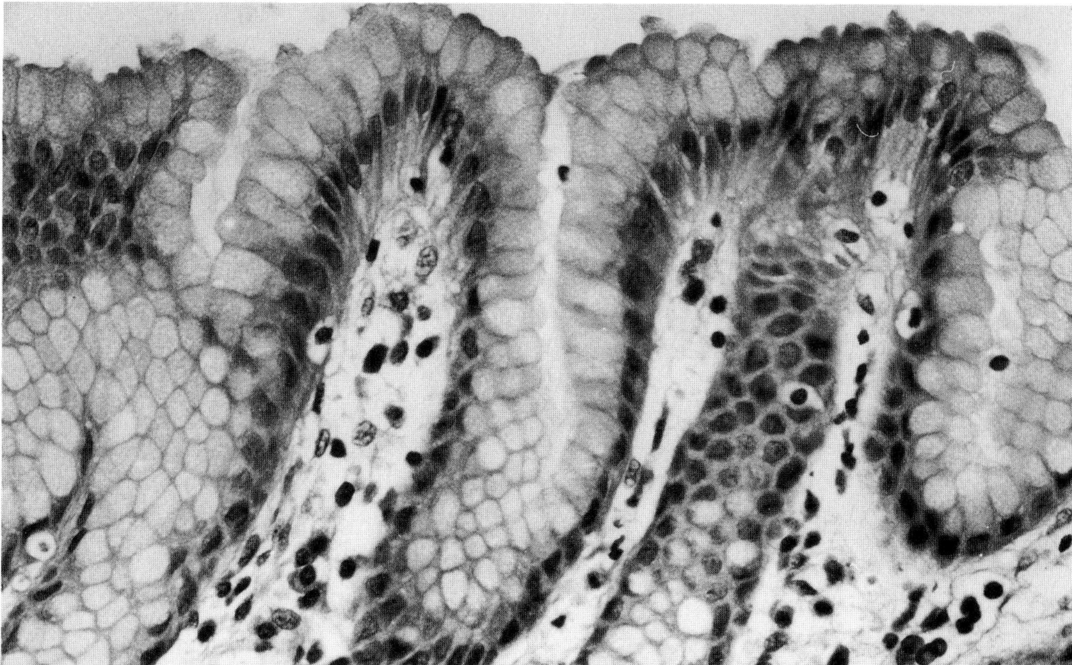

Fig. 4-1. Luminal aspect of the normal stomach. The surface (top) and gastric pits (foveolae) are lined by a continuous layer of tall columnar mucous cells. The mucus granules are concentrated in the superficial portion of the cells. There is a small amount of inflammatory cells in the lamina propria (× 425).

tric pits (Fig. 4-5). The mucosa throughout the fundus and corpus is generally the same, revealing a diffuse surface of mucous cells and relatively short gastric pits, to each of which are connected three to five glands. Overall the glands are about three to five times longer than the pits in the normal stomach. The gastric glands contain two major differentiated cells: the parietal cells, which are concentrated in the midportion of the mucosa and are responsible for the secretion of both acid and intrinsic factor of vitamin B_{12} in humans; and the chief cells, which are mainly in the lower portion of the mucosa, and release the class of pepsinogens. The parietal cells are large and polygonal, pink, and finely granular due to the numerous mitochondria within the cytoplasm. The chief cells are more basophilic, reflecting the major component of rough endoplasmic reticulum responsible for protein formation. Unlike the cardia and antrum, the lamina propria in the normal fundic and corpus region tends to be scant due to the relative lack of inflammatory cells. With aging, there develops a mild increase of mononuclear inflammatory cells within the lamina propria in the superficial portion separating the gastric pits, but there is usually no extension of this inflammation into the region between the specialized glands.

Antral Mucosa

The antral mucosa is characterized by longer gastric pits and by the presence in the lower two-thirds of the mucosa of the antral or pyloric-type mucous glands, similar to those seen in the gastric cardia (Fig. 4-6). There are many more mucous glands in the antral region. As in the cardia, these stain with the PAS reaction for neutral glycoproteins but not for acid mucins. They are typi-

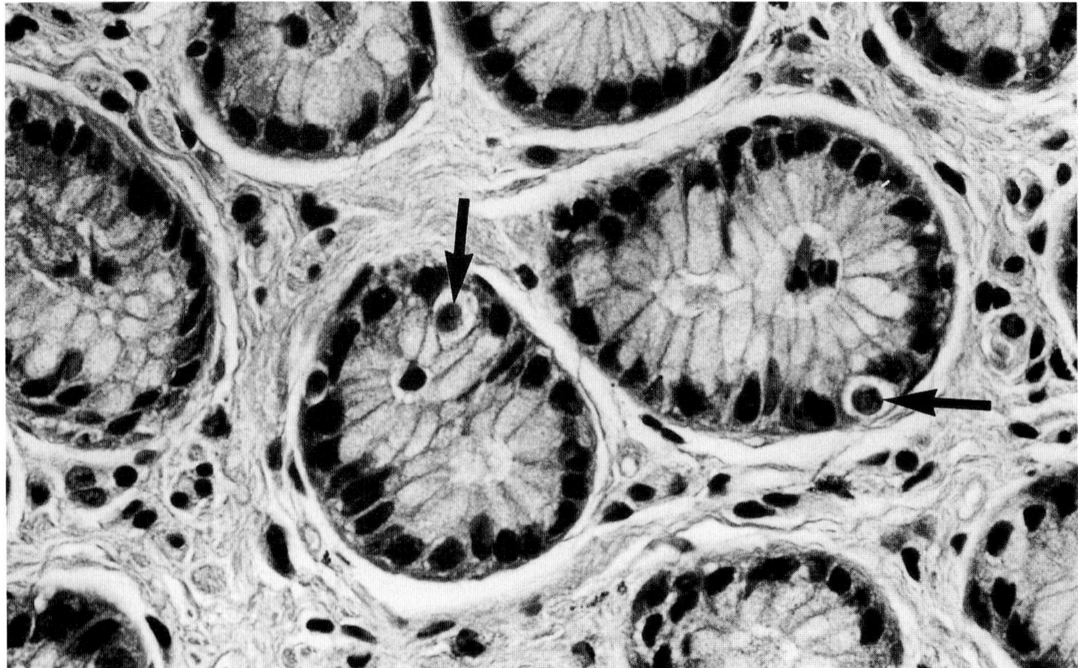

Fig. 4-2. Cross section of normal gastric antral glands. Interspersed between the mucous cells are scattered neuroendocrine cells (arrows), which have central nuclei and clear cytoplasm (× 635).

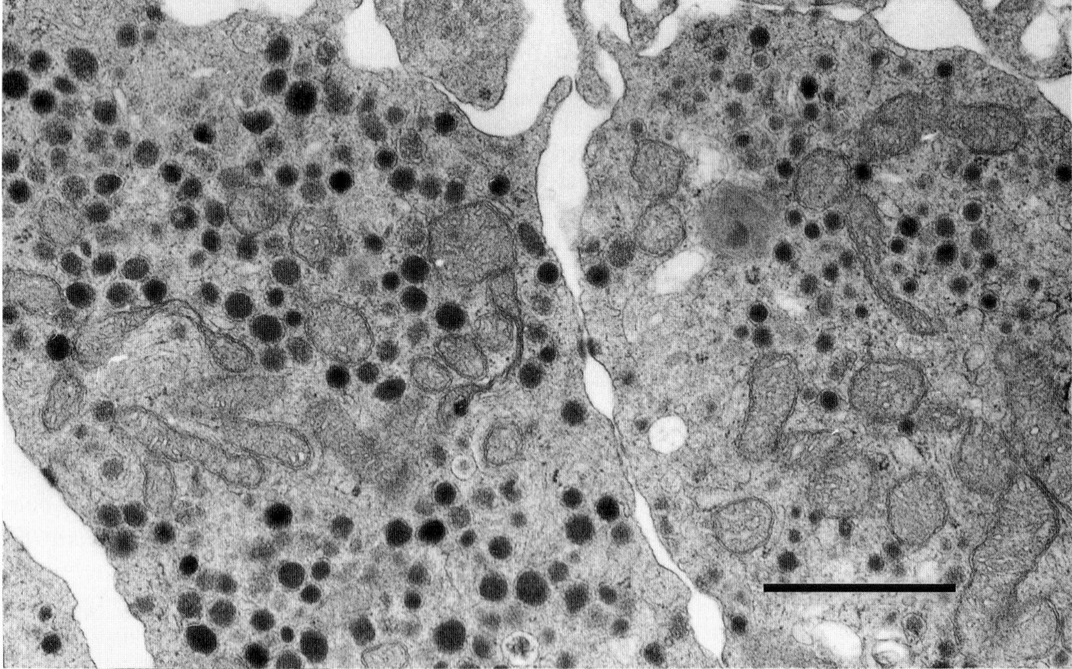

Fig. 4-3. Electron micrograph of gastrin (G) cells taken from a tumor. The cytoplasm contains numerous membrane-bound granules that measure an average of 150 nm in diameter and have electron-dense cores. The G-cell granules in the normal antrum are slightly larger (× 25,000; bar = 1 μm).

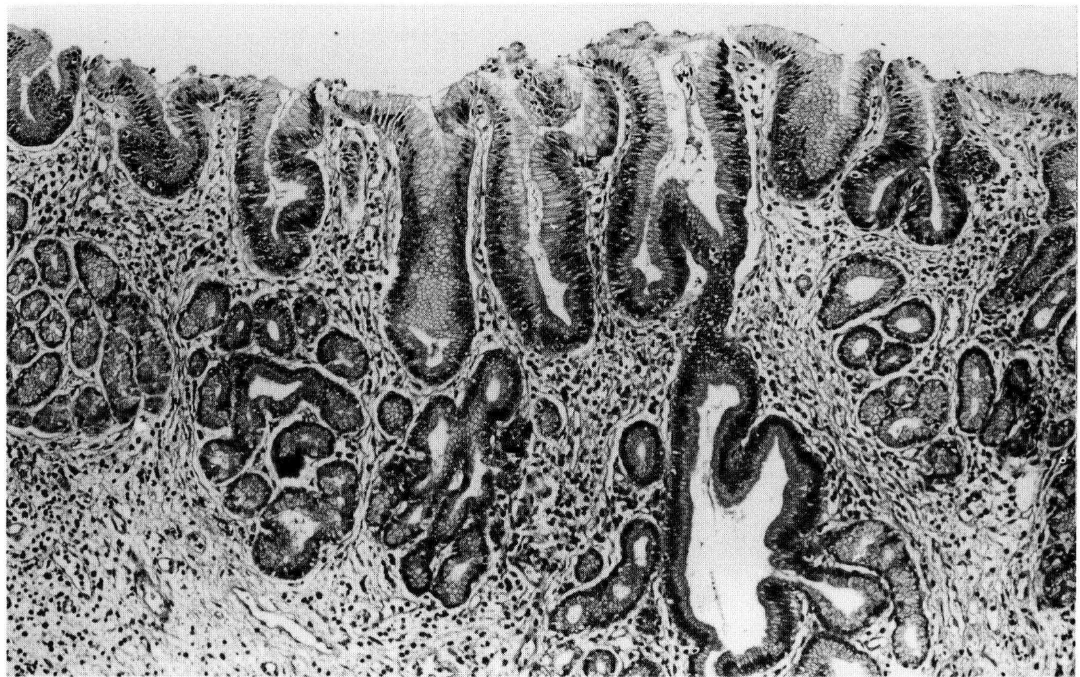

Fig. 4-4. Normal gastric cardiac mucosa, with surface at top. The gastric pits are relatively short and are connected to the cardiac glands that contain mucous cells. Compared to the surface mucous cells, the mucous cells of the cardiac and antral glands are more distended with mucus. There is normally a prominent amount of inflammatory cells in the lamina propria of the cardia (× 105).

cally confined to the mucosa and do not extend beneath the muscularis mucosae, in contrast to the Brunner's glands in the duodenum. Compared to the corpus, there is more evident lamina propria seen in the biopsies, due to a greater component of muscular tissue and also of an increased inflammatory cell population. The muscle cells are present in infants, whereas the number inflammatory cells increases decidedly with age, and most are of the mononuclear cell type. Given their presence, one should require considerable increases in the number of inflammatory cells or in the presence of lymphoid nodules or neutrophils as more certain evidence of disease.

Other Features

The endoscopic biopsies usually provide only a portion of the mucosa in adult populations. The full mucosa is revealed in cases with atrophy or other major alterations, such as may be associated with a tumor, and in children with a thinner mucosa. In situations in which the full mucosa or underlying submucosa is needed for the evaluation, aspiration-type biopsies can be obtained. These are particularly useful for morphometric studies in which all of the cells of the glands need to be counted, or for the detection of substances that are concentrated in the submucosa, such as amyloid material, or certain tumors.

At the junction of the corpus and antrum, the mucosa typically reveals a mixture of features, with specialized gastric cells associated with the gastric antral glands.[14] These cells tend to fade out over a few centimeters but occasional parietal cells are seen throughout the antrum and even in the duodenal mucosa.[15] Some of the gastric glands, particularly in the corpus/fundic region, show mild cystic change; these may be lined in part by mucous cells with short cilia.[16] The lamina

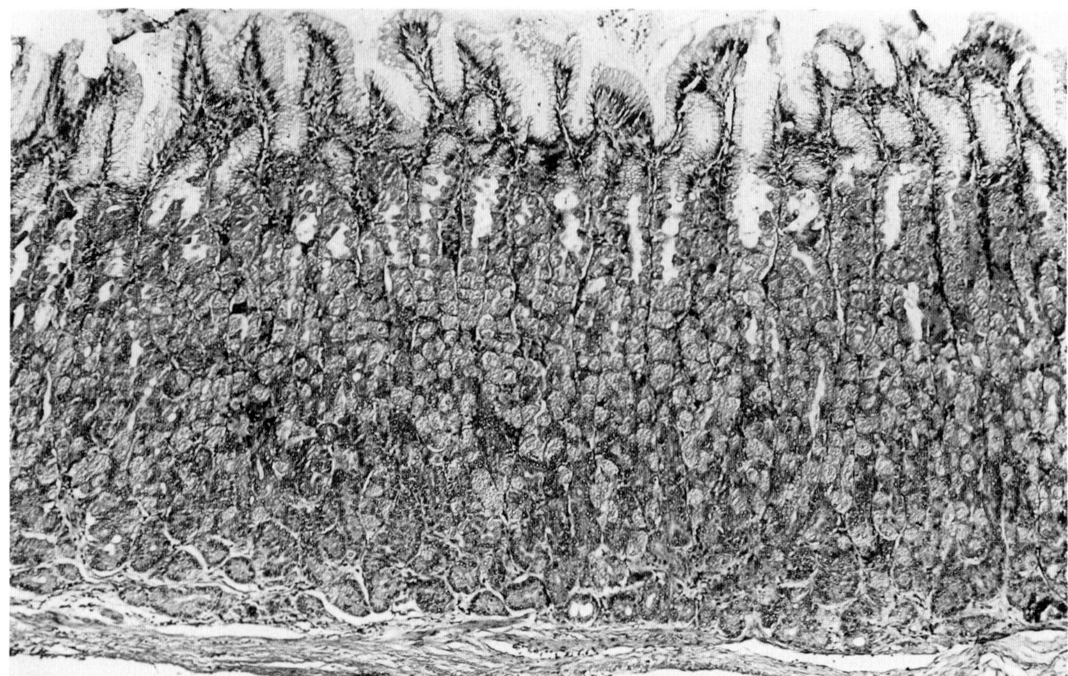

Fig. 4-5. Normal gastric mucosa of the corpus and fundic regions. Short pits lined by mucous cells are at top. Most mucosa comprises glands with specialized cells: paler parietal cells mostly in the midportion; denser chief cells at the base. Minimal lamina propria is seen, reflecting lack of inflammation. The muscularis mucosae is at the bottom (× 68).

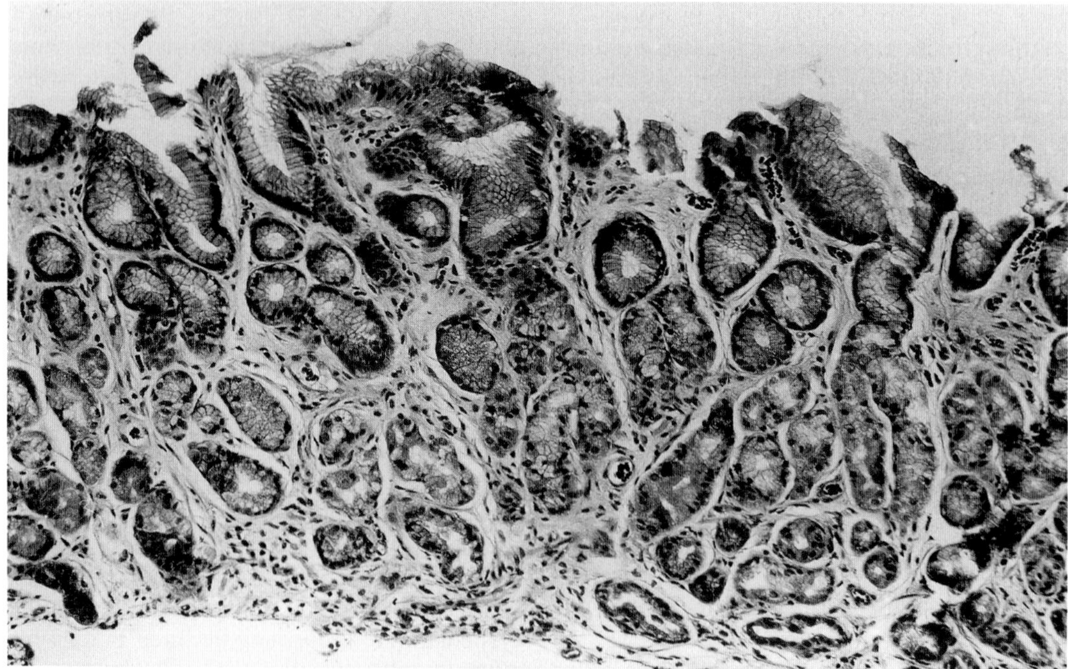

Fig. 4-6. Normal gastric antral mucosa. Compared with the corpus, gastric pits are longer and connected to the antral glands with distended mucous cells. Scattered amidst the glands are endocrine and parietal cells. The lamina propria has fibromuscular tissue and inflammatory cells (× 140).

propria throughout the normal stomach lacks lymphatics except in the basal region next to the muscularis mucosae.[17,18] A proliferation of lymphatics is seen, however, in the chronic inflammatory conditions.

Effects of Procedure

As a result of the patient preparation and especially of the endoscopic procedure itself, there can be traumatic effects in the biopsy (Fig. 4-7). These must be discounted before confirming that there is actual disease. Most of these are of a mechanical nature, including edema and hemorrhages of the lamina propria in the absence of any damage to the epithelium; flattening of the surface epithelial cells unassociated with inflammation; and simple distortion of the biopsy due to compression from the endoscopic forceps.

Effects of Aging

Over time, mild injury and increasing inflammation affect the stomach, particularly the antral portion. Thus, by age 50, practically all gastric antral mucosae show a considerable amount of mononuclear inflammatory cells within the lamina propria as well as occasional foci of intestinal metaplasia involving the gastric pits and glands. In the absence of active inflammation or glandular destruction, this is probably not significant.

General Pathologic Features

Details of the pathologic features associated with acute and chronic inflammation, and with active and inactive disease, are presented in the section titled "General Pathologic Features" in Chapter 2. They are summarized here with special reference to the

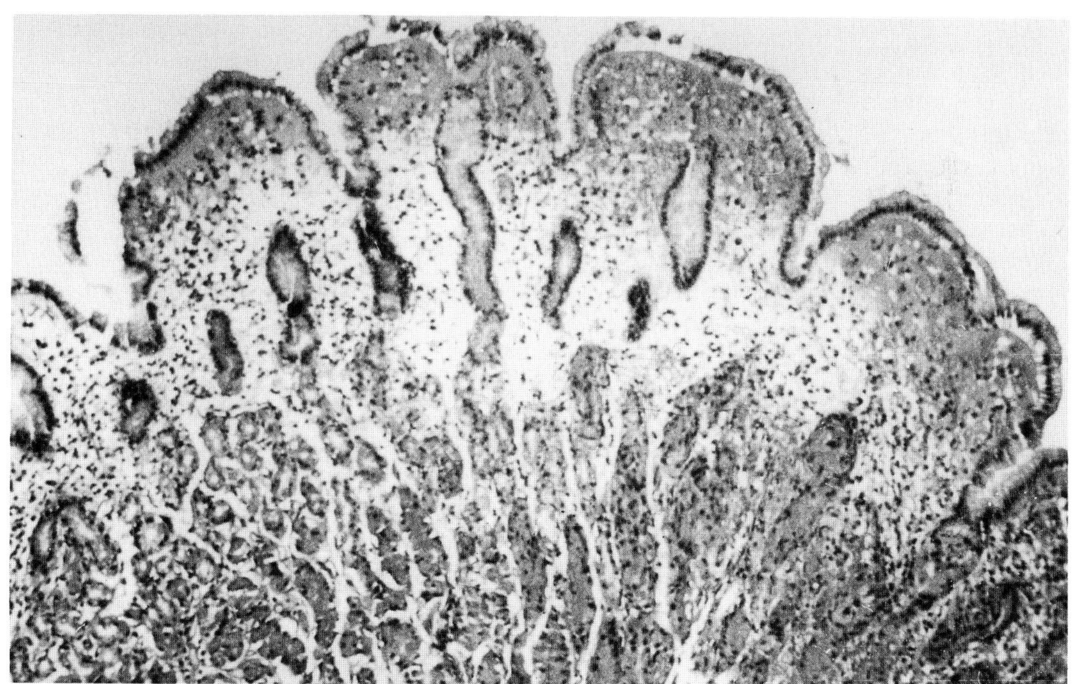

Fig. 4-7. Gastric corpus mucosa, showing the traumatic effects of the endoscopic procedure. There is fresh hemorrhage and edema in the lamina propria of the superficial part without a neutrophilic reaction.

gastric mucosa, and are further presented in a later section in this chapter, "General Features of Gastritis."

Acute or active inflammation is characterized by the presence of degeneration of the surface and pit mucous cells in association with edema, congestion, and neutrophils, the amounts of which depend on the particular etiology (Table 4-3). For example, in many injuries related to drugs and chemicals, there is often considerable edema but relatively little neutrophilic reaction, this in contrast to infections where inflammatory cells are particularly pronounced. The features of chronic gastritis include a great increase in the amount of mononuclear-type inflammatory cells and the appearance of lymphoid nodules within the lamina propria; atrophy of the indigenous glands and cells of the particular area; a change or metaplasia to intestinal-type epithelium throughout the stomach and to pyloric-type in the corpus region; and varying effects on the local neuroendocrine cells.

Other features of inflammatory disorders include an increase in the number of mitoses, which are ordinarily rare in the normal stomach; this can reflect a simple healing of an acute gastritis or an ongoing proliferation in a chronic disorder. Also noted are varying degrees of necrosis and ulceration with granulation tissue and fibrosis, when the lesions are more severe. More specific features are seen in many of the disorders affecting the stomach, including prominent vascular pattern in some of the ectasia disorders, the presence of granulomas in a variety of conditions, and the occurrence of recognizable microorganisms or their inclusions. More often, however, the features observed in the stomach indicate that the patient has an acute or chronic gastritis affecting a particular part of the stomach, with the specific etiology provided in the historical information.

Table 4-3. Histologic Features of Gastritis

Acute
Edema, congestion, and hemorrhage
Neutrophils and eosinophils
Erosion and ulcer
Repair
Hyperplasia of gastric pits
Granulation tissue
Chronic
Mononuclear inflammatory cells
Lymphoid nodules
Atrophy of specialized glands
Hyperplasia of gastric pits
Intestinal and pyloric metaplasia

Special Studies

The hematoxylin and eosin (H & E) sections are ordinarily sufficient for most biopsy diagnoses. Various histochemical stains can be employed to accent the areas of intestinal metaplasia since the mucous cells in these regions are particularly rich in acid mucins; most often used are Alcian Blue and high-iron diamine stains to demonstrate the less acidic and the sulfated mucins, respectively. Special stains including histochemical and immunocytochemical types are also employed to identify the particular neuroendocrine cells, specific deposits such as amyloid and minerals, and microorganisms.

DEVELOPMENTAL DISORDERS

Cysts and Diverticula

Cysts and diverticula of the stomach are rarely observed; they usually concentrate in the gastric wall without mucosal prominence.[19–22] Exceptionally, there is extension of a duplication cyst into the lumen, and these lesions often have aberrant epithelium such as squamous- or pancreatic-type tissues.[23] Biopsy may also be useful in identifying cysts that are confined to the mucosa[24]; such lesions are possibly increased in cases of gastric adenocarcinoma.

Hypertrophic Pyloric Stenosis

Hypertrophic pyloric stenosis typically develops in young infants and is represented by hypertrophy of the pyloric musculature together with inadequate opening of this region. The children develop gastric distention and episodes of esophageal reflux and pneumonia. The diagnosis is ordinarily made by the history and radiographic study with mucosal examination limited to uncertain cases. The endoscopy serves to rule out any tumors or inflammatory strictures in the pyloric region, and biopsies are rarely obtained.[25]

Conversely, some cases of gastritis can be associated with marked edema and narrowing of the pyloric region, simulating pyloric stenosis in infants and children. This is particularly seen in cases of allergic gastritis, which can affect the younger population.[26] Mucosal biopsy in such cases is helpful by demonstrating the active gastritis and marked infiltration of eosinophils within the lamina propria and gastric epithelium. Such features are not seen in the congenital form of hpertrophic pyloric stenosis.

Another condition that can be associated with pyloric stenosis is *Behçet's disease.*[27] This is usually seen in older children and is associated with lesions in the esophagus and intestines (see Chs. 2, 8, and 9).

Heterotopic Tissues

The aberrant presentation of a variety of tissues may occur in the gastrointestinal tract, including ectopic foci of gastric corpus, of pancreatic tissues with or without associated muscle, and of *Brunner's glands.*

Stomach

The heterotopic stomach is the most frequently encountered example at endoscopy and is mainly found in the upper portion of the esophagus and in the duodenum.[28–30] The tissue consists of well formed gastric corpus mucosa, and can occur almost anywhere in the gut, being also noted in *Meckel's diverticula* and in the rectal mucosa (see Table 2-5). This topic is detailed in Chapter 2.

Pancreas

Heterotopic pancreatic tissue is also common but typically limited to the wall of the stomach and duodenum, and extending in most cases only into the submucosa.[31–33] Exceptionally, it may reach the mucosa and be associated with a small nodule of tissue, which can have an indented or dimpled area representing the opening of a ductal structure. These are most commonly observed in the duodenum and less often in the stomach, particularly the distal portion. The foci are readily recognized by the presence of ductal and acinar pancreatic tissue, alone or together with varying degrees of muscle and fibrous tissue (Fig. 4-8A). When the latter is pronounced, the lesion has been interpreted as an adenomyoma but still probably represents a developmental rather than a neoplastic condition.[34]

It has recently been noted that foci of pancreatic metaplasia can be frequently seen in cases of chronic gastritis and this must be distinguished from the heterotopic presence of pancreatic tissue.[35] The metaplastic tissue consists of mature acinar tissue that is present in a focal region within the gastric mucosa, similar to the development of intestinal metaplasia (Fig. 4-8B). It is not associated with a large nodule but rather is assimilated into the rest of the mucosa. It is important for biopsies to distinguish between the two entities, because the identification of the metaplastic foci may help to define the presence of an associated chronic gastritis.

Brunner's Glands

Also occasionally noted in the stomach, particularly in the distal portion, are Brunner's glands. These are distinguished from pyloric glands by the larger size of the mucous cells and by their presence within the submucosa. They rarely cause a significant clinical lesion, and it may be difficult in a biopsy to distinguish between an ectopic fo-

A

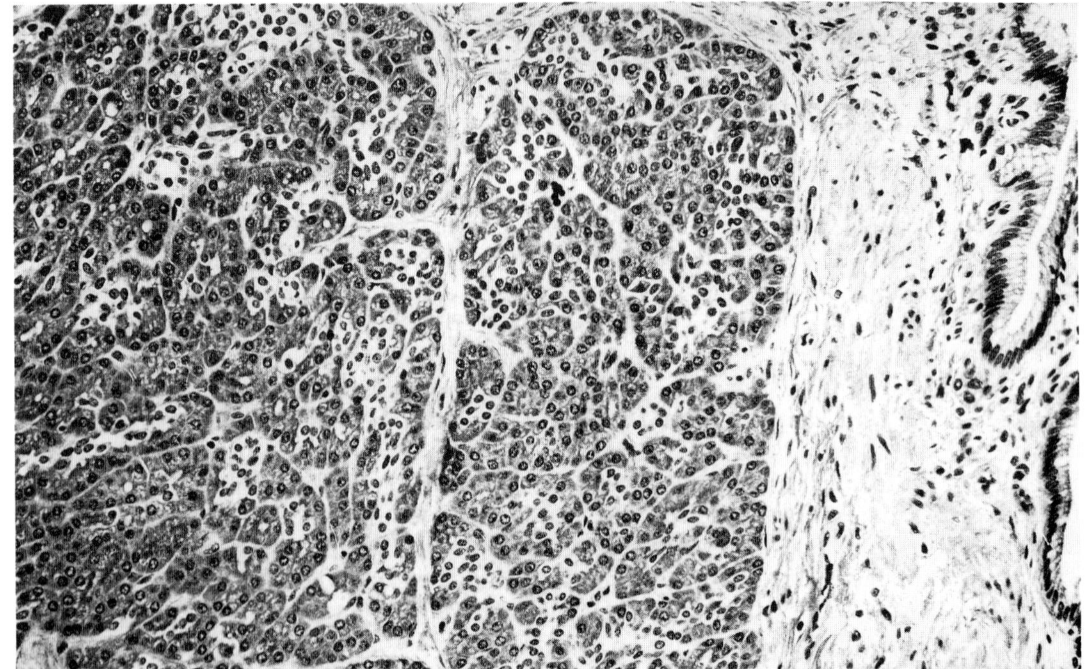

B

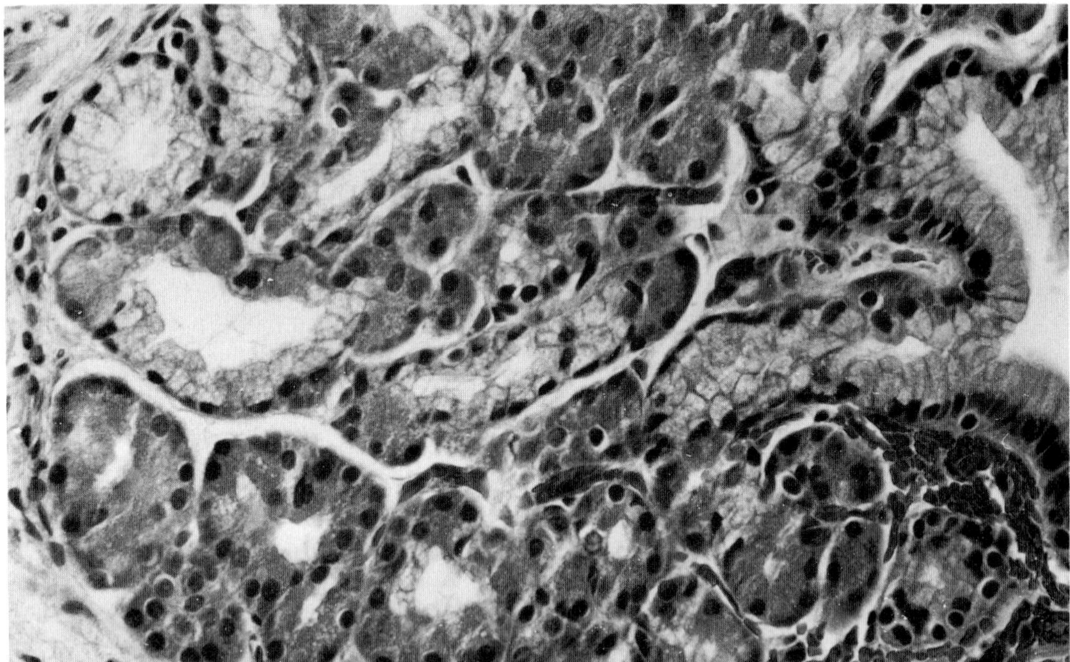

Fig. 4-8. (A) Nodule of heterotopic pancreas in the stomach. There is well formed exocrine pancreatic tissue, fibrous stroma, and part of ducts at the right (× 105). **(B)** Pancreatic metaplasia in the gastric mucosa. Mature pancreatic acinar tissue with prominent zymogen cells is attached to the gastric pits (× 425).

cus and the inadvertent taking of a duodenal sample. In all of these instances of heterotopic tissues, there is usually no major necrosis or inflammation. The biopsies mainly recognize the tissue and help to explain the aberrant appearance of the mucosa or identify the nature of a nodule.

MOTOR AND MECHANICAL DISORDERS

Obstruction of the stomach typically occurs in the naturally narrow regions, such as the cardia and pyloric antrum, and these are typically due to either chronic inflammatory or tumorous conditions. Biopsies are routinely obtained to identify their nature. Effects on the overall musculature and nervous supply in the stomach are relatively mild compared to other portions of the gut, perhaps reflecting the large diameter and easy distensibility of the stomach.

NEUROMUSCULAR CONDITIONS

Systemic sclerosis can involve all parts of the gastrointestinal tract, but lesions and effects in the stomach are exceedingly rare. In most conditions leading to loss of peristaltic activity, the functional and clinical alterations are more pronounced and notable in the esophagus and in the intestinal tract, probably reflecting the lesser diameter of the lumen in these areas. When there is pronounced distention of the stomach, as may occur in uncontrolled diabetes mellitus, there can develop secondary pressure or ischemic injury of the mucosa, leading to hemorrhages and superficial necrosis.[36, 37] Mucosal biopsy of the stomach in these conditions is ordinarily not obtained.

MALLORY-WEISS SYNDROME

This syndrome is represented by longitudinal ulcers at the junction of the esophagus and stomach, and is seen in patients following severe retching and vomiting.[38, 39] The lesion is usually evident by gross endoscopy, and biopsies are only obtained if there is more extensive ulceration to exclude an infection or tumor. This topic is detailed in Chapter 2.

VASCULAR DISORDERS

There are many conditions associated with dilation of the small or large vessels that affect the gastric mucosa and wall, and which can lead to significant hemorrhage (Table 4-4). In addition, there can develop destructive lesions as a result of inadequate blood supply. Endoscopic examination is commonly used to sort out these various conditions and to distinguish them from other causes of gastric hemorrhage and of gastritis.

VARICES AND CONGESTIVE GASTROPATHY

Both esophageal and gastric varices commonly occur in patients with cirrhosis and other causes of portal hypertension. The dilated veins typically involve the proximal half of the stomach, where they project into the lumen and are readily visualized by radiographic and gross endoscopic examinations. In some cases, there is less pronounced dilation of the larger veins and more extensive ectasia of the smaller veins together with a variable degree of fibrosis that involves both

Table 4-4. Vascular Disorders of the Stomach

Varices and congestive gastropathy
Vascular malformations
Osler–Weber–Rendu disease
Dieulafoy's ulcer
Gastric antral vascular ectasia
Ischemic (stress) lesions
Hemorrhage
Acute ulcer
Small vessel diseases
Vasculitis
Atheromatous emboli
Amyloid deposition

the submucosa and the mucosa (Fig. 4-9).[40–44] These cases can also be the source of significant bleeding, and biopsies are occasionally needed to identify the vascular ectasia and to exclude other forms of hemorrhage, in these patients. It should be noted that there are multiple sources of hematemesis in these patients, including bleeding from esophageal or gastric varices, from Mallory-Weiss lesions, from gastritis associated with ethanol or with various drugs, and from chronic peptic ulcers.

Vascular Malformations

Several vascular alterations involve the stomach, and can bleed and be the source of both acute and chronic hemorrhagic disorders. The term *angiodysplasia* has been applied at a collective level,[45, 46] but this should not be confused with the entity in the right side of the colon, also termed *vascular ectasia,*[47] which is largely limited to older persons and is probably related to progressive constipation.

Telangiectasia

In the *Osler-Weber-Rendu syndrome,* there are multiple telangiectasias that involve medium-size veins located in the submucosa and mucosa in all parts of the gastrointestinal tract.[48] These can occur in the stomach, where they are typically multiple and readily appreciated on gross endoscopic examination. Mucosal biopsy of these lesions is not ordinarily obtained; when done, it simply shows prominent veins and venules within the mucosa. Multiple telangiectasias affecting the gastric mucosa are also seen in patients with renal failure, particularly those on hemodialysis.[49]

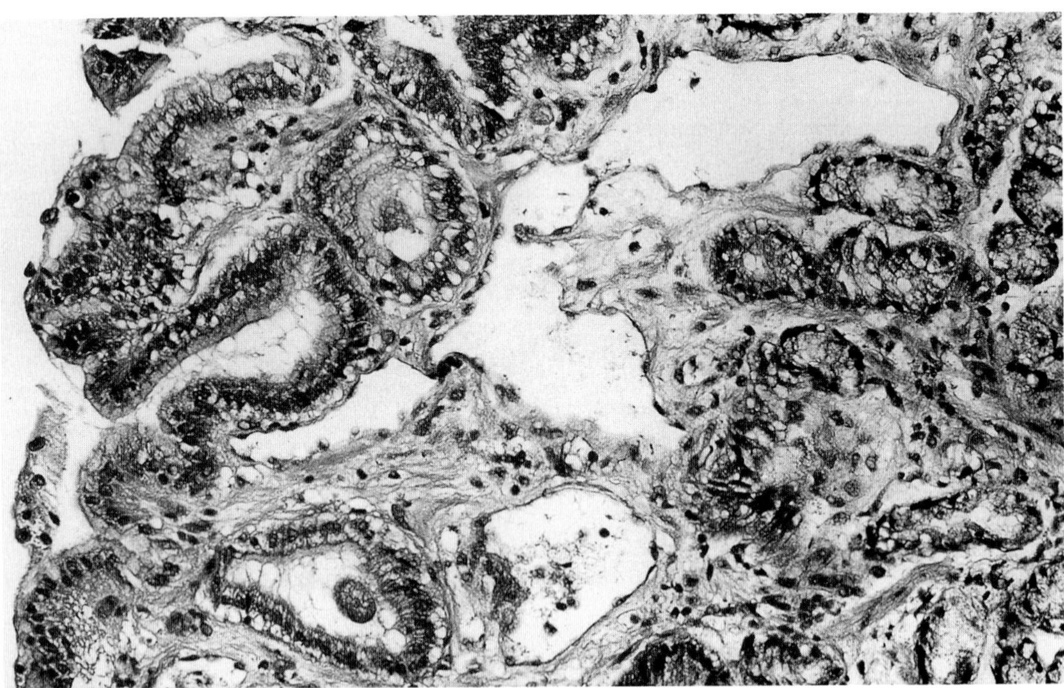

Fig. 4-9. Congestive gastropathy, with mucosal surface at left. There are markedly dilated venules in the lamina propria (× 42).

Dieulafoy's Ulcer

A more striking vascular lesion is noted in the caliber-persistent artery, or *Dieulafoy's ulcer.*[50–53] This typically occurs in a younger person and presents as an ulcer in the proximal part of the stomach, with major hemorrhage from a prominent central artery in the submucosa. The lesion is usually recognized grossly, and the diagnosis is confirmed by examination of the operative specimen.

Gastric Antral Vascular Ectasia

Gastric antral vascular ectasia (GAVE) is a more diffuse abnormality involving the lower part of the stomach, most frequently in older women.[54–58] Such lesions usually present with chronic bleeding that leads to iron-deficiency anemia. These cases formerly required antral resection but now can be successfully treated by endoscopic laser in most cases.[59] They have a striking gross appearance with streaks of hemorrhage likened to and called a *watermelon stomach.* Biopsies reveal numerous dilated venules containing recent thrombi together with variable edema and fresh hemorrhage in the lamina propria (Fig. 4-10). Some earlier studies had also noted a prominence of muscle within the lamina propria, but it is not certain whether this is increased over the normal in the antral area.

Ischemic Lesions

Because of the excellent collateral circulation to the stomach, major infarction with involvement of the wall is rarely seen.[60, 61] However, lesions associated with shock and other stress situations are common, mainly affecting the mucosal lining.[62, 63] These are seen in patients who have experienced either major trauma, multiple organ failure, or increased intracranial pressure. It is probable that reduced mucosal blood flow is a dominant pathogenetic factor and that lesions are facilitated by the presence of normal or increased acid secretion.

Most commonly noted at endoscopy are patches of fresh hemorrhage and multiple small erosions. Examination of early lesions suggests an evolution from hemorrhage to superficial mucosal infarction, resulting in the acute erosions or ulcers.

Endoscopy is often done to exclude other causes of bleeding in these patients, and the ischemic (stress) lesions are readily appreciated on gross examination. Mucosal biopsy is usually not needed; when obtained, largely to exclude other causes, they reveal the patchy hemorrhages alone or in association with superficial necrosis and erosion of the mucosa (Fig. 4-11). The earliest lesions typically show no inflammation. During the healing phase, which typically occurs rapidly over the next few days, there can be noted a prominent neutrophilic reaction, marked mitotic activity, and rapid restoration of the mucosa.[64] Because of the superficial nature of the lesions, there is usually no significant granulation tissue or fibrosis.

The lesions can be found in all parts of the stomach, including the corpus and fundic regions, which helps to differentiate them from other causes of gastritis that are often concentrated in the distal portion. Similarly, the acute stress ulcers may be present in the proximal or distal region, whereas chronic peptic ulcers are invariably limited to the antral region. Overall, biopsies are not commonly obtained in these conditions but do serve to identify the lesion in its active and healing phases and to exclude other causes of gastric injury in these critical patients. (See the later section "Acute Stress Ulcer" for further details.)

Small Vessel Diseases

There are several other conditions in which the small vessels of the stomach can be injured, resulting in hemorrhage or the

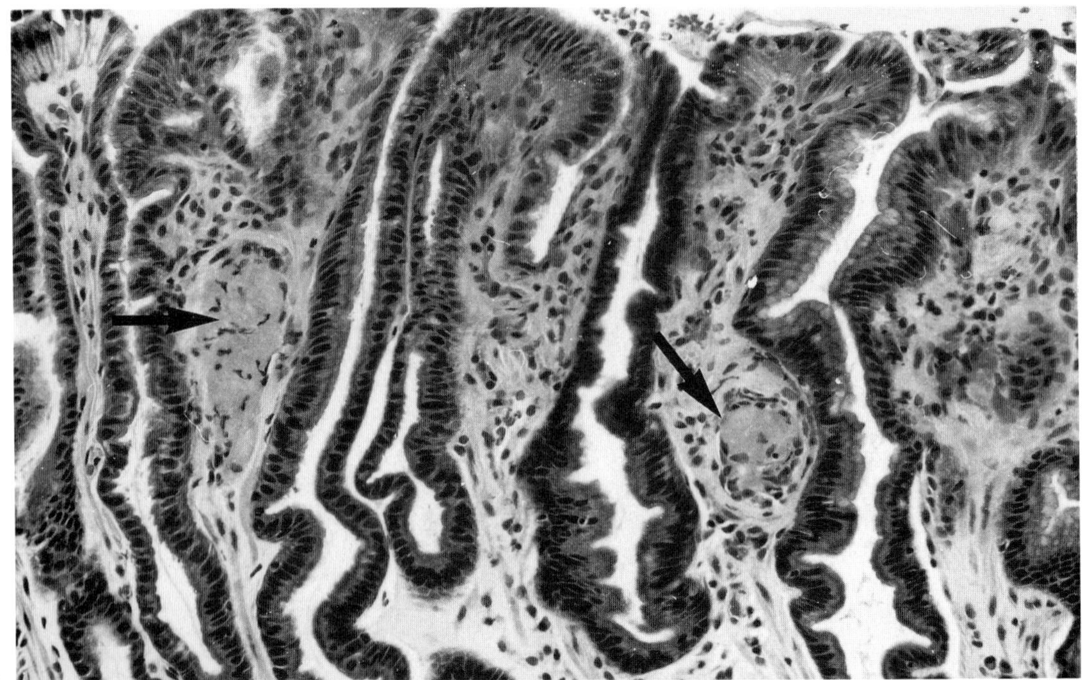

A

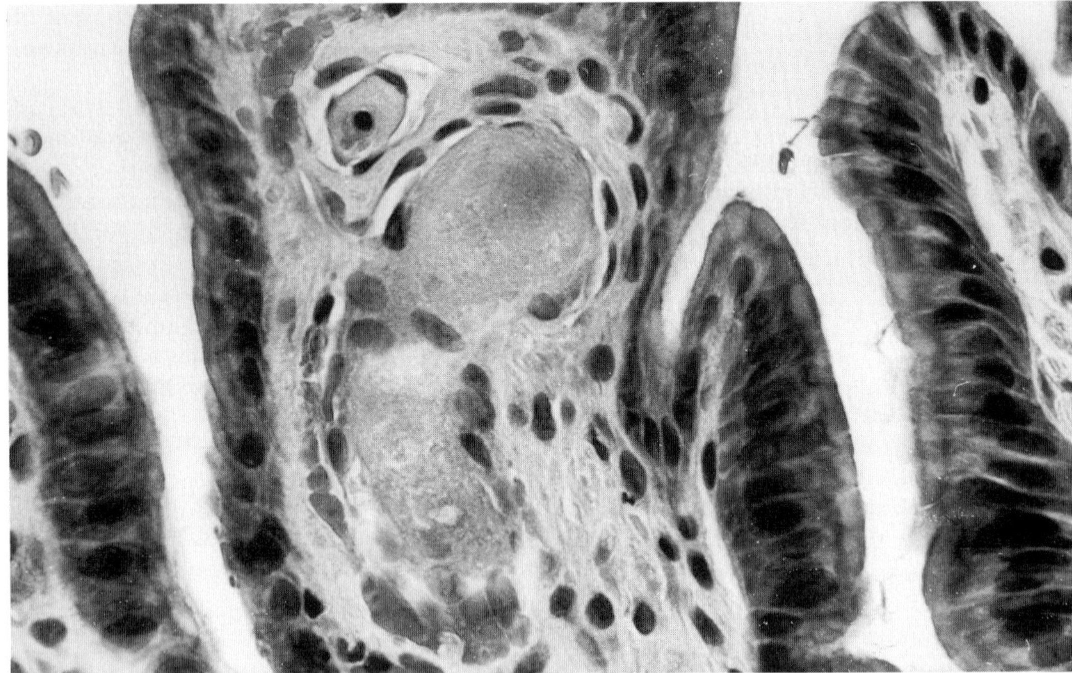

B

Fig. 4-10. Gastric antral vascular ectasia, with surface at top. **(A)** The lamina propria reveals venules that are distended with thrombi (arrows) (× 210). **(B)** Closer view of thrombi (× 635).

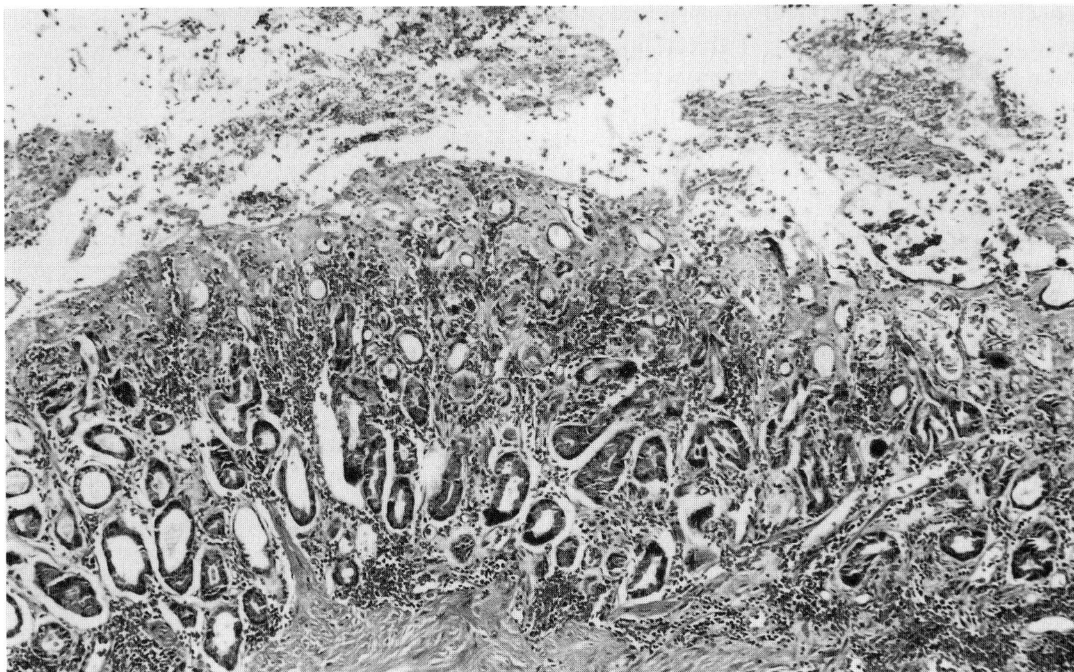

Fig. 4-11. Ischemic gastritis in the antral mucosa. There is diffuse hemorrhage, necrosis, and erosion involving the upper part of the mucosa. The lumen contains acute inflammatory exudate (× 105).

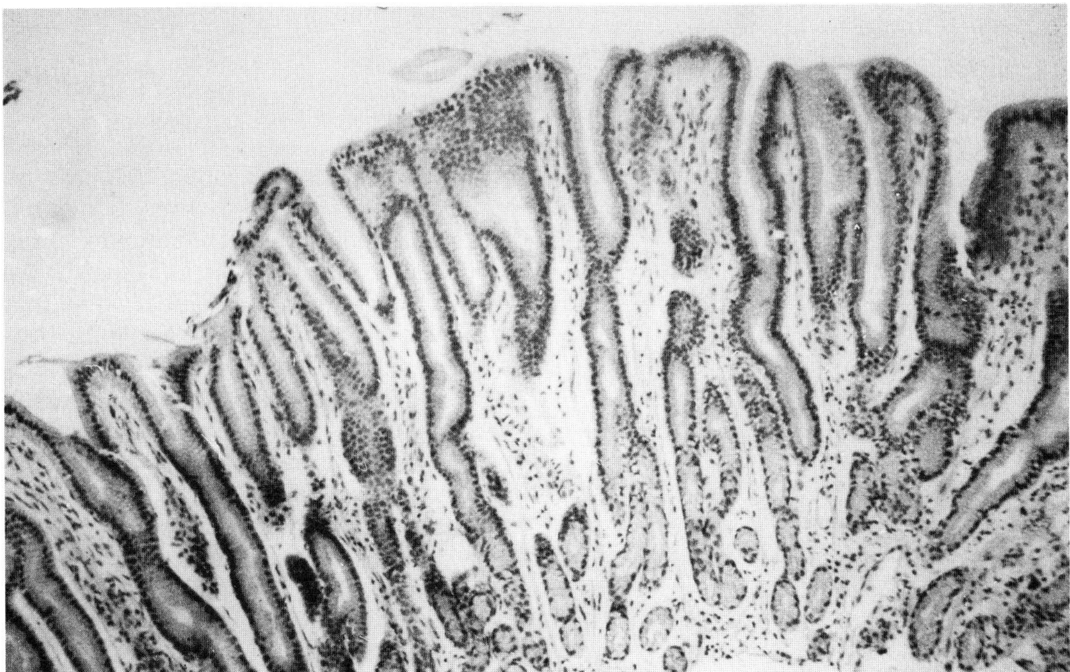

Fig. 4-12. Healing gastritis in the antral mucosa. There is a marked elongation of the gastric pits, with scattered mitoses in the mucous cells.

development of local ulcerations. These include vasculitis, which is relatively uncommon in the stomach[65]; the occurrence of atheromatous emboli, causing obstruction of submucosal vessels[66] (see Fig. 9-15); and the deposition of amyloid material,[67] which is presented in a later section of this chapter.

GENERAL FEATURES OF GASTRITIS

There are many etiologies and conditions that can lead to injury of the gastric mucosa, alone or together with damage of other parts of the alimentary tract[68–71] (Table 4-5). Biopsies are typically obtained at endoscopy, because they are considered much more sensitive than simple gross inspection.[72–76] These cases of gastritis can generally be separated into acute and chronic forms, based largely on their duration and expected outcomes. The general features of the various forms of gastritis are presented here, and the detailed descriptions in the subsequent sections of this chapter are related to specific causes.

Acute Gastritis

Acute gastritis is defined as injury of the gastric mucosa that is characterized by short duration and usually complete recovery. The onset tends to be rapid and related to a specific cause; the morphologic lesions and clinical course are generally predictable; and there is typically prompt recovery following elimination of the cause and other appropriate therapy.

Table 4-5. Causes of Gastritis

Chemical and drug injury
Infections and allergic conditions
Immunologic disorders
Ischemic (stress) lesions
Radiation and trauma
Granulomatous conditions
Neuromuscular and metabolic disorders

Causes

Most cases of acute gastritis are due to chemical or toxic substances, including ethanol, aspirin, nonsteroidal anti-inflammatory drugs (NSAIDs), and reflux of duodenal contents into the stomach.[77, 78] Stress lesions, as described above, can also cause acute gastric injury, typically in the form of hemorrhages or ulcers with relatively scant inflammation. Other causes, such as infections and allergic conditions, are less frequent.

Gross Features

At a gross endoscopic level, the lesions in acute gastritis are separated into hemorrhagic and nonhemorrhagic, and also into erosive and nonerosive forms. These generally reflect severity, with cases of gross hemorrhage or erosion representing more advanced lesions; however, they also provide some clues as to etiology, since some causes more dominantly present with hemorrhage as opposed to others with ulceration.

Biopsy Features

Mucosal biopsies are often obtained in cases of suspected acute gastritis to identify or confirm the lesion, to exclude other specific conditions such as infections, and, occasionally, to monitor the patient following therapy. There have been extensive human and experimental studies to demonstrate the early features of acute gastritis, which mainly consist of edema and variable hemorrhage of the lamina propria, together with variable damage to the epithelial cells. The amount of acute inflammatory cells, including neutrophils and eosinophils, appears to relate to the specific etiology. For example, there are relatively few granulocytes in cases of reflux gastritis, prominent neutrophils in most infections, and dominance of eosinophils in allergic and some chronic conditions.

Once the offending agent, such as a toxic substance, is eliminated, there is typically a very prompt renewal of the epithelium and a return to the normal state. If biopsies are taken during this phase, they show lesser or no damage to the surface and pit mucous cells and no acute inflammatory cells, but rather increased mitoses and transient lengthening or hyperplasia of the gastric pits (Fig. 4-12). It should be recalled that mitoses are rare in the normal state, and their presence together with the appearance of regenerative cells should serve as a clue that the patient has a healing gastritis. There are usually no sequellae in cases of acute gastritis. Although it has been supposed that cases of acute gastritis after multiple episodes could develop into a chronic disorder, this has rarely been established.

Chronic Gastritis

Cases of chronic gastritis are characterized by the lack of a clear inciting event, protracted duration, and probable irreversible disease affecting the mucosa. Depending on the particular etiology, the condition can mainly affect the antrum, corpus–fundic mucosa, or both areas[79, 80] (Table 4-6). As with all chronic disorders, cases of chronic gastritis are subject to episodes of relapses, or active disease, alternating with remissions, or inactive disease; and the frequency and severity of the active lesions appears to depend on the particular cause, being greater with infections than with immunologic lesions. Aside from the functional and clinical effects of chronic active disease, there are further complications that include the increased potential for the development of gastric carcinoma.

Table 4-6. Types of Chronic Gastritis*

Chronic antral gastritis
Chronic fundic/corpus gastritis
Chronic infections
Post-gastrectomy gastritis
Chronic erosive gastritis
Chronic hypertrophic gastritis

* From Goldman,[70] with permission.

Causes

The major causes of chronic gastritis are infections, particularly due to *Helicobacter pylori,* and the immunologic disorder of primary pernicious anemia. It is possible that the various chemical and drug injuries may, if sustained, lead to a small fraction of chronic gastritis, but this has not been clearly proven. Nevertheless, there are almost certainly other genetic and environmental etiologic factors, since the causes of all cases of chronic gastritis are not established.

Gross Features

Endoscopy and biopsy are often done in patients with suspected chronic gastritis to establish the lesion, its major location (such as antrum or corpus), and its extent; to determine whether there is active or inactive disease; to follow the patients after treatment; and to survey the cases for complications, particularly for the development of epithelial dysplasia and carcinoma. At a gross level, there may be atrophy, as evidenced by a simplification of the gastric rugae and the ready appearance of the submucosal vessels through the thinned-out mucosa. Also noted grossly are signs of active disease in the form of hemorrhages, friability, and erosions.

Biopsy Features

In evaluating the mucosal biopsy, one should look for markers of chronic disease, such as lymphoid nodules, atrophy of indigenous elements, and the appearance of metaplastic epithelium (Fig. 4-13); for features of active disease, typically in the form of degeneration of the mucous cells and neutrophil reaction (Fig. 4-14), with more severe cases

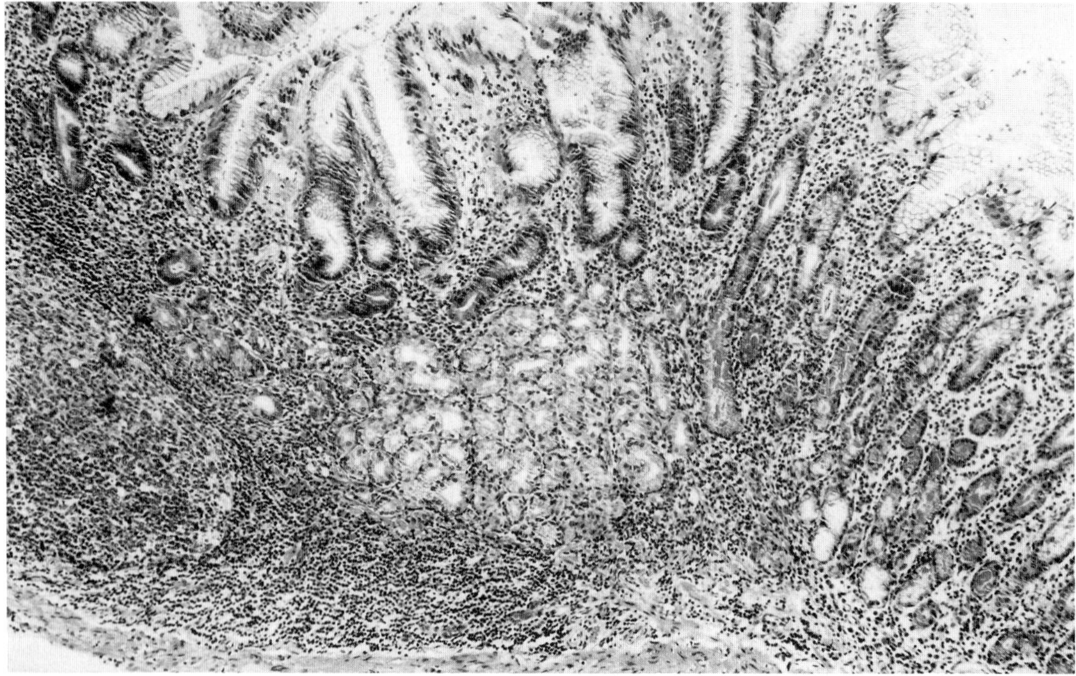

Fig. 4-13. Chronic gastritis in the antral mucosa. There is a marked loss of antral glands with residual foci at the center. Noted are a diffuse lymphoid reaction in the lamina propria with nodules (lower left) and foveolar hyperplasia (lower right). A portion of the muscularis mucosae appears at the bottom (× 105).

showing overt erosion or ulceration; and for the development of any additional lesions, such as polyps and dysplastic epithelium.[70] The features of chronic gastritis differ somewhat depending on the location and particular cause.[71, 81]

In all types of chronic gastritis there is a considerable increase of mononuclear inflammatory cells and of eosinophils within the lamina propria, and the appearance of numerous well formed lymphoid nodules (Fig. 4-15). Such lymphoid tissues are not ordinarily present in the normal stomach, and their detection in a mucosal biopsy serves to identify a case of chronic gastritis in whatever location. In cases in which there is marked or complete loss of the specialized glands, the term *chronic atrophic gastritis* has been applied. This is especially used in the cases involving the corpus and fundus where the functional effect of the loss of parietal and chief cells is so striking. The term serves to indicate the marked severity of the lesion and identifies the patients at increased risk for the development of complications such as carcinoma.

Another variable finding is the appearance of the neuroendocrine cells. They may be reduced but more often show a hyperplasia. It is not known whether this increase in cells is a simple reflection of the chronic gastritis leading to extra proliferation, or whether there are other functional stimuli. This has been most studied in cases of primary pernicious anemia and atrophic gastritis involving the gastric fundus and corpus. In such cases there is noted an increase in the amount of G cells in the antrum, thought to be a secondary response to the reduced acid production (Fig. 4-16). In turn, this can lead to a stimulation of the ECL cells in the gastric corpus. In both sites the increase in cells may appear as a simple hyperplasia where there are greater numbers of cells in otherwise

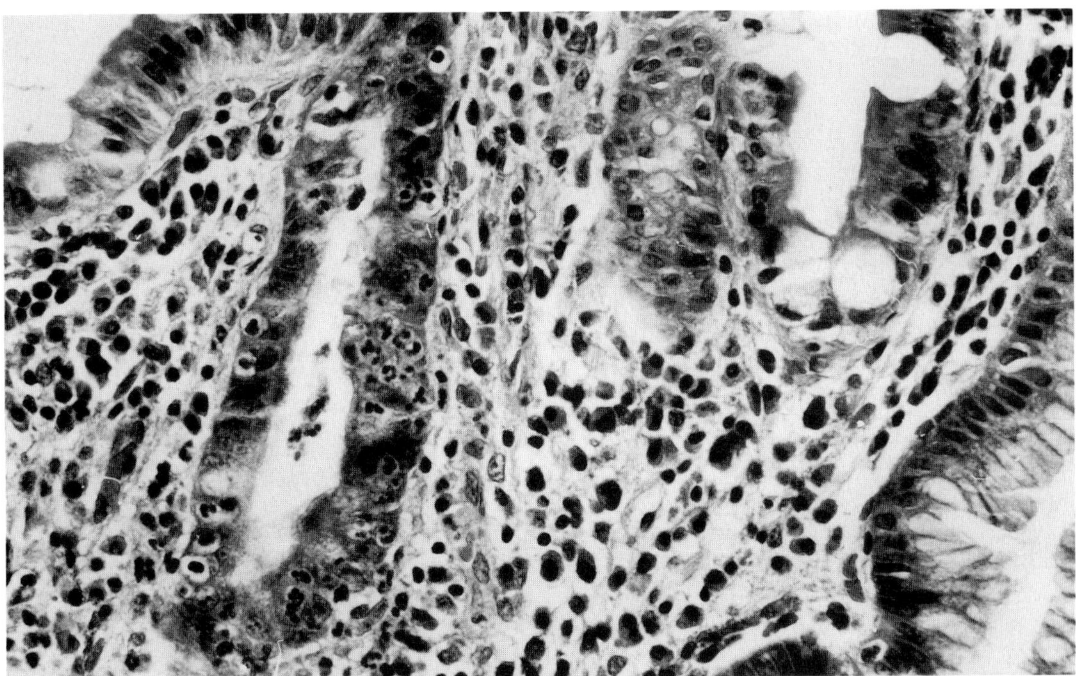

Fig. 4-14. Chronic active gastritis in the antral mucosa. The gastric pit at the left shows degeneration of the lining epithelial cells and a marked neutrophilic infiltrate. There is also an increase in plasma cells in the lamina propria (× 425).

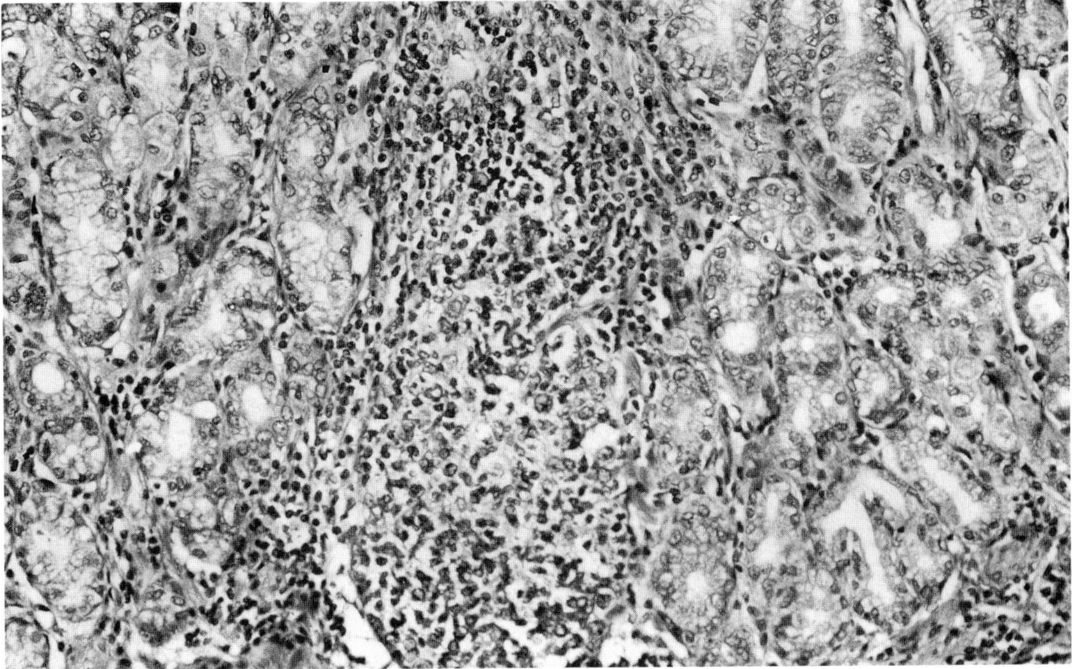

Fig. 4-15. Chronic active gastritis, showing well formed lymphoid nodule with follicle in the center (× 105).

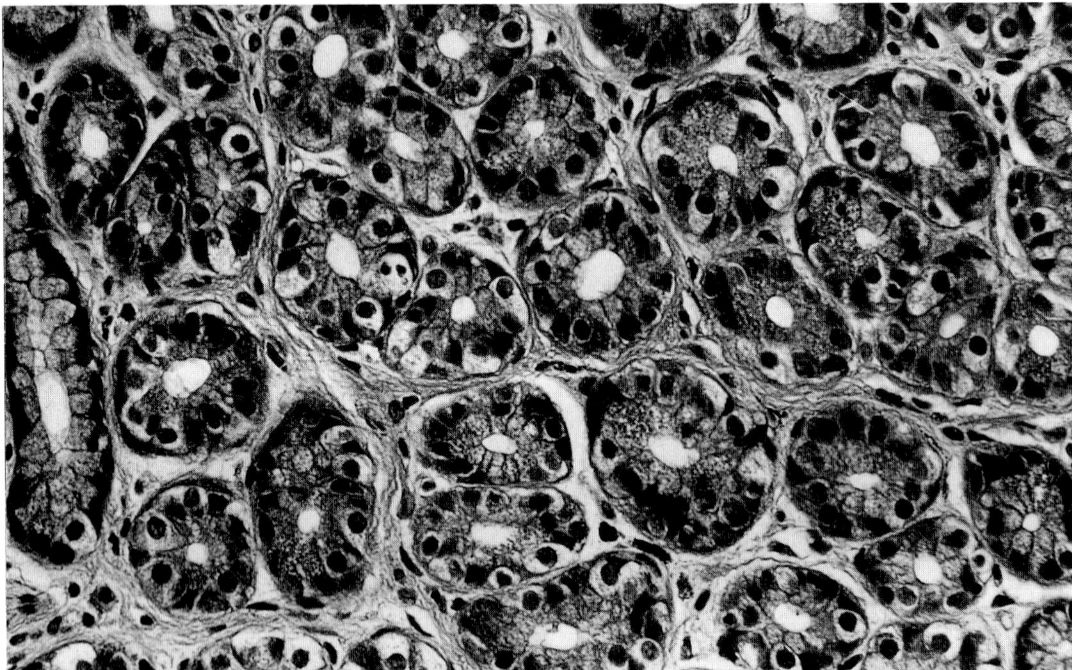

Fig. 4-16. G-cell hyperplasia in the gastric antrum. A cross section of the antral glands reveals a marked increase of neuroendocrine cells (see Fig. 4-2). The cells stained positively for gastrin (× 425).

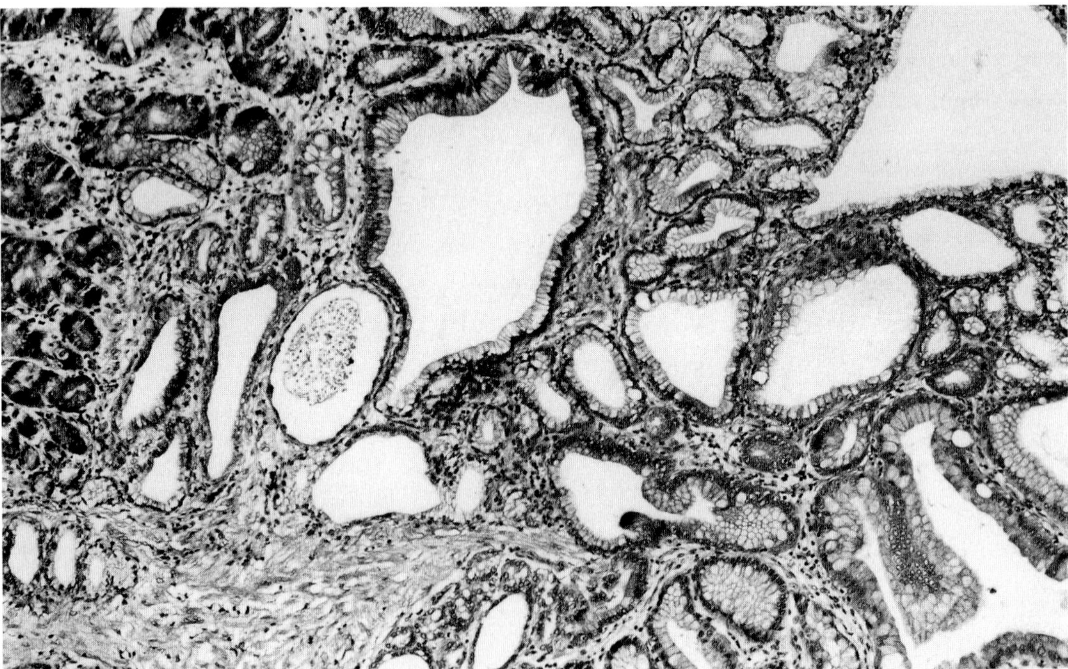

Fig. 4-17. Chronic gastritis of the gastric corpus, following antral resection. Much of the mucosa is replaced by hyperplastic gastric pits and pyloric-type glands with cystic change. There is a small amount of intestinal metaplasia in the lower right (× 105).

ordinary-appearing glands; the presence of nests of cells termed microcarcinoids; and the development of larger tumor nodules.[82–85] This is discussed further in Chapter 5.

TYPES OF CHRONIC GASTRITIS

Chronic Antral Gastritis

This form of chronic gastritis is mainly due to chronic infection with *H. pylori* and is frequently associated with active disease. There is usually a pronounced degree of intestinal metaplasia, and atrophy of the pyloric glands occurs only late in the disorder (see the section in this chapter on "Infections"). There probably is also a reduction in the local neuroendocrine cells, mainly of the G-cell type, but this is rarely documented or a problem.

Chronic Fundic Gastritis

This is the form of chronic gastritis that has an immunologic cause and is related to primary pernicious anemia. There is a progressive loss of the specialized glands and cells, leading to a state of atrophy of the mucosa together with prominent intestinal and pyloric types of metaplasia[86] (see the section in this chapter on "Immunologic Disorders").

Post-Gastrectomy Gastritis

In patients who have had a resection of their distal stomach, usually for peptic ulcer disease, there regularly develops a chronic gastritis in the residual proximal stomach.[87, 88] This is presumably due to the ready reflux of pancreatic and biliary substances through the gastrojejunostomy into the gastric stump; this subject is discussed later in this chapter under "Reflux Gastritis." The lesions typically develop in the region immediately adjacent to the gastrojejunostomy stoma, and over time extend more proximally but rarely involve the entire residual stomach. Noted are an atrophy of the specialized glands, prominent cystic glandular change, and variable pyloric glandular metaplasia (Fig. 4-17). Of interest, there is usually little intestinal metaplasia in these cases.

Chronic Erosive Gastritis

In this type of chronic gastritis, there is the presence of alternating areas of erosions and hyperplasia of the mucosa, which can create a very irregular surface and be confused with tumors.[89–91] Biopsies can also be difficult to evaluate because of the considerable degeneration and regeneration of the epithelial cells, alternating with relatively normal forms. Such lesions can be misconstrued as showing dysplasia. This form of gastritis is more prominent in the proximal half of the stomach, may be associated with prominent protein loss,[92] and has also been termed *varioliform gastritis.*[93]

Often noted in these cases is an increase in the amount of lymphocytes within the epithelial layer, including the surface and pit mucous cells. Accordingly, this has recently been called *lymphocytic gastritis,*[94] and it has been suggested that there is an increased association between some of these cases and other conditions of the gut in which there are increased lymphocytes in surface endothelial cells, such as in celiac disease and in lymphocytic colitis.[95] Alternatively, the presence of increased intraepithelial lymphocytes may be an entirely nonspecific finding, noted in many cases including gastritis due to *H. pylori* and to celiac disease[96] (Fig. 4-18). In summary, biopsies from cases of chronic erosive gastritis typically reveal the erosions, the prominent regeneration

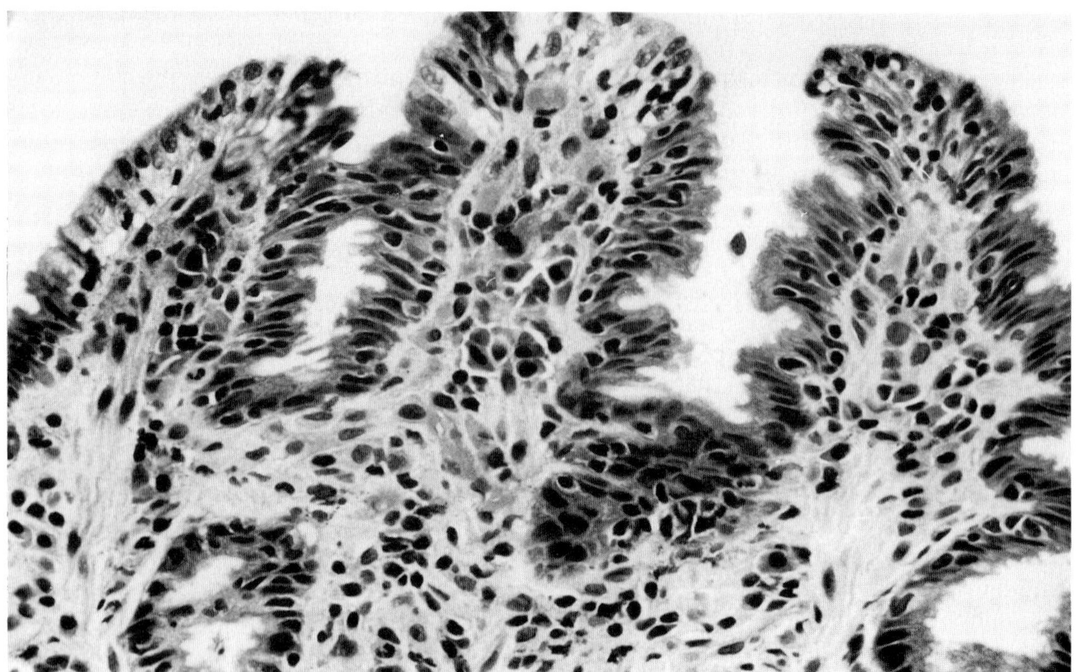

Fig. 4-18. Gastric antral mucosa in a case of active celiac disease, with surface appearing at top. There is a marked increase of intraepithelial lymphocytes involving the surface and pit mucous layer (× 425).

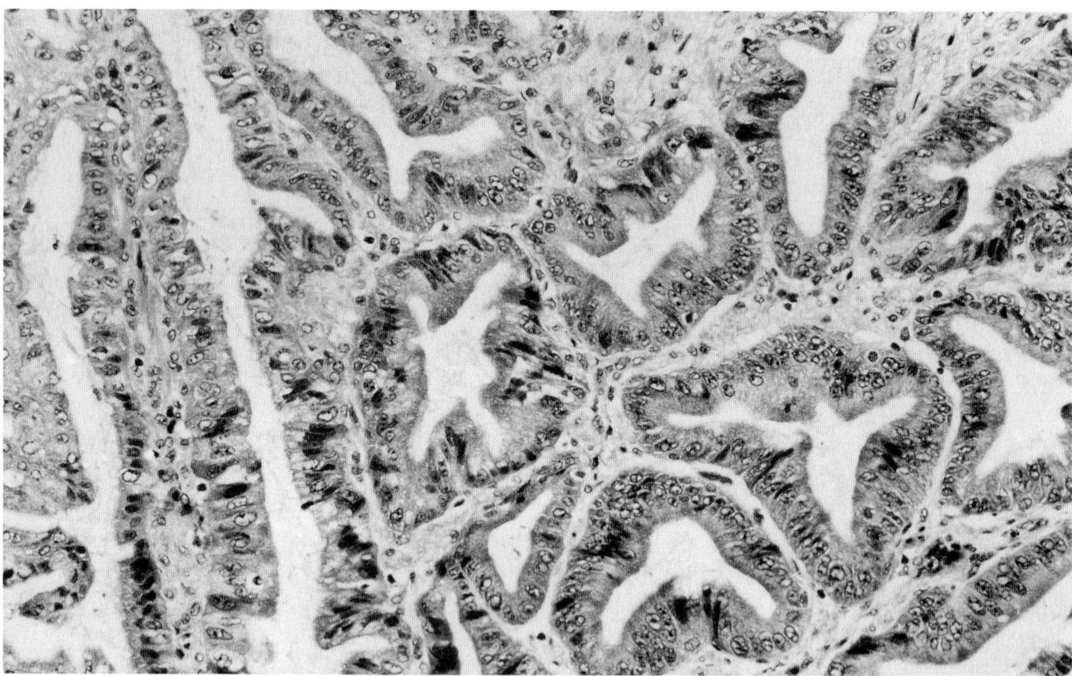

Fig. 4-19. Marked regeneration of gastric pits. There is nuclear enlargement and lack of cytoplasmic mucin. The nuclei tend to have a similar size, shape, and position within the cells, and lack prominent palisading and hyperchromatism (× 210).

that must be distinguished from neoplasia, and the variable presence of increased lymphocytes in the surface and pit epithelial mucous cells.

Chronic Hypertrophic Gastritis

This type of chronic gastritis has an unusual degree of hypertrophy of the mucosa, either polypoid or diffuse, due to a hyperplasia of the gastric pits.[97, 98] Such cases must be distinguished from the purer forms of mucosal hypertrophy that are seen in *Ménétrier's disease* and in the *Zollinger-Ellison syndrome.*[99, 100] The latter conditions reveal hyperplasia of the pits and specialized cells, respectively, and typically a scant amount of inflammation (see Ch. 5). Indeed, much of the information that suggests an increase in the frequency of carcinoma complicating Ménétrier's disease may be due to confusion with cases of chronic hypertrophic gastritis. The most helpful feature that distinguishes chronic hypertrophic gastritis is the presence of increased inflammatory cells in the lamina propria together with more mitoses and regenerative-type cells in the gastric pits.

Summary of Chronic Gastritis

The biopsy in chronic gastritis is much more variable than in cases of acute gastritis. Potential findings include chronic disease with variable atrophy and metaplasia but no activity; the presence of acute or active disease superimposed on the chronic condition; the appearance of prominent regeneration, typically evidenced in the gastric pits in the form of enlarged but similar-sized nuclei with prominent nucleoli and with reduced mucin and overall cytoplasm (Fig. 4-19); and the development of complicating lesions such as xanthomas, hyperplastic polyps, neuroendocrine cell proliferations, and genuine dysplastic epithelium.

METAPLASIA

A common feature of chronic gastritis is the appearance of metaplastic epithelium, particularly of intestinal-type cells, in all portions of the stomach, and of pyloric glandular–type cells in the corpus and fundus.[70] A small amount of this occurs with ordinary aging, best seen with foci of intestinal metaplasia in the gastric antrum, but it is greatly heightened in cases of chronic gastritis. Recently noted is metaplasia directed to the development of pancreatic acinar tissue.[35] This has been described in the gastric antrum and cardia, and it is probable that this also is a sign of chronic disease, but more studies are needed. Rarely seen are foci of mature squamous epithelium, mainly in cases of extreme atrophy.

Intestinal Metaplasia

There have been extensive studies dealing with the appearance of intestinal metaplasia and with their classification.[101–105] There are two major forms, similar in appearance to small intestinal and to colonic epithelium, respectively (Fig. 4-20). The former has also been termed *type I, complete,* or *small intestinal–type metaplasia* and is characterized by the presence of scattered goblet type mucous cells, absorptive cells with brush borders, Paneth cells, and an occasional villiform surface. The mucin cells contain acid forms, evidenced by positive stains for Alcian Blue at pH 2.5 and weaker stains with the PAS reaction when compared to the normal stomach. The other major form of intestinal metaplasia is the *colonic, incomplete,* or *type III metaplasia* with appearances simulating normal colonic epithelium in the form of a greater number of goblet mucus cells, less or no absorptive cells, and absence of Paneth cells. The goblet cell mucus in this form contains sulfated types and stains strongly with both the Alcian Blue and with high-iron diamine stains. Many cases have *intermediate*

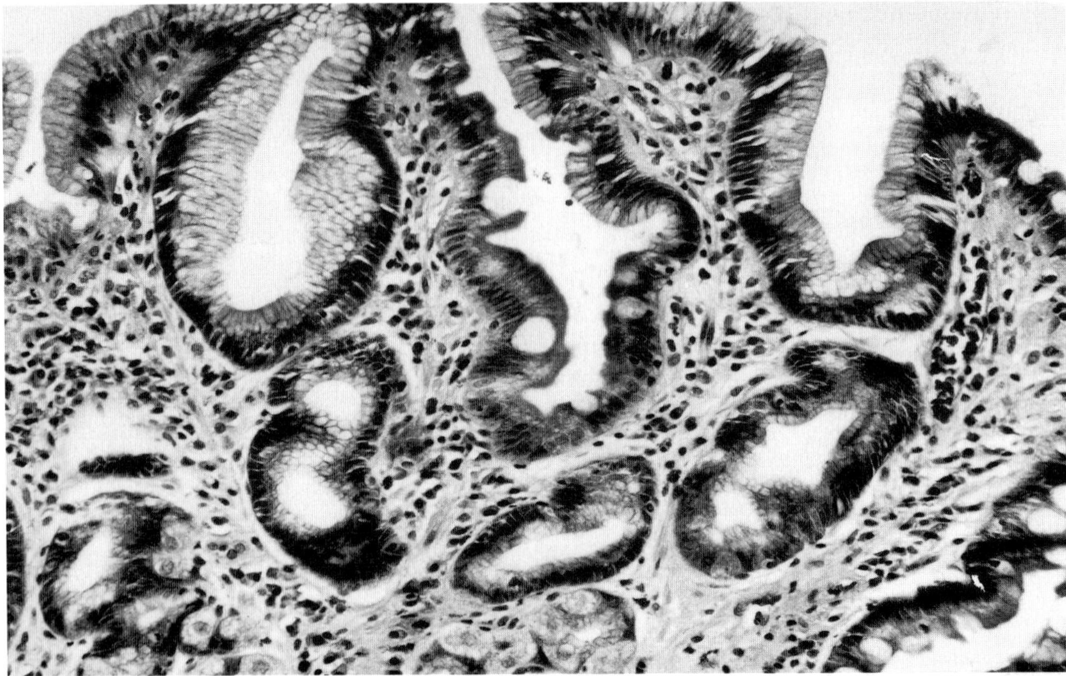

Fig. 4-20. Intestinal metaplasia in the gastric mucosa. The glands appearing in the center and at the lower right reveal numerous goblet mucous cells. Compare with the other gastric pits containing columnar-type mucous cells (× 210).

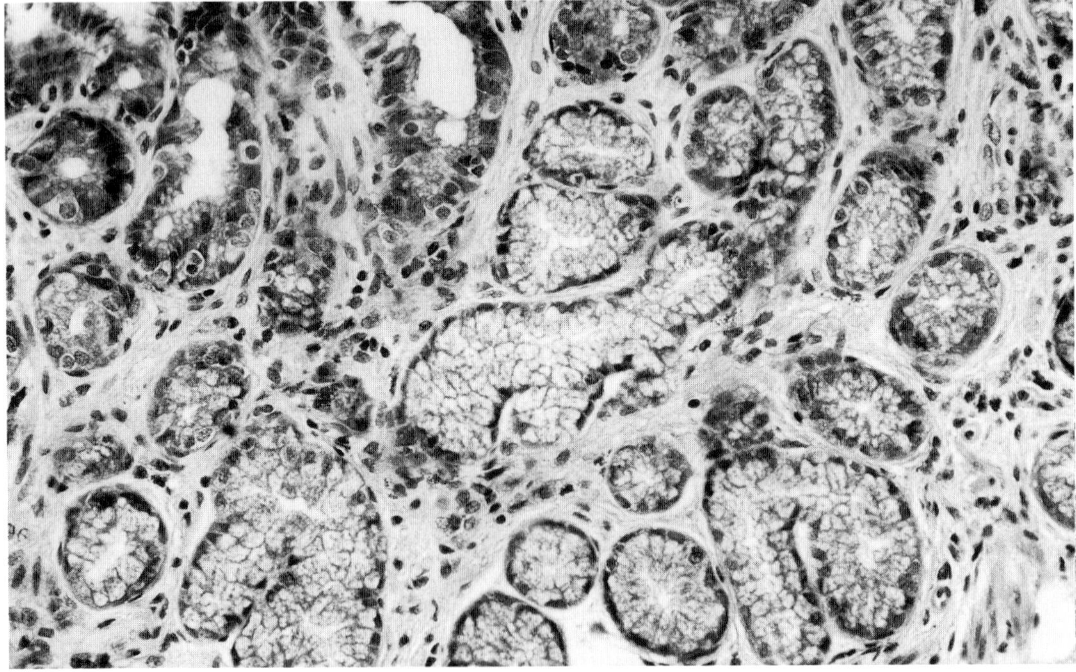

Fig. 4-21. Pyloric metaplasia in gastric corpus. Specialized glands replaced by mature pyloric glands. Pits with increased endocrine cells are seen in the upper left (× 280).

or *type II* forms of metaplasia in which there are columnar mucous cells containing acid mucin in addition to the goblet forms. Also present in all forms of metaplasia are neuroendocrine cells of the intestinal types.[106, 107]

The finding of the intestinal metaplasia, particularly when prominent, helps to identify that a patient has a chronic gastritis. In addition, it had been supposed that this could serve as a marker for increased development of tumors.[108–110] Indeed, most cases of carcinoma are associated with the colonic form of metaplasia, but this lesion remains too common to be a helpful marker.[111, 112] Rather, one needs to find an alteration of the nuclei in the form of dysplasia, as discussed below. It should be re-emphasized that the finding of small foci of intestinal metaplasia in otherwise normal gastric antra is a common feature of aging and not a certain sign of significant chronic disease.

Pyloric Gland Metaplasia

The other major form of epithelial metaplasia is a transformation to pyloric glands (Fig. 4-21). This typically occurs in the fundus and corpus of the stomach, where it replaces the specialized glands. Accordingly, it is seen in the cases of chronic fundic gastritis and of post-gastrectomy gastritis. Because such pyloric glands are normally present in the gastric antrum, there may be difficulties in distinguishing a native location from an area in which the metaplasia has developed. For example, in a patient with a prior distal gastric resection, in which the subsequent biopsy is presumed to be coming from the corpus, the finding of the pyloric glands could either represent a metaplastic phenomena in support of a chronic gastritis involving the gastric stump, or it could indicate that there remains a portion of the gastric antrum in the patient. To assist in this distinction other features of chronic disease are sought, in the form of an increase in the amount of inflammatory cells in the lamina propria, and of regeneration or hyperplasia of the gastric pits.

Table 4-7. Examples of Metaplasia in the Alimentary Tract

Location	Type of Metaplasia
Esophagus	Glandular (Barrett's)
Stomach	Intestinal
Gastric corpus	Pyloric glandular
Duodenum	Gastric mucous cell
Small intestine	Pyloric glandular
Colon	Paneth cell

Throughout the alimentary tract, chronic injury is characterized by regeneration and hyperplasia of the local elements and by metaplasia to embryologically similar epithelia (Table 4-7). Only the latter is recognized as abnormal for the site and, therefore, serves as a marker for chronic disease. Examples include the glandular metaplasia of Barrett's esophagus, the intestinal metaplasia in the stomach, the pyloric glandular metaplasia in the proximal stomach and in the small intestine, and Paneth cell metaplasia in the distal colon.

Complications of Chronic Gastritis

Aside from adverse functional effects due to the atrophy of the indigenous tissues to an area, there can develop persistent hyperplasia of the gastric pits leading to hypertrophy of the mucosa, localized deposits of lipids within the macrophages (termed *xanthomas*),[113–115] hyperplastic polyps,[116] neuroendocrine cell hyperplasia and neoplasia[82–85] (see the section "Biopsy Features" under "Chronic Gastritis"), and the potential for epithelial dysplasia[117–120] and adenocarcinoma[121, 122] (Table 4-8). These are dis-

Table 4-8. Complications of Chronic Gastritis

Atrophy of local tissue
Xanthoma
Hyperplastic polyp
Glandular dysplasia and adenocarcinoma
Neuroendocrine cell hyperplasia and neoplasia

cussed in later parts of this chapter and in Chapter 5.

CHEMICAL AND DRUG INJURY

Some of the most common causes of gastric mucosal injury are due to the ingestion of toxic chemicals and drugs and to the reflux of duodenal contents into the gastric lumen[123] (Table 4-9). These largely cause acute gastritis, with defects ranging from minimal to life-threatening hemorrhage, but are probably not a major cause of chronic disease.

Corrosive Gastritis

This is a relatively rare cause of gastric injury that is due to the accidental or suicidal ingestion of strong acids, alkali, and other highly toxic substances.[124–125] Whereas the alkaline solutions tend to cause major effects in the esophagus, the acids more regularly affect the stomach presumably due to less spasm and retention of the material in the esophagus. This can result in extensive areas of hemorrhage and ulceration, the potential for perforation, and the possible development of late strictures. The diagnosis is typically provided by the history, and gross endoscopic inspection may be done to determine the extent of the lesion and the appearance of any complications.[126, 127] Mucosal biopsy is not ordinarily obtained in these cases.

Table 4-9. Chemical and Drug Gastritis

Common causes
Reflux of bile salts
Ethanol
Aspirin
NSAIDs
Mechanism
Damage to membranes of surface/pit mucous cells, promoting increased back diffusion of hydrogen ions
Major effects
Edema and congestion
Hemorrhage and erosion
Mild inflammation

Chemotherapy Effects

Various chemotherapeutic agents that are used alone or in conjunction with radiotherapy may damage any part of the alimentary tract including the stomach.[128] The lesions are typically nonspecific, consisting of focal ulcerations with neutrophilic reaction, of granulation tissue in their repair, and of variable but usually slight fibrosis. Significant stricture formation is uncommon in the stomach. Biopsy examination may be done to identify the lesions and to rule out other problems, such as the development of infections or the spread of tumor. Marked epithelial atypism has been noted in cases receiving intrarterial infusions, usually for hepatic tumors, and these changes must be distinguished from neoplasia.[129–130]

Reflux Gastritis

Reflux gastritis results from the reflux of duodenal contents through the pylorus into the stomach.[131] The potential toxic elements are the bile salts and possibly the pancreatic enzymes, and the effects are principally on the gastric antral mucosa. The lipid-soluble substances, such as the bile salts, are absorbed by the luminal ends of the surface mucous cells in the stomach, causing them to permit increased back diffusion of acid ions. The acid in turn, either by direct cellular damage or by local vasoconstriction, can lead to injury of the mucosa and the development of an acute gastritis. The overall incidence of this lesion is not unknown nor is it established why the pyloric sphincter should be intermittently incompetent.

The biopsy features are fairly characteristic, revealing edema and hemorrhage of the lamina propria, elongated gastric pits, minimal degeneration of the surface and pit epithelial cells, and a relative paucity of acute inflammatory cells[132] (Fig. 4-22). As noted above, there may be a modest amount of mononuclear inflammatory cells in the lamina propria and even foci of intestinal metaplasia, which are features of aging and do not signify chronic disease. The features in reflux and in most chemical or drug gastritis are distinguished from cases due to infections by the lesser amount of neutrophils present in the damaged gastric pits. The lesions appear to subside rapidly with nonspecific therapy, and biopsies taken during the healing phase may simply show some increased mitoses and regeneration of the gastric pits with no other abnormality (see Fig. 4-12). It is not possible on the biopsy features to distinguish reflux gastritis from most causes of toxic or drug-induced gastritis.

Reflux of bile salts also regularly occurs in patients with a prior antrectomy and gastrojejunostomy and is responsible for the gastritis seen in those cases [133] (see Fig. 4-17) (see above "Post-Gastrectomy Gastritis").

Alcohol Gastritis

Alcohol gastritis regularly develops after the consumption of excessive amounts of ethanol. It is believed that the same mechanism of absorption of alcohol into the surface membranes, leading to increased back diffusion of acid, applies in these cases. Depending on the severity, the mucosa may reveal congestion or hemorrhages, friability, and overt erosions or ulcerations.[134–136] The lesions are typically diffuse, involving the antrum and occasionally extending into the middle part of the stomach. There also may be slight changes in the duodenal mucosa but this is usually not a dominant feature.

The biopsy features in alcohol-associated gastritis are nonspecific and similar to those noted in reflux gastritis, revealing prominent congestion, edema, and hemorrhage in the lamina propria. There is only mild dilation and damage of the gastric pits and relatively little acute inflammation. The lesions rapidly subside following removal of the toxic agent, and later biopsies reveal only the gastric pit regeneration. There is no definite proof that these cases proceed to a chronic atrophic gastritis of the antrum.

Drug-Induced Gastritis

Practically every medication can cause gastric irritation.[123, 137, 138] Some antibiotics induce prompt nausea and vomiting or pain, and the patients are immediately intolerant to and cannot use the drug; these cases are not typically associated with the development of any morphologic injury or inflammation of the mucosa, and biopsies are not obtained. Other drugs act by interfering with the normal development or maturation of the cells that line the gastric mucosa, leading to a reduced resistance to other factors and the potentiation of gastritis and ulcer formation. Corticosteroids and antimetabolites probably act in this way.[139] There are no specific features in the gastric mucosa with any of these drugs.

Aspirin

Most cases of drug-induced gastric injury are due to aspirin and to other anti-inflammatory drugs. These also mainly act by damaging the surface membranes of the mucous cells and potentiating the back diffusion of acid to the gastric mucosa.[140, 141] The greatest amount of investigations has been with aspirin, and it is acknowledged that the injury is of a dose-dependent nature and that virtually all patients taking this medication will develop at least a microscopic degree of acute gastritis.[142–145] Nevertheless, the benefits of the drug, especially in small doses, probably dictate its continued use provided the patient is monitored for symptoms of gastric irritation or hemorrhage. Biopsy in cases due to aspirin are similar to all the

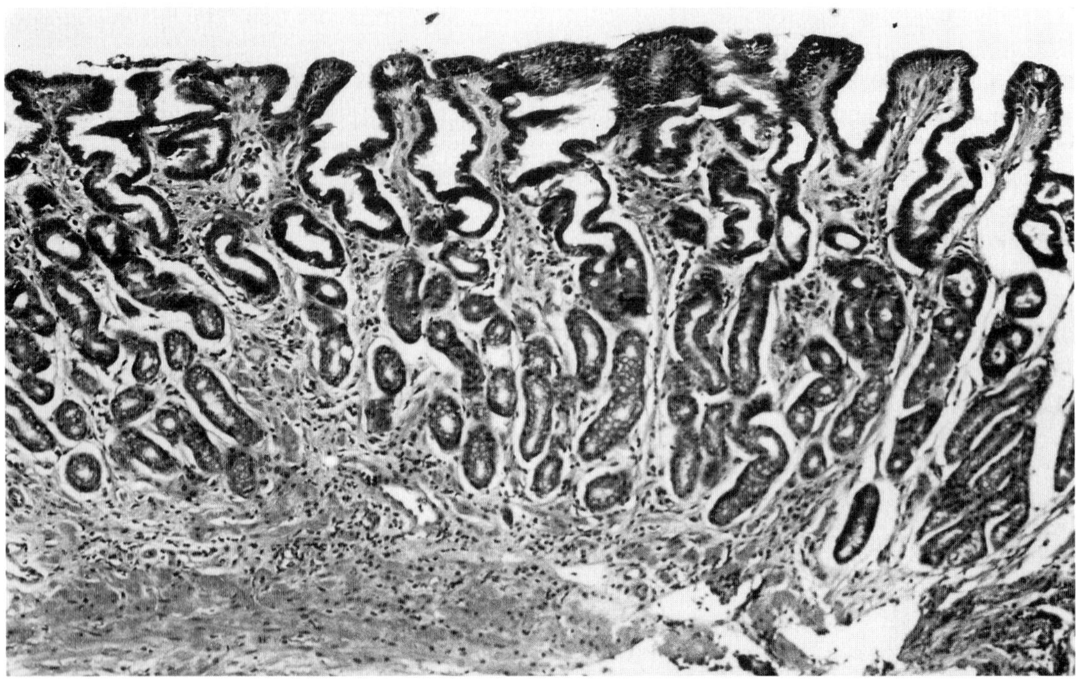

Fig. 4-22. Reflux gastritis in the gastric antrum (surface at top). Marked hyperplasia of the gastric pits and relatively little inflammation in the lamina propria (× 105). Compare with chronic active gastritis due to *H. pylori* (Fig. 4-13).

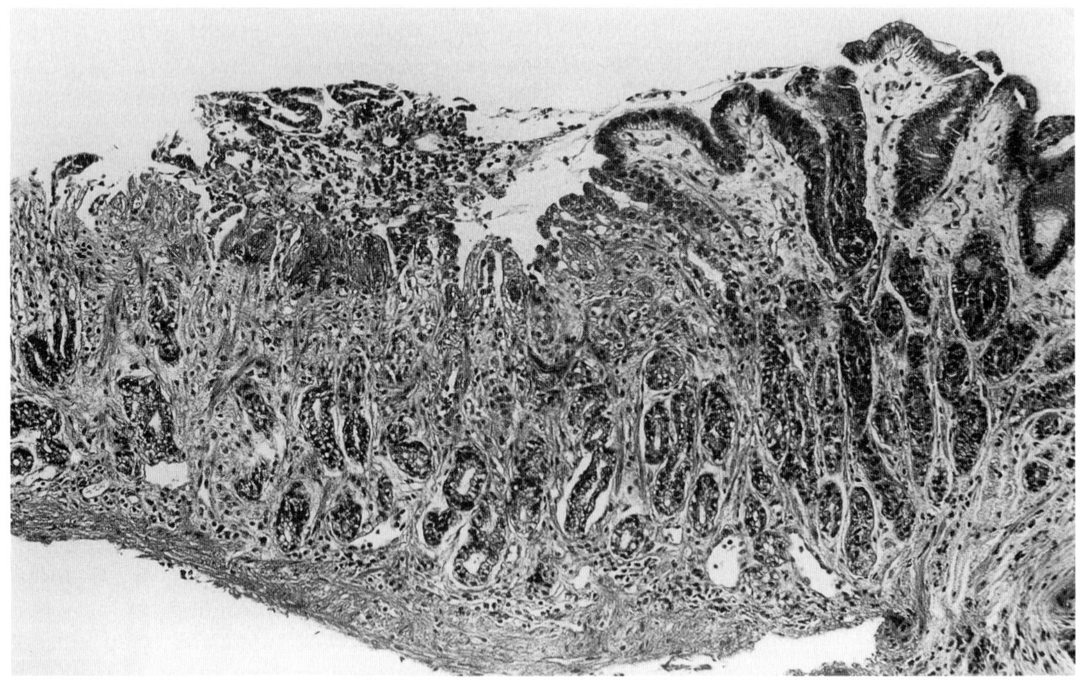

Fig. 4-23. Erosive gastritis due to nonsteroidal anti-inflammatory drugs. Hemorrhage, necrosis, and erosion but no features of chronic disease. Fovelar hyperplasia evident at the edge on the right (× 105).

other chemical agents, revealing the congestion, hemorrhage, and edema without prominent acute inflammation in the acute stages. During the healing phase there may be pronounced regeneration of the gastric pits, including the presence of numerous mitoses. Some cases develop more extensive hemorrhage that leads to superficial ulcers, and both increased neutrophils as well as greater regeneration are present in such instances.

Nonsteroidal Anti-Inflammatory Drugs

The development of the many agents in the NSAID group reflects an effort to find medicines that are less damaging to the gastrointestinal tract. Nevertheless, practically every agent in this category has ultimately been shown to be injurious,[146–150] with increased frequency related to patient age and to female gender.[151] There are additive effects with aspirin and with alcohol but an inverse correlation with *H. pylori* infection.[152] The effects are most often seen in the stomach but exceptionally may affect the duodenum and more distal parts of the small and large intestine, leading to inflammation, ulceration, and rare strictures in those sites. The lesions in the stomach are similar to those observed with aspirin, alcohol, and reflux of duodenal contents. Noted in the acute stage are edema and variable hemorrhage of the lamina propria; injury of the gastric pits ranging from minor dilation to superficial ulcerations (Fig. 4-23); and the relative paucity of inflammatory cells except in those instances with prominent ulceration. The mucosal biopsy can identify the lesion of acute gastritis but cannot distinguish the particular drug or other etiologic agent that is responsible. All of the drugs can cause acute ulceration as part of the acute gastritis and can promote the activation of a chronic peptic ulcer.

Other Causes and Summary

Less common causes of acute drug gastritis include iron and potassium salts.[153–155] These are occasionally associated with greater ulceration and fibrous strictures, both in the stomach and intestines. Overall, endoscopic examination and mucosal biopsy are done in cases of suspected drug-induced gastritis to verify the lesion, to determine its severity and distribution, and to exclude other causes, particularly if ulcers are present. In a chronic peptic ulcer, the adjacent mucosa is always inflamed, whereas cases of acute gastritis reveal relatively little or no inflammation.[156,157] Accordingly, the finding in support of an acute ulcer helps to direct attention to a particular drug rather than to an underlying chronic disorder.

INFECTIONS

General Features of Infections

The stomach has potent mechanisms to prevent the development of infection. The most important is the exceptionally low pH which would be incompatible for the growth of most microorganisms. This acid shower probably helps in reducing the microorganism load that reaches the small intestine. Nevertheless, infections can occur in the stomach when there is a compromise of other factors, such as in immunodeficiency states (Table 4-10). Also, *H. pylori* thrives in this environment, presumably due to specific receptors in the gastric mucous cells.

The pathologic effects of infections are largely detailed in Chapter 2 and are briefly summarized here. Most cases are associated with necrosis and ulceration together with a neutrophilic reaction in the acute stage; variable features include the presence of granulomas in a limited number of infections, and of granulation tissue and fibrosis in those cases with greater necrosis. The biopsies are largely obtained to identify the

Table 4-10. Infections of the Stomach

Viral	Bacterial	Fungal	Protozoan	Helminthic
Herpes Cytomegalovirus	*Helicobacter pylori* *Gastrospirillum hominis* *Mycobacteria tuberculosis* and *m. avium* Pyogenic bacteria in phlegmonous gastritis Rare: *Treponema pallidum, Actinomyces*	*Candida* *Aspergillus* *Phycomyces* *Histoplasma* *Blastomyces*	*Cryptosporidia* *Giardia*	*Anisakis marina* *Ascaris*

lesions and the infectious agents or their products. Selected special stains and immunocytochemical stains are often added to enhance the detection and to provide specificity. (See Chapter 2 for further details related to the general features and to the descriptions of the individual microorganisms.)

Viral Infections

In most cases designated as viral gastroenteritis, the lesion is solely present in the small intestine with no abnormalities noted in the stomach; such conditions should preferably be termed *viral enteritis.* In many inflammatory conditions involving all parts of the body, the patient may develop nausea and vomiting and upper abdominal pain as part of the constitutional symptoms, but such cases do not reveal abnormalities in the gastric tissues. Infections due to viruses are largely limited to patients with immunodeficiency, this due to either drugs or diseases.

Herpes Simplex

Infection due to herpes simplex is rare since the agents more characteristically involve the squamous epithelium, such as in the esophagus and anal canal.[158, 159] In immunocompromised patients, there is the rare appearance of herpes inclusions within gastric epithelial cells, mainly in the nuclei of pit or pyloric gland mucous cells. Biopsies reveal the characteristic intranuclear inclusions, and there is usually no associated ulceration or inflammation in the gastric cases (Fig. 2-15 and Plate 1A).

Cytomegalovirus

More often noted in immunocompromised patients are the presence of the inclusions of cytomegalovirus. These may occur alone or in association with ulceration.[160–163] When seen without necrosis, the inclusions are typically present in the epithelial cells, mainly in the gastric pits and in the pyloric glands (Fig. 4-24). In contrast, in cases with necrosis, the inclusions are more characteristically found in the mesenchymal cells, including endothelial cells and macrophages. The inclusions can be enhanced by immunocytochemical stains,[164] and are described in Chapter 2 (Fig. 2-17 and Plate 1B).

Helicobacter pylori Infection

H. pylori infection is probably the leading cause of chronic active gastritis involving the antrum, and also either a major cause or potentiating factor in the development of chronic peptic ulcers involving the stomach and the duodenum.[165–169] Limited human and animal transmission studies have shown the rapid development of a gastritis,[170, 171] but this is not a major form of clinical presentation. Rather, the patients appear with evidence of gastritis symptoms for a longer period, and biopsies disclose features of chronic as well as of active gastritis.[172]

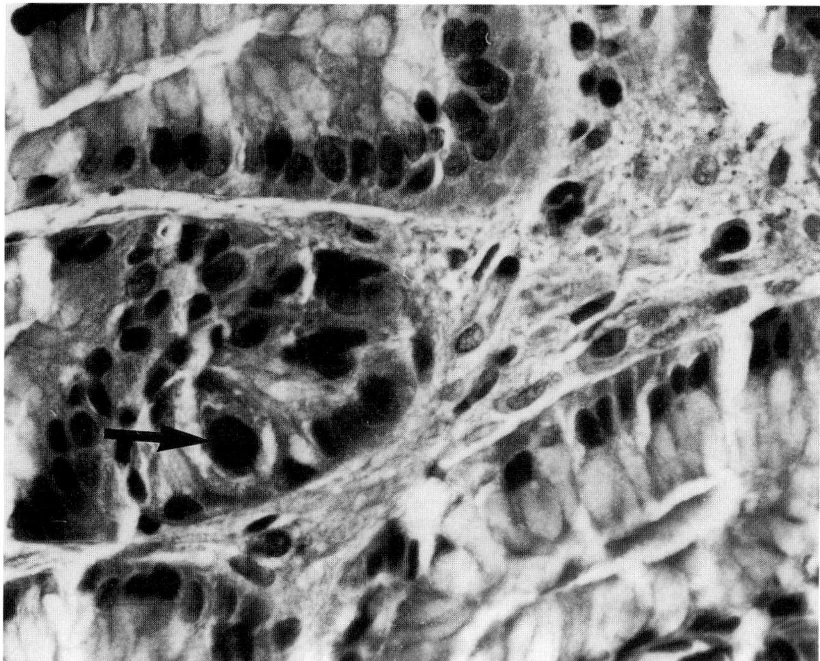

Fig. 4-24. Cytomeglovirus inclusion in the nuclei (arrow) of gastric antral mucous glands. This was an isolated finding without associated ulcer or inflammation (× 635).

Location of Organisms

The lesions invariably involve the antrum and may extend to affect the corpus and cardiac mucosae.[70, 76] The organisms are also found in areas of Barrett's esophagus and in cases with peptic duodenitis but only in association with their presence in the gastric antrum.[173, 174] It is believed that the gastric surface mucous cells possess receptors for the helicobacter, which are needed for their colonization.[175] This is the natural in the gastric antrum and probably, but to a lesser degree, in the corpus and cardia; in contrast, there must develop a gastric mucous cell metaplasia in the esophagus or duodenum before the bacteria appear in those sites.[176] The diagnosis of *H. pylori* infection involving the stomach is characteristically made by the biopsy showing the features of chronic active gastritis and by the identification of the organism.

The bacteria are readily seen at high magnification with the regular hematoxylin and eosin stain (Fig. 4-25); they are concentrated on the surface of the mucous cells and within the lumen of the gastric pits. Their appearance can be accented by histochemical stains, particularly the Giemsa stain and Dieterle's silver stain[177](Fig. 4-26 and Plate 1C), and also by immunocytochemical techniques.[178,179] By ultrastructural examination, they are mostly adherent to the luminal surface membranes of the mucous cells.[180–182] Other methods for their detection include simple smears of the gastric mucosa, measurement of urease production by the organisms, breath tests reflecting such urease activity, and specific antibody serologies.[183–185] The sensitivity can be further enhanced by the use of a polymerase chain reaction assay.[186]

Biopsy Features

The biopsies typically reveal evidence of a chronic active gastritis (see Fig. 4-13). The chronic features include an increase in the

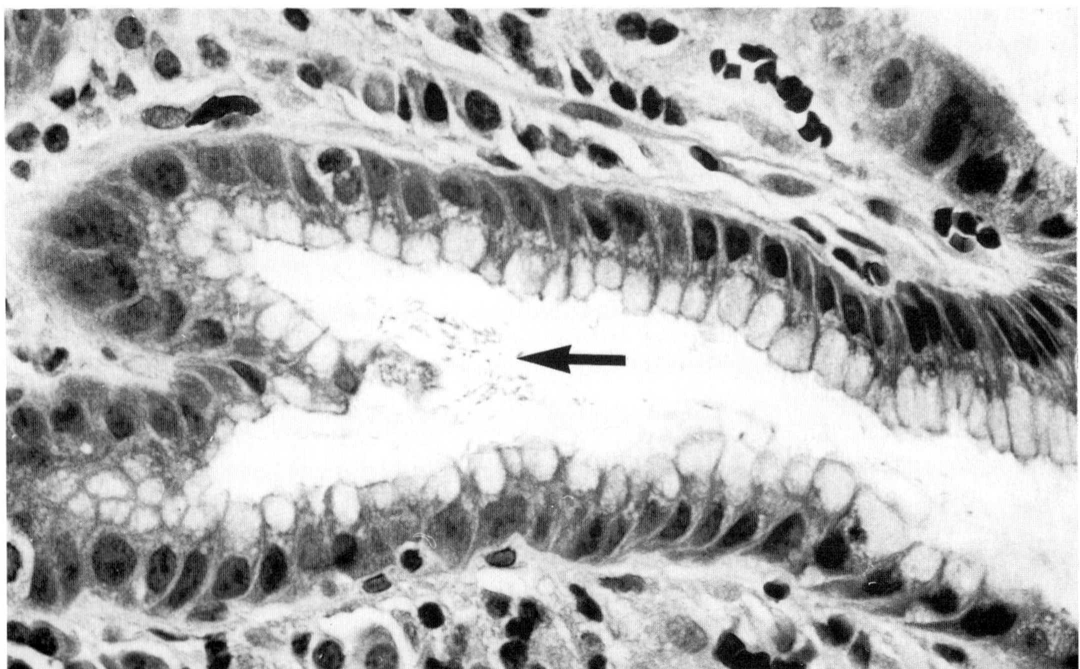

Fig. 4-25. *Helicobacter pylori* in gastric pits. There are many bacteria in the pit lumen in the center (arrow), seen with the H & E stain (× 635).

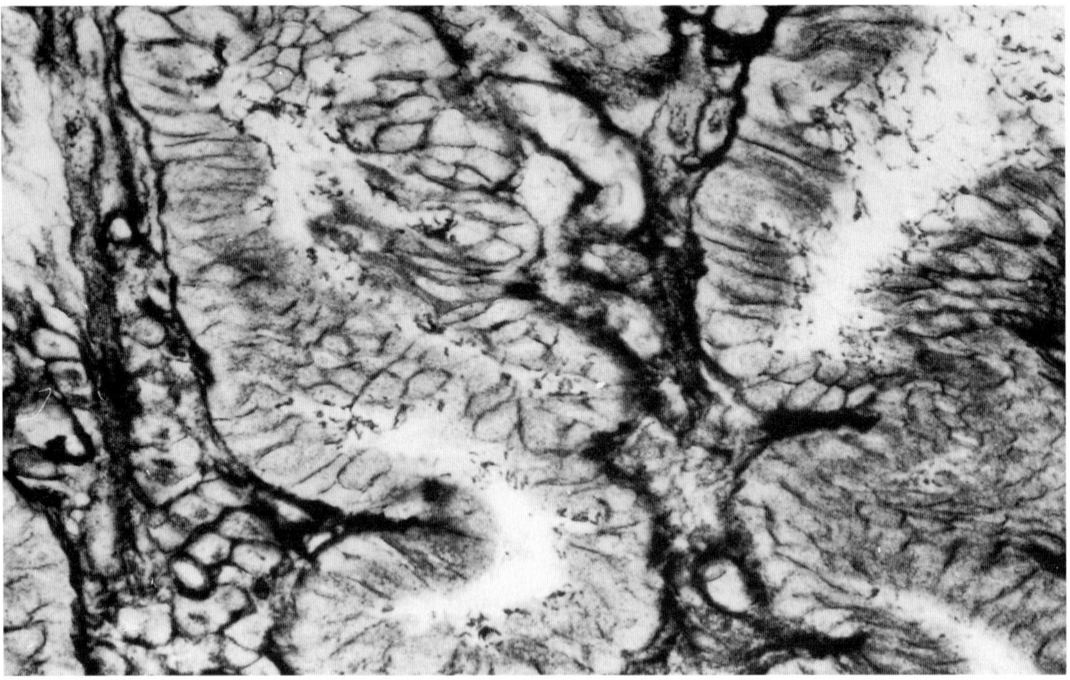

Fig. 4-26. *Helicobacter pylori* in gastric pits. The visualization of the bacteria is greatly enhanced by Dieterle's silver stain (× 635) (See Plate 1C).

amount of mononuclear inflammatory cells in the lamina propria and the presence of well formed lymphoid nodules with follicle centers[187–189] (see Fig. 4-15). The nodules tend to be concentrated in the lower portion of the mucosa. An increase of lymphocytes is also noted in the surface epithelial layer, but is distinguished from lymphocytic gastritis by its limitation to the antrum.[190] There is a variable amount of intestinal metaplasia. The features of active disease are in the form of damaged surface and pit mucous cells together with the presence of neutrophils, which occur as clusters within the lumen of the pits and extend into the epithelial cell area and into the region of the lamina propria[191–193] (see Fig. 4-14). A variable amount of eosinophils are often present as well, probably reflecting the chronic nature of the disease.

In cases showing the chronic features without the active inflammation, there are usually no bacteria present; these are considered cases in remission or of inactive chronic gastritis.[191, 194, 195] Occasionally noted are samples with bacteria but lacking the acute inflammation, and it has been estimated that this occurs in about 5 percent of the asymptomatic population.[196, 197] Whether these represent carriers or subclinical levels of chronic gastritis is not clear, but decisions on therapy are largely dictated by the presence of the neutrophils as evidence of injury to the mucosa.

Associated Conditions and Clinical Course

The presence of chronic active gastritis and of *H. pylori* is very common, and it is important in biopsies to exclude other associated or complicating conditions. For example, the bacteria have been seen in the mucosa adjacent to lesions of chronic peptic ulcer, of hyperplastic polyps, of early forms of gastric lymphoma, and of both dysplasia and carcinoma.[198–200] Despite the strong association, the exact relation of chronic *H. pylori* infection to the development of gastric neoplasia is not settled.[201, 202] A reduced frequency of infection is noted in patients with NSAID gastritis, with pernicious anemia, and with AIDS.[152, 203, 204]

Treatment with antibiotics and with bismuth compounds leads to the resolution of most cases of chronic active gastritis and the healing of peptic ulcers, as well as the elimination of the bacteria.[194, 195, 205] In such instances, mucosal biopsies are often obtained to evaluate the therapeutic response; there persist the features of the chronic gastritis but a diminution or absence of the active inflammation and bacteria.

Other Bacterial Infections

Gastrospirillum Hominis

Uncommonly noted in cases of chronic active gastritis is the presence of a longer spiral bacterium, *Gastrospirillum hominis,* which is thought to be the causative agent.[206–208] It is probably present in less than 1 percent of the cases, and the full behavior is not known. The organism has also been found in children and in normal persons.[209, 210] Because of their large size, the organisms can be readily appreciated with the routine H & E stain. Biopsy is otherwise similar to cases due to *H. pylori,* showing features of both chronic and of active gastritis.

Phlegmonous and Emphysematous Gastritis

Acute phlegmonous gastritis can be caused by a variety of staphlococcal and streptococcal agents, leading to extensive necrosis of the stomach and sloughing of the mucosa.[211, 212] Also rarely noted is acute emphysematous gastritis in which there is significant necrosis together with much gas-forming bacteria or with infarction.[213, 214]

These conditions are mainly limited to very debilitated or immunocompromised patients but are rarely seen in the modern antibiotic era.

Actinomycosis

Actinomycosis can affect immunocompromised patients, with lesions maximally in the distal ileum and colon. Infection is rarely seen in the stomach and is associated with extensive ulceration and neutrophils.[215] The diagnosis is dependent on the finding of the sulfur granules and long thin rods, best seen with the Gram stain.

Syphilis

Syphilitic infection of the stomach is generally rare,[216–218] but occurs more frequently in AIDS patients.[219] The lesion is characterized by a pronounced degree of fibrosis of the submucosa and a thickening of the inner lining with relatively little necrosis and no granuloma formation.[220] The diagnosis is dependent on a positive serology or stain for *Treponema pallidum* in the tissues.[221]

Mycobacterial Infections

M. tuberculosis is characteristically located in the distal ileum and in the colon. Gastric lesions reveal ulcerations and thickening of the mucosa, more striking in the antrum, together with well formed granulomas that typically show caseation.[222–224] The diagnosis depends on the finding of the organisms by acid-fast stain and confirmation by culture. More often seen in immunocompromised patients are infections due to *M. avium intracellulare.*[70, 225] These patients usually have less well formed granulomas without necrosis, but acid-fast stains reveal numerous organisms both within the macrophages and lying free in the lamina propria (Fig. 4-27 and Plate 1D). It is recommended that patients with severe immunocomprised disorders such as AIDS should routinely have acid-fast stains of mucosal biopsies to look for these organisms. (See "Infections" in Ch. 2 for further details about these infections.)

Fungal Infections

The presence of *Candida albicans* overlying ulcerative disorders of the stomach has been noted (Fig. 4-28 and Plate 1E), with the suggestion that this was enhanced since the appearance of potent H_2-blocking agents.[226, 227] It was thought that this might promote the ulcer disease, leading to deeper involvement and other complications, but this concept has not been confirmed. Additional infections by *Candida*[228, 229] and by other fungal agents including *Aspergillus*[230] and *Phycomyces*[231, 232] are rarely seen in the stomach and almost always limited to patients with a severe immunocompromised state (Plates 1F and 1G). The infections are usually associated with lesions in other parts of the alimentary tract, including the esophagus and the intestine. All of these fungal infections are associated with necrosis and prominent neutrophilic reaction; the specific diagnosis is provided by identification of the particular organism, enhanced by the use of the PAS reaction or the methenamine silver stain, and by culture. Infections by the pathogenic fungi, including *Histoplasma* and *Blastomyces,* are usually part of a more generalized infection.[233, 234] (See "Infections" in Ch. 2 for further details about these fungal infections and the features of the microorganisms.)

Parasitic Infections

Protozoa

Protozoal infections of the stomach are generally rare.[235] Noted in patients with AIDS is an extension of infection due to

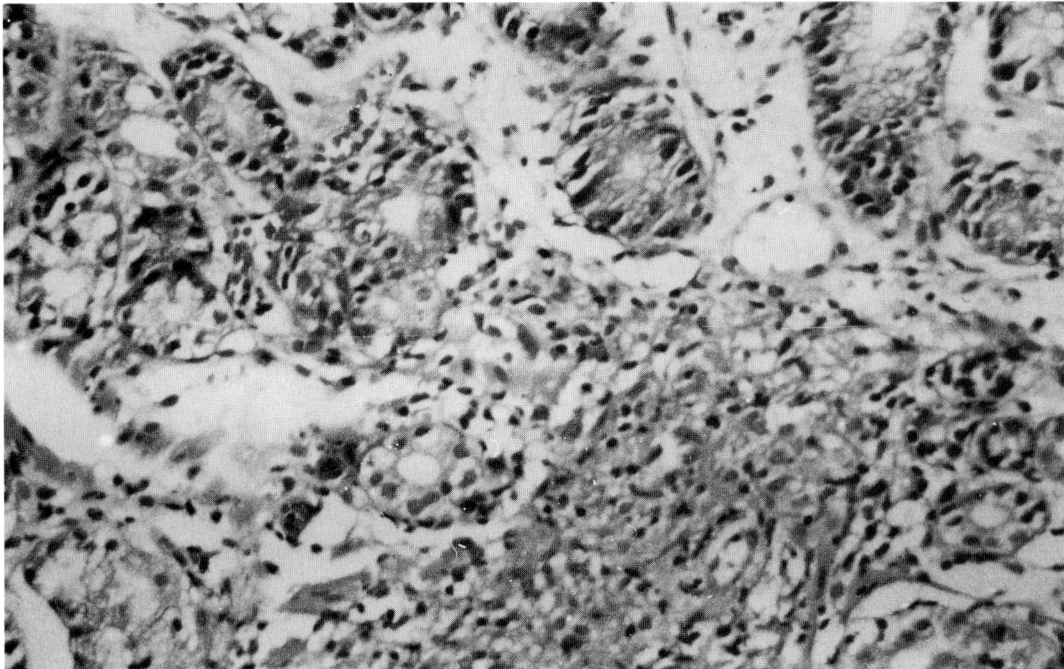

Fig. 4-27. Gastritis due to *Mycobacterium avium intracellulare.* There is a poorly formed granuloma in the lamina propria at the lower right. Acid-fast stain revealed numerous bacteria (see Plate 1D).

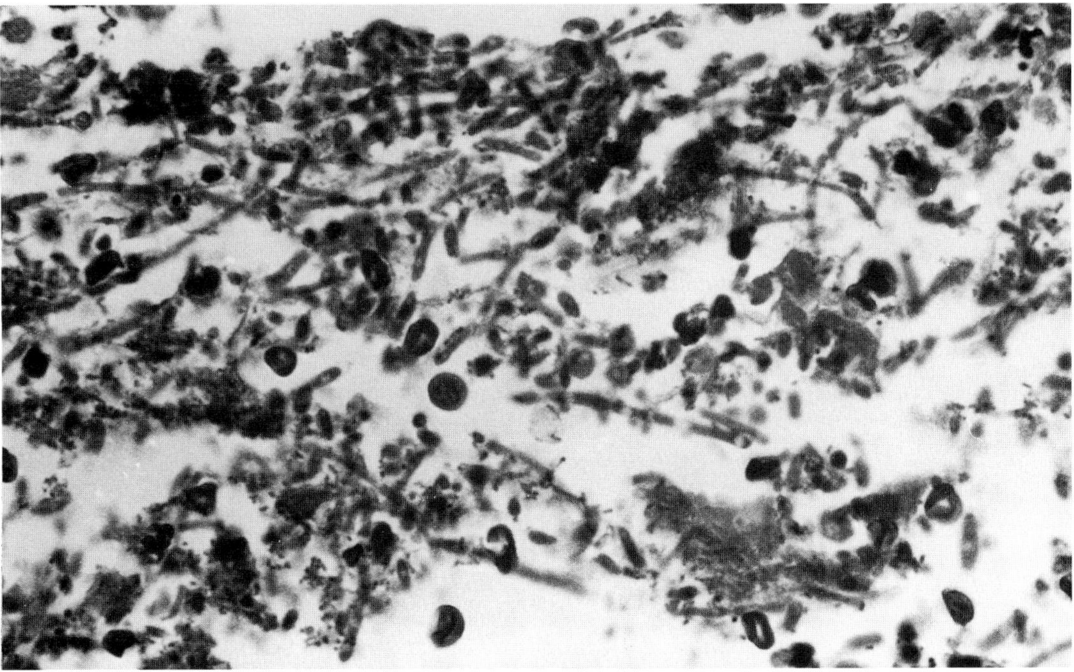

Fig. 4-28. Candidal infection of stomach, showing the characteristic spores and pseudohyphae in the exudate overlying an ulcer (methenamine silver stain; × 840) (see Plate 1E).

Cryptosporidia.[236, 237] This infection largely involves the small intestine in such patients (Plate 2B), but the organism may be found in the stomach and in the biliary tract as well. The organisms are seen as small spherical bodies attached to the surface membranes of the mucous cells. There is usually minimal or no necrosis or inflammation in these cases. It is probable that the functional effect is more directly related to the infection involving the small intestine. In immunocompetent persons, *Cryptosporidia* can cause an infection of the colon; this does not affect the stomach in such persons.

Rarely seen are *Giardia,* which may be enhanced in patients with reduced acid secretion.[238]

Helminths

The major helminthic infection that is encountered in the stomach is anisakiasis. *Anisakis marina* is a round worm whose ova can elicit a marked destructive and granulomatous reaction, mainly in the small intestine, that mimics Crohn's disease.[239, 240] Exceptionally, the adult worms can be located in the gastric mucosa and cause an ulceration and a localized inflammatory reaction.[241, 242] This probably develops soon after the ingestion of the uncooked fish. The diagnosis depends on the finding of segments of the worm.

There are also rare cases of *Ascaris*[243, 244] and *Necator*[245] present in the lumen, without effects on the gastric mucosa; and of amoebic infection in the stomach.[246]

IMMUNOLOGIC DISORDERS

Included in this section are those disorders affecting the stomach in which the injury is a result of a primary immunologic effect.

Pernicious Anemia/Atrophic Gastritis

Definition and Pathogenesis

This is the entity of chronic fundic gastritis, which is due to a primary immunologic injury of the specialized glands in that area.[70, 86] Over time, there is the destruction and eventual loss of the parietal and chief cells, resulting in a generalized atrophy of the area and the functional state of primary pernicious anemia. The anemia results from the loss of the intrinsic factor that is located in the membranes of the human parietal cells, resulting ultimately in inadequate B_{12} absorption. The diagnosis is typically suspected by noting the marked anemia in an older patient, characterized by megaloblastosis, and typically confirmed by the *Schilling test.* The patients also have an absence of gastric acid secretion, both at the basal and stimulated levels.

The exact immunologic mechanism has not been established. Antibodies to the parietal cells can be detected both within the gastric lumen and in the serum, but these are thought to be of a secondary nature. Associated in some of these patients are chronic injury and atrophy affecting other endocrine organs, particularly the thyroid and the adrenal cortex.[247, 248]

Location and Gross Features

At one time, this was referred to as *type A gastritis* and distinguished from the antral form, which was called *type B,* with the impression that immunologic factors were responsible for the fundic and environmental factors for the antral forms.[79] It is now evident that there may be a mixture, related either to extension of one type to the other area or of different etiologies affecting both regions.[80] In the classical form of primary pernicious anemia due to the chronic fundic gastritis, the disease may ultimately extend into the antrum, whereas chronic active *H. pylori* infection starting in the antrum may eventually move into the corpus.

As a result of the atrophy, gross endoscopic examination may reveal reduced or absent rugae in the fundus and corpus and the easy visibility of the submucosal vessels through the thin mucosa. There are typically no erosions or ulcers because of the lack of gastric acid; if such occur one should suspect the development of a complication such as a tumor or some other superimposed disease. Other gross alterations that may be present include the appearance of xanthomas secondary to localized hemorrhages, and of hyperplastic polyps representing focal nodules of inflammatory and regenerative mucosa. (See "Complications of Chronic Gastritis" above and Ch. 5 for discussions.)

Stages and Biopsy Features

These cases have also been referred to as *chronic atrophic gastritis,* but it should be appreciated that this is a generic term that can be applied to any form of gastritis. Based on the evolution of the lesions, cases of chronic fundic gastritis are separated into the following three stages: superficial inflammation with partial glandular atrophy; transmucosal inflammation with marked atrophy; and gastric atrophy showing total loss of glands and minimal inflammation.

The biopsy abnormalities are primarily in the fundic and corpus regions.[69–72] The earlier lesions show inflammation mainly of mononuclear cells involving the superficial mucosa between the gastric pits, and only mild and patchy loss of the specialized glands and cells (Fig. 4-29). In the advanced lesions there is diffuse loss of the specialized glands throughout the corpus and fundus, and their replacement by a mixture of intestinal and pyloric gland metaplasia together with hyperplasia of the gastric pits (Fig. 4-30). Although the biopsies may show the glandular atrophy, one needs a functional estimate to appreciate the widespread effect throughout the corpus and fundic mucosa, which is readily evident by the observed megaloblastosis and low acid secretion.

Also evident are marked increases in the amount of mononuclear inflammatory cells and of eosinophils together with numerous enlarged lymphoid nodules. There is usually only scant fibrosis in the mucosa. Active inflammation in the form of degeneration of gastric pits together with neutrophilic infiltrate is relatively slight and limited to the superficial regions. There may also be proliferation of the neuroendocrine cells, involving mainly the indigenous ECL cells but occasionally the EC cells in areas of intestinal metaplasia. (See "Chronic Gastritis" above for details.)

The biopsy features in the antrum are highly variable. They are most often normal except for the effects of aging but may reveal hyperplasia of the G cells due to the low acid secretion (see Fig. 4-16), extension of the primary disease into the antrum, or an antral gastritis due to some other cause. Of interest, cases of *H. pylori* infection are reduced in patients with pernicious anemia.[203]

Clinical Course

Mucosal biopsy is largely employed in cases of chronic fundic gastritis to evaluate for complications, particularly to survey patients for the development of glandular dysplasia and of early adenocarcinoma.[117–120, 249–252] As noted above, patients who develop dysplasia and carcinoma are more apt to have associated intestinal metaplasia of the incomplete or colonic type, but this feature is so common that it does not select cases that need surveillance. At the present time, only patients in countries with a higher prevalence of gastric carcinoma are involved with such surveillance programs, which look for the features of dysplasia in the glands. (This topic is primarily presented in Ch. 5.)

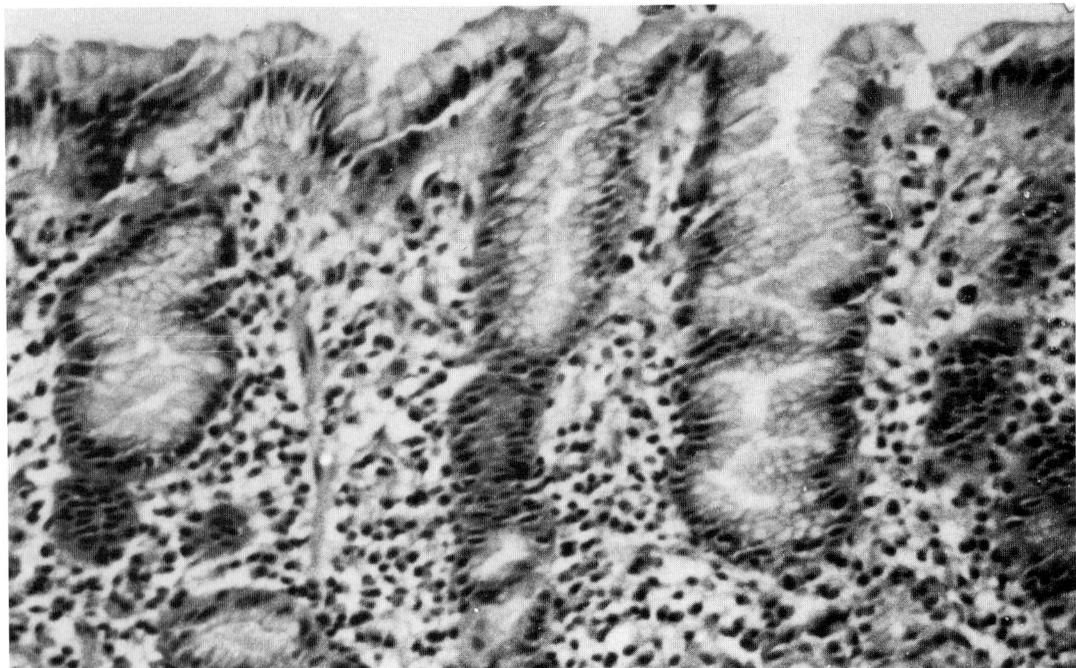

Fig. 4-29. Chronic superficial gastritis of corpus mucosa (surface at top). Increase of mononuclear inflammatory cells in the lamina propria but only minimal damage to the specialized glands (not shown). Gastric pits are normal.

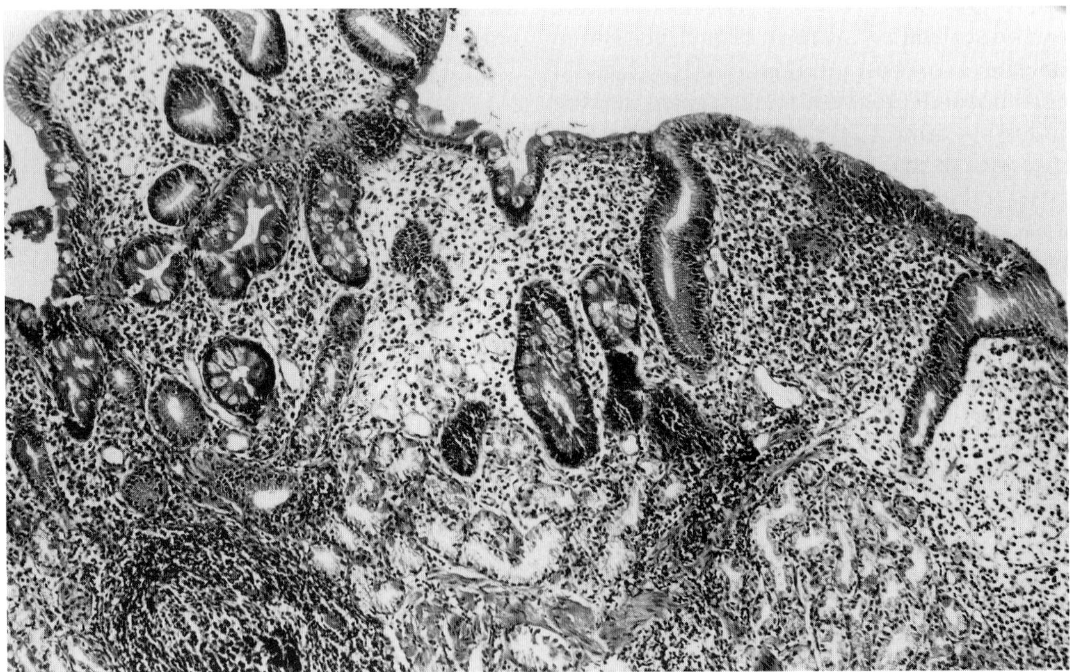

Fig. 4-30. Chronic atrophic gastritis of corpus mucosa. Total loss of the specialized glands associated with the presence of intestinal metaplasia (left), elongated pits and pyloric glands (right), and prominent lymphoid nodule (left bottom) (× 105).

Allergic (Eosinophilic) Gastroenteritis

Allergic or eosinophilic gastroenteritis is more commonly seen in children and young adults, presenting with iron-deficiency anemia due to bleeding, with protein loss due to oozing lesions, and occasionally with signs of malabsorption.[253–255] The lesions are more prominent in the upper portions of the gut from esophagus to small intestine and are especially marked in the gastric antrum (Table 4-11.) Practically all cases of allergic gastroenteritis affect the gastric antrum, and the lesions in this area are usually very striking.[256] Prominent lesions are also noted in the esophageal and small intestinal mucosa, whereas there is usually no involvement or only mild disease in the gastric corpus and large intestine.[257]

Grossly, there can be hypertrophic folds or vesicles, typically concentrated in the antrum, which are visualized by radiographic and gross endoscopic examinations.[258] Biopsies reveal marked infiltrate by eosinophils of the lamina propria and of the gastric pit and surface epithelium (Fig. 4-31). The lesions are not entirely specific, since prominent eosinophils can also be noted in any chronic disorder, including patients with chronic peptic ulcers. Nevertheless, the finding in a young person of gastritis with a pronounced amount of eosinophils should alert one to the possibility of an allergic disorder. In such cases, the peripheral eosinophil count is often elevated as well. In children this is an important distinction, since both celiac disease and allergic gastroenteritis can result in an abnormal small intestinal mucosa; in such cases, biopsy of the gastric antrum can be discriminatory since it typically shows alterations in allergic disease, whereas it is usually normal or shows only increased lymphocytes in celiac disease.

Other Immunologic Effects

In acute graft-versus-host disease, lesions can develop in the alimentary tract and are ordinarily most pronounced in the small intestine.[259, 260] Focal lesions can occur in the stomach, as revealed by mononuclear cell increases adjacent to and within the surface epithelial layer. The features are nonspecific and are not usually the cause of a significant gastritis. As noted above, immunocompromised patients are also subject to a large variety of opportunistic infections.

PHYSICAL DISORDERS

Radiation Injury

This topic is discussed in Chapter 2 (see Table 2-11) and the findings are briefly summarized here. Low-dose radiotherapy had been tried to reduce the parietal cell mass in cases of peptic ulcer but proved to be ineffective.[261] More sustained damage to the stomach can result from larger quantities of radiation, typically in the form of radiotherapy alone or together with chemotherapeutic agents.[262–264] Noted in the acute stage are edema and variable ulceration, which may proceed to granulation tissue and fibrosis (see Fig. 2-22).[265, 266] The naturally narrow areas

Table 4-11. Mucosal Biopsy in Allergic Gastroenteritis*

Tissue	Cases (%)	Positive (%)	Marked Change (%)
Esophagus	39	60	53
Gastric corpus	55	52	10
Gastric antrum	58	100	73
Small intestine	89	79	12
Rectum	21	13	0

* Modified from Goldman and Proujansky.[257]

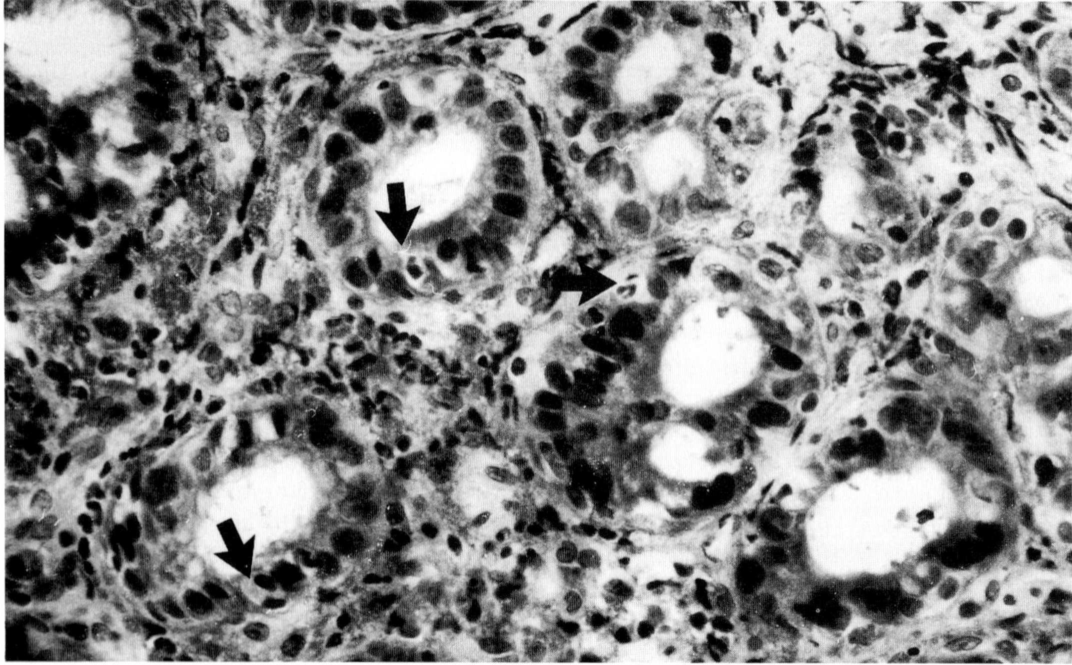

Fig. 4-31. Allergic gastroenteritis in the antral mucosa. There is a marked infiltrate of esoinophils in the lamina propria that extends into the epithelial layer of the gastric pits (arrows) (× 425).

of the cardia and pylorus are potentially subject to stenosis. Overall, lesions due to radiation are rarely a major problem in the stomach. Biopsies may be performed to identify the lesion but are more often aimed at excluding opportunistic infections or recurrent tumor.

Gastric Freezing

At one time, the installation of ice solutions was used to damage the parietal cell mass, in an effort to reduce acid secretion in patients who were poor risks for surgery.[267, 268] This resulted in temporary injury to the parietal cells, but there was ultimately restoration of the function. This technique is no longer applied, and mucosal biopsies were never of use.

Trauma and Foreign Bodies

Endoscopy may be performed to determine the presence or extent of traumatic lesions and to identify and help extricate any foreign materials.[269, 270] There may develop secondary ulcerations and fibrotic strictures, for which biopsy can be employed to identify their nature.

ULCER DISEASES

Most of the cases of acute and of chronic gastritis can be associated with ulceration. This section deals with those disorders in which the ulcers are the major and constant event.

Acute Stress Ulcer

Acute stress ulcers are those that develop following a major stressful situation, such as significant trauma, intracranial increase of pressure, a large burn of the body, and probably any shock situation.[62, 63, 271] The pathogenesis is thought to be a reduction in blood flow that, coupled with acid secretion, leads to the ulcerations. As noted above, these same situations can be associated with patchy hemorrhages and more superficial erosions (see "Ischemic Lesions" under "Vascular Disorders" for details).

Gross and Clinical Features

The ulcers are often multiple and may involve any portion of the stomach including both the corpus and antrum, and they also frequently affect the proximal portion of the duodenum. Although usually superficial, they may exceptionally perforate. The ulcers lead to major hemorrhage in patients who are already very sick, particularly those with coagulopathy or pulmonary problems, and this can be a critical or terminal event.[272] The diagnosis is largely established by the clinical situation, and endoscopy may be done to provide confirmation and to rule out other causes of hemorrhage.

Histologic Features

Mucosal biopsies are not ordinarily obtained. From studies of specimens, the expected findings are localized hemorrhagic infarctions of the mucosa that can lead to ulceration with little inflammation in the early stages.[64] In the reparative phase, there are neutrophils and prompt cellular renewal. Since the lesions are typically superficial, later findings of granulation tissue and fibrosis do not ordinarily occur. There are also no features of chronicity that help to distinguish acute ulcers from chronic peptic ulcer disease. The differential diagnosis mainly includes other types of acute gastritis due to chemicals, drugs, and stress situations.

Chronic Peptic Ulcer

Chronic peptic ulcer is a major cause of ulceration that affects the gastric antrum and the first portion of the duodenum.

Pathogenesis

The pathogenesis appears to be different in the two areas, with chronic active gastritis largely due to *H. pylori* in the stomach,[165–169] and probably the dominance of a hypersecretory state in the initial lesions of the duodenum.[273] In either case, the bacterium is present in over three-quarter of the cases and is thought to play at least a potentiating role. An increased frequency of chronic peptic ulcers is noted in many conditions, including chronic pulmonary disease, uremia, and hyperparathyroidism.[274–276] The lesions are chronic, and activation of the ulcers may also be associated with the ingestion of drugs such as aspirin or NSAID.

Gross Features

The ulcers are usually single and confined to the gastric antrum or the first part of the duodenum.[271] They may be of any size and usually reveal sharply demarcated edges that may be slightly raised. There are often signs of more diffuse inflammation in the form of hemorrhages and friability throughout the mucosa.

Endoscopic examination and biopsy are commonly obtained in patients with chronic ulcers of the stomach, mainly to distinguish between a benign peptic ulcer and a malignant tumor with secondary ulceration. It is recommended in such cases that at least four to five mucosal biopsies and brush cytology be obtained, which permits the detection of practically all malignant tumors[251, 252, 277–279] (Fig. 4-32).

Biopsy Features

Except for the presence of *H. pylori* in most cases, the histologic features are generally nonspecific and reflect the chronic and active nature of the lesions.[280] Revealed are a mixture of necrosis in the central ulcer area; acute and chronic inflammation together

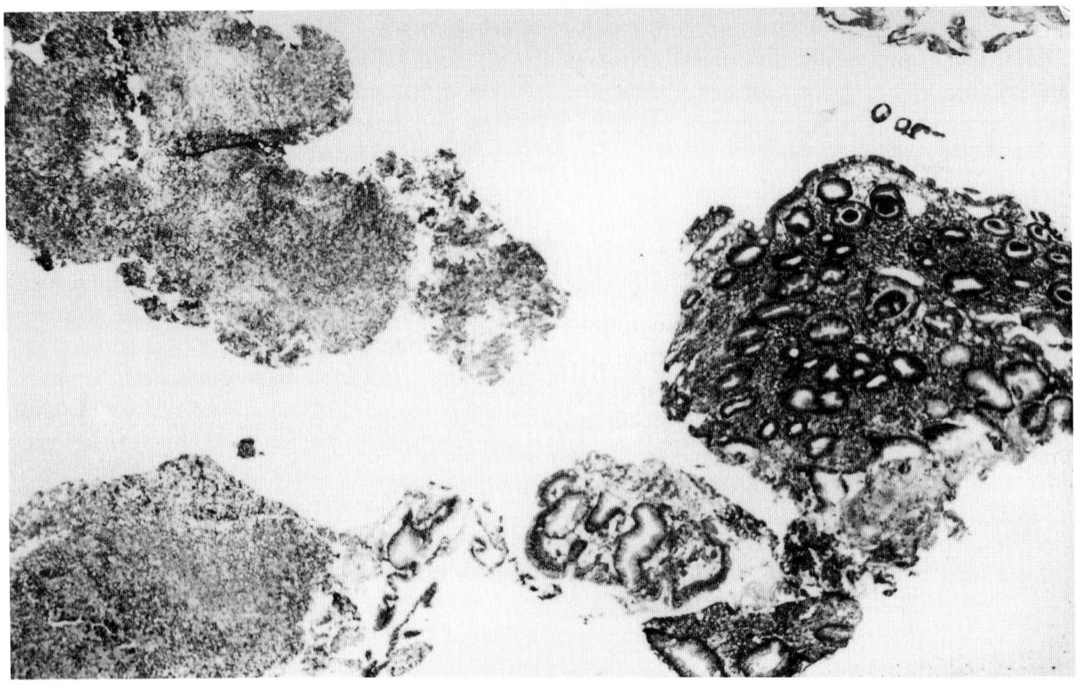

Fig. 4-32. Multiple mucosal biopsies taken from a chronic ulcer in the stomach. Included are samples from the necrotic area (left) and from the adjacent mucosa (right).

with glandular regeneration in the ulcer edges; and granulation tissue and fibrosis at the base of the ulcer[281] (Figs. 4-33 and 4-34). Also present are the other features of chronic gastritis including prominent mononuclear cells and metaplasia.[282]

Biopsies from the peripheral portion of the ulcer should be included to capture the adjacent mucosa. This helps to distinguish between the acute ulcers and chronic peptic ulcer.[156, 157] In the latter, the mucosa invariably shows evidence of chronic inflammation in the form of increased mononuclear inflammatory cells and prominent intestinal metaplasia. Biopsies of the edges of acute ulcers of whatever cause, but mainly related to drug ingestion, usually show sparse or no inflammation. As noted previously, some cases of peptic ulcer develop fungal overgrowth, particularly of *Candida,* and it is possible that this leads to greater destruction in such cases.[226, 227]

In the biopsy samples of chronic peptic ulcers, there should be considerable caution to avoid overrating some of the inflammatory changes. In particular, there can be very exuberant granulation tissue containing vessels with enlarged endothelial cells. The glandular tissue at the edge of the ulcer shows prominent regeneration together with ongoing damage to these cells, resulting in a very tattered appearance to the gastric pits. Nevertheless, the regenerative nature can be appreciated by noting that the enlarged nuclei are practically of all the same size and shape as well as position within the cell (cf. Fig. 4-19). In addition, the nuclei tend to have very fine chromatin and large central nucleoli, in contrast to dysplastic cell nuclei that are more irregular and hyperchromatic. There has been a tendency in the past to rate many of these samples as showing epithelial atypism or even designating such cases as mild dysplasia, but this practice should be

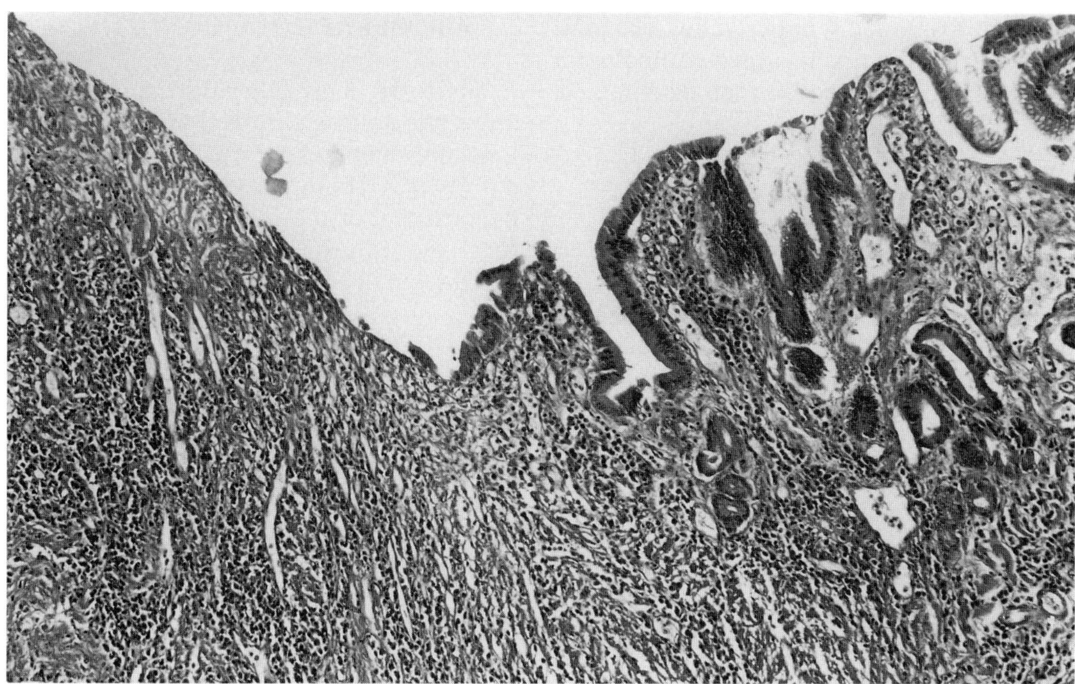

Fig. 4-33. Chronic peptic ulcer of the gastric antrum. Under the ulcer base appearing at the left is prominent granulation tissue and fibrosis. The adjacent mucosa appearing at the right is markedly inflamed (× 105).

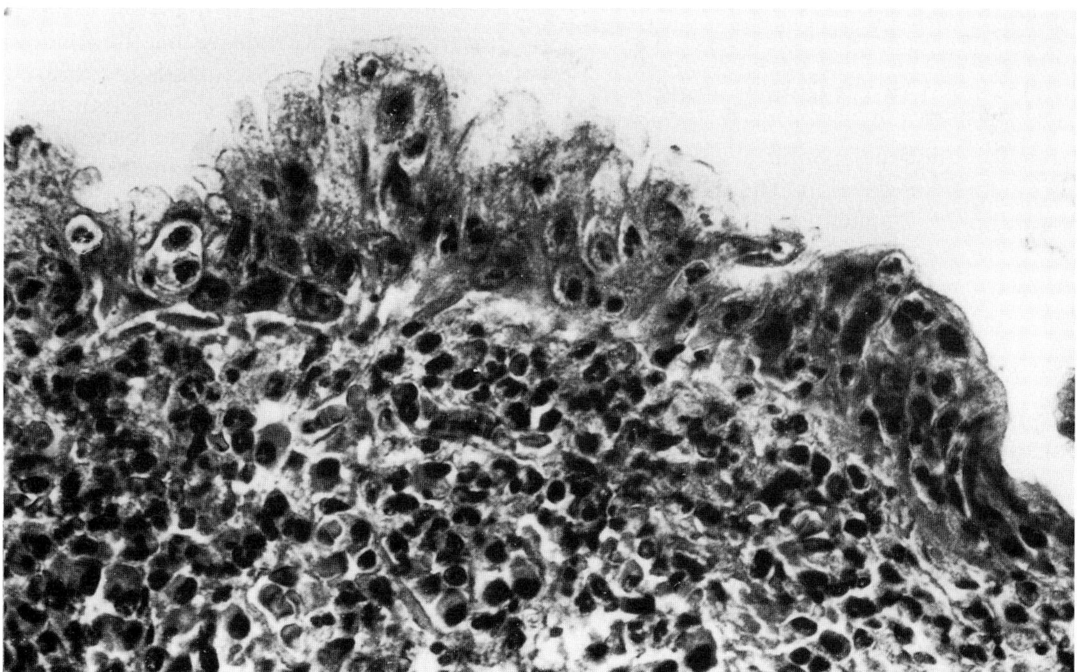

Fig. 4-34. Edge of chronic peptic ulcer of the stomach, showing marked inflammation in lamina propria with many plasma cells; and epithelial layer with signs of degeneration and regeneration together with neutrophilic infiltrate (× 680).

avoided. Overall, it is important to recognize that regeneration is an expected finding; if needed, additional biopsies can be obtained.

Associated Conditions and Complications

Aside from the overt ulcers, peptic disease can be associated with a more diffuse injury and inflammation, mainly involving the distal esophagus and proximal duodenum; these entities are discussed in Chapters 2 and 6. More extensive peptic disease and ulceration can occur in patients with hypergastrinemia, whether due to retained antrum or to hyperplasia or neoplasia of the G cells.[283] In such cases injury, including ulceration, can be found in more distal portions of the duodenum and jejunum, but the proximal stomach still remains relatively immune to the action of the acid.

Endoscopy and biopsy can also help in the evaluation of complications of peptic ulcer disease, such as hemorrhage, obstruction, and penetration into adjacent organs. The samples may reveal tissue from the liver or spleen.[284, 285] Following distal gastric resection for duodenal peptic ulcer, recurrence is low but can develop. The ulcers typically occur on the jejunal side of the gastrojejunostomy stoma. These lesions can be readily seen by radiographic and gross endoscopic examinations, and biopsies are usually not obtained.

Overall, endoscopy and biopsies are performed in patients with chronic peptic ulcer of the stomach to confirm the presence of the lesions, to distinguish them from tumors, to detect complications, and to follow the patients after therapy. It is not thought that the lesion of chronic peptic ulcer is premalignant, but the underlying state of chronic active gastritis is such a condition that may require further surveillance.

MISCELLANEOUS CONDITIONS

There are many other disorders that can affect the stomach, either singly or in conjunction with other parts of the gastrointestinal tract.[286] Those diseases associated with hypertrophy of the mucosa, including both focal and diffuse conditions, are presented in Chapter 5.

DEPOSITIONS

Amyloidosis

In the systemic form of amyloidosis, including both primary and secondary cases, the amyloid is commonly deposited in the gastrointestinal tract.[287, 288] This occurs particularly in the walls of small vessels within the submucosa, and aspiration biopsy of the rectal mucosa is frequently obtained in such cases.[289] It has been noted as well that the amyloid can be found in the upper portions of the tract, including the stomach, and positive yields are especially high in sites of ulcerations.[67, 290–292] It is probable that the amyloid involvement of the vessels leads to localized vascular compromise and the ulceration, resulting in selected areas for the biopsy.

The amyloid material is characteristic, revealing acellular pink material that appears fractured (cf. Fig. 9-46). It is concentrated in the walls of small vessels in the submucosa at the base of the ulcers, and exceptionally extends in a more diffuse fashion into the surrounding tissues. Specificity is provided by demonstrating green birefrigence in Congo Red–stained sections (Plate 4D); or by recognizing the specific fibrils and their measurements by ultrastructural examination (Fig. 4-35).[293, 294]

Rarely noted are diffuse areas of edema in the lamina propria that may stain deeply eosinophilic and initially resemble amyloid (Fig. 4-36). This can be readily excluded by the special stains.

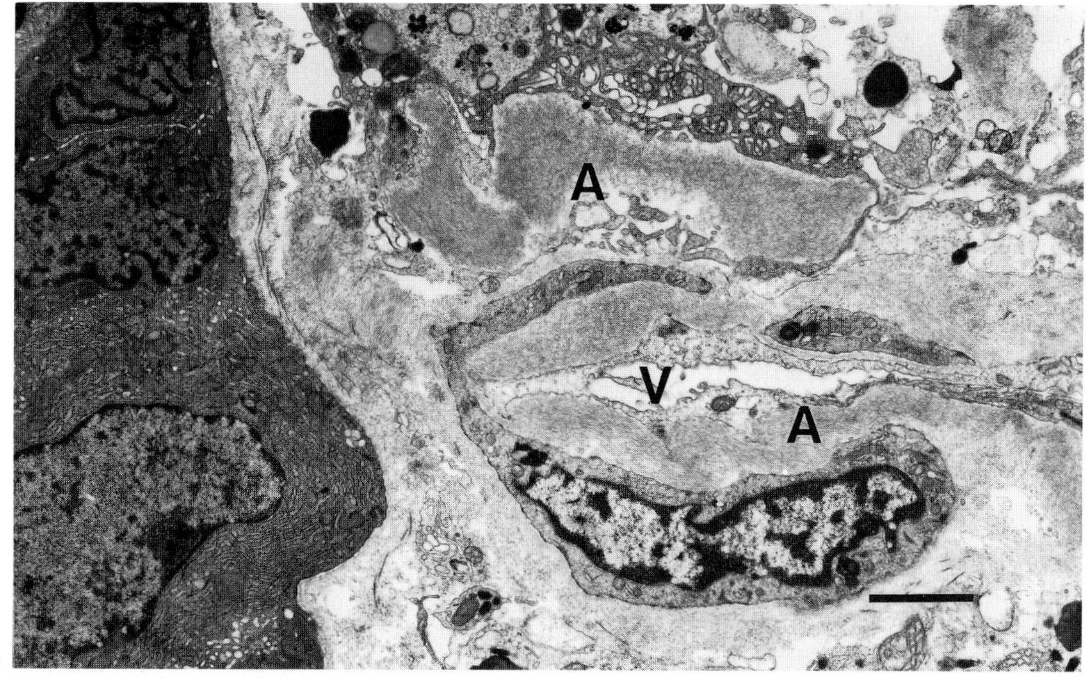

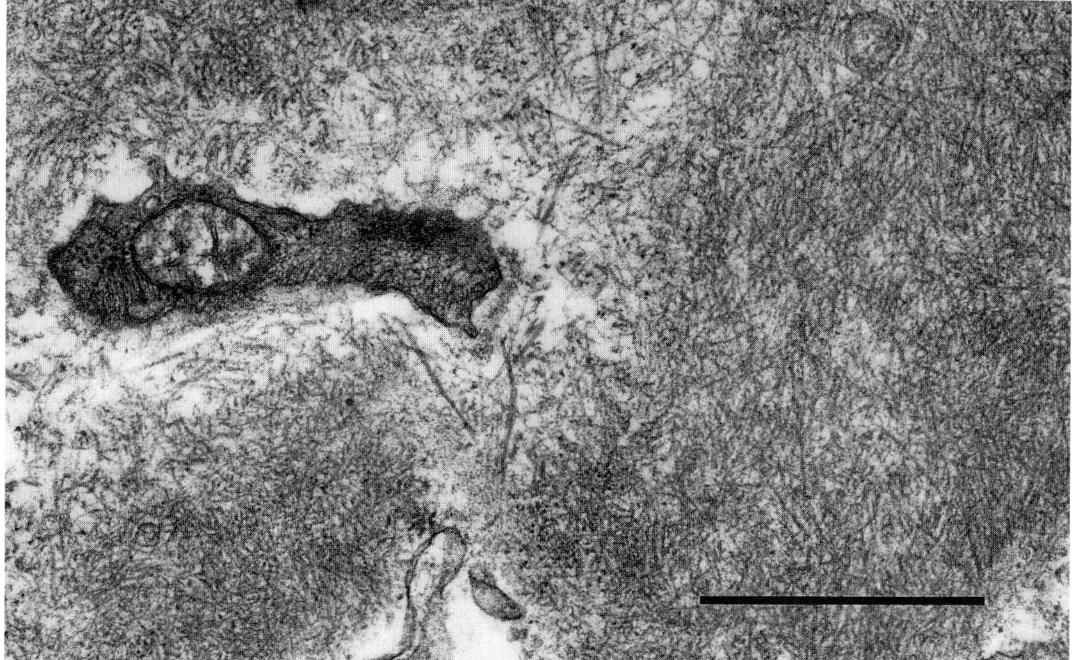

Fig. 4-35. Electron micrographs of amyloidosis from a bowel biopsy. **(A)** Large areas of amyloid (A) adjacent to vascular space (V) below epithelial cells (× 6,700; bar = 2 μm). **(B)** Higher magnification of amyloid fibrils that are disoriented, measure an average 10 nm in diameter, and are of variable length (× 37,500; bar = 1 μm).

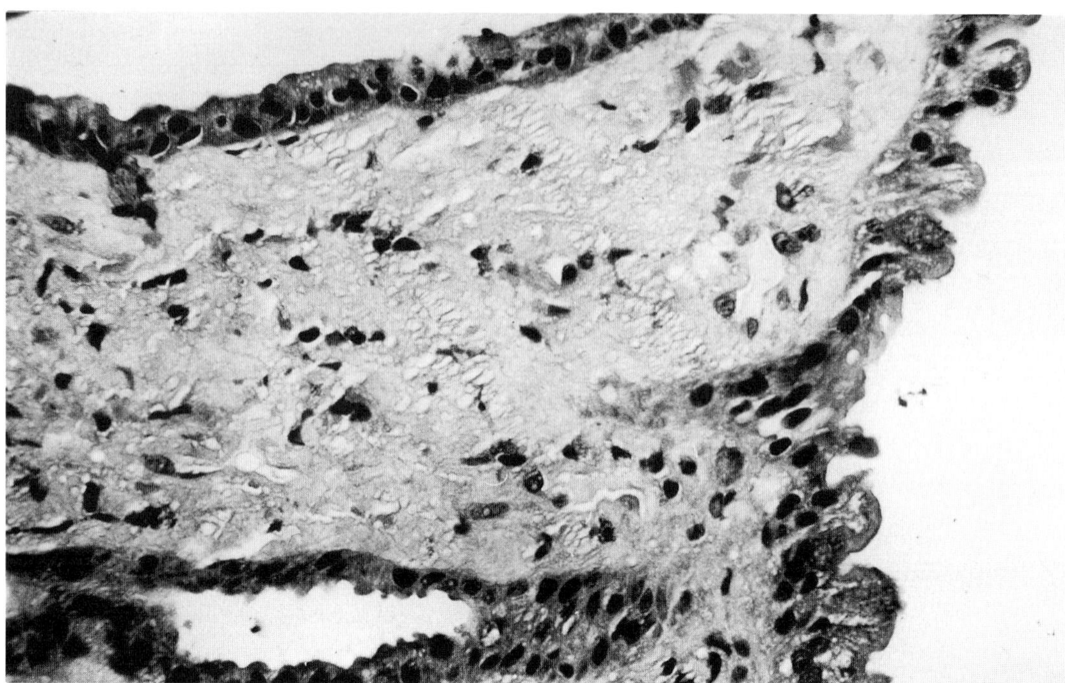

Fig. 4-36. Marked edema of the lamina propria in the gastric mucosa, with the surface appearing at the right. The appearance of the fluid may be unusually eosinophilic and condensed, resembling other proteinaceous substances such as amyloid.

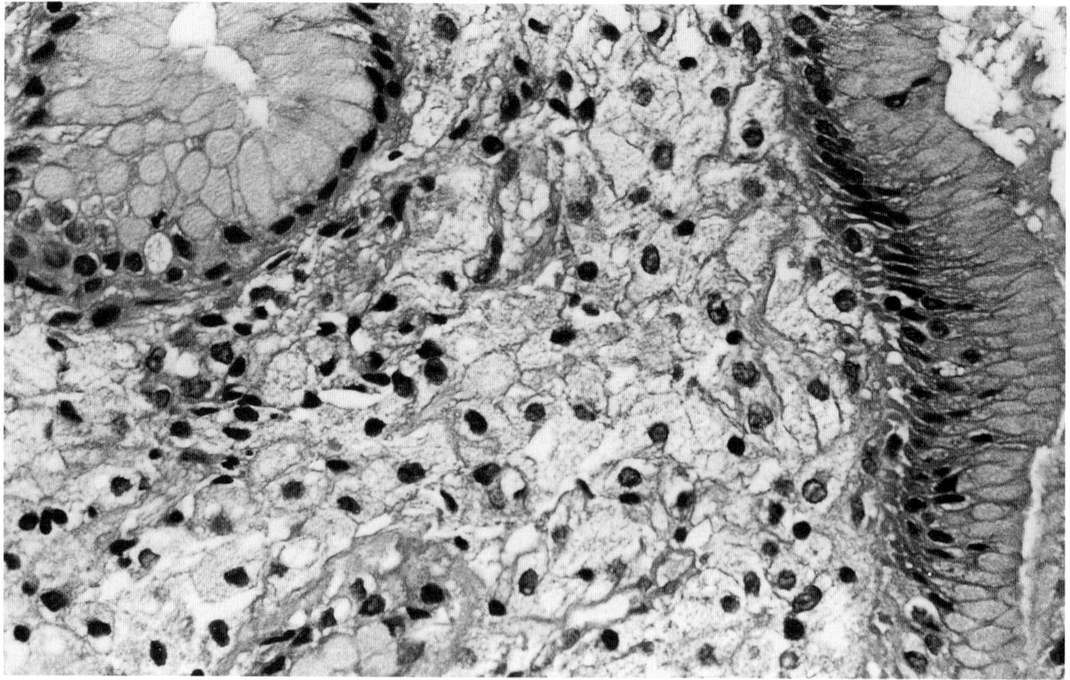

Fig. 4-37. Xanthoma of gastric mucosa. The lamina propria is mainly composed of macrophages with foamy cytoplasm and small nuclei. There is no damage of the gastric pits (× 425).

Xanthoma (Xanthelasma)

These are small, barely raised yellow nodules that are found on the surface of the mucosa.[113–115] They represent localized collections of macrophages that are filled with neutral lipids, and are mainly a consequence of prior hemorrhage. They are more often seen in cases with gastric remnants.

Biopsies are done to confirm the lesions, revealing closely packed clusters of foamy macrophages in the lamina propria and absence of other inflammation (Fig. 4-37). The differential principally includes macrophages and epithelial cells with other vacuolated material such as mucin, which appear as more irregular and larger granules; this can be selectively stained if there is doubt.

Histiocytosis

Cases of Langerhans' cell histiocytosis uncommonly affect the stomach, presenting with tiny nodules of macrophage-like cells in the lamina propria.[295, 296] Contained with the cytoplasm are pigmented, lipofuscin-like material. The exact nature of the cells as Langerhans' type can be determined by selective immunohistochemical stains and particularly by the ultrastructure detection of Birbeck granules (Fig. 4-38). An example of benign and reversible histiocytosis was also reported in the stomach.[297] Other disorders that can be associated with such localized collections of pigment-containing cells include chronic granulomatous disease and some rare metabolic disorders; these are more typically present in the colonic mucosa and are associated with other features (see "Granulomatous Diseases" below).

Cases of the chronic form of histiocytosis, termed *eosinophilic granuloma,* can also be seen in the stomach. They usually appear as localized lesions in the gastric wall and ordinarily are not accessed by mucosal biopsy.

Mineral Deposits

Increases in iron within the macrophages in the lamina propria are noted in cases with hemosiderosis, and major deposition of iron in the parietal cells is noted in patients with hemochromatosis[298] (Plate 4A). Ulcers can also show depositions of calcium, ranging from scattered granules to diffuse plaques, which has been termed *calcinosis*[299] (Fig. 4-39). These appear to be more common in patients with chronic renal disease but are not absolutely related to the level of the serum calcium.

Granulomatous Diseases

There are many disorders that can be associated with granulomas in the gastric mucosa[70, 300] (Table 4-12). These tend to be concentrated in the antral portion, resulting in a thickened mucosa and occasional stenosis of the pyloric region. This can be confused with diffuse tumor, but the diagnosis of the granulomatous lesion is readily made by the mucosal biopsy.

Isolated Granulomatous Gastritis

Isolated granulomatous gastritis is the most common form of granulomatous disorder affecting the stomach.[301–304] It tends to occur in older persons with an insidious onset, leading to partial gastric obstruction. Biopsy reveals many granulomas without necrosis, and special studies fail to demonstrate a particular etiology (Fig. 4-40). The lesions

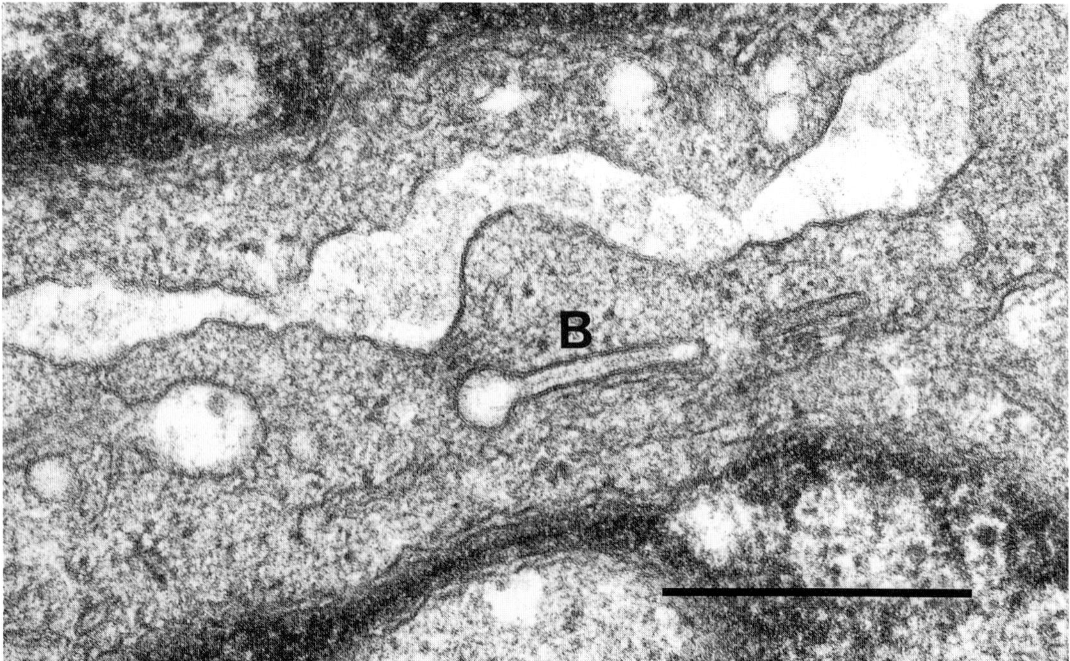

Fig. 4-38. Electron micrograph showing a Birbeck granule (B), which is characteristic and unique to the Langerhans' histiocytes, both normal and neoplastic. The rod-shaped structure is of variable length, has a core with periodicity, and one end is often dilated (× 81,000; bar = 0.5 μm).

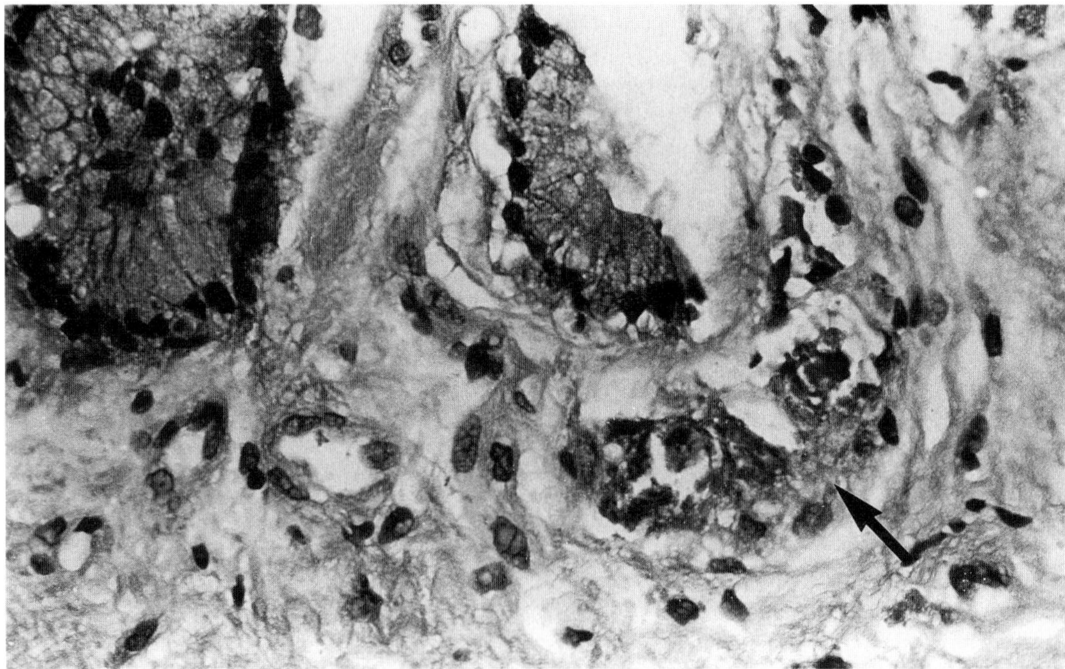

Fig. 4-39. Calcinosis of the stomach. Noted is a deposit of calcium in the base of the mucosa (arrow) (× 560).

Table 4-12. Granulomatous Diseases of the Stomach

Isolated granulomas
Sarcoidosis
Crohn's disease
Infections
Tuberculosis
Mycobacterium avium
Histoplasmosis
Foreign body reaction
Rare
Whipple's disease
Malakoplakia
Lymphoma

usually last for a few months and ultimately resolve without specific therapy.[305] It is important not to ascribe granulomas of the stomach to any particular cause unless there is solid evidence, considering this condition with reversible granulomas.

Crohn's Disease

Crohn's disease can affect any part of the alimentary tract, showing ulcers, granulomas, or fistulae within the stomach.[306, 307] However, isolated involvement to this area is very rare,[308] and one should seek evidence of disease in a more common spot such as in the intestines. Biopsies of the cases with Crohn's disease usually show just nonspecific inflammation, with or without ulceration, but granulomas without necrosis are exceptionally found[309–311] (Fig. 4-41).

Sarcoidosis

Sarcoidosis rarely affects the gastrointestinal tract. In the stomach[312–314] there can be multiple granulomas without necrosis (Fig. 4-42), but the diagnosis depends on the finding of classical lesions in some other areas, such as in the lungs, hilar lymph nodes, or liver. Gastric sarcoidosis mainly affects the antrum, and the lesions are identical to those seen in isolated granulomas of the stomach.

Chronic Granulomatous Disease

Cases of chronic granulomatous disease usually involve the colon but can exceptionally affect the stomach, leading to antral mucosal thickening.[315, 316] Biopsy reveals poorly formed granulomas that are mainly due to nodular collections of macrophages containing lipofuscin pigment. Occasionally noted are ulcers due to secondary infections.

Other Causes

Granulomas in the stomach are also observed in infections due to *M. tuberculosis,*[222–224] *Mycobacterium avium,*[225] and *Histoplasma*[233, 234] (see section on "Infections"); in reactions to suture and other foreign material[317] (Fig. 4-43); and rarely in association with lymphoma,[318] Whipple's disease,[319] and with malakoplakia[320, 321] (see Chs. 7 and 9).

Metabolic Disorders

The effects of many other diseases can lead to alterations in the gut mucosa, including the stomach. Most of these are discussed in other sections and are briefly summarized here (Table 4-13).

Endocrine Disorders

Cases of chronic atrophic fundic gastritis leading to pernicious anemia may be associated with immunologic injury that affects other endocrine organs, resulting in chronic thyroiditis and in atrophy of the adrenal cortex.[247, 248] Patients with diabetes mellitus can develop a marked distention of the stomach, and this can lead to secondary ischemic damage of the mucosa.[36, 37]

Hematologic Disorders

In any case with megaloblastic anemia, the nuclear maturation arrest can also be appreciated in epithelial tissues, including the

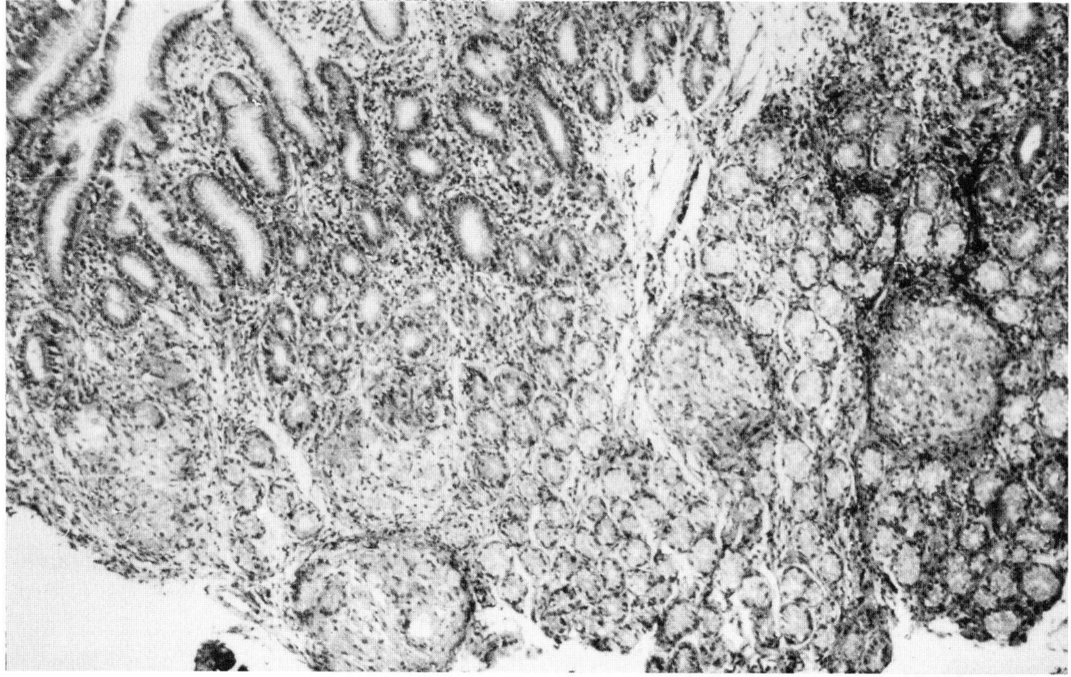

Fig. 4-40. Isolated granulomatous gastritis in the antrum, with surface appearing at top. There are several well formed granulomas without necrosis.

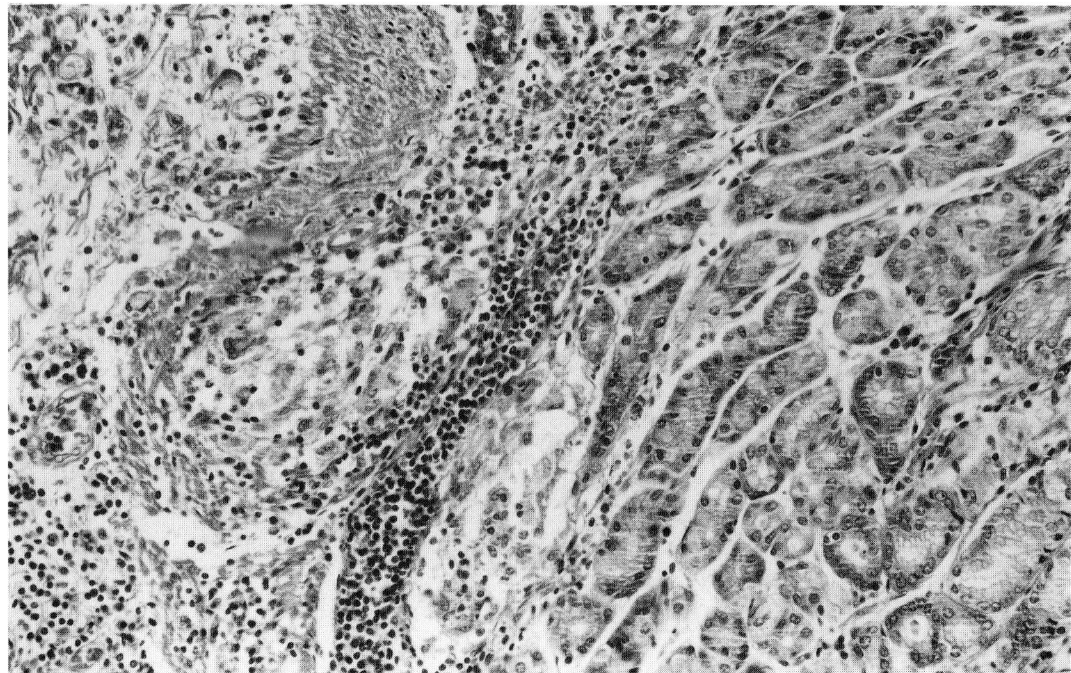

Fig. 4-41. Crohn's disease of the stomach, showing a small granuloma without necrosis at the base of the mucosa. This is surrounded by mononuclear inflammatory cells that extend into the submucosa appearing at the left.

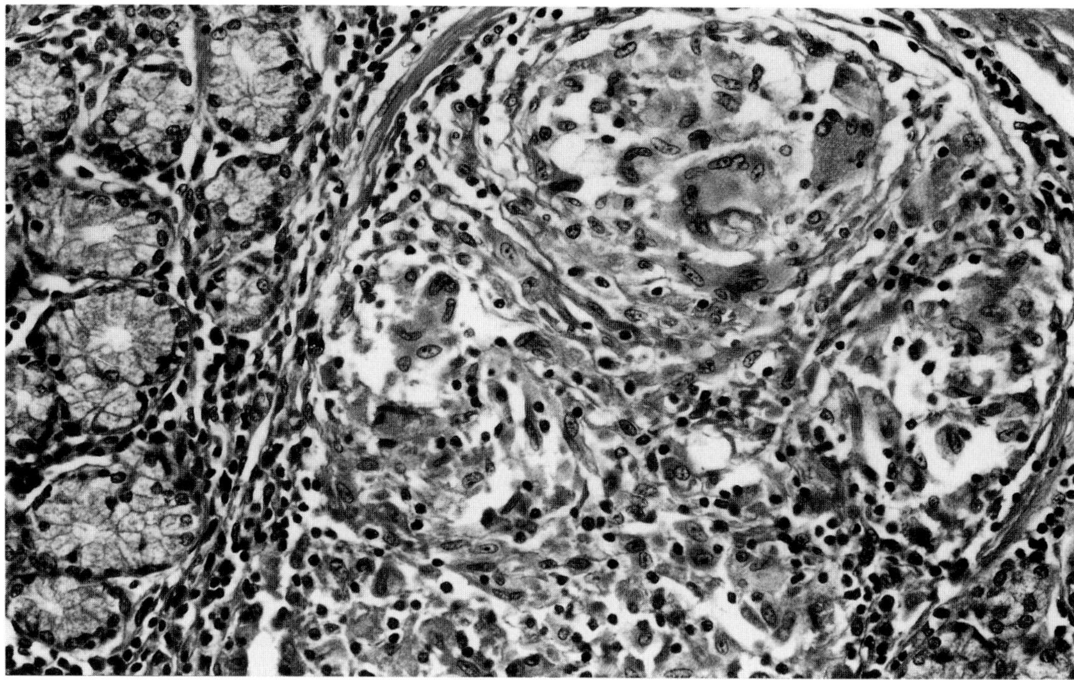

Fig. 4-42. Sarcoidosis of the stomach. Close view of typical granuloma without necrosis, composed of enlarged (epithelioid) macrophages and multinucleated cells (× 210).

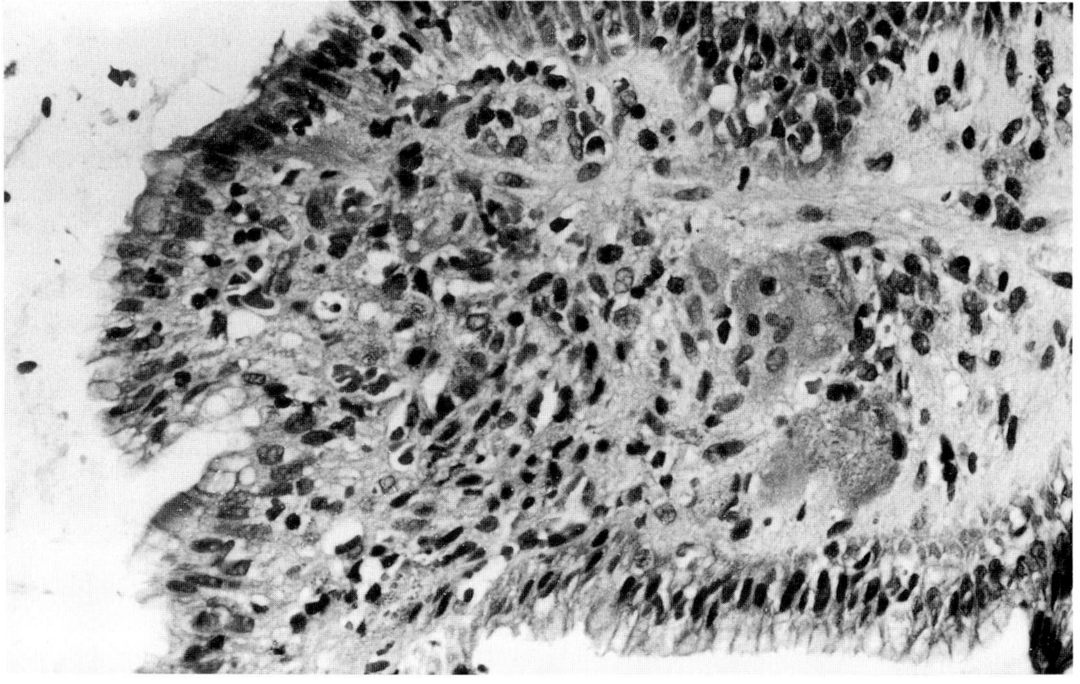

Fig. 4-43. Foreign body giant cells in lamina propria of the stomach (× 425).

Table 4-13. Effects of Other Disorders on the Stomach

Disorder	Effect on the Stomach
Diabetes mellitus	Distention and pressure necrosis
Megaloblastic anemia	Enlarged nuclei in gastric pits
Respiratory acidosis	Promote ulcers
Uremia	Hemorrhages and ulcers
Hemochromatosis	Iron deposition in parietal cells
Celiac disease	Lymphocytic gastritis

gastric pits. Biopsies reveal enlargement of the cells and their nuclei without apparent reason, simply reflecting the megaloblastic alteration in the renewing cells.[322] This is usually not a prominent finding since gastric epithelial cells undergo only slight renewal. As indicated above, cases of hemochromatosis can reveal increased iron in practically all eptithelial cells, and this is especially pronounced in the parietal cells within the gastric fundus and body.[298]

Pulmonary and Renal Disorders

Patients with chronic pulmonary disease and respiratory acidosis have an increased association of peptic ulcer disease, which is probably mediated by effects on acid secretion. Cases of uremia develop assorted lesions of the gastrointestinal mucosa, mainly in the form of patchy hemorrhages and ulcerations[323, 324]; these can be associated with calcium deposits in the lesions.

Celiac Disease

An increase in intraepithelial lymphocytes within the surface and pit mucous cells of the antrum has been noted in over 60 percent of cases of active celiac disease[96] (cf. Fig. 4-18). This is similar to the increased epithelial lymphocytes seen in the small intestine and may represent expression of the same immunologic injury to the stomach. Furthermore, there is loss of the lymphocytes with successful treatment of the disorder by a gluten-free diet. As noted previously, this feature should not be confused with the lymphocytic gastritis that tends to be located in the proximal part of the stomach.[94]

Gastritis Cystica

Gastritis cystica represents a chronic proliferative lesion that can result in a polypoid mass and in extension of the glands into the submucosa and deeper parts of the gastric wall.[325–327] These have been termed, respectively, *gastritis cystica polyposa* and *gastritis cystica profunda.* The condition is probably a reflection of a severe gastritis, analogous to the enteritis and colitis cystica lesions seen in the intestines of patients with longstanding inflammatory bowel disease. The lesions in the stomach are most commonly observed in gastric remnants following partial resection.

Biopsies are obtained to exclude recurrent or new cancer. In the polyposa form they reveal marked hypertrophy of the mucosa, due to hyperplasia and cystic change of the gastric pits and to considerable acute and chronic inflammation within the lamina propria (Fig. 4-44). There may also be superficial erosions due to the large size of the lesions. The profunda type reveals extension of mature glands into the submucosa (Fig. 4-45). This must be distinguished from invasive carcinoma, which is usually easy in view of the lack of any atypism in the cells. In addition, the mature glands are usually surrounded by connective tissue resembling lamina propria rather than by submucosal elements or by tumor-type stroma.

Other Disorders

There are rare reports of gastric biopsies with a prominent degree of collagen in the lamina propria, termed *collagenous gastritis;*

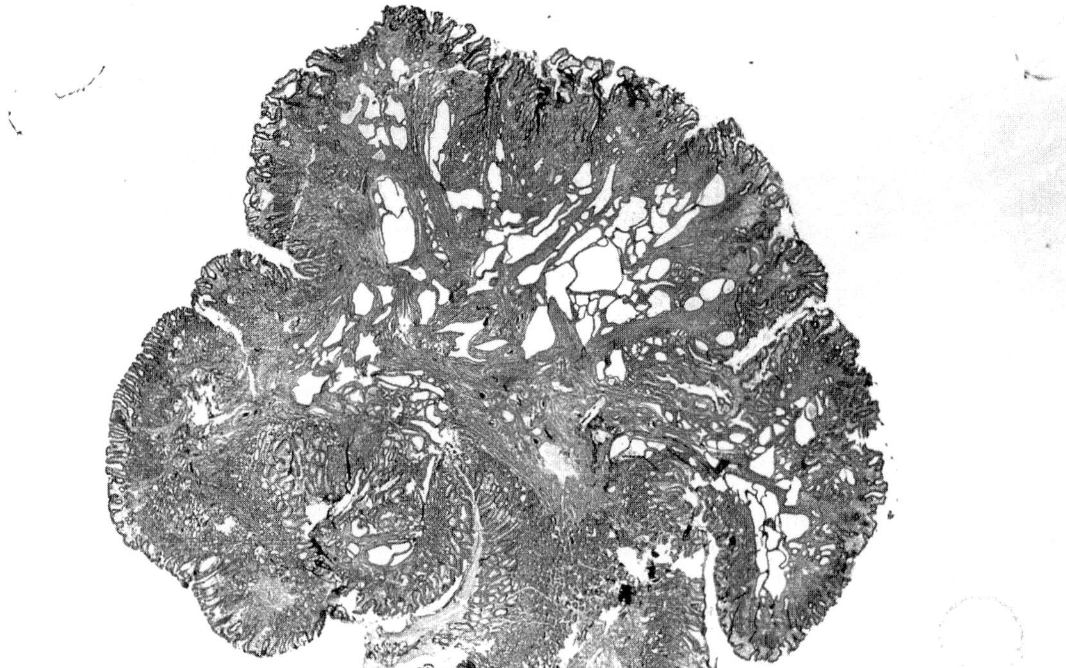

Fig. 4-44. Gastritis cystica polyposa. Polypoid area of inflamed and hyperplastric mucosa, with prominent cystic changes, in a gastric stump. Small fragment of normal stalk mucosa (bottom) (× 11).

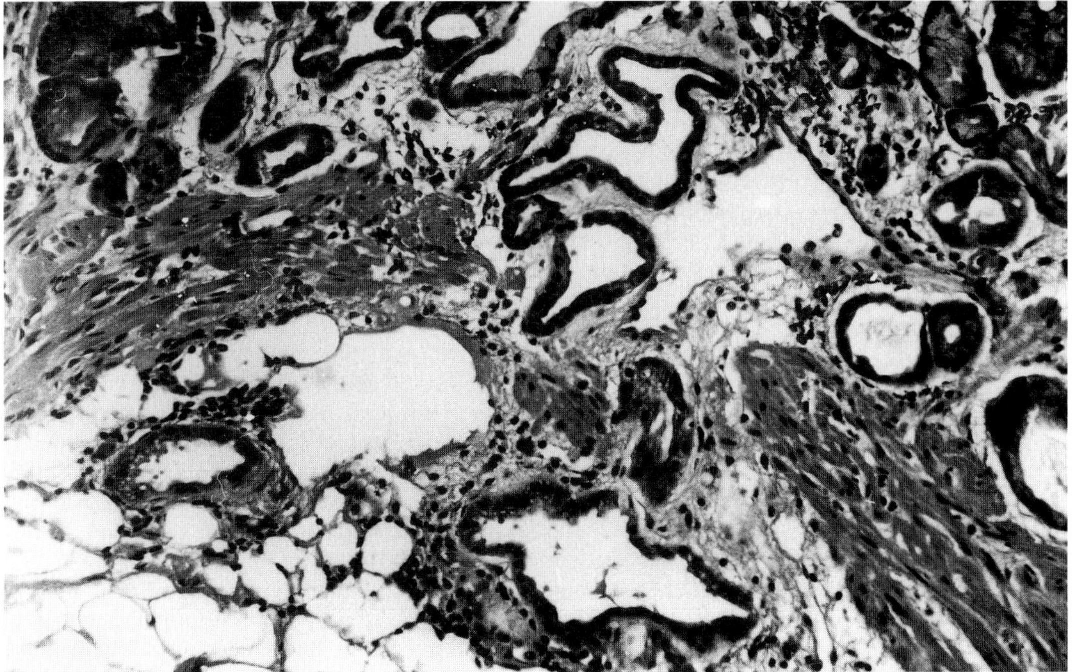

Fig. 4-45. Gastritis cystica profunda in the proximal stomach after an antral resection. Cystic glands at the base of the mucosa extend through the muscularis mucosae into the submucosa (bottom center). Misplaced glands have fragments of lamina propria; epithelial cells show no atypism (× 210).

both an isolated form[328] and a case associated with collagenous colitis[329] have been described. Occasionally noted are inflammatory conditions with extremely florid lymphoid proliferation, either diffuse or in the form of nodules. These have been termed *pseudolymphoma* and must be distinguished from actual neoplasms of the lymphoid tissue. This subject together with the other causes of mucosal hypertrophy are discussed in Chapter 5.

REFERENCES

1. Goldman H, Antonioli DA: Mucosal biopsy of the esophagus, stomach and proximal duodenum. Human Pathol 13:423–448, 1982
2. Whitehead R: Mucosal Biopsy of the Gastrointestinal Tract. 4th Ed. pp. 41–157. WB Saunders, Philadelphia, 1990
3. Rotterdam H: Stomach. pp. 62–255. In Rotterdam H, Sheahan DG, Sommers SC: Biopsy Diagnosis of the Digestive Tract. 2nd Ed. Raven Press, New York, 1993
4. Owen DA: Normal histology of the stomach. Am J Surg Pathol 10:48–61, 1986
5. Kreunig J, Bosman FT, Kuiper G et al: Gastric and duodenal mucosa in healthy individuals. J Clin Pathol 31:69–77, 1978
6. Helander HF: The cells of the gastric mucosa. Int Rev Cytol 70:217–289, 1981
7. Rubin W, Ross LL, Sleisenger MH et al: The normal human gastric epithelia: a fine structural study. Lab Invest 19:598, 1968
8. Lev R: The mucin histochemistry of normal and neoplastic gastric mucosa. Lab Invest 14:2080, 1965
9. Goldman H, Ming S-C: Mucins in normal and metaplastic gastrointestinal epithelium: histochemical distribution. Arch Pathol 85:580, 1968
10. Filipe MI: Mucins in the human gastrointestinal epithelium: a review. Invest Cell Pathol 2:195–216, 1979
11. Rubin W: Endocrine cells in the normal stomach: a fine structural study. Gastroenterology 62:784, 1972
12. Lechago J: The endocrine cells of the digestive tract. General concepts and historic perspective. Am J Surg Pathol II (suppl 1):63–70, 1987
13. Solcia E, Bordi C, Creutzfeldt W et al: Histopathological classification of nonantral gastric endocrine growths in man. Digestion 41:185–200, 1988
14. Kimura K: Chronological transition of the fundic pyloric border determined by stepwise biopsy of the lesser and greater curvatures of the stomach. Cancer 63:584–592, 1972
15. Tominaga K: Distribution of parietal cells in the antral mucosa of human stomachs. Gastroenterology 69:1201, 1975
16. Rubio C, Hayashi T, Stemmermann G: Ciliated gastric cells: a study of their phenotypic characteristics. Modern Pathol 3:720–723, 1990
17. Lehnert T, Erlandson RA, Decosse JJ: Lymph and blood capillaries of the human gastric mucosa. A morphologic basis for metastasis in early gastric carcinoma. Gastroenterology 89:939–950, 1985
18. Listrom MB, Fenoglio-Preiser CM: Lymphatic distribution of the stomach in normal, inflammatory, hyperplastic and neoplastic tissue. Gastroenterology 93:506–514, 1987
19. Shireman PK: Intramural cyst of the stomach. Hum Pathol 18:857–858, 1987
20. Sung ME: Histopathological study of mucosal and submucosal cysts of stomach. Acta Pathol Jpn 41:31–40, 1991
21. Eras P, Beranbaum S: Gastric diverticula: congenital and acquired. Am J Gastroenterol 57:120, 1972
22. Schweiger F, Noonan JS: An unusual case of gastric diverticulosis. Am J Gastroenterol 86:1817–1819, 1991
23. Chen YM, Teaque RS, Ott DJ et al: Gastric duplication cyst simulating leiomyoma. Gastrointest Endosc 33:250–252, 1987
24. Kato Y, Sugano H, Rubio CA: Classification of intramucosal cysts of the stomach. Histopathology 7:931–938, 1983
25. Batcup G, Spitz L: A histopathological study of gastric mucosal biopsies in infantile hypertrophic pyloric stenosis. J Clin Pathol 32:625–628, 1979
26. Snyder JD, Rosenblum N, Wershil B et al: Pyloric stenosis and eosinophilic gastroenteritis in infants. J Pediatr Gastroenterol Nutr 6:543–547, 1987
27. Satake K, Yada K, Ikehara T et al: Pyloric stenosis: an unusual complication of Beh-

çet's disease. Am J Gastroenterol 81:816–818, 1986
28. Goldman H: Other inflammatory disorders of the intestine. pp. 713–715. In Ming S-C, Goldman H (eds): Pathology of the Gastrointestinal Tract. WB Saunders, Philadelphia, 1992
29. Jabbari M, Goresky CA, Lough J et al: The inlet patch: heterotopic gastric mucosa in the upper esophagus. Gastroenterology 89:352–356, 1985
30. Franzin G, Musola R, Negri A et al: Heterotopic gastric (fundic) mucosa in the duodenum. Endoscopy 14:166–167, 1982
31. Barbosa JC, Dockerty MB, Waugh JM: Pancreatic heterotopia: review of literature and report of 41 authenticated surgical cases, of which 25 were clinically significant. Surg Gynecol Obstet 85:527–542, 1946
32. Theoni RF, Gedgaudas RK: Ectopic pancreas: usual and unusual features. Gastrointest Endosc 5:37–42, 1980
33. Kaneda M, Yano T, Yamamoto T et al: Ectopic pancreas on the stomach presenting as an inflammatory abdominal mass. Am J Gastroenterol 84:663–666, 1989
34. Zarling EJ: Gastric adenomyoma with coincidental pancreatic rest: a case report and review of the literature. Gastrointest Endosc 27:175–177, 1981
35. Doglioni C, Laurino L, Dei Tos A et al: Pancreatic (acinar) metaplasia of the gastric mucosa. Histology, ultrastructure, immunocytochemistry, and clinicopathologic correlations of 101 cases. Am J Surg Pathol 17:1134–1143, 1993
36. Feldman M, Schiller LR: Disorders of gastrointestinal motility associated with diabetes mellitus. Ann Intern Med 98:378–384, 1983
37. Rothstein RD: Gastrointestinal motility disorders in diabetes mellitus. Am J Gastroenterol 85:782–785, 1990
38. Knauer CM: Mallory–Weiss syndrome. Characterization of 75 Mallory–Weiss lacerations in 528 patients with upper gastrointestinal hemorrhage. Gastroenterology 71:5–8, 1976
39. Graham DY, Schwartz JT: The spectrum of the Mallory–Weiss tear. Medicine (Baltimore) 57:307–318, 1978
40. McCormack TT, Sims J, Eyre-Brook I et al: Gastric lesions in portal hypertension: inflammatory gastritis or congestive gastropathy? Gut 26:1226–1232, 1985
41. Papazian A, Braillon A, Dupas JL et al: Portal hypertensive gastric mucosa: an endoscopic study. Gut 27:1199–1203, 1986
42. Tarnowski AS, Sarfeh LG, Stachura J et al: Microvascular abnormalities of the portal hypertensive gastric mucosa. Hepatology 8:1488–1494, 1988
43. D'Amico G, Montabano L, Traina M et al: Natural history of congestive gastropathy in cirrhosis. Gastroenterology 99:1558–1564, 1990
44. Parikh SS, Desai SB, Prabhu SR et al: Congestive gastropathy: factors influencing development, endoscopic features, Helicobacter pylori infection, and microvessel changes. Am J Gastroenterol 89:1036–1042, 1994
45. Gunnlaugsson O:Angiodyplasia of the stomach and duodenum. Gastrointest Endosc 31:251–254, 1985
46. Gilmore PR: Angiodysplasia of the upper gastrointestinal tract. J Clin Gastroenterol 10:386–394, 1988
47. Boley SJ, Brandt LJ: Vascular ectasias of the colon—1986. Dig Dis Sci 31:26S–42S, 1986
48. Ona FV, Ahluwalia M: Endoscopic appearance of gastric angiodysplasia in hereditary hemorrhagic telangiectasia. Am J Gastroenterol 73:148–149, 1980
49. Marmaduke DP, Greenson JK, Cunningham I et al: Gastric vascular ectasia in patients undergoing bone marrow transplantation. Am J Clin Pathol 102:194–198, 1994
50. Van Zanten SJOV, Boifelsman JFWM, Schipper ME, Tytgat GNJ: Recurrent massive haematemesis from Dieulafoy vascular malformation—a review of 101 cases. Gut 27:213–222, 1986
51. Pointner R, Schwab G, Konigsrainer A, Dietze O: Endoscopic treatment of Dieulafoy's disease. Gastroenterology 94:563–566, 1988
52. Miko TL, Thomazy VA: The caliber persistent artery of the stomach: a unifying approach to gastric aneurysm, Dieulafoy's lesion, and submucosal arterial malformation. Hum Pathol 19:914–921, 1988

53. Eidus LB, Rosali P, Manion D, Heringer R: Caliber-persistent artery of the stomach (Dieulafoy's vascular malformation). Gastroenterology 99:1507–1510, 1990
54. Jabbari M, Cherry R, Lough JO et al: Gastric antral vascular ectasia. The watermelon stomach. Gastroenterology 87:1165–1170, 1984
55. Kruger R, Ryan ME, Dickson KB, Nunez JR: Diffuse vascular ectasia of the gastric antrum. Am J Gastroenterol 82:421–426, 1987
56. Suit PF, Petras RE, Bauer TW, Petrini JL Jr: Gastric antral vascular ectasia. A histologic and morphometric study of "the watermelon stomach". Am J Surg Pathol 11:750–757, 1987
57. Ma CK, Behrle KM, Rosenberg BF et al: Gastric antral vascular ectasia: the watermelon stomach. Surg Pathol 1:231–239, 1988
58. Gouldesbrough DR, Pell ACH: Gastric antral vascular ectasia: a problem of recognition and diagnosis. Gut 32:954–955, 1991
59. Potamiano S, Carter CR, Anderson JR: Endoscopic laser treatment of diffuse gastric antral vascular ectasia. Gut 35:461–463, 1994
60. Cherry RD, Jabbari M, Goresky CA et al: Chronic mesenteric vascular insufficiency with gastric ulceration. Gastroenterology 91:1548–1552, 1986
61. Hojgaard L, Krag E: Chronic ischemic gastritis reversed after revascularization operation. Gastroenterology 92:226–228, 1987
62. Skillman JJ, Silen W: Stress ulcers. Lancet 2:1303, 1972
63. Lev R: "Stress" ulcers following war wounds in Vietnam: a morphologic and histochemical study. Lab Invest 25:471, 1971
64. Skillman JJ, Bushnell LS, Goldman H et al: Respiratory failure, hypotension, sepsis and jaundice: a clinical syndrome associated with lethal hemorrhage from acute stress ulceration of the stomach. Am J Surg 117:523, 1969
65. Burke AP, Sobin LH, Virmani R: Localized vasculitis of the gastrointestinal tract. Am J Surg Pathol 19:338–349, 1995
66. Taylor NS, Gueft B, Lebowich RJ: Atheromatous embolization: a cause of gastric ulcers and small bowel necrosis. Gastroenterology 47:97, 1964
67. Yamada M, Hatakeyama S, Tsukagoshi H: Gastrointestinal amyloid deposition in AL (primary or myeloma-associated) and AA (secondary) amyloidosis. Diagnostic value of a gastric biopsy. Hum Pathol 16:1206–1211, 1985
68. Weinstein WM: The diagnosis and classification of gastritis and duodenitis. J Clin Gastroenterol 3(suppl 2):7–16, 1981
69. Owen DA: Gastritis and duodenitis. pp. 37–77. In Appelman HD (ed): Pathology of the Esophagus, Stomach and Duodenum. Churchill Livingstone, New York, 1984
70. Goldman H: Gastritis. pp. 481–516. In Ming S-C, Goldman H (eds): Pathology of the Gastrointestinal Tract. WB Saunders, Philadelphia, 1992
71. Appelman HD: Gastritis: terminology, etiology, and clinicopathological correlations: another biased view. Hum Pathol 25:1006–1019, 1994
72. Whitehead SC, Truelove SC, Gear MWL: The histological diagnosis of chronic gastritis in fiberoptic gastroscope biopsy specimens. J Clin Pathol 25:1, 1972
73. Fung WP, Papadimitriou JM, Matz LR: Endoscopic, histologic and ultrastructural correlations in chronic gastritis. Am J Gastroenterol 71:269–279, 1979
74. Elta GH, Appelman HD, Behler EM et al: A study of the correlation between endoscopic and histological diagnoses in gastroduodenitis. Am J Gastroenterol 82:749–753, 1987
75. Carpenter HA, Talley NJ: Gastroscopy is incomplete without biopsy: clinical relevance of distinguishing gastropathy from gastritis. Gastroenterology 108:917–924, 1995
76. Yardley JH: Pathology of chronic gastritis and duodenitis. pp. 69–143. In Goldman H, Appelman HD, Kaufman N (eds): Gastrointestinal Pathology. Williams & Wilkins, Baltimore, 1990
77. Borch K, Jansson L, Sjodahl R et al: Hemorrhagic gastritis. Incidence, etiologic factors, and prognosis. Acta Chir Scand 154:211–214, 1987
78. Laine L, Weinstein WM: Subepithelial hemorrhages and erosions of human stomach. Dig Dis Sci 33:490–503, 1988
79. Strickland RG, Mackay IR: A reappraisal of the nature and significance of chronic atrophic gastritis. Am J Dig Dis 18:426, 1973

80. Correa P: Chronic gastritis: a clinico-pathological classification. Am J Gastroenterol 83:504–509, 1988
81. Andrew A, Wyatt JI, Dixon MF: Observer variation in the assessment of chronic gastritis according to the Sydney system. Histopathology 25:317–322, 1994
82. Harvey RF, Davidson CM, Bradshaw MJ et al: Multifocal gastric carcinoid tumors, achlorrhydria, and hypergastrinemia. Lancet 1:951–954, 1985
83. Muller J, Kirchner T, Muller-Hermelink HK: Gastric endocrine cell hyperplasia and carcinoid tumors in atrophic gastritis type A. Am J Surg Pathol 11:909–917, 1987
84. Itsuno M, Watanabe H, Iwafuchi M et al: Multiple carcinoids and endocrine cell micronests in type A gastritis. Their morphology, histogenesis, and natural history. Cancer 63:881–890, 1989
85. Berendt RC, Jewell LD, Shnitha TK et al: Multicentric gastric carcinoids complicating pernicious anemia. Origin from the metaplastic endocrine cell population. Arch Pathol Lab Med 113:399–403, 1989
86. Glass GBJ, Pitchumoni CS: Atrophic gastritis. Hum Pathol 6:219, 1975
87. Geboes K, Rutgeerts P, Broeckaert L et al: Histologic appearances of endoscopic gastric mucosal biopsies 10–20 years after partial gastrectomy. Ann Surg 192:179, 1980
88. Pickford IR, Craven JL, Hall R et al: Endoscopic examination of the gastric remnant 31–39 years after subtotal gastrectomy for peptic ulcer. Gut 25:393–397, 1984
89. Green PHR, Gold RP, Marboe CC et al: Chronic erosive gastritis: clinical, diagnostic and pathological features in nine patients. Am J Gastroenterol 77:543–547, 1982
90. Elta Gh, Fawaz KA, Dayal Y et al: Chronic erosive gastritis—a recently recognized disorder. Dig Dis Sci 28:7–12, 1983
91. Gallagher CG, Lennon JR, Crowe JP: Chronic erosive gastritis: a clinical study. Am J Gastroenterol 82:302–306, 1987
92. Wolber RA, Owen DA, Anderson FH, Freeman HJ: Lymphocytic gastritis and giant gastric folds associated with gastrointestinal protein loss. Modern Pathol 4:13–15, 1991
93. Haot J, Jouret A, Willette M et al: Lymphocytic gastritis—prospective study of its relationship with varioliform gastritis. Gut 31:282–285, 1990
94. Haot J, Hamicki L, Walley L, Mainquet P: Lymphocytic gastritis: a newly described entity: a retrospective endoscopic and histological study. Gut 29:1258–1264, 1988
95. Wolber R, Owen D, Del Buona L et al: Lymphocytic gastritis in patients with celiac sprue or sprue-like intestinal disease. Gastroenterology 98:310–315, 1990
96. Alsaigh N, Odze R, Antonioli D et al: Gastric and esophageal inflammatory changes in pediatric celiac disease. Modern Pathol 8:57A, 1995
97. Stamp GWH, Palmer K, Misiewicz JJ: Antral hypertrophic gastritis: a rare cause of iron deficiency. J Clin Pathol 38:390–392, 1985
98. Komorowski RA, Caya JG: Hyperplastic gastropathy. Clinicopathologic correlation. Am J Surg Pathol 15:577–585, 1991
99. Wolfsen HC, Carpenter HA, Talley NJ. Ménétrier's disease: a form of hypertrophic gastropathy or gastritis? Gastroenterology 104:1310–1319, 1993
100. Goldman H: Mucosal hypertrophy and hyperplasia of the stomach. pp. 537–546. In Ming S-C, Goldman H (eds): Pathology of the Gastrointestinal Tract. WB Saunders, Philadelphia, 1992
101. Goldman H, Ming S-C: Find structure of intestinal metaplasia and adenocarcinoma of the human stomach. Lab Invest 18:203, 1968
102. Teglbjaerg PS, Nielson HO: "Small intestinal type" and "colonic type" intestinal metaplasia of the human stomach. Acta Pathol Microbiol Scand A 86:351, 1978
103. Iida F, Kusama J: Gastric carcinoma and intestinal metaplasia. Significance of types of intestinal metaplasia upon development of gastric carcinoma. Cancer 501:2854–2858, 1982
104. Stockton M, McCall I: Comparative electron microscopic features of normal, intermediate and metaplastic pyloric epithelium. Histopathology 7:859–871, 1983
105. Craenen ME, Blok P, Dekher W et al: Prevalence of subtypes of intestinal metaplasia in gastric antral mucosa. Dig Dis Sci 36: 1529–1536, 1991
106. Rubin W: A fine structural characterization of the proliferated endocrine cells in

atrophic gastric mucosa. Am J Pathol 70:109, 1973

107. Bordi C, Ravazzola M: Endocrine cells in the intestinal metaplasia of gastric mucosa. Am J Pathol 90:391–395, 1979
108. Jass JR, Filipe MI: Sulphamucins and precancerous lesions of the human stomach. Histopathology 4:271, 1980
109. Huang C-B, Xu J, Huang J-T et al: Sulphomucin colonic type intestinal metaplasia and carcinoma of the stomach. Cancer 57:1370–1375, 1986
110. Rokkas T, Filipe MI, Sladen GE: Detection of an increased incidence of early gastric cancer in patients with intestinal metaplasia type III who are closely followed up. Gut 32:1110–1113, 1991
111. Bramesar KCR, Sanders DSA, Hopwood D: Limited value of type III intestinal metaplasia in predicting risk of gastric carcinoma. J Clin Pathol 40:1287–1290, 1987
112. Mutsukuma A, Mori M, Enjoji M: Sulphamucin-secreting intestinal metaplasia in the human gastric mucosa. An association with intestinal-type gastric carcinoma. Cancer 66:689–694, 1990
113. Domellof L, Erickson S, Helander HF et al: Lipid islands in the gastric mucosa after resection for benign ulcer disease. Gastroenterology 72:14, 1977
114. Drude RB, Balart LA, Herrington JP et al: Gastric xanthoma: histological similarity to signet ring cell carcinoma. J Clin Gastroenterol 4:217–221, 1982
115. Kunze KC, Baum RA, Nasrallah SM: Gastric xanthoma. Gastrointest Endosc 33:114–115, 1987
116. Stemmermann GN, Hayashi T: Hyperplastic polyps of the gastric mucosa adjacent to gastroenterostomy stomas. Am J Clin Pathol 71:341, 1979
117. Morson BC, Sobin LH, Grundmann E et al: Precancerous conditions and epithelial dysplasia in the stomach. J Clin Pathol 33:711, 1980
118. Jass JR: A classification of gastric dysplasia. Histopathology 7:181–193, 1983
119. Ming S-C, Bajtai A, Correa P et al: Gastric dysplasia. Significance and pathologic criteria. Cancer 54:1794–1801, 1984
120. Di Gregorio C, Morandi P, Fante R, De Gaetani C: Gastric dysplasia. A follow-up study. Am J Gastroenterol 88:1714–1719, 1993
121. Offerhaus GJA, Stadt J, Hurbregtse K et al: The mucosa of the gastric remnant harboring malignancy. Histologic findings in the biopsy specimens of 504 asymptomatic patients 15 to 46 years after partial gastrectomy with emphasis on nonmalignant lesions. Cancer 64:698–703, 1989
122. von Holstein CS, Hammar E, Eriksson S, Huldt B: Clinical significance of dysplasia in gastric remnant biopsy specimens. Cancer 72:1532–1535, 1993
123. Goldman H, Szabo S: Chemical and physical disorders. pp. 141–170. In Ming S-C, Goldman H (eds): Pathology of the Gastrointestinal Tract. WB Saunders, Philadelphia, 1992
124. Allen R, Thoshinsky M, Stallone R et al: Corrosive injuries of the stomach. Arch Surg 100:409–413, 1970
125. Poelman JR, Hausman RH, Holtsma HFW: Endoscopy in lye burns of oesophagus and stomach. Endoscopy 9:172, 1977
126. Lowe JE, Graham DY, Bolsaubin EV Jr, Lanza FL: Corrosive injury to the stomach: the natural history and role of fiberoptic endoscopy. Am J Surg 137:803–806, 1979
127. Sugawa C, Mullins RJ, Lucas CE, Leibold WC: The value of early endoscopy following caustic ingestion. Surg Gynecol Obstet 153:553–556, 1981
128. Mitchell EP, Schein PS: Gastrointestinal toxicity of chemotherapeutic agents. Semin Oncol 9:52–64, 1982
129. Weidner N, Smith JG, La Vanway JM: Peptic ulceration with marked epithelial atypia following hepatic arterial infusion chemotherapy. Am J Surg Pathol 7:261–268, 1983
130. Petras RE, Hart WR, Bukowski RM: Gastric epithelial atypia associated with hepatic arterial infusion chemotherapy: its distinction from early gastric carcinoma. Cancer 56: 745–750, 1985
131. Meshkinpour H, Marks JW, Schoenfield LJ et al: Reflux gastritis syndrome: mechanism of symptoms. Gastroenterology 79:1283, 1980
132. Dixon MF, O'Connor HJ, Axon ATR et al: Reflux gastritis: a distinct histopathological entity? J Clin Pathol 39:524–530, 1986
133. Niemela S, Kaittanen T, Heikkila J, Lehtola J: Characteristics of bile gastritis. Scand J Gastroenterol 22:349–354, 1987

134. Gottfried EB, Korsten MA, Lieber CS: Alcohol-induced gastric and duodenal lesions in man. Am J Gastroenterol 70:587–592, 1978
135. Valencia-Parparcen J: Alcoholic gastritis. Clin Gastroenterol 10:389–399, 1981
136. Laine L, Weinstein WM: Histology of alcoholic hemorrhagic "gastritis": a prospective evaluation. Gastroenterology 94:1254–1262, 1988
137. Riddell RH: The gastrointestinal tract. pp. 515–606. In Riddell RH (ed): Pathology of Drug-Induced and Toxic Diseases. Churchill Livingstone, New York, 1982
138. Lewis JH: Gastrointestinal injury due to medicinal agents. Am J Gastroenterol 81: 819–834, 1986
139. Messer J, Reitman D, Sacks HS et al: Association of adrenocorticosteroid therapy and peptic ulcer disease. N Engl J Med 309: 21–24, 1983
140. Smith BM: Permeability of the human gastric mucosa: alteration by acetylsalicylic acid and ethanol. N Engl J Med 285:216, 1971
141. Ritchie WJ: Acute gastric mucosal damage induced by bile salts, acid and ischemia. Gastroenterology 68:699–707, 1975
142. Metzger WH, McAdam L, Bluestone R, Guth PH: Acute gastric mucosal injury during continuous or interrupted aspirin ingestion in humans. Am J Dig Dis 21:963–968, 1976
143. Silvoso GR, Ivey KJ, Butt et al: Incidence of gastric lesions in patients with rheumatic disease on chronic aspirin therapy. Ann Intern Med 91:517–520, 1979
144. Piper DW, McIntosh JH, Ariotti DE et al: Analgesic ingestion and chronic peptic ulcer. Gastroenterology 80:427, 1981
145. Graham DY, Smith JL, Dobbs SM: Gastric adaptation occurs with aspirin administration in man. Dig Dis Sci 28:1–6, 1983
146. McIntyre RL, Irani MS, Piris J: Histological study of the effects of three anti-inflammatory preparations on the gastric mucosa. J Clin Pathol 34:836–841, 1981
147. Larkai EN, Smith JL, Lidsky MD, Graham DY: Gastroduodenal mucosa and dyspeptic symptoms in arthritic patients during chronic nonsteroidal anti-inflammatory drug use. Am J Gastroenterol 82:1153–1158, 1987
148. Graham DY, Smith JL: Gastroduodenal complications of chronic NSAID therapy. Am J Gastroenterol 83:1081–1084, 1988
149. Allison MC, Howatson AG, Torrance CJ et al: Gastrointestinal damage associated with the use of nonsteroidal anti-inflammatory drugs. N Engl J Med 327:749–754, 1992
150. Lanza FL: Gastrointestinal toxicity of newer NSAID. Am J Gastroenterol 88:1318–1323, 1993
151. Henry D, Dobson A, Turner C: Variability in the risk of major gastrointestinal complications from non-aspirin non-steroidal anti-inflammatory drugs. Gastroenterology 105: 1078–1088, 1993
152. Quinn CM, Bjarnason I, Price AB: Gastritis in patients on non-steroidal anti-inflammatory drugs. Histopathology 23:341–348, 1993
153. Filpi RG, Majd M, LoPresto JM: Reversible gastric stricture following iron ingestion. South Med J 66:845–846, 1973
154. Carne-Ross IP: Pyloric stenosis and sustained-release iron tablets. Br Med J 2:642–643, 1976
155. Weiss SM, Rutenberg HL, Paskin DL, Zeren HA: Gut lesions due to slow-release KCl tablets. N Engl J Med 296:111–112, 1977
156. McDonald WC: Correlation of mucosal histology and aspirin intake in chronic gastric ulcer. Gastroenterology 65:381, 1973
157. Hamilton SR, Yardley JH: Endoscopic biopsy diagnosis of aspirin-associated chronic gastric ulcers. Gastroenterology 78:1178, 1980
158. Howiler W, Goldberg HI: Gastroesophageal involvement in herpes simplex. Gastroenterology 70:775, 1976
159. Sperling HV, Reed WG: Herpetic gastritis. Am J Dig Dis 22:1034, 1977
160. Allen JI, Silvis SE, Summer HW, McClain CJ: Cytomegalic inclusion disease diagnosed endoscopically. Dig Dis Sci 26:133, 1981
161. Andrade JS, Bambirra EA, Lima GF et al: Gastric cytomegalic inclusion bodies diagnosed by histologic examination of endoscopic biopsies in patients with gastric ulcer. Am J Clin Pathol 79:493–496, 1983
162. Hinnant KL, Rotterdam HZ, Bell ET, Tapper ML: Cytomegalovirus infection of the alimentary tract: a clinicopathological correlation. Am J Gastroenterol 81:944–950, 1986

163. Cheung ANY, Ng IOL: Cytomegalovirus infection of the gastrointestinal tract in non-AIDS patients. Am J Gastroenterol 88: 1882–1886, 1993
164. Wu G-D, Shintaku IP, Chien K, Geller SA: A comparison of routine light microscopy, immunohistochemistry, and in-situ hybridization for the detection of cytomegalovirus in gastrointestinal biopsies. Am J Gastroenterol 84:1517–1520, 1989
165. Blaser MJ: Gastric Campylobacter-like organisms, gastritis, and peptic ulcer disease. Gastroenterology 93:371–382, 1987
166. Graham DY. Campylobacter pylori and peptic ulcer disease. Gastroenterology 96:615–625, 1989
167. Peterson WL: Helicobacter pylori and peptic ulcer disease. N Engl J Med 324: 1043–1048, 1991
168. Marshall BJ: Helicobacter pylori. Am J Gastroenterol 89:S116–S128, 1994
169. NIH Consensus Conference. Helicobacter pylori in peptic ulcer disease. JAMA 272:65–69, 1994
170. Warren JR, Marshall BJ: Unidentified curved bacilli on gastric epithelium in active chronic gastritis. Lancet 1:1273, 1983
171. Dubois A, Fiala N, Heman-Ackah IM et al: Natural gastric infection with Helicobacter pylori in monkeys: a model for spiral bacteria infection in humans. Gastroenterology 106:1405–1417, 1994
172. Leung KM, Hui PK, Chan WY, Thomas TMM: Helicobacter pylori–related gastritis and gastric ulcer. A continuum of progressive epithelial degeneration. Am J Clin Pathol 98:569–574, 1992
173. Paull G, Yardley JH: Gastric and esophageal Campylobacter pylori in patients with Barrett's esophagus. Gastroenterology 95: 216–218, 1988
174. Loffeld RJ, Ten Tije BJ, Arends JW: Prevalence and significance of Helicobacter pylori in patients with Barrett's esophagus. Am J Gastroenterol 87:1598–1600, 1992
175. Boren T, Falk P, Roth KA et al: Attachment of Helicobacter pylori to human gastric epithelium mediated by blood group antigens. Science 262:1892–1896, 1993
176. Noach LA, Rolf TM, Bosma NB et al: Gastric metaplasia and Helicobacter pylori infection. Gut 34:1510–1514, 1993
177. Madan E, Kemp J, Westblam TU et al: Evaluation of staining methods for identifying Campylobacter pylori. Am J Clin Pathol 90:450–453, 1988
178. Barbosa AJA, Queiroz DMM, Mendes EN et al: Immunocytochemical identification of Campylobacter pylori in gastritis and correlation with culture. Arch Path Lab Med 112:523–525, 1988
179. Cortun RW, Kryzmowski GA, Pederson CA et al: Immunocytochemical identification of Helicobacter pylori in formalin-fixed gastric biopsies. Modern Pathol 4:498–502, 1991
180. Chen XG, Correa P, Offerhaus J et al: Ultrastructure of the gastric mucosa harboring Campylobacter-like organisms. Am J Clin Pathol 86:575–582, 1986
181. Caselli M, Aleotti A, Boldrini P et al: Ultrastructural patterns of Helicobacter pylori. Gut 34:1507–1509, 1993
182. Noach LA, Rolf TM, Tytgat GNJ: Electron microscopic study of association between Helicobacter pylori and gastric and duodenal mucosa. J Clin Pathol 47:695–699, 1994
183. Nichols L, Sughayer M, DeGirolami PC et al: Evaluation of diagnostic methods for Helicobacter pylori gastritis. Am J Clin Pathol 95:769–773, 1991
184. Graham DY, Klein PD, Evans DJ Jr et al: Campylobacter pylori detected noninvasively by the ^{13}C-urea breath test. Lancet 1:1174–1177, 1987
185. Loffeld RJ, Stobberingh E, Flendrig JA, Arends JW: Helicobacter pylori in gastric biopsy specimens. Comparison of culture, modified giemsa stain, and immunohistochemistry—a retrospective study. J Pathol 165:69–75, 1991
186. Fabre R, Sobhani I, Laurent-Puig P et al: Polymerase chain reaction assay for the detection of Helicobacter pylori in gastric biopsy specimens: comparison with culture, rapid urease test, and histopathological tests. Gut 35:905–908, 1994
187. Genta RM, Hamner HW, Graham DY: Gastric lymphoid follicles in Helicobacter pylori infection: frequency, distribution, and response to triple therapy. Hum Pathol 24:577–583, 1993
188. Eidt S, Stolte M: Prevalence of lymphoid follicles and aggregates in Helicobacter pylori gastritis. J Clin Pathol 46:832–836, 1993

189. Wyatt JI: Histopathology of gastroduodenal inflammation: the impact of Helicobacter pylori. Histopathology 26:1–15, 1995
190. Dixon MF, Wyatt JI, Burke DA et al: Lymphocytic gastritis—relationship to Campylobacter pylori infection. J Pathol 154:125–132, 1988
191. Hansing RZ, D'Amico H, Levy M, Guillan RA: Prediction of Helicobacter pylori in gastric specimens by inflammatory and morphological histological evaluation. Am J Gastroenterol 87:1125–1131, 1992
192. Hui PK, Chan WY, Cheung PS et al: Pathologic changes of gastric mucosa colonized by Helicobacter pylori. Hum Pathol 23: 548–556, 1992
193. Chan WY, Hui PK, Leung KM, Thomas TMM: Modes of Helicobacter colonization and gastric epithelial damage. Histopathology 21:521–528, 1992
194. Valie J, Seppala K, Sipponen P, Kosunen T: Disappearance of gastritis after eradication of Helicobacter pylori—a morphometric study. Scand J Gastroenterol 26:1057–1065, 1991
195. Genta RM, Lew GM, Graham DY: Changes in the gastric mucosa following eradication of Helicobacter pylori. Modern Pathol 6: 281–289, 1993
196. Dooley CP, Cohen H, Fitzgibbons PL et al: Prevalence of Helicobacter pylori infection and histologic gastritis in asymptomatic persons. N Engl J Med 321:1562–1566, 1989
197. Meyer B, Werth B, Beglinger C et al: Helicobacter pylori infection in healthy people: a dynamic process? Gut 32:347–350, 1991
198. Hussell T, Isaacson PG, Crabtree JE, Spenser J: The response of cells from low-grade B-cell gastric lymphomas of mucosa-associated lymphoid tissue to Helicobacter pylori. Lancet 342:571–575, 1993
199. Tatsuta Nm Iishi H, Okuda S et al: The association of Helicobacter pylori with differentiated-type early gastric cancer. Cancer 72:1841–1845, 1993
200. Hansson L-E, Engstrand L, Nyren O et al: Helicobacter pylori infection: independent risk indicator of gastric andenocarcinoma. Gastroenterology 105:1098–1103, 1993
201. Wee A, Kang JY, Teh M: Helicobacter pylori and gastric cancer correlation with gastritis, intestinal metaplasia, and tumor histology. Gut 33:1029–1032, 1992
202. Parsonnet J, Hansen S, Rodriguez L et al: Helicobacter pylori infection and gastric lymphoma. N Engl J Med 330:1267–1271, 1994
203. Fong T-L, Dooley CP, Dehesa M et al: Helicobacter pylori infection in pernicious anemia: a prospective controlled study. Gastroenterology 100:328–332, 1991
204. Edwards PD, Carrick J, Turner J et al: Helicobacter pylori–associated gastritis is rare in AIDS: antibiotic effects or a consequence of immunodeficiency? Am J Gastroenterol 86:1761–1764, 1991
205. Sung JJY, Chung SCS, Ling TKW et al: Antibacterial treatment of gastric ulcers associated with Helicobacter pylori. N Engl J Med 332:139–142, 1995
206. McNulty CAM, Dent JC, Curry A et al: New spiral bacterium in gastric mucosa. J Clin Pathol 42:585–591, 1989
207. Morris A, Ali MR, Thomsen L, Hollis B: Tightly spiral-shaped bacteria in the human stomach: another cause of active chronic gastritis? Gut 31:139–143, 1990
208. Heilman KL, Borchard F: Gastritis due to spiral-shaped bacteria other than Helicobacter pylori: clinical, histological, and ultrastructural findings. Gut 32:137–140, 1991
209. Oliva MM, Lazenby AJ, Perman JA: Gastritis associated with Gastrospirillum hominis in children. Comparison with Helicobacter pylori and review of the literature. Modern Pathol 6:513–515, 1993
210. Mazzucchelli L, Wildersmith CH, Ruchti C et al: Gastrospirillum hominis in asymptomatic, healthy individuals. Dig Dis Sci 38: 2087–2090, 1993
211. Miller AI, Smith M, Rogers AI: Phlegmonous gastritis. Gastroenterology 68:231, 1975
212. O'Toole PA, Morris JA: Acute phlegmonous gastritis. Postgrad Med J 64:315–316, 1988
213. Gonzalez L, Schowengerdt C, Skinner H, Lynch P: Emphysematous gastritis. Surg Gynecol Obstet 116:79, 1963
214. Binmoeller KF, Benner KG: Emphysematous gastritis secondary to gastric infarction. Am J Gastroenterol 87:526–529, 1992
215. Van Olmen G, Larmuseau MF, Geboes K et al: Primary gastric actinomycosis: a case

report and review of the literature. Am J Gastroenterol 79:512–516, 1984

216. Butz WC, Watts JC, Rosales-Quintana S, Hicklin MD: Erosive gastritis as a manifestation of secondary syphilis. Am J Clin Pathol 63:895–900, 1975
217. Fyfe B, Poppiti RJ Jr, Lubin J, Robinson MJ: Gastric syphilis. Primary diagnosis by gastric biopsy: report of four cases. Arch Pathol Lab Med 117:820–823, 1993
218. Atten MJ, Attar BM, Teopengco E et al: Gastric syphilis: a disease with multiple manifestations. Am J Gastroenterol 89: 2227–2229, 1994
219. Kasmin F, Riddy S, Mathur-Wagh U et al: Syphilitic gastritis in an HIV-infected individual. Am J Gastroenterol 87:1820–1822, 1992
220. Morin ME, Tan A: Diffuse enlargement of gastric folds as a manifestation of secondary syphilis. Am J Gastroenterol 74:170–172, 1980
221. Besses C, Sans-Sabrofen J, Badia X et al: Ulceroinfiltrative syphilitic gastropathy: silver stain diagnosis from biopsy specimen. Am J Gastroenterol 82:773–774, 1987
222. Mathis G, Dirschmid K, Sutterlutti G: Tuberculous gastric ulcer. Endoscopy 19:133–135, 1987
223. Subei I, Attar B, Schmitt G, Levendoglu H: Primary gastric tuberculosis: a case report and literature review. Am J Gastroenterol 82:769–772, 1987
224. Tromba JL, Inglese R, Rieders B, Todaro R: Primary gastric tuberculosis presenting as pyloric outlet obstruction. Am J Gastroenterol 86:1820–1822, 1991
225. Rotterdam H, Tsang P: Gastrointestinal disease in the immunocompromised patient. Hum Pathol 25:1123–1140, 1994
226. Katzenstein ALA, Maksen J: Candidal infection of gastric ulcers: histology, incidence and clinical significance. Am J Clin Pathol 71:137, 1979
227. Loffeld RJ, Loffeld BC, Arends JW et al: Fungal colonization of gastric ulcers. Am J Gastroenterol 83:730–733, 1988
228. Knoke M, Bernhardt H: Endoscopic aspects of mycosis in the upper digestive tract. Endoscopy 12:295, 1980
229. Young JA, Elias E: Gastro-oesophageal candidiasis: diagnosis by brush cytology. J Clin Pathol 38:293–296, 1985
230. Young RC, Bennett JE, Vogel CL et al: Aspergillosis: the spectrum of the disease in 98 patients. Medicine 49:147, 1970
231. Lyon DT, Schubert TT, Mantia AG, Kaplan MH: Phycomycosis of the gastrointestinal tract. Am J Gastroenterol 72:379–394, 1979
232. Whiteway DE, Virata RL: Mucormycosis. Arch Intern Med 139:944, 1979
233. Miller DP, Everett ED: Gastrointestinal histoplasmosis. J Clin Gastroenterol 1:233, 1979
234. Cappell MS, Mandell W, Grimes MM, Neu HC: Gastrointestinal histoplasmosis. Dig Dis Sci 33:353–360, 1988
235. Guerrant RL, Bobak DA: Bacterial and protozoal gastroenteritis. N Engl J Med 325:327–340, 1991
236. Garone MA, Winston BJ, Lewis JH: Cryptosporidiosis of the stomach. Am J Gastroenterol 81:465–470, 1986
237. Godwin TA: Cryptosporidiosis in the acquired immunodeficiency syndrome: a study of 15 autopsy cases. Hum Pathol 22:1215–1224, 1991
238. Doglioni C, Deboni M, Cielo R et al: Gastric giardiasis. J Clin Pathol 45:964–967, 1992
239. Watt IA, McLean NR, Girdwood RWA et al: Eosinophilic gastroenteritis associated with a larval anisakine nematode. Lancet 2:893–894, 1979
240. McKerrow JH, Sakanari J, Deerdorff TL: Anisakiasis: revenge of the sushi parasites. N Engl J Med 319:1228–1229, 1988
241. Sugimachi K, Inokuchi K, Ooiwa T, Fujino T et al: Acute gastric anisakiasis. Analysis of 178 cases. JAMA 253:1012–1013, 1985
242. Hsiu J-G, Gamsey AJ, Ives CE et al: Gastric anisakiasis: report of a case with clinical, endoscopic, and histological findings. Am J Gastroenterol 81:1185–1187, 1986
243. Jacob GS, Al Nakeb B, Al Ruwaih A: Ascariasis producing upper gastrointestinal hemorrhage. Endoscopy 15:67, 1983
244. Chondkuri G, Saha SS, Tandon RK: Gastric ascariasis. Am J Gastroenterol 81:788–790, 1986
245. Dumont A, Sefevon, Barbier P: Endoscopic discovery and capture of Necator Americanus in the stomach. Endoscopy 15:65–66, 1983
246. Otrakji CL, Albores-Saavedra J, Martinex AJ: Gastric malignant lymphoma with su-

perimposed amebiasis. Am J Gastroenterol 85:72–75, 1990
247. Irvine WJ: The association of atrophic gastritis with autoimmune thyroid disease. Clin Endocrinol Metab 4:351, 1975
248. Tobin MV, Aldridge SA, Morris AI et al: Gastrointestinal manifestations of Addison's disease. Am J Gastroenterol 84:1302–1305, 1989
249. Sipponen P, Kekki M, Siuralla M: Atrophic chronic gastritis and intestinal metaplasia in gastric carcinoma. Comparison with representative population sample. Cancer 52:1062–1068, 1983
250. Armbrecht U, Stockbrugger RW, Rode J et al: Development of gastric dysplasia in pernicious anemia: a clinical and endoscopic follow up study of 80 patients. Gut 31:1105–1109, 1990
251. Gupta JP, Jain AK, Agrawal BK et al: Gastroscopic cytology and biopsies in diagnosis of gastric malignancies. J Surg Oncol 22:62–64, 1983
252. Tatsuta M, Iishi H, Okuda S et al: Prospective evaluation of diagnostic accuracy of gastrofiberscopic biopsy in diagnosis of gastric cancer. Cancer 63:1415–1420, 1989
253. Klein NC, Hargrove RL, Sleisenger MH et al: Eosinophilic gastroenteritis. Medicine (Baltimore) 40:299–319, 1970
254. Talley NJ, Shorter RG, Phillips SF et al: Eosinophilic gastroenteritis: a clinicopathological study of patients with disease of the mucosa, muscle layers and subserosal tissues. Gut 31:54–58, 1990
255. Goldman H: Allergic disorders. pp. 171–187. In Ming S-C, Goldman H (eds): Pathology of the Gastrointestinal Tract. WB Saunders, Philadelphia, 1992
256. Katz AJ, Goldman H, Grand RJ: Gastric mucosal biopsy in eosinophilic (allergic) gastroenteritis. Gastroenterology 73:705–709, 1977
257. Goldman H, Proujansky R: Allergic proctitis and gastroenteritis in children: clinical and mucosal biopsy features in 53 cases. Am J Surg Pathol 10:75–86, 1986
258. Teele RL, Katz AJ, Goldman H et al: The radiographic features of eosinophilic gastroenteritis (allergic gastroenteropathy) of childhood. Am J Radiol 132:575, 1979
259. Snover DC, Weisdorf SA, Vercolotti GM et al: A histopathologic study of gastric and small intestinal graft-versus-host disease following allogeneic bone marrow transplantation. Hum Pathol 16:387–392, 1985
260. Ferrara JLM, Deeg HJ: Graft-versus-host disease. N Engl J Med 324:667–674, 1991
261. Goldgraber MB, Rubin CE, Palmer WL et al: The early gastric response to irradiation: a serial biopsy study. Gastroenterology 27:1–20, 1954
262. Warren S, Friedman B: Pathology and pathologic diagnosis of radiation lesions in the gastrointestinal tract. Am J Pathol 18:499–507, 1942
263. Novak JM, Collins JT, Donowitz M et al: Effects of radiation on the human gastrointestinal tract. J Clin Gastroenterol 1:9, 1979
264. Berthrong M, Fajardo LF: Radiation injury in surgical pathology. Part II. Alimentary tract. Am J Surg Pathol 5:153–178, 1981
265. Hamilton FE: Gastric ulcer following radiation. Arch Surg 55:394–399, 1947
266. Kellum JM, Jaffe BM, Calhoun T, Ballinger WF: Gastric complications after radiotherapy for Hodgkin's disease and other lymphomas. Am J Surg 134:314–317, 1977
267. McIlrath DC, Hallenbeck GA: Review of gastric freezing. JAMA 190:715, 1964
268. Barner HB, Collins CH, Jones TI, Garlick TB: Morphology of human stomach after therapeutic freezing. Arch Surg 90:358, 1965
269. Kadian RS, Rose JF, Mann NS: Gastric bezoars—spontaneous resolution. Am J Gastroenterol 70:79–80, 1978
270. Holloway W, Lee S, Nicholson G: The composition and dissolution of phytobezoars. Arch Pathol Lab Med 104:159, 1980
271. Goldman H: Stress ulcer and chronic peptic ulcer disease. pp. 517–536. In Ming S-C, Goldman H (eds): Pathology of the Gastrointestinal Tract. WB Saunders, Philadelphia, 1992
272. Cook DJ, Fuller HD, Guyatt GH et al: Risk factors for gastrointestinal bleeding in critically ill patients. N Engl J Med 330: 377–381, 1994
273. Szabo S: Biology of disease: pathogenesis of duodenal ulcer disease. Lab Invest 51:121–147, 1984
274. Langman MJS, Cooke AR: Gastric and duodenal ulcer and their associated diseases. Lancet 1:680–683, 1976

275. Shepard AMM, Stewart WK, Wormsley KG: Peptic ulceration in chronic renal failure. Lancet 1:1357–1359, 1973
276. Linos Da, van Heerden JA, Abboud CF, Edis AJ: Primary hyperparathyroidism and peptic ulcer disease. Arch Surg 113:384–386, 1978
277. Graham DY, Schwartz JT, Cain GT, Gyorkey F: Prospective evaluation of biopsy number in the diagnosis of esophageal and gastric carcinoma. Gastroenterology 82:228–231, 1982
278. Lal N, Bhasin DK, Malik AK et al: Optimal number of biopsy specimens in the diagnosis of carcinoma of the esophagus. Gut 33: 724–726, 1992
279. Marshall JB, Diaz-arias AA, Barthel JS et al: Prospective evaluation of optimal number of biopsy specimens and brush cytology in the diagnosis of cancer of the colorectum. Am J Gastroenterol 88:1352–1354, 1993
280. Price AB, Levi J, Dolby JM et al: *Campylobacter pyloridis* in peptic ulcer disease: microbiology, pathology, and scanning electron microscopy. Gut 26:1183–1188, 1985
281. Shimazu H, Koniski T, Yamogishi T et al: A histopathological study on pyloric ulcer. Gastroenterol Jpn 15:362, 1980
282. Oohara T, Tohma H, Aono G et al: Intestinal metaplasia of the regenerative epithelia in 549 gastric ulcers. Hum Pathol 14: 1066–1071, 1983
283. Wolfe MM, Jensen RT: Zollinger–Ellison syndrome: current concepts in diagnosis and management. N Engl J Med 317:1200–1209, 1987
284. Guerrieri C, Waxman M: Hepatic tissue in gastroscopic biopsy: evidence of hepatic penetration by peptic ulcer. Am J Gastroenterol 82:890–893, 1987
285. Joffe H, Antonioli DA: Penetration into spleen by benign peptic ulcers. Clin Radiol 32:177–181, 1981
286. Goldman H: Systemic and miscellaneous conditions. pp. 351–380. In Ming S-C, Goldman H (eds): Pathology of the Gastrointestinal Tract. WB Saunders, Philadelphia, 1992
287. Gilat T, Spiro HM: Amyloidosis and the gut. Am J Dig Dis 13:619–633, 1968
288. Rocken C, Saeger W, Linke RP: Gastrointestinal amyloiid deposits in old age—report on 110 consecutive autopsical patients and 98 retrospective bioptic specimens. Pathol Res Pract 190:641–649, 1994
289. Coughlin GP, Remer, RG, Grant AK: Endoscopic diagnosis of amyloidosis. Gastrointest Endosc 26:154, 1980
290. Ohno F, Numata Y, Yamono T et al: Gastroscopic biopsy of the stomach for the diagnosis of amyloidosis. Gastroenterol Jpn 17:415–421, 1982
291. Brom B, Bunk S, Marks IN: Ischemic colitis, gastric ulceration, and malabsorption in a case of primary amyloidosis. Gastroenterology 57:319–323, 1969
292. Walley VM: Amyloid deposition in a gastric arteriovenous malformation. Arch Pathol Lab Med 110:69–71, 1986
293. Shousha S, Lowdell CP, Bull TB, Parkins RA: Secondary amyloidosis of the gastrointestinal tract: an electron microscopic study. Hum Pathol 16:596–601, 1985
294. Balazs M: Amyloidosis of the stomach. Report of a case with ultrastructure. Virchows Arch A Pathol Anat Histopathol 391: 227–240, 1981
295. Wada R, Yagihashi S, Konta R et al: Gastric polyposis caused by multifocal histiocytosis X. Gut 33:994–996, 1992
296. Groisman GM, Rosh JR, Harpaz N: Langerhans cell histiocytosis of the stomach. Arch Pathol Lab Med 118:1232–1235, 1994
297. Iwofuchi M, Watanabe H, Shiratsuka M: Primary benign histiocytosis of the stomach: a report of a case showing spontaneous remission after 5 1/2 years. Am J Surg Pathol 14:489–496, 1990
298. Conte D, Velio P, Brunelli L et al: Stainable iron in gastric and duodenal mucosa of primary hemochromatosis patients and alcoholics. Am J Gastroenterol 82:237–240, 1987
299. Tim LO, Hurwitz S, Tuch P: The endoscopic diagnosis of gastric calcification. J Clin Gastroenterol 4:213–215, 1982
300. Haggitt RC: Granulomatous diseases of the gastrointestinal tract. pp. 257–305. In Joachim HL (ed): Pathology of Granulomas. Raven Press, New York, 1983
301. Fahimi HD, Deren JJ, Gottleib LS et al: Isolated granulomatous gastritis. Gastroenterology 45:161–175, 1963
302. Khan MH, Lam R, Tamoney HJ: Isolated granulomatous gastritis. Am J Gastroenterol 71:90–94, 1979

303. Brown KM, Kass M, Wilson R: Isolated granulomatous gastritis. Treatment with corticosteroids. J Clin Gastroenterol 9:442–446, 1987
304. Ectors EL, Dixon MF, Geboes KJ et al: Granulomatous gastritis: a morphological and diagnostic approach. Histopathology 23:55–61, 1993
305. Weinstock JV: Idiopathic isolated granulomatous gastritis: spontaneous resolution without surgical intervention. Dig Dis Sci 25:233–235, 1980
306. Haggitt RC, Meissner WA: Crohn's disease of the upper gastrointestinal tract. Am J Clin Pathol 59:613–622, 1973
307. Rutgeerts P, Onette E, Vantrappen G et al: Crohn's disease of the stomach and duodenum: a clinical study with emphasis on the value of endoscopy and endoscopic biopsies. Endoscopy 12:288, 1980
308. Oren R, Harats N, Polak A et al: Granulomatous colitis 10 years after presentation with isolated Crohn's gastritis. Am J Gastroenterol 84:449–450, 1989
309. Korelitz BI, Waye JD, Kreuning J et al: Crohn's disease in endoscopic biopsies of the gastric antrum and duodenum. Am J Gastroenterol 76:103–109, 1981
310. Tanaka M, Kimura K, Sakai H et al: Long-term follow-up for minute gastroduodenal lesions in Crohn's disease. Gastrointest Endosc 32:206–209, 1986
311. Gad A: The diagnosis of gastroduodenal Crohn's disease by endoscopic biopsy. Scand J Gastroenterol (suppl) 167:23–28, 1989
312. Konda J, Ruth M, Sassaris M et al: Sarcoidosis of the stomach and rectum. Am J Gastroenterol 73:516, 1980
313. Chinitz MA, Brandt LJ, Frank MS et al: Symptomatic sarcoidosis of the stomach. Dig Dis Sci 30:682–688, 1985
314. Panella VS, Katz S, Kahn E, Ulberg R: Isolated gastric sarcoidosis. Unique remnant of disseminated disease. J Clin Gastroenterol 10:327–331, 1988
315. Ament ME, Ochs HD: Gastrointestinal manifestations of chronic granulomatous disease. N Engl J Med 288:382–387, 1973
316. Griscom NT, Kirkpatrick JA, Girdany JA et al: Gastric antral narrowing in chronic granulomatous disease of childhood. Pediatrics 54:456–460, 1974
317. Harned RK, Anderson JC, Owen DR: Suture granuloma of the stomach following splenectomy. Am J Gastroenterol 72: 302–305, 1979
318. Leach IH, Maclennon KA: Gastric lymphoma associated with mucosal and nodal granulomas: a new differential diagnosis in granulomatous gastritis. Histopathology 17:87–88, 1990
319. Ectors N, Geboes K, Wynants P, Desmet V: Granulomatous gastritis and Whipple's disease. Am J Gastroenterol 87:509–513, 1992
320. Yunis EJ, Estevez JM, Pinson GJ et al: Malakoplakia: discussion of pathogenesis and report of three cases including one of fatal gastric and colonic involvement. Arch Pathol 83:180, 1967
321. Nakabayashi H, Ito T, Izutsu K et al: Malakoplakia of the stomach: report of a case and review of the literature. Arch Pathol Lab Med 102:136, 1978
322. Graham RM, Rheault MH: Characteristic cellular changes in epithelial cells in pernicious anemia. J Lab Clin Med 43:235–245, 1954
323. Franzin G, Musola R, Mencarelli R: Morphological changes of the gastroduodenal mucosa in regular dialysis in uremic patients. Histopathology 6:429–437, 1982
324. Wee A, Kang JY, Choong HL et al: Gastroduodenal mucosa in uraemia: endoscopic and histological correlation and prevalence of Helicobacter-like organisms. Gut 31: 1093–1096, 1990
325. Littler ER, Gleibermann E: Gastritis cystica polyposa (gastric mucosal prolapse at gastroenterostomy site, with cystic and infiltrative epithelial hyperplasia). Cancer 29:205, 1972
326. Franzin G, Novelli P: Gastritis cystica profunda. Histopathology 5:535–547, 1981
327. Fonde EC, Rodning CB: Gastritis cystica profunda. Am J Gastroenterol 81:459–464, 1986
328. Colletti Rb, Trainer TD: Collagenous gastritis. Gastroenterology 97:1552–1555, 1989
329. Stolte M, Ritter M, Borchard F, Koch-Scheuer G: Collagenous gastroduodenitis in collagenous colitis. Endoscopy 22:186–187, 1990

5

Tumors of the Stomach

This chapter presents material on disorders that are characterized by mucosal hypertrophy and hyperplasia, and discusses gastric polyps, adenocarcinoma, and other tumors that occur in the stomach (Table 5-1).

GENERAL ASPECTS

Rigid gastroscopes largely limited the use of endoscopic examination and biopsy to the identification of mass lesions. The development of flexible scopes led to a great increase in the number of procedures involving examination of the stomach, and these have included the follow up of conditions that predispose to tumors.[1–3] Accordingly, there has been much more attention to the early lesions that precede the development of carcinoma and its invasion.[4–6] Extensive studies in regions with a high frequency of gastric carcinoma, such as in Japan, have led to precise classification and early detection of many tumors, with attendant improvements in therapy and prognosis.

Biopsy Material

The general uses and potential limitations of biopsy material in the examination of the upper gastrointestinal tract for tumors are mainly presented in Chapter 3 (see Table 3-2). These principles largely apply to the examination of the stomach as well. Endoscopy and biopsy of the stomach are commonly obtained to evaluate persistent ulcers or mass lesions, to follow patients with premalignant conditions in an effort to detect dysplasia or early carcinoma, and to monitor patients following therapy.[7–9] The diagnostic accuracy is enhanced by the addition of cytologic material, most often obtained by brushings at the time of endoscopic visualization.[10–14] A combination of four to six mucosal samples and cytologic material permits the detection of practically all malignant tumors.[15] Specimens should be obtained from any mucosal irregularity, including raised or depressed areas. Further attempts to improve detection include the uses of fine-needle aspiration of tumors at endoscopy[16, 17] and of endoscopic ultrasound to outline the extent of the lesions.[18, 19]

Special Studies

The routine H & E stains are sufficient for most diagnoses. There have been extensive studies employing histochemical stains for mucins and other substances, in efforts to better define the pathogenesis of the lesions

Table 5-1. Tumors of the Stomach

Inflammatory and heterotopic nodules
Benign gastric polyps
Adenocarcinoma
Endocrine tumors
Lymphoid tumors
Mesenchymal tumors
Secondary and metastatic tumors

and, potentially, to enhance the diagnoses[20–24] (Table 5-2). More recently, there has occurred the application of many immunocytochemical stains for similar purposes, and a variety of antibody stains are now used to improve on the diagnosis or to provide prognostic information, particularly in the analysis of gastric adenocarcinomas.[25] There have been several studies identifying the presence of proliferating cell nuclear antigen (PCNA) in the nuclei of various tumors.[26] In particular, there are suggestions that increases in this expression are associated with more aggressive gastrointestinal stromal tumors and possibly with worse prognosis in adenocarcinomas.[27, 28] There have also been efforts to help identify the earlier lesion of dysplasia by such techniques. For example, it has been shown that sucrase–isomaltase is commonly present in the cytoplasm of dysplastic cells, in contrast to normal or inflammatory gastric epithelial cells.[29]

For highly cellular tumors such as lymphomas, the use of metal-containing fixatives such as B5 are preferred, as these produce much clearer slides for examination. In addition, cell markers are often needed to establish monotypicality in malignant lymphomas.[30] There has also been considerable application of flow cytometry to gastric tumors of all sorts in efforts to relate to the prognosis. This has been limited by heterogeneity of the tumors, but the presence of aneuploidy has roughly correlated with the development of malignancy and with more advanced stage of development.[31, 32]

Table 5-2. Special Studies of Gastric Tumors

Mucin and enzyme histochemistry
Immunocytochemical markers
Ultrastructure
Flow cytometry and image analysis
Oncogenes and tumor suppressor genes
Gene restriction

Most recently, many studies have searched for oncogenes or for overexpression of aberrant tumor suppressor genes in gastric tumors and in adjacent mucosa.[33–38] Most of these studies are helping to define the sequence of tumor development and have not as yet reached the stage of practical use in diagnosis and in determination of therapy.

MUCOSAL HYPERTROPHY AND HYPERPLASIA

Focal Disorders

Localized thickenings of the mucosa can be due to inflammatory lesions and to ectopic tissue such as pancreas[39–41] (described in Ch. 4), and to a variety of polyps (presented later in this chapter) (Table 5-3). When the lesions are very large, they can produce mucin, protein, and electrolyte losses, simulating some of the diffuse mucosal disorders. However, their limited distribution can usually be identified by endoscopy and their nature determined by multiple mucosal biopsies. Probably any case of persistent or chronic gastritis can have transient, localized areas of foveolar hyperplasia, and these must be distinguished from the diffuse mucosal hyperplasia disorders that are not associated with such inflammation, principally Ménétrier's disease and Zollinger-Ellison syndrome.

Table 5-3. Mucosal Hypertrophy and Hyperplasia of the Stomach

Focal disorders
Heterotopic tissues
Gastric polyps
Inflammatory nodules
Diffuse disorders
Ménétrier's disease
Zollinger-Ellison syndrome
Chronic gastritis
Carcinoma and lymphoma

DIFFUSE DISORDERS

A variety of inflammatory and tumorous conditions can be associated with a thickening of the mucosal layer, involving either a large part of or the entire stomach surface.[42–44] Based on the principal localization, such as the antrum or the corpus, an initial estimate of the disorder can be made and a precise diagnosis determined by the biopsy. Ménétrier's disease and Zollinger-Ellison syndrome are concentrated in the proximal stomach, most of the inflammatory conditions are in the antrum, and tumors often involve both portions.

There is variation in the size of the normal gastric rugae, and probably the leading cause for simple prominence of these folds is a normal variation. Such enlarged rugae are encountered at the time of endoscopy or radiographic examination and their normality suspected by the lack of any irregularity or of any functional, secretory problem. Biopsies in such patients simply reveal a normal mucosa as the enlarged rugae are probably the result of more prominent submucosal tissue.

Ménétrier's Disease

Ménétrier's disease is an uncommon disorder characterized by a pure hyperplasia of the gastric pit mucous cells.[43–47] There results a diffuse and occasionally polypoid thickening of the mucosa, principally beginning in and largely remaining in the fundus and corpus regions. In the later stages the lesion may progress into the antrum; rarely, cases are seen in which the antrum is equally involved in the early stages of the disease. The cause of the disorder is unknown, and its natural course is highly variable, particularly in adults. The lesion may be associated with prominent mucus and protein loss, resulting in reduced serum albumin and in edema formation.

The diagnosis is suspected by the clinical information and by the gross appearance at endoscopic and radiographic examinations. Biopsies of the diffuse and polypoid areas are similar, revealing simple hyperplasia of the gastric pit mucous cells with variable cyst formation[48] (Fig. 5-1). There is characteristically very little inflammation or active regeneration of the cells. Most of the cells appear to be distended with the mucus granules. These granules are normally present only in the apical portion of normal cells, but in this hyperplastic state the granules are present in larger portions of the cytoplasm. The mucin stains strongly with the PAS reaction for neutral glycoproteins and weakly or not at all with acid mucin stains. The absence of inflammation, of prominent regeneration of the cells in the form of enlarged nuclei with prominent nucleoli, and of many mitoses help to distinguish Ménétrier's from a chronic gastritis with secondary hyperplasia of the gastric pits.[43, 49] Patients with the chronic erosive or chronic lymphocytic form of gastritis can have marked hyperplasia of the gastric pits leading to protein loss.[50, 51] These cases should be carefully distinguished from the pure Ménétrier's disease, which lacks the associated inflammation. Similarly, examples of extensive gastritis cystica can lose protein but are readily recognized by the appearance of a more limited mass and by the presence of pronounced inflammation and glandular regeneration.[52–54]

The development of carcinoma has been claimed in cases of Ménétrier's disease,[55] but it is probable that this involves cases of chronic gastritis of the hypertrophic and erosive types. In the pure Ménétrier's cases, there is no certain increase in tumor development. The potential importance is whether such patients would need surveillance to look for dysplasia and early carcinoma, but this is not established.

Ménétrier's disease also occurs in children where it has a more characteristic course.[56–58] It typically develops shortly after a respiratory infection, is more easily recognized be-

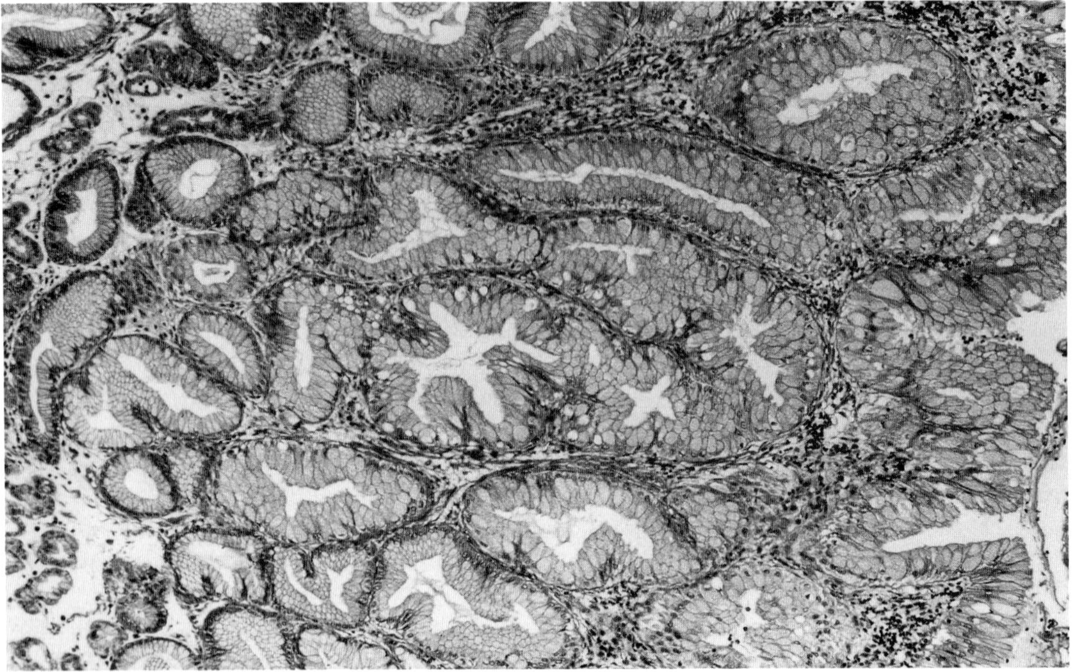

Fig. 5-1. Ménétrier's disease involving the gastric corpus, with surface appearing at right. There is a marked hyperplasia of the gastric pits. The lining cells are enlarged and distended with mucus. Mitoses are rare, the epithelial cell nuclei lack features of active regeneration, and there is only slight inflammation in the lamina propria (× 105).

cause of the prominence of the proximal gastric folds in patients who do not have chronic gastritis, and is largely a reversible lesion. Children are also prone to develop allergic gastritis that can be associated with prominent mucosal folds and protein loss, but these are typically confined to the antral region.[59, 60]

In all cases of Ménétrier's disease, the biopsy is not specific but does provide the features of pure hyperplasia that are supportive of the diagnosis. In particular, the biopsy serves to rule out a chronic gastritis and other lesions, such as tumors, which can be causing the thickened folds in this area.

Zollinger-Ellison Syndrome

Zollinger-Ellison syndrome results from an autonomous proliferation of gastrin-producing cells, usually in the form of a hyperplasia or tumor of the pancreatic islets, and less often involving the duodenal or gastric mucosa.[43, 61, 62] There is a sustained and maximal stimulation of the parietal cells, which undergo profound hyperplasia resulting in excess acid and water secretions. This results in intractable ulcer disease and the potential for malabsorption due to dilution and acidification of the duodenal contents. The ulcers develop in the gastric antrum, in all parts of the duodenum, and may even extend into the proximal jejunum.

The diagnosis is typically made by the acid secretion studies, demonstrating maximal production at a basal and stimulated level, as well as by elevated gastrin levels in the blood. Morphologic studies are ordinarily not obtained but are characteristic. There is a marked thickening of the mucosa of the gastric fundus and corpus that is principally due to a great increase in the number of parietal cells. Accordingly, the mucosa reveals normal-sized gastric pits overlying specialized glands that may be double or triple the normal length. As a result, regular endoscopic biopsies may obtain only a fraction of the mucosa, and aspiration-type samples would be needed to realize the full thickness of the mucosa and the extent of the glands. The parietal cells extend into the neck and lower pit region, but their appearance in this location is not a reliable criterion to document hyperplasia since they are frequently seen in this site in otherwise normal mucosa.

As mentioned above, most cases are due to tumors or hyperplasias involving the pancreas or duodenum. Exceptionally, a lesion may be due to a hyperplasia of the antral G cells, and aspiration-type biopsies might be used to count the number of cells in this area.[63] The aspiration biopsies are needed to be sure that the full thickness of the mucosa is obtained to get precise numbers. As pointed out above, blood and tissue levels of hormones are more often used for ordinary diagnoses instead of these morphometric studies.

Endoscopy and biopsy are commonly obtained in patients with Zollinger-Ellison syndrome to chart the ulcers and to monitor the patients following therapy. As discussed, because of the large amount of acid secretion, the ulcers are not limited to the antrum and first position of the duodenum but can extend into the further parts of the small intestine. Otherwise, the biopsy features are similar to those seen in any ulcer, showing necrosis and both acute and chronic inflammation. There is no special relationship between the cases of Zollinger-Ellison syndrome and the presence of *Helicobacter pylori.*

Other Secretory Disorders

There are rare cases of mucosal hypertrophy due to a mixture of hyperplasia of the pit mucous cells and the specialized glands.[43, 44] These may be associated with excess protein loss and, less often, with increased acid secretion. It is probable that they represent variants of the other hyperplastic disorders, and their precise analysis requires complete examination of a gastric specimen. Biopsies are largely used to rule out other significant inflammatory or tumor conditions.

Inflammatory Conditions

As noted, many of the inflammatory conditions, particularly the chronic disorders, can be associated with a thickening of the mucosa, due in part to edema and inflammatory cells and also to a hyperplasia of the gastric pit mucous cells. All of these features are temporary and eventually resolve. Biopsy during the active phase reveals the inflammatory and regenerative features. Most inflammatory lesions tend to be concentrated in the antrum, and this helps to distinguish the thickening from the proximal disorders such as Ménétrier's disease and Zollinger–Ellison syndrome. The diseases that are mainly in the antrum include the cases of allergic gastritis, as part of eosinophilic or allergic gastroenteritis, many of the chronic infections, and most of the granulomatous conditions.[64] The special selection of the antrum may simply reflect the existence of a looser lamina propria in this region.

Tumors

Both adenocarcinomas of the diffuse or signet ring cell type and malignant lymphomas can present with diffuse rather than localized polypoid lesions. The classic example is the linitis plastica lesion of diffuse carcinoma. In these tumor cases, there may be diffuse and polypoid nodules involving any portion of the stomach with variable erosions and ulcers. The irregularity of the surface and the variable distribution usually serve to distinguish these cases grossly from the more regular examples of Ménétrier's and

Zollinger-Ellison, and the diagnosis is readily secured by multiple biopsies revealing the tumor cells.

GASTRIC MUCOSAL POLYPS

Presented in this section are the localized polyps that develop from the mucosa of the stomach (Table 5-4). Most of these appear as single or as multiple nodules, and included are a variety of inflammatory lesions as well as rare neoplasms. Exceptionally, the stomach is involved in a patient with a polyposis syndrome, in which there is the development of many more polyps.

Single and Multiple Polyps

Hyperplastic (Regenerative) Polyp

Hyperplastic polyps are probably the most common polyps noted in the stomach, but occur much less frequently than polyps seen in the large intestine.[65–69] An incidence of approximately 1 in 1000 has been estimated, with most lesions considered incidental findings at the time of endoscopic, radiographic, or gross examination of the stomach. The frequency of the hyperplastic polyps is increased in any sustained inflammatory condition, and as many as 10 percent of cases of chronic gastritis may reveal such lesions. They have been seen in all forms of chronic gastritis, including chronic antral disease, pernicious anemia and chronic fundic gastritis, and the post-gastrectomy form of gastritis. Since the lesions are largely of an inflammatory and reparative nature, the polyps can be considered analogous to the inflammatory pseudopolyps seen in cases of chronic colitis.

Table 5-4. Benign Mucosal Polyps of the Stomach

- Single and Multiple Polyps
  - Hyperplastic (regenerative) polyp
  - Cystic fundic gland polyp
  - Inflammatory fibroid polyp
  - Other non-neoplastic polyps
  - Adenoma
- Polyposis syndromes
  - Adenomatous polyposis coli
  - Juvenile polyposis
  - Peutz-Jeghers syndrome
  - Cronkhite-Canada syndrome

The polyps are usually single but may be multiple in up to one-quarter of the cases. They are of variable size, with the smaller being sessile and the larger assuming a short stalk. Most are smooth surfaced. They are composed of a mixure of hyperplastic gastric pits with variable regenerative activity, considerable edema and inflammation of the lamina propria, and a relative paucity of intestinal metaplasia (Fig. 5-2). The hyperplastic polyps may contain *H. pylori,* particularly in cases complicating chronic antral gastritis due to this agent.[70] Occasionally noted within the stroma of a hyperplastic polyp are islands of macrophages containing lipid material,[71] identical to the xanthomas that can be seen in the gastric mucosa.[72–74] These appear to be related to the foci of resolving hemorrhage. The biopsy material is often in the form of fragments of tissue, and the analysis typically requires the recognition of the inflammatory and hyperplastic tissue, which would be compatible with the hyperplastic polyps. In the biopsy interpretation it is equally important to exclude some other form of polyp, particularly an adenoma; the latter shows dysplastic glands, as described below.

Most cases of hyperplastic polyps are asymptomatic, probably representing localized areas of excess regeneration in a region of injury or prolonged inflammation. When multiple polyps are encountered, it is important to examine the intervening mucosa as well to determine whether there is an underlying chronic gastritis. Such cases of gastritis in turn require more analysis and potential surveillance to rule out any future dysplasia or carcinoma. The hyperplastic polyp itself may cause difficulty by virtue of enlargement and twisting on a stalk, leading to superficial erosion and bleeding; by location in the antrum with the potential to prolapse through the pylorus, causing intermittent obstruction; by a very large size that would require multiple samples to exclude neoplasia; and by multiple recurrences.[75] In addition, there are exceptional cases where there are literally too many polyps to evaluate, leading to the need for segmental resection. Finally, those cases with multiple and recurring hyperplastic polyps can develop foci of dysplastic or adenomatous change and carcinoma within the hyperplastic polyps[76, 77] (Fig. 5-3). It is probable that such cases simply represent samples of chronic gastritis in which the dysplasia and carcinoma is developing in the polyp as well as in the flat mucosa.[78, 79] They should be treated as any case with dysplasia and early cancer, requiring not only removal of the involved polyp but also systematic examination of the rest of the stomach to exlude more extensive neoplasia.

It may be difficult to distinguish the solitary or multiple hyperplastic polyps from other lesions occurring in the stomach that have an inflammatory or hamartomatous nature. Indeed, they may share a common pathogenesis in the form of the excess growth of inflammatory tissue. Thus, the lesion of gastritis cystica polyposa may represent an unusually large hyperplastic polyp that is concentrated in the gastric stump near a stoma[80] (see Fig. 4-44). Similarly, examples of inflammatory fibroid polyps, of juvenile polyps, and of polyps seen in the Peutz–Jeghers syndrome may be indistinguishable histologically from the ordinary hyperplastic polyp. The differentation in such cases depends on other findings in the alimentary tract.

Cystic Fundic Gland Polyp

Cystic fundic gland polyp is a very common polyp, possibly more frequent than the hyperplastic polyp, but without known incidence figures.[81–83] These lesions were recognized in patients with adenomatous polyposis coli and were initially considered to be a potential marker of that syndrome.[84] However, it became evident that they could occur as well in otherwise normal persons and could disappear over time. The lesions are typically tiny (in the range of a few millimeters), have a smooth surface, and are sessile.

They are composed of normal gastric fundic-corpus mucosa, with prominent cystic change of the specialized glands that results in the mucosal enlargement and polyp formation (Fig. 5-4). There is typically no other feature such as inflammation, metaplasia, or dysplasia of the cells. They are readily encompassed by the biopsy, and the diagnostic features are specific. There are no known sequellae.

Inflammatory Fibroid Polyp

The inflammatory fibroid polyp is an uncommon inflammatory-type polyp that is seen most often in the stomach and in the distal ileum.[85–89] The gastric lesions tend to be larger and develop a stalk, and they can cause obstruction if located in the pyloric region, where they may prolapse through the sphincter area. The lesions typically involve not only the mucosa but often extend into the upper portion of the submucosa, suggesting that they may arise from an ulcerated lesion in that area. They are comprised of a mixture of hyperplastic pits, collagen and smooth muscle strands, and extensive inflammatory tissue with prominent edema and eosinophils. The larger lesions can have superficial erosions, probably due to the twisting of stalks. Biopsies typically reveal fragments of tissue with the evident connective tissue elements, edema, and eosinophils, but without any epithelial dysplasia (see Figs. 8-11 and 10-7). This permits a diagnosis that is consistent with an inflammatory fibroid polyp. It should be stressed that the histological features seen in the ordinary hyperplastic polyp and in the inflammatory fibroid polyp greatly

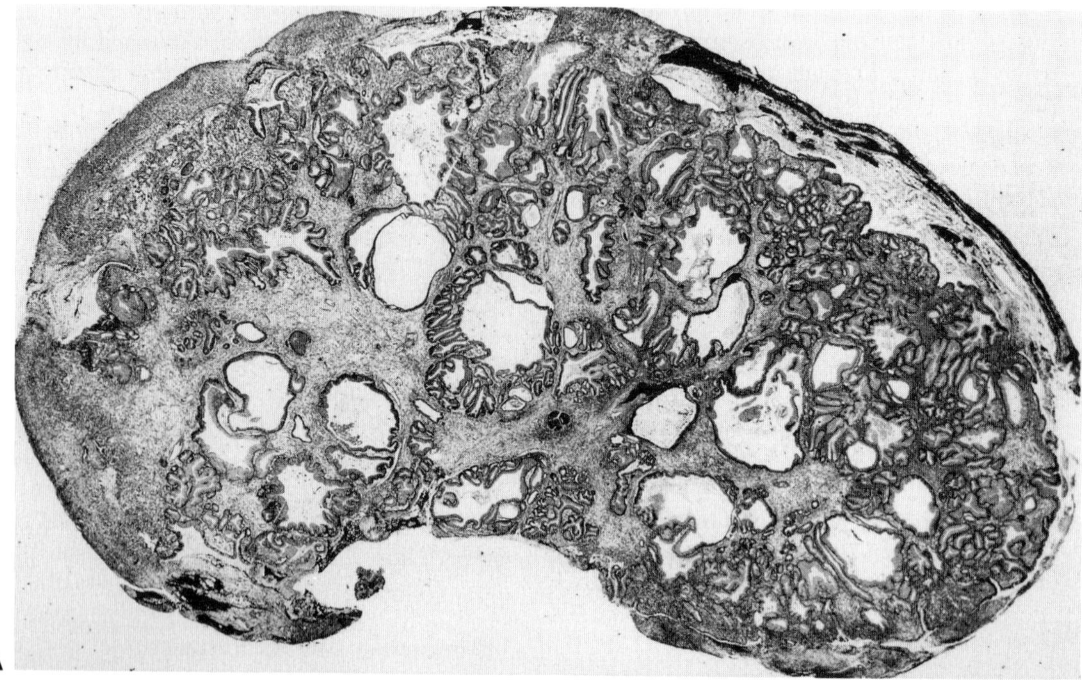

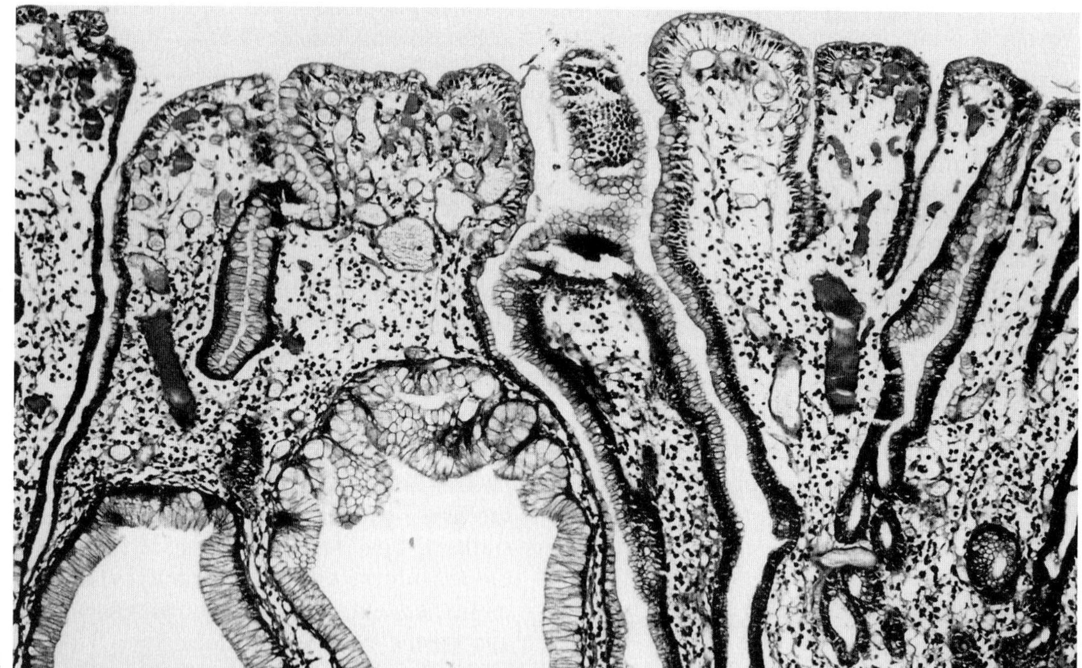

Fig. 5-2. Hyperplastic polyp of the stomach. (**A**) The polyp has a smooth surface and is composed of a mass of cystic and proliferative glands together with edematous stroma (× 11). (**B**) Surface of polyp, showing the hyperplastic pits without any cellular atypism and the inflammatory cells in the stroma (× 105). (*Figure continues.*)

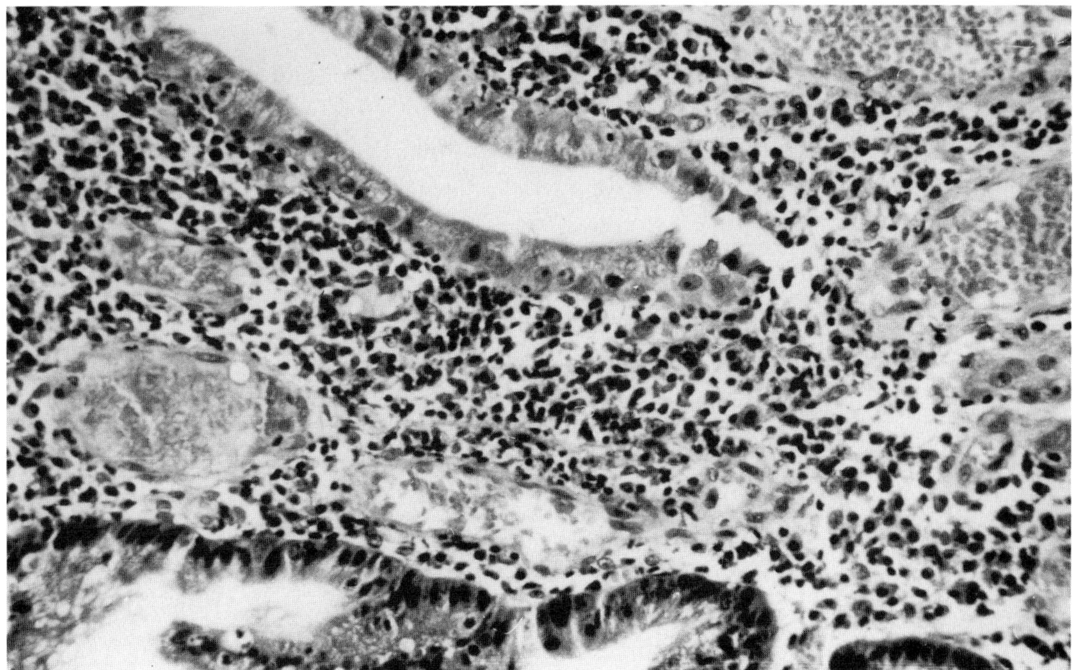

C

Fig. 5-2. (*Continued*). (**C**) Area of polyp adjacent to erosion, revealing degeneration and regeneration of the epithelial cells and marked inflammation.

overlap. One of the more important functions of the biopsy is to exlude a neoplastic growth such as an adenoma or an adenocarcinoma.

Other Non-Neoplastic Polyps

There are various other inflammatory and hamartomatous lesions that can result in localized polyp formation in the stomach. Those related to the several polyposis syndromes are described below. Any area of localized inflammation may transiently persist, causing the appearance of an inflammatory-type polyp; these are typically comprised of edematous and inflamed tissue or of prominent granulation tissue, and they ultimately subside. Biopsies show the inflammatory or reparative component, and they are best diagnosed as simple inflammatory-type polyps. A polyp designated as focal foveolar hyperplasia probably represents a variant of the hyperplastic polyp in which there is mainly the feature of the elongated gastric pits without much associated inflammation in the lamina propria. In such cases one should also consider the possibility of a localized area of regeneration and a healing gastritis.

Adenoma

Adenoma of the stomach represents a localized benign neoplasm of the gastric epithelium.[65, 66, 90, 91] In contrast to the colon, adenomas of the stomach in otherwise normal persons are rare. They are increased in patients with chronic gastritis and in those with adenomatous polyposis syndromes that affect the colon. In the non-polyposis cases the lesions tend to be single, and most are larger than 1 to 2 cm. The isolated adenomas have a variable gross appearance, ranging from those that are polypoid or papillary to

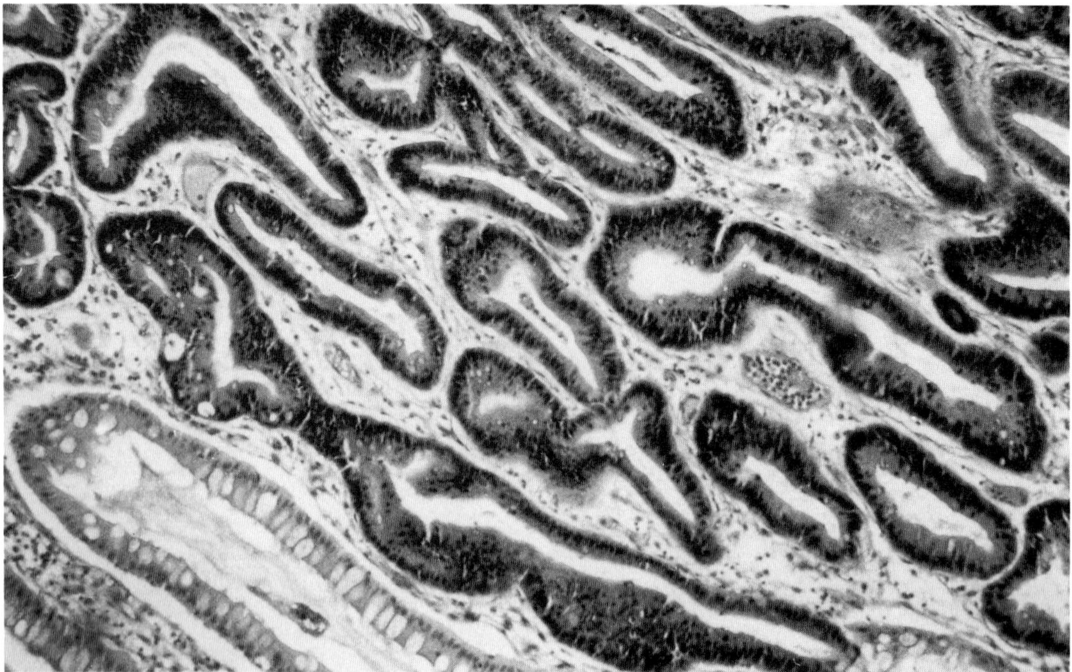

Fig. 5-3. Adenomatous (dysplastic) epithelium in a hyperplastic polyp of the stomach. This occurred in a patient with multiple recurring polyps. The dysplastic epithelium shows nuclear enlargement, palisading, and hyperchromatism. A small part of the original hyperplastic polyp appears at the lower left.

lesions that are flat or depressed. As with adenomas in any part of the alimentary tract, they are prone to transformation to adenocarcinoma.[92] Accordingly, the lesions once diagnosed require endoscopic or segmental excision.

The diagnosis can be suspected grossly by the larger size and papillary surface, and it is confirmed readily by the microscopic analysis. Revealed are the typical features of dysplastic cells with evident elongation and palisading of the nuclei, variation in their size and shape, and hyperchromatism (Fig. 5-5). The degree of dysplasia can vary within the adenoma, tending to be more severe, or high grade, in the larger lesions. Based on the dominant gross features, the adenomas have been divided into those that are polypoid or papillary and the less common ones that are relatively flat. All are prone to malignancy, and multiple samples should be obtained to exclude the coexistence of intramucosal or invasive adenocarcinoma.

Summary of Isolated Gastric Polyps

In the analysis of a mucosal polyp of the stomach, one should exclude any lesion that extends from the submucosa as well as a variety of other nodules that can appear in the mucosa, such as mucosal cysts,[93] pancreatic or other heterotopic tissues,[39–41, 94] and xanthomas.[72–74] All of these lesions are readily recognized by their distinctive features, and they are described in Chapter 4.

In the analysis of a mucosal polyp, the major distinction is between a neoplasm, including adenoma or polypoid adenocarcinoma, as opposed to all the other conditions. If the latter, it may be possible to render a highly specific diagnosis, such as a cystic fundic gland polyp, or to indicate that the features are compatible with one or another polyp, such as a hyperplastic polyp. In some instances, particularly with the polyposis syndromes, it is necessary to relate the features to the clinical information. If the biopsies

A

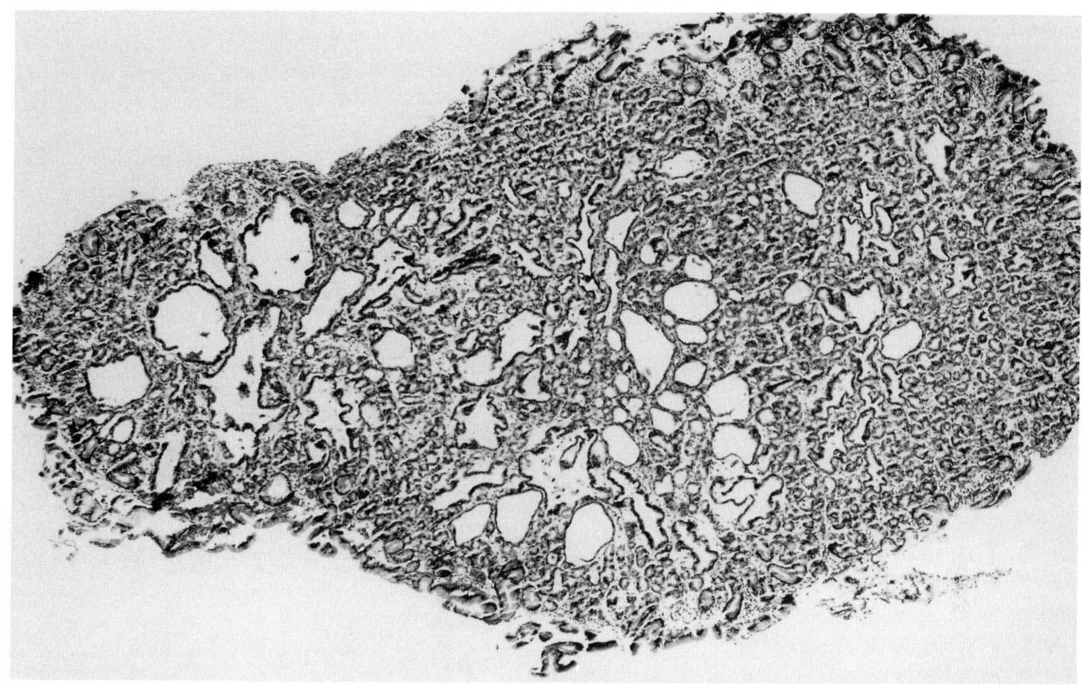

B

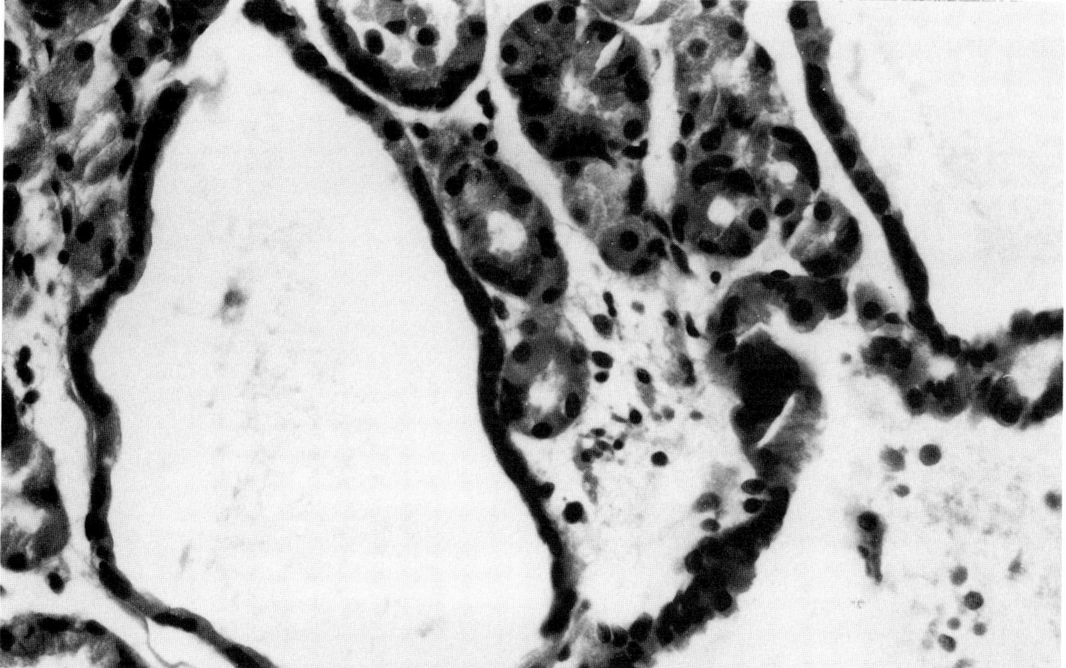

Fig. 5-4. Cystic fundic gland polyp of the stomach. (**A**) The polyp is small, only slightly raised, and has a smooth surface. Cystic glands and lack of inflammation are characteristic (× 11). (**B**) The cystic spaces typically involve the specialized glands and are lined by the parietal and chief cells (× 425).

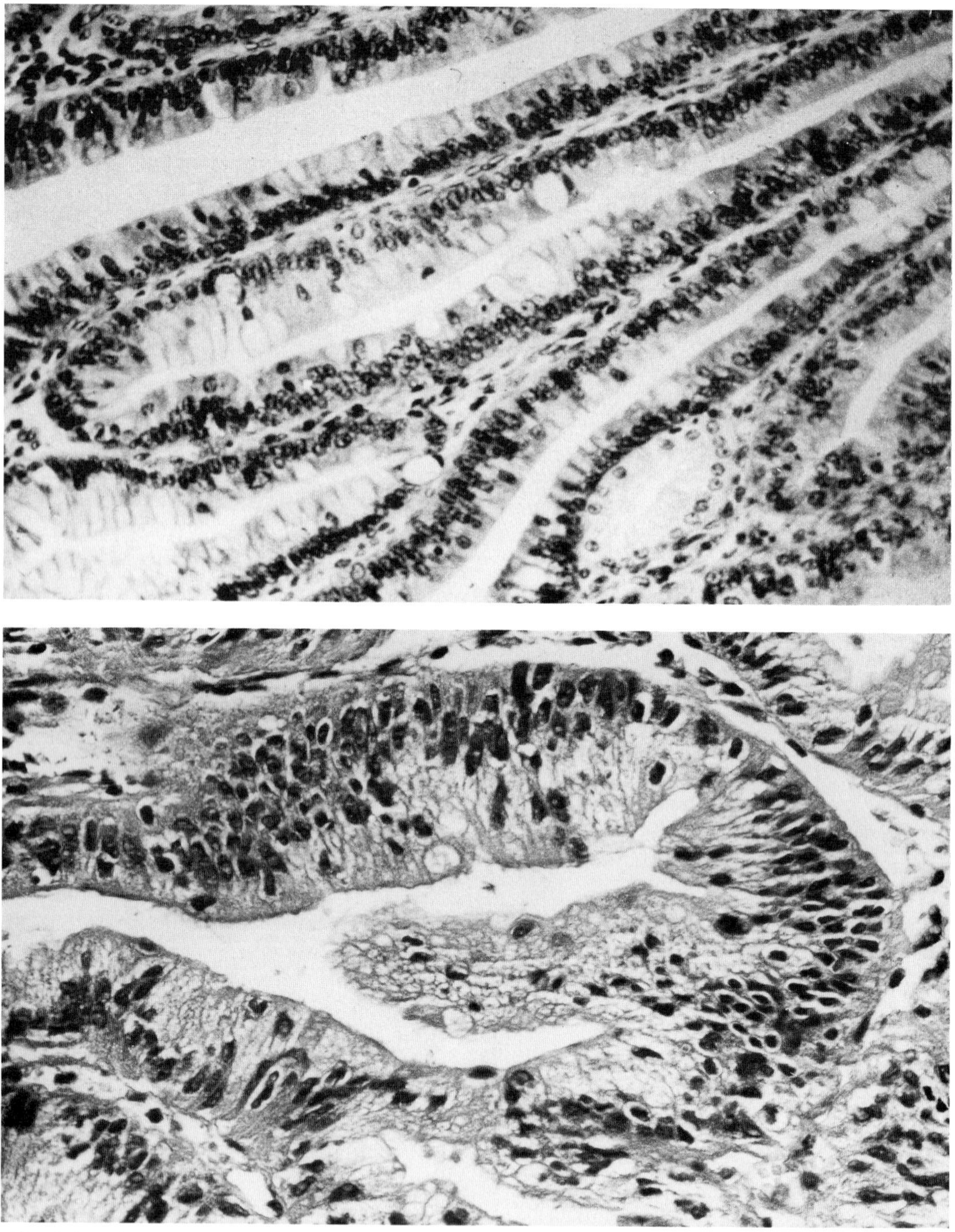

A

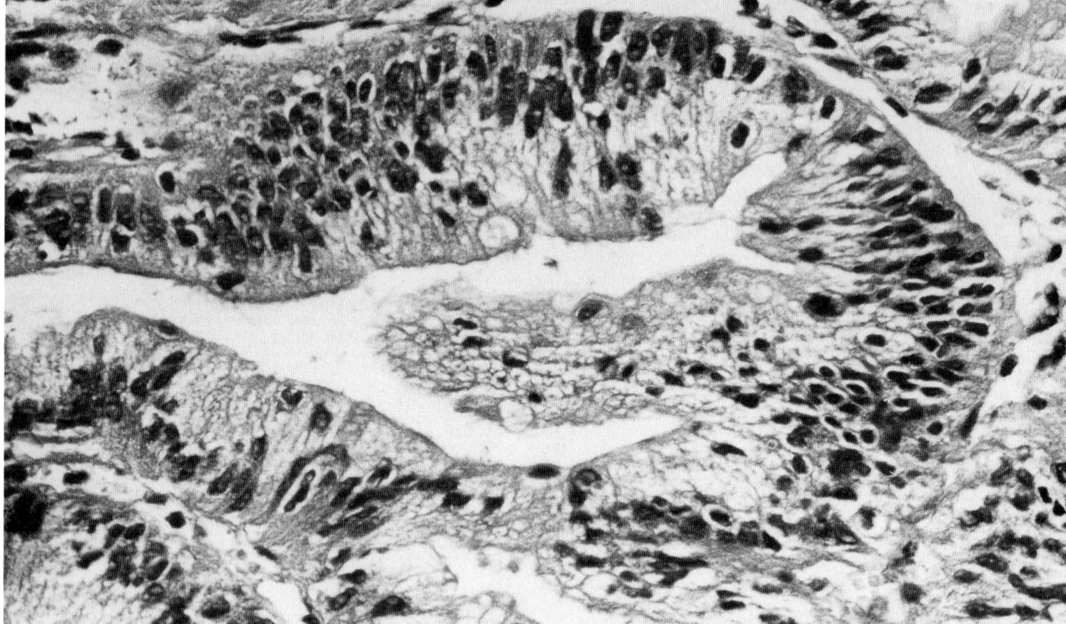

B

Fig. 5-5. Adenoma of the stomach. (**A**) The polyp is composed of dysplastic cells, including both gastric- and intestinal-type cells. (From Goldman,[1] with permission.) (**B**) Gland in adenoma, showing the pronounced palisading of the nuclei and irregularly reduced mucin content (× 425).

reveal an adenoma, it becomes important to look as well for areas of carcinoma, either limited to the mucosa or extending into the submucosal tissue, if such material is provided. This subject is discussed further in this chapter under "Adenocarcinoma."

Polyposis Syndromes

There are several syndromes in which multiple polyps can develop in the stomach.[95–97] As with the isolated cases, it is most important to sort out those that are of an inflammatory or a hamartomatous nature and not at immediate risk for associated carcinoma, as opposed to the adenomas. Also, it is important to distinguish between cases that have multiple or recurrent polyps but are not part of a generalized polyposis syndrome. This is particularly so in cases with chronic gastritis, which can develop multiple hyperplastic polyps.[75]

Adenomatous Polyposis Coli

Patients with adenomatous polyposis coli develop extensive adenomas of the rectum and colon and have a risk of carcinoma for that area that approaches 100 percent. Accordingly, they are treated at a young age by a prophylactic proctocolectomy. Gardner's syndrome represents a variant in which the patients also develop a variety of proliferative and hamartomatous lesions involving their soft tissues, skin, and teeth. In Gardner's syndrome there are often a lesser number of adenomas in the colon, but there is no easy separation with the rest of the adenomatous polyposis cases.

In patients with adenomatous polyposis coli there is an increased incidence of adenomas and of carcinomas affecting the other parts of the gastrointestinal tract. These have been particularly noted in the stomach, in the duodenum with major concentration in the ampullary region, and in distal ileal segments including both ileostomy and reservoir tissues. The polyps develop in patients with the full polyposis syndrome[98–104] and also in those with the Gardner's variant[105, 106] and the flat adenoma syndrome of the colon.[107]

Accordingly, these areas are surveyed for the appearance of such lesions. They typically present in patients from the third decade on with small but multiple adenomas. These patients can also develop other types of polyps in the stomach, including hyperplastic and cystic fundic gland polyps.[84, 108, 109] Therefore biopsy is needed to secure the diagnosis as well as to remove the polyps. In the stomach the cases can usually be controlled by repeated endoscopy and removal of the lesions. If it becomes more extensive leading to marked formation of polyps, resection would be required. As noted, these lesions also affect the duodenal mucosa, including especially the ampullary region, and require very close surveillance and removal of all adenomas to prevent the development of invasive carcinoma.

Juvenile Polyposis

Juvenile polyps are rarely seen in the stomach except as part of a polyposis syndrome.[69] The most common form of juvenile polyposis is limited to the large intestine.[110] The stomach can be affected by an isolated form that is exceedingly rare, more so in a subset of cases of generalized gastrointestinal juvenile polyposis.[111, 112] The polyps are mainly small, sessile, and are comprised of inflammatory tissue with prominent cystic dilation of the gastric pits (see Ch. 10). At both a gross and histologic level, the lesions are practically identical to the ordinary hyperplastic polyps, and the particular diagnosis almost always requires the historical information that the patient has many polyps or similar lesions in the colon. In cases of juvenile polyposis of the colon, there is a small risk of development of dysplasia and carcinoma in the colon.[113] Rarely observed are foci of dysplastic epithelium in juvenile polyps of the stomach, which can presage the development of carcinoma similar to that seen in the colon. In such cases, the polyp needs to be completely excised and the patient requires continued surveillance.

Peutz-Jeghers Syndrome

Peutz-Jeghers syndrome is a disorder with generalized polyps of the alimentary tract, most pronounced in the small intestine, with variable lesions in the colon and in the stomach.[114, 115] The features are most characteristic in the small bowel, showing a hamartoma that involves all components of the mucosa as revealed by irregularly dilated indigenous and metaplastic glands together with broad bands of smooth muscle (see Figs. 6-23 and 10-17). Any polyp may have a small amount of muscle proliferation, but the quantitiy in the Peutz-Jeghers polyp is especially striking, presumbly due to proliferation that emanates from the muscularis mucosae. These polyps may occasionally be associated with an extension of mature glands and stroma into the underlying submucosa, and even into the muscularis propria. This is most prominently seen in the polyps that affect the small bowel. When present, there is the need to distinguish the misplaced epithelium from an invasive carcinoma. The precise features of these polyps are usually not present in the gastric lesions, which more often resemble the ordinary hyperplastic polyps. It is, therefore, necessary to link the biopsy findings with the historical information to make the particular diagnosis. An increase in carcinoma of various organs has been noted in this syndrome,[116, 117] including rare examples in the stomach.[118]

Cronkhite-Canada Syndrome

Cronkhite-Canada syndrome is associated with polyps throughout the gastrointestinal tract, with the stomach involved in about 90 percent of the cases.[119–122] There is a marked transformation of the mucosa that results in alternating areas of relatively atrophic and polypoid types of mucosa. Principal clinical problems are protein loss from the damaged mucosal surface, variable malabsorption, and involvement of the integument with skin pigmentation, nail abnormalities, and hair loss. The differential is often with a variety of inflammatory conditions in any part of the alimentary tract.

Biopsies show the edematous mucosa with inflammatory cells, and the lack of any significant ulceration, metaplasia, or other epithelial alterations (see Fig. 10-18). The features resemble a gastritis or case of inflammatory polyps, and the particular diagnosis of the Cronkhite-Canada syndrome requires the information related to the findings outside of the gastrointestinal tract.

An additional problem is the potential for malignant transformation, which most commonly affects the colon and the stomach, with estimates as high as 20 percent of cases.[123] Accordingly, given a patient with this syndrome in whom the lesion persists, surveillance biopsies might be considered. This does not, however, appear to be an important contributor to gastric carcinoma.

ADENOCARCINOMA

Although there has been a continuous decline of incidence of adenocarcinoma in the United States, it remains the leading malignant neoplasm of the human stomach.

Epidemiology

Gastric carcinoma continues to be highly prevalent in Chile, in the Scandanavian countries, and especially in Japan and other parts of the Orient.[124–126] The tumors are typically encountered in middle-aged and older persons and are more frequent in men. Two major changes in distribution and types of tumors have been noted over the past 20 years. There has been a decided increase in the percentage of tumors that involve the gastric cardia, which now encompass about one-quarter of the cases of gastric cancer.[127–130] These cardiac cases continue to involve relatively older patients, with a male predominance. In addition, there has been noted a marked increase in the number of cases of gastric carcinoma of the diffuse or signet ring cell type, which now approaches one-half of all of the carcinomas affecting the non-cardiac portion of the stomach.[127] This appears to be a relative increase, due to a reduction in the amount of the intestinal or glandular types of carcinomas occurring in this region. In concert with this cellular change, the cases with the distal carcinomas present at an earlier age and have an equal involvement of men and women.[131–133] Again, this suggests a reduction in a subset of cases involving older men with glandular-type carcinoma in the antral region. The reason for this decline is not known.

The cause of gastric carcinoma is not known.[124–126] Both dietary and genetic factors have been encountered (Table 5-5). One major theory suggests that in cases of chronic gastritis there is less acid, leading to increased bacteria and to more conversion of dietary nitrates to nitrites, which appear experimentally to favor cancer development. It has also been noted that populations consuming large amounts of smoked and salted foods are at an increased risk for gastric cancer development. Of considerable interest is the association with patients who have blood group O, since it has been recently recognized that these patients are probably at an increased risk for the development of chronic antral gastritis due to *H. pylori,* possibly due to the increased association of receptors for the bacterium in such people.[134] Despite all of these observations, a unified mechanism for the development of gastric carcinoma has not been established.

Table 5-5. Risk Factors and Conditions in Gastric Adenocarcinoma

Geographic distribution
Dietary components
Chronic gastritis
Chronic *H. pylori* infection
Immunodeficiency disorders
Polyposis syndromes

Premalignant Conditions and Lesions

Chronic Gastritis

It is generally accepted that patients with chronic gastritis are at some increased risk for the development of gastric carcinoma, but the frequency is probably highly variable in different populations.[135–137] Thus, the indigenous Japanese population seems to be at risk for this tumor without any other antecedent inflammatory marker. In contrast, the finding of a chronic gastritis serves in other areas to identify populations that are at an increased risk and that might benefit from a surveillance program. The increase in tumor has been noted in patients with chronic fundic gastritis and pernicious anemia,[138–140] with chronic antral gastritis due to *H. pylori,*[141–144] and with post-gastrectomy gastritis involving the stumps.[4, 5, 145–150] The frequency of carcinoma development in gastric remnants has been especially variable, being relatively high in most Scandinavian series and less prominent in the United States.[151–153] In many of these cases, endoscopy can detect dysplastic lesions before the frank appearance of carcinoma.[154–156] It has been noted that bile diversion techniques can reduce the inflammation in gastric stumps and potentially decrease the likelihood of cancer formation.[157]

This has led to extensive study of the patients with these various forms of chronic gastritis. As noted previously, there is a strong association between the development of carcinoma and the appearance of the type III, or colonic form, of intestinal metaplasia in contrast to the type I, or small intestinal form.[158–164] Nevertheless, this marker of colonic metaplasia is so common in the patients with chronic gastritis that it has not been possible to use it in a prospective fashion. (This subject is discussed in Ch. 4 under "Chronic Gastritis".)

Other Premalignant Conditions

A smaller increase of gastric cancer formation has been noted in patients with a variety of immunodeficiency and other immunologic disorders, including patients with AIDS and with celiac disease.[165, 166] There is no support for tumor development following radiation or chemical exposure to the stomach. There is a potential link to cases with long-standing infection due to *H. pylori*[141, 142] and possibly also to chronic syphilitic infection of the stomach. The latter has been associated with marked mucosal atrophy, squamous metaplasia, and squamous cell carcinoma. An increase in gastric carcinoma also occurs in the various polyposis syndromes, particularly those that are composed of adenomas (see "Polyposis Syndromes", above). As described above, the alleged relationship to Ménétrier's disease is probably due to confusion of the pure cases with those of hypertrophic and of erosive chronic gastritis. There is also no established proof of an association of carcinoma in patients with chronic peptic ulcer or with isolated hyperplastic polyps. In the cases with ulcer the underlying chronic gastritis may serve as a promoting factor but the ulcer itself is not a premalignant lesion. The same applies to the hyperplastic-type polyps that may also be seen in patients with chronic gastritis.

Premalignant Lesions

As in other parts of the alimentary tract, the essential premalignant lesion in the stomach is represented by epithelial dysplasia.[167–170] This involves the gastric pits and is recognized by the alterations in the nuclei. This dysplasia occurs in the flat mucosa in cases with chronic gastritis and allows for the use of endoscopy and biopsy to search for its presence in high-risk patients. The adenoma represents a gross lesion of dysplastic tissue. This can be seen as an isolated finding in an otherwise normal person but is very rare; can develop in association with other dysplastic lesions in patients with chronic gastritis; and is increased in patients with adenomatous polyposis coli, as described above. Many of the lesions labeled as early gastric carcinoma represent highly dysplastic lesions that are limited to the mucosa. They probably represent the simple extension of dysplasia or adenoma to early carcinoma, beginning within the mucosa and ultimately extending into the submucosa. This continuum has been well established in high-risk populations, such as in the Japanese and in patients with chronic gastritis, including, particularly, pernicious anemia and those with gastric remnants.

In all of the patient groups with increased risk for carcinoma, surveillance endoscopy and biopsy has been considered and is most useful if the frequency of the tumors is relatively high, such as in Scandinavian and Asian countries as opposed to the United States. In the gross examination, areas of early carcinoma, described below, should be sought. In addition, it is necessary to sort out the residual inflammatory lesions largely in the form of erosions or polyps. In cases with gastric remnants and with chronic fundic gastritis, there frequently are prominent areas of hyperplastic polyps and cyst formation within the mucosa. The examples of chronic antral gastritis often harbor a great deal of active disease, including the presence of erosions and ulcers. Biopsies are often needed in these polypoid and ulcerated areas to exclude overt carcinoma, while looking for the preceding changes of dysplasia and early cancer.

Glandular Dysplasia

Classification

Areas of epithelial dysplasia are seen at the edges of most glandular- or intestinal-type carcinomas in the stomach (Table 5-6), whereas they tend to be less prominent in the cases with the diffuse or signet ring cell type of cancers.[170–180] There have been many studies of the dysplasia, leading to a classification with the 3 principal grades of *mild, moderate,* and *severe.* There are recent efforts to collate some of these groups and relate them more to the classifications used in the esophagus and the colon, employing just the 2 categories of low-grade and high-grade dysplasia[181] (see Table 3-9). On a rough scale, cases of mild and, probably, most of the moderate dysplasias in the stomach would correlate with low grade; and there is a close assimilation of the severe and high-grade categories.[182, 183] In contrast to the other areas of the gut, intramucosal carcinoma is seemingly much more common in the stomach and deserves a clear separation because of the large amount of information pertaining to its behavior and treatment.

Biopsy Features

The architectural and cytologic features of dysplasia are generally well described and may involve native gastric pits or those that have been converted into intestinal glands by metaplasia. In either case, the features are similar to those described in the esophagus in cases of Barrett's esophagus (see Ch. 3). In the mild/moderate (low-grade) degrees of dysplasia there is very little or no architectural alteration, but there is a presence of abnormal and unexplained cellular nuclei with some variation in size and shape, usually palisading and elongation of the nuclei, and variable presence and location of the nucleoli (Fig. 5-6). In this lesser degree of dysplasia, there is usually no prominent pleomorphism or hyperchromatism.

The cases of severe (high-grade) dysplasia show even greater abnormalities, including more variation in the size and shape of the pits, and greater differences in the size and shape of the nuclei with more evident hyperchromatism and loss of polarity (Fig. 5-7). Examples of *adenocarcinoma in-situ,* meaning highly dysplastic cells that are still contained within the gland, are best considered within the realm of high-grade dysplasia. These should be distinguished from examples of tumor infiltration into the lamina propria in the form of either single cells or highly irregular and dilated glands, which corresponds to intramucosal adenocarcinoma. The latter is the characteristic histologic feature seen in early gastric carcinoma rather than in high-grade dysplasia. There is probably a continuum, and one should designate the case by the worst feature.

Table 5-6. Types of Glandular Tumors in the Stomach

Glandular dysplasia and adenoma
Adenocarcinoma
Early
Advanced
Variants of adenocarcinoma
Adenosquamous cell carcinoma
Squamous cell carcinoma and mucoepidermoid carcinoma
Lymphoepithelioma-like carcinoma
Hepatoid carcinoma and parietal cell carcinoma

Diagnosis and Behavior

The finding of dysplasia is mainly in patients with the established premalignant conditions, particularly with chronic gastritis. Most work has been done in patients with pernicious anemia and in those with gastric stumps. In both areas it is extremely important to exclude inflammatory and regenerative features that persist in these patients. This may be grossly evident in the form of polyps or more subtle in the way of promi-

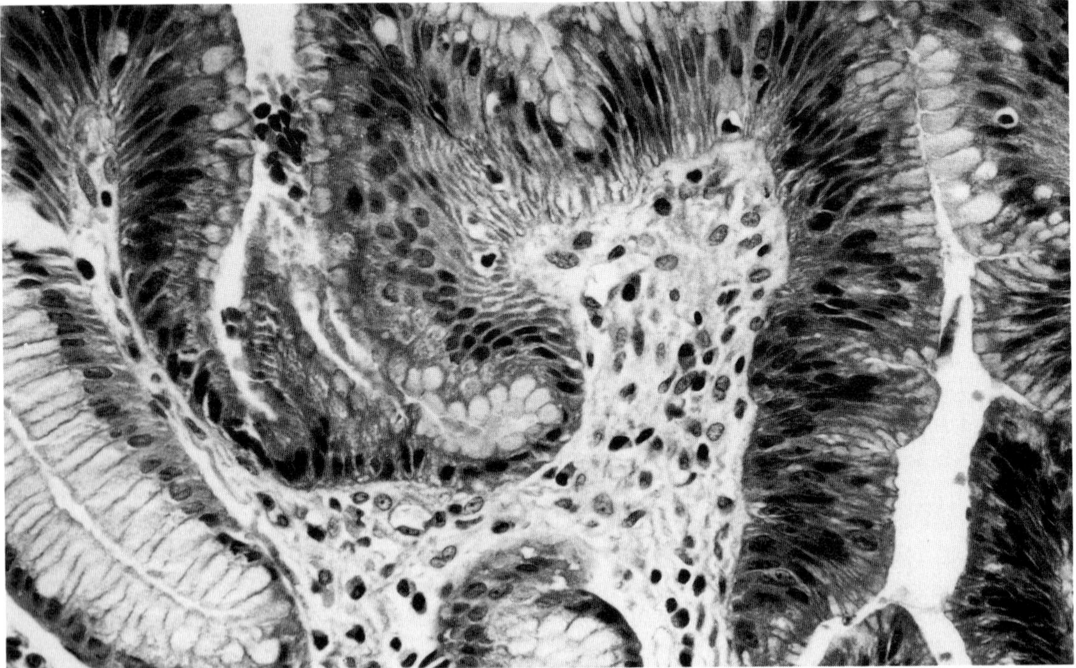

Fig. 5-6. Low-grade dysplasia of the stomach, seen in the gland appearing at the right. The dysplastic cells have elongated and slightly hyperchromatic nuclei that are mainly present in the lower portion of the cells. Compare with the normal surface and pit mucous cell at the left and center (× 425).

nent regeneration of the gastric pits. The latter can be readily appreciated by noting the regularity of the enlarged nuclei, the relative fineness of the chromatin pattern, and the presence but regular central location of the nucleoli (see Fig. 4-19). In the past there were several series with a mild dysplasia that was noted to disappear or not to progress to more severe forms, probably reflecting an excess in diagnosis of this form.[184, 185] It is best to demand considerable conservatism in the stomach for the diagnosis of dysplasia.

There is greater support for the significance of high-grade dysplasia in the evolution of cancer, based on regularly finding the lesion next to carcinomas and also by the follow-up studies. Of patients with low-grade dysplasia, including mild and moderate cases, only 5 to 9 percent proceeded to cancer development over 2 years in contrast to 31 to 54 percent of the severe or high-grade cases.[173] Accordingly, it is probably best to continue to closely follow cases with low-grade dysplasia and to consider more biopsies and possible resection in those with high-grade lesions. In all of these instances, it is particularly important to survey the entire surface for examples of early gastric carcinoma, as described below.

Because of the relatively lesser frequency of gastric carcinoma development in the United States, there has been less attention to surveillance programs in this area in contrast to the patients with esophageal and colonic diseases. It will be important to watch the progression of these patients with chronic gastritis to determine whether surveillance programs might be indicated at later dates. Certainly, the use of endoscopy and biopsy in countries with a higher frequency of gastric

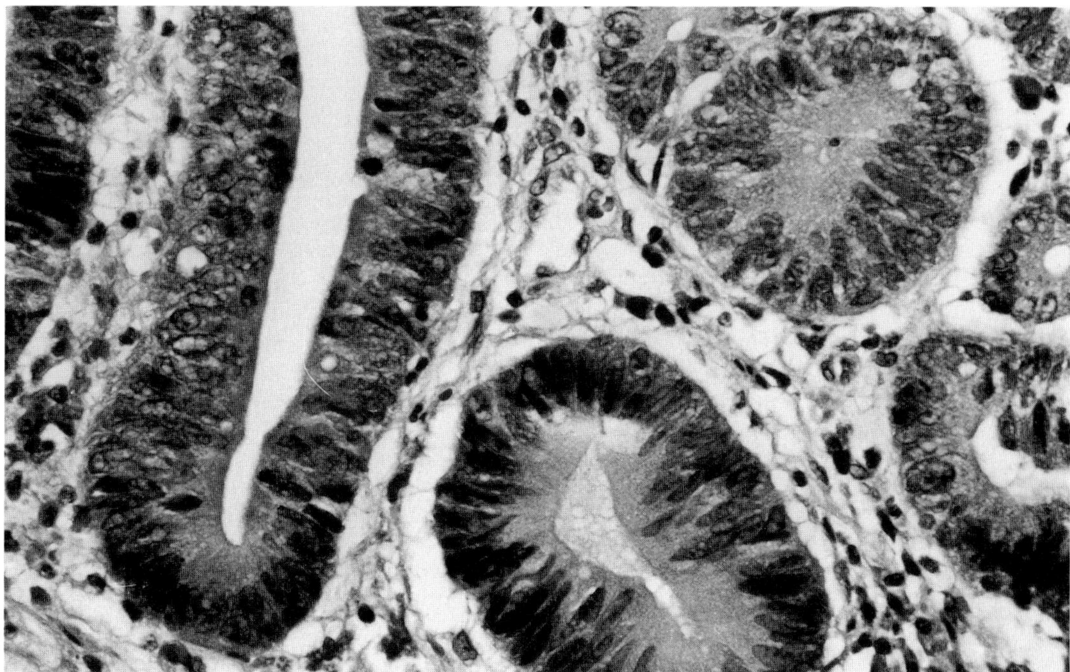

Fig. 5-7. High-grade dysplasia of the stomach. There is marked variation in size and shape of the epithelial cell nuclei as well as prominent palisading and hyperchromatism. Many of the nuclei extend into the superficial part of the cells (× 635).

cancer, particularly in patients with established chronic gastritis or with gastric remnants, seems justified.

Types and Features of Adenocarcinoma

Classifications and General Types

The carcinomas of the stomach are classified based on their principal location, glandular differentiation, and mode of spread (Table 5-7). As mentioned above, about one-quarter of the cases now originate in the cardia and proximal stomach.[186,187] These cases share attributes with those of the lower esophagus and junctional region by involving older patients, with a higher frequency of men. There is also an increased association with smoking and with ethanol consumption as opposed to patients with more distal gastric carcinomas.

The tumors are broadly divided into those with glandular formation, often with differentiation to intestinal cells, presumably due to prior intestinal metaplasia; and tumors in which there are broad sheets of cells with variable signet ring cell formation.[188] These have been termed *intestinal* or *glandular* as opposed to *diffuse* or *signet ring cell* types. As noted above, there is a stronger correlation of the intestinal type with the antecedent development of dysplasia. There appears to be a decline in the percent of glandular cases that formerly were the majority, whereas now the diffuse tumors are of equal frequency in the lower part of the stomach. Tumors can also be separated based on their growth pattern (spread), whether *infiltrative* or *expansile,* with the latter associated with an improved prognosis.[189]

Based on the dominant histologic feature the carcinomas are further characterized as *papillary,* in which there is a prominent villous surface; as *tubular,* where there is well formed gland formation; and as *mucinous* (or colloid), where there is extensive extracellular mucin in association with the carcinoma.[190] Of the tumors with glandular formation, they also can be separated into those that are *well, moderately,* or *poorly* differentiated, based on the degree of gland formation. Both the presence of excess mucin production and the lack of differentiation predict a poorer prognosis.[191–193] Overall, the staging of the tumor serves to best define the prognosis and survival.[194]

Table 5-7. Classifications of Gastric Adenocarcinoma

Classification
Location
Cardia
Corpus/antrum
Depth
Early
Advanced
Differentiation
Glandular (intestinal)
Signet ring cell (diffuse)
Spread
Expansile
Infiltrative
Histologic patterns
Papillary
Tubular
Mucinous

Biopsy Indications and Features

Endoscopic examination and biopsy are largely performed to identify the carcinoma and to determine its spread within the mucosa. In particular, biopsies may be needed in extensive tumors to find any lesions in the adjacent esophagus or duodenum as well as in the stomach. Radiographic scans are often added to determine the mural extent of the tumor, whether it is limited to the gastric wall or extends externally. This information can help in determinations about surgery.

Multiple biopsy samples are taken from the edges and central portion of the major tumor together with cytologic brushings (Plate 3E–H). Details of the cytologic features are provided in Chapter 3 (see Table 3-7). Compared to regenerative cells, the cancers show greater variation in size and shape of cells and nuclei; denser and more irregular chromatin patterns with heavy condensation along the nuclear membrane; and greater variation in the size and position of the nucleoli. The glandular nature of the tumor cells is defined by the eccentric localization of the nuclei within the cells.

The appearance of the neoplastic glands resembles either those of the gastric pits or of the intestinal-type glands. These features are evident with routine light microscopy, with mucin stains showing neutral glycoproteins in the native gastric pits as opposed to prominent acid and, particularly, sulfated mucins in the intestinal-type tumor glands. In addition, ultrastructural features support the appearance of both gastric and intestinal-type glands in the various tumors.[20] There does not appear to be any definite correlation between the type of tumor cell, whether gastric or intestinal in appearance, and the overall spread of tumor or ultimate prognosis.

Early Adenocarcinoma

Extensive studies, largely in Japan, have permitted the fine definition of early gastric carcinoma at the level of tumors that are just millimeters in size.[195, 196] These have been referred to as *early* or *minute* cancers. There is a gross classification, revealing tumors that are polypoid, relatively flat, and depressed. The cases are concluded to be early if the cancer is limited to the mucosa or invades at most into the submucosa at a microscopic but not a gross level. If ulceration is present it may extend beyond the tumor but there is no carcinoma at its base. The lesion of early carcinoma has been noted in all regions of the stomach, including the cases involving the cardia and gastric remnants.[197, 198] Particularly in cases of carcinoma complicating chronic gastritis, there is often the presence of both dysplasia and early carcinoma.

The diagnosis of early gastric carcinoma is largely related to detection at a gross level. This is commonly successful in populations with a high frequency of gastric carcinoma, such as in many parts of Europe,[199–202] whereas it is often an incidental finding in the North American countries.[203–205] At a biopsy level the features are straightforward, revealing overt adenocarcinoma. This takes the form of highly irregular and dilated glands comprised of markedly atypical cells (Fig. 5-8). Less differentiated adenocarcinomas can also be seen at this early stage. In the biopsy analysis there is the identification of the tumor and also a search for any infiltration of cells into the lamina propria, which helps to establish the diagnosis of intramucosal adenocarcinoma as opposed to high-grade dysplasia.[206, 207] In examining many of the samples from the Japanese studies rated as type I early gastric adenocarcinoma, some of the cases could be construed as high-grade dysplasia without invasive carcinoma. As a rough estimate, when the dysplastic glands extend to the base of the mucosa, there is the tendency to rate the case as an early carcinoma rather than just dysplasia.

As with the diagnosis of dysplasia, it is important to rule out exuberant granulation tissue with enlarged endothelial cells, as well as prominent regeneration and irregular glands at the edge of the ulcers, in the diagnosis of invasive carcinoma.[208, 209] In general, the regenerative tissue lacks hyperchromatic nuclei and there is less variation in size and shape of the cells. It is also necessary to distinguish early gastric carcinoma from peptic ulcers that may have similar gross findings of relatively flat lesions with sharply demar-

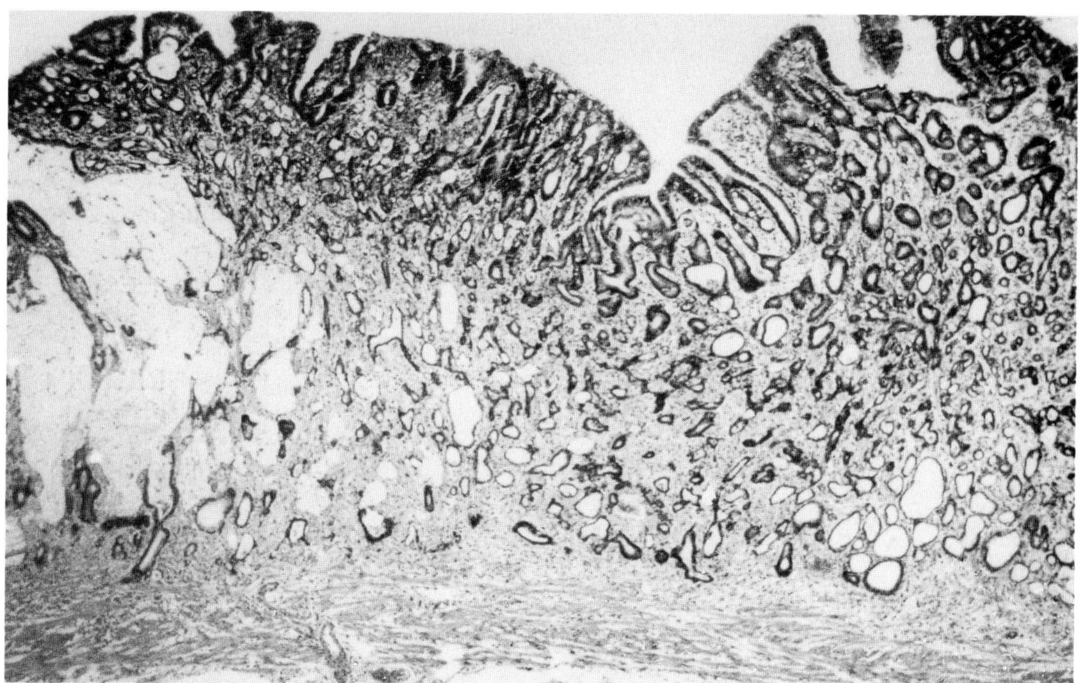

Fig. 5-8. Intramucosal adenocarcinoma of the stomach. The mucosa is largely converted into an irregular mass of malignant glands, many of which are dilated. The muscularis mucosae appearing at the bottom shows no invasion.

cated ulcers. It may be impossible to separate these at a gross or radiographic level, emphasizing the need for biopsies. Furthermore, cases of early gastric carcinoma can develop secondary peptic ulceration that can even partially heal. These are not examples of the conversion of a benign ulcer into a carcinoma. Whatever the response rate of the ulcer is in the stomach, endoscopic biopsy to exclude an early carcinoma is highly desirable for any persistent lesion.

The biopsies in cases of early gastric carcinoma serve to provide the diagnosis of malignancy. Only the larger samples include submucosal tissue that would permit statements regarding invasion into that layer.[210] Overall, the patients with early carcinoma do very well, with 5-year survival rates over 90 percent.[211,212] The lymphatics in the normal gastric mucosa are limited to the most basal region adjacent to the muscularis mucosae, and this factor may contribute to the delayed extension of tumors from this area.[213,214]

Advanced Adenocarcinoma

Advanced adenocarcinoma represents the cases with gross evidence of tumor extending into the submucosa or beyond. Of interest, tumors that are limited to the mucosal layer and associated with lymph nodal metastases still do much better than the advanced carcinomas. Most of the advanced lesions present with an overt mass in the form of a large irregular polyp, an ulcerated lesion, or a more infiltrative tumor that may involve a large part of the stomach, termed the *linitis plastica* form. Several histologic patterns can be seen, including tumors with prominent gland formation (Fig. 5-9); with extensive extracellular mucin; with diffuse sheets of cells containing minimal cytoplasmic mucin (Figs. 5-10 and 5-11); and with signet ring cells (Fig. 5-12). Biopsies should be obtained from the edges of any lesions that best show the glandular formation; and from the central regions that are preferred for the areas with diffuse tumor and also other neoplasms. A combination of 4 to 6 biopsies together with cytologic brushings detect malignancy in practically all cases.[15]

Potential problems occur when there is extensive ulceration or when the tumor is largely beneath the surface. In such cases, multiple samples, larger and deeper biopsies, and local aspiration cytology can be of assistance. Conversely, there must be caution in interpreting irregular glands at the edges of ulcerated lesions as well as prominent granulation tissue at their bases.[208,209] These may reveal cells with very enlarged nuclei, but they tend to be regular in appearance and to lack a constant degree of hyperchromatism. It may be particularly difficult to distinguish the chronic erosive form[215–217] of chronic gastritis from carcinoma,[218] because of the very prominent regenerative glands that are present in the gastritis cases.

In the recognition of signet ring cells, one must exclude the potential for clusters of macrophages containing either fatty substances or mucins. Ultimately the distinction is made by the appearance of the nuclei, which appear bland in macrophages as opposed to the carcinoma cells. In exceptional cases, immunocytochemical stain might be employed to distinguish the macrophages from epithelial cells, with the latter revealing positive stains for cytokeratins and for epithelial membrane antigen. Such stains may also help in identifying scattered tumor cells within the biopsy stroma. The finding of signet ring–type cells can be mimicked by other tumors, notably seen in malignant lymphomas and in sarcomas. In these cases, the cytoplasm appears particularly clear in contrast to the fragmented nature of the mucus within the signet ring cells. Nevertheless, if there is any doubt, mucin stains can be done to confirm the type of material within the cytoplasm.

Special Studies

There have been many efforts at utilizing modern techniques to gain additional information related to the expected behavior of

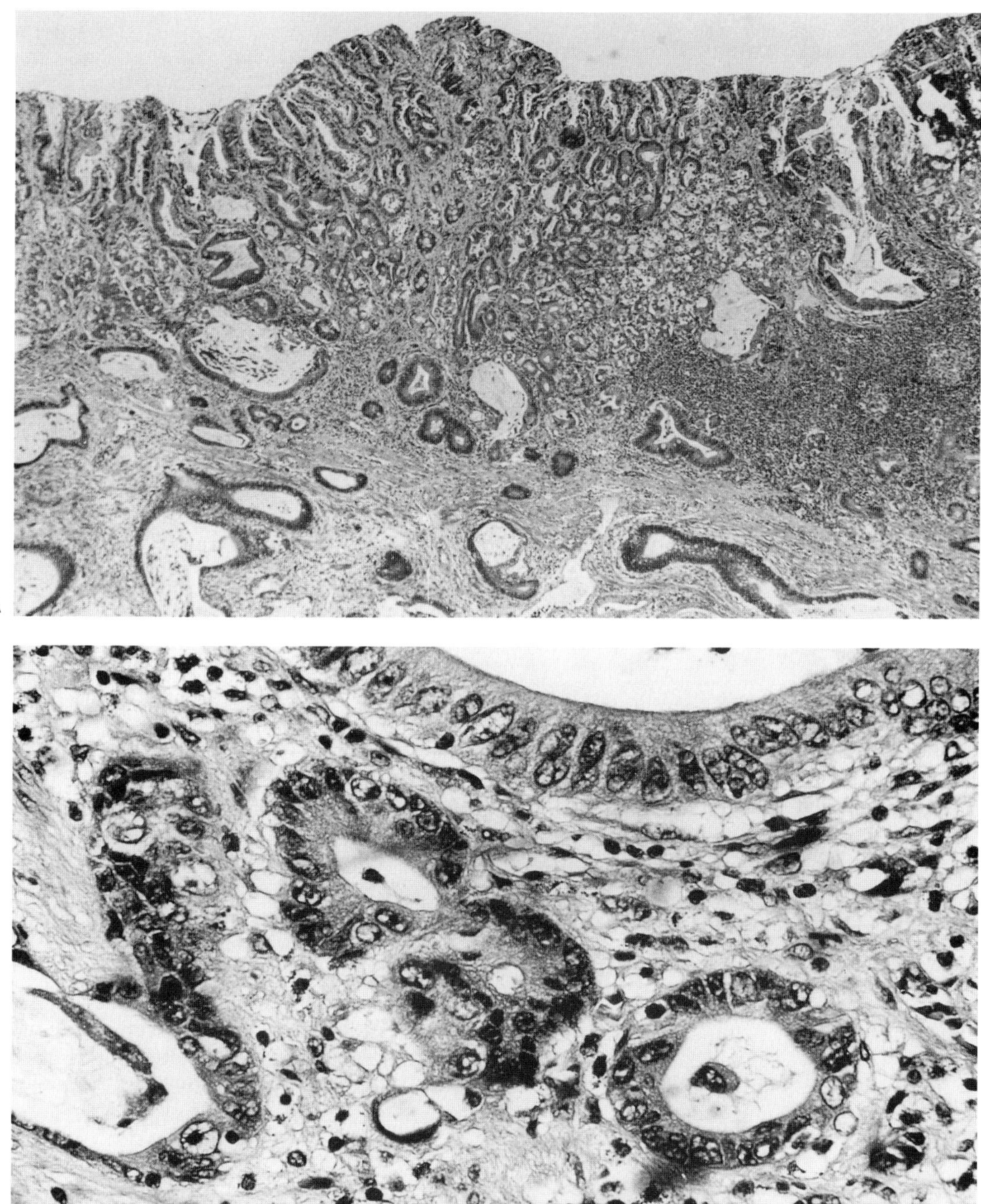

Fig. 5-9. Well differentiated adenocarcinoma of the stomach. (**A**) Area of mucosal carcinoma with invasion into the underlying submucosa, appearing at the bottom (× 42). (**B**) Malignant glands with markedly atypical cells (× 425).

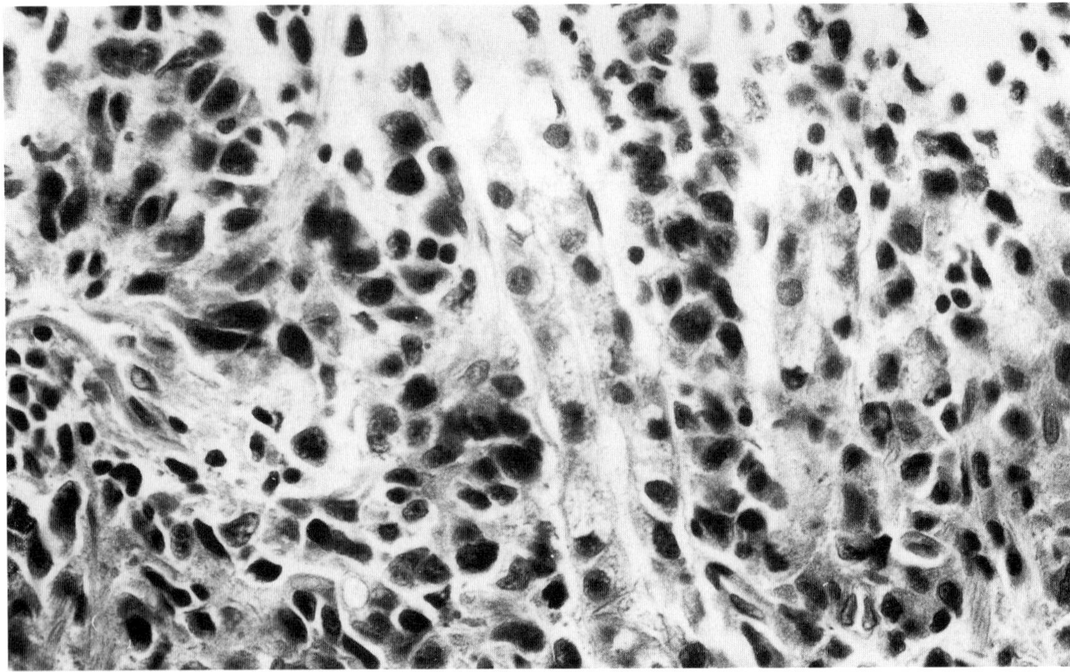

Fig. 5-10. Poorly differentiated adenocarcinoma of the stomach. There are mainly sheets of malignant cells with prominent cytoplasm and occasional glands (× 425).

the carcinomas. These include the use of stains for PCNA localization[28, 219, 220] and p53 expression[33–36, 221–224] in tumor cells as well as flow cytometry to detect aneuploidy. [31, 32, 225–228] In general, the malignant cells tend to reveal stronger stains and greater chromosomal abnormalities, but there remains considerable overlap and heterogeneity that limit their application. Current efforts are directed to apply these studies to prognosis rather than to primary diagnosis.

Summary

Mucosal biopsies are essentially used to detect the carcinoma and to chart its mucosal spread. Whether the tumor is early and superficial or more advanced is ultimately determined by other studies, including examination of the resected specimen. In general, the majority of early carcinomas are well differentiated, but many of the advanced tumors will also show such features. Conversely, the simple presence of a diffuse or signet ring cell carcinoma does not signify an advanced tumor.

In contrast to the esophagus and to the colon, endoscopic examination of the stomach appears to be better at detecting early carcinoma. Whether this relates to the large and easily visualized lumen of the stomach or to the growth rate of the tumor in this locale is not known. Nevertheless, this has proven to be of considerable assistance in identifying early cases. It has probably also tended to inhibit some of the efforts in detecting cases at the high-grade dysplastic level.

Variant Forms of Adenocarcinoma

Tumors with Squamous Elements

Adenosquamous cell carcinoma, also called adenocanthoma, accounts for about 1 percent of gastric carcinomas[229–231]

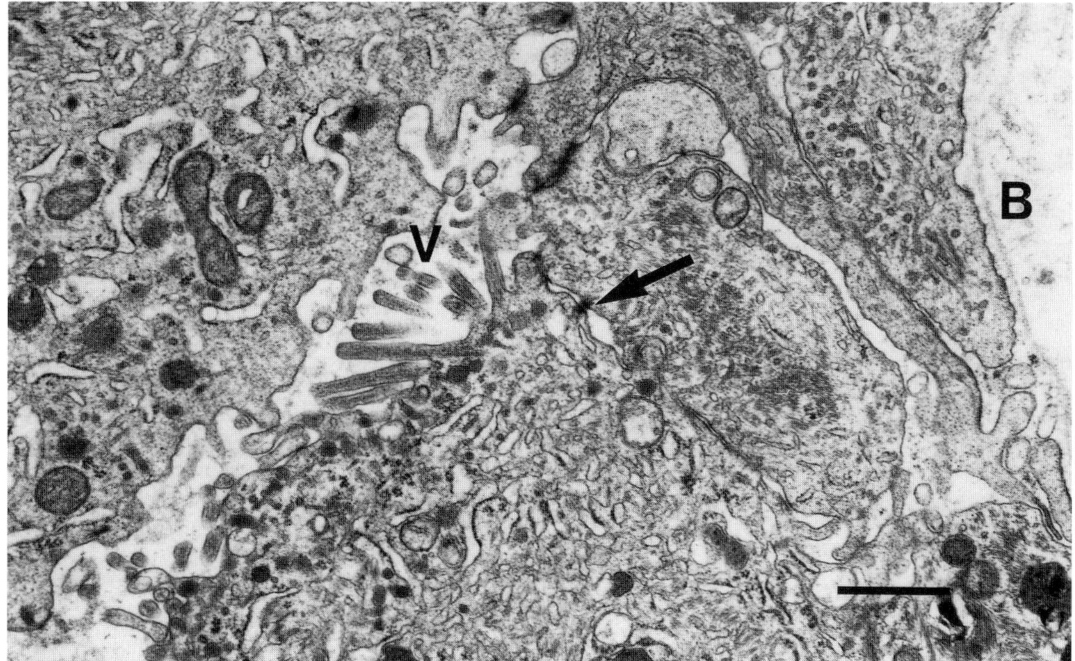

Fig. 5-11. Electron micrograph of a poorly differentiated adenocarcinoma. Groups of cells form lumen-like spaces lined by a few microvilli (V), are joined by primitive junctions (arrow), and are surrounded by a partial basal lamina (B). Nonspecific secretory granules are mostly seen in the apical part of the cells (× 15,000; bar = 1 μm).

(Table 5-6) (see Fig. 3–17). These tend to be located in the prominal part of the stomach and are probably derived from cells that are capable of both squamous and glandular differentiation. More rarely seen are pure squamous cell carcinomas.[232–235] In such cases one needs to exclude a cancer that is extending from the esophagus or one that is developing in a duplication cyst that may have aberrant epithelium. They appear to be more frequent in gastric remnants and, exceptionally, can also occur following a long-standing infection, such as with syphilis affecting the mucosa. All of these squamous tumors tend to behave in an aggressive fashion similar to the adenocarcinomas. Biopsy simply shows the squamous as well as the glandular elements. In biopsies that reveal just the squamous tissue, additional samples should be sought to localize the tumor in the stomach, if needed. Also rarely observed in the stomach are mucoepidermoid carcinomas that reveal more definite squamous tumor together with foci of glands[236] (see Fig. 11-15). These are thought to arise from heterotopic pancreas or ectopic submucosal glands.

In most instances, the biopsy serves to identify the tumor and possibly the aberrant component. In such cases multiple sections should be obtained to look for the more distinctive features (e.g., a glandular component in a biopsy showing squamous carcinoma).

Lymphoepithelioma-like Carcinoma

Lymphoepithelioma-like carcinoma resembles the tumors seen in the nasopharynx, revealing sheets of large and otherwise undifferentiated epithelial cells together with huge amounts of lymphoid stroma[237–240] (Fig. 5-13). Of great interest, they have re-

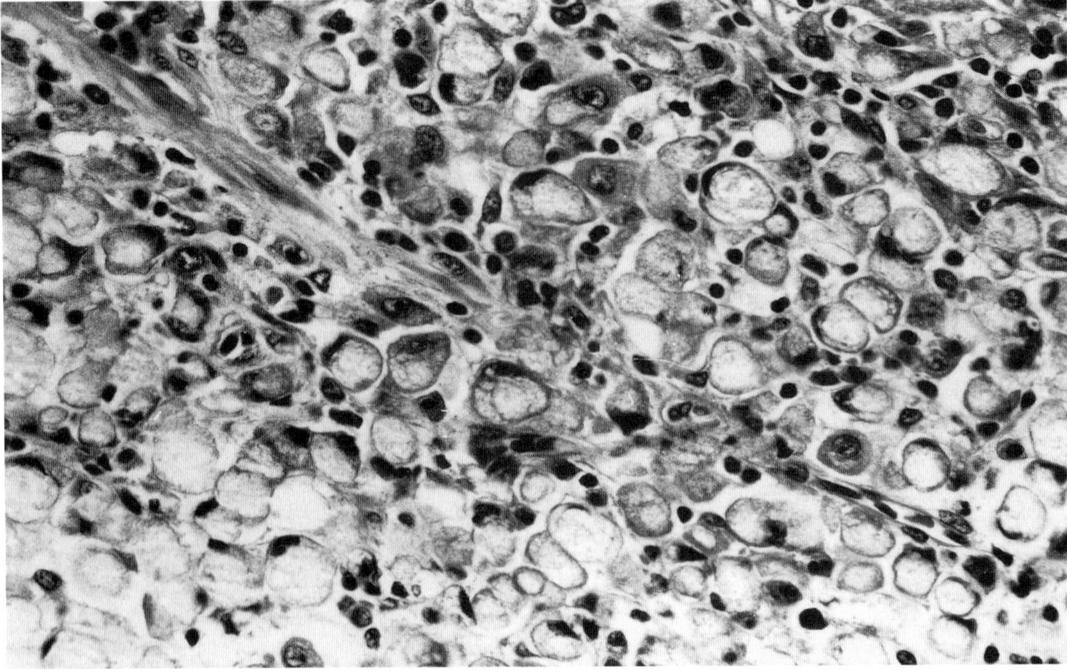

Fig. 5-12. Signet ring cell type of adenocarcinoma in the stomach. Noted are a sheet of malignant cells with nuclei at the edges of the cells and the cytoplasm distended with mucus (× 425).

cently been associated with identification of the Epstein–Barr virus in the tumors. It is probable that EBV is a major etiologic agent. The exact frequency of this tumor in the stomach is not known, but it is likely that it will behave in a fashion similar to nasopharyngeal carcinoma with increased radiosensitivity, compared to other gastric carcinomas. But, this needs to be tested. Biopsies have not played a major role in defining this tumor. If such a lesion is suspected, special insitu hybridization techniques can be employed to identify the viral antigens.

Hepatoid Carcinoma

Hepatoid carcinoma tumors are composed of large polygonal cells with prominent eosinophilic cytoplasm, resembling liver cells.[241–243] They reveal positive stains for alpha-fetoprotein and other liver markers such as albumin and transferrin. There are also prominent eosinophilic globules within the cytoplasm. The biopsy features are distinctive and should permit the identification of this particular type of tumor, which appears to have a bad prognosis.

Parietal Cell Carcinoma

Parietal cell carcinoma is a very rare tumor, representing an adenocarcinoma with focal or more extensive differentiation to parietal cells.[244–246] These appear as large, rounded pink cells, with prominent mitochondria and intracellular canaliculi revealed by electron microscopy. It has been suggested that they may have a better prognosis, but this is not fully established.

Paneth Cells in Tumors

Occasionally noted are Paneth cells in both adenomas and adenocarcinomas of the stomach.[247–249] This is probably a conse-

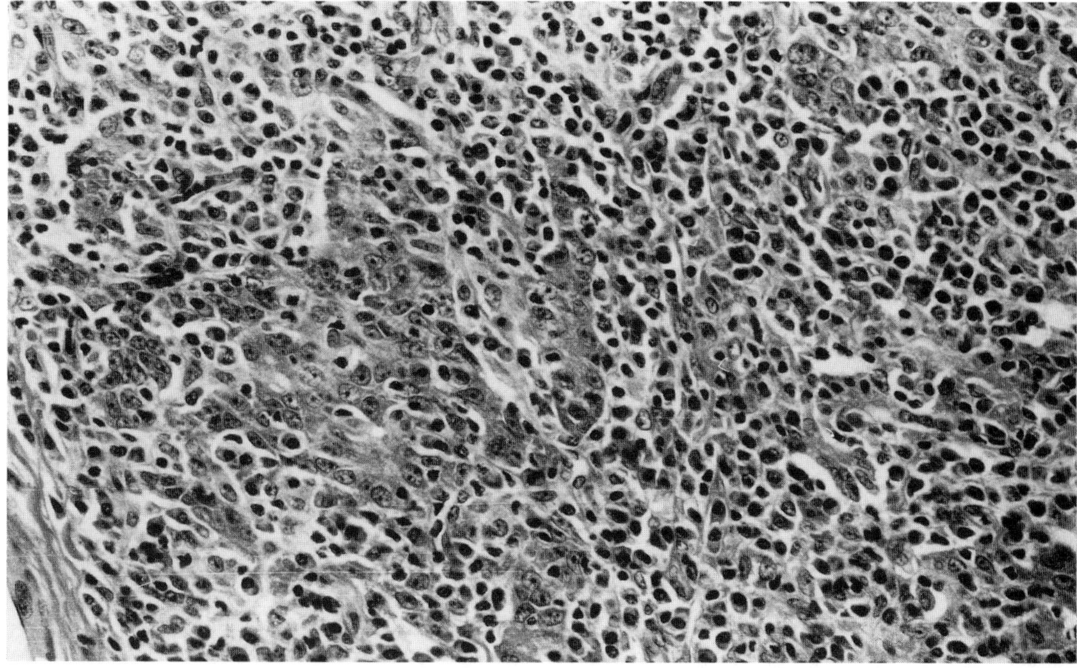

Fig. 5-13. Lymphoepithelioma-like adenocarcinoma of the stomach. There are irregular sheets and ribbons of malignant epithelial cells together with an intense lymphocytic infiltrate. These cases are associated with Epstein-Barr virus (× 210).

quence of the prior intestinal metaplasia in these patients. This feature has no influence in the behavior of the tumors.

OTHER TUMORS

There are many other primary tumors that can affect the stomach (Table 5-8). They are often associated with mucosal extension leading to polyps or ulcers that can be biopsied. In many instances the biopsy is able to identify a neoplasm but is not always capable of providing the specific type of tumor. This is readily obtained by additional samples or by examination of the surgical specimens.

Endocrine Tumors

Carcinoid Tumors

Carcinoid tumors represent a few percent of the gastric tumors. They can develop as large masses and present with late lesions,[250–252] but with modern endoscopy they are now more often detected at an early polypoid stage[253–256] (Fig. 5-14). The tumors arise from the foregut and are mostly non-

Table 5-8. Other Tumors of the Stomach

Endocrine Tumors
Carcinoid tumor
Composite tumor
Small cell carcinoma
Lymphoid tumors
Benign hyperplasia (pseudolymphoma)
Malignant lymphoma
Mesenchymal tumors
Stromal tumors
Leiomyoma, leiomyoblastoma, schwannoma
Undifferentiated
Vascular tumors
Kaposi's sarcoma
Angioma and glomus tumor
Other benign tumors
Granular cell tumor
Lipoma
Other sarcomas
Other primary tumors
Choriocarcinoma and teratoma
Carcinosarcoma
Secondary and metastatic tumors

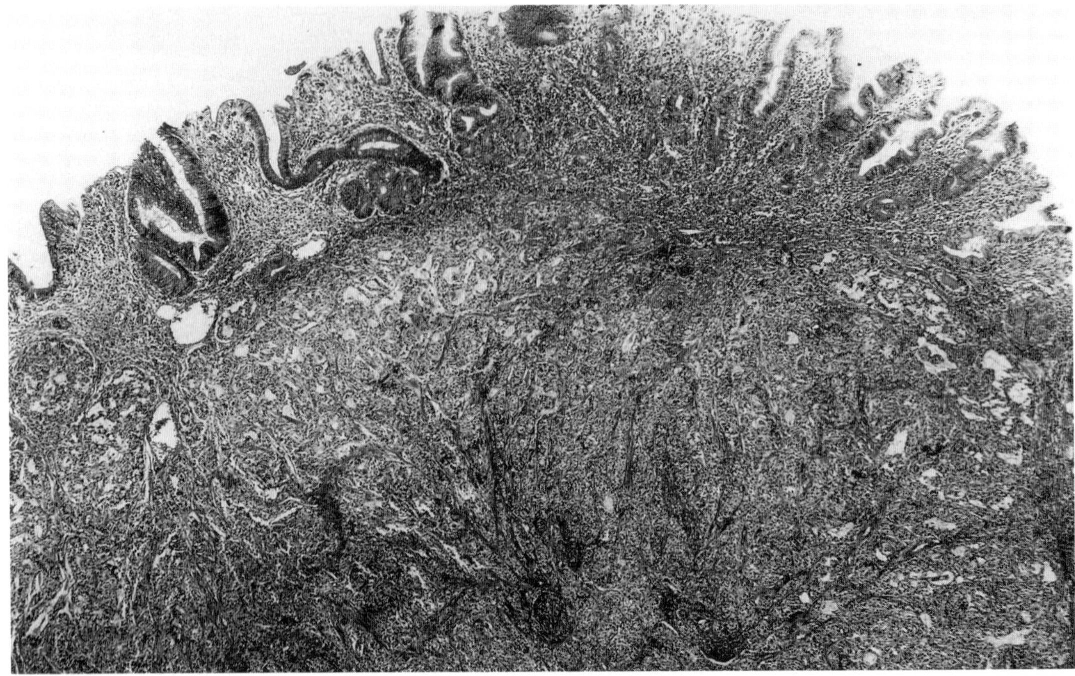

Fig. 5-14. Carcinoid tumor of the stomach. Shown is a polypoid tumor, occurring mainly in the submucosa with focal extension into the mucosa. The mucosal surface with residual gastric glands appears at the top (× 42).

functional, producing mainly the symptoms of a mass. Accordingly, their particular nature is usually identified at the time of the biopsy, and the therapy is determined by the extent of the tumor.

The biopsies are highly distinctive, revealing the ribbons or small nests of very uniform cells with regular central nuclei and prominent cytoplasm (Fig. 5-15). The neuroendocrine nature of the cells is readily established by special stains, and particularly used are chromogranin and synaptophysin. They also mostly stain for argyrophilic substances by Grimelius' stain, but are usually argentaffinic-negative.

Endocrine Cell Hyperplasia and Tumors in Chronic Gastritis

An increase in endocrine cells is noted in cases of chronic gastritis, particularly in those with pernicious anemia.[257–260] This can appear as simple hyperplasia, as microscopic nests of cells, and as multiple carcinoids[261–267] (Fig. 5-16). The cells most often involved are the G cells in the antrum, but there can also develop a secondary hyperplasia of the ECL cells in the gastric body[268, 269] (see "Features of Chronic Gastritis" in Ch. 4 for further details).

Composite Tumors

Composite tumors are lesions that represent mixtures of adenoma or adenocarcinoma together with foci of neuroendocrine cells.[270–272] The dominant lesion is usually the glandular one, and the presence of the endocrine cells does not appear to affect the overall behavior of the adenoma or carcinoma. Biopsies reveal mainly the glandular lesion with a relatively small portion of neuroendocrine cells, which can be selectively stained as described above.

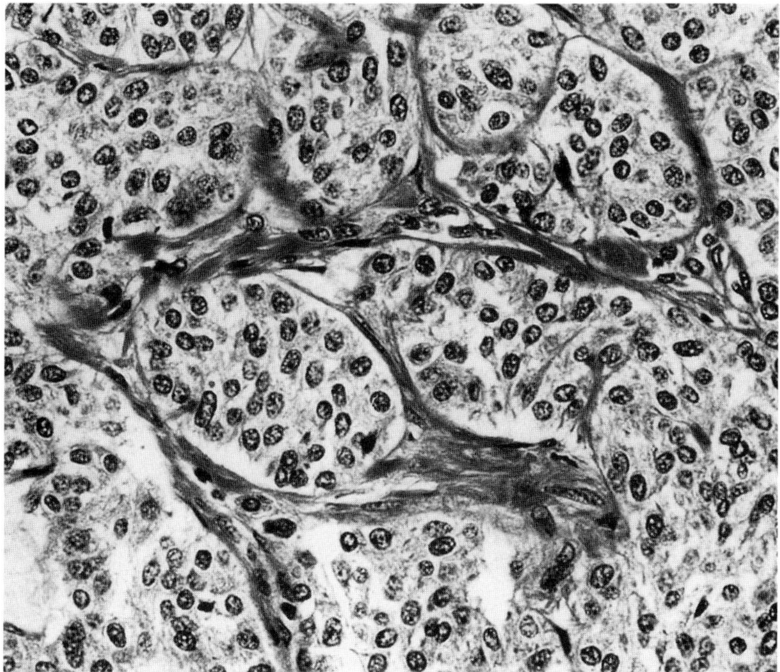

Fig. 5-15. Characteristic appearance of a carcinoid tumor, showing nests of monomorphic cells with stippled nuclei and lack of gland formation (× 425).

Occasionally seen are tumors with a greater admixture of the glandular and endocrine elements[273–276] or stomachs containing separate carcinomas and carcinoid tumors.

Small Cell Carcinoma

Small cell carcinomas are very rare tumors in the stomach, analogous to the undifferentiated oat cell carcinomas seen in the lung.[277–279] They are composed of dense oval cells with prominent nuclei, often stain positively with neuroendocrine markers, and contain sparse granules by electron microscopy (Fig. 5-17). They are usually associated with other areas of adenocarcinoma, and the overall behavior is poor. Biopsy has rarely been done and would show the small dense cells (see Fig. 3-19). If necessary, marker studies can be done to support a carcinoma over a lymphoma in such cases.

Lymphoid Tumors

Benign Lymphoid Hyperplasia (Pseudolymphoma)

There is a prominent proliferation of benign lymphoid nodules in cases of chronic gastritis, and these are readily seen on biopsy. In some instances, particularly in cases associated with chronic peptic ulcer, there can be a marked amount of lymphoid tissue involving large parts of the gastric wall.[280] These have been termed *pseudolymphoma* and are said to account for about 10 percent of all lymphoid proliferations in the stomach.[281–285] (The author is not fond of this term because it tends to imply an entity and

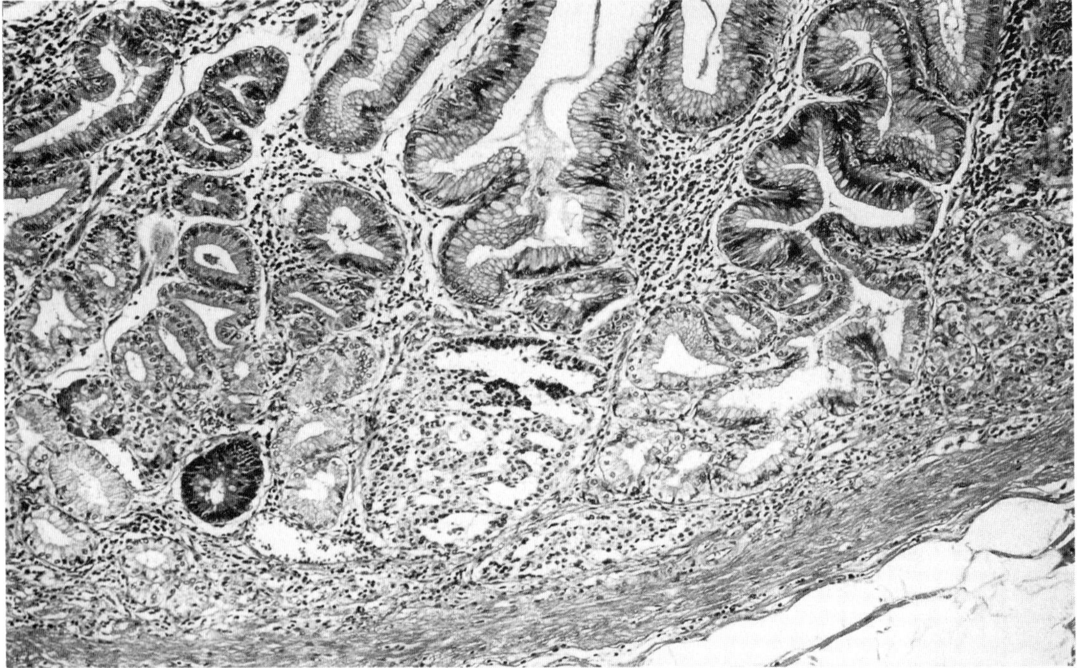

Fig. 5-16. Neuroendocrine cell hyperplasia and microcarcinoid formation, present in the base of the mucosa. The muscularis mucosa appears at the bottom. This developed in the antrum of a patient with pernicious anemia (× 105).

obscures the absolute need to distinguish an inflammatory from a tumor condition.) The benign lesions reveal prominent follicle formation, and any diffuse area typically reveals an admixture of small lymphocytes and many plasma cells (Fig. 5-18). In contrast, although the well differentiated lymphomas may show preservation of follicles in focal areas, other follicles may be converted to lymphoma, and the more solid areas show a greater uniformity of lymphoid cells without associated plasma cells. Transitional cases illustrating the overlap of pseudolymphoma and malignant lymphoma features have been reported.[286–288]

Improvements in separating benign and malignant lymphoid lesions are provided by obtaining larger samples, by fixing in solutions such as B5, by cutting at thinner levels, and by performing marker studies. In most cases with the florid benign hyperplasia, the cells are relatively small. Special stains can serve to identify their blood cell nature as opposed to neuroendocrine or epithelial cells. To assist in the distinction of benign versus malignant, larger samples studied for monoclonality are often needed.

Malignant Lymphoma

The stomach can be involved with malignant lymphoma as part of an isolated lesion, in the form of a single mass or a more diffuse tumor[289–292]; together with other parts of the alimentary tract, particularly of the small intestine[293–298]; and as part of a systemic spread.[299] The stomach is one of the most common extranodal sites for malignant lymphoma, with most lesions presenting as a polypoid or ulcerated mass, similar grossly to adenocarcinoma. There appears to be an overall increase in gastric lymphoma noted over the past 2 decades, with probable increases in patients with AIDS and possibly in those with inflammatory bowel

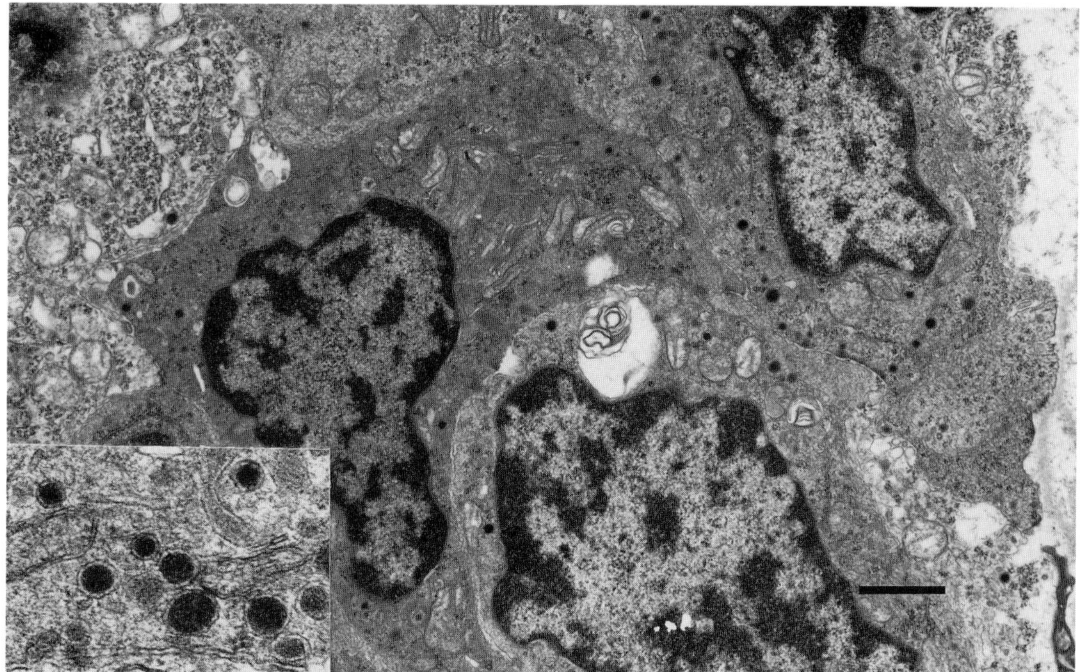

Fig. 5-17. Electron micrograph of a small cell (neuroendocrine) carcinoma. The cells have irregular nuclei and the cytoplasm contains small granules, usually few in number (× 11, 250; bar = 1 μm). **(Inset)** High magnification of granules that are round, membrane bound with dense cores, and measure an average of 100 nm in diameter (× 42,500).

disease.[165, 300, 301] Most of these tumors are non-Hodgkin's of the B cell type. There is also an increase in patients with celiac disease, characterized by the prominence of T-cell lymphoma, as described below.[166, 302, 303] A strong association has recently been noted between the presence of *H. pylori* and the earliest type of mucosa-associated lymphoid tissue (MALT) lymphomas.[304–306] It has even been suggested that aggressive antibiotic therapy might be used for the early MALT-type tumors.[307, 308]

There has been considerable improvement in the mucosal biopsy diagnosis of malignant lymphoma, based on the obtaining of larger samples and the utilization of better fixatives and of marker studies. About 55 percent of the gastric lymphomas are of the high grade or large cell types, and their malignant features are usually evident on the routine sections (Fig. 5-19). Revealed are sheets of cells with enlarged, irregular, and variably hyperchromatic nuclei, and there is an absence of glands or mucin production in the tumor cells. The gastric pits are mainly destroyed and not selectively infiltrated by the lymphoma cells. In such cases the differential often includes a diffuse type of carcinoma that can be readily distinguished by immunocytochemical stains, using leukocyte common antigen for the lymphoma and cytokeratins for the carcinoma.[309] These can also be distinguished by ultrastructural examination (Fig. 5-20). Occasionally noted are signet ring cells that must be distinguished from those seen in carcinomas; this by the absence of mucin granules in the lymphoma cells.[310]

Difficulties more often arise in the lymphomas composed of the smaller cells of the low or intermediate grade. In such cases, it is necessary to distinguish the lymphoma from a florid inflammatory reaction. It has recently been appreciated that many of these tumors are derived from the mucosa-

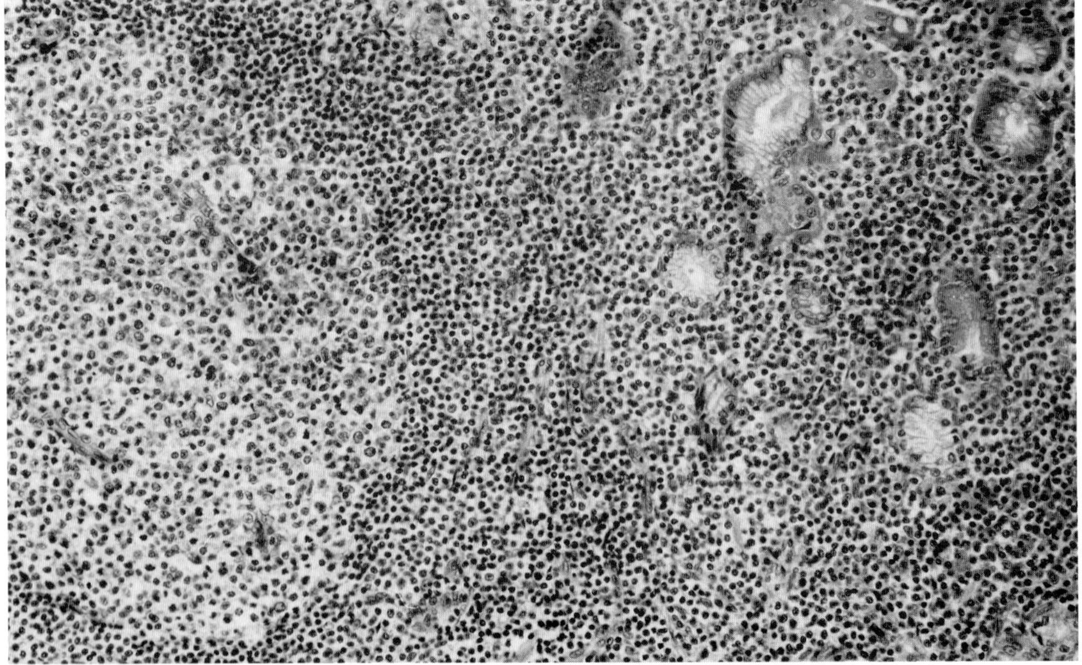

Fig. 5-18. Lymphoid hyperplasia of the stomach. There is a dense infiltrate of mature lymphocytes in the lamina propria together with a well formed lymphoid nodule containing a central follicle (appearing at the left). The epithelial cells show no lymphocytic penetration. Compare with lymphoma of Figure 5-21A (× 210).

associated lymphoid tissue, and these have been termed MALT-related lymphomas.[311, 312] Helpful clues to make the diagnosis of malignancy in the mucosal biopsy include the presence of sheets of slightly immature cells without many plasma cells, and, particularly, the presence of the lymphoepithelial lesion, which is characterized by a prominent infiltrate of the immature lymphoid cells into the preserved epithelial glands[313, 314] (Fig. 5-21). Scattered, well preserved lymphoid follicles with centers can be seen in both benign and malignant conditions.[315] In most of the inflammatory disorders there is usually more complete destruction of the glands together with greater neutrophilic reaction. Nevertheless, it is not always possible to make the distinction on histologic grounds. In such cases, the suspicion should be made and additional material in the form of larger samples should be provided for study of monoclonality. In many instances there is an evident mass lesion that is symptomatic, and surgery is ultimately required, at which time the tissue can be provided for the special studies.

In summary, biopsy in a case of suspected lymphoma of the stomach may reveal overt, large malignant cells that need to be separated from carcinoma; or small cells that require distinction from inflammatory conditions.[316–320] For the latter, additional samples for marker studies and for determination of monotypicality are eventually needed in about one-quarter of the cases.[30, 321–324] The cases of lymphoma seen in patients with AIDS are more often of the high-grade type and are associated with lesions in other parts of the gut, principally in the small intestine. Lymphoma also complicates celiac disease and tends to be more often of the T-cell type.[303, 325] These lesions

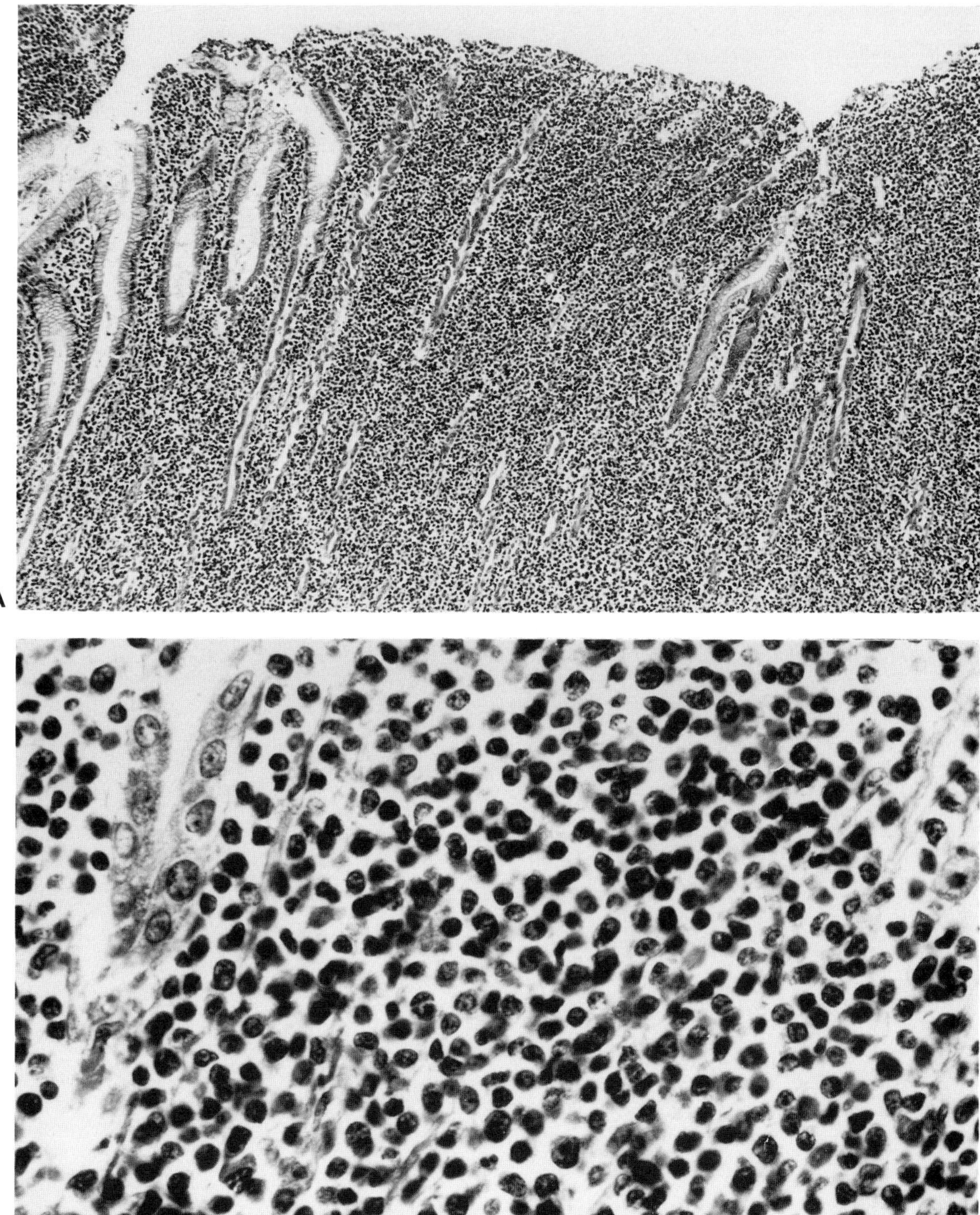

Fig. 5-19. Malignant lymphoma of the stomach. (**A**) There is a monomorphic infiltrate of lymphoid cells largely replacing the mucosa. Residual pits are present at the left (× 105). (**B**) Closer view showing enlarged and irregular lymphoid cells and entrapped gastric pit (upper left) (× 425).

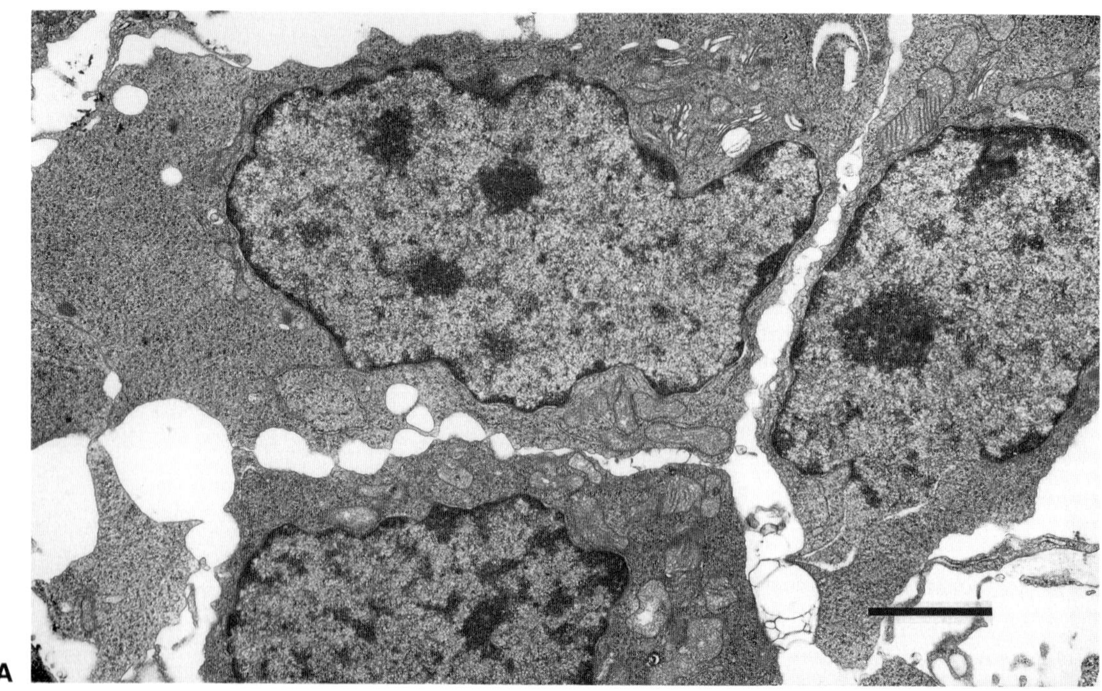

A

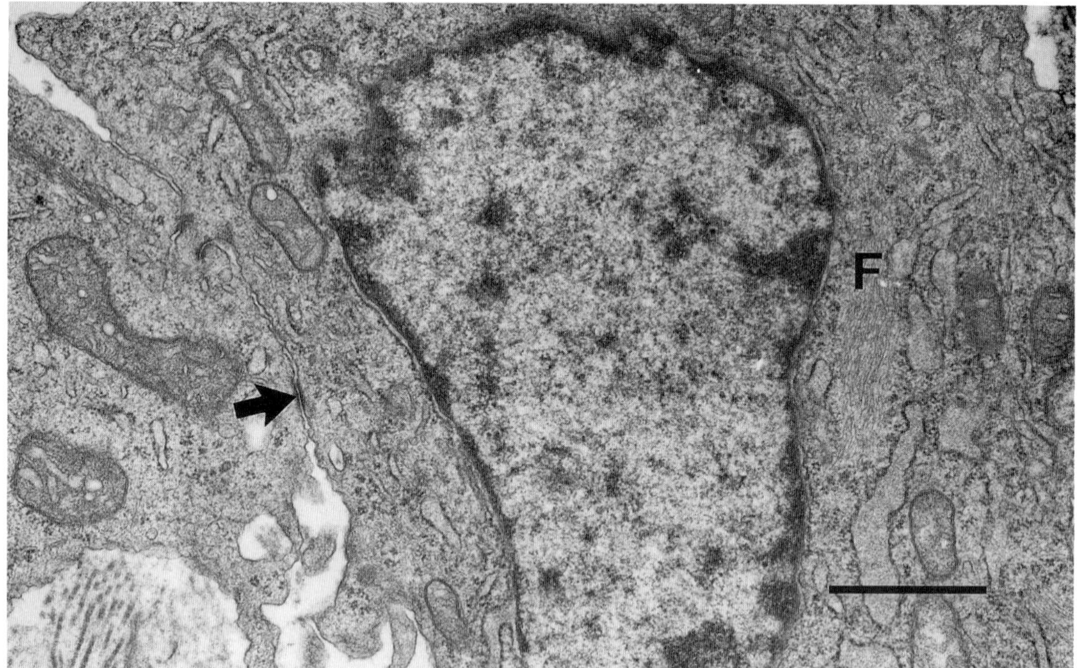

B

Fig. 5-20. (**A**) Electron micrograph of malignant lymphoma. Note that the cells are closely apposed without the presence of any junctions and that the cytoplasm has few organelles (× 7,900; bar = 2.5 μm). (**B**) Electron micrograph of anaplastic carcinoma. In comparison to the lymphoma, small primitive junctions (arrow) are present, and the cytoplasm is rich in organelles, including filaments (F). These point to some epithelial differentiation (× 20,000; bar = 1 μm).

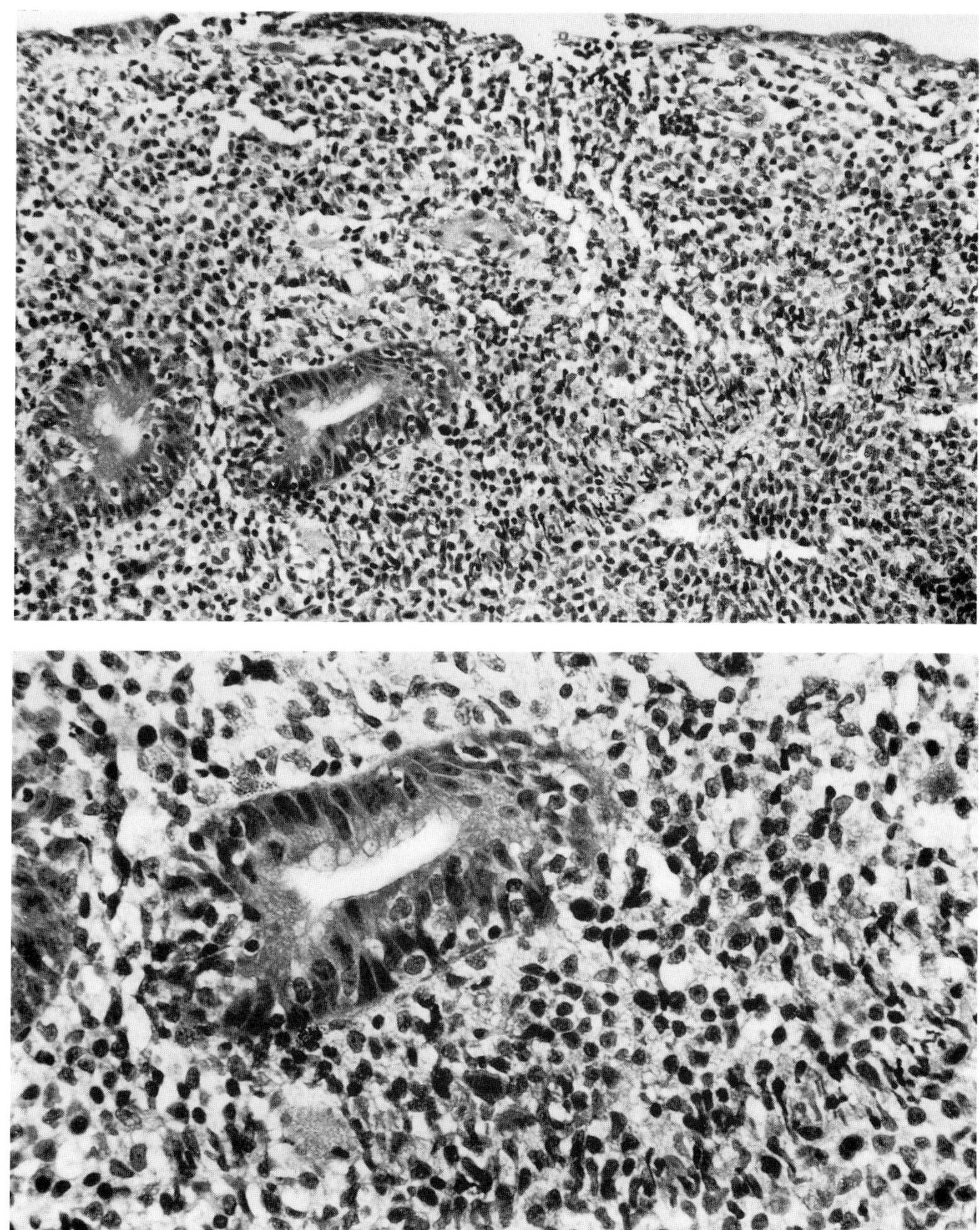

Fig. 5-21. Malignant lymphoma of the MALToma type in the stomach. (**A**) There is a diffuse infiltrate of small lymphoid cells in the mucosa, which extend into the gastric pits appearing at the lower left (× 210). (**B**) Closer view of lymphoepithelial lesion that is characteristic of MALToma, showing invasion of many atypical lymphoid cells into the epithelial layer (× 425).

are mainly in the small intestine but may exceptionally involve the stomach, presenting with ulceration.[326] The tumors usually reveal large cells, and marker studies are needed to identify the particular type. They are highly aggressive and not responsive to simple resection. Most cases of B-cell lymphoma, in contrast, are well managed by resection, with or without associated chemotherapy.[327] Much less noted in the stomach are other lymphoid tumors, including pure plasmacytomas[328, 329] and rare examples of Hodgkin's disease.[330, 331]

Overall, biopsies are obtained in patients with lymphomatous conditions to provide the initial diagnosis, to determine the extent of the disease, and to monitor the patient following therapy, particularly for the development of recurrent tumor and of opportunistic infections.

Mesenchymal Tumors

There is a wide array of mesenchymal-type tumors, both benign and malignant, that can arise from all portions of the wall of the stomach and other parts of the gastrointestinal tract.[232, 332, 333] They are most commonly comprised of muscle, which is the largest component of the wall.

Differentiated Muscle and Nervous Tumors

Readily identifiable are small and well formed tumors that are derived from smooth muscle and from schwann cells. These include the well differentiated muscle tumors with dominant spindle cells called *leiomyoma*[334, 335] (see Fig. 3-20) and those with rounded, epithelial-like cells termed *leiomyoblastoma*[336] (Fig. 5-22); well developed tumors of the nerve sheath[337]; and neurofibromas in cases of von Recklinghausen's disease.[338, 339] All of these samples tend to be small, well circumscribed, and usually limited to the wall, with uncommon mucosal extension. Most diagnoses are evident on routine histologic sections. In cases of doubt, immunocytochemical stains can be employed, revealing desmin, and actin and myosin in the muscle tumors as opposed to S-100 and neurone-specific enolase in most nervous tissue lesions. Electron microscopy can also assist by the identification of specific myofibrils (Fig. 5-23).

Stromal Tumors

More difficult to define are the larger tumors that are seemingly derived from the same tissues but lack the specific histologic features, and these have been collectively grouped under the generic term of *gastrointestinal stromal tumors (GISTs)*.[340–343] The tumors tend to be less circumscribed and frequently extend into the submucosa and even the mucosa (Fig. 5-24). Most are comprised of spindle cells with wide variation in overall cellularity, presence of nuclear atypism, and mitoses (Fig. 5-25). Occasional tumors are seen with rounded, epithelial-like cells and signet ring forms, but they can be readily separated from carcinomas by the lack of staining for mucin or epithelial antigens. Many marker and ultrastructural studies have favored differentiation to muscle or nerve, but also to neither[334–347] (Fig. 5-26). In particular, the presence of CD34, a mesenchymal cell antigen, has been noted in most GISTs but not in pure leiomyomas or schwannomas.[348] Additionally, electron microscopy reveals in a small proportion of these cases elements of the autonomic nervous system in the form of electron-dense granules within many of the cells (Fig. 5-27); they have been called *gastrointestinal autonomic nervous system tumors (GANT.)*[349, 350.]

Whatever their nature, the stromal tumors tend to be most common in the stomach and the more significant question relates to their behavior. Tumors of large size, probably over 5 cm, and those associated with necrosis

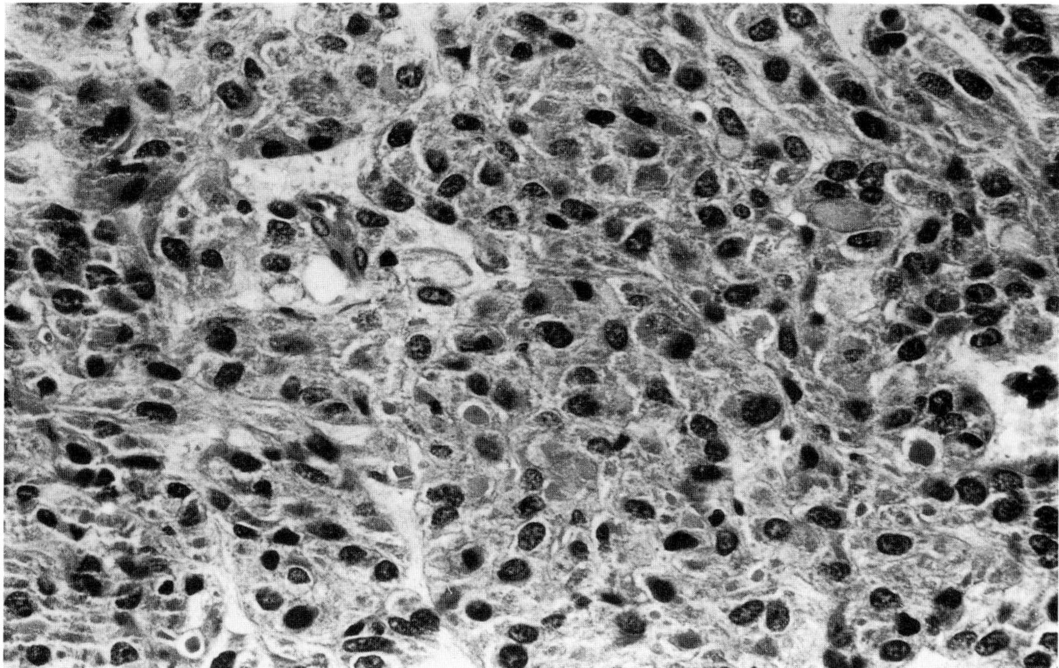

Fig. 5-22. Leiomyoblastoma of the stomach. The tumor is comprised of sheets of large cells with round and regular nuclei, and abundant granular or clear cytoplasm (× 425).

tend to behave in an aggressive fashion even if there is very little cellular atypism. These large tumors can compress and cause ulceration of the overlying mucosa, at which time the tumor may be biopsied. Biopsy samples ordinarily reveal spindle cells or a mixture with rounded ones containing clear cytoplasm, and immunocytochemical stains serve to exclude carcinoma and lymphoma. The ultimate diagnosis of a stromal tumor often requires examination of the resected mass. The tumors regularly contain vimentin and, variably, other markers of muscle or nervous derivation. As noted above, determination of malignancy is based in part on cytologic atypism but also on large size and presence of necrosis. The biopsy is mainly helpful in detecting the tumor. Aggressive behavior has been noted in those tumors that are larger than 5 to 6 cm, that reveal more than 3 mitoses per 10 high-power fields, and which show aneuploidy by flow cytometry.[351–354] It has also been suggested that increased staining for PCNA may be predictive of a poor prognosis.[27]

Vascular Tumors

There are a variety of well formed vascular lesions, including telangiectasias, persistent caliber artery of an ulcer, and antral vascular ectasia[355–365]; these are described under the section "Vascular Disorders" in Chapter 4.

Patients with AIDS often develop Kaposi's sarcoma, which frequently affects the gastrointestinal tract.[366–368] Lesions can be seen in any portion from stomach to colon and appear as ragged ulcerated areas on endoscopy. Biopsies taken from these depressed or ulcerated areas typically show small fragments of the tumor, which are recognizable by their compact, spindly nature and prominent hemorrhage together with numerous mitoses (see Figs. 6-28 and 10-36). The major differential is with granulation tis-

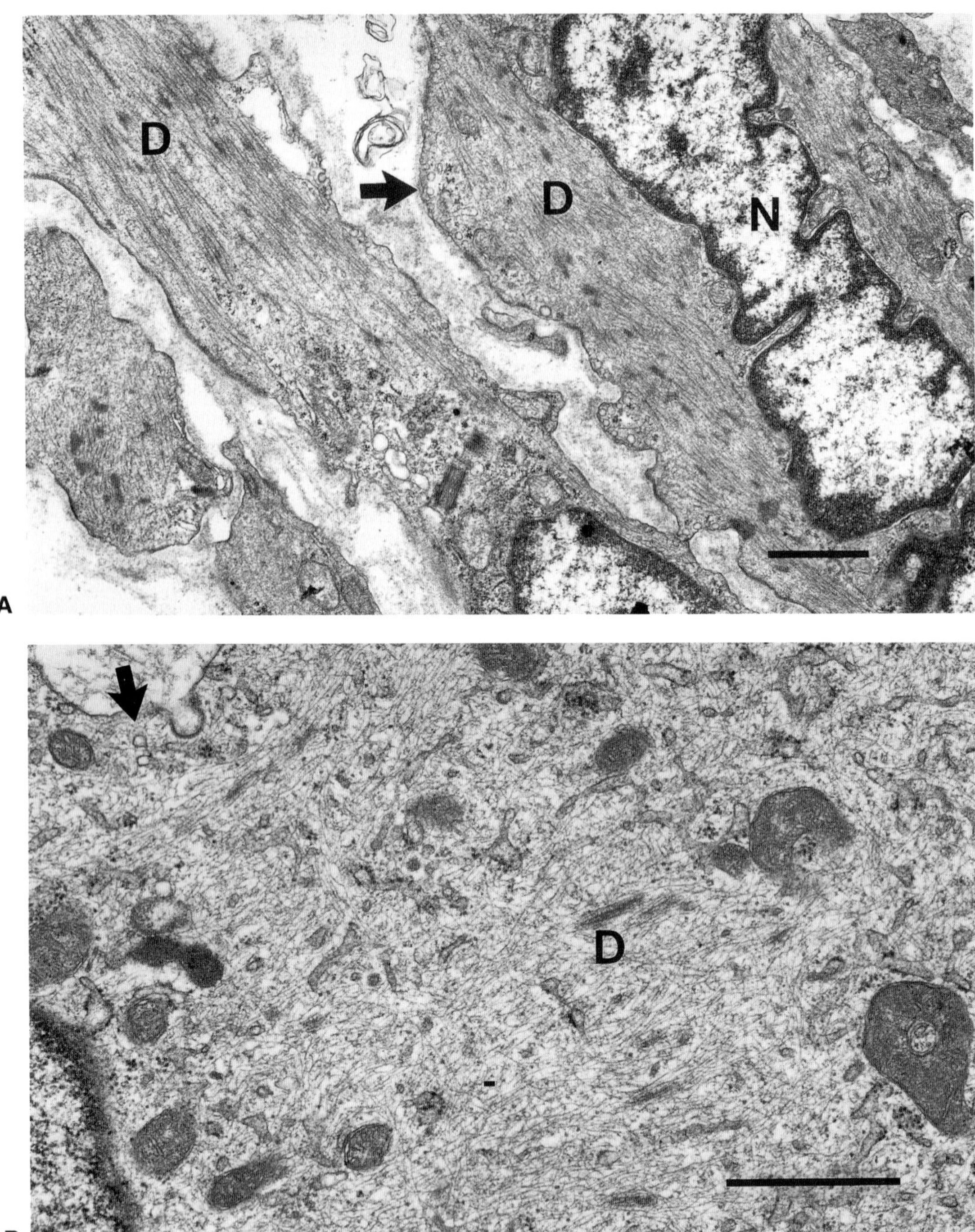

Fig. 5-23. (**A**) Electron micrograph of a differentiated smooth muscle tumor. There are characteristic spindle-shaped cells with convoluted nuclei (N), oriented filaments with dense bodies (D), pinocytotic vesicles (arrow), and external lamina (× 15,000; bar = 1 μm). (**B**) Electron micrograph of gastric leiomyoblastoma with abundant cytoplasmic, nonoriented filaments, associated dense bodies (D), and rare pinocytotic vesicles (arrow) that indicate a degree of smooth muscle differentiation (× 25,000; bar = 1 μm).

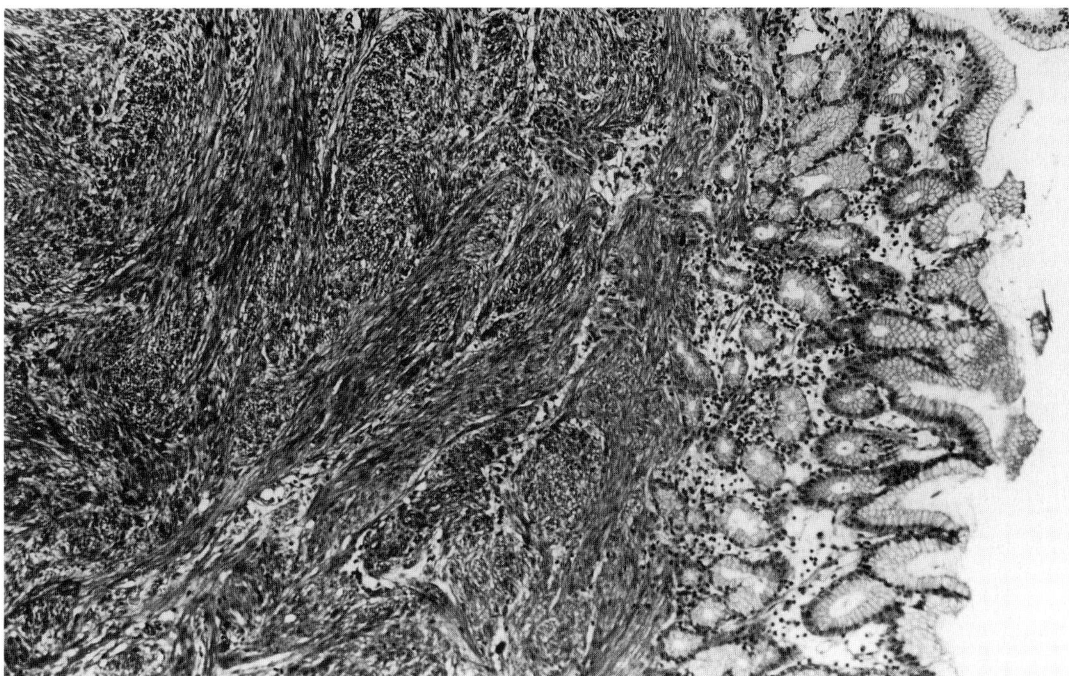

Fig. 5-24. Stromal tumor of the stomach, with mucosal surface appearing at the right. The tumor is comprised of spindle cells and extends into the base of the mucosa (× 105).

sue, which tends to show a much looser stroma. In cases with AIDS, there is a strong index of suspicion that helps to identify the Kaposi tumors. Other rare vascular tumors affecting the stomach include the glomus tumor that has a highly distinctive histology, showing regular, rounded cells enwrapped by reticulum sheaths[369–371] (Fig. 5-28). These are typically confined to the wall and ordinarily do not present on mucosal biopsy.

Other Benign Tumors

Granular cell tumors are benign lesions, probably of nervous origin, which can affect many parts of the body, including the alimentary tract[372–375] (see Fig. 3-21). They tend to be more common in the esophagus and colon but may also involve the stomach. The lesions are in the wall but can extend into the mucosa; they are readily appreciated by their large cells with granular cytoplasm, which can be accented by the PAS reaction (Fig. 5-29) (see Ch. 3 for further details). Lipomas also regularly occur in the stomach in the form of well circumscribed nodules of mature adipose tissue that are confined to the submucosa.[376] These can project into the lumen but do not ulcerate. The diagnosis is usually apparent on radiographic and gross endoscopic examination, and biopsies are uncommonly obtained; they reveal an atrophic mucosa and possibly the underlying mature adipose tissue.

Other Sarcomas

Aside from the malignant stromal tumors there are scattered reports of malignancy involving most elements of the gut wall in the stomach.[376–378] These include examples of leiomyosarcoma,[379–381] liposarcoma,[382] malignant fibrous histiocytoma,[383] and alveolar soft part sarcoma.[384] In all of these exam-

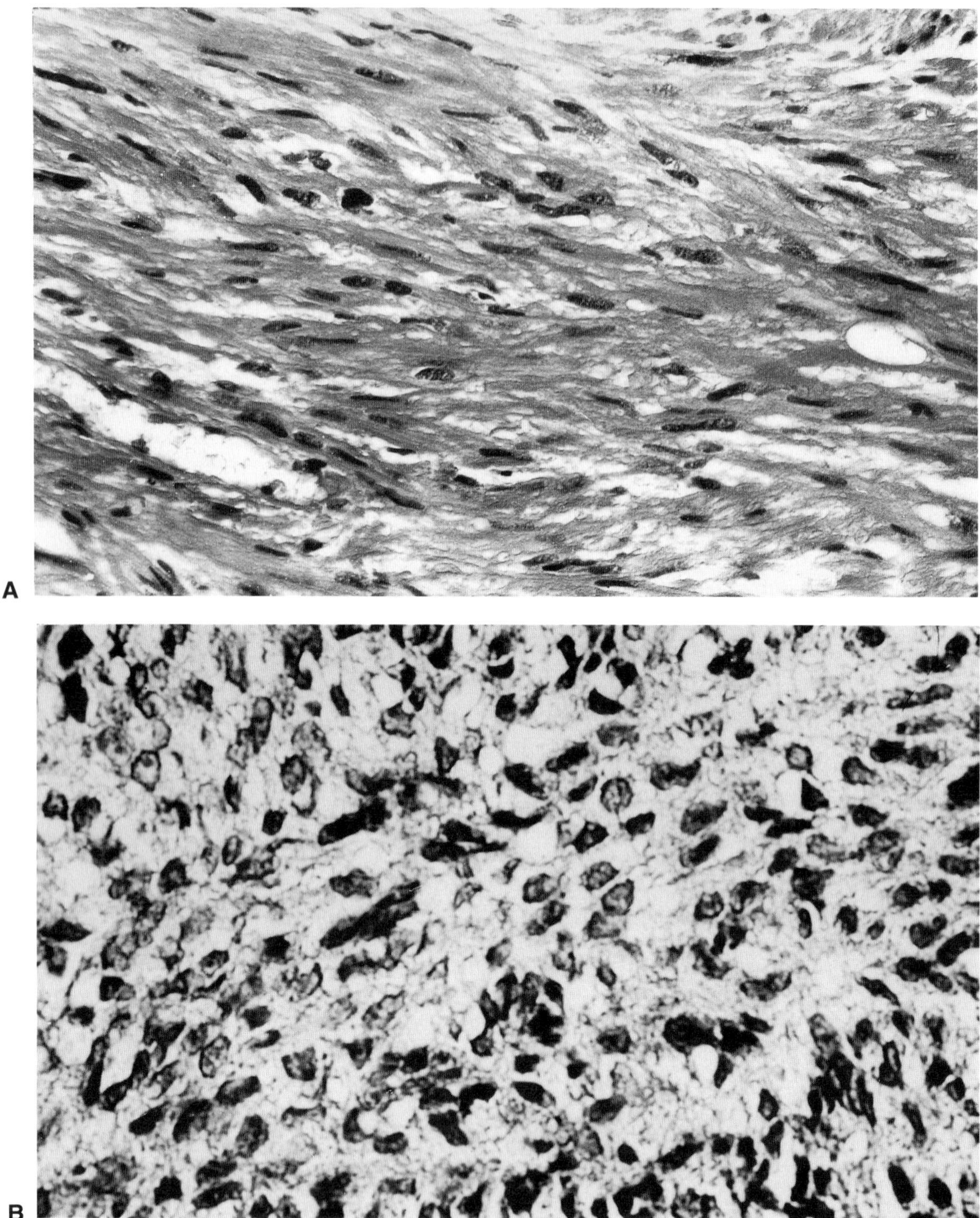

Fig. 5-25. Stromal tumor of the stomach, showing range of histologic appearance. (**A**) Spindle cells with abundant cytoplasm and thin nuclei without atypism (× 425). (**B**) Tumor showing marked pleomorphism and prominent hyperchromatism, features that strongly suggest a malignant lesion. (From Goldman,[1] with permission).

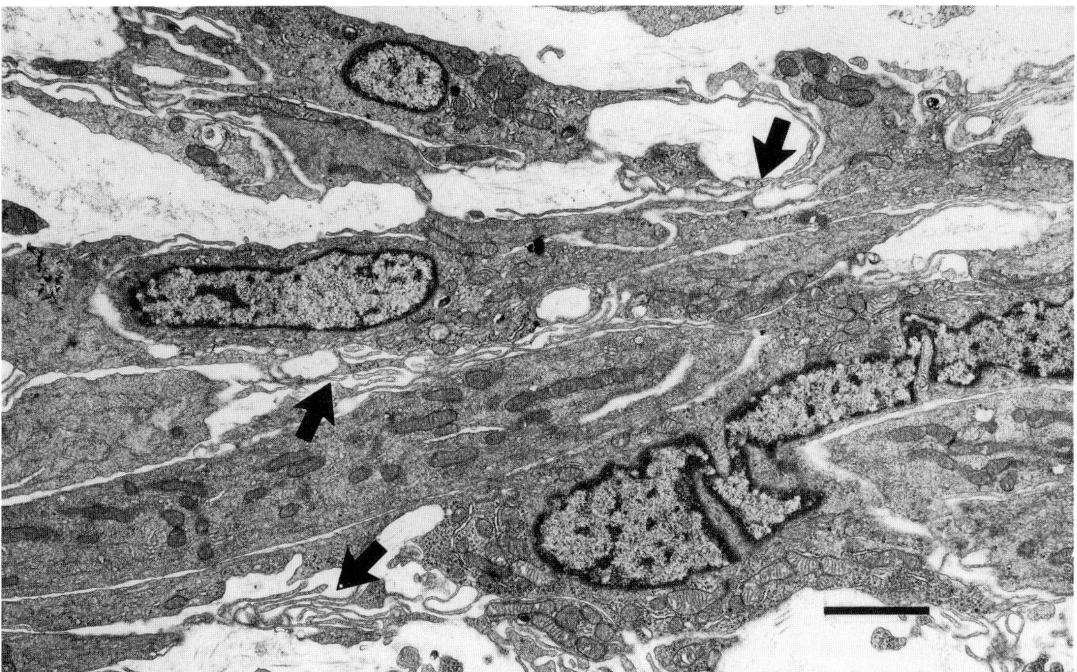

Fig. 5-26. Electron micrograph of gastrointestinal stromal tumor of the duodenum. It is composed of spindle-shaped cells that have interdigitating thin cell processes (arrow) but no specific differentiating features (× 6,750; bar = 2 μm).

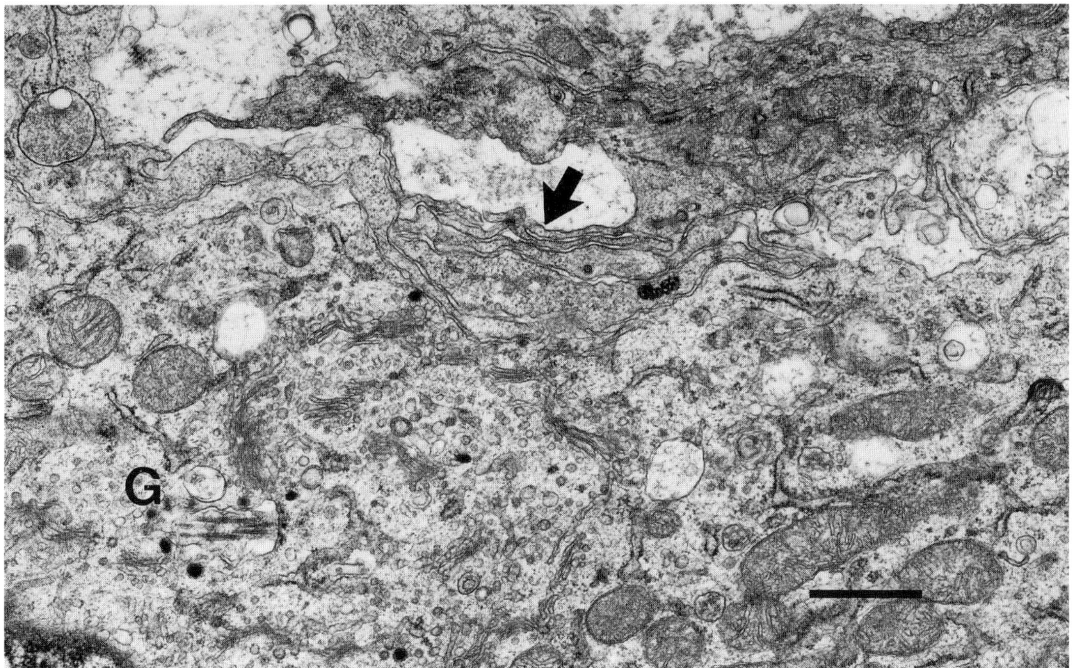

Fig. 5-27. Electron micrograph of gastrointestinal stromal tumor of the stomach. The cells contain granules with dense cores (G), a background of filaments and microtubules in the cytoplasm (top right), and interdigitating processes (arrow) that indicate some neural differentiation (× 15,000; bar = 1 μm).

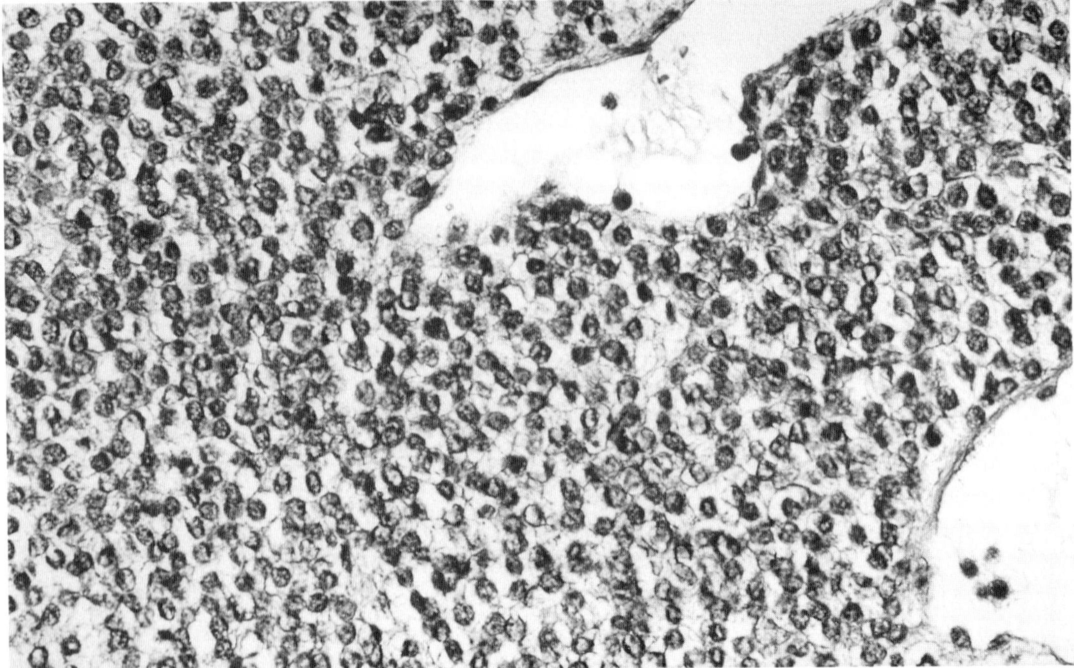

Fig. 5-28. Glomus tumor of the stomach, showing sheet of monomorphic cells apposed to vessels (× 425).

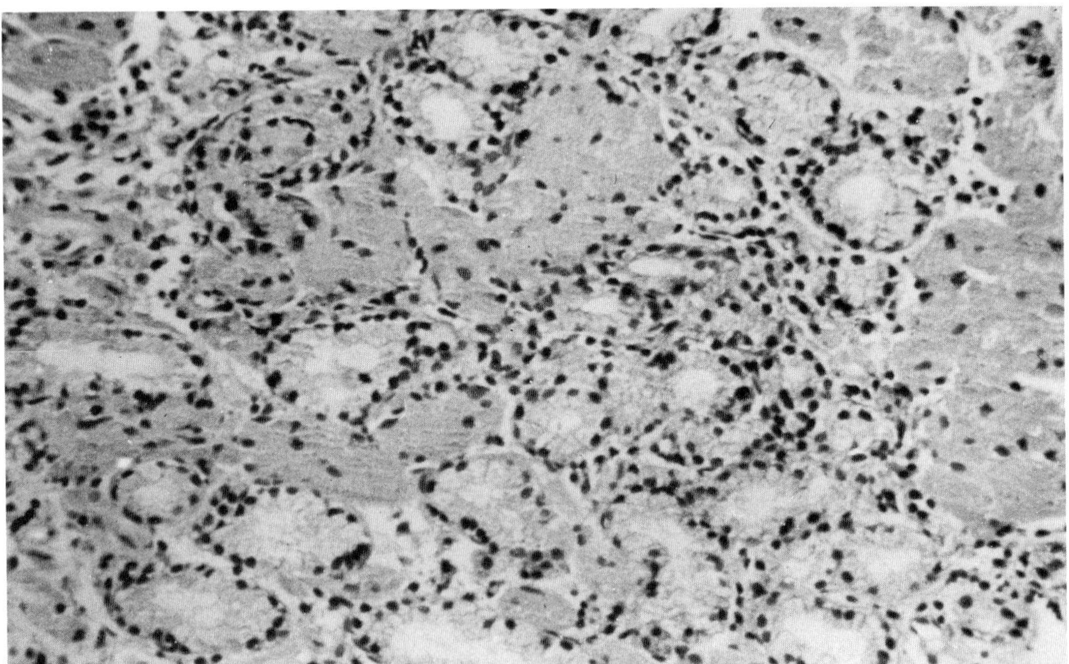

Fig. 5-29. Granular cell tumor of the stomach. The granular cells have infiltrated the mucosa, separating the antral mucous glands. (See Figure 3-21 for fine details of tumor cells).

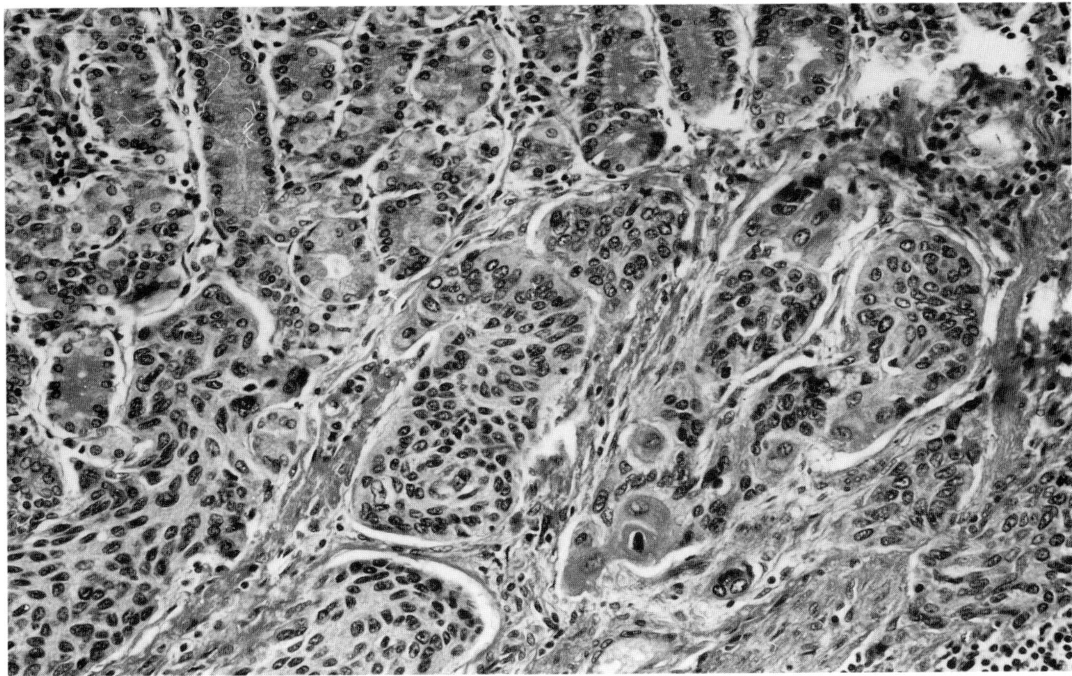

Fig. 5-30. Metastatic squamous cell carcinoma (of the lung) in the stomach. The base of the gastric specialized glands appears at the top. Sheets of malignant squamous cells are noted in the vascular spaces in the region of the muscularis mucosae (× 210).

ples, mucosal biopsy reveals the overlying atrophic mucosa or fragments of malignant tumor but without specific differentiation in most instances, because of the small size of the samples.

OTHER PRIMARY TUMORS

Choriocarcinoma and Teratoma

Choriocarcinoma and teratoma are rare germ cell tumors that can affect the stomach. The choriocarcinomas can appear as a pure lesion or, more often, associated with an adenocarcinoma.[385–387] The lesions involve the mucosa and are readily sampled by biopsy, revealing the characteristic syncytial and cytotrophoblasts (see Fig. 3-26). The cells are also rich in chorionic gonadotrophin, which may be elevated in the serum. The tumors overall tend to be aggressive. Rarely associated with the choriocarcinomas are other elements of germ cell differentiation, such as endodermal sinus tumor portions.[388, 389] The teratomas are much rarer, are more often seen in children, and typically present with a mural mass rather than a mucosal lesion.[390]

Carcinosarcoma

Carcinosarcomas are tumors that demonstrate cytologic features of both epithelial and spindle cell differentiation.[391–394] Epithelial markers such as cytokeratins can be found, however, in most of the spindle areas, suggesting that they are mainly carcinomas with areas of spindle cell appearance, similar to that observed in the esophagus (see Figs. 3-9 and 3-10). In addition, heterologous mesenchymal elements in the form of muscle

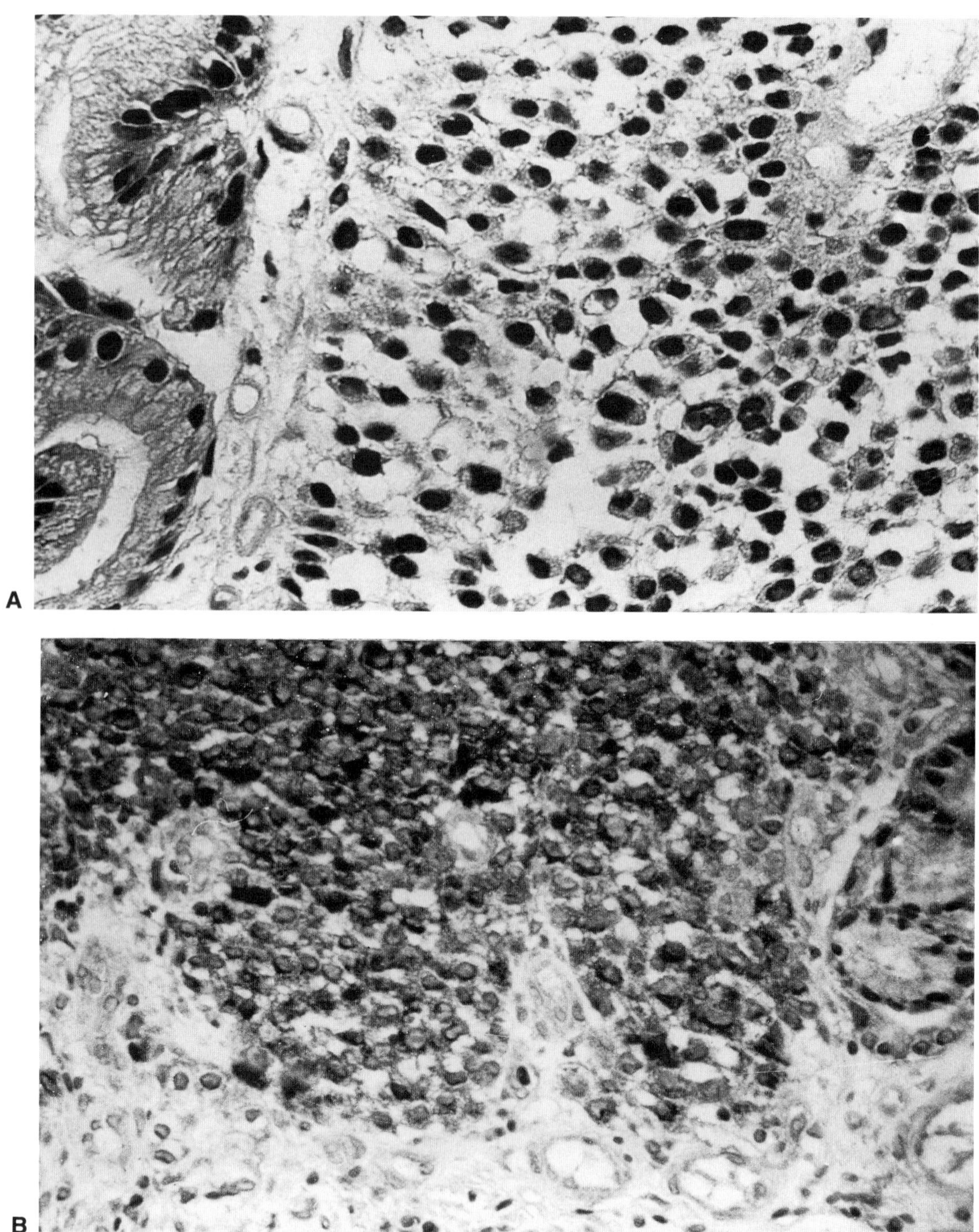

Fig. 5-31. Metastatic malignant melanoma (of the skin) in the stomach. (**A**) There is a large sheet of melanoma cells in the mucosa. Residual gastric pits appear at the left (× 425). (**B**) Immunoperoxidase stain for HMB-45, showing strong staining in the melanoma tumor cells. Residual gland appears at the right.

or cartilage can also be observed in these tumors. Since the mesenchymal elements are typically in the deeper portions, these do not ordinarily present in mucosal biopsies.

Secondary and Metastatic Tumors

Tumors readily extend into the stomach from adjacent organs, particularly both squamous and glandular lesions of the esophagus,[395] pancreatic carcinomas, hepatomas, and adenocarcinomas from the transverse colon. These are typically late findings that result in masses or ulcers within the stomach. Biopsy can readily identify the tumor, and determination of the original source is dependent on the overall clinical and gross information.

Metastases to the stomach occur in a fraction of 1 percent of the tumor cases involving the stomach,[396–399] with most samples coming from the lung[400, 401] (Fig. 5-30), the pancreas, the esophagus, the colon, and the breast.[402, 403] Metastatic breast tumors occur in 8 to 15 percent of cases and can reveal almost any appearance from scattered nodules to a linitis plastica pattern. Other tumors that commonly invade the alimentary tract mucosa, including that of the stomach, are the leukemias and malignant melanoma[404] (Fig. 5-31). These typically present as multiple flat and umbilicated nodules that are usually hemorrhagic.

REFERENCES

1. Goldman H, Antonioli DA: Mucosal biopsy of the esophagus, stomach, and proximal duodenum. Human Pathol 13:423–448, 1982
2. Whitehead R: Mucosal Biopsy of the Gastrointestinal Tract. 4th Ed. pp. 41–157. WB Saunders, Philadelphia, 1990
3. Rotterdam H: Stomach. pp. 62–255. In Rotterdam H, Sheahan DG, Sommers SC: Biopsy Diagnosis of the Digestive Tract. 2nd Ed. Raven Press, New York, 1993
4. Geboes K, Rutgeerts P, Broeckaert L et al: Histologic appearances of endoscopic gastric mucosal biopsies 10–20 years after partial gastrectomy. Ann Surg 192:179, 1980
5. Pickford IR, Craven JL, Hall R et al: Endoscopic examination of the gastric remnant 31–39 years after subtotal gastrectomy for peptic ulcer. Gut 25:393–397, 1984
6. Armbrecht U, Stockbrugger RW, Rode J et al: Development of gastric dysplasia in pernicious anemia: a clinical and endoscopic follow up study of 80 patients. Gut 31:1105–1109, 1990
7. Tatsuta M, Iishi H, Okuda S et al: Prospective evaluation of diagnostic accuracy of gastrofiberscopic biopsy in diagnosis of gastric cancer. Cancer 63:1415–1420, 1989
8. Winawar SJ, Sherlock P, Hajdu SI: The role of upper gastrointestinal endoscopy in patients with cancer. Cancer 37:440, 1976
9. Hunt RH, Cotton PB, Crespi M et al: Role of endoscopy in the diagnosis of cancer. Cancer Res 49:6822–6827, 1989
10. Gupta JP, Jain AK, Agrawal BK et al: Gastroscopic cytology and biopsies in diagnosis of gastric malignancies. J Surg Oncol 22:62–64, 1983
11. Witzel L, Halter F, Gretillat PA et al: Evaluation of specific value of endoscopic biopsies and brush cytology for malignancies of the esophagus and stomach. Gut 17:375, 1976
12. Halter F, Witzel L, Gretillat PA et al: Diagnostic value of biopsy, guided lavage, and brush cytology in esophagogastroscopy. Am J Dig Dis 22:129–131, 1977
13. Hanson JT, Thorenson C, Morrissey JF: Brush cytology in the diagnosis of upper gastrointestinal malignancy. Gastrointest Endosc 26:33, 1980
14. Qizilbash AH, Casteli M, Kowalski MA et al: Endoscopic brush cytology and biopsy in the diagnosis of cancer of the upper gastrointestinal tract. Acta Cytol 24:313, 1980
15. Graham DY, Schwartz JT, Cain GT, Gyorkey F: Prospective evaluation of biopsy number in the diagnosis of esophageal and gastric carcinoma. Gastroenterology 82:228–231, 1982
16. Iishi H, Yamamoto R, Tatsuta M, Okuda S: Evaluation of fine needle aspiration biopsy under direct vision gastro-fiberoscopy in di-

agnosis of diffusely infiltrative carcinoma of the stomach. Cancer 57:1365–1369, 1986
17. Zargar SA, Khuroo MS, Mahajan R et al: Endoscopic fine needle aspiration cytology in the diagnosis of gastro-esophageal and colorectal malignancies. Gut 32:745–748, 1991
18. Mitsunaga A: Diagnosis of submucosal tumors of the upper gastrointestinal tract by endoscopic ultrasonography. Gastrointest Endosc 29:3–15, 1987
19. Nickl NJ, Cotton PB: Clinical application of endoscopic ultrasonography. Am J Gastroenterol 85:675–682, 1990
20. Goldman H: Mucosal hypertrophy and hyperplasia of the stomach. pp. 537–546. In Ming S-C, Goldman H (eds): Pathology of the Gastrointestinal Tract. WB Saunders, Philadelphia, 1992
21. Teglbjaerg PS, Nielson HO: "Small intestinal type" and colonic type" intestinal metaplasia of the human stomach. Acta Pathol Microbiol Scand A 86:351, 1978
22. Iida F, Kusama J: Gastric carcinoma and intestinal metaplasia. Significance of types of intestinal metaplasia upon development of gastric carcinoma. Cancer 501:2854–2858, 1982
23. Stockton M, McCall I: Comparative electron microscopic features of normal, intermediate and metaplastic pyloric epithelium. Histopathology 7:859–871, 1983
24. Craenen ME, Blok P, Dekher W et al: Prevalence of subtypes of intestinal metaplasia in gastric antral mucosa. Dig Dis Sci 36:1529–1536, 1991
25. Mori M, Ambe k, Adachi Y et al: Prognostic value of immunohistochemically identified CEA, SC, AFP, and S-100 protein-positive cells in gastric carcinoma. Cancer 62:534–540, 1988
26. Amin MB, Ma CK, Linden MD et al: Prognostic value of proliferating cell nuclear antigen index in gastric stromal tuomrs. Correlation with mitotic count and clinical outcome. Am J Clin Pathol 100:428–432, 1993
27. Ray R, Tahan SR, Andrews C, Goldman H: Stromal tumors of the stomach: prognostic value of the PCNA index. Modern Pathol 7:26–30, 1994
28. Maeda K, Chung Y-S, Onoda N et al: Proliferating cell nuclear antigen labelling index of preoperative biopsy specimens in gastric carcinoma with special reference to prognosis. Cancer 73:528–533, 1994
29. Nikulasson S, Andrews CA Jr, Goldman H et al: Sucrase–isomaltase expression in gastric dysplasia and in dysplasia associated with Barrett's esophagus and chronic gastritis and in adenocarcinomas of the gastrointestinal tract. Int J Surg Pathol 2:281–286, 1995
30. Grody WW, Gatti RA, Naeim F: Diagnostic molecular pathology. Modern Pathol 2: 533–568, 1990
31. Odegaard S, Hostmark J, Skogen DW et al: Flow cytometric DNA studies in human gastric cancer and polyps. Scand J Gastroenterol 22:1270–1276, 1987
32. Rugge M, Sonego F, Panozzo M et al: Pathology and ploidy in the prognosis of gastric cancer with no extranodal metastases. Cancer 73:1127–1133, 1994
33. Chang F, Syrjanen S, Kurinen K, Syrjanen K: The p53 tumor suppressor gene as a common cellular target in human carcinogenesis. Am J Gastroenterol 88:174–186, 1993
34. Lauwers GY, Wahl SJ, Melamed J, Rojas-Corona R: p53 expression in precancerous gastric lesions: an immunohistochemical study of PAb 1801 monoclonal antibody on adenomatous and hyperplastic gastric polyps. Am J Gastroenterol 88:1916–1919, 1993
35. Imazeki F, Omata M, Nose H et al: p53 gene mutations in gastric and esophageal cancers. Gastroenterology 103:892–896, 1992
36. Joypaul BV, Newman EL, Hopwood D et al: Expression of p53 protein in normal, dysplastic, and malignant gastric mucosa: an immunohistochemical study. J Pathol 170: 279–283, 1993
37. Wright PA, Quirke P, Attanoos R, Wilkins GT: Molecular pathology of gastric carcinoma: progress and prospects. Hum Pathol 23:848–859, 1992
38. Stemmermann G, Heffelfinger SC, Noffsinger A et al: The molecular biology of esophageal and gastric cancer and their precursors. Hum Pathol 25:968–981, 1994
39. Barbosa JC, Dockerty MB, Waugh JM: Pancreatic heterotopia: review of literature and report of 41 authenticated surgical cases, of which 25 were clinically significant. Surg Gynecol Obstet 85:527–542, 1946

40. Theoni RF, Gedgaudas RK: Ectopic pancreas: usual and unusual features. Gastrointest Endosc 5:37–42, 1980
41. Kaneda M, Yano T, Yamamoto T et al: Ectopic pancreas on the stomach presenting as an inflammatory abdominal mass. Am J Gastroenterol 84:663–666, 1989
42. Komorowski RA, Caya JG: Hyperplastic gastropathy. Clinicopathologic correlation. Am J Surg Pathol 15:577–585, 1991
43. Goldman H: Mucosal hypertrophy and hyperplasia of the stomach. pp. 537–546. In Ming S-C, Goldman H (eds): Pathology of the Gastrointestinal Tract. WB Saunders, Philadelphia, 1992
44. Appelman HD: Localized and extensive expansions of the gastric mucosa: mucosal polyps and giant folds. pp. 79–119. In Appelman HD (ed): Pathology of the Esophagus, Stomach, and Duodenum. Churchill Livingstone, New York, 1984
45. Scharschmidt BF: The natural history of hypertrophic gastropathy (Ménétrier's disease). Am J Med 63:644, 1977
46. Fieber SS, Rickert RR: Hyperplastic gastropathy. Analysis of 50 selected cases from 1955–1980. Am J Gastroenterol 76:321, 1981
47. Meuwissen SGM, Ridwan BU, Hasper HJ, Innernee G: Hypertrophic protein-losing gastropathy. A retrospective analysis of 40 cases in the Netherlands. Scand J Gastroenterol 194(suppl 27):1–8, 1992
48. Bjork JT, Geenen JE, Komorowski RA et al: Ménétrier's disease diagnosed by electrosurgical snare biopsy. JAMA 238:1755, 1977
49. Wolfsen HC, Carpenter HA, Talley NJ: Ménétrier's disease: a form of hypertrophic gastropathy or gastritis? Gastroenterology 104:1310–1319, 1993
50. Wolber RA, Owen DA, Anderson FH, Freeman HJ: Lymphocytic gastritis and giant gastric folds associated with gastrointestinal protein loss. Modern Pathol 4:13–15, 1991
51. Haot J, Bogomoletz WV, Jouret A, Mainquet P: Ménétrier's disease with lymphocytic gastritis: an unusual association with possible pathogenic implications. Hum Pathol 22:379–386, 1991
52. Littler ER, Gleibermann E: Gastritis cystica polyposa (gastric mucosal prolapse at gastroenterostomy site, with cystic and infiltrative epithelial hyperplasia). Cancer 29:205, 1972
53. Franzin G, Novelli P: Gastritis cystica profunda. Histopathology 5:535–547, 1981
54. Fonde EC, Rodning CB: Gastritis cystica profunda. Am J Gastroenterol 81:459–464, 1986
55. Mosnier JF, Flejou JF, Amouyal G et al: Hypertrophic gastropathy with gastric adenocarcinoma: Ménétrier's disease and lymphocytic gastritis. Gut 32:1565–1567, 1991
56. Sandberg DH: Hypertrophic gastropathy (Ménétrier's disease) in childhood. J Pediatr 78:866, 1971
57. Chouraqui JP, Roy CC, Brocha P et al: Ménétrier's disease in children: report of a patient and review of sixteen other cases. Gastroenterology 80:1042–1047, 1981
58. Baker A, Volberg F, Sumner T, Moran R: Childhood Ménétrier's disease: four new cases and discussion of the literature. Gastrointest Radiol 11:131–134, 1986
59. Goldman H, Proujansky R: Allergic proctitis and gastroenteritis in children: clinical and mucosal biopsy features in 53 cases. Am J Surg Pathol 10:75–86
60. Teele RL, Katz AJ, Goldman H et al: The radiographic features of eosinophilic gastroenteritis (allergic gastroenteropathy) of childhood. Am J Radiol 132:575, 1979
61. Wolfe MM, Jensen RT: Zollinger–Ellison syndrome: current concepts in diagnosis and management. N Engl J Med 317:1200–1209, 1987
62. Creutzfeldt W, Arnold R, Creutzfeldt C et al: Pathomorphologic, biochemical and diagnostic aspects of gastrinomas (Zollinger-Ellison syndrome). Hum Pathol 6:47, 1975
63. McIntyre RLE, Piris J: A method for the quantification of human gastric G cell density in endoscopic biopsy specimens. J Clin Pathol 34:514, 1981
64. Goldman H: Gastritis. pp. 481–516. In Ming S-C, Goldman H (eds): Pathology of the Gastrointestinal Tract. WB Saunders, Philadelphia, 1992
65. Ming S-C, Goldman H: Gastric polyps. A histologic classification and its relation to carcinoma. Cancer 18:721–726, 1965
66. Tomasulo J: Gastric polyps. Histologic types and their relationship to gastric carcinoma. Cancer 27:1346–1355, 1971

67. Neimark S, Rogers AI: Gastric polyps: a review. Am J Gastroenterol 77:543–547, 1982
68. Snover DC: Benign epithelial polyps of the stomach. Pathol Annu 20:303–329, 1985
69. Ming S-C: Epithelial polyps of the stomach. pp. 547–569. In Ming S-C, Goldman H (eds): Pathology of the Gastrointestinal Tract. WB Saunders, Philadelphia, 1992
70. Wauters GV, Ferrell L, Ostroff JW, Heyman MB: Hyperplastic gastric polyps associated with persistent Helicobacter pylori infection and active gastritis. Am J Gastroenterol 85:1395–1397, 1990
71. Lin PY, Brown DB, Deppisch LM: Gastric xanthelasma in hyperplastic gastric polyposis. Arch Pathol Lab Med 112:428–430, 1989
72. Domellof L, Ericksson S, Helander HF et al: Lipid islands in the gastric mucosa after resection for benign ulcer disease. Gastroenterology 72:14, 1977
73. Drude RB, Balart LA, Herrington JP et al: Gastric xanthoma: histological similarity to signet ring cell carcinoma. J Clin Gastroenterol 4:217–221, 1982
74. Kunze KC, Baum RA, Nasrallah SM: Gastric xanthoma. Gastrointest Endosc 33: 114–115, 1987
75. Joffe N, Goldman H, Antonioli DA: Recurring hyperplastic gastric polyps following subtotal gastrectomy. Am J Roentgenol 130:301, 1978
76. Hattori T: Morphological range of hyperplastic polyps and carcinomas arising in hyperplastic polyps of the stomach. J Clin Pathol 38:622–630, 1985
77. Daibo M, Hirota T: Malignant transformation of gastric hyperplastic polyps. Am J Gastroenterol 82:1016–1025, 1987
78. Carneiro F, David L, Seruca R et al: Hyperplastic polyposis and diffuse carcinoma of the stomach. A study of a family. Cancer 72:323–329, 1993
79. Laxen F, Kekki M, Sipponen P, Surala M: The gastric mucosa in stomach with polyps: morphologic and dynamic evaluation. Scand J Gastroenterol 18:503–511, 1983
80. Stemmerman GN, Hayashi T: Hyperplastic polyps of the gastric mucosa adjacent to gastroenterostomy stomas. Am J Clin Pathol 71:341, 1979
81. Iida M, Yao T, Watanabe H et al: Fundic gland polyposis in patients without familial adenomatosis coli: its incidence and clinical features. Gastroenterology 86:1437–1442, 1984
82. Lee RG, Burt RW: The histopathology of fundic gland polyps of the stomach. Am J Clin Pathol 86:498–503, 1986
83. Marcial MA, Villafana M, Hernandez-Denton J, Colon-Pagan JR: Fundic gland polyps: prevalence and clinicopathologic features. Am J Gastroenterol 88:1711–1713, 1993
84. Iida M, Yao T, Itoh H et al: Natural history of fundic gland polyposis in patients with familial adenomatosis coli/Gardner's syndrome. Gastroenterology 89:1021, 1985
85. Kim YI, Kim WH: Inflammatory fibroid polyps of gastrointestinal tract. Am J Clin Pathol 89:721–727, 1988
86. Helwig EB, Raider A: Inflammatory fibroid polyps of stomach. Surg Gynecol Obstet 96:355, 1953
87. Navas-Palacios JJ, Colima-Ruizdelgado F, Sanchez-Larrea, Cortes-Consino J. Inflammatory fibroid polyps of the gastrointestinal tract. An immunohistochemical and electron microscopic study. Cancer 51: 1682–1690, 1983
88. Kolodziejczyk P, Yao T, Tsuneyoshi M: Inflammatory fibroid polyp of the stomach. A special reference to an immunohistochemical profile of 42 cases. Am J Surg Pathol 17:1159–1168, 1993
89. Tada S, Iida M, Yao T et al: Endoscopic removal of inflammatory fibroid polyps of the stomach. Am J Gastroenterol 86: 1247–1250, 1991
90. Ito H, Hata J, Yokozaki H et al: Tubular adenoma of the stomach. An immunohistochemical analysis of gut hormones, serotonin, carcinoembryonic antigen, secretory component, and lysozyme. Cancer 58: 2264–2272, 1986
91. Nakomura K, Sakoquchi H, Enjoji M: Depressed adenoma of the stomach. Cancer 62:2197–2202, 1988
92. Kolodziejczyk P, Yao T, Oya M et al: Long term follow-up study of patients with gastric adenomas with malignant transformation. An immunohistochemical and histochemical analysis. Cancer 74:2896–2907, 1994
93. Kato Y, Sugano H, Rubio CA: Classification of intramucosal cysts of the stomach. Histopathology 7:931–938, 1983

94. Zarling EJ: Gastric adenomyoma with coincidental pancreatic rest: a case report and review of the literature. Gastrointest Endosc 27:175–177, 1981
95. Erbe RW: Inherited gastrointestinal polyposis syndromes. N Engl J Med 294:1101–1104, 1976
96. Haggitt RC, Reid BJ: Hereditary gastrointestinal polyposis syndromes. Am J Surg Pathol 10:871–877, 1986
97. Listron MB, Fenoglio-Preiser C: Short course. Gastrointestinal polyps. Modern Pathol 2:161–181, 1989
98. Watanabe H, Enjoji M, Yao T et al: Gastric lesions in familial adenomatous polyposis coli: their incidence and histological analysis. Hum Pathol 9:269, 1978
99. Jarvinen H, Nyberg M, Peltokallio P: Upper gastrointestinal tract polyps in familial adenomatosis coli. Gut 24:333–339, 1983
100. Nishiura M, Hirota T, Itabashi M et al: A clinical and histopathological study of gastric polyps in familial polyposis coli. Am J Gastroenterol 79:98–103, 1984
101. Shemesk E, Bat L: A prospective evaluation of the upper gastrointestinal tract and periampullary region in patients with Gardner syndrome. Am J Gastroenterol 80:825–827, 1985
102. Kurtz RC, Sternberg SS, Miller HH, DeCosse JJ: Upper gastrointestinal neoplasia in familial polyposis. Dig Dis Sci 32: 459–465, 1987
103. Iida M, Yao T, Itoh H et al: Natural history of gastric adenomas in patients with familial adenomatosis coli/Gardner's syndrome. Cancer 61:605–611, 1988
104. Domizio P, Talbort IC, Spigelman AD et al: Upper gastrointestinal pathology in familial adenomatous polyposis—results from a prospective study of 102 patients. J Clin Pathol 43:738–743, 1990
105. Burt RW, Berenson MM, Lee RG et al: Upper gastrointestinal polyps in Gardner's syndrome. Gastroenterology 86:295–301, 1984
106. Coffey RJ, Knight CD, von Heerden JA, Weiland LH: Gastric adenocarcinoma complicating Gardner's syndrome in a North American woman. Gastroenterology 88: 1263–1266, 1985
107. Lynch HT, Smyrk TC, Lanspa SJ et al: Upper gastrointestinal manifestations in families with hereditary flat adenoma syndrome. Cancer 71:2709–2714, 1993
108. Sarre RG, Frost AG, Jagelman DG et al: Gastric and duodenal polyps and familial adenomatous polyposis: a prospective study of the nature and prevalence of upper gastrointestinal polyps. Gut 28:306–314, 1987
109. Odze RD, Quinn PS, Terrault NA et al: Advanced gastroduodenal polyposis with ras mutations in a patient with familial adenomatous polyposis. Hum Pathol 24:442–448, 1993
110. Roth SI, Helwig EB: Juvenile polyps of the colon and rectum. Cancer 16:468–479, 1963
111. Watanabe A, Nagashima H, Motoi M et al: Familial juvenile polyposis of the stomach. Gastroenterology 77:146, 1979
112. Sachatello CR, Pickren JW, Grace JT: Generalized juvenile gastrointestinal polyposis. Gastroenterology 58:669, 1970
113. Stemper TJ, Kent TH, Summers RW: Juvenile polyposis and gastrointestinal carcinoma: a study of a kindred. Ann Intern Med 83:639–646, 1975
114. Williams GT, Bussey HJR, Morson BC: Hamartomatous polyps in Peutz–Jeghers syndrome. N Engl J Med 299:101, 1978
115. Foley TR, McGarrity TJ, Abt AB: Peutz–Jeghers syndrome: a clinicopathologic survey of the "Harrisburg Family" with a 49-year follow-up. Gastroenterology 95:1535–1540, 1988
116. Dodds WJ, Schulte WJ, Hensley Gt, Hogan WJ: Peutz–Jeghers syndrome and gastrointestinal malignancy. AJR 115:374–377, 1972
117. Giardiello FM, Welsh SB, Hamilton SR et al: Increased risk of cancer in the Peutz–Jeghers syndrome. N Engl J Med 316: 1511–1514, 1987
118. Halbert RE: Peutz–Jeghers syndrome with metastasizing gastric adenocarcinoma: report of a case. Arch Pathol Lab Med 106:517–520, 1982
119. Ali M, Weinstein J, Biempica J et al: Cronkhite–Canada syndrome: report of a case with bacteriologic, immunologic, and electron microscopic studies. Gastroenterology 79:731, 1980
120. Daniel ES, Ludwig SL, Lewin KJ et al: The Cronkhite–Canada syndrome. An analysis of clinical and pathological features and

therapy in 55 patients. Medicine 61:293–309, 1982

121. Burke AP, Sobin LH: The pathology of Cronkhite–Canada polyps: a comparison to juvenile polyposis. Am J Surg Pathol 13:940–946, 1989
122. Nardone G, D'Armiento F, Carlomagno P et al: Cronkhite–Canada syndrome: case report with some features not previously described. Gastrointest Endosc 36:150–152, 1990
123. Sagara K, Fujiyama S, Kamuro Y et al: Cronkhite–Canada syndrome associated with gastric cancer: report of a case. Gastroenterol Jpn 18:260–266, 1983
124. Ming S-C: Adenocarcinoma and other malignant epithelial tumors of the stomach. pp. 584–617. In Ming S-C, Goldman H (eds): Pathology of the Gastrointestinal Tract. WB Saunders, Philadelphia, 1992
125. Correa P, Haenszel W, Tannenbaum S: Epidemiology of gastri carcinoma: review and future prospects. Natl Cancer Inst Monogr 62:129–134, 1982
126. Lauren PA, Nevalainen TJ: Epidemiology of intestinal and diffuse types of gastric carcinoma. A time-trend study in Finland with comparison between studies from high- and low-risk areas. Cancer 71:2926–2933, 1993
127. Antonioli DA, Goldman H: Changes in location and type of gastric adenocarcinoma. Cancer 50:755–781, 1982
128. Cady B, Rossi RL, Silverman ML et al: Gastric adenocarcinoma: a disease in transition. Arch Surg 124:303–308, 1989
129. Craanen ME, Dekher W, Bloh P et al: Time trends in gastric carcinoma: changing patterns of type and location. Am J Gastroenterol 87:572–579, 1992
130. Thomas RM, Sobin LH: Gastrointestinal cancer. Cancer 75:154–170, 1995
131. Grabiec J, Owen DA: Carcinoma of the stomach in young persons. Cancer 56: 388–396, 1985
132. Radi MJ, Fenoglio-Preiser CM, Bartow SA et al: Gastric carcinoma in the young: a clinicopathological and immunohistochemical study. Am J Gastroenterol 81:747–756, 1986
133. Tso PL, Bringaze WL, Dauterine AH et al: Gastric carcinoma in the young. Cancer 59:1362–1365, 1987
134. Boren T, Falk P, Roth KA et al: Attachment of Helicobacter pylori to human gastric epithelium mediated by blood group antigens. Science 262:1892–1896, 1993
135. Correa P: Precursors of gastric and esophageal cancer. Cancer 50:2554–2565, 1982
136. Ming S-C: Precancerous states of the esophagus and stomach. pp. 192. In Carter RL (ed): Precancerous states. Oxford University Press, London, 1984
137. Antonioli DA: Precursors of gastric carcinoma: a critical review with a brief description of early (curable) gastric cancer. Hum Pathol 25:994–1005, 1994
138. Sipponen P, Kekki M, Siuralla M: Atrophic chronic gastritis and intestinal metaplasia in gastric carcinoma. Comparison with representative population sample. Cancer 52: 1062–1068, 1983
139. Armbrecht U, Stockbrugger RW, Rode J et al: Development of gastric dysplasia in pernicious anemia: a clinical and endoscopic follow up study of 80 patients. Gut 31:1105–1109, 1990
140. Sipponen P, Riihela M, Hyvarinen H, Seppala K: Chronic nonatrophic ("superficial") gastritis increases the risk of gastric carcinoma. A case-control study. Scand J Gastroenterol 29:336–341, 1994
141. Tatsuta NM, Iishi H, Okuda S et al: The association of Helicobacter pylori with differentiated-type early gastric cancer. Cancer 72:1841–1845, 1993
142. Hansson L-E, Engstrand L, Nyren O et al: Helicobacter pylori infection: independent risk indicator of gastric adenocarcinoma. Gastroenterology 105:1098–1103, 1993
143. Wee A, Kang JY, Teh M: Helicobacter pylori and gastric cancer correlation with gastritis, intestinal metaplasia, and tumor histology. Gut 33:1029–1032, 1992
144. Hu PJ, Mitchell HM, Li YY et al: Association of Helicobacter pylori with gastric cancer and observations on the detection of this bacterium in gastric cancer cases. Am J Gastroenterol 89:1806–1810, 1994
145. Offerhaus GJA, Stadt J, Hurbregtse K et al: The mucosa of the gastric remnant harboring malignancy. Histologic findings in the biopsy specimens of 504 asymptomatic patients 15 to 46 years after partial gastrectomy with

emphasis on nonmalignant lesions. Cancer 64:698–703, 1989
146. von Holstein CS, Hammar E, Eriksson S, Huldt B: Clinical significance of dysplasia in gastric remnant biopsy specimens. Cancer 72:1532–1535, 1993
147. Domellof L, Eriksson S, Janunger KG: Carcinoma and possible precancerous change in the gastric stump after Billroth II resection. Gastroenterology 73:462–468, 1977
148. Savage A, Jones S: Histological appearances of the gastric mucosa 15 to 27 years after partial gastrectomy. J Clin Pathol 32:179, 1979
149. Viste A, Opheim P, Thunold J et al: Risk of carcinoma following gastric operations for benign disease. A historical cohort study of 3470 patients. Lancet 2:502–505, 1986
150. Northfield TC, Hall CN: Carcinoma of the gastric stump: risks and pathogenesis. Gut 31:1217–1219, 1990
151. Giarelli L, Melato M, Stanta G et al: Gastric resection. A cause of high frequency of gastric carcinoma. Cancer 52:1113–1116, 1983
152. Schafer LW, Larson DE, Melton J et al: The risk of gastric carcinoma after surgical treatment for benign ulcer disease. A population-based study in Olmsted County, Minnesota. N Engl J Med 309:1210–1213, 1983
153. Sandler RS, Johnson MD, Holland KL: Risk of stomach cancer after gastric surgery for benign conditions. A case-control study. Dig Dis Sci 29:703–708, 1984
154. Farrands PA, Blake JRS, Ansell ID et al: Endoscopic review of patients who have had gastric surgery. Br Med J 286:755–758, 1983
155. Graem N, Fischer AB, Beck H: Dysplasia and carcinoma in the Billroth II resected stomach 27–35 years post-operatively. Acta Pathol Microbiol Scand 92:185–188, 1984
156. Bogomoletz WV, Potet F, Borge J et al: Pathological features and mucin histochemistry of primary gastric stump carcinoma associated with gastritis cystica polyposa. A study of six cases. Am J Surg Pathol 9:401–410, 1985
157. Luukhonen P, Kalima T, Kwilookso E: Decreased risk of gastric stump carcinoma after partial gastrectomy supplemented with bile diversion. Hepatogastroenterology 37:392–394, 1990
158. Jass JR, Filipe MI: Sulphamucins and precancerous lesions of the human stomach. Histopathology 4:271, 1980
159. Huang C-B, Xu J, Huang J-T et al: Sulphomucin colonic type intestinal metaplasia and carcinoma of the stomach. Cancer 57:1370–1375, 1986
160. Rokkas T, Filipe MI, Sladen GE: Detection of an increased incidence of early gastric cancer in patients with intestinal metaplasia type III who are closely followed up. Gut 32:1110–1113, 1991
161. Bramesar KCR, Sanders DSA, Hopwood D: Limited value of type III intestinal metaplasia in predicting risk of gastric carcinoma. J Clin Pathol 40:1287–1290, 1987
162. Mutsukuma A, Mori M, Enjoji M: Sulphamucin-secreting intestinal metaplasia in the human gastric mucosa. An association with intestinal-type gastric carcinoma. Cancer 66:689–694, 1990
163. Ming S-C, Goldman H, Freiman DG: Intestinal metaplasia and histogenesis of carcinoma in human stomach: light and electron microscopic study. Cancer 20:1418, 1967
164. Filipe MI, Potet F, Bogomoletz WV et al: Incomplete sulphomucin-secreting intestinal metaplasia for gastric cancer. Preliminary data from a prospective study from three centres. Gut 26:1319–26, 1985
165. Danzig JB, Brandt LJ, Reinus JF, Klein RS: Gastrointestinal malignancy in patients with AIDS. Am J Gastroenterol 86:715–718, 1991
166. Cooper BT, Holmes GK, Ferguson R, Cooke WT: Celiac disease and malignancy. Medicine (Baltimore) 59:249–261, 1980
167. Morson BC, Sobin LH, Grundman E et al: Precancerous conditions and epithelial dysplasia in the stomach. J Clin Pathol 33:711, 1980
168. Jass JR: A classification of gastric dysplasia. Histopathology 7:181–193, 1983
169. Ming S-C, Bajtai A, Correa P et al: Gastric dysplasia. Significance and pathologic criteria. Cancer 54:1794–1801, 1984
170. Di Gregorio C, Morandi P, De Gaetani C: Gastric dysplasia. A follow-up study. Am J Gastroenterol 88:1714–1719, 1993
171. Cuello C, Correa P, Zamara G et al: Histopathology of gastric dysplasias. Correlation with gastric juice chemistry. Am J Surg Pathol 3:491–500, 1979

172. Saraga E-P, Gardiol D, Costa J: Gastric dysplasia. A histological follow-up study. Am J Surg Pathol 11:788–796, 1987
173. del Corral MJM, Pardo-Mindon FJ, Razquin S, Ojeda C: Risk of cancer in patients with gastric dysplasia. Follow-up study of 67 patients. Cancer 65:2078–2085, 1990
174. de Dombal FT, Price AB, Thompson H et al: The British Society of Gastroenterology early gastric cancer/dysplasia survey; an interim report. Gut 31:115–120, 1990
175. Burke AP, Sobin LH, Shekita KM, Helwig EB: Dysplasia of the stomach and Barrett esophagus: a follow-up study. Modern Pathol 4:386–441, 1991
176. Farinati F, Rugge M, Dimario F et al: Early and advanced gastric cancer in the follow-up of moderate and severe gastric dysplasia. A prospective study. Endoscopy 25:261–264, 1993
177. Fertitta AM, Comin U, Terruzzi V et al: Clinical significance of gastric dysplasia. A multicenter follow-up study. Endoscopy 25:265–268, 1993
178. Ghondur-Monaymneh L, Paz J, Rolden E, Jassady J: Dysplasia of non-metaplastic gastric mucosa. A proposal for its classification and its possible relationship to diffuse-type gastric carcinoma. Am J Surg Pathol 12:96–114, 1988
179. Bearzi I, Brancorsini D, Santinelli A et al: Gastric dysplasia—a 10 year follow-up study. Pathol Res Pract 190:61–68, 1994
180. Rugge M, Farinati F, Baffa R et al: Gastric epithelial dysplasia in the natural history of gastric cancer: a multicenter prospective follow-up study. Gastroenterology 107: 1288–1296, 1994
181. Riddell RH, Goldman H, Ransohoff DF et al: Dysplasia in inflammatory bowel disease: standardized classification with provisional clinical applications. Hum Pathol 14: 931–968, 1983
182. Tosi P, Boak JPA, Luzi P et al: Morphometric distinction of low- and high-grade dysplasia in gastric biopsies. Hum Pathol 20: 839–844, 1989
183. Lansdown M, Quirke P, Dixon MF et al: High grade dysplasia of the gastric mucosa: a marker for gastric carcinoma. Gut 31:977–983, 1990
184. Farini R, Leandro G, Farinati F et al: Epithelial dysplasia in endoscopic gastric mucosal biopsies. Tumori 67:589–598, 1981
185. Farini R, Arslan Pagnini C, Farinati F et al: Is mild gastric epithelial dysplasia an indication for follow-up? J Clin Gastroenterol 5:307–310, 1983
186. Wang HH, Antonioli DA, Goldman H: Comparative features of esophageal and gastric adenocarcinomas: recent changes in type and frequency. Hum Pathol 17:482–487, 1986
187. MacDonald WC, MacDonald JB: Adenocarcinoma of the esophagus and/or gastric cardia. Cancer 60:1094–1098, 1987
188. Lauren P: The two histological main types of gastric carcinoma: diffuse and so-called intestinal type carcinoma. An attempt at a histochemical classification. Acta Pathol Microbiol Scand 64:31, 1965
189. Ming S-C: Gastric carcinoma. A pathobiological classification. Cancer 39:2475–2485, 1977
190. Adachi Y, Mori M, Kido A et al: A clinicopathologic study of mucinous gastric carcinoma. Cancer 69:866–871, 1992
191. Dixon MF, Martin IG, Sue-Ling HM et al: Goseki grading in gastric cancer: comparison with existing systems of grading and its reproducibility. Histopathology 25:309–316, 1994
192. Martin IG, Dixon MF, Sue-Ling H et al: Goseki histological grading of gastric cancer is an important predictor of outcome. Gut 35:758–763, 1994
193. Ikeda Y, Mori M, Kamakura T et al: Increased incidence of undifferentiated type of gastric cancer with tumor progression in 912 patients with early gastric cancer and 1245 with advanced gastric cancer. Cancer 73:2459–2463, 1994
194. Adachi Y, Mori M, Maehara Y, Sugimachi K: Duke's classification: a valid prognostic indicator for gastric cancer. Gut 35:1368–1371, 1994
195. Arema S, Shimura H: Clinicopathological study on 100 early gastric cancer cases. Gastroenterol Jpn 13:244, 1978
196. Hirota T, Ming S-C: Early gastric carcinoma. pp. 570–583. In Ming S-C, Goldman H (eds): Pathology of the Gastrointestinal Tract. WB Saunders, Philadelphia, 1992

197. Mori M, Kitagawa S, Iida M et al: Early carcinoma of the gastric cardia. A clinicopathologic study of 21 cases. Cancer 59:1758–1766, 1987
198. Pointner R, Schwab G, Konigsrainer A et al: Early cancer of the gastric remnant. Gut 29:298–301, 1988
199. Grigioni WF, Alampi G, Bondi A et al: Retrospective studies of early gastric cancer in a high incidence area in Italy. Histopathology 4:533, 1980
200. Rubio CA, Slezak P, Ohman U, Emos S: The histological classification of early gastric cancer (Micro-invasive carcinoma of the stomach). Acta Pathol Microbiol Scand 90:311–316, 1982
201. Bogomoletz WV: Early gastric cancer. Am J Surg Pathol 8:381–391, 1984
202. Eckardt VF, Giessler W, Kanzler G et al: Clinical and morphological characteristics of early gastric cancer. A case-control study. Gastroenterology 98:708–714, 1990
203. Qizilbash A: Early gastric carcinoma. Arch Pathol Lab Med 101:610–614, 1977
204. Green PHR, O'Toole KM, Weinberg IM et al: Early gastric cancer. Gastroenterology 81:247–256, 1981
205. Goldstein F, Kline TS, Kline IK et al: Early gastric cancer in a United States hospital. Am J Gastroenterol 78:715–719, 1983
206. Kodama Y, Inokuchi K, Soejima K et al: Growth patterns and prognosis in early gastric carcinoma. Superficially spreading and penetrating growth types. Cancer 51:320–326, 1983
207. Mori M, Adachi Y, Kakeji Y et al: Superficial flat-type early carcinoma of the stomach. Cancer 69:306–313, 1992
208. Isaacson P: Biopsy appearances easily mistaken for malignancy in gastrointestinal endoscopy. Histopathology 6:377–389, 1982
209. Shekitka KM, Helwig EB: Deceptive bizarre stromal cells in polyps and ulcers of the gastrointestinal tract. Cancer 67:2111–2117, 1991
210. Sino T, Okuyoma Y, Kobori O et al: Early gastric cancer. Endoscopic diagnosis of depth of invasion. Dig Dis Sci 35:1340–1344, 1990
211. Houghton PWJ, Mortensen NJMcC, Allan A et al: Early gastric cancer: the case for long term surveillance. Br Med J 291: 305–308, 1985
212. Sue-Ling HM, Martin J, Griffith J et al: Early gastric cancer: 46 cases in one surgical department. Gut 33:1318–1322, 1992
213. Lehnert T, Erlandson RA, Decosse JJ: Lymph and blood capillaries of the human gastric mucosa. A morphologic basis for metastasis in early gastric carcinoma. Gastroenterology 89:939–950, 1985
214. Listrom MB, Fenoglio-Preiser CM: Lymphatic distribution of the stomach in normal, inflammatory, hyperplastic and neoplastic tissue. Gastroenterology 93:506–514, 1987
215. Green PHR, Gold RP, Marboe CC et al: Chronic erosive gastritis: clinical, diagnostic and pathological features in nine patients. Am J Gastroenterol 77:543–547, 1982
216. Elta GH, Fawaz KA, Dayal Y et al: Chronic erosive gastritis—a recently recognized disorder. Dig Dis Sci 28:7–12, 1983
217. Gallagher CG, Lennon JR, Crowe JP: Chronic erosive gastritis: a clinical study. Am J Gastroenterol 82:302–306, 1987
218. Capella MS, Green PHR, Marboe C: Neoplasia in chronic erosive (varioliform) gastritis. Dig Dis Sci 33:1035–1038, 1988
219. Jain S, Filipe MI, Hall PA et al: Prognostic value of proliferating cell nuclear antigen in gastric carcinoma. J Clin Pathol 44:655–659, 1991
220. Yonemura Y, Kimura H, Fushida S et al: Analysis of proliferating activity using anti-proliferating cell nuclear antigen antibody in gastric cancer tissue specimens obtained by endoscopic biopsy. Cancer 71:2448–2453, 1993
221. Brito MJ, Williams GT, Thompson H, Filipe MI: Expression of p53 in early (T1) gastric carcinoma and precancerous adjacent mucosa. Gut 35:1697–1700, 1994
222. Fukunaga M, Monden T, Nakanishi H et al: Immunohistochemical study of p53 in gastric carcinoma. Am J Clin Pathol 101:177–180, 1994
223. Hurlimann J, Saraga EP: Expression of p53 protein in gastric carcinomas. Association with histologic type and prognosis. Am J Surg Pathol 18:1247–1253, 1994
224. Shiao Y-H, Rugge M, Correa P et al: p53 alteration in gastric precancerous lesions. Am J Pathol 144:511–517, 1994

225. Macortney JC, Camplejohn RS, Powell G: DNA flow cytometry of histological material from human gastric cancer. J Pathol 148:273–277, 1986
226. Sowa M, Yoshino H, Kato Y et al: An analysis of the DNA ploidy patterns of gastric cancer. Cancer 62:1325–1330, 1988
227. Brito MJ, Filipe MI, Williams GT et al: DNA ploidy in early gastric carcinoma (T1): a flow cytometric study of 100 European cases. Gut 34:230–234, 1993
228. Lee KH, Lee JS, Suh C et al: DNA flow cytometry of stomach cancer. Prospective correlation with clinicopathologic findings. Cancer 72:1819–1826, 1993
229. Watanabe H, Jass JR, Sobin LH: WHO Histological Typing of Oesophageal and Gastric Tumors. Springer-Verlag, Berlin, 1990
230. Mingazzini PL, Barsotti P, Albedi FM: Adenosquamous carcinoma of the sotmach: histological, histochemical and ultrastructural observations. Histopathology 7:433–443, 1983
231. Mori M, Iwashita A, Enjoji M: Adenosquamous carcinoma of the stomach. A clinicopathologic analysis of 28 cases. Cancer 57:333–339, 1986
232. Bonnheim DC, Sarac OK, Fett W: Primary squamous cell carcinoma of the stomach. Am J Gastroenterol 80:91–94, 1985
233. Mori M, Iwashita A, Enjoji M: Squamous cell carcinoma of the stomach: report of three cases. Am J Gastroenterol 81: 339–342, 1986
234. Ruck P, Wehrmann M, Campbell M et al: Squamous cell carcinoma of the gastric stump. A case report and review of the literature. Am J Surg Pathol 13:317–324, 1989
235. Piper MH, Ross JM, Benes FN et al: Primary squamous cell carcinoma of a gastric remnant. Am J Gastroenterol 86:1080–1082, 1991
236. Hayashi I, Muto Y, Fujii Y, Morimatsu M: Mucoepidermoid carcinoma of the stomach. J Surg Oncol 34:94–99, 1987
237. Shibata D, Weiss LM: Epstein–Barr virus-associated gastric adenocarcinoma. Am J Pathol 140:769–774, 1992
238. Oda K, Tamaru J, Takenouchi T et al: Association of Epstein–Barr virus with gastric carcinoma with lymphoid stroma. Am J Pathol 143:1063–1071, 1993
239. Fukayama M, Hayashi Y, Iwski Y et al: Epstein–Barr virus-associated gastric carcinoma and Epstein–Barr virus infection of the stomach. Lab Invest 71:73–81, 1994
240. Nakamura S, Ueki T, Yao T et al: Epstein–Barr virus in gastric carcinoma with lymphoid stroma. Cancer 73:2239–2249, 1994
241. Ishikura H, Kirimoto K, Shamoto M et al: Hepatoid adenocarcinomas of the stomach: an analysis of seven cases. Cancer 58: 119–126, 1986
242. de Lorimier A, Park F, Aranha GV, Reyes C: Hepatoid carcinoma of the stomach. Cancer 71:293–296, 1993
243. Nagai E, Ueyama T, Yao T, Tsuneyoshi M: Hepatoid adenocarcinoma of the stomach. A clinicopathologic and immunohistochemical analysis. Cancer 72:1827–1835, 1993
244. Capella C, Frigerio B, Cornaggia M et al: Gastric parietal cell carcinoma—a newly recognized entity: light microscopic and ultrastructural features. Histopathology 8:813–824, 1984
245. Byrne D, Holley MP, Cuschieri A: Parietal cell carcinoma of the stomach: association with long-term survival after curative resection. Br J Cancer 58:85–87, 1988
246. Robey-Cafferty SS, Ro JY, McKee EG: Gastric parietal cell carcinoma with an unusual, lymphoma-like histologic appearance: report of a case. Modern Pathol 2:536–540, 1989
247. Lev R, DeNucci TD: Neoplastic Paneth cells in the stomach. Report of two cases and review of the literature. Arch Pathol Lab Med 113:129–133, 1989
248. Rubio CA: Paneth cell adenoma of the stomach. Am J Surg Pathol 13:325–328, 1989
249. Kazzaz BA, Eulderink F: Paneth cell–rich carcinoma of the stomach. Histopathology 15:303–305, 1989
250. Lattes R, Grossi C: Carcinoid tumors of the stomach. Cancer 9:698, 1977
251. Wilander E, El-Salky M, Putkanen P: Histopathology of gastric carcinoids: a survey of 42 cases. Histopathology 8:183–193, 1984
252. Rindi G, Luinetti O, Cornaggia M et al: Three subtypes of gastric argyrophil carcinoid and the gastric neuroendocrine carcinoma: a clinicopathologic study. Gastroenterology 104:994–1006, 1993

253. Guellar R, Haddad JK: Gastric carcinoids simulating benign polyps: two cases diagnosed by endoscopic biopsy. Gastrointest Endosc 21:153, 1975
254. Goldfarb JP, Gross F, Maxfield R et al: Gastric carcinoid: two unusual presentations. Am J Gastroenterol 78:332–334, 1983
255. DeSchryver-Kecshemeti K, Clouse RE, Kraus FT: Surgical pathology of gastric and duodenal neuroendocrine tumors masquerading clinically as common polyps. Sem Diagn Pathol 1:5–12, 1984
256. Thomas RM, Baybick JH, Elsayed AM, Sobin LH: Gastric carcinoids. An immunohistochemical and clinicopathologic study of 104 patients. Cancer 73:2053–2058, 1994.
257. Dayal Y, DeLellis RA, Wolfe HJ: Hyperplastic lesions of the gastrointestinal endocrine cells. Am J Surg Pathol 87 (suppl 1):87–101, 1987
258. Mendelsohn G, de la Monte S, Dunn JL, Yardley JH: Gastric carcinoid tumors, endocrine cell hyperplasia, and associated intestinal metaplasia. Histologic, histochemical, and immunohistochemical findings. Cancer 60:1022–1031, 1987
259. Solcia E, Capella C, Fiocca R et al: Disorders of the endocrine system. pp. 240–263. In Ming S-C, Goldman H (eds): Pathology of the Gastrointestinal Tract. WB Saunders, Philadelphia, 1992
260. Lechago J: Gastrointestinal neuroendocrine cell proliferations. Hum Pathol 25:1114–1122, 1994
261. Harvey RF, Davidson CM, Bradshaw MJ et al: Multifocal gastric carcinoid tumors, achlorrhydria, and hypergastrinemia. Lancet 1:951–954, 1985
262. Muller J, Kirchner T, Muller-Hermelink HK: Gastric endocrine cell hyperplasia and carcinoid tumors in atrophic gastritis type A. Am J Surg Pathol 11:909–917, 1987
263. Itsuno M, Watanabe H, Iwafuchi M et al: Multiple carcinoids and endocrine cell micronests in type A gastritis. Their morphology, histogenesis, and natural history. Cancer 63:881–890, 1989
264. Berendt RC, Jewell LD, Shnitha TK et al: Multicentric gastric carcinoids complicating pernicious anemia. Origin from the metaplastic endocrine cell population. Arch Pathol Lab Med 113:399–403, 1989
265. Morgan JE, Kaiser CW, Johnson W et al: Gastric carcinoid (gastrinoma) associated with achlorhydria (pernicious anemia). Cancer 51:2332–2340, 1983
266. Borch K, Renvall H., Liedberg G: Gastric endocrine cell hyperplasia and carcinoid tumors in pernicious anemia. Gastroenterology 88:638–648, 1985
267. Bordi C, Yu J-Y, Boggi MT, et al: Gastric carcinoids and their precursor lesions. A histologic and immunohistochemical study of 23 cases. Cancer 67:663–672, 1991
268. Hodges JR, Isaacson P, Wright R: Diffuse enterochromaffin-like (ECL) cell hyperplasia and multiple gastric carcinoids: A complication of pernicious anemia. Gut 22: 237–241, 1981
269. Gilligan CJ, Lawton GP, Tang LH et al: Gastric carcinoid tumors: the biology and therapy of an enigmatic and controversial lesion. Am J Gastroenterol 90:338–352, 1995
270. Watanabe H: Argentaffin cells in adenomas of the stomach. Cancer 30:1267, 1972
271. Azzopardi JG, Polloch DJ: Argentaffin and argyrophil cells in gastric carcinoma. J Pathol Bacteriol 86:443, 1963
272. Bonar SF, Sweeney EC: The prevalence, prognostic significance and hormonal content of endocrine cells in gastric cancer. Histopathology 10:53–63, 1986
273. Klappenbach RS, Kurman RJ, Sinclair CF, James LP: Composite carcinoma—carcinoid tumors of the gastrointestinal tract. A morphologic, histochemical and immunocytochemical study. Am J Clin Pathol 84:137–143, 1985
274. Lewin K: Carcinoid tumors and the mixed (composite) glandular–endocrine cell carcinomas. Am J Surg Pathol 11(suppl 1):71–86, 1987
275. Caruso ML, Pilato FP, D'Adda T, et al: Composite carcinoid–adenocarcinoma of the stomach associated with multiple gastric carcinoids and nonantral gastric atrophy. Cancer 64:1534–1539, 1989
276. Yang GCH, Rotterdam H: Mixed (composite) glandular–endocrine cell carcinoma of the stomach. Report of a case and review of literature. Am J Surg Pathol 15:592–598, 1991
277. Eimoto T, Hayakawa H: Oat cell carcinoma of the stomach. Pathol Res Pract 168: 229–236, 1980

278. Hussein AM, Otrakji CL, Hussein BT: Small cell carcinoma of the stomach: case report and review of the literature. Dig Dis Sci 35:513–518, 1990
279. Matsui K, Kitagawa M, Miwa A et al: Small carcinoma of the stomach: a clinicopathologic study of 17 cases. Am J Gastroenterol 86:1167–1175, 1991
280. Ranchod M, Lewin KJ, Dorfman RF: Lymphoid hyperplasia of the gastrointestinal tract. Am J Surg Pathol 2:383, 1978
281. Saraga P, Hurlimann J, Ozzello L: Lymphomas and pseudolymphomas of the alimentary tract: an immunohistochemical study with clinicopathologic correlations. Hum Pathol 12:713–723, 1981
282. Hyjek E, Kelenyi G: Pseudolymphomas of the stomach: a lesion characterized by progressively transformed germinal centers. Histopatholoy 6:61–68, 1982
283. Brooks JJ, Enterline HT: Gastric pseudolymphoma. Its three subtypes and relation to lymphoma. Cancer 51:476–486, 1983
284. Tokunaga O, Watanabe T, Morimatsu M: Pseudolymphoma of the stomach. Cancer 59:1320–1327, 1987
285. Schwartz MS, Sherman H, Smith T, Janis R: Gastric pseudolymphoma and its relationship to malignant gastric lymphoma. Am J Gastroenterol 84:1555–1559, 1989
286. Wolf JA Jr, Spjut HJ: Focal lymphoid hyperplasia of the stomach preceding gastric lymphoma: case report and review of the literature. Cancer 48:2518–2523, 1981
287. Scoazer J-Y, Brousse N, Potet F, Jeulain J-F: Focal malignant lymphoma in gastric pseudolymphoma. Histologic and immunohistochemical study of a case. Cancer 57:1330–1336, 1986
288. Burke JS, Sheiboni K, Nathwoni BN et al: Monoclonal (well-differentiated) lymphocytic proliferations of the gastrointestinal tract resembling lymphoid hyperplasia: a neoplasm of uncertain malignant potential. Hum Pathol 18:1238–1245, 1987
289. Heule BV, Kehem CV, Herman R: Benign and malignant lymphoid lesions of the stomach. A histologic reappraisal in the light of the Kiel classification for non-Hodgkin's lymphoma. Histopathology 3:309–320, 1979
290. Dworkin B, Lightdale CJ, Weingrad DN: Primary gastric lymphoma. A review of 50 cases. Dig Dis Sci 27:986–992, 1982
291. Brooks JJ, Enterline HT: Primary gastric lymphoma. A clinicopathologic study of 58 cases with long-term follow-up and literature review. Cancer 51:701–711, 1983
292. Isaacson PG, Spencer J, Finn T: Primary B-cell gastric lymphoma. Hum Pathol 17: 72–82, 1986
293. Lewin KJ, Ranchod M, Dorfman RF: Lymphomas of the gastrointestinal tract: a study of 117 cases presenting with gastrointestinal disease. Cancer 42:693, 1978
294. Weingrad DN, DeCosse JJ, Sherlock P et al: Primary gastrointestinal lymphoma: a 30-year review. Cancer 49:1258–1265, 1982
295. Filippa DA, Lieberman PH, Weingrad DN et al: Primary lymphoma of the gastrointestinal tract. Analysis of prognostic factors with emphasis on histological type. Am J Surg Pathol 7:363–372, 1983
296. Dragosics B, Bauer P, Radaszkiewicz T: Primary gastrointestinal non-Hodgkin's lymphoma. A retrospective clinicopathologic study of 150 cases. Cancer 55:1060–1073, 1985
297. Appelman HD, Hirsch SD, Schnitzer B, Coon WW: Clinicopathologic overview of gastrointestinal lymphomas. Am J Surg Pathol 9(3)(suppl):71–83, 1985
298. Isaacson PG: Gastrointestinal lymphoma. Hum Pathol 25:1020–1029, 1994
299. Katz S, Klein MS, Winawer SJ, Sherlock P: Disseminated lymphoma involving the stomach. Correlation of endoscopy with directed cytology and biopsy. Am J Dig Dis 18:370–374, 1973
300. Hayes J, Dunn E: Has the incidence of primary gastric lymphoma increased? Cancer 63:2073–2076, 1989
301. Severson RK, Davis S: Increasing incidence of primary gastric lymphoma. Cancer 66:1283–1287, 1990
302. Swinson CM, Slavin G, Coles EC, Booth CC: Celiac disease and malignancy. Lancet 1:111–115, 1983
303. Isaacson PG, Spencer J, Connolly CE et al: Malignant histiocytosis of the intestine: a T-cell lymphoma. Lancet 2:688–691, 1985
304. Hussell T, Isaacson PG, Crabtree JE, Spenser J: The response of cells from low-grade B-cell gastric lymphomas of mucosa-

associated lymphoid tissue to Helicobacter pylori. Lancet 342:571–575, 1993
305. Parsonnet J, Hansen S, Rodriguez L et al: Helicobacter pylori infection and gastric lymphoma. N Engl J Med 330:1267–1271, 1994
306. Eidt S, Stolte M, Fisher R: Helicobacter pylori gastritis and primary gastric non-Hodgkin's lymphoma. J Clin Pathol 47:436–440, 1994
307. Wotherspoon AC, Doglioni C, Diss TC et al: Regression of primary low-grade B-cell gastric lymphoma of mucosa-associated lymphoid tissue type after eradication of Helicobacter pylori. Lancet 342:575–578, 1993
309. Dean RJ, Moinuddin SM, Emerson LD: Application of anti-leukocyte common antigen and anti-cytokeratin antibodies to the biopsy diagnosis of gastric large cell lymphoma. Hum Pathol 18:918–923, 1987
310. Tungekar MF: Gastric signet-ring cell lymphoma with alpha heavy chains. Histopathology 10:725–733, 1986
311. Isaacson PG, Spencer J: Malignant lymphoma of mucosa-associated tissues. Histopathology 11:445–462, 1987
312. Castrillo JM, Montalban C, Obeso G et al: Gastric B-cell mucosa associated lymphoid tissue lymphoma: a clinicopathological study in 56 patients. Gut 33:1307–1311, 1992
313. Papadaki L, Wotherspoon AC, Isaacson PG: The lymphoepithelial lesion of gastric low-grade B-cell lymphoma of mucosa-associated lymphoid tissue (MALT): an ultrastructural study. Histopathology 21:415–421, 1992
314. Radasykiewicz T, Dragosics B, Bauer P: Gastrointestinal malignant lymphomas of the mucosa-associated lymphoid tissue: factors relevant to prognosis. Gastroenterology 102:1628–1638, 1992
315. Isaacson PG, Wotherspoon AC, Pan A: Follicular colonization in B-cell lymphoma of mucosa-associated lymphoid tissue. Am J Surg Pathol 15:819–828, 1991
316. Spineli P, Guillo L, Pizzetti P: Endoscopic diagnosis of gastric lymphomas. Endoscopy 12:211, 1980
317. Zuckerberg LR, Ferry JA, Southern JF, Harris NL: Lymphoid infiltrates of the stomach. Evaluation of histologic criteria for the diagnosis of low-grade gastric lymphoma on endoscopic biopsy specimens. Am J Surg Pathol 14:1087–1099, 1990
318. Arista-Najr J, Jimenez A, Keirns C et al: The role of the endoscopic biopsy in the diagnosis of gastric lymphoma. A morphologic and immunohistochemical reappraisal. Hum Pathol 22:339–348, 1991
319. Suekane H, Iida M, Kuwano Y et al: Diagnosis of primary early gastric lymphoma. Usefulness of endoscopic mucosal resection for histologic evaluation. Cancer 71:1207–1213, 1993
320. Seifert E, Schulte F, Weismuller J et al: Endoscopic and bioptic diagnosis of malignant non-Hodgkin's lymphoma of the stomach. Endoscopy 25:497–502, 1993
321. Mir R, Kahn LB, Selzer G: Immunohistochemistry of primary gastrointestinal lymphomas: a study of 76 cases. Histopathology 10:391–403, 1986
322. Spies CM, Miller TP, Recher LC et al: Immunophenotyping endoscopic biopsies in gastric lymphomas. Surg Pathol 1:113–121, 1988
323. Osborne BM, Pugh WC: Practicality of molecular studies to evaluate small lymphocytic proliferations in endoscopic gastric biopsies. Am J Surg Pathol 16:838–844, 1992
324. Algara P, Martinez P, Sanchez L et al: The detection of B-cell monoclonal populations by polymerase chain reaction: accuracy of approach and application in gastric endoscopic biopsy specimens. Hum Pathol 24:1184–1188, 1993
325. Yatabe Y, Mori N, Oka K et al: Primary gastric T-cell lymphoma. Morphological and immunohistochemical studies of two cases. Arch Pathol Lab Med 118:547–550, 1994
326. Roehrkasse RL, Roberts IM, Wald A et al: Celiac sprue complicated by lymphoma presenting with multiple gastric ulcers. Gastroenterology 91:740–745, 1986
327. Amer MH, El-Akkad S: Gastrointestinal lymphoma in adults: clinical features and management of 300 cases. Gastroenterology 106:846–858, 1994
328. Nahanishi I, Kajikawa K, Migita S et al: Gastric plasmacytoma: an immunologic and immunohistochemical study. Cancer 49: 2025–2028, 1982

329. Ooi A, Nakanishi I, Hashiba A: Gastric plasmacytoma: an early lesion diagnosed with the aid of immunoperoxidase and immunogold techniques. Am J Gastroenterol 82:572–578, 1987
330. Soderstrom K-O, Joensuu H: Primary Hodgkin's disease of the stomach. Am J Clin Pathol 89:806–809, 1988
331. Mori N, Yatabe Y, Narita M et al: Primary gastric Hodgkin's disease. Morphologic, immunohistochemical, and immunogenetic analyses. Arch Pathol Lab Med 119: 163–166, 1995
332. Kiefer ED, Christiansen PA: Benign tumors of the stomach and duodenum. Med Clin North America 40:381, 1956
333. Grafe W, Thorbjarnarson B, Pearch JM: Benign neoplasms of stomach. Am J Surg 100:561, 1960
334. Meissner WA: Leiomyoma of the stomach. Arch Pathol 38:207–209, 1944
335. Yameda Y, Kato Y, Yanogisawa A et al: Microleiomyomas of human stomach. Hum Pathol 19:569–572, 1988
336. Appelman HD, Helwig EB: Gastric epithelioid leiomyoma and leiomyosarcoma (leiomyoblastoma). Cancer 38:708–728, 1976
337. Daimaru Y, Kido H, Hashimoto H, Enjoji M: Benign schwannoma of the gastrointestinal tract: a clinicopathologic and immunohistochemical study. Hum Pathol 19:257–264, 1988
338. Petersen JM, Ferguson DR: Gastrointestinal neurofibromatosis. J Clin Gastroenterol 6:529–534, 1984
339. Fuller CE, Williams GT: Gastrointestinal manifestations of type-1 neurofibromatosis (von Recklinghausen's disease). Histopathology 19:1–12, 1991
340. Appelman HD: Mesenchymal tumors of the gut: historical perspectives, new approaches, new results, and does it many any difference? pp. 220–246. In Goldman H, Appelman HD, Kaufman N (eds): Gastrointestinal Pathology. Williams & Wilkins, Baltimore, 1990
341. Miettinen M: Gastrointestinal stromal tumors. An immunohistochemical study of cellular differentiation. Am J Surg Pathol 89:601–610, 1988
342. Lerma E, Oliva E, Tugues D, Prat J: Stromal tumours of the gastrointestinal tract: a clinicopathological and ploidy analysis of 33 cases. Virchows Archiv A Pathol Anat Histophatol 424:19–24, 1994
343. Franquemont DW: Differentiation and risk assessment of gastrointestinal stromal tumors. Am J Clin Pathol 103:41–47, 1995
344. Saul SH, Rast ML, Brooks JJ: The immunohistochemistry of gastrointestinal stromal tumors. Am J Surg Pathol 11:464–473, 1987
345. Pike AM, Lloyd RV, Appelman HD: Cell markers in gastrointestinal stromal tumors. Hum Pathol 19:830–834, 1988
346. Newman PL, Wadden C, Fletcher CDM: Gastrointestinal stromal tumors. Correlation of immunophenotype with clinicopathological features. J Pathol 164:107–118, 1991
347. Ma CK, Amin MB, Kintanor E: Immunohistologic characterization of gastrointestinal stromal tumors: a study of 82 cases compared with 11 cases of leiomyoma. Modern Pathol 6:139–144, 1993
348. Miettinen M, Virolainen M, Rikala M-S: Gastrointestinal stromal tumors—value of CD34 antigen in their identification and separation from true leiomyomas and schwannomas. Am J Surg Pathol 19:207–216, 1995
349. Walker P, Dvorak AM: Gastrointestinal autonomic nerve (GAN) tumor. Ultrastructural evidence for a newly recognized entity. Arch Path Lab Med 110:309–316, 1986
350. Lauwers GY, Erlandson RA, Casper ES et al: Gastrointestinal autonomic nerve tumors. A clinicopathological, immunohistochemical, and ultrastructural study of 12 cases. Am J Surg Pathol 17:887–897, 1993
351. Flint A, Appelman HD, Beckwith AL: DNA analysis of gastric stromal neoplasms: correlation with pathologic features. Surg Pathol 2:117–124, 1989
352. El-Naggar AK, Ro JY, McLemore D et al: Gastrointestinal stromal tumors: DNA flowcytometric study of 58 patients with at least five years of follow-up. Modern Pathol 2:511–515, 1989
353. Cooper PN, Quirke P, Hardy GJ, Dixon MF: A flow cytometric, clinical, and histological study of stromal neoplasms of the gastrointestinal tract. Am J Surg Pathol 16:163–170, 1992
354. Cunningham RE, Federspiel BH, McCarthy WF et al: Predicting prognosis of gastrointes-

tinal muscle tumors. Role of clinical and histologic evaluations, flow cytometry, and image cytometry. Am J Surg Pathol 17: 588–594, 1993

355. Ona FV, Ahluwalia M: Endoscopic appearance of gastric angiodysplasia in hereditary hemorrhagic telangiectasia. Am J Gastroenterol 73:148–149, 1980
356. Marmaduke DP, Greenson JK, Cunningham I et al: Gastric vascular ectasia in patients undergoing bone marrow transplantation. Am J Clin Pathol 102:194–198, 1994
357. Van Zanten SJOV, Boifelsman JFWM, Schipper ME, Tytgat GNJ: Recurrent massive haematemesis from Dieulafoy vascular malformation—a review of 101 cases. Gut 27:213–222, 1986
358. Pointer R, Schwab G, Konigsrainer A, Dietze O: Endoscopic treatment of Dieulafoy's disease. Gastroenterology 94:563–566, 1988
359. Miko TL, Thomazy VA: The caliber persistent artery of the stomach: a unifying approach to gastric aneurysm, Dieulafoy's lesion, and submucosal arterial malformation. Hum Pathol 19:914–921, 1988
360. Eidus LB, Rosali P, Manion D, Heringer R: Caliber-persistent artery of the stomach (Dieulafoy's vascular malformation). Gastroenterology 99:1507–1510, 1990
361. Jabbari M, Cherry R, Lough et al: Gastric antral vascular ectasia. The watermelon stomach. Gastroenterology 87:1165–1170, 1984
362. Kruger R, Ryan ME, Dickson KB, Nunex JF: Diffuse vascular ectasia of the gastric antrum. Am J Gastroenterol 82:421–426, 1987
363. Suit PF, Petras RE, Bauer TW, Petrini JL Jr: Gastric antral vascular ectasia. A histologic and morphometric study of "the watermelon stomach." Am J Surg Pathol 11:750–757, 1987
364. Ma CK, Behrle KM, Rosenberg BF et al: Gastric antral vascular ectasia: the watermelon stomach. Surg Pathol 1:231–239, 1988
365. Gouldesbrough DR, Pell ACH: Gastric antral vascular ectasia: a problem of recognition and diagnosis. Gut 32:954–955, 1991
366. Freedman SL, Wright TL, Altman DE: Gastrointestinal Kaposi's sarcoma in patients with acquired immunodeficiency syndrome. Endoscopic and autopsy findings. Gastroenterology 89:102–108, 1985
367. Boyd GD, Shabot JM, Pollard RB, Gourley WK: Endoscopic evolution of gastric Kaposi's sarcoma. Gastrointest Endosc 33:450–453, 1987
368. Parente F, Cernuschi M, Orlando G et al: Kaposi's sarcoma and AIDS—frequency of gastrointestinal involvement and its effect on survival—a prospective study in a heterogeneous population. Scand J Gastroenterol 26:1007–1012, 1991
369. Almagro UA, Schulte WJ, Norback DH, Turcotte JK: Glomus tumor of the stomach: histologic and ultrastructural features. Am J Clin Pathol 75:415–419, 1981
370. Haque S, Modlin I, West AB: Multiple glomus tumors of the stomach with intravascular spread. Am J Surg Pathol 16:291–299, 1992
371. Imamura A, Tochihara M, Natsui K et al: Glomus tumor of the stomach: endoscopic ultrasonographic findings. Am J Gastroenterol 89:271–272, 1994
372. Khansur T, Balducci L, Tavassoli M: Granular cell tumor. Cancer 60:220–222, 1987
373. Schwartz DT, Gaetz HP: Multiple granular cell myoblastomas of the stomach. Am J Clin Pathol 44:453–457, 1965
374. Goodman MD, Cooper PH: Granular cell tumor (myoblastoma) of the stomach. A case report with ultrastructural findings and review of the literature. Am J Dig Dis 17:1117–1125, 1972
375. White JG, El-Newihi HM, Hauser CJ: Granular cell tumor of the stomach presenting as gastric outlet obstruction. Am J Gastroenterol 89:2259–2260, 1994
376. Appelman HD: Mesenchymal tumors of the gastrointestinal tract. pp. 310–350. In Ming S-C, Goldman H (eds): Pathology of the Gastrointestinal Tract. WB Saunders, Philadelphia, 1992
377. Appelman HD, Helwig EB: Sarcomas of the stomach. Am J Clin Pathol 67:2–10, 1977
378. Bedekian AY, Khankhanian N, Valdizieso M: Sarcoma of the stomach: clinicopathologic study of 43 cases. J Surg Oncol 13:121–127, 1980
379. Ranchod M, Kempson RL: Smooth muscle tumors of the gastrointestinal tract and ret-

roperitoneum: a pathologic analysis of 100 cases. Cancer 39:255, 1977
380. Lindsay PC, Ordonez N, Raff JH: Gastric leiomyosarcoma: clinical and pathologic review of fifty patients. J Surg Oncol 18:399–421, 1981
381. Evans HL: Smooth muscle tumors of the gastrointestinal tract. A study of 56 cases followed for a minimum of 10 years. Cancer 56:2242–2250, 1985
382. Lakey D, Stoica T: Gastric liposarcoma: a case report. Pathol Res Pract 181: 112–115, 1986
383. Wright JR, Kyriakos M, DeSchrywer-Kerskemeti K: Malignant fibrous histiocytoma of the stomach. A report and review of malignant fibrohistiocytic tumors of the alimentary tract. Arch Pathol Lab Med 112: 251–258, 1988
384. Yagihaski S, Yagihaski N, Hase Y et al: Primary alveolar soft-part sarcoma of stomach. Am J Surg Pathol 15:399–406, 1991
385. Mori H, Soeda O, Kamano T, et al: Choriocarcinomatous change with immunocytochemically HCG-positive cells in the gastric carcinoma of the males. Virchows Arch A Pathol Anat Histopathol 396:141–153, 1982
386. Ramponi A, Angeli G, Arceci F, Pozzuoli R: T1 Gastric choriocarcinoma: an immunohistochemical study. Pathol Res Pract 181:390–396, 1986
387. Krulewski T, Cohen LB: Choriocarcinoma of the stomach: pathogenesis and clinical characteristics. Am J Gastroenterol 83:1172–1175, 1988
388. Garcia RL, Ghali VS: Gastric choriocarcinoma and yolk sac tumor in a man: observations about its possible origin. Hum Pathol 16:955–958, 1985
389. Zamecnik M, Patrikova J, Gomolcak P: Yolk sac carcinoma of the stomach with gastric positivity. Hum Pathol 24:927–928, 1993
390. Moriuchi A, Nakayama I, Muta H et al: Gastric teratoma of children: a case report with review of the literature. Acta Pathol Jpn 27:749–758, 1977
391. Siegal A, Freund U, Gal R: Carcinosarcoma of the stomach. Histopathology 13:350–353, 1988
392. Robey-Cafferty SS, Grignon DJ, Ro JY et al: Sarcomatoid carcinoma of the stomach: a report of three cases with immunohistochemical and ultrastructural observations. Cancer 65:1601–1606, 1990
393. Aiba M, Hirayama A, Suzuki T et al: Carcinosarcoma of the stomach: report of a case with review of the literature of gastrectomized patients. Surg Pathol 4:75–83, 1991
394. Kallakury BVS, Bui HX, del Rosario A et al: Primary gastric adenosarcoma. Arch Pathol Lab Med 116:299–301, 1992
395. Saito T, Iizuka T, Kato H, Watanabe H: Esophageal carcinoma metastatic to the stomach: a clinicopathologic study of 35 cases. Cancer 56:2235–2241, 1985
396. Menuck LS, Amberg JR: Metastatic disease involving the stomach. Dig Dis Sci 20: 903–913, 1975
397. Walker Q, Bilous M, Tiver KW, Langlands AO: Breast cancer metastases masquerading as primary gastric carcinoma. Aust N Z J Surg 56:395–398, 1986
398. Esaki Y, Hirajama R, Hirokawa K: A comparison of patterns of metastasis in gastric cancer by histologic type and age. Cancer 65:2086–2090, 1990
399. Kadakia S, Parker A, Canales L: Metastatic tumors of the upper gastrointestinal tract: Endoscopic experience. Am J Gastroenterol 87:1418–1423, 1992
400. Antler AS, Ough Y, Pitchumoni CS et al: Gastrointestinal metastases from malignant tumors of the lungs. Cancer 49:170–172, 1982.
401. Green LK: Hematogenous metastases to the stomach. A review of 67 cases. Cancer 65:1596–1600, 1990
402. Choi SH, Sheehan FR, Pickren JW: Metastatic involvement of the stomach by breast cancer. Cancer 17:791–797, 1964
403. Cormie WJ, Gaffey TA, Welch JM, Edmonson JH: Linitis plastica caused by metastatic lobular carcinoma of the breast. Mayo Clin Proc 55:747–753, 1980
404. Klausner JM, Skornick Y, Lelcuk S et al: Acute complications of metastatic melanoma to the gastrointestinal tract. Br J Surg 69:195–196, 1982

6

Disorders of the Duodenum

This chapter concentrates on the inflammatory disorders and tumors that are mainly limited to the duodenum or that often present in this region at upper endoscopy. Those conditions shared with the stomach, such as stress lesions, chronic peptic ulcer disease, and the polyposis syndromes, are primarily presented in Chapters 4 and 5. The many conditions that can affect the overall small intestine, such as most infections and the malabsorptive disorders, are largely presented in Chapter 7. The salient features of the conditions detailed in Chapters 4, 5, and 7 are briefly discussed in this chapter.

GENERAL ASPECTS

Following the appearance of flexible endoscopes, endoscopic examination of the duodenum tended to be neglected, with attention to the upper tract mostly applied toward the esophagus and the stomach. It ultimately became evident, however, that the proximal part, particularly the first two portions, could also be readily visualized, leading to extensive examinations of the duodenum at the present time.[1–4]

The biopsies are largely obtained to identify cases of duodenitis, to determine their particular etiology, and to monitor patients following therapy (Table 6-1). In addition, the endoscopy and samples are used to assess ulcers and mass lesions,[5–7] and to help in the evaluation of malabsorptive disorders.[8–11] The latter conditions more often require biopsies from the distal duodenum or, preferably, from the jejunum where the lesions tend to be more evident.

NORMAL STRUCTURE

Distal Part

The appearance of the duodenal mucosa varies depending on its location[12–15] (Table 6-2). In its distal half, it most closely resembles the mucosa seen in the jejunum and in the rest of the small intestine (Fig. 6-1). The villous : crypt ratio is on the order of 3 : 1 to 5 : 1. The villi are long, thin, and tapered at

Table 6-1. Uses of Duodenal Mucosal Biopsy

Duodenitis
Identification and cause
Acute versus chronic
Monitor patient after therapy
Peptic ulcer disease
Malabsorptive disorders
Tumors

the surface, and the principal epithelial cells are the columnar absorptive ones together with scattered goblet mucous cells. The mucus is largely in the form of mildly acidic types, which stain weakly with the PAS reaction and strongly with Alcian Blue at pH 2.5.[16, 17] There is usually only scant sulfated mucin in contrast to the colonic mucous cells.

The crypts contain the less differentiated forms of the absorptive and mucous cells, Paneth cells with their large and refractile eosinophilic granules in the cytoplasm, and the dividing cells with mitoses (Fig. 6-2). There are also scattered neuroendocrine cells at the base of the epithelium, largely in the crypts and occasional ones in the lamina propria.[18, 19] Their appearance is suspected by either clear cytoplasm or the presence of fine red granules within the cytoplasm, and they are often interposed between the other crypt cells and the basement membrane, with the cytoplasm directed away from the crypt lumina (Fig. 6-3). These endocrine cells are best visualized with special stains such as chromogranin and synaptophysin, as well as the immunocytochemical demonstration of antibodies directed to a specific substance like gastrin or somatostatin (Fig. 6-4).

There is a relatively slight amount of lamina propria in the normal state, interspersed between the crypts and also forming the core of the villi.[20] This contains a scant amount of collagen and muscular tissue, and mainly monomuclear-type inflammatory cells, including lymphocytes, plasma cells, and macrophages. Also present are a variable number of eosinophils but only rare or no neutrophils in this area. The lymphocytes are present as well in the epithelial area, particularly in the villous region; these intraepithelial lymphocytes are largely of the T-cell class in contrast to the lymphocytes in the lamina propria that are mostly of the B-cell type. The B-cells and plasma cells secrete all types of immunoglobulins including IgA, IgG, and IgM in the normal state. Scattered throughout the duodenum and the rest of the small intestine are well formed lymphoid nodules that extend from the surface to the base of the mucosa. They have discrete germinal centers, and the epithelium overlying the lymphoid follicles is flattened and contains the M cells that are responsible for antigen collection.[21] These structures are noted throughout the small and large intestine and are most highly concentrated in the ileum. They undergo hyperplasia in many disease states, but their occasional presence in mucosal biopsies is not an abnormal finding. At the base of the mucosa is a well formed muscularis mucosae that consists of two layers of smooth muscle cells.

Table 6-2. Biopsy Features of Normal Duodenal Mucosa

Feature	Proximal	Distal
Villous: crypt ratio	1:1 to 3:1	3:1 to 5:1
Crypt branching	Occasional	Absent
Mononuclear cells in lamina propria	Moderate	Mild
Brunner's glands		
Submucosa	Marked	Slight
Mucosa	Focal, slight	Absent

Other features are the same, including the presence of absorptive and goblet mucous cells in villi; mitoses, Paneth cells, and neuroendocrine cells in the crypts.

Proximal Part

The duodenal mucosa differs in the proximal part, particularly in the first portion (Fig. 6-5). This is due in part to the distortion caused by the Brunner's glands in the underlying submucosa, which tend to compress the mucosa. Probably of greater significance is the regular mild injury that occurs in this part due to the appearance of gastric acid,

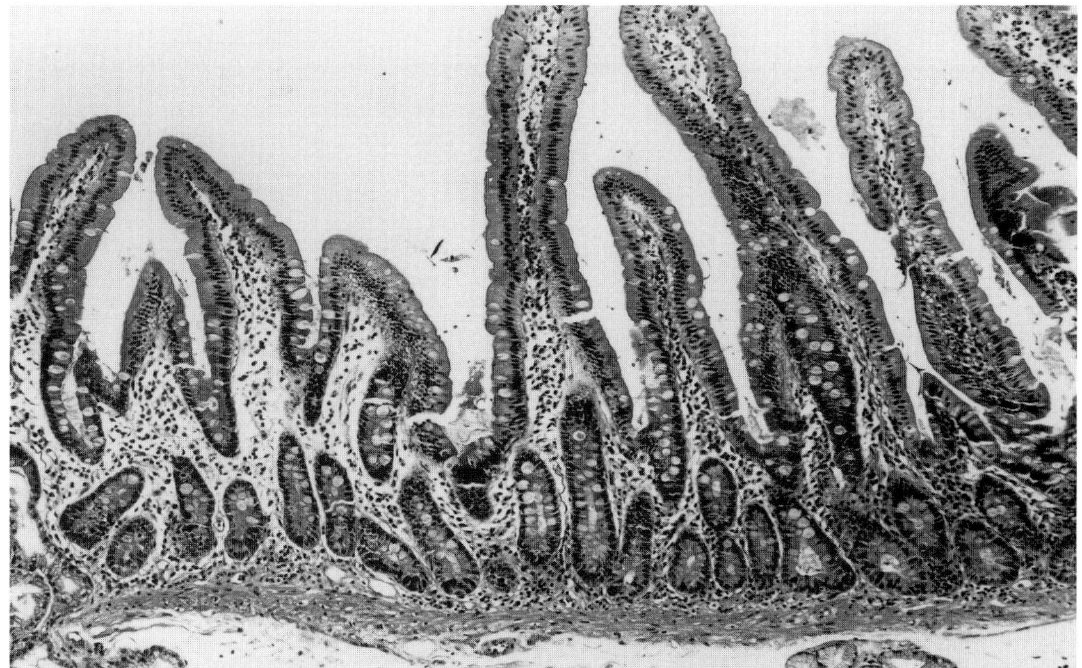

Fig. 6-1. Normal mucosa of the distal duodenum, similar to the jejunum, showing tall villi and short crypts. Villi are slender and mainly covered by columnar absorptive cells with scattered goblet mucous cells. Small amount of inflammatory cells in lamina propria. Muscularis mucosae and adjacent submucosa with a few Brunner glands appear at bottom (× 105).

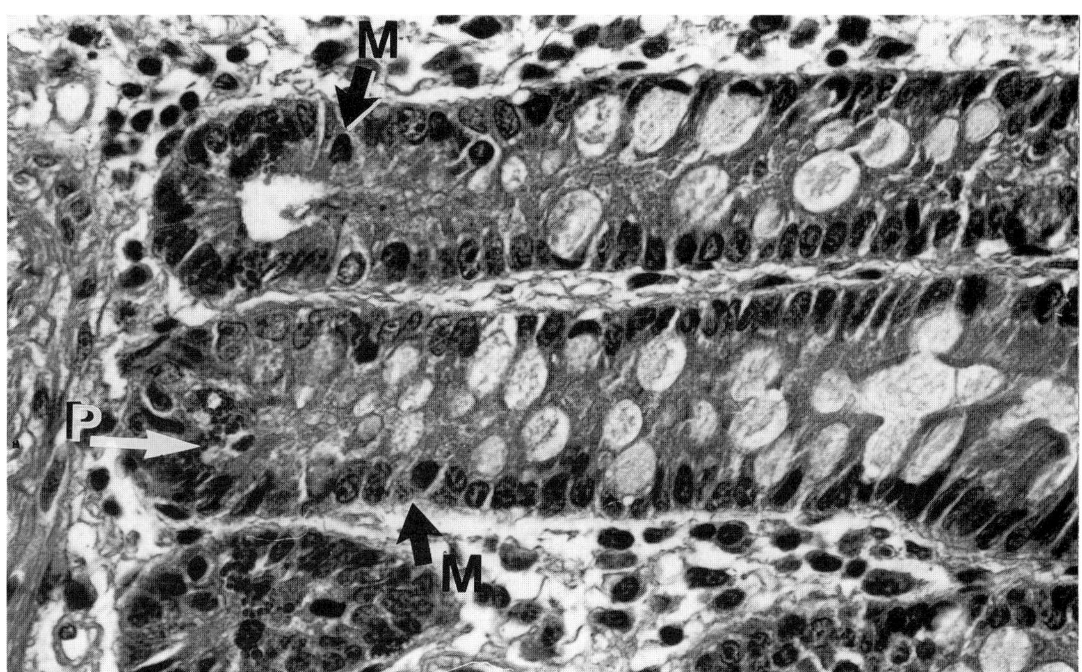

Fig. 6-2. Normal crypt in the duodenum, with base and muscularis mucosae at left. Crypts contain goblet mucous cells and immature absorptive cells. Several mitoses, appearing as dense and fragmented nuclei, are present (M). Paneth cells with large cytoplasmic granules are seen at crypt base (P) (× 635).

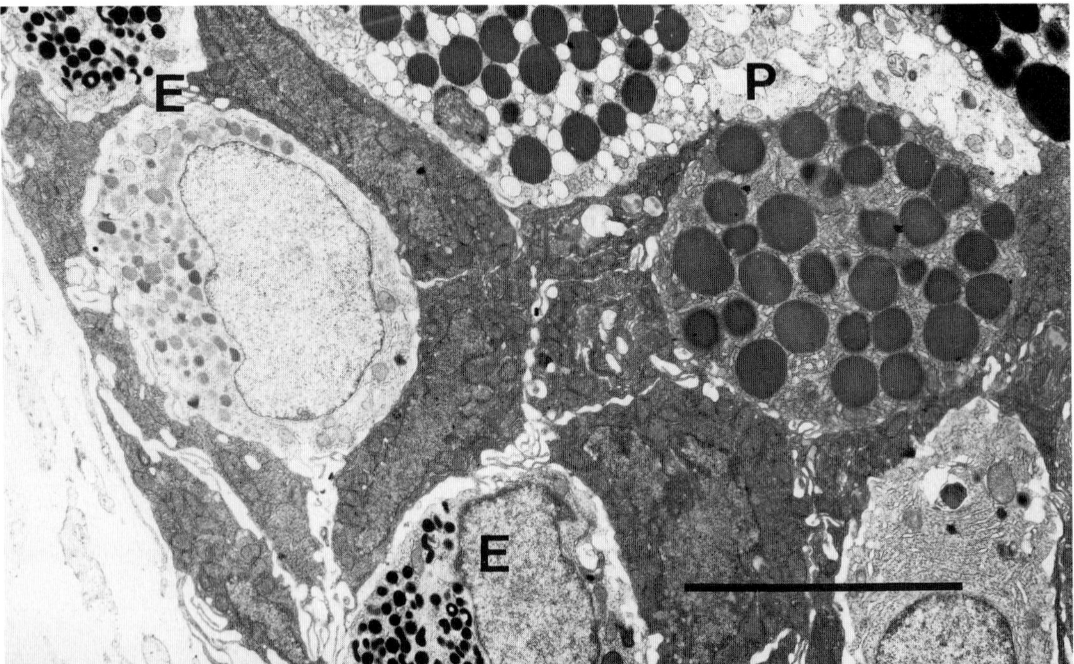

Fig. 6-3. Electron micrograph of epithelia in a duodenal crypt. Seen are Paneth cells (P) containing large electron-dense granules; and endocrine cells (E) with smaller granules of varying densities, suggesting different secretory products (× 3,600; bar = 10 μm).

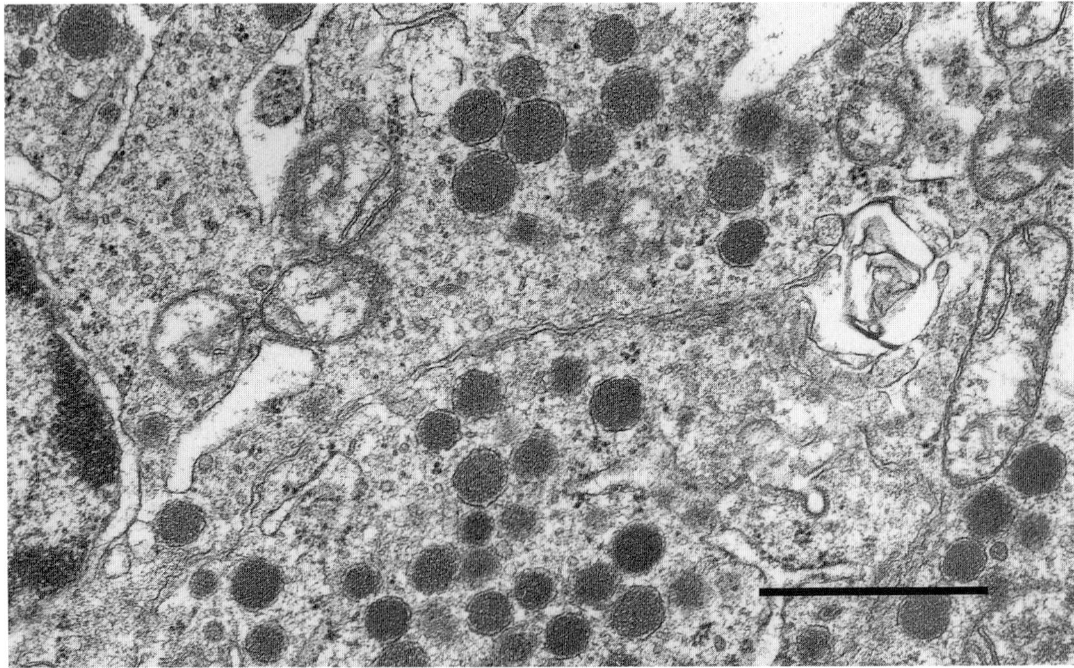

Fig. 6-4. Electron micrograph of somatostatin-secreting cells. The secretory granules are round, membrane bound, have moderately electron dense contents, and measure an average of 200 nm in diameter (× 30,000; bar = 1 μm).

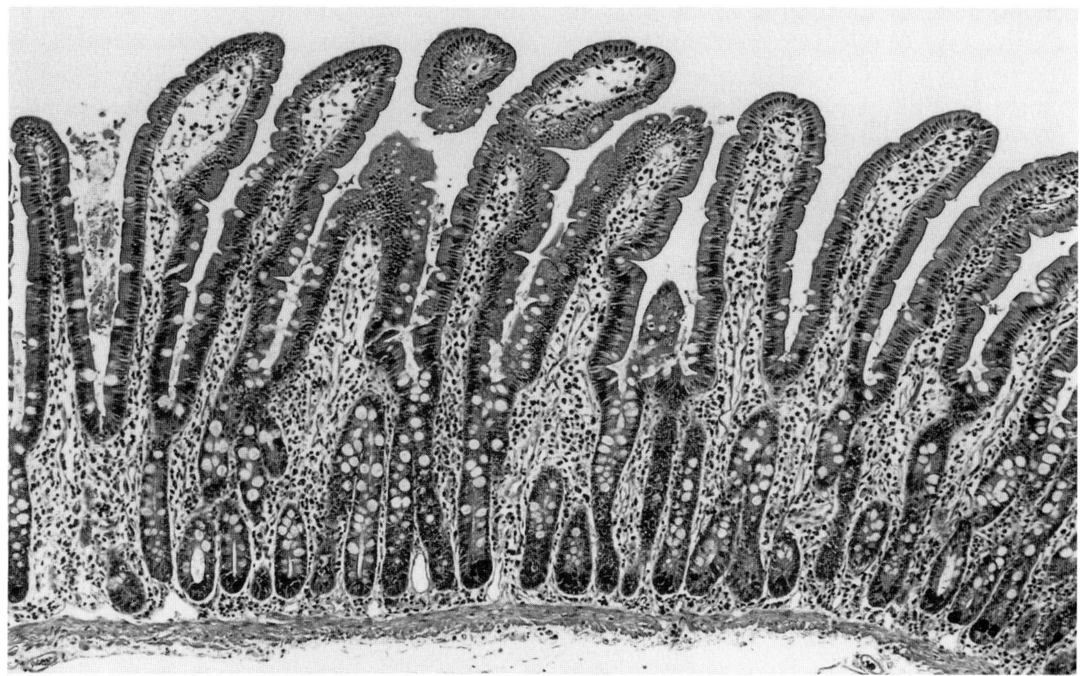

Fig. 6-5. Normal mucosa of the proximal duodenum. Compared to the distal part (see Fig. 6-1), the villi are slightly shorter and the crypts longer. The epithelial cells are otherwise normal, and there is no increase of inflammatory cells in the lamina propria in ths example. The muscularis mucosae appears at the bottom (× 105).

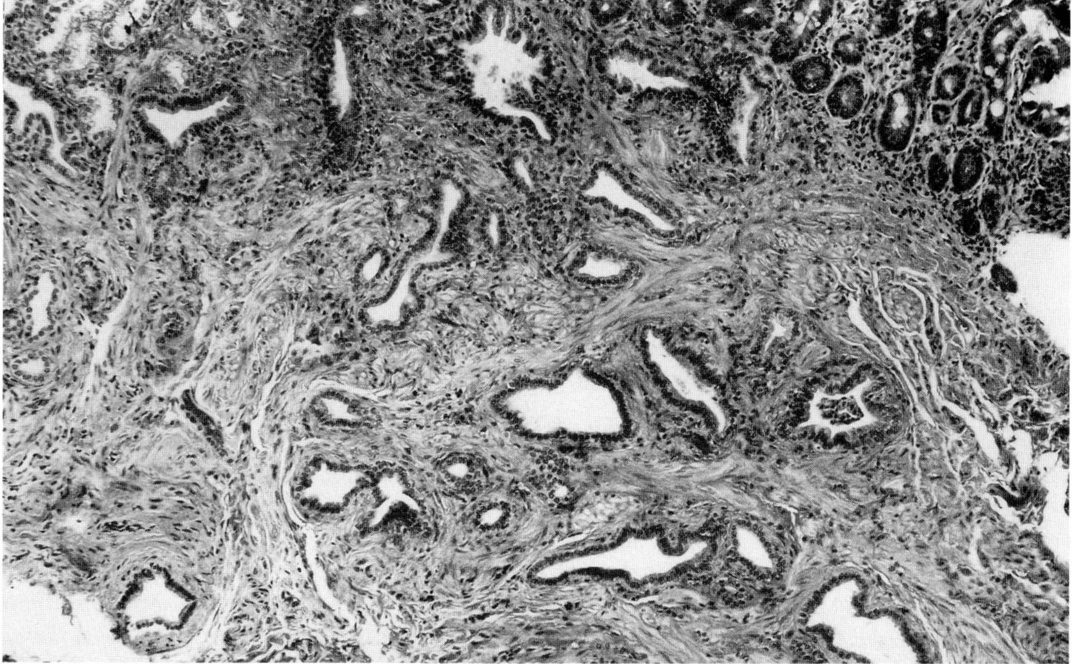

Fig. 6-6. Normal ampulla, with mucosal surface appearing at top. Just beneath the mucosa are numerous ducts surrounded by a prominent fibromuscular stroma (× 105).

leading to mild shortening of the villi and reactive crypt elongation, yielding ratios of 2 : 1 or 3 : 1 in this area. This is often accompanied by mild degrees of Brunner's gland hyperplasia, noted by their extension into the mucosal region. The end result is a greater distortion of the mucosa and the appearance of a chronic but inactive injury. It is important to appreciate this typical and perhaps universal finding in this area so that one avoids assigning any significance in the form of documenting a diseased state. To identify a definite alteration in this area, there should be even greater loss of the villi and signs of damage to the epithelial cells together with a neutrophilic infiltrate.

Aside from the mild hyperplasia that may be present, the crypts in the proximal duodenum are generally similar to the rest of the small intestine. Also noted in this area are occasional parietal cells.

Ampullary Region

Located in the second portion of the duodenum is the papilla of Vater, through which the common bile duct and major pancreatic duct ordinarily enter their excretions. The duodenal mucosa over this area is usually atrophic, and most of the region is composed of the bile duct together with periductal glands and a loose stroma (Fig. 6-6). It is important to recognize this normal region and to avoid confusing the prominent ductal and glandular tissue with invasive tumor.[4] The latter would reveal cytologic atypism and a tumor-like stroma.

Biopsy Material

Most of the material used for the evaluation of duodenal mucosa is obtained by direct endoscopic visualization, similar to that in the esophagus and stomach. Cytologic material may be added in the evaluation of tumors.[22, 23] Larger samples can be taken if there is a need to witness the submucosa, to better evaluate a cellular tumor such as a lymphoma that may need additional tissue for cell markers and study of monoclonality,[24] or to remove a polyp. The standard H & E stain is adequate for the great majority of diagnoses. As with other parts of the gut, there is a large array of immunocytochemical stains that can help in the identification of particular tumors and of their spread in the tissues (see Table 5-2). Except for the ampullary region, there is a much lower incidence of malignant tumors in the duodenum and, therefore, much less attention paid in this area to stains and cytometric techniques for the evaluation of cell growths.

DEVELOPMENTAL DISORDERS

Diverticula and Cysts

Diverticula

Most diverticula develop as a consequence of the healing of a deep and penetrating chronic peptic ulcer of the duodenum.[25–27] The ulcer leads to destruction of the muscle wall and the reparative connective tissue is less able to withstand the peristaltic wave, yielding the localized diverticulum. These are typically present in the first part of the duodenum, corresponding to the location of the chronic peptic ulcer. Other diverticula of the duodenum are rare and are related either to congenital defects or to other muscle deficits; in either case, they are often seen in conjunction with diverticula in other parts of the small bowel. The diverticula can serve as pockets of stasis but rarely cause any significant problem unless they are extensive in the jejunum, favoring bacterial proliferation. In the localized lesions of the proximal duodenum, they may cause some confusion at the time of gross endoscopic examination but there is usually no active inflammation. Biopsies are rarely obtained but would simply show the atrophic mucosa overlying an area of prior ulceration.

Cysts

Cysts are rare and mainly related to Brunner's glands or to ectopic pancreas.[28] The ducts or glands of the Brunner's area can become obstructed, yielding cystic change, and such lesions may protrude into the lumen. Biopsy shows the many well formed Brunner's glands with cystic change and typically no cytologic atypism.

HETEROTOPIC TISSUES

The major tissues that are abnormally located in the duodenum are well formed pancreas and gastric corpus-fundic mucosa.

Pancreatic Tissue

Heterotopic pancreatic tissue is most commonly seen in the stomach and in the duodenum and presents as single or multiple nodules that tend to be small and to have a central dimple corresponding to a duct[29–31] (see Fig. 4-8A). The ectopic foci should be distinguished from the normal pancreas, which is intimately attached to the deeper portions of the duodenal wall. Pancreatic tissue can occasionally be associated with a prominence of muscle, yielding lesions termed *adenomyoma;* these probably represent hamartomas rather than true neoplasms. The heterotopic tissue should also be separated from foci of pancreatic acinar metaplasia. The latter has recently been described in the stomach in cases of chronic gastritis, and it probably can occur in areas of duodenitis as well (see Ch. 4).

Gastric Tissue

Heterotopic stomach can involve all portions of the gut, being especially prominent in the upper esophagus, the duodenum, and in Meckel's diverticula.[32–37] The lesions present in the duodenum as either single or few discrete nodules that are almost always less than 1 cm in diameter. They are formed by gastric corpus-fundic mucosa without any other alteration (Fig. 6-7). These lesions should be distinguished from the appearance of other gastric tissues that are signs of chronic inflammation in the small intestine, including the occurrence of gastric mucous cell metaplasia in cases of chronic duodenitis, and of pyloric metaplasia in cases of any chronic enteritis. The metaplastic changes are comprised of the limited tissue elements and lack the well formed gastric glands that contain the parietal and chief cells. Biopsies are often taken of nodules seen at endoscopy in the duodenum, and the diagnosis of heterotopic stomach is easily made by the pathogenomonic features. *Helicobacter pylori* may be present but there is typically no active inflammation, and the lesions are not associated with localized ulcer formation, because any secretions are promptly diluted by the alkaline substances in the duodenal lumen.

MOTOR AND MECHANICAL DISORDERS

MECHANICAL OBSTRUCTION

Localized obstructions of the duodenum can result from congenital atresias but are more often related to inflammatory strictures.[38] The most common site is at the place of a chronic peptic ulcer, leading to obstruction mainly of the stomach. The rest of the duodenum can be affected from drug-induced lesions and, particularly, from chronic inflammatory disorders such as Crohn's disease. The duodenum proximal to the stricture shows dilation, and there is a potential for bacterial proliferation leading to poor absorption and to secondary damage of the mucosa. The effects on the mucosa from the obstruction itself are usually not

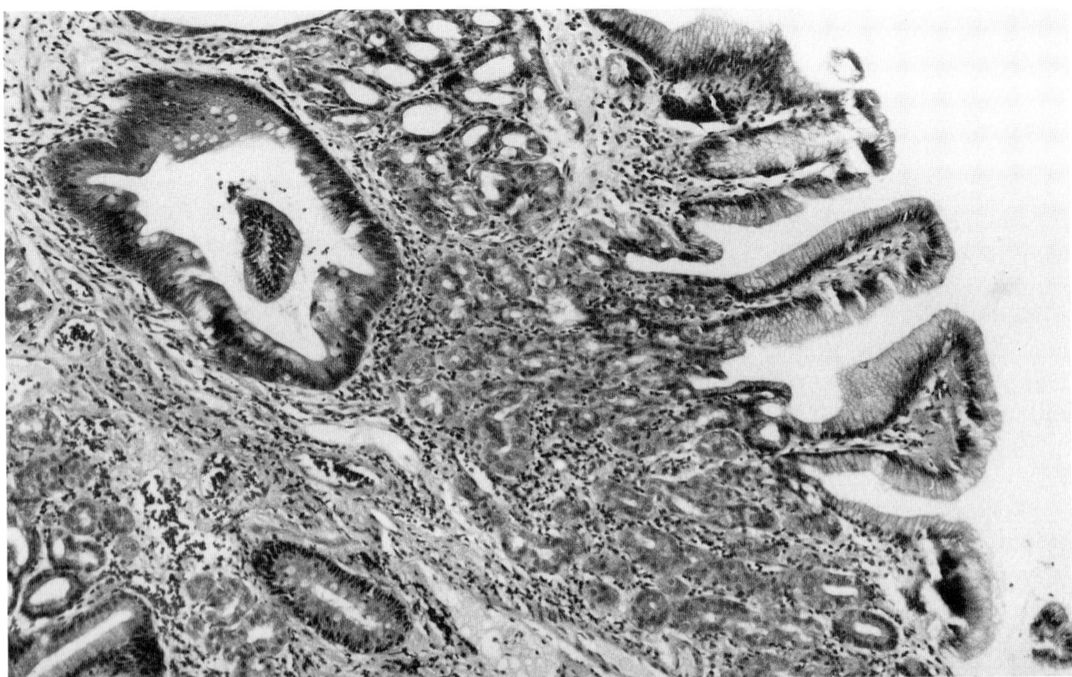

Fig. 6-7. Nodule of heterotopic stomach in the duodenum. The lesion is composed of the specialized glands of the corpus-fundic region (center) and covered by the gastric surface and pit type of mucous cells (right). Compare with the intestinal gland (upper left). This case shows mild inflammation, but most examples lack this feature (× 105).

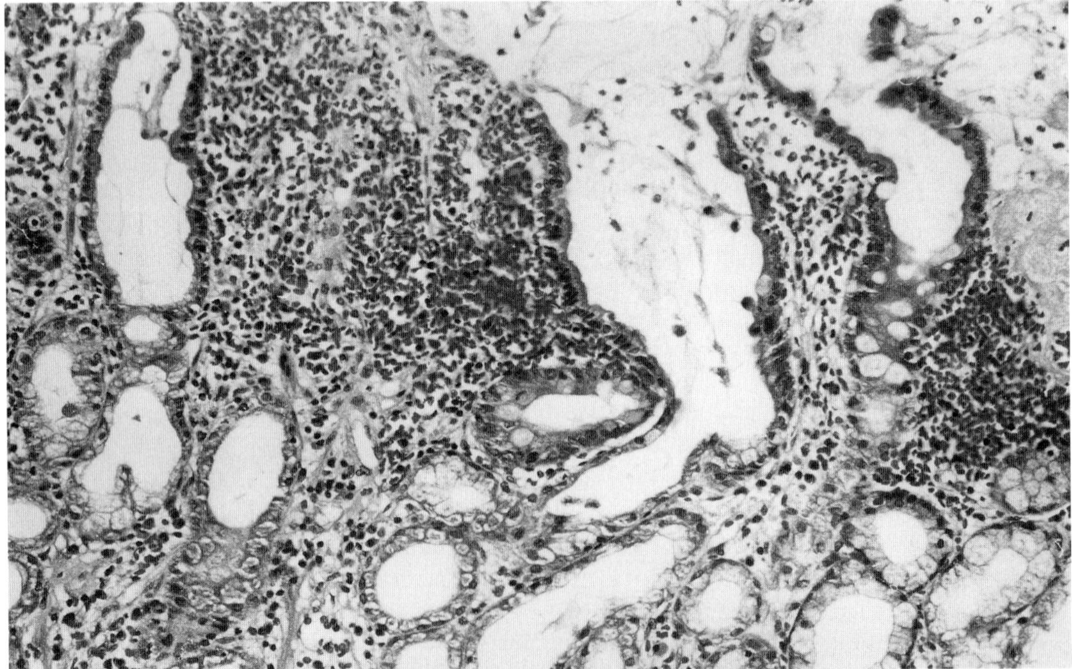

Fig. 6-8. Acute duodenitis, with surface at the top. There is a diffuse hemorrhage and erosion of the superficial mucosa leading to loss of villi and a neutrophilic reaction. Hyperplastic Brunner's glands are present at the base (× 210).

pronounced, and biopsies are rarely needed in these cases.

Pseudo-obstructive Disorders

There are many familial and acquired conditions that can lead to poor motility of the small intestine and can affect the duodenum.[39–41] These conditions include cases of scleroderma, amyloidosis, drug effects, diabetes mellitus and other metabolic disorders, many neurologic diseases, and idiopathic conditions termed *hollow visceral myopathy* and *neuropathy* (see Table 7-3). These can be associated with extreme dilation termed *megaduodenum.* The problems are those of poor motility, of bacterial overgrowth leading to malabsorption, and only minimally of injury involving the mucosa. Diagnoses are typically suggested by the radiographic studies, and biopsies are ordinarily obtained to exclude conditions with more extensive mucosal damage such as celiac disease. The biopsies show only slight shortening of the villi with mild active inflammation that usually does not correlate in intensity with the overall clinical problem.

VASCULAR DISORDERS

Varices and Vascular Malformations

Varices and Telangiectasia

Varices due to cirrhosis and other causes of portal hypertension are more commonly observed in the esophagus and stomach but may extend into the duodenum, particularly if there has been prior injury and adhesions in this area.[42–44] The lesions appear as discrete enlarged veins that may protrude into the lumen, or as multiple smaller venules occupying the lamina propria. These are a rare source of significant hemorrhage. The more extensive presence of dilated venules, termed *telangiectasia,* has also been noted in other groups of patients, particularly in the Osler–Weber–Rendu syndrome and in those with renal failure, either alone or in conjunction with dialysis or transplantation[45–48] (see Fig. 4-9). The actual cause for the renal association is not known, but the lesions may ooze in these patients. Overall, the lesions are typically suspected at the time of gross endoscopy, and biopsies are often not taken because of the fear of excess hemorrhage. Intact lesions show the prominent dilation of venules within the lamina propria, identical to that seen in the equivalent lesion of congestive gastropathy in the stomach (see Table 4-4).

Dieulafoy's Ulcer

Occasional lesions noted in the duodenum are similar to the Dieulafoy's ulcer that is more typically present in the proximal stomach.[49] These are persistent ulcers with a central conspicuous artery, and the vessel is thought to be a sign of an arteriovenous malformation. The lesions often differ from the ordinary chronic peptic ulcer by their more variable location within the duodenum. Biopsies may be obtained from the edge of the ulcer, largely to exclude tumor, but are otherwise nonspecific, revealing necrosis and and inflammation.

Ischemic Lesions

Because of the exceptional vascular supply to the duodenal area ordinary infarction is rarely seen, even in cases of extensive small bowel ischemia. Nevertheless, in efforts to contain the hemorrhage from duodenal ulcers, there had been attempts to inject material such as Gelfoam or preformed clots in the major arteries to this area, and this resulted in localized areas of marked infarction and to perforation.[50] These are typically very sick patients and endoscopic examination is usually not needed.

Small Vessel Diseases

The small vessels in the wall of the duodenum and small intestine can be affected by amyloid material or by vasculitis, leading to localized vascular compromise and to areas of both hemorrhage and ulcers in the overlying mucosa.[51, 52] These also can occur as a result of atheromatous emboli affecting these arteries[53] (cf. Fig. 9-15). The mucosal lesions are nonspecific and show necrosis and inflammation, and deeper samples are often needed to identify the specific disorder affecting the artery.

PEPTIC DUODENITIS

Definition, Etiology, and Pathogenesis

Peptic duodenitis is probably the most common disorder affecting the duodenum, and is largely related to the presence of excess acid and peptic enzymes[54–57] (Table 6-3). The primary cause in most cases is not known, but patients often reveal increases in the basal and the maximal stimulated acid production. This leads to greater amounts of acid present within the duodenal lumen, presumably exceeding the local defenses of the alkaline substances produced by the Brunner's glands and bile secretions. There results a damage to the surface of the duodenal mucosa that leads to a primary villous-type injury.[58–60.]

Table 6-3. Causes of Duodenitis

- Acid-peptic disease
- Stress hemorrhages and ulcers
- Chemical and drug effects
- Infections
- Immunologic disorders
- Miscellaneous conditions
  - Radiation
  - Granulomatous diseases
  - Effects of depositions and metabolic diseases

Clinical Features

The patient typically presents with signs and symptoms similar to those with chronic peptic ulcer of the duodenum. There is burning pain in the mid-epigastric area that is associated with an empty stomach. Indeed, there is considered to be a continuum of peptic duodenitis and peptic ulcer, with the same factors present in both disorders, and the patients presenting with one or the other malady at different times.

Gross and Biopsy Features

The duodenal mucosa reveals congestion, petechiae, and friability, without overt ulceration. The lesions are most striking in the first and second portions of the duodenum, where there is the greatest amount of acid effect. Beyond this region, there is dilution and protection by the alkaline duodenal content. Biopsies are distinctive and reveal marked shortening of the villi, damage to the surface epithelium, and a heavy infiltrate of neutrophils in the acute or active phase[61–68] (Table 6-4 and Fig. 6-8). Features of chronic

Table 6-4. Biopsy Features of Duodenitis

- Acute (active) duodenitis
  - Shortening of villi and elongation of crypts
  - Presence of neutrophils in lamina propria and epithelial layer
  - Variable increase of eosinophils and mononuclear cells
  - Erosions and ulcers in severe cases
- Chronic duodenitis
  - Persistence of villous shortening and crypt hyperplasia
  - Increase of eosinophils and mononuclear inflammatory cells in lamina propria
  - Variable increase of lymphoid nodules
  - Hyperplasia of Brunner's glands with extension into mucosa
  - Gastric mucous cell metaplasia involving villi
  - Pyloric gland metaplasia

duodenitis, due to repeated episodes of acute disease, include a persistence of the shortened villi, an increase in the amount of Brunner's glands that extend from the submucosa into the mucosa to a varying degree[69, 70] (Fig. 6-9), and a metaplasia principally involving the villous epithelial area, with a switch from the absorptive and goblet mucous cells of the intestine to the gastric surface-type mucous cells[71–74] (Fig. 6-10). These appear as thin columnar cells with the mucus granules concentrated in the apical portion, and stain like the stomach with a marked PAS reaction and a negative stain for acid mucins. As noted above, this metaplastic effect representing chronic duodenitis must be distinguished from gastric heterotopia, which is composed of mature fundic mucosa.

Once there is the appearance of the gastric surface mucous cells, there is also the presence of *H. pylori* that probably require this structure for their attachment and persistence.[75, 76] Whether the cases of chronic duodenitis with the gastric surface mucous cell metaplasia and secondary *H. pylori* infection are more prone to greater destruction has been seriously considered in the evolution of duodenal ulcers. Nevertheless, most cases of ordinary peptic duodenitis without ulcer formation do not show conspicuous presence of the bacteria. Some cases of persistent or chronic peptic duodenitis develop an increase in the amount of lymphoid tissue that can cause numerous small nodules grossly; this has been termed *nodular duodenitis.*[77, 78] There does not appear to be any direct relationship of this lesion to the development of lymphoma.

In the healing of the duodenitis, there is loss of the neutrophilic infiltrate from the lamina propria and epithelial layer and a restoration of the villous epithelial cells. There may persist varying degrees of the chronic features, notably the Brunner's gland hyperplasia and gastic mucous cell metaplasia together with increased number of mononuclear inflammatory cells in the lamina propria.[79, 80] It is hard to evaluate the architecture for signs of chronic disease in this proximal part of the duodenum, because it is so variable in the normal state in this area. The features of the chronic and active duodenitis that are seen in peptic duodenitis are identical in appearance at a microscopic level with that seen in the mucosa adjacent to a chronic peptic ulcer. Indeed, the overall features of the inflammation are entirely nonspecific and can be seen in any other inflammatory condition affecting the duodenum.

ULCER DISEASES

Ulcer diseases are largely discussed in Chapter 4, and are briefly mentioned here in reference to duodenal involvement.

Acute Stress Ulcer

Following highly stressful lesions such as examples of multiple trauma, burns, increased intracranial pressure, and probably any shock state, there can develop foci of hemorrhage and multiple acute ulcers that affect the mucosa of the stomach and duodenum.[81] These are thought to represent ischemic lesions due mainly to vasoconstriction and enhanced by local acid, and they are usually superficial.[82, 83] However, more extensive lesions leading to performation can occur, and major efforts are made in intensive care units to prevent their development in otherwise very sick patients. These stress lesions are most commonly noted in patients with coagulopathy and pulmonary conditions.[84] The diagnosis is characteristically made by consideration of the clinical information and is supported by gross endoscopic examination, if done. Biopsies are uncommonly obtained and show superficial erosion with acute inflammation and typically no signs of chronic disease (Fig. 6-11).

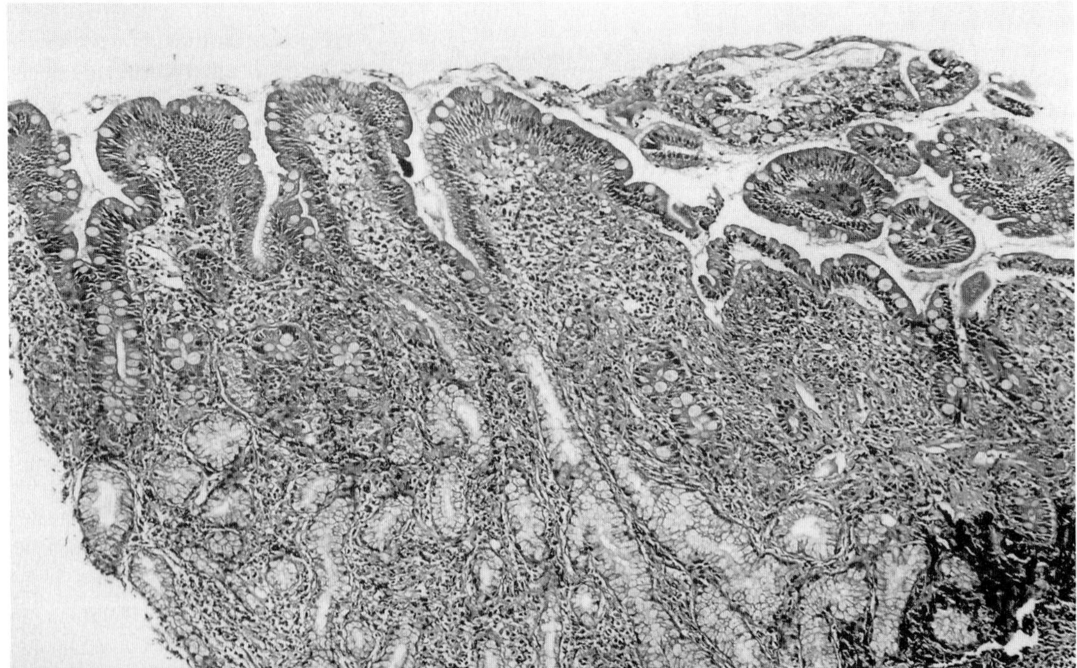

Fig. 6-9. Chronic duodenitis, with Brunner's gland hyperplasia. Noted are shortened villi, increased inflammatory cells in the lamina propria, and a prominent proliferation of the Brunner's glands that extend into the mucosal region (bottom) (× 105).

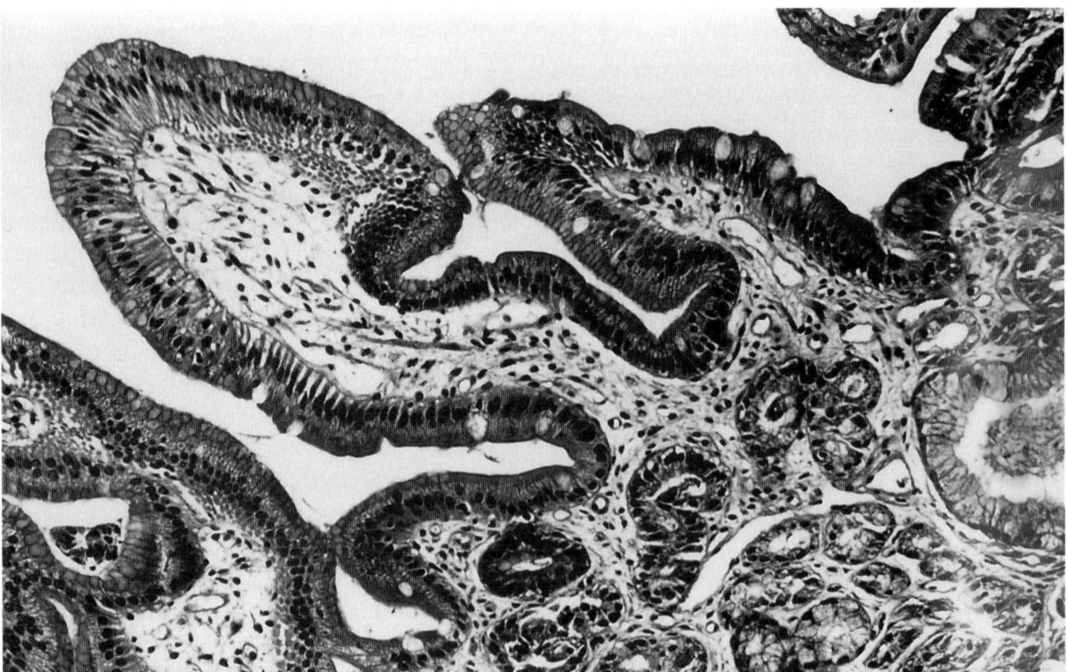

Fig. 6-10. Chronic duodenitis, with gastric mucous cell metaplasia. The surface of the villi (left) is covered with a layer of columnar mucous cells of the gastric surface/foveolar type. Compare with the intestinal-type goblet mucous cells appearing at the top right (× 210).

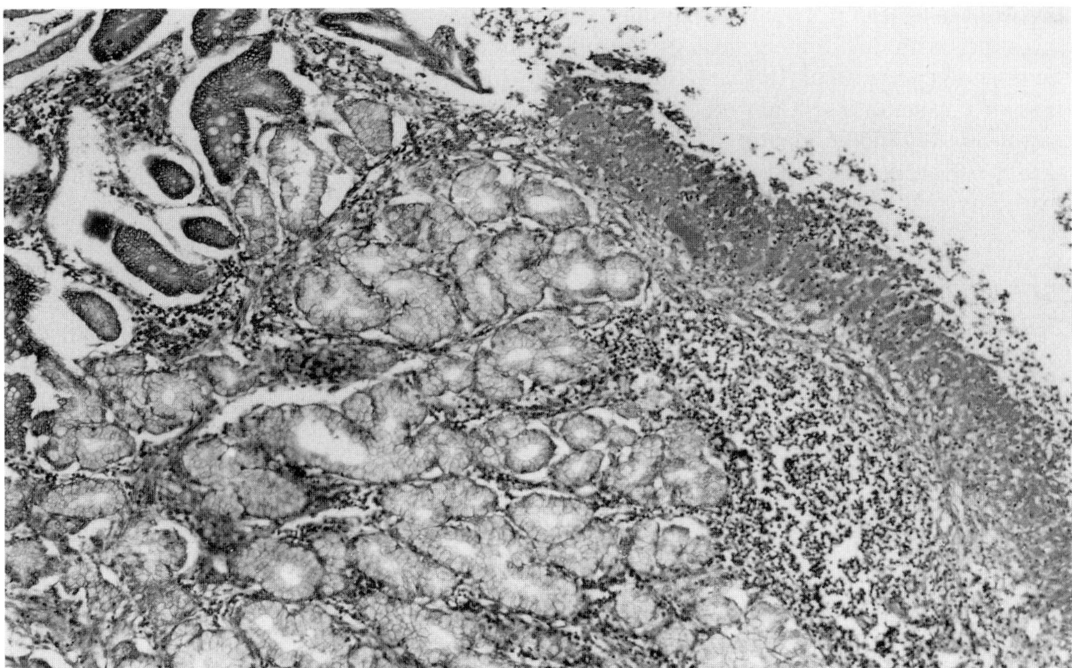

Fig. 6-11. Acute stress ulcer of the duodenum, with surface appearing at right. Noted is an ulcer of the mucosa associated with marked acute inflammation, overlying an area of hyperplastic Brunner's glands. There is no fibrosis (× 105).

Chronic Peptic Ulcer

Over one-half of the cases of chronic peptic ulcer (and reaching three-quarters in some series) occur in the first portion of the duodenum. It is currently thought that these develop from excess acid leading to injury of the duodenum that favors secondary *H. pylori* colonization, and the combination results in the ulcer. This pathogenesis is greatly supported by the successful use of antibiotics together with anti-secretory agents in the treatment and prevention of ulcer recurrence.[85] The bacteria have been found in 80 to 90 percent of these cases; of interest, the bacteria are largely present in the stomach as evidence of a more generalized infection in this area. Cases associated with increased gastrin production, such as Zollinger-Ellison syndrome and retained antrum, can show ulcers in the more distal portions of the duodenum as well, and these cases are less often associated with the presence of bacteria.[86]

Endoscopic examination and biopsy of chronic peptic ulcers that affect the duodenum are less often obtained because of the much less likelihood of cancer formation in this region compared to the stomach (see Fig. 4-33). The endoscopy may be done to follow the ulcer in response to therapy but biopsies are not always obtained. Whenever there is an unusual appearance or, particularly, location of ulcer, the possibility of an underlying mass lesion should be considered and multiple samples obtained as in other parts of the gut. This is discussed further in later sections of this chapter on tumors.

CHEMICAL AND DRUG INJURY

Chemotherapy Effects

The small intestinal mucosa is exquisitely sensitive to most chemicals used in the treatment of tumors.[87, 88] The duodenum may be involved as well as any other part of the small intestine, with the appearance of multiple hemorrhages and ulcers. Indeed, the destruction of the small intestinal mucosa is often a rate-limiting step in the use of the particular therapeutic regimen. Many of the drugs, such as methotrexate and other antimetabolites, act on the crypt epithelial cells resulting in shortened villi and a lack of crypt hyperplasia. With time, there can be complete loss of these cells and secondary ulceration with the threat of secondary infection. The findings are mainly self-limited, but cases of deeper ulceration can result in perforation or the later presence of fibrosis and strictures.

Biopsy features are nonspecific, showing the mucosal atrophy or necrosis, together with inflammation. Biopsies are also done to look for the effects of radiation if employed, for secondary infections, and for residual or recurrent tumor.

Injections of chemotherapeutic drugs into the hepatic artery, largely to control malignant tumors in the liver, can cause localized ulcers in the duodenum.[89, 90] The mucosa adjacent to the ulcers often shows marked cytologic atypism, which has been confused with tumor. This effect appears to have lessened in more recent studies.

Alcohol Duodenitis

The major effects of excess ethanol consumption are on the stomach but lesions are occasionally seen in the duodenal mucosa.[91–93] Noted are foci of hemorrhage and erosions together with nonspecific acute and chronic inflammation of the mucosa. The changes are largely of an acute nature, and chronic disease in this area from alcohol is not established. Practically all cases are associated with the presence of more extensive changes in the stomach.

Drug-Induced Duodenitis

All of the nonsteroidal anti-inflammatory drugs (NSAIDs) can cause damage to the gastric and small intestinal mucosa[94, 95] (see Table 7-4). The lesions are probably more universal in the stomach, but effects on the duodenal mucosa or more distal parts of the small bowel are seen in one-quarter to one-third of the cases.[96–101] Typically noted are patchy hemorrhages and erosions with acute inflammation, which rapidly resolve following elimination of the medication. Exceptionally, there can develop deeper ulcers with the formation of fibrous strictures and of fibromuscular diaphragms that can partially obstruct the lumen.[102, 103] Of interest, the strictures and diaphragms due to NSAIDS and to other agents such as potassium chloride are more common in the jejunum and ileum than in the duodenum.[104]

Most of these lesions, whether acute or move advanced, are identified by the historical information and gross endoscopic examination, and biopsies are uncommonly obtained. The alterations seen microscopically are entirely nonspecific but serve to exclude infections and granulomatous diseases, if needed. (See Chs. 4 and 7 for further discussion.)

INFECTIONS

Practically all of the infections that occur in the duodenum affect the other parts of the small intestine as well (see Table 7-6). These are discussed in Chapter 7, and are mentioned here with special reference to their presentation and detection in the duodenum (Table 6-5).

General Features

The effects of the infections are largely related to the microorganism and are not tissue specific. Most of the features are described in the other chapters, notably in Chapters 2 and 4. There are the expected ulcers and acute inflammation in cases caused by highly chemotactic organisms, such as most pyogenic bacteria and fungi; the presence of marked mononuclear cell in-

Table 6-5. Infections of the Duodenum

Viral
Common agents
Herpes simplex
Cytomegalovirus
Human immunodeficiency virus (HIV)
Bacterial
Helicobacter pylori
Common enteric pathogens
Mycobacterium
Bacterial proliferation syndrome
Rare
Syphilis
Whipple's disease
Fungal
Candida
Aspergillus
Phycomyces
Histoplasma
Cryptococcus
Protozoal
Giardia
Cryptosporidium
Microsporidia
Less common
Isospora
Cyclospora
Pneumocystis
Leishmania
Heiminthic
Hookworms
Flatworms
Schistosoma
Strongyloides
Capillaria

filtrate with many of the organisms requiring a delayed hypersensitivity reaction, such as viruses and protozoa; and the nonspecific features of ulcers, granulation tissue, and fibrosis reflecting the extent of disease and healing processes. The diagnoses are established by identifying the organism through stains and specific cultures.

Viral Infections

Several viruses can cause an acute and reversible enteritis that affects all parts of the small intestine including the duodenum, resulting in nonspecific villous injury and secondary crypt hyperplasia. Included are the rotaviruses, enteroviruses, adenoviruses, and Norwalk group,[105] and they are described in Chapter 7.

Herpes and Cytomegalovirus Infections

As in any part of the gut, the presence of the various immunodeficiency disorders favors the development of infection with herpes simplex and with cytomegalovirus[106, 107] (Plates 1A and 1B). The viral inclusions are seen in the epithelial cells, particularly of the Brunner's glands, and more often in the reactive mesenchymal elements. Cytomegalovirus is more frequently seen in the small intestine and especially in cases with ulceration. They have also been observed in immunocompetent patients, where their significance in causing disease is less well established.[108]

Human Immunodeficiency Virus Infection

There has been considerable investigation of the duodenal and other small intestinal mucosa in patients with AIDS, particularly in those with diarrhea who lack an identifiable opportunistic infection.[109–111] Viral particles corresponding to HIV have been demonstrated in the mucosal epithelial cells by electron microscopy, but the toxic actions and direct relation to the clinical symptoms are still not established (see Fig. 7-7).

Bacterial Infections

There are many bacteria that can cause disease in the small or large intestines by a variety of pathophysiologic mechanisms.[112] These mechanisms include excess proliferation of bacteria in static or fistulous segments, resulting in destruction of bile salts and maldigestion; growth of bacteria in the lumen and their release of toxins that are absorbed, causing several food poisoning states; attachment of bacteria to the surface cells causing interference with absorption and a prominent watery diarrhea; and invasion of the tissues together with release of toxic enzymes resulting in a purulent or dysenteric disorder. These are mainly presented in Chapters 7 and 9.

Helicobacter pylori Infection

As noted above, *H. pylori* is frequently present in cases of chronic peptic ulcer of the duodenum and may play a role in its development and progression. Current therapy is directed against the bacteria as well as the acid, with favorable results.[85]

Mycobacterial Infections

Tuberculosis is more commonly seen in the distal ileum and colon but may occasionally affect the stomach and duodenum.[113–115] Present are ulcers with extensive necrosis, granuloma formation, and often fibrosis. The diagnosis requires specific stain or culture. More commonly observed in immunocompromised patients are infections with *Mycobacterium avium intracellulare* and other species.[116, 117] These cases show less ulceration and poorly formed granulomas but a superabundance of organisms as revealed by acid-fast stain in the lamina propria (Figs. 6-12 and 6-13, and Plate 1D). There are so many organisms that they are readily seen in stool smears as well.

Other Bacterial Infections

Rarely affecting the duodenum alone are syphilis and the several disorders associated with defective monocyte reaction to bacteria, such as chronic granulomatous disease and malakoplakia.[118, 119] Whipple's disease is more chacteristically present in the jejunum but can also affect the duodenum, often in a focal fashion.[120] Such cases can be detected by endoscopy and biopsy revealing the distinctive PAS-positive macrophages that contain the numerous bacteria, best visualized by ultrastructure. All of these rare infections are discussed in Chapter 7.

Fungal Infections

Candidal infections are seen as a secondary problem in some chronic peptic ulcer cases, and more diffuse disease appears in immunosuppressed patients.[121, 122] Other fungal infections that affect the small intestine, including the duodenum, result form *Phycomyces, Aspergillus, Histoplasma,* and *Cryptococcus*[123–126] (see Plates 1E–F). These are rarely seen alone in the duodenum.[127]

Protozoal Infections

There is an ever increasing list of protozoal agents responsible for human disease, mostly occurring in patients with AIDS and with other immunodeficiency disorders of a primary or acquired nature[128, 129] (see Table 6-6). The patients typically present with chronic diarrhea, but the exact mechanism responsible for the mucosal injury is not known. Practically all of these organisms act throughout the small intestine and can frequently be detected by duodenal samples obtained at endoscopy.

Biopsies are mainly obtained for the identification of the organisms, which can be readily distinguished by their individual characteristics and location in the mucosal sample. There is frequently no constant degree of necrosis or inflammation and only the organisms are found. Multiple samples with special stains and ultrastructure are recommended to achieve the greatest yield. It has also been suggested that direct smears or brushings be taken from the surface of the small intestinal epithelium to increase the detection of *Giardia* and possibly other protozoal agents.

Giardial Infection

The responsible organism, *Giardia lamblia,* represents a pathogen and can cause disease in immunocompetent persons, often following exposure to contaminated wells or other water supplies.[130, 131] The patients usually present with watery diarrhea, cramps and prominent flatulence, and the blood eosinophil count is variably elevated. The diagnosis is mainly secured by looking for the organism in the duodenal fluid and mucosa, obtained by smears or biopsy; they may also be noted in the stools.[132–134] *Giardia* are almost always located on the surface of the mucosa and in the spaces between the villi (Fig. 6-14 and Plate 2A), although invasion into the tissue has been seen in extremely malnourished and immunodeficient patients. The organisms appear as pear-shaped structures with prominent nuclei; they can be readily recognized by H & E and accented by the Giemsa stain. The mucosa is otherwise normal in most immunocompetent patients, whereas it more often shows signs of enteritis in the compromised patients. Of interest, recent studies suggest a lesser prevalence of *Giardia,* with yields as low as 1 positive case in 144 patients examined.[135]

Cryptosporidial Infection

The species of Cryptosporidium are indigenous to many animals and cause two forms of disease in humans: a reversible colitis in immunocompetent children, and an intractable diarrhea due to small bowel involvement in immunocompromised patients.[136–139] Infection has also been noted in the stomach and biliary tract. The organisms are spherical, measure a few micrometers in diameter, and contain a nucleoid structure (Figs. 6-15 and 6-16, and Plate 2B). In biopsy samples, they are concentrated on the surface of the villi where they appear to be intimately related to the cellular membranes, as revealed by ultrastructure.[134,140,141] The duodenal mucosa often reveals evidence of active enteritis, in the form of shortened villi, damaged epithelial cells, and infiltrate with neutrophils.

Microsporidial Infections

Recently noted in AIDS patients are infections due to agents of the microsporidial group, including *Enterocytozoon bieneusi* and *Septata intestinalis* (a member of the Encephalitozoon class).[142–144] The patients present with a watery diarrhea, and duodenal biopsies are performed to look for the organism and to identify the particular type. Of interest, the duodenal mucosa usually has a normal appearance, without evidence of a chronic or active enteritis.

In contrast to species of *Giardia* and *Cryptosporidium,* the Microsporidia are typically localized within the cytoplasm of the epithelial cells on the villi (Figs. 6-17 and 6-18, and Plate 2C). The organisms of the Enterocytozoon class appear as tiny vacuoles or granules in the apical portion of the cells, depending on the stage of the protozoa. They are best seen in the shed epithelial cells at the tips of the villi. The larger Microsporidia of the *Septata intestinalis* type are present both in the epithelial cells and in the macrophages within the lamina propria.[145] They have also been found in the colonic and gallbladder epithelia, in Kupffer cells of the liver, and in renal tubular epithelial cells. The organisms are present in tissue and brush preparations, are doubly refractile in paraffin sections, and can be best visualized with the modified Gram, trichrome, and specific flurochrome stains.[146–148] Ultrastructural study is particularly helpful because it enhances the sensitivity and allows for easy separation of the various types.

Other Protozoal Infections

More rarely observed in the duodenum are infections due to *Isospora,*[149, 150] *Pneumocystis,*[151, 152] *Leishmania,*[153] and the newly

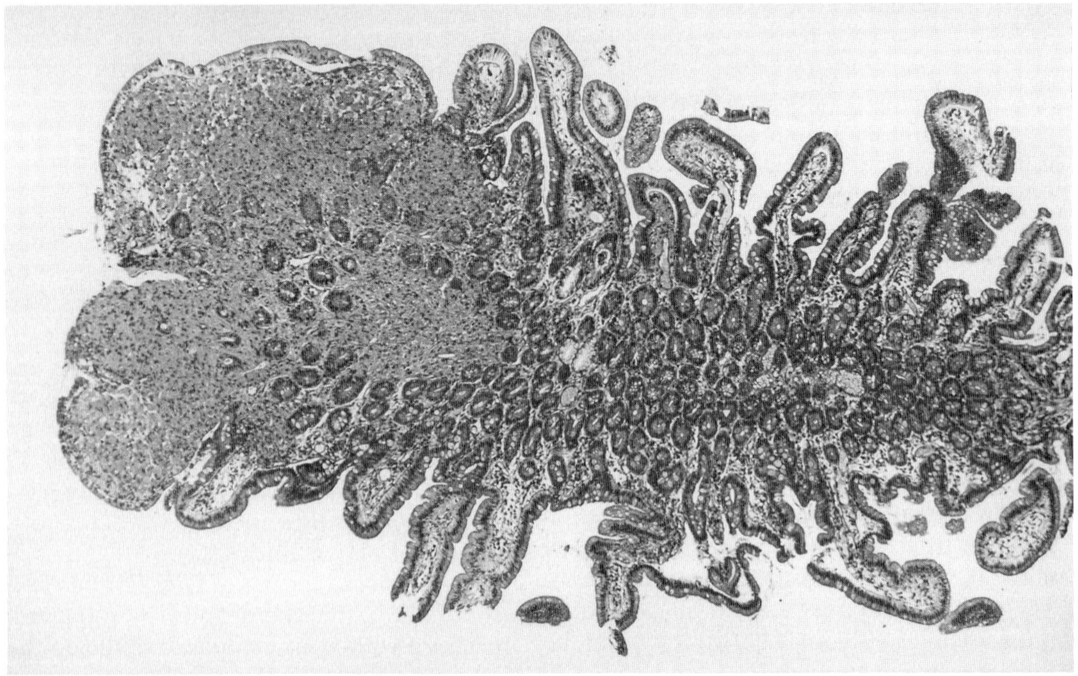

A

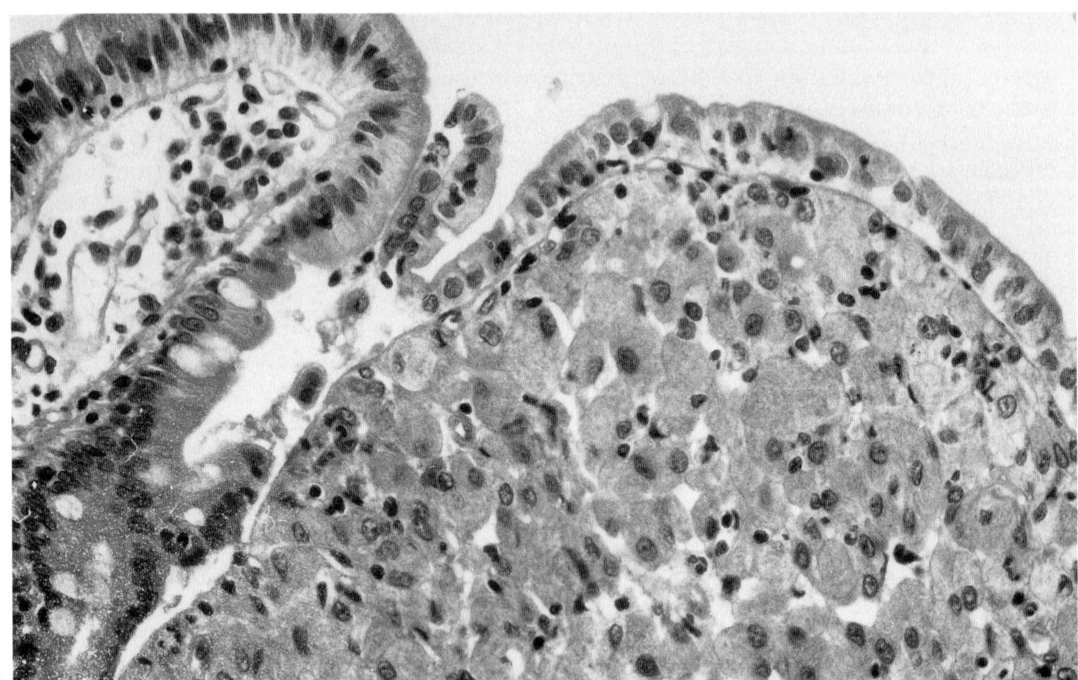

B

Fig. 6-12. Duodenal infection due to *Mycobacterium avium intracellulare.* **(A)** Biopsy of duodenal mucosa showing a nodule at the left (× 42). **(B)** The lamina propria (right) is stuffed with macrophages that have a granular cytoplasm (× 425). (*Figure continues.*)

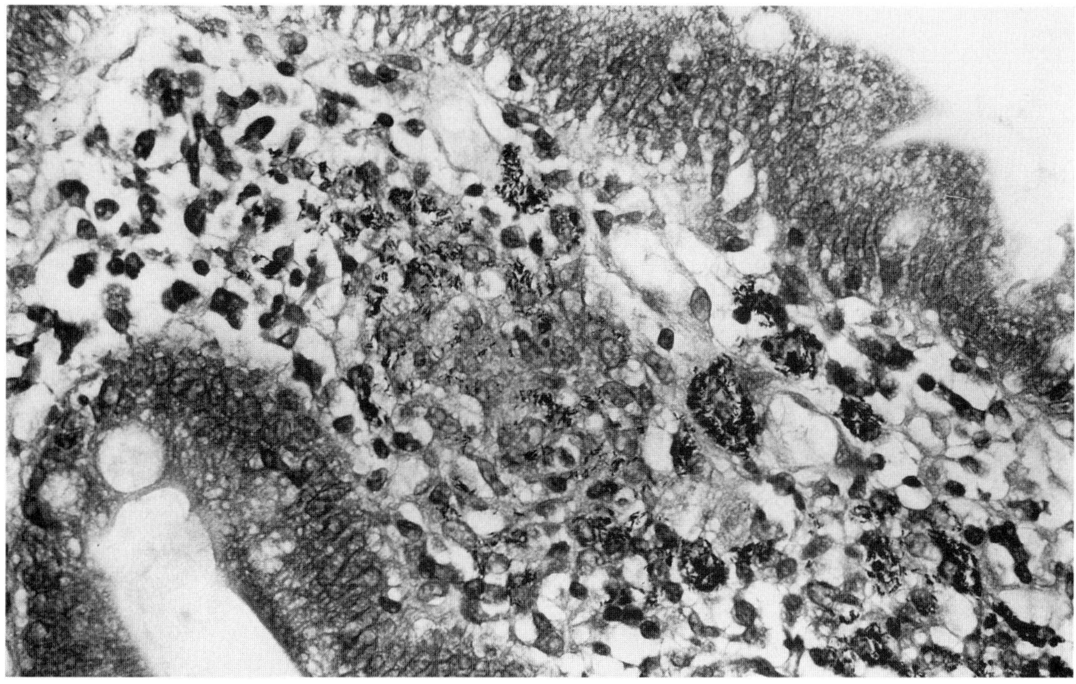

C

Fig. 6-12 (*Continued*). (C) Acid-fast stain revealing a huge number of organisms within the macrophages in the lamina propria (× 425).

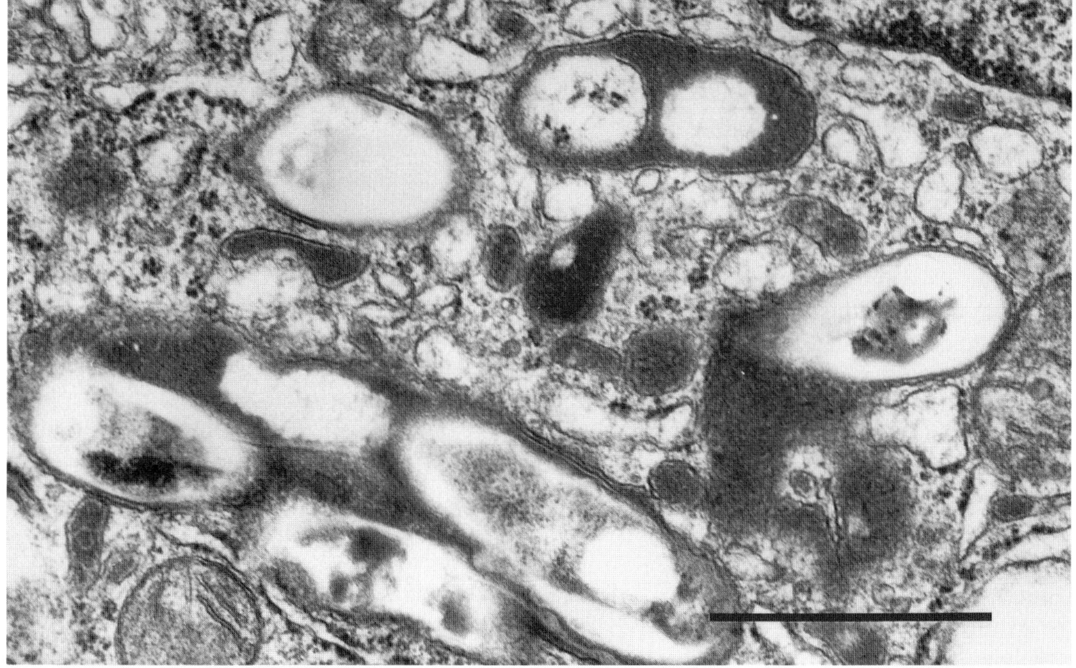

Fig. 6-13. Electron micrograph of duodenum, showing *Mycobacterium avium intracellulare* in a macrophage (× 37, 500; bar = 1 μm).

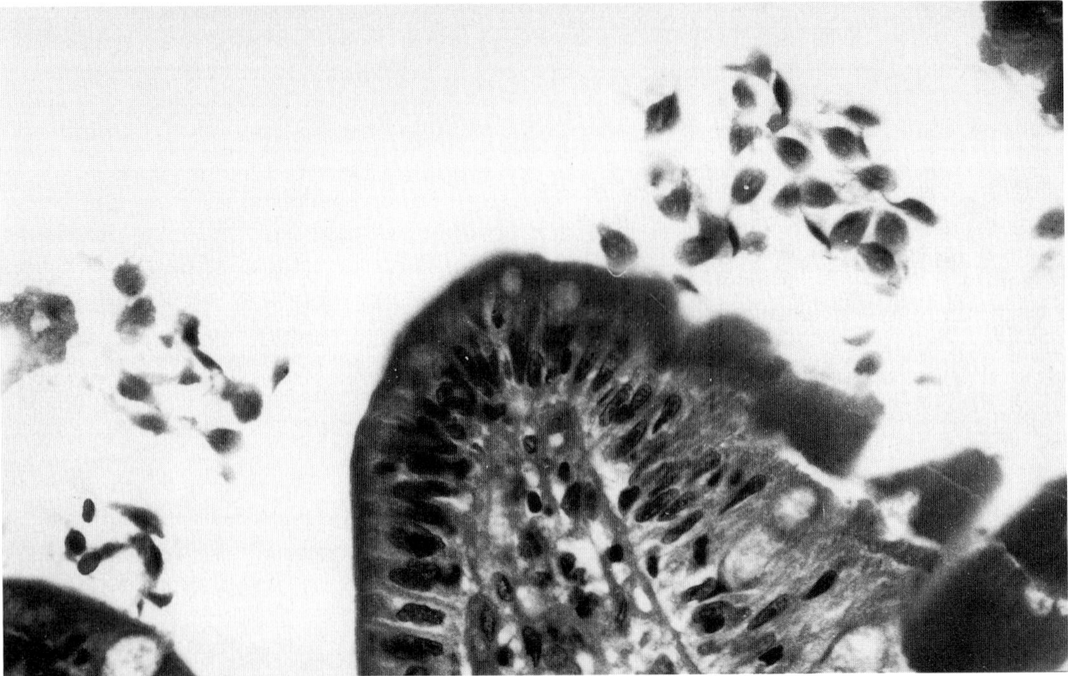

Fig. 6-14. Giardiasis in the duodenum. There are a large number of the protozoa on the surface of the mucosa. The villous tip shows no signs of injury (× 425).

described organism of *Cyclospora.*[154] The *Cyclospora* are best seen in smears, and the other protozoa in biopsy sections (Plate 4D).

Helminthic Infections

Helminthic infections also involve the jejunum but often present with problems in the duodenum. Potential lesions include foci of hemorrhage from hookworms[155]; nutritional deficit such as reduced folate from flatworms[156]; localized inflammatory nodules and granulomas from the eggs of *Schistosoma* and *Strongyloides*[157–161]; and more diffuse inflammation and mild erosion from *Capillaria.*[162]

Many of these disorders are diagnosed by smears of stools to identify the particular ova. Direct visualization and biopsy of the duodenal mucosa is especially helpful in those instances where there is an inflammatory lesion. The cases with *Strongyloides* show the fragments of worm or ova together with many eosinophils (Fig. 6-19), and lesions due to schistosomiasis reveal granuloma formation and varying fibrosis, which may be in the form of a flat or polypoid lesion (see Fig. 9-23 and Plate 2F).

MALABSORPTIVE DISORDERS

Examination of the duodenum is helpful in two ways, as a screening test in those diseases that are diffuse, such as celiac disease; and to evaluate localized lesions that can be related to malabsorptive states such as focal areas of Whipple's disease and of lymphangectasia.[8–11] In addition, the functional problems in many cases of malabsorption are directly related to the occurence of infections, either primarily or complicating an immunodeficiency disorder. Duodenal mucosal biopsy can be especially helpful in identifying the infectious agent as well as the underlying mucosal disorder. [The malabsorptive disorders are principally presented in Ch. 7[163, 164] (see Table 7-7).]

General Considerations

Since celiac disease, also termed *gluten sensitive enteropathy* and *non-tropical sprue,* is typically a diffuse disorder, endoscopic examination of the duodenum can be employed as a screening test. If the biopsy is negative, it serves to rule out an untreated case of celiac disease. Conversely, if the biopsy shows reduced folds and the features of active celiac disease, there is the potential for lack of specificity since there are other causes of duodenitis, notably acid-peptic disease.[165, 166] In general, peptic duodenitis is associated with only partial loss of the villi whereas the most florid examples of celiac disease reveal complete loss and the greatest degree of crypt hyperplasia. Accordingly, an estimate can be made of a probable case of celiac disease justifying an attempt at a gluten-free diet. If there is any doubt in the lesion, biopsies taken from the distal duodenum or from the jejunum would be needed to provide support.

There are no specific features to help in distinguishing celiac disease from most of the other forms of duodenitis, including the peptic type. In general, cases of peptic duodenitis tend to be associated with a greater amount of neutrophils in the lamina propria and surface epithelium, to be limited to the most proximal portions of the duodenum, to have lesser degrees of villous shortening, and to show fewer lymphocytes in the surface epithelium. In contrast, cases of celiac disease reveal more marked lymphocytic infiltrates and lesser amounts of neutrophils together with a greater loss of the villi in the advanced cases (see Ch. 7).

Specific Disorders

Most of these lesions are best expressed in the jejunum. As noted, the diffuse disorders can also be present in the duodenum; included are celiac disease,[167–169] tropical sprue,[170, 171] many of the immunodeficiency states, viral enteritis, and the large number of opportunistic infectious disorders. Also, focal lesions may be present in the duodenum in cases of Whipple's disease and of intestinal lymphangiectasia.[120, 172–175] It is probable that many of the other disorders can also be found in the duodenum, including mastocytosis,[176, 177] amyloidosis and other depositions, the many storage diseases (see "Miscellaneous Conditions" below), and microvillous inclusion disease.[178–181] These are presented in Chapter 7.

IMMUNOLOGIC DISORDERS

Allergic (eosinophilic) Enteritis

Allergic enteritis is a disorder that primarily affects children and young adults with multiple lesions in the esophagus, stomach (particularly the antral region), and the small intestine[182–185] (see Table 4-11). The gastric corpus and large intestine tend to be less involved. Milder cases are associated with a single allergen, such as cows milk or soy protein, and these patients usually have more focal lesions scattered in the stomach and small intestine.[186–189] In the cases of allergic (or eosinophilc) gastroenteritis, there is probably reaction to multiple antigens that cannot be easily identified and eliminated, and the consequence is a greater extent of injury in these regions.

The characteristic lesion is a focal area of epithelial damage associated with an infiltrate of eosinophils[190] (Fig. 6-20). In the small intestine, there are normally a fair number of eosinophils in the lamina propria, and these must be greatly increased to appreciate their abnormality. Helpful is the finding of a large number of eosinophils extending into the epithelium of the overlying villi or into the underlying muscularis mucosae. The lesions are focal in those cases with a single allergen and also in most examples due to more generalized eosinophilic gastroenteritis, with only

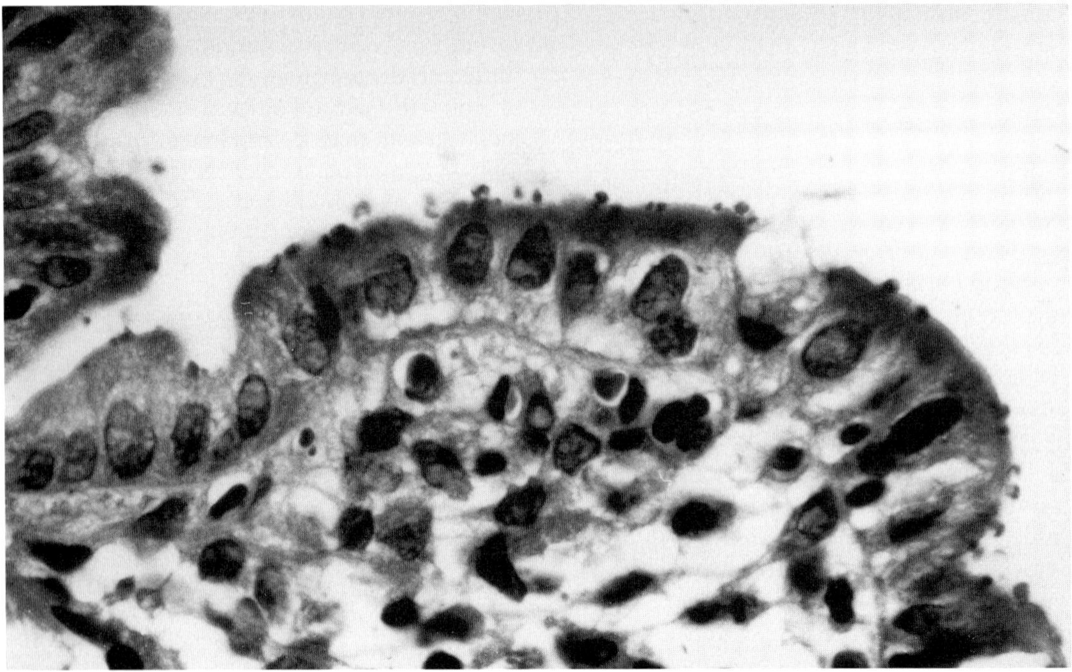

Fig. 6-15. Cryptosporidiosis in the duodenum. Numerous spherical organisms are present on the surface of the villous epithelial cells. There is no penetration into the cytoplasm or lamina propria (× 1060).

one-quarter of the patients showing a more diffuse lesion. In the latter it may be difficult to distinguish from other diffuse lesions such as celiac disease, and gastric antral biopsies may be particularly helpful since they reveal the allergic lesions but no constant effects from the celiac disease.

With treatment by elimination diets or by corticosteroids, there is typically resolution of the inflammation and restoration of the epithelium without chronic changes. The features, however, can recur, showing the same active lesions. These also affect the jejunum, but most biopsies are currently obtained at the time of endoscopy of the duodenum and probably reflect the jejunal involvement as well (see Ch. 4).

Immunodeficiency Disorders

Immunodeficiency disorders may be due to a variety of inherited or acquired conditions that lead to alterations of the immune mechanisms and occasionally of the mucosal structure[191] (Table 6-6). The functional effects are largely related to the promotion of opportunistic infections, and their eradication can help in maintaining stability in these patients. Most of the immunologic disorders are diagnosed by characterizing the elements of the immune system, particularly the features of the lymphocytes, macrophages, and antibody production. Biopsy can assist in the diagnosis by showing certain alterations, but they are largely employed to identify or exclude the secondary infections or tumors.

Primary Conditions

The primary conditions include selected IgA deficiency, transient hypogammaglobulinemia of infancy, inherited agammaglobulinemia, congenital hypogammaglobulinemia with or without nodular lymphoid hyperplasia, and a variety of other conditions charac-

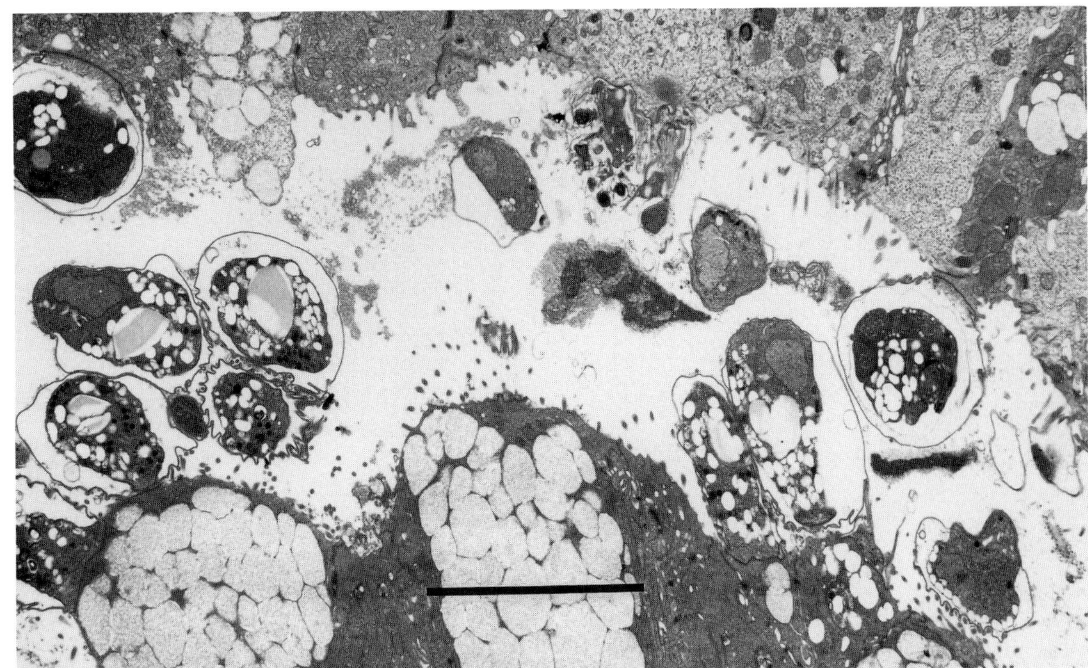

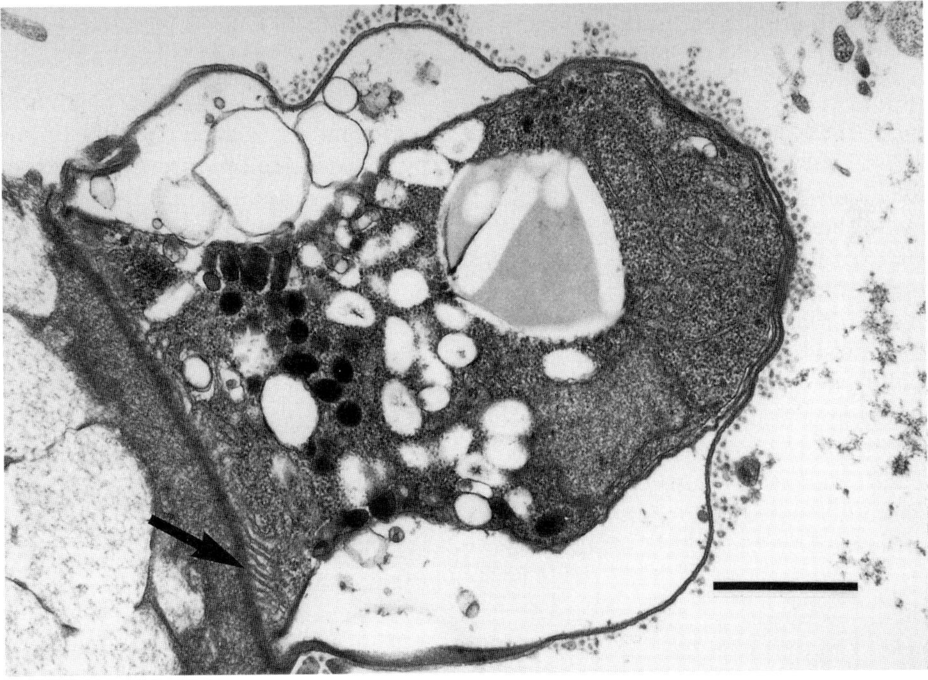

Fig. 6-16. (A) Electron micrograph of numerous cryptosporidia in various stages of development, present in the lumen and on the surface of the intestinal crypt epithelia (× 4,750; bar = 5 μm). **(B)** Macrogamete of *Cryptosporidium* on the surface of an intestinal epithelial cell, showing electron-dense and electron-lucent granules. The parasite membrane forms complex folds (arrow) at the attachment site, and a membrane of host cell origin surrounds the organism (× 19,000; bar = 1 μm).

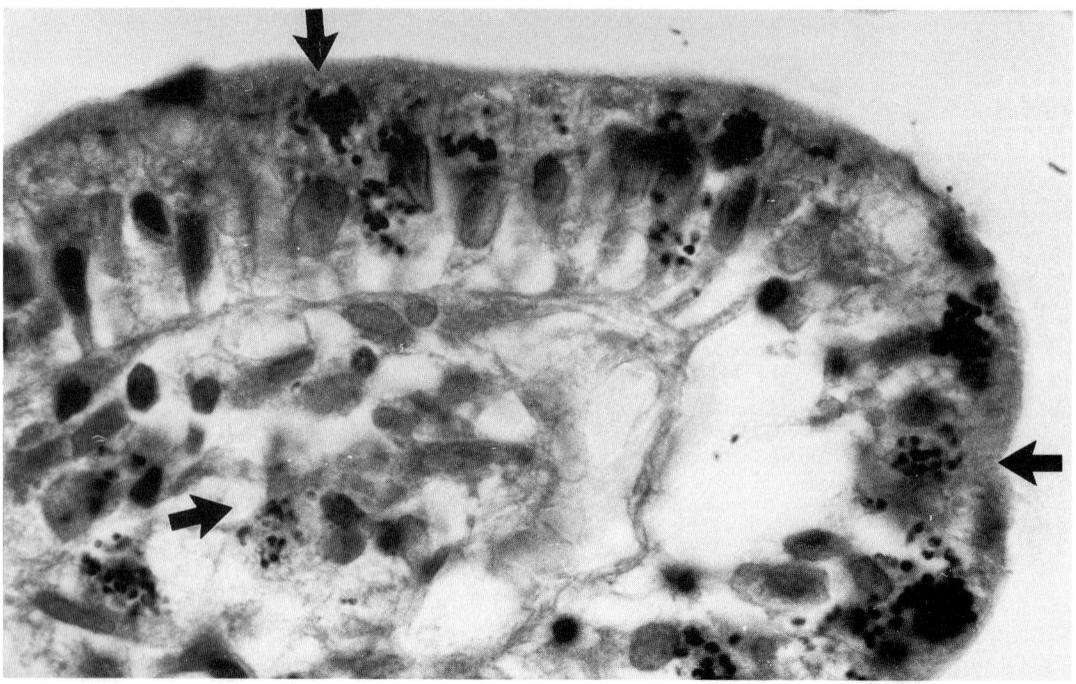

Fig. 6-17. Microsporidiosis in the duodenum, due to *Septata intestinalis.* Numerous spores, seen as dense granules, are present in the absorptive cells of the villi and also in macrophages within the lamina proporia (arrows) (Gram stain, × 1060).

terized by defects in the B and/or T lymphocytes.[191–193] As mentioned above, many of these patients present with secondary infections, and these are often appreciated in endoscopic examination of the duodenum. Most notable are those due to *Giardia, Cryptosporidium,* Microsporidia, and mycobacterial infections. The biopsy can help in identifying the particular immune disorder, such as demonstrating reduced plasma cells, and also can provide the identification of the particular organism. These conditions have been mainly studied in the jejunum and are thus principally presented in Chapter 7.

Acquired Conditions

Acquired conditions include patients who have received anti-inflammatory or immunosuppressive therapy for various inflammatory and tumor conditions as well as for transplant preservation; cases of AIDS; patients with tumors, particularly lymphomas, that may be associated with immune suppression; and those receiving bone marrow or small bowel transplants.[129, 194–198] The effects on the small bowel are highly variable, but a major development is the presence of opportunistic infections, as described above. These eventually limit the use of immunosuppressive therapy or chemotherapy in many patients, and are often the determining factor in the prognosis of the AIDS cases. In all of these patients, mucosal biopsy of the duodenum and other parts of the gut are commonly obtained to look for the organisms as well as evidence of injury.

With the bone marrow transplants, the problem is mainly of a graft-versus-host reaction.[195–197] In the early stages there are the effects of the radiation and immunosuppressive drugs used, resulting in focal ulcers that largely heal. After about 3 weeks, the

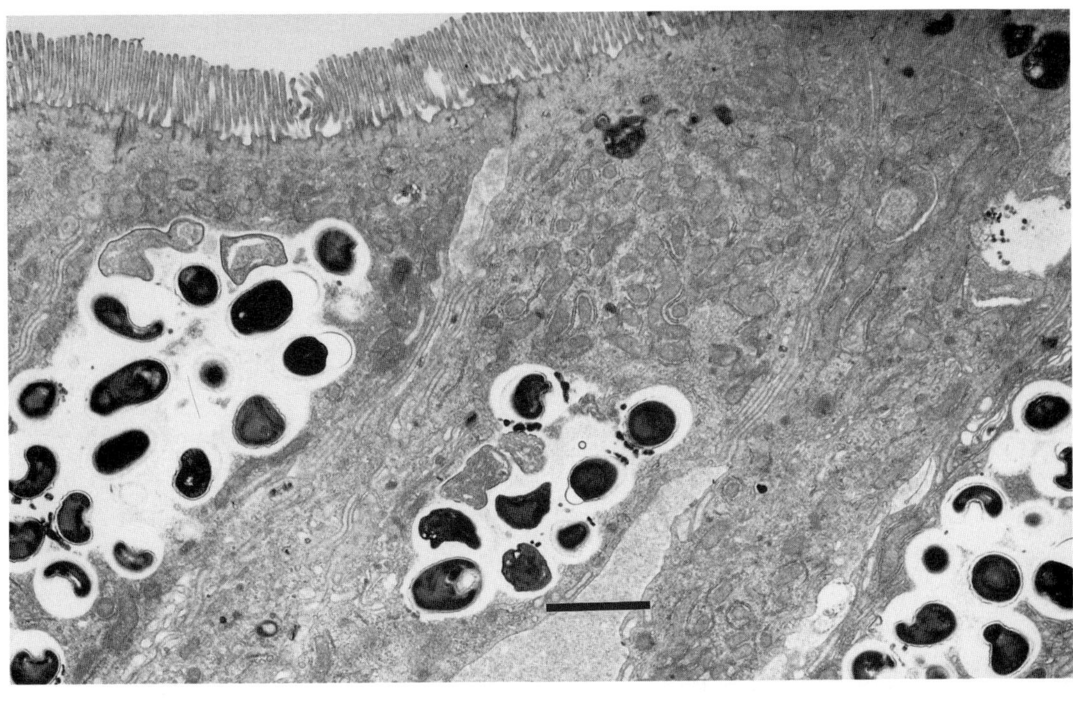

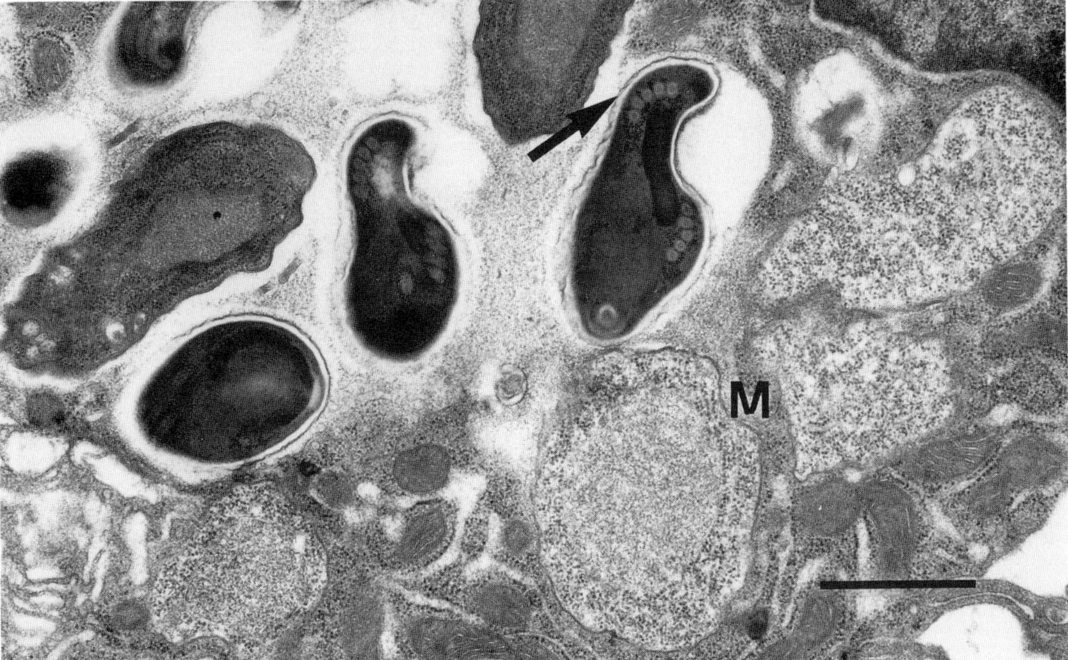

Fig. 6-18. (A) Electron micrograph of *Septata intestinalis* in the villous epithelial cells of the duodenum. Various stages of the organism are seen in the parasitophorous vacuoles with honeycomb-like chambers (× 6,250; bar = 2 μm). **(B)** Electron micrograph of *Septata intestinalis* spores, showing single row of cross sections of polar filament coil (arrow), which is characteristic of this species of Microsporidia. Meront stages (M) are also seen in this micrograph (× 20,000; bar = 1 μm). (*Figure continues.*)

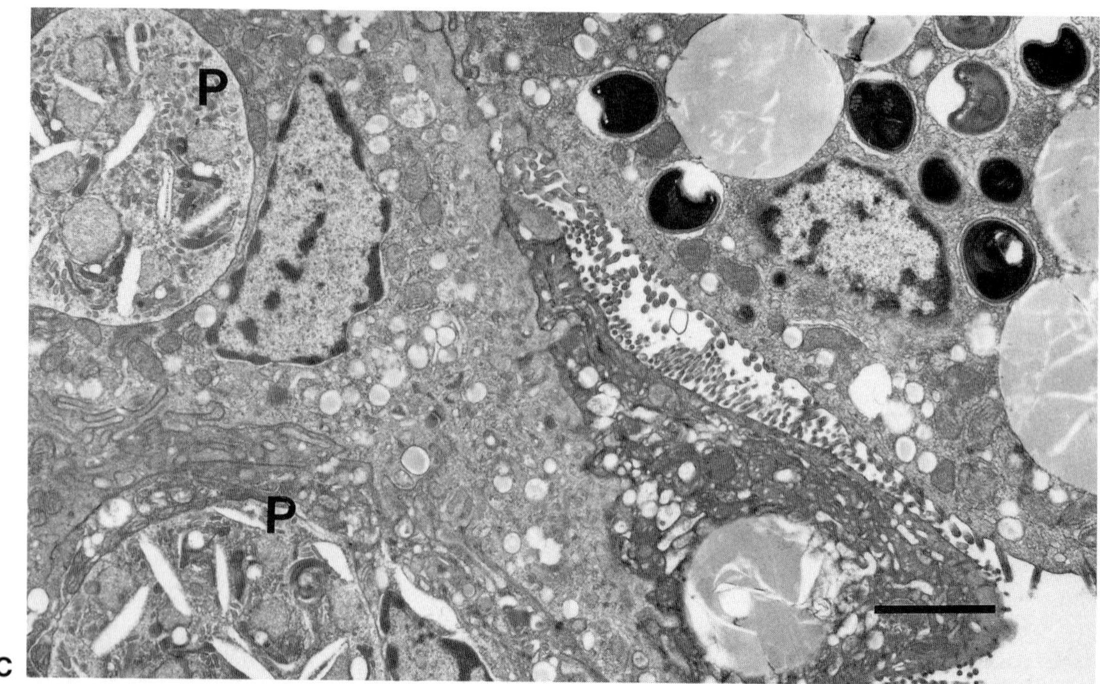

C

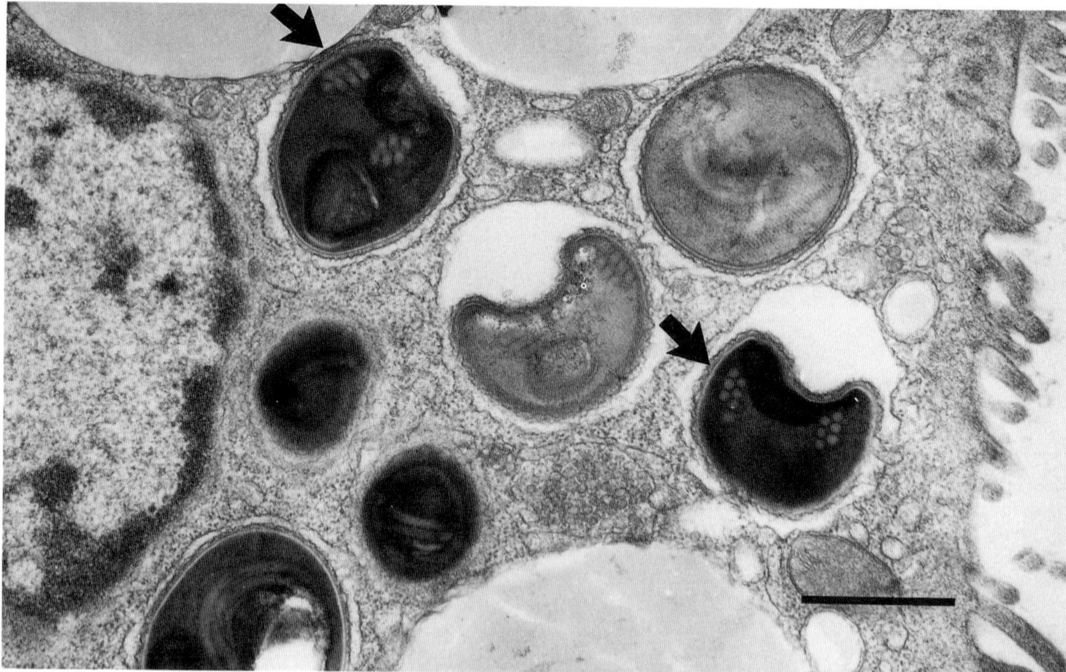

D

Fig. 6-18 (*Continued*). **(C)** Electron micrograph of the Microsporidia, *Enterocytozoon bieneusi* in the villous epithelial cells of duodenum. The plasmodium stage (P) shows polar tube formation, and spores are seen singly in the cytoplasm without vacuole formation (× 7,500; bar = 2 μm). **(D)** Electron micrograph of *Enterocytozoon bieneusi* spores with characteristic double rows of cross sections of polar filament coil (arrows) (× 20,000; bar = 1 μm).

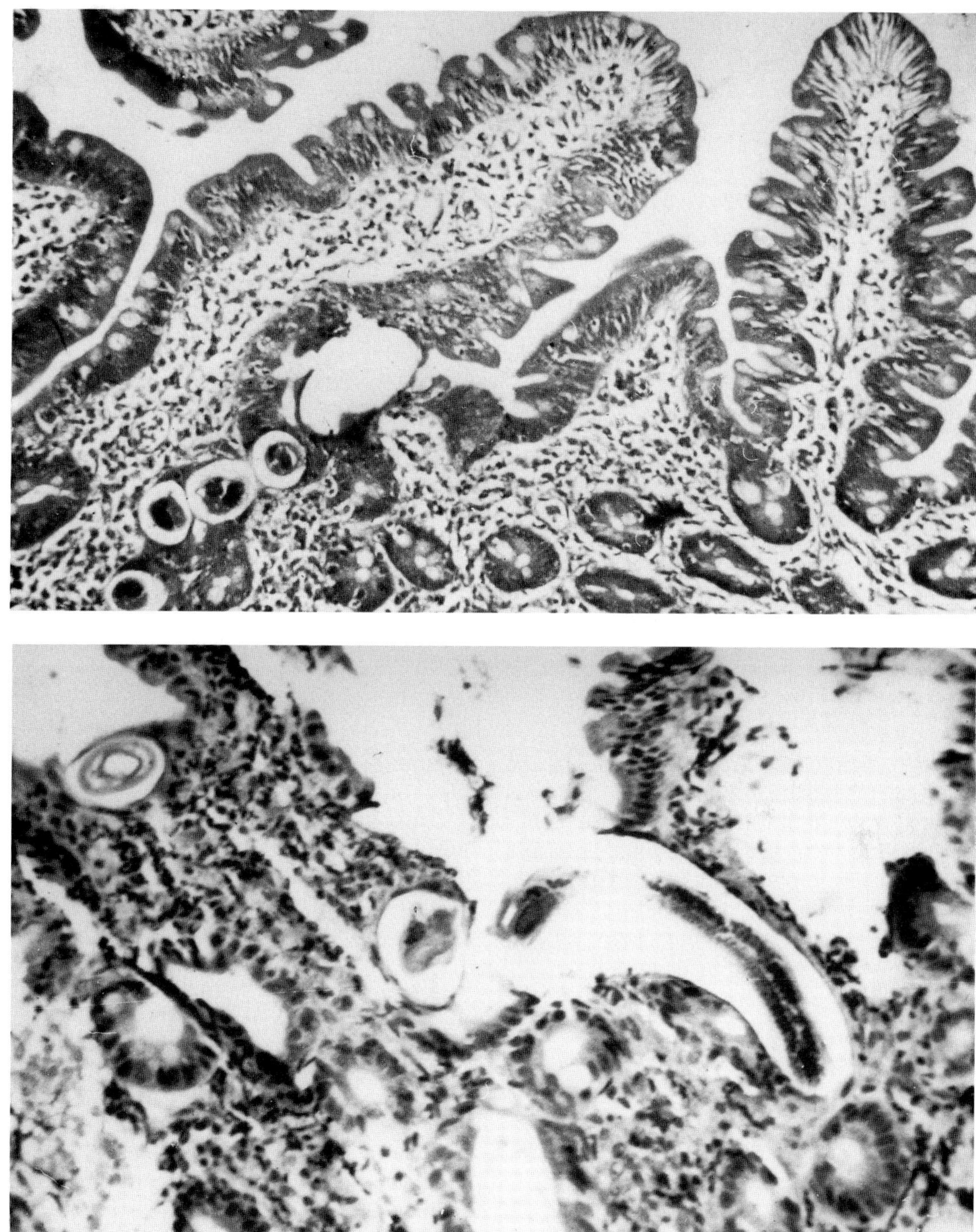

Fig. 6-19. *Strongyloides* infection in the duodenum. **(A)** Several eggs are present in the crypt region appearing at the lower left. **(B)** Fragments of larvel forms are seen in the mucosa, associated with a marked eosinophilic infiltrate.

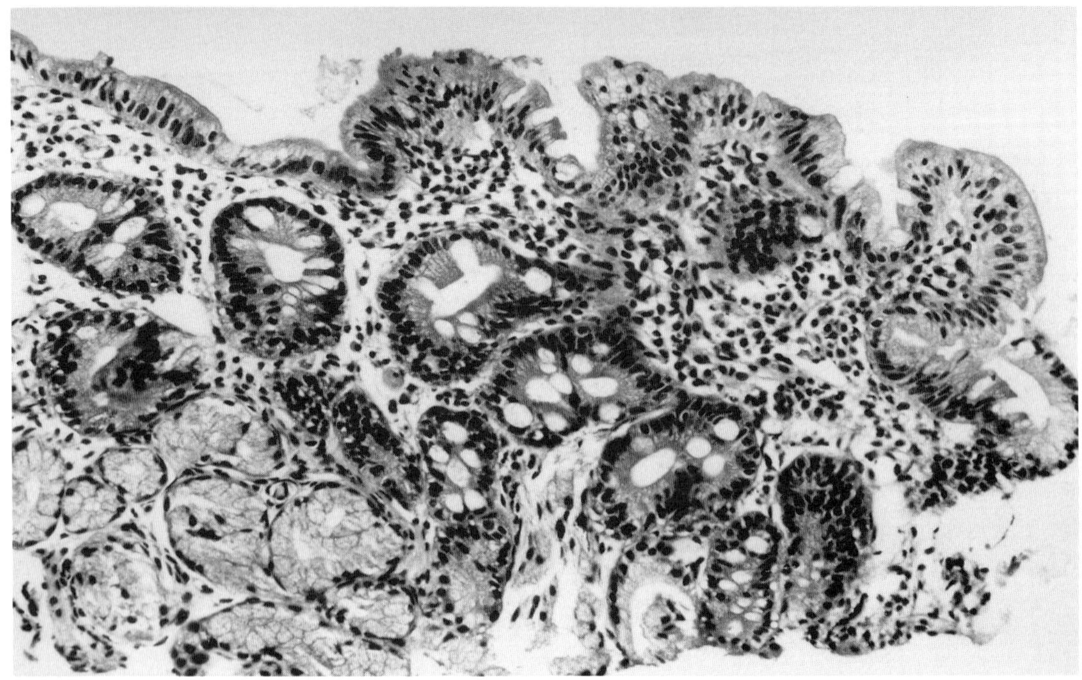

Fig. 6-20. Allergic enteritis in the duodenum. Seen are areas of villous shortening and a prominent infiltrate of eosinophils, mainly in the lamina propria with focal extension into the epithelial layer (top center and right) (× 210).

changes that occur are mainly due to the graft-versus-host reaction. These are characterized by the infiltrate of mononuclear cells largely into the crypt region, leading to loss of villous development, ulcer formation, and secondary infections. The features can be seen in any part of the small intestine and are often associated with prominent fungal infections.

Table 6-6. Immunologic Disorders of the Duodenum

Allergic (eosinophilic) gastroenteritis
Primary immunodeficiency conditions
Selective IgA deficiency
Transient hypogammaglobulinemia of infants
X-linked agammaglobulinemia
Hypogammaglobulinemia with nodular lymphoid hyperplasia
Other defects in B and/or T lymphocytes
Acquired immunodeficiency conditions
Prolonged treatment with anti-inflammatory and immunosuppressive drugs
Acquired immunodeficiency syndrome
Tumors (mainly lymphomas)
Bone marrow transplant leading to graft-versus-host reaction
Small intestinal transplant

There have been initial studies on small bowel transplants, and biopsy surveillance is largely from the distal end through an ileostomy area.[198] The features range from the monuclear infiltrate in classic rejection to more extensive hemorrhagic necrosis. Duodenal biopsy is not employed in these cases as yet.

BENIGN MUCOSAL TUMORS

Compared to the other parts of the gut, lesions of the small intestine, including the duodenum, are much less common (Table 6-7). Except for certain polyposis cases, the nodules are largely non-neoplastic. Nevertheless, practically all sorts of tumors can occur, and they tend to be more easily detected in the duodenum (probably because of the ease of access by upper endoscopy) as compared to the jejunum and ileum (see Table 3-2).

Table 6-7. Tumors of the Duodenum

Benign mucosal tumors
Non-neoplastic nodules
Adenoma
Polyposis syndromes
Adenocarcinoma
Endocrine tumors
Carcinoid and composite tumors
Neuroendocrine carcinoma
Lymphoid tumors
Benign hyperplasia
Malignant lymphomas
Mesenchymal tumors
Benign tumors
Undifferentiated stromal tumors
Sarcomas
Other primary tumors
Choriocarcinoma and melanoma
Adenosquamous cell carcinoma
Sarcomatoid carcinoma
Secondary and metastatic tumors

Hyperplastic and Heterotopic Nodules

When encountering a small nodule in the duodenal mucosa, the likely diagnoses are Brunner's gland hyperplasia, a hyperplastic lymphoid nodule, or a focus of heterotopic stomach.[199, 200] Less often are ectopic pancreatic tissue and cysts mostly of the Brunner's gland tissue. The nodules of Brunner's gland hyperplasia have been erroneously termed *adenomas,* but lack any cytologic atypism. They are comprised of compact cells that are greatly distended with neutral mucin, and there is virtually no dysplasia (Fig. 6-21). Occasional Brunner's gland nodules are seen with less conspicuous mucus, with more prominent ductal proliferation, or with cyst formation. An actual adenoma of the Brunner's gland, however, has not been adequately described.

Inflammatory and Hamartomatous Polyps

Single and multiple lesions composed of inflammatory tissue can be found, probably representing excess regenerative tissue in cases of duodenitis. Some of these have prominent fibromuscular stroma, edema, and eosinophils, and have been termed *inflammatory fibroid polyps*[201, 202] (see Fig. 8-11). In contrast to the lesions in the more distal small intestine, the inflammatory fibroid tumors tend to be small in the duodenum. Solitary polyps with admixture of mucosal tissue suggesting a hamartomatous nature have also been described but are less frequently seen than in a polyposis syndrome.[203, 204] Biopsy in all of these cases serves to distinguish the lesion from a neoplasm, either an adenoma or a malignant tumor.

Adenoma

Solitary adenomas of the tubular, or villous, type can occur in all parts of the small bowel including the duodenum.[205–208] They tend to be congregated in the region of the ampulla and only cause problems when they get large. Such lesions may cause partial obstruction of the bile ductal region or develop secondary carcinoma leading to ulceration and bleeding. There are examples of very large villous adenomas occupying several centimeters. These lesions can produce protein loss, whereas any electrolyte seepage is reabsorbed in the distal small intestine.

The adenomas are suspected grossly by their larger size and papillary surface. Histologic features are characteristic and similar to adenomas in any other part of the gut, revealing the composition of dysplastic cells. These show elongation and palisading of the nuclei with varying degrees of hyperchromasia and loss of polarity (Fig. 6-22). As in other parts of the tract, the smaller lesions tend to show lesser degrees of dysplasia, and the larger lesions tend toward high grade. Paneth cell differentiation is very common, probably reflecting their normal presence in this area. The adenomas are definitely premalignant and require excision; when multiple tumors are encountered, the

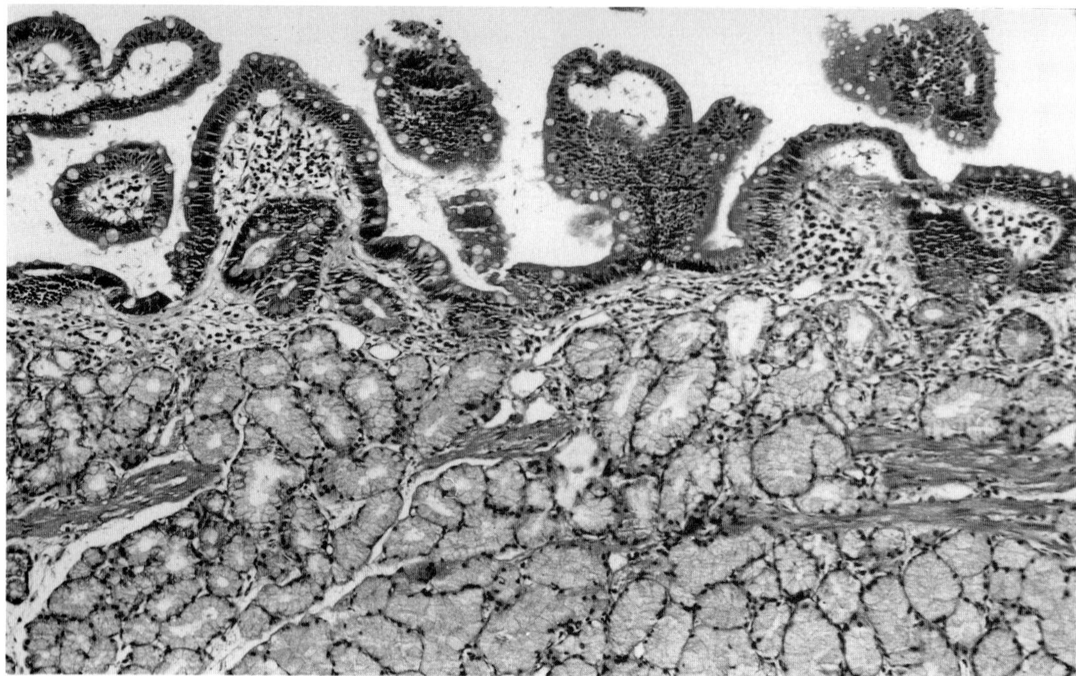

Fig. 6-21. Nodule of Brunner's gland hyperplasia in the duodenum. There is a marked proliferation of mature Brunner's glands in the submucosa (bottom) and extending into the mucosa. The overlying villi (top) are compressed and atrophic. The cells in the Brunner's glands show no cytologic atypism (× 105).

potential for an associated polyposis syndrome should be explored.

Polyposis Syndromes

Non-Neoplastic

The duodenum is commonly involved in all of the polyposis syndromes.[209,210] Less frequent are the lesions of juvenile polyps and of the Cronkhite-Canada syndrome, which are described in Chapter 5. The polyps of the Peutz-Jeghers syndrome are more characteristic, revealing hamartomas of the entire mucosa and showing a mixture of glands with broad bands of muscle tissue[211–214] (Fig. 6-23). These are seen in the small intestine in almost 90 percent of the cases, and can affect the duodenum as well. They present problems by the large size causing twisting around stalks and secondary ulceration; by obstruction due to simple mass or to intussusception; by extension into the underlying wall, causing a localized area of enteritis cystica profunda; and by developing secondary areas of carcinoma in the polyps or in other sites in the body. Overall, the syndrome is relatively rare, and polyps are removed that are causing clinical problems.

Neoplastic

The more significant polyposis syndrome is related to the development of multiple adenomas (Fig. 6-24). These are seen in the classical cases of adenomatous polyposis coli,[215–218] in the Gardner's variant,[219, 220] and in the flat adenoma of the colon syndrome.[221] In all of these cases multiple adenomas form

A

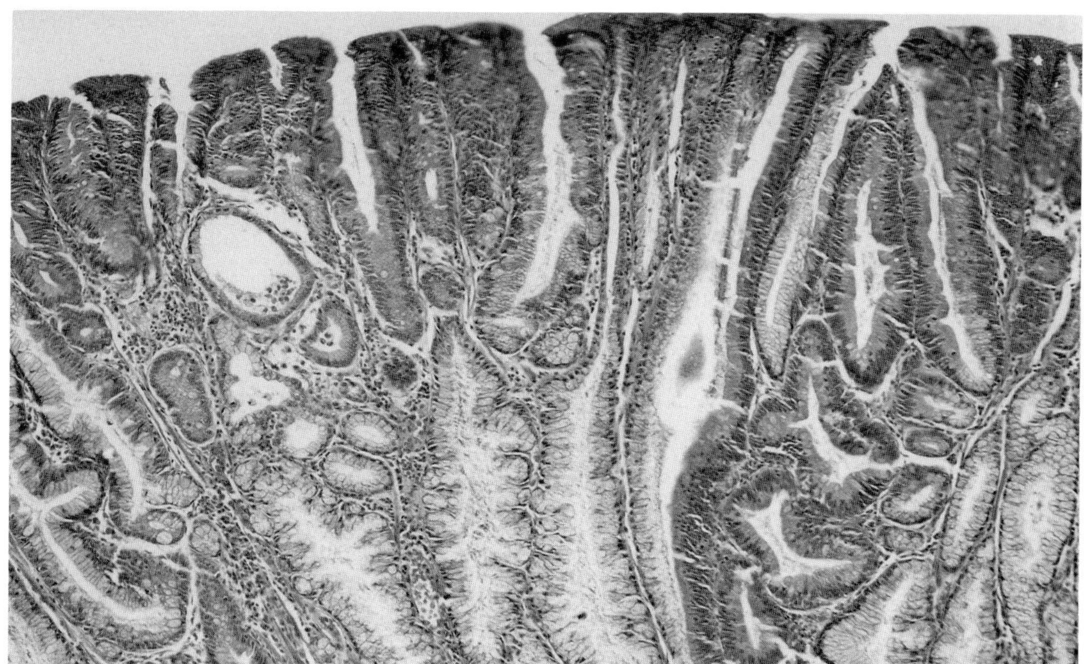

B

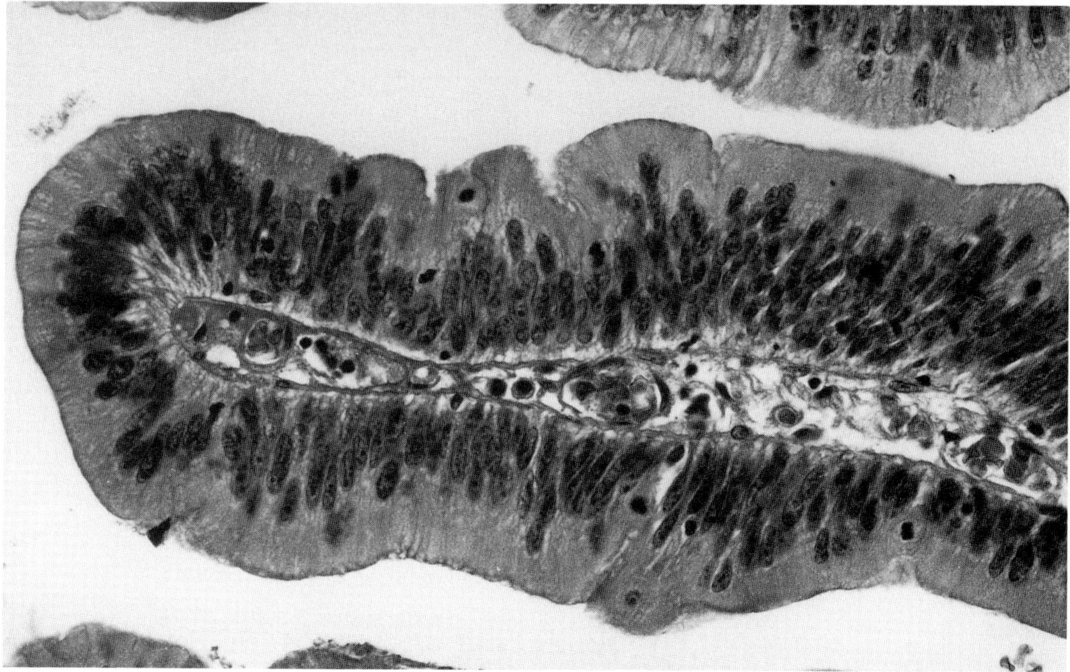

Fig. 6-22. Adenoma of the duodenum. **(A)** Example of tubular adenoma, composed of dysplastic epithelium (× 105). **(B)** Surface fronds showing the characteristic epithelium. There are elongation and palisading of the nuclei (× 425).

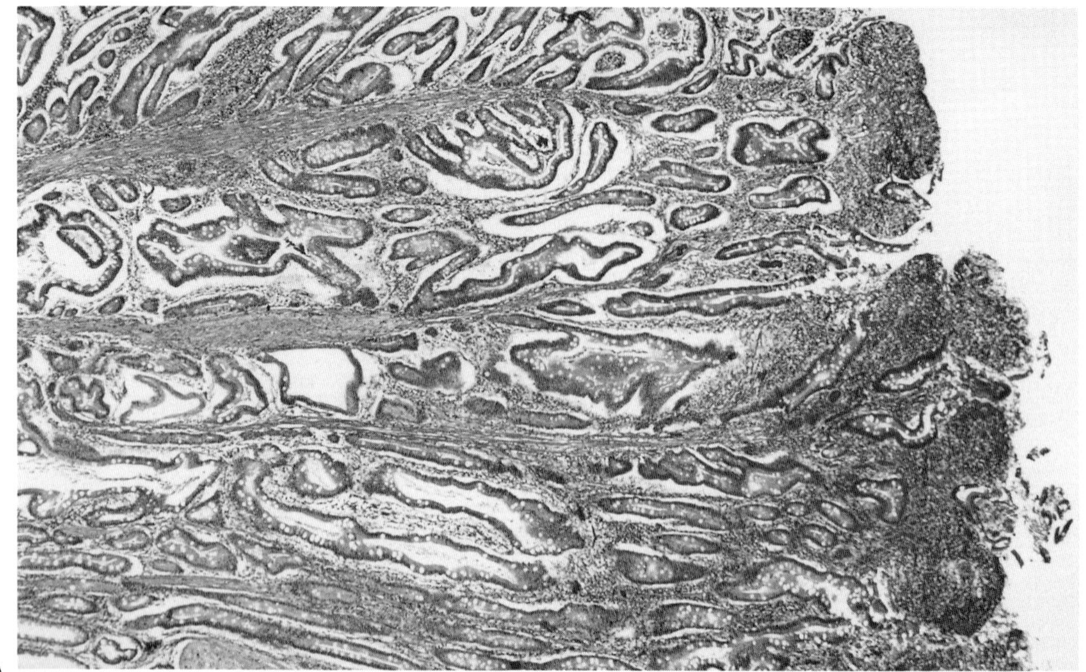

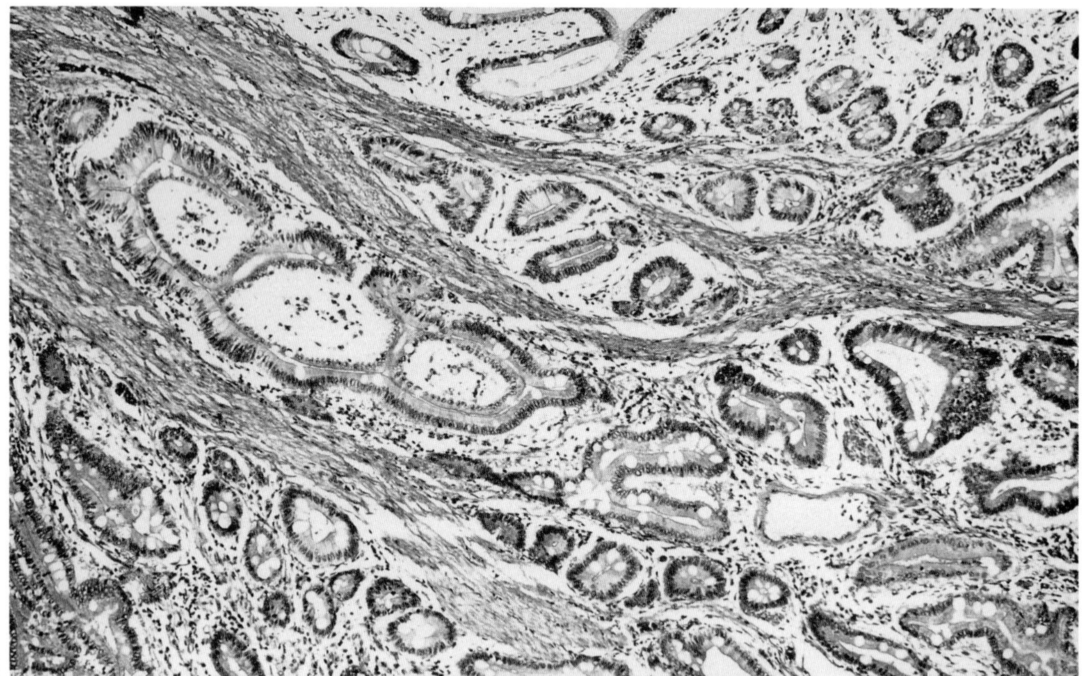

Fig. 6-23. Peutz-Jeghers polyp in the duodenum. **(A)** The polyp is composed of markedly elongated glands and a fibromuscular stroma. An erosion is seen on the surface appearing at the right; these may develop in the larger lesions (× 42). **(B)** The epithelia in the glands are mainly of the intestinal type and lack cytologic atypism. Noted is the prominent smooth muscle tissue in the lamina propria (× 105).

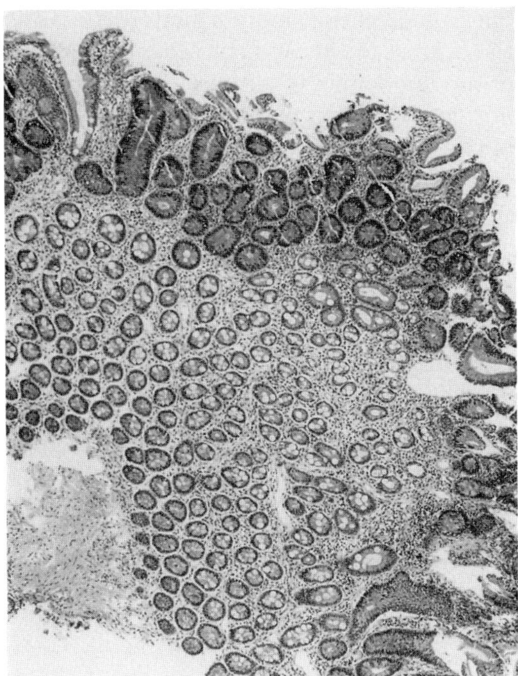

Fig. 6-24. Duodenal mucosal biopsy in a case of Gardner's syndrome. The surface (top) shows adenomatous change in the glands (× 42).

later in the stomach and duodenum, including the ampullary region, and they are prone to the further development of adenocarcinoma.[222–224] The lesions need to be removed either by polypectomy or by a larger operation. This becomes a bigger problem in the duodenum where the resection may require a Whipple-type of resection. (See discussion in Ch. 5 for further details.)

OTHER TUMORS

The benign lesions are more common, relatively small, and mostly incidental, whereas the malignant tumors of the small bowel vary in frequency. Although adenocarcinomas are relatively uncommon, there has been more attention recently on tumors derived from the endocrine, lymphoid, and mesenchymal elements. With the availability of endoscopy there has been greater detection of these tumors, but the effect on overall prognosis has not greatly improved. This may reflect the fact that many of these tumors arise in the wall and that their finding in the mucosal biopsies is a relatively late feature.

ADENOCARCINOMA

Frequency and Premalignant Conditions

Compared to other parts of the gut, adenocarcinoma of the small bowel is decidedly uncommon to rare.[225–229] Most lesions in the duodenum occur in association with prior adenomas, either of the duodenal mucosa proper or, particularly, in the ampullary region. There is an increased development in the patients with adenomatous polyposis and with the Lynch syndromes. A greater frequency of carcinoma has also been noted in patients with celiac disease,[230–232] with AIDS,[233] and with other chronic inflammatory conditions involving the small intestine including, in particular, Crohn's disease. There have been claims of an increase in cases due to other chronic infections, such as tuberculosis and schistosomiasis, affecting the intestinal tract, but these are now rare. Of interest, and unlike other parts of the gut, there is no increase in dysplasia or adenocarcinoma development in the common cases of chronic peptic duodenitis. There is also no relation of carcinoma to chronic peptic ulcer. Indeed, whereas the ulcer tends to be in the first portion of the duodenum, the carcinoma is preferentially in other portions of the duodenum.

Biopsy Features

Most tumors present in association with adenomas or as separate ulcerated lesions. They can be suspected grossly, and biopsy readily confirms their nature, revealing the irregular and dysplastic glands together with invasion[224, 234] (Fig. 6-25A). Less commonly seen are tumors mainly comprised of signet ring cells, [235] like those in the stomach, and the presence of prominent Paneth cells in the neoplastic glands.[236] It is important to look for evidence of adenoma in the biopsies, which, if present, secures that the lesion is primary in the duodenal mucosa. Adenocarcinomas from the pancreas and bile duct can extend into the duodenum; these are more common than the primary carcinomas, and the external ones would not show the associated adenoma. This might be helpful information in planning for any possible surgery. Biopsies are largely done to identify the tumor and to determine its extent.

Adenosquamous Cell Carcinoma

Adenosquamous cell carcinoma is a rare variant that contains both glandular and squamous elements[225, 237] (see Fig. 3-17). These tend to be aggressive lesions, and are typically detected at a late stage.

Ampullary Carcinoma

In identifying tumors of the duodenum, it is necessary to sort out those that arise in the ampullary region, which more commonly present with earlier symptoms because of their proximity to the bile duct lumen[238–240] (Fig. 6-25B). Accordingly, the carcinomas in the ampullary region tend to have a much better prognosis than the other carcinomas. They have been broadly separated into those arising in the ampulla, which have the best prognosis; tumors affecting the periampullary region, with an intermediate behavior; and the lesions arising from the rest of the duodenum and adjacent tissues, all of which have generally poor prognoses. Histologic examination is not helpful in distinguishing the tumors from the various locales, since all are adenocarcinomas with varying degrees of differentiation. Most are well differentiated, but this does not imply a better prognosis. In contrast to the stomach, adenocarcinoma of the duodenum is still rare, and there does not need to be as active a concern over the peptic ulcers in this region.

Endocrine Tumors

The duodenum is one of the sites where there is a relatively greater amount of endocrine tumors.[241] It is estimated that about 5 percent of the gastrinomas responsible for the Zollinger–Ellison syndrome occur in the wall of the duodenum.[242–245] These are typically small, on the order of 1 to 2 cm in diameter, and it is important to consider this location in a case without an evident pancreatic mass.

Carcinoid Tumors

Also observed in the duodenum are other forms of neuroendocrine tumors that are well differentiated and associated with multiple syndromes.[246–248] The tumors may present as polyps or as infiltrative masses but are usually small (Fig. 6-26). They are comprised of mature cells in the form of nests and ribbons with a monomorphic appearance, and most behave in a relatively benign fashion. Most common of the functional types are the tumors producing somatostatin, and these frequently have concentric whorls of calcium resembling psammoma bodies.[249–252] These tumors may or may not be associated with the syndrome leading to diarrhea and a rash. Rarer tumors produce glucagon, insulin, or vasoactive intestinal polypeptide.

In all of these cases the biopsy readily identifies the tumor and provides a suspicion of a neuroendocrine lesion, based on the epithelial character with little dysplasia. Immunocytochemical stains for chromogranin and synaptophysin can help established the neuroendocrine nature, and further specific

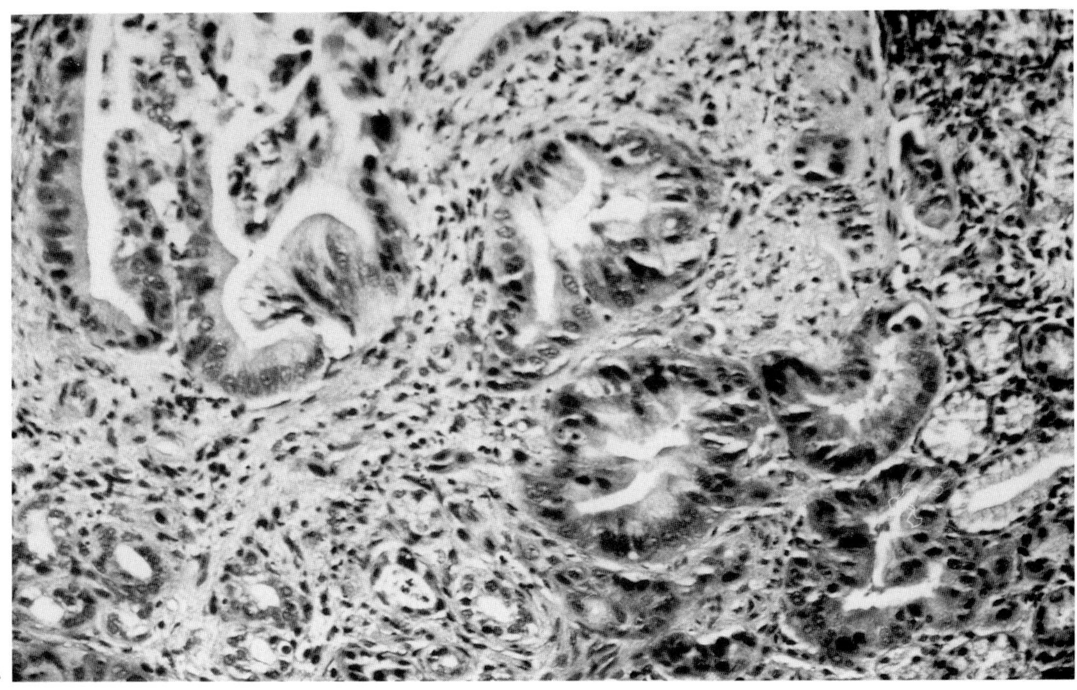

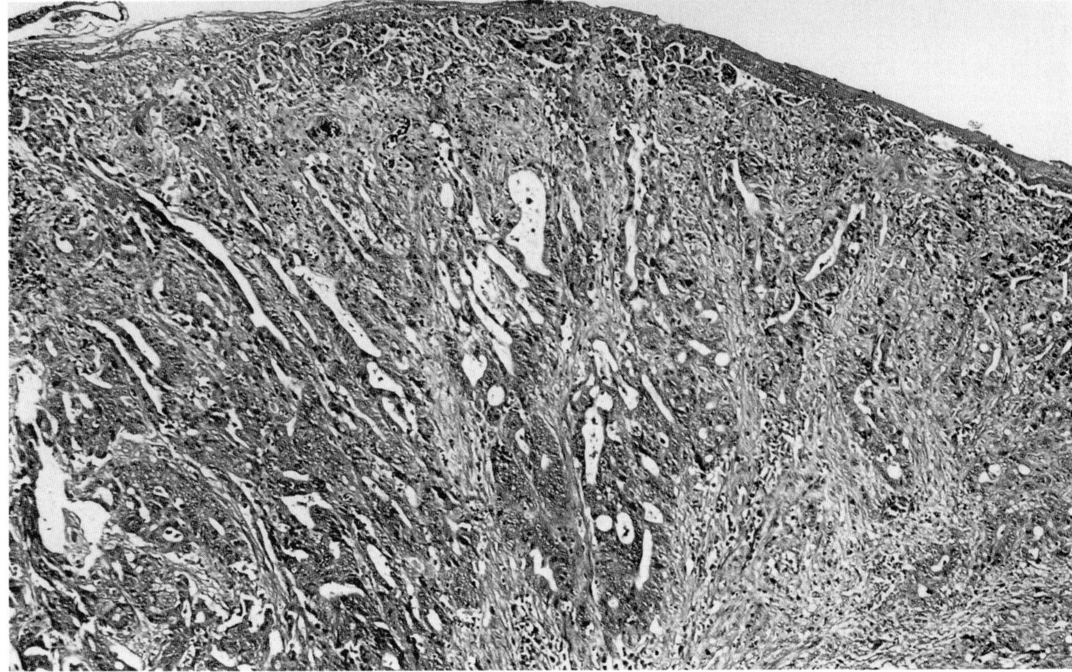

Fig. 6-25. (A) Adenocarcinoma of the duodenum in a mucosal biopsy. The tumor is composed of glands of variable size. There are compressed normal glands appearing at the right (× 210). **(B)** Adenocarcinoma of the ampullary region in the duodenum. There is a tumor mass composed of highly irregular glands, with invasion into the stroma (× 85).

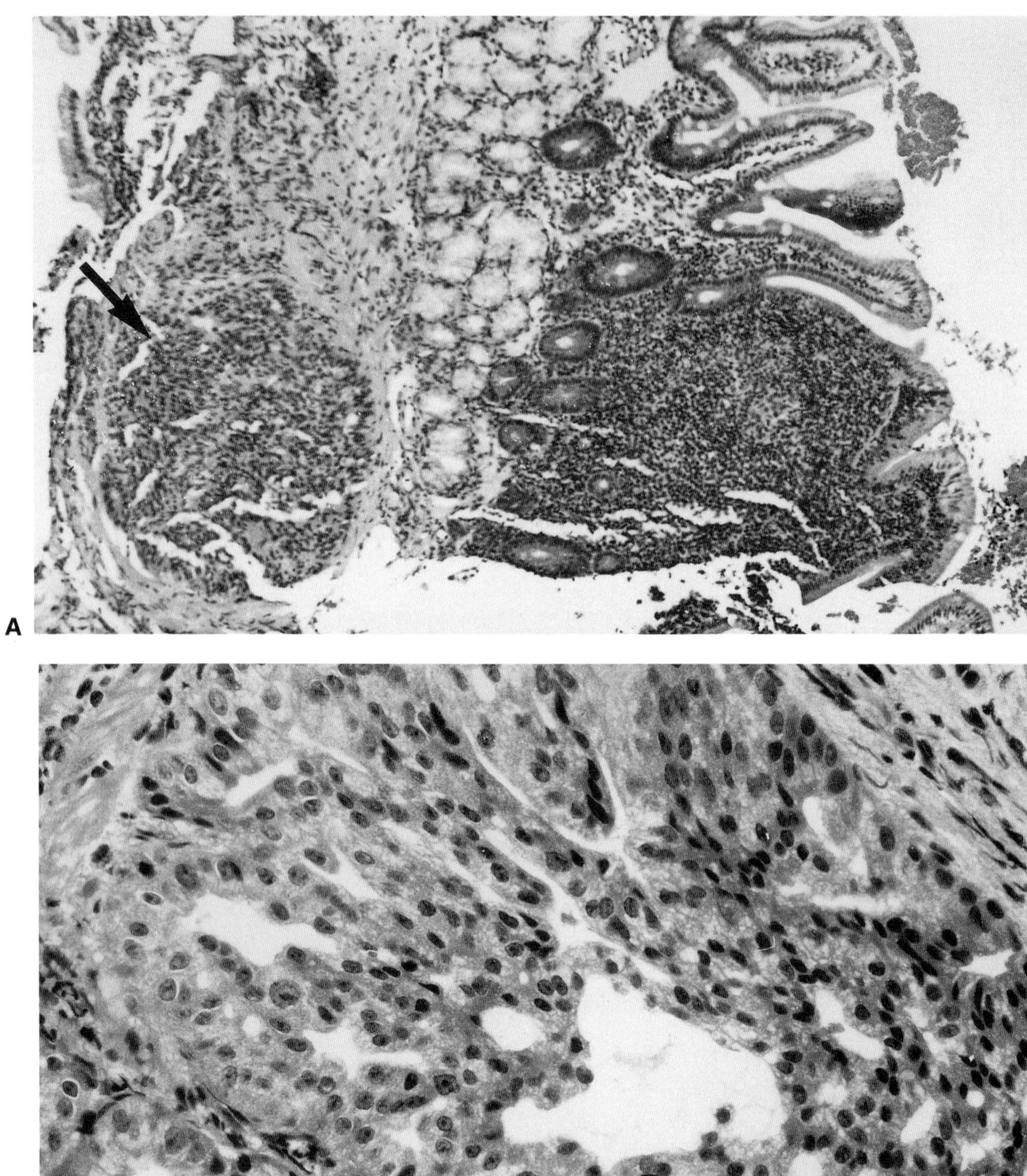

Fig. 6-26. Carcinoid tumor in the duodenum. **(A)** Duodenal biopsy, with surface appearing at right. A tumor nodule is present in the upper part of the submucosa (arrow at lower left). The overlying mucosa at the right reveals a lymphoid nodule and hyperplastic Brunner's glands (× 105). **(B)** Nodule of carcinoid tumor showing trabeculae and microglands composed of regular cells with little atypism (× 425).

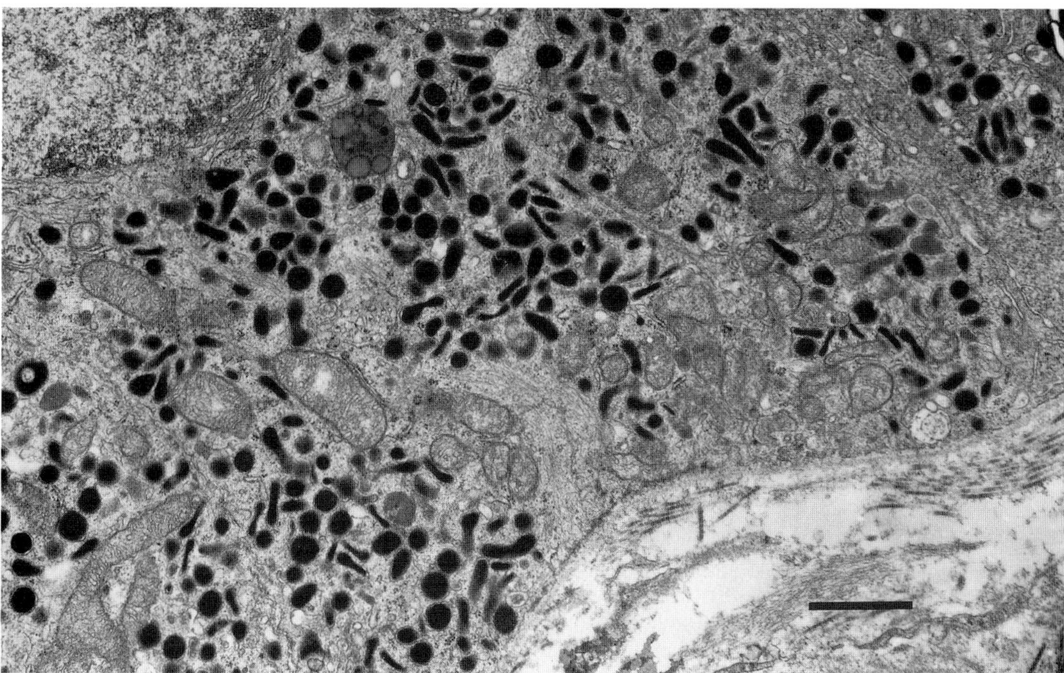

Fig. 6-27. Electron micrograph of a carcinoid tumor. The cytoplasm contains numerous pleomorphic, elliptical membrane-bound granules with electron-dense cores characteristic of a mid-gut carcinoid. These features are more typical of tumors seen in a distal duodenum, jejunum, and ileum (× 12,500; bar = 1 μm).

stains for gastrin, somatostatin, and other hormones can be done. The specific features that are noted in the ultrastructure of these cells can also help in their definition (Figs. 6-4 and 6-27).

Composite Tumors

Composite tumors are adenomas and adenocarcinomas in which there is a portion comprised of neuroendocrine cells.[237, 253] The latter tends to be the minor part, and the prognosis is largely related to the presence of carcinoma and its stage. There are rarer tumors in this area with a greater admixture of cells, termed *adenocarcinoid tumors.*[254, 255] Most of these composite lesions are nonfunctional. The biopsy readily shows the two components, which can be sorted out by special stains.

Neuroendocrine carcinoma

Small cell carcinomas are rarely noted in the small bowel, including the duodenum.[256] These are comprised of small oval cells with scant cytoplasm and hyperchromatic nuclei, equivalent in appearance to the oat cell carcinomas of the lung (see Fig. 3-19). Their nature can be supported by immunocytochemical stains and by ultrastructure showing scattered electron-dense granules. They rarely cause functional syndromes and are highly aggressive tumors, but are exceptionally rare in this area.

Lymphoid Tumors

This subject is more extensively covered in Chapters 5 and 7 and is briefly mentioned here.

Benign Hyperplasia

There are scattered, well formed lymphoid nodules in the normal duodenal mucosa, and these are often increased in cases of chronic peptic duodenitis and of other chronic inflammatory conditions that affect this area, such as Crohn's disease. More prominent degrees of lymphoid hyperplasia can be seen in a focal or more diffuse fashion throughout the duodenum and jejunum.[257, 258] These tend to be more common in children, can be appreciated by radiographic as well as by endoscopic study, and most eventually subside. In adults, there is greater concern when there is a persistence of a diffuse lymphoid lesion, raising the possibility of a lymphoproliferative disorder and of an early lymphoma. Such cases require multiple samples for histology and usually material for cell clonality as well to make a definitive diagnosis[259] (see Ch. 5).

Malignant Lymphoma

These can present in the small bowel as localized masses,[260–263] as diffuse or multinodular tumors, and as multiple polyposis.[264, 265] In all instances, multiple samples are desirable to make the diagnosis.[266] As in the stomach, the high-grade lesions are readily recognized as neoplasms because of the large irregular cells, and stains may help in sorting out carcinoma from lymphoma. In the small bowel, the likelihood of carcinoma is so low that the great majority of these cases prove to be lymphoma. Greater difficulties are encountered with the low-grade tumors because of the relatively small size of the cells, and studies of clonality are often needed. The lymphomas tend to be characterized by diffuse infiltrates of relatively monomorphic cells that extend from the surface epithelium through the muscularis mucosae into the submucosa. The Mediterranean type of lymphoma, also termed *immunoproliferative small intestinal disease (IPSID),* is typically associated with a preexisting chronic enteritis characterized by a marked proliferation of plasma cells that eventually become monotypic, and many of these cases are associated with alpha-chain disease.[267–272] The biopsy features have been best characterized in the jejunum and are described in that chapter.

There are several conditions that appear to predispose to the development of intestinal lymphoma, including celiac disease,[273–276] immunodeficiency states,[277, 278] the IPSID, and possibly chronic idiopathic inflammatory bowel disease.

Probably the most difficult diagnosis of lymphoma is that associated with celiac disease.[279] Most of these cases appear to be of the T-cell vintage, and they typically present as very focal lesions. Alarm signals in the patient are the presence of nonresponsiveness to therapy, the appearance of ulcers in the small intestine or stomach,[275, 276] and the presence of unusually atypical cells in the lamina propria. Such cases call for more extensive sectioning as well as examination of the bone marrow. Other types of malignant lymphoma that can be encountered in the small bowel include MALT-associated lesions,[280, 281] follicular lymphomas,[282] histiocytic tumors,[283, 284] and Hodgkin's disease.[285] All of these lymphomatous disorders are presented in more detail in Chapter 7.

Mesenchymal Tumors

Nearly all mesenchymal tumors can affect the small intestine, including the duodenum, and they may exceptionally be sampled in a biopsy. (The general presentation of this subject is given in Ch. 5).

Benign Tumors

Well formed leiomyomas are typically small and mural lesions without mucosal extension[286] (see Fig. 3-20). Rarely observed are granular cell tumors (cf. Fig. 3-21), hemangiomas, and lipomas.[287–289] The latter may be biopsied, revealing an overlying atrophic mucosa and the characteristic mature adipose tissue. They tend to be more common in the ileum but can occur in the proximal small intestine as well.

Uncommonly noted in the mucosa are gangliocytic paragangliomas, which tend to be congreated in the ampullary region.[290, 291] These are often associated with cases of neurofibromatosis or with other duodenal tumors such as adenocarcinoma. The tumors show irregular nests of clear cells in a stroma that appears to be of neural origin and that contains ganglion cells. Special stains support a neuroendocrine nature for the epithelial cells. These are positive with Grimelius' argyrophilic stain and with several of the other more specific antibody stains. There are also paragangliomas that lack the neurofibromatous type of stroma.[292]

Undifferentiated Stromal Tumors

Undifferentiated stromal tumors are the gastrointestinal tumors arising in the wall that fail to show regular muscle or nerve differentiation and that may or may not be associated with elements of the autonomic nervous system[293] (see Figs. 5-24 and 5-25). They are described in more detail in Chapter 5. Tumors in the small intestine, including the duodenum, tend to be more aggressive with greater likelihood of invasion and metastases than those in the stomach. Biopsies are only helpful when the tumor extends into and causes erosion of the overlying mucosa, at which time samples of the tumors can be obtained.[294]

Sarcomas

Kaposi's sarcoma is frequently seen in patients with AIDS.[295–299] This can affect all parts of the alimentary tract, and the lesions are highly distinctive grossly, revealing a ragged vascular surface. The biopsies are also typical, showing the compact proliferation of the enlarged spindle cells with fresh areas of hemorrhage (Fig. 6-28). This needs to be distinguished from ordinary granulation tissue, which has a looser stroma and is often associated with an ulcer and acute inflammation. Other sarcomas are mainly of muscle origin and overlap with the topic of stromal tumors.[300, 301]

OTHER PRIMARY TUMORS

Rarely observed in the duodenum are choriocarcinomas,[302, 303] malignant melanomas,[304] and carcinomas with sarcomatoid elements.[305] These are similar to the tumors described in other organs (see Chs. 3 and 5). All of these lesions tend to behave in an aggressive fashion. Considering their distinctive features, biopsy should provide the specific diagnosis in most cases. It is important, however, to exclude metastases, since these lesions are more apt to be a primary tumor in some other site.

SECONDARY AND METASTATIC TUMORS

Many tumors can spread to the duodenum; the most likely are those coming from adjacent organs, including the stomach carcinomas and lymphomas that cross the pylorus, the pancreatic adenocarcinomas, and the lesions arising from the ampulla and periampullary tissues.[306–308] Cancers can also spread to the retroperitoneal portion of the duodenum from the back of the colon and from the kidney. The diagnosis is largely established by the gross distribution of the tumor and is supported by biopsy material.

There can be metastatic disease from practically any tumor, but most common are malignant melanoma and carcinomas from

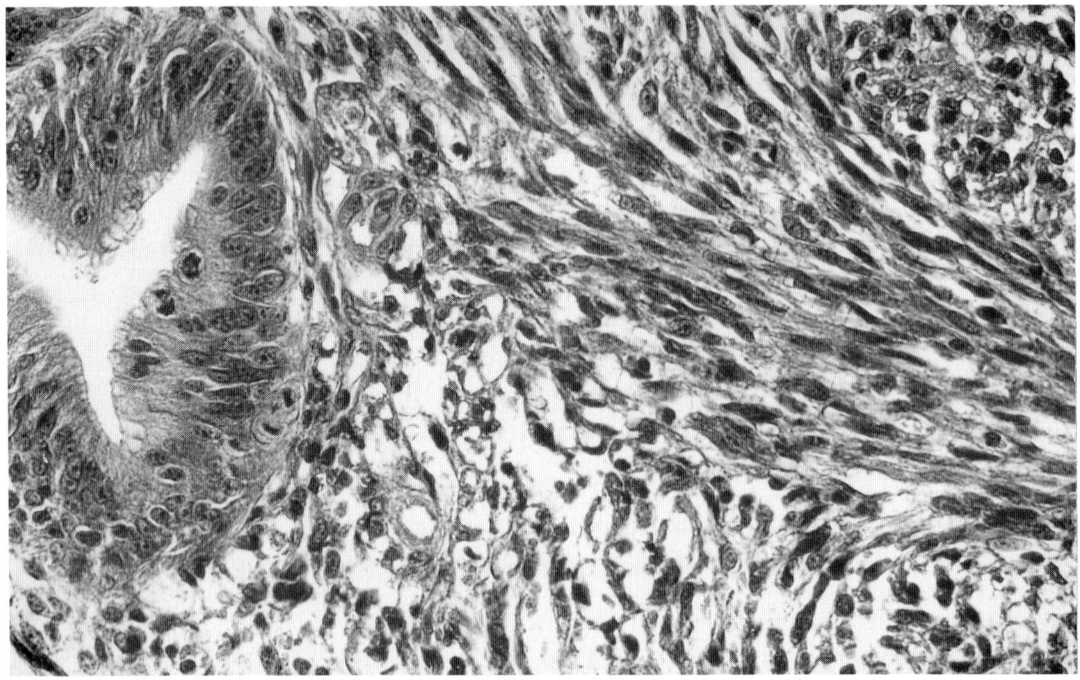

Fig. 6-28. Kaposi's sarcoma in the duodenum. The tumor is composed of compact spindle-shaped cells showing some variation in nuclear size and form. A gland appears at the left (× 425).

the lung and breast.[309–311] Rare sources include the cervix, ovaries, and kidneys.[312]

MISCELLANEOUS CONDITIONS

Physical Disorders

The major physical disorder is from the effects of radiation (see Table 7-5). This is principally provided in the form of therapy of primary or adjacent tumors, mainly lymphomas and retroperitoneal sarcomas. The mucosa is very sensitive to radiation, and there can result prompt arrest of crypt activity leading to necrosis and ulceration.[313–315] Chronic changes can result in an atrophy of the mucosa, which is further described in Chapter 7. The overall effects require more extensive small bowel disease to lead to poor absorption. Localized problems from stricture or fistula can occur but are rare.

Depositions

Melanosis

Melanosis is represented by a variety of dark pigments within the macrophages of the lamina propria.[316–319] Included are iron, sulfur, and other metal substances, and the lesion has also been termed *pseudomelanosis* because of the lack of true melanin material in most instances. Some cases are associated with lipofuscin substances similar to that seen in the colon. However, there is no relationship to laxative use. Rather, there appears to be an increase in this deposition in patients with chronic renal disease, but the connection is not known. The lesions are readily recognized grossly by their dark appearance and microscopically by the pigment. Stains may be needed to exclude hemosiderin. There is no known clinical problem.

Other Substances

Increases in iron can be seen in the macrophages in instances of hemosiderosis and in the epithelial cells in cases of hemochromatosis[320, 321] (Plate 4A). As with all parts of the small bowel, there can be amyloid deposition in the small vessels, which may lead to localized areas of hemorrhage and ulceration.[322] This is not a common site to employ biopsy to look for amyloid; rather, greater yields are seen in the stomach and in the rectum (Plate 4D and Fig. 9-46). The deposits seen in the many storage diseases may exceptionally be found in the duodenal mucosa,[323] and these are discussed in Chapter 7.

Granulomatous Diseases

Granulomatous diseases are usually due to chronic infections, including tuberculosis, other mycobacterial diseases, and schistosomal lesions; and to Crohn's disease. The lesions of Crohn's disease can be highly variable, ranging from microscopic foci of increased inflammation with rare granulomas to cases of extensive ulceration and fistula formation.[324–327] The diagnosis typically needs the finding in some other established area, such as the distal small intestine and colon, for confidence. Of patients with established Crohn's disease, microscopic findings can be found in the duodenum and stomach in almost one-half of the patients, but these do not necessarily presage eventual gross disease.[328–331]

Rarer cases of granuloma formation in the duodenum include examples of chronic granulomatous disease and of sarcoidosis[332–334] (see Table 4-12).

Metabolic Disorders

In patients with megaloblastic anemia, the altered cells can be appreciated in the epithelium of the small intestinal villi as well as in the blood cells.[335, 336] This has no clinical significance. Cases of myeloid metaplasia may show hematopoietic elements in the duodenal mucosa.[337, 338]

As mentioned previously, patients with chronic renal disease develop an assortment of lesions in the duodenum, including depositions of pseudomelanin, telangiectasias, hemorrhages, and ulcers.[339–341] The exact relation to the renal disease is not clear.

Other Disorders

Foci of macrophages containing fatty substances, termed *xanthomas,* can rarely be found in the duodenum and are probably related to localized areas of prior hemorrhage.[342] There have also been examples of deposition of collagen in the small bowel beneath the surface epithelium similar to that seen in the colon, and at least one instance of a combined finding of a collagenous enterocolitis.[343] These cases should be distinguished from the so-called collagenous sprue that probably represents a late and potentially refractory form of celiac disease.[344] The latter is not associated with the colonic disease.

REFERENCES

1. Goldman H, Antonioli DA: Mucosal biopsy of the esophagus, stomach and proximal duodenum. Hum Pathol 13:423–448, 1982
2. Sheahan DG, Rotterdam H: Duodenum. pp. 256–313. In Rotterdam H, Sheahan DG, Sommers SC (eds): Biopsy Diagnosis of the

Digestive Tract. 2nd Ed. Raven Press, New York, 1993

3. Chang MH, Wang TH, Hsu JY et al: Endoscopic examination of the upper gastrointestinal tract in infancy. Gastrointest Endosc 29:15–17, 1983
4. Komorowski RA, Beggs BK, Geenan JE, Venu RP: Assessment of ampulla of Vater pathology. An endoscopic approach. Am J Surg Pathol 15:1188–1196, 1991
5. Wald A, Milligan FD: The role of fiberoptic endoscopy in the diagnosis and management of duodenal neoplasms. Am J Dig Dis 20:499–505, 1975
6. Sharon P, Stalnikovicz R, Rachmilewitz D: Endoscopic diagnosis of duodenal neoplasms causing upper gastrointestinal bleeding. J Clin Gastroenterol 4:35–38, 1982
7. Blackman E, Nash SV: Diagnosis of duodenal and ampullary epithelial neoplasms by endoscopic biopsy: a clinicopathologic and immunohistochemical study. Hum Pathol 16:901–910, 1985
8. Scott BB, Jenkins D: Endoscopic small intestinal biopsy. Gastrointest Endosc 27:162–187, 1981
9. Gillberg R, Kastrup W, Mobachen H et al: Endoscopic duodenal biopsy compared with biopsy with the Watson capsule from the upper jejunum in patients with dermatitis herpetiformis. Scand J Gastroenterol 17:305–308, 1982
10. Mee AS, Burke M, Vallon AG et al: Small bowel biopsy for malabsorption: comparison of the diagnostic accuracy of endoscopic forceps and capsule biopsy specimens. Br Med J 291:769–772, 1985
11. Achkar E, Carey WD, Petras R et al: Comparison of suction capsule and endoscopic biopsy of small bowel mucosa. Gastrointest Endosc 32:278–281, 1986
12. Gear EV, Dobbins WO: The histologic spectrum of proximal duodenal biopsy in adult males. Am J Med Sci 257:90–99, 1969
13. Korn ER, Foroozan P: Endoscopic biopsies of normal duodenal mucosa. Gastrointest Endosc 21:51, 1974
14. Roca M, Truelove SD, Whitehead R: The histological state of the gastric and duodenal mucosa in healthy volunteers. Gut 16:404, 1975
15. Kreuning J, Bosman FT, Kuiper G et al: Gastric and duodenal mucosa in healthy individuals. J Clin Pathol 31:69–77, 1978
16. Goldman H, Ming S-C: Mucins in normal and metaplastic gastrointestinal epithelium: histochemical distribution. Arch Pathol 85:580–586, 1968
17. Filipe MI: Mucins in the human gastrointestinal epithelium: a review. Invest Cell Pathol 2:195–216, 1979
18. Sjolund K, Sanden G, Hakonson R, Sundler F: Endocrine cells in human intestine: an immunocytochemical study. Gastroenterology 85:1120–1130, 1983
19. Lechago J: The endocrine cells of the digestive tract. General concepts and historic perspective. Am J Surg Pathol 11(suppl 1): 63–70, 1987
20. Keren F: Structure and function of the immunologic system of the gastrointestinal tract. pp. 69–80. In Ming S-C, Goldman H (eds): Pathology of the Gastrointestinal Tract. WB Saunders, Philadelphia, 1992
21. Owen RL, Jones AL: Epithelial cell specialization within human Peyer's patches: an ultrastructual study of intestinal lymphoid follicles. Gastroenterology 66:189, 1974
22. Hanson JT, Thorenson C, Morrissey JF: Brush cytology in the diagnosis of upper gastrointestinal malignancy. Gastrointest Endosc 26:33, 1980
23. Qizilbash AH, Casteli M, Kowalski MA et al: Endoscopic brush cytology and biopsy in the diagnosis of cancer of the upper gastrointestinal tract. Acta Cytol 24:313, 1980
24. Grody WW, Gatti RA, Naeim F: Diagnostic molecular pathology. Modern Pathol 2:553–568, 1990
25. Mathieu B, Salducci J, Remacle J-P et al: Intraluminal duodenal diverticulum: report of a case investigated by fiberoptic endoscopy. Dig Dis Sci 23:15–55, 1978
26. Eggert A, Teichmann G, Wiltman DH: The pathological implications of duodenal diverticula. Surg Gynecol Obstet 154:62–64, 1982
27. Navab F, Coleman M, Caldwell F: Resection for intra-luminal duodenal diverticulum. Am J Gastroenterol 83:761–764, 1988
28. Edison H, Miyawaki T, Straehley CJ: Mucoceles of Brunner's glands. Am J Surg 126:688–690, 1973

29. Thoeni RF, Gedgaudas RK: Ectopic pancreas: usual and unusual features. Gastrointest Endosc 5:37–42, 1980
30. Tanemura H, Uno S, Suzuki M et al: Heterotopic gastric mucosa accompanied by aberrant pancreas in the duodenum. Am J Gastroenterol 82:685–688, 1987
31. Gal R, Rathwolfson L, Ginzburg M, Kessler E: Adenomyomas of the small intestine. Histopathology 18:369–371, 1991
32. Franzin G, Musola R, Negri A et al: Heterotopic gastric (fundic) mucosa in the duodenum. Endoscopy 14:166–167, 1982
33. Vizcarrondo FJ, Wang T-Y, Brady PG: Heterotopic gastric mucosa: presentation as a rugose duodenal mass. Gastrointest Endosc 29:107–111, 1983
34. Tsadilas T: Duodenal polyp composed of ectopic gastric mucosa. Dig Dis Sci 29:475–477, 1984
35. Tsubone M, Kozura S, Taki T et al: Heterotopic gastric mucosa in the small intestine. Acta Pathol Jpn 34:1425–1431, 1984
36. Jabbori M, Goresky CA, Lough J et al: The inlet patch: heterotopic gastric mucosa in the upper esophagus. Gastroenterology 89:352–356, 1985
37. Shah KK, DeRidder PH, Shah KK: Ectopic gastric mucosa in proximal esophagus. Its clinical significance and hormonal profile. J Clin Gastroenterol 8:509–513, 1986
38. Fonkalsrud EW, Delorimier AA, Hays DM: Congenital atresia and stenosis of the duodenum. A review compiled from the members of the Surgical Section of the American Academy of Pediatrics. Pediatrics 43:70–83, 1968
39. Rodriques CA, Shepherd NA, Lennard-Jones JE et al: Familial visceral myopathy: a family with at least six involved members. Gut 30:1285–1292, 1989
40. Krishnamurthy S, Heng Y, Schuffler MD: Chronic intestinal pseudo-obstruction in infants and children caused by diverse abnormalities of the myenteric plexus. Gastroenterology 104:1398–1408, 1993
41. Tada S, Iida M, Yao T et al: Intestinal pseudo-obstruction in patients with amyloidosis: clinicopathologic differences between chemical types of amyloid protein. Gut 34:1412–1417, 1993
42. Rappazzo JA, Kozarek RA, Altman M: Duodenal varices: endoscopic diagnosis of an unusual source of upper gastrointestinal hemorrhage. Gastrointest Endosc 27:227–228, 1981
43. Vigneri S, Termini R, Piraino A et al: The duodenum in liver cirrhosis. Endoscopic, morphologic and clinical findings. Endoscopy 23:210–213, 1991
44. Viggiano TR, Gostout CJ: Portal hypertensive intestinal vasculopathy. A review of the clinical endoscopic, and histopathologic features. Am J Gastroenterol 87:944–954, 1992
45. Farup PG, Rosseland AR, Stray N et al: Localized telangiopathy of the stomach and duodenum diagnosed and treated endoscopically: case reports and review. Endoscopy 13:1, 1981
46. Cunningham JT: Gastric telangiectasias in chronic hemodialysis patients: a report of six cases. Gastroenterology 81:1131–1133, 1981
47. Sassaris M, Pang G, Hunter F: Telangiectasias of the gastrointestinal tract. Report of six cases and review. Endoscopy 15:85–88, 1983
48. Tai D-I, Chou F-F, Lee T-Ym, Lin C-C: Vascular ectasia of the duodenum detected by duodenoscopy. Am J Gastroenterol 82: 1071–1073, 1987
49. McClave SA, Goldschmid S, Cunningham JT, Boyd WP Jr: Dieulafoy's cirsoid aneurysm of the duodenum. Dig Dis Sci 33:801–805, 1988
50. Shapiro N, Brandt L, Sproyregan S et al: Duodenal infarction after therapeutic gelfoam embolization of bleeding duodenal ulcer. Gastroenterology 80:176–180, 1981
51. Shepherd HA, Patal C, Bamforth J, Isaacson P: Upper gastrointestinal endoscopy in systemic vasculitis presenting as an acute abdomen. Endoscopy 15:307–311, 1983
52. Camilleri M, Pusey CD, Chadwick VS, Rees AJ: Gastrointestinal manifestations of systemic vasculitis. Q J Med 206:141–149, 1983
53. Taylor NS, Gueft B, Lebowich RJ: Atheromatous embolization: a cause of gastric ulcers and small bowel necrosis. Gastroenterology 47:97, 1964
54. Goldman H: Other inflammatory disorders of the intestines. pp. 689–696. In Ming S-C, Goldman H (eds): Pathology of the Gastro-

intestinal Tract. WB Saunders, Philadelphia, 1992
55. Weinstein WM: The diagnosis and classification of gastritis and duodenitis. J Clin Gastroenterol 3(suppl 2):7–16, 1981
56. Owen DA: Gastritis and duodenitis. pp. 37–77. In Appelman HD (ed): Pathology of the Esophagus, Stomach and Duodenum. Churchill Livingstone, New York, 1984
57. Yardley JH: Pathology of chronic gastritis and duodenitis. pp. 69–143. In Goldman H, Appelman HD, Kaufman N (eds): Gastrointestinal Pathology. Williams & Wilkins, Baltimore, 1990
58. Hasan M, Sirius W, Ferguson A: Duodenal mucosal architecture in non-specific and ulcer-associated duodenitis. Gut 22:637–641, 1981
59. Venables CW: Duodenitis. Scand J Gastroenterol 20(suppl 109): 91–97, 1985
60. Odeida G, Forni M, Farina L et al: Duodenitis in children: clinical, endoscopic and pathological aspects. Gastrointest Endosc 33:366–369, 1987
61. Whitehead R, Roca M, Meihl DD et al: The histological classification of duodenitis in fiberoptic biopsy specimens. Digestion 13:129, 1975
62. Paoluzi P, Pallone F, Palazzesi P et al: Frequency and extent of bulbar duodenitis in duodenal ulcer, endoscopic and histological study. Endoscopy 14:193–195, 1982
63. Shousha S, Spiller RC, Parkins RA: The endoscopically abnormal duodenum in patients with dyspepsia: biopsy findings in 60 cases. Histopathology 7:23–34, 1983
64. Schmitz-Moormann P, Pittner PM, Reichmann L, Massarat S: Quantitative histological study of duodenitis in biopsies. Pathol Res Pract 178:499–507, 1984
65. Jenkins D, Goodall A, Gille FR, Scott BB: Defining duodenitis: quantitative histological study of mucosal responses and their correlations. J Clin Pathol 38:1119–1126, 1985
66. Sircus W: Duodenitis: a clinical, endoscopic and histopathologic study. Q J Med 56:593–600, 1985
67. Elta GH, Appelman HD, Behler EM et al: A study of the correlation between endoscopic and histological diagnoses in gastroduodenitis. Am J Gastroenterol 82:749–753, 1987
68. Kreuning J, Wal AM, Kuiper G et al: Chronic non specific duodenitis. A multiple biopsy study of the duodenal bulb in health and disease. Scand J Gastroenterol 167(suppl):16–20, 1989
69. Maratka Z, Kocianova J, Kudrmann J, Jirk P: Hyperplasia of Brunner's glands. Radiology, endoscopy and biopsy. HepatoGastroenterology 26:64–69, 1979
70. Franzin G, Musola R, Ghidini O et al: Nodular hyperplasia of Brunner's glands. Gastrointest Endosc 31:374–378, 1985
71. James AH: Gastric epithelium in the duodenum. Gut 5:285, 1964
72. Shousha S, Parkins RA, Bille TB: Chronic duodenitis with gastric metaplasia: electron microscopic study including comparison with normal. Histopathology 7:873–885, 1983
73. Wyatt JI, Rathbone BJ, Dixon MF, Heatley RV: Campylobacter pyloridis and acid induced gastric metaplasia in the pathogenesis of duodenitis. J Clin Pathol 40:841–848, 1987
74. Fitzgibbons PL, Dooley CP, Cohen H, Appleman MD: Prevalence of gastric metaplasia, inflammation, and Campylobacter pylori in the duodenum of members of a normal population. Am J Clin Pathol 90:711–714, 1988
75. Frierson HF, Caldwell SH, Marshall BJ: Duodenal biopsy findings for patients with non-ulcer dyspepsia with or without Campylobacter pylori gastritis. Modern Pathol 3:271–276, 1990
76. Noach LA, Rolf TM, Bosma NB et al: Gastric metaplasia and Helicobacter pylori infection. Gut 34:1510–1514, 1993
77. Zukerman GR, Mills BA, Koehler RE et al: Nodular duodenitis: pathologic and clinical characteristics in patients with end-stage renal disease. Dig Dis Sci 28:1018–1024, 1983
78. Triadafilopoulos G: Clinical and pathologic features of the nodular duodenum. Am J Gastroenterol 88:1058–1064, 1993
79. Hasan M, Hay F, Sircus W, Ferguson A: Nature of the inflammatory cell infiltrate in duodenitis. J Clin Pathol 36:280–288, 1983
80. Scott BB, Goodall A, Stephenson P, Jenkins D: Duodenal bulb plasma cells in duodenitis and duodenal ulceration. Gut 26:1032–1037, 1985

81. Goldman H: Stress ulcer and chronic peptic ulcer disease. pp. 517–536. In Ming S-C. Goldman H (eds): Pathology of the Gastrointestinal Tract. WB Saunders, Philadelphia, 1992
82. Skillman JJ, Silen W: Stress ulcers. Lancet 2:1303, 1972
83. Skillman JJ, Bushnell LS, Goldman H et al: Respiratory failure, hypotension, sepsis and jaundice: a clinical syndrome associated with lethal hemorrhage from acute stress ulceration of the stomach. Am J Surg 117:523–530, 1969
84. Cook DJ, Fuller HD, Guyett GH et al: Risk factors for gastrointestinal bleeding in critically ill patients. N Engl J Med 330:377–381, 1994
85. Pan S, Liao C-H, Lien G-S, Chen S-H: Histological maturity of healed duodenal ulcers and ulcer recurrence after treatment with colloidal bismuth subcitrate or cimetidine. Gastroenterology 101:1187–1191, 1991
86. Wolfe MM, Jensen RT: Zollinger–Ellison syndrome: current concepts in diagnosis and management. N Engl J Med 317:1200–1209, 1987
87. Cunningham D, Morgan RJ, Mills PR et al: Functional and structural changes of the human proximal small intestine after cytotoxic therapy. J Clin Pathol 38:265–270, 1985
88. Trier JS: Morphologic alterations induced by methotrexate in the mucosa of the human proximal intestine. Gastroenterology 42:295–305, 1962
89. Jewell LD, Fields AL, Murray CJW, Thomson ABR: Erosive gastroduodenitis with marked epithelial atypia after hepatic infusion chemotherapy. Am J Gastroenterol 80:421–424, 1985
90. Schuger L, Peretz T, Goldin E et al: Duodenal epithelial atypia. A specific complication of hepatic arterial infusion chemotherapy. Cancer 61:663–666, 1988
91. Gottried EB, Korsten MA, Lieber CS: Alcohol-induced gastric and duodenal lesions in man. Am J Gastroenterol 70:587–592, 1978
92. Millan MS, Morris GP, Beck IT et al: Villous damage induced by suction biopsy and by acute ethanol intake in normal human small intestine. Dig Dis Sci 75:513, 1980
93. Draper LR, Gyure LA, Hall JG, Robertson D: Effect of alcohol on the integrity of the intestinal epithelium. Gut 24:399–404, 1983
94. Riddell RH: The gastrointestinal tract. pp. 515–606. In Riddell RH (ed): Pathology of Drug-Induced and Toxic Diseases. Churchill Livingstone, New York, 1982
95. Lewis JH: Gastrointestinal injury due to medicinal agents. Am J Gastroenterol 81:819–834, 1986
96. Eliakim R, Ophis M, Rachmilewitz D: Duodenal mucosal injury with nonsteroidal anti-inflammatory drugs. J Clin Gastroenterol 9:395–399, 1987
97. Graham DY, Smith JL: Gastroduodenal complications of chronic NSAID therapy. Am J Gastroenterol 83:1081–1084, 1988
98. Allison MC, Howatson AG, Torrance CJ et al: Gastrointestinal damage associated with the use of nonsteroidal anti-inflammatory drugs. N Engl J Med 327:749–754, 1992
99. Henry D, Dobson A, Turner C: Variability in the risk of major gastrointestinal complications from non-aspirin non-steroidal anti-inflammatory drugs. Gastroenterology 105:1078–1088, 1993
100. Bjornason I, Hayllar J, Macpherson AJ, Russell AS: Side effects of nonsteroidal anti-inflammatory drugs on the small and large intestine in humans. Gastroenterology 104:1832–1847, 1993
101. Lee FD: Drug-related pathological lesions of the intestinal tract. Histopathology 25:303–308, 1994
102. Morris AJ, Madhok R, Sturrock RD et al: Enteroscopic diagnosis of small bowel ulceration in patients receiving non-steroidal anti-inflammatory drugs. Lancet 1:520, 1991
103. Matsukashi N, Yamada A, Hiraishi M et al: Multiple strictures of the small intestine after long-term nonsteroidal anti-inflammatory drug therapy. Am J Gastroenterol 87: 1183–1186, 1992
104. Weiss SM, Rutenberg HL, Paskin DL, Zeren HA: Gut lesions due to slow-release KCI tablets. N Engl J Med 296:111–112, 1977
105. Kapikian AZ: Viral gastroenteritis. JAMA 269:627–630, 1993
106. Hinnant KL, Rotterdam HZ, Bell ET, Tapper ML: Cytomegalovirus infection of the alimentary tract: a clinicopathological correlation. Am J Gastroenterol 81:944–950, 1986

107. Chetty R, Roskell DE: Cytomegalovirus infection in the gastrointestinal tract. J Clin Pathol 47:968–972, 1994
108. Cheung ANY, Ng IOL: Cytomegalovirus infection of the gastrointestinal tract in non-AIDS patients. Am J Gastroenterol 88:1882–1886, 1993
109. Cummins AG, LaBrooy JT, Stanley DP et al: Quantitative histological study of enteropathy associated with HIV infection. Gut 31:317–321, 1990
110. Ehrenpreis ED, Patterson BK, Brainer JA et al: Histopathologic findings of duodenal biopsy specimens in HIV-infected patients with and without diarrhea and malabsorption. Am J Clin Pathol 97:21–28, 1992
111. Fontana M, Boldorini R, Zulin G et al: Ultrastructural changes in the duodenal mucosa of HIV-infected children. J Ped Gastroenterol Nutr 17:255–260, 1993
112. Guerrant RL, Bobak DA: Bacterial and protozoal gastroenteritis. N Engl J Med 325:327–340, 1991
113. Gleason T, Prinz RA, Kirsch EP et al: Tuberculosis of the duodenum. Am J Gastroenterol 72:36–40, 1979
114. Misra D, Rai RR, Nundy S et al: Duodenal tuberculosis presenting as bleeding peptic ulcer. Am J Gastroenterol 83:203–204, 1988
115. Nair KV, Pai CG, Rajagopal KP et al: Unusual presentations of duodenal tuberculosis. Am J Gastroenterol 86:756–760, 1991
116. Gray JR, Rabeneck L: Atypical mycobacterial infections of the gastrointestinal tract in AIDS patients. Am J Gastroenterol 84: 1521–1524, 1989
117. Mascheck H, Georgil A, Schmidt RE et al: Mycobacterium genavense. Autopsy findings in three patients. Am J Clin Pathol 101:95–99, 1994
118. Schlossberg D, Rudy FR, Jackson FW, Dumalag LB: Syphilitic enteritis. Arch Intern Med 144:811–812, 1984
119. McClure J: Malakoplakia of the gastrointestinal tract. Postgrad Med J 57:95, 1981
120. Volpicelli NA, Salyer WR, Milligan FD et al: The endoscopic appearance of the duodenum in Whipple's disease. Johns Hopkins Med J 138:19, 1976
121. Eras P, Goldstein MJ, Sherlock P: Candida infection of the gastrointestinal tract. Medicine (Baltimore) 51:367–379, 1972
122. Peters M, Weiner J, Whelan G: Fungal infection associated with gastroduodenal ulceration: endoscopic and pathologic appearances. Gastroenterology 78:350–354, 1980
123. Lyon DT, Schubert TT, Mantia AG, Kaplan MH: Phycomycosis of the gastrointestinal tract. Am J Gastroenterol 72:379–394, 1979
124. Young RC, Bennett JE, Vogel CL et al: Aspergillosis: the spectrum of the disease in 98 patients. Medicine (Baltimore) 49:147, 1970
125. Cappell MS, Mandell W, Grimes MM, Neu HC: Gastrointestinal histoplasmosis. Dig Dis Sci 33:353–360, 1988
126. Washington K, Gottfried MR, Wilson ML: Gastrointestinal cryptococcosis. Modern Pathol 4:707–711, 1991
127. Knoke M, Bernhardt H: Endoscopic aspects of mycosis in the upper digestive tract. Endoscopy 12:295, 1980
128. Simon D, Brandt LJ: Diarrhea in patients with the acquired immunodeficiency syndrome. Gastroenterology 105:1238–1242, 1993
129. Rotterdam H, Tsang P: Gastrointestinal disease in the immunocompromised patient. Hum Pathol 25:1123–1140, 1994
130. Sun T: The diagnosis of giardiasis. Am J Surg Pathol 4:256–271, 1980
131. Oberhuber G, Stolte M: Giardiasis—analysis of histological changes in biopsy specimens of 80 patients. J Clin Pathol 43:641–643, 1990
132. Thornton SA, West AH, DuPont HL, Pickering LK: Comparison of methods for identification of Giardia lamblia. Am J Clin Pathol 80:858–860, 1983
133. Marshall JB, Kelley DH, Vogele K: Giardiasis: diagnosis by endoscopic brush cytology of the duodenum. Am J Gastroenterol 79:517–519, 1984
134. Lager DJ, Landos SK: Correlative light and scanning electron microscopy of intestinal giardiasis, cryptosporidiosis, and spirochetosis. Ultrastruct Pathol 15:585–592, 1991
135. McHenry R, Bartlett MS, Lehman GA, O'Connor KW: The yield of routine duodenal aspiration for Giardia lamblia during esophagogastroduodenoscopy. Gastrointest Endosc 33:425–426, 1987
136. Guarda LA, Stein SA, Cleary KA, Ordonez NG: Human cryptosporidiosis in the ac-

quired immune deficiency syndrome. Arch Pathol Lab Med 107:562–566, 1983

137. Godwin TA: Cryptosporidiosis in the acquired immunodeficiency syndrome: a study of 15 autopsy cases. Hum Pathol 22:1215–1224, 1991
138. Phillips AD, Thomas AG, Walker-Smith JA: Cryptosporidium, chronic diarrhea and the proximal small intestinal mucosa. Gut 33:1057–1061, 1992
139. Genta RM, Chappell CL, White AC et al: Duodenal morphology and intensity of infection in AIDS-related intestinal cryptosporidiosis. Gastroenterology 105:1769–1775, 1993
140. Lefkowitch JH, Krumholz S, Feng Chen KC et al: Cryptosporidiosis of the human small intestine: a light and electron microscopic study. Hum Pathol 15:746–752, 1984
141. Marcial MA, Madara JL: Cryptospordium: cellular localization, structural analysis of absorptive cell–parasite membrane–membrane interaction in guinea pigs, and suggestion of protozoan transport by M cells. Gastroenterology 90:83–94, 1986
142. Orenstein JM, Chiang J, Steinberg W et al: Intestinal microsporidiosis as a cause of diarrhea in human immunodeficiency virus–infected patients: a report of 20 cases. Hum Pathol 21:475–481, 1990
143. Peacock CS, Blanchard C, Tovey DG et al: Histological diagnosis of intestinal microsporidiosis in patients with AIDS. J Clin Pathol 44:558–563, 1991
144. Shadduck JA, Orenstein JM: Comparative pathology of microsporidiosis. Arch Pathol Lab Med 117:1215–1219, 1993
145. Orenstein JM, Tenner M, Cali A, Kotler DP: A microsporidian previously undescribed in humans, infecting enterocytes and macrophages, and associated with diarrhea in an acquired immunodeficiency syndrome patient. Hum Pathol 23:722–728, 1992
146. Weber R, Bryan RT, Owen RL et al: Improved light-microscopic detection of microsporidia spores in stool and duodenal aspirates. N Engl J Med 326:161–166, 1992
147. Giang TT, Kotler DP, Garro ML, Orenstein MD: Tissue diagnosis of intestinal microsporidiosis using the chromotrope-2R modified trichrome stain. Arch Pathol Lab Med 117:1149–1251, 1993
148. Vangool T, Snijdoors F, Reiss P et al: Diagnosis of intestinal and disseminated microsporidial infections in patients with HIV by a new rapid fluorescence technique. J Clin Pathol 46:694–700, 1993
149. Shein R, Gelb A: Isospora belli in a patient with acquired immunodeficiency syndrome. J Clin Gastroenterol 6:525–528, 1984
150. DeHovitz JA, Pape JN, Boncy M, Johnson WD Jr: Clincial manifestations and therapy of Isospora belli infection in patients with the acquired immunodeficiency syndrome. N Engl J Med 315:87–90, 1986
151. Carter TR, Cooper PH, Petri WA et al: Pneumocystic carinii infection of the small intestine in a patient with acquired immune deficiency syndrome. Am J Clin Pathol 89:679–683, 1988
152. Dieterich DT, Lew EA, Bacon DJ et al: Gastrointestinal pneumocystosis in HIV-infected patients on aerosolized pentamidine: report of five cases and literature review. Am J Gastroenterol 87:1763–1770, 1992
153. Muigai R, Shaunak S, Gatei DG et al: Jejunal function and pathology in visceral leishmoniasis. Lancet 2:476–479, 1983
154. Ortega YR, Sterling CR, Gilman RH et al: Cyclospora species: a new protozoan pathogen of humans. N Engl J Med 328:1308–1312, 1993
155. Croese J, Loukas A, Opdebeeck J, Provic P: Occult enteric infection by Ancylostoma caninum: a previously unrecognized zoonosis. Gastroenterology 106:3–12, 1993
156. Descombes P, Dupar JL, Capron JP: Endoscopic discovery and capture of Taenia saginata. Endoscopy 13:44, 1981
157. Witham RR, Mosser RS: An unusual presentation of schistosomiasis duodenitis. Gastroenterology 77:1316, 1979
158. Thatcher BS, Fleischer D, Rankin GB, Petras R: Duodenal schistosomiasis diagnosed by endoscopic biopsy of an isolated polyp. Am J Gastroenterol 79:927–929, 1984
159. Contractor QQ, Benson L, Schultz TB et al: Duodenal involvement in Schistosoma mansoni infection. Gut 29:1011–1012, 1988
160. Bone MF, Chesner IM, Oliver R, Asquith P: Endoscopic appearances of duodenitis due to strongyloidiasis. Gastrointest Endosc 28:190–191, 1982

161. Ainley CC, Clarke DG, Timothy AR, Thompson RPH: Strongyloides stercoralis hyperinfection associated with cimetidine in an immunosuppressed patient: diagnosis by endoscopic biopsy. Gut 27:337–338, 1986
162. Whalen GE, Rosenberg EB, Strickland GT et al: Intestinal capillariasis. A new disease in man. Lancet 1:13–16, 1969
163. Perera DR, Weinstein WM, Rubin CE: Small intestinal biopsy. Human Pathol 6:157–217, 1975
164. Dobbins WO III: Small bowel biopsy in malabsorptive states. pp. 121–165. In Norris HT (ed): Pathology of the Colon, Small Intestine, and Anus. Churchill Livingstone, New York, 1983
165. Holdstock G, Eade OE, Isaacson P, Smith CL: Endoscopic duodenal biopsy in coeliac disease and duodenitis. Scand J Gastroenterol 14:717–720, 1979
166. Corazza GR, Brocchi E, Caletti G, Gasborrini G: Loss of duodenal folds allows diagnosis of unsuspected coeliac disease. Gut 31:1080–1081, 1990
167. Yardley JH, Bayless TM, Norton JH et al: Celiac disease: a study of the jejunal epithelium before and after a gluten-free diet. N Engl J Med 267:1173, 1962
168. Falchuk ZM: Update on gluten-sensitive enteropathy. Am J Med 67:50, 1979
169. Trier JS, Falchuk ZM, Carey MC et al: Celiac sprue and refractory sprue. Gastroenterology 75:307–316, 1978
170. Schenk EA, Samloff IM, Klipstein FA: Morphologic characteristics of jejunal biopsy in celiac disease and tropical sprue. Am J Pathol 47:765–781, 1965
171. Cook GC: Aetiology and pathogenesis of postinfective tropical malabsorption (tropical sprue). Lancet 1:721–723, 1984
172. Comer GM, Brandt LJ, Abissi CJ: Whipple's disease: a review. Am J Gastroenterol 78:107–114, 1983
173. Relman DA, Schnidt TM, Mac Dermott RP, Falkow S: Identification of the uncultured bacillus of Whipple's disease. N Engl J Med 327:193–301, 1992
174. Gangl A, Polterauer P, Krepler R et al: A further case of submucosal lymphangioma of the duodenum during endoscopy. Endoscopy 12:188, 1980
175. Salata HH, Mercader J, Navarro A et al: Lymphangioma of the duodenum. Endoscopy 16:30–32, 1984
176. Ammann RW, Vetter D, Deyhle P et al: Gastrointestinal involvement in systemic mastocytosis. Gut 17:107–112, 1976
177. Braverman DZ, Dollberg L, Shiner M: Clinical histological and electron microscopic study of mast cell disease of the small bowel. Am J Gastroenterol 80:30–37, 1985
178. Phillips AD, Jenkins P, Rafat F, Walker-Smith JA: Congenital microvillous atrophy: specific diagnostic features. Arch Dis Child 60:135–140, 1985
179. Schofield DE, Agostini RM, Yunis EJ: Gastrointestinal microvillus inclusion disease. Am J Clin Pathol 98:119–124, 1992
180. Groisman GM, Ben-Izhak O, Schwersenz A et al: The value of polyclonal carcinoembryonic antigen immunostaining in the diagnosis of microvillous inclusion disease. Hum Pathol 24:1232–1237, 1993
181. Bell SW, Kerner JA Jr, Sibley RK: Microvillous inclusion disease. The importance of electron microscopy for diagnosis. Am J Surg Pathol 15:1157–1164, 1991
182. Klein NC, Hargrove RL, Sleisenger MH et al: Eosinophilic gastroenteritis. Medicine (Baltimore) 40:299–319, 1970
183. Talley NJ, Shorter RG, Phillips SF et al: Eosinophilic gastroenteritis: a clinicopathological study of patients with disease of the mucosa, muscle layers and subserosal tissues. Gut 31:54–58, 1990
184. Goldman H: Allergic disorders. pp. 171–187. In Ming S-C, Goldman H (eds): Pathology of the Gastrointestinal Tract. WB Saunders, Philadelphia, 1992
185. Lee D-M, Changchien C-S, Chen, P-C et al: Eosinophilic gastroenteritis: 10 years experience. Am J Gastroenterol 88:70–74, 1993
186. Shiner M, Ballard J, Brook CGD et al: Intestinal biopsy in the diagnosis of cow's milk protein intolerance without acute symptoms. Lancet 2:1060–1063, 1975
187. Ament M, Rubin CE: Soy protein—another cause of the flat intestinal lesion. Gastroenterology 62:227–234, 1972
188. Perkkio M, Savilahti E, Kuitunen P: Morphometric and immunohistochemical study of jejunal biopsies from children with intesti-

nal soy allergy. Fin Eur J Pediatr 137:63–69, 1981

189. Rosekrans PCM, Meijer CJLM, Cornelisse CJ et al: Use of morphometry and immunohistochemistry of small intestinal biopsy specimens in the diagnosis of food allergy. J Clin Pathol 33:125–130, 1980
190. Goldman H, Proujansky R: Allergic proctitis and gastroenteritis in children: clinical and mucosal biopsy features in 53 cases. Am J Surg Pathol 10:75–86, 1986
191. Keren DF: Gastrointestinal immune system and its disorders. pp. 247–285. In Goldman H, Appelman HD, Kaufman N (eds): Gastrointestinal Pathology. Williams & Wilkins, Baltimore, 1990
192. Perlmutter PH, Leichtner AM, Goldman H, Winter HS: Chronic diarrhea associated with hypogammaglobulinemia and enteropathy in infants and children. Dig Dis Sci 30:1149–1155, 1985
193. Ament ME, Rubin CE: Relation of giardiasis to abnormal intestinal structure and function in gastrointestinal immunodeficiency syndromes. Gastroenterology 62: 216–226, 1972
194. Dworkin B, Wormser GP, Rosenthal WS et al: Gastrointestinal manifestations of the acquired immunodeficiency syndrome: a review of 22 cases. Am J Gastroenterol 80:774–778, 1985
195. Snover DC, Weisdorf SA, Vercolotti GM et al: A histopathologic study of gastric and small intestinal graft-versus-host disease following allogeneic bone marrow transplantation. Hum Pathol 16:387–392, 1985
196. Spencer GD, Shulman HM, Mayerson D et al: Diffuse intestinal ulceration after marrow transplantation: a clinicopathologic study of 13 patients. Hum Pathol 17:621–633, 1986
197. Ferrara JLM, Deeg HJ: Graft-versus-host disease. N Engl J Med 324:667–674, 1991
198. Hansmann M-L, Deltz E, Gundloch M et al: Small bowel transplantation in a child. Morphologic, immunohistochemical and clincal results. Am J Clin Pathol 92:686–692, 1989
199. Jepsen JM, Persson M, Jakobsen NO et al: Epidemiology. Prospective study of prevalence and endoscopic and histopathologic characteristics of duodenal polyps in patients submitted to upper endoscopy. Scand J Gastroenterol 29:483–488, 1994
200. Levine JA, Burgart LJ, Batts KP, Wang KK: Brunner's gland hamartomas: clinical presentations and pathological features of 27 cases. Am J Gastroenterol 90:290–294, 1995
201. Kim YI, Kim WH: Inflammatory fibroid polyps of gastrointestinal tract. Am J Clin Pathol 89:721–727, 1988
202. Ott DJ, Wu WC, Shiflett DW, Pennell TC: Inflammatory fibroid polyp of the duodenum. Am J Gastroenterol 73:62–64, 1980
203. Blott SJ, Hanks JB, Stone DD: Solitary hamartomatous polyp of the duodenum in the absence of familial polyposis. Am J Gastroenterol 81:993–994, 1986
204. Matsui K, Kitagawa M: Biopsy study of polyps in the duodenal bulb. Am J Gastroenterol 88:253–257, 1993
205. Perzin KH, Bridge MF: Adenomas of the small intestine: a clinicopathologic review of 51 cases and a study of their relationship to carcinoma. Cancer 48:799, 1981
206. Batra SK, Schuman BM, Reddy RR: The endoscopic variety of duodenal villous adenoma: an experience with ten cases. Endoscopy 15:89–92, 1983
207. Siegel JH, Xatto RP: Endoscopic evaluation and therapy of periampullary adenoma. Am J Gastroenterol 78:225–226, 1983
208. Yamaguchi K, Enjoji M: Adenoma of the ampulla of Vater: putative precancerous lesion. Gut 32:1558–1561, 1991
209. Haggitt RC, Reid BJ: Hereditary gastrointestinal polyposis syndromes. Am J Surg Pathol 10:871–877, 1986
210. Listron MB, Fenoglio-Preiser C: Short course. Gastrointestinal polyps. Modern Pathol 2:161–181, 1989
211. Williams GT, Bussey HJR, Morson BC: Hamartomatous polyps in Peutz–Jeghers syndrome. N Engl J Med 299:101, 1978
212. Foley TR, McGarrity TJ, Abt AB: Peutz-Jeghers syndrome: a clinicopathologic survey of the "Harrisburg Family" with a 49-year follow-up. Gastroenterology 95:1535–1540, 1988
213. Dodds WJ, Schulte WJ, Hensley GT, Hogan WJ: Peutz-Jeghers syndrome and gastrointestinal malignancy. AJR 115:374–377, 1972
214. Giardiello FM, Welsh SB, Hamilton SR et al: Increased risk of cancer in the Peutz-

Jeghers syndrome. N Engl J Med 316: 1511–1514, 1987

215. Jarvinen H, Nyberg M, Peltokallio P: Upper gastrointestinal tract polyps in familial adenomatosis coli. Gut 24:333–339, 1983
216. Sarre RG, Frost AG, Jagelman DG et al: Gastric and duodenal polyps and familial adenomatous polyposis: a prospective study of the nature and prevalence of upper gastrointestinal polyps. Gut 28:306–314, 1987
217. Domizio P, Talbort IC, Spigelman AD et al: Upper gastrointestinal pathology in familial adenomatous polyposis—results from a prospective study of 102 patients. J Clin Pathol 43:738–743, 1990
218. Odze R, Gallinger S, So K, Antonioli D: Duodenal adenomas in familial adenomatous polyposis: relation of cell differentiation and mucin histochemical features to growth pattern. Modern Pathol 7:276–384, 1994
219. Burt RW, Berenson MM, Lee RG et al: Upper gastrointestinal polyps in Gardner's syndrome. Gastroenterology 86:295–301, 1984
220. Shemesk E, Bat L: A prospective evaluation of the upper gastrointestinal tract and periampullary region in patients with Gardner syndrome. Am J Gastroenterol 80:825–827, 1985
221. Lynch HT, Smyrk TC, Lanspa SJ et al: Upper gastrointestinal manifestations in families with hereditary flat adenoma syndrome. Cancer 71:2709–2714, 1993
222. Noda Y, Watanabe H, Iida M et al: Histologic follow-up of ampullary adenomas in patients with familial adenomatous coli. Cancer 70:1847–1856, 1992
223. Offerhaus GJA, Giardiello FM, Krush AJ et al: The risk of upper gastrointestinal cancer in familial adenomatous polyposis. Gastroenterology 102:1980–1982, 1992
224. Spigelman AD, Talbot IC, Penna C et al: Evidence for adenomacarcinoma sequence in the duodenum of patients with familial adenomatous polypsosis. J Clin Pathol 47:705–709, 1994
225. Fenoglio-Preiser CM, Pascal RR, Perzin KH: Tumors of the intestines. Atlas of Tumor Pathology, second series, fascicle 27. Armed Forces Institute of Pathology, Washington DC, 1990
226. Spira IA, Ghazi A, Wolff WI: Primary adenocarcinoma of the duodenum. Cancer 39:1721–1726, 1977
227. Gaddy M, Max MH: Carcinoma of the duodenum. South Med J 78:150–152, 1985
228. Lien G-S, Mori M, Enjoji M: Primary carcinoma of the small intestine. A clinicopathologic and immunohistochemical study. Cancer 61:316–323, 1988
229. Lynch HT, Smgrk TC, Lynch PM et al: Adenocarcinoma of the small bowel in Lynch syndrome II. Cancer 64:2178–2183, 1989
230. Fishman MJ, Jeejeebhoy N, Gopinath N et al: Small intestinal villous adenoma and celiac disease. Am J Gastroenterol 85:748–751, 1990
231. Javier J, Lukie B: Duodenal adenocarcinoma complicating celiac sprue. Dig Dis Sci 25:150–153, 1980
232. Levine ML, Dorf BS, Bank S: Adenocarcinoma of the duodenum in a patient with non-tropical sprue. Am J Gastroenterol 81:800–802, 1986
233. Danzig JB, Brandt LJ, Reinus JF, Klein RS: Gastrointestinal malignancy in patients with AIDS. Am J Gastroenterol 86:715–718, 1991
234. Sellner F: Investigations on the significance of the adenoma-carcinoma sequence in the small bowel. Cancer 66:702–715, 1990
235. Gardner HAR, Matthews J, Ciano PS: A signet-ring cell carcinoma of the ampulla of Vater. Arch Pathol Lab Med 114:1071–1072, 1990
236. London NJM, Leese T, Bingham P et al: Invasive Paneth cell–rich adenocarcinoma of the duodenum. Br J Hosp Med 40:222–223, 1988
237. Barnhill M, Hess E, Guccion JG et al: Tripartite differentiation in a carcinoma of the duodenum. Cancer 73:266–272, 1994
238. Yamaguchi K, Enjoji M: Carcinoma of the ampulla of Vater. A clinicopathology study and pathologic staging of 109 cases of carcinoma and 5 cases of adenoma. Cancer 59:506–515, 1987
239. Talbot IC, Neoptolemos JP, Shaw DE, Carr-Locke D: The histopathology and staging of carcinoma of the ampulla of Vater. Histopathology 12:156–165, 1988
240. Seifert E, Schulte F, Stolte M: Adenoma and carcinoma of the duodenum and papilla of Vater: a clinicopathologic study. Am J Gastroenterol 87:37–42, 1992
241. Solcia E, Capella C, Fiocca R et al: Disorders of the endocrine system. pp. 240–263. In

Ming S-C, Goldman H (eds): Pathology of the Gastrointestinal Tract. WB Saunders, Philadelphia, 1992
242. Hofmann JW, Fox PS, Wilson SD: Duodenal wall tumors and the Zollinger–Ellison syndrome. Arch Surg 17:334–339, 1973
243. Gilhoal WJ: Endoscopic diagnosis and removal of a duodenal wall gastrinoma. Am J Gastroenterol 79:679–683, 1984
244. Thompson NW, Vinik AI, Eckhauser FE: Microgastrinomas of the duodenum: a cause of failed operations of the Zollinger–Ellison syndrome. Ann Surg 209:396–404, 1989
245. Pipeleers-Marichal M, Somers G, Willens G et al: Gastrinomas in the duodenum of patients with multiple endocrine neoplasia type 1 and the Zollinger–Ellison syndrome. N Engl J Med 322:723–727, 1990
246. Dayal Y, Tallberg KA, Nunnemacher G et al: Duodenal carcinoids in patients with and without neurofibromatosis. A comparative study. Am J Surg Pathol 10:348–357, 1986
247. Burke AR, Federspiel BH, Sobin LH et al: Carcinoids of the duodenum. A histologic and immunohistochemical study of 65 tumors. Am J Surg Pathol 13:828–837, 1989
248. Noda Y, Watanabe H, Iwafuchi M et al: Carcinoids and endocrine cell micronests of the minor and major duodenal papillae. Their incidence and characteristics. Cancer 70:1825–1833, 1992
249. Dayal Y, Doos WG, O'Brien MJ et al: Psammomatous somatostatinomas of the duodenum. Am J Surg Pathol 7:653–665, 1983
250. Griffiths DFR, Jasani B, Newman GR et al: Glandular duodenal carcinoid—a somatostatin rich tumor with neuroendocrine association. J Clin Pathol 37:163–169, 1984
251. Taccogni GL, Carlucci M, Sironi M et al: Duodenal somatostatinoma with psammoma bodies: an immunohistochemical and ultrastructural study. Am J Gastroenterol 81:33–37, 1986
252. Albrecht S, Gardiner GW, Kovac SK et al: Duodenal somatostatinoma with psammoma bodies. Arch Pathol Lab Med 113:517–520, 1989
253. Iwafuchi M, Watanabe H, Iishihara N et al: Neoplastic endocrine cells in carcinomas of the small intestine: histochemical and immunohistochemical studies of 24 tumors. Hum Pathol 18:185–194, 1987
254. Jones MA, Griffith LM, West AB: Adenocarcinoid tumor of the periampullary region. A novel duodenal neoplasm presenting as biliary tract obstruction. Hum Pathol 20: 198–200, 1989
255. Burke A, Lee YK: Adenocarcinoid (goblet cell carcinoid) of the duodenum presenting as gastric outlet obstruction. Hum Pathol 21:238–239, 1990
256. Toker C: Oat cell carcinoma of the small bowel. Am J Gastroenterol 61:481–483, 1976
257. Saraga P, Hurlimann J, Ozzello L: Lymphomas and pseudolymphomas of the alimentary tract: an immunohistochemical study with clinicopathologic correlations. Hum Pathol 12:713–723, 1981
258. Levendoglu H, Rosen Y: Nodular lymphoid hyperplasia of gut in HIV infection. Am J Gastroenterol 87:1200–1202, 1992
259. Mir R, Kahn LB, Selzer G: Immunohistochemistry of primary gastrointestinal lymphomas: a study of 76 cases. Histopathology 10:391–403, 1986
260. Dragosics B, Bauer P, Radaszkiewicz T: Primary gastrointestinal non-Hodgkin's lymphoma. A retrospective clinicopathologic study of 150 cases. Cancer 55:1060–1073, 1985
261. Appelman HD, Hirsch SD, Schnitzer B, Coon WW: Clinicopathologic overview of gastrointestinal lymphomas. Am J Surg Pathol 9(3)(suppl):71–83, 1985
262. Netto D, Nowak JA, Balaban EP, Demian SDE: Primary lymphoma of the duodenum. Surg Pathol 4:57–67, 1991
263. Isaacson PG: Gastrointestinal lymphoma. Hum Pathol 25:1020–1029, 1994
264. Fernandes BJ, Amato D, Goldfinger M: Diffuse lymphomatous polyposis of the gastrointestinal tract. A case report with immunohistochemical studies. Gastroenterology 88:1267–1270, 1985
265. Stessens L, Van Den Oord JJ, Geboes K et al: Gastrointestinal lymphomatous polyposis. Gastroenterology 90:2041–2042, 1986
266. Halphen M, Najjar T, Jaofoura H et al: Diagnostic value of upper intestinal fiber endoscopy in primary small intestinal lymphoma. A prospective study by the Tunision–French intestinal lymphoma group. Cancer 58: 2140–2145, 1986
267. Al-Bahrani ZR, Al-Mondhiry H, Bakir F, Al-Saleem T: Clinical and pathologic sub-

types of primary intestinal lymphoma. Experience with 132 patients over a 14-year period. Cancer 52:1666–1672, 1983

268. Khojasteh A, Haghehenass M, Haghighi P: Immunoproliferative small intestinal disease. A "third-world lesion". N Engl J Med 308:1401–1405, 1983
269. Tabbone F, Mourali N, Cammoun M, Najjar T: Results of laparotomy in immunoproliferative small intestinal disease. Cancer 61:1699–1706, 1988
270. Price SK: Immunoproliferative small intestine disease: a study of 13 cases with alpha heavy-chain disease. Histopathology 17:7–18, 1990
271. Helmy I: Endoscopic diangosis of immunoproliferative small intestinal disease (IPSID). Endoscopy 12:114–116, 1980
272. Gilinsky NH, Novis BH, Mee AS et al: Immunoproliferative small intestinal disease: follow-up of an alpha-chain negative, lymphoma-free group. J Clin Gastroenterol 5:421–428, 1983
273. Cooper BT, Holmes GK, Ferguson R, Cooke WT: Celiac disease and malignancy. Medicine (Baltimore) 59:249–261, 1980
274. Swinson CM, Slavin G, Coles EC, Booth CC: Celiac disease and malignancy. Lancet 1:111–115, 1983
275. Robertson DAF, Dixon MF, Scott BB et al: Small intestinal ulceration: diagnostic difficulties in relation to coeliac disease. Gut 24:565–574, 1983
276. Collin P, Reunala T, Pukkala E et al:Coeliac disease—associated disorders and survival. Gut 35:1215–1218, 1994
277. Matuchansky C, Touchard G, Lemaire M et al: Malignant lymphoma of the small bowel associated with diffuse nodular lymphoid hyperplasia. N Engl J Med 313:166–172, 1985
278. Steinberg JJ, Bridges N, Feiner HD, Valensi Q: Small intestinal lymphoma in three patients with acquired immune deficiency syndrome. Am J Gastroenterol 8:21–26, 1985
279. Isaacson PG, Spencer J, Connolly CE et al: Malignant histiocytosis of the intestine: a T-cell lymphoma. Lancet 2:688–691, 1985
280. Isaacson PG, Spencer J: Malignant lymphoma of mucosa-associated tissues. Histopathology 11:445–462, 1987
281. Radasykiewicz T, Dragosics B, Bauer P: Gastrointestinal malignant lymphomas of the mucosa-associated lymphoid tissue: factors relevant to prognosis. Gastroenterology 102:1628–1638, 1992
282. LeBrun DP, Kamel OW, Cleary ML et al: Follicular lymphomas of the gastrointestinal tract. Pathologic features in 31 cases and bcl-2 oncogenic protein expression. Am J Pathol 140:1327–1335, 1992
283. Milchgrub S, Kamel OW, Wiley E et al: Malignant histiocytic neoplasms of the small intestine. Am J Surg Pathol 16:11–20, 1992
284. Miettinen M, Fletcher CDM, Lasota J: True histiocytic lymphoma of the small intestine. Analysis of two S-10 protein-positive cases with features of interdigitating reticulum cells sarcoma. Am J Clin Pathol 100:285–292, 1993
285. Devaney K, Jaffe ES: The surgical pathology of gastrointestinal Hodgkin's disease. Am J Clin Pathol 95:794–801, 1991
286. Appelman HD: Mesenchymal tumors of the gastrointestinal tract. pp. 310–350. In Ming S-C, Goldman H (eds): Pathology of the Gastrointestinal Tract. WB Saunders, Philadelphia, 1992
287. Khansur T, Balducci L, Tavassoli M: Granular cell tumor. Cancer 60:220–222, 1987
288. Boyle L, Lack EE: Solitary cavernous hemangioma of small intestine. Case report and literature review. Arch Pathol Lab Med 117:939–941, 1993
289. Imamura K, Fuchigami T, Iida M et al: Duodenal lipoma—a report of three cases. Dig Dis Sci 29:223–224, 1983
290. Hamid QA, Bishop AE, Rode J et al: Duodenal gangliocytic paragangliomas. A study of 10 cases with immunocytochemical neuroendocrine markers. Hum Pathol 17: 1151–1157, 1986
291. Anders KH, Glasgow BJ, Lewin KJ: Gangliocytic paraganglioma associated with duodenal adenocarcinoma. Arch Pathol Lab Med 111:49–52, 1987
292. Kheir SM, Halpern NB: Paraganglioma of the duodenum in association with congenital neurofibromatosis. Cancer 53:2491–2496, 1984
293. Goldblum JR, Appelman HD: Stromal tumors of the duodenum. A histologic and immunohistochemical study of 20 cases. Am J Surg Pathol 19:71–80, 1995

294. Holst L, Burstein S, Moranker V, Goldberg M: Leiomyosarcoma of the duodenum recognized preoperatively. J Clin Gastroenterol 5:447–451, 1983
295. Saltz RK, Kurtz RC, Lightdale CJ et al: Kaposi's sarcoma. Gastrointestinal involvement and correlation with skin findings and immunologic function. Dig Dis Sci 29:817–823, 1984
296. Bernal A, del Junco GW, Gibson SR: Endoscopic and pathologic features of gastrointestinal Kaposi's sarcoma: a report of four cases in patients with the acquired immune deficiency syndrome. Gastrointest Endosc 31:74–77, 1985
297. Freedman SL, Wright TL, Altman DF: Gastrointestinal Kaposi's sarcoma in patients with acquired immunodeficiency syndrome. Endoscopic and autopsy findings. Gastroenterology 89:102–108, 1985
298. Parents F, Cernuschi M, Orlando G et al: Kaposi's sarcoma and AIDS—frequency of gastrointestinal involvement and its effect on survival—a prospective study in a heterogeneous population. Scand J Gastroenterol 26:1007–1012, 1991
299. Rose HS, Balthazar EJ, Megibow AJ et al: Alimentary tract involvement in Kaposi's sarcoma: radiographic and endoscopic findings in 25 homosexual men. Am J Radiol 39:661–666. 1982
300. Ranchod M, Kempson RL: Smooth muscle tumors of the gastrointestinal tract and retroperitoneum: a pathologic analysis of 100 cases. Cancer 39:255, 1977
301. Evans HL: Smooth muscle tumors of the gastrointestinal tract. A study of 56 cases followed for a minimum of 10 years. Cancer 56:2242–2250, 1985
302. Engle JM, Deitch EA, Risch J: Extragenital choriocarcinoma in the duodenum. Am J Radiol 133:933–935, 1979
303. Matthews TH, Haton GH, Christopherson WM: Primary duodenal choriocarcinoma. Arch Pathol Lab Med 110:550–552, 1986
304. Raymond AR, Rorat E, Goldstein D et al: AN unusual case of malignant melanoma of the small intestine. Am J Gastroenterol 79:689–692, 1984
305. Robey-Cafferty SS, Silva EG, Cleary KR: Anaplastic and sarcomatoid carcinoma of the small intestine. A clinicopathologic study. Hum Pathol 20:858–863, 1989
306. Menuck L: Transpyloric extension of gastric carcinoma. Dig Dis Sci 23:269–274, 1978
307. Cronstedt JI, Kalczynski J, Jonsson NGE: Involvement of the duodenum by gastric carcinoma. Gastrointest Endosc 28:44–45, 1982
308. Hricak T, Theoni RF, Margulis AR et al: Extension of gastric lymphoma into the esophagus and duodenum. Radiology 135:309–312, 1980
309. Kadakia S, Parker A, Canalels L: Metastatic tumors of the upper gastrointestinal tract: endoscopic experience. Am J Gastroenterol 87:1418–1423, 1992
310. Adair C, Ro JY, Sahin AA et al: Malignant melanoma metastatic to gastrointestinal tract. Int J Surg Pathol 2:3–10, 1994
311. Raijman I: Duodenal metastases from lung cancer. Endoscopy 26:752–753, 1994
312. Gurian L, Ireland K, Petty W et al: Carcinoma of the cervix involving the duodenum: case report and review of the literature. J Clin Gastroenterol 3:291–294, 1981
313. Trier JS, Browning TH: Morphologic response of the mucosa of human small intestine to x-ray exposure. J Clin Invest 45:194, 1966
314. Berthrong M, Fajardo LF: Radiation injury in surgical pathology. Part II. Alimentary tract. Am J Surg Pathol 5:153–178, 1981
315. Case records of the MGH. Radiation enteritis. N Engl J Med 330:627–632, 1994
316. Yamare H, Norris M, Gillies C: Pseudomelanosis duodeni: a clinicopathologic entity. Gastrointest Endosc 31:83–86, 1985
317. Gupta TP, Weinstock JV: Duodenal pseudomelanosis associated with chronic renal failure. Gastrointest Endosc 32:358–360, 1986
318. West B: Pseudomelanosis duodeni. J Clin Gastroenterol 10:127–129, 1988
319. Rex DK, Jersild RA Jr: Further characterization of the pigment in pseudomelanosis duodeni in three patients. Gastroenterology 95:177–182, 1988
320. Steckman M, Bozymski EM: Hemosiderosis of the duodenum. Gastrointest Endosc 29:326–327, 1983
321. Conte D, Velio P, Brunelli L et al: Stainable iron in gastric and duodenal mucosa of primary hemochromatosis patients and alcoholics. Am J Gastroenterol 82:237–240, 1987

322. Rocken C, Saeger W, Linke RP: Gastrointestinal amyloid deposits in old age–report on 110 consecutive autopsical patients and 98 retrospective bioptic specimens. Pathol Res Pract 190:641–649, 1994
323. Goldman H: Systemic and miscellaneous disorders. pp. 351–380. In Ming S-C, Goldman H (eds): Pathology of the Gastrointestinal Tract. WB Saunders, Philadelphia, 1992
324. Haggitt RC, Meissner WA: Crohn's disease of the upper gastrointestinal tract. Am J Clin Pathol 59:613–622, 1973
325. Rutgeerts P, Onette E, Vantrappen G et al: Crohn's disease of the stomach and duodenum: a clinical study with emphasis on the value of endoscopy and endoscopic biopsies. Endoscopy 12:288, 1980
326. Korelitz BI, Waye JD, Kreuning J et al: Crohn's disease in endoscopic biopsies of the gastric antrum and duodenum. Am J Gastroenterol 76:103–109, 1981
327. Tanaka M, Kimura K, Sakai H et al: Long-term follow-up for minute gastroduodenal lesions in Crohn's disease. Gastrointest Endosc 32:206–209, 1986
328. Schuffler MD, Chaffee RE: Small intestinal biopsy in a patient with Crohn's disease of the duodenum. (The spectrum of abnormal findings in the absence of granulomas.) Gastroenterology 76:1009–1014, 1979
329. Gad A: The diagnosis of gastroduodenal Crohn's disease by endoscopic biopsy. Scand J Gastroenterol 167(suppl):23–28, 1989
330. Alcantara M, Rodriguez R, Potenciano JLM et al: Endoscopic and bioptic findings in the upper gastrointestinal tract in patients with Crohn's disease. Endoscopy 25:282–286, 1993
331. Lescut D, Vanco D, Bonniere P et al: Perioperative endoscopy of the whole small bowel in Crohn's disease. Gut 34:647–649, 1993
332. Ament ME, Ochs HS: Gastrointestinal manifestations of chronic granulomatous disease. N Engl J Med 288:382–387, 1973
333. Rauf A, Davis P, Levendoglu H: Sarcoidosis of the small intestine. Am J Gastroenterol 83:187–189, 1988
334. Stampfl DA, Grimm IS, Barbot DJ et al: Sarcoidosis causing duodenal obstruction. Case report and review of gastrointestinal manifestations. Dig Dis Sci 35:526–532, 1990
335. Graham RM, Rheault MH: Characteristic cellular changes in epithelial cells in pernicious anemia. J Lab Clin Med 43:235–245, 1954
336. Foroozan P, Trier JS: Mucosa of the small intestine in pernicious anaemia. N Engl J Med 277:553–559, 1967
337. Sharma BK, Pounder RE, Cruse JP et al: Extramedullary haemopoiesis of the small bowel. Gut 27:873–875, 1986
338. Schreibman D, Brenner B, Jacobs R et al: Small intestinal myeloid metaplasia. JAMA 259:2580–2582, 1988
339. Gupta S, Walker DL, Keshavarzian A, Hodgson HJF: Upper endoscopy for occult bleeding in renal failure. J Clin Gastroenterol 9:43–45, 1987
340. Franzin G, Musola R, Mencarelli R: Morphological changes of the gastroduodenal mucosa in regular dialysis in uremic patients. Histopathology 6:429–437, 1982
341. Musola R, Franzin G, Mora R, Manfrini C: Prevalence of gastroduodenal lesions in uremic patients undergoing dialysis and after renal transplantation. Gastrointest Endosc 30:343–346, 1984
342. Coletta U, Sturgill BC: Isolated xanthomatosis of the small bowel. Hum Pathol 16:422–424, 1985
343. Eckstein RP, Dowsett JF, Riley JW: Collagenous enterocolitis: a case of collagenous colitis with involvement of the small intestine. Am J Gastroenterol 83:767–771, 1988
344. Weinstein WM, Saunders DR, Tytgat GN, Rubin CE: Collagenous sprue: an unrecognized type of malabsorption. N Engl J Med 283:1297–1301, 1970

7

Disorders of the Jejunum

This chapter concentrates on the diseases that primarily affect or are concentrated in the jejunum. In these instances, there is often the need for a mucosal biopsy examination of the area to secure the diagnosis. Since many of the diseases can affect all parts of the small intestine, they also may present in the duodenum at upper endoscopy and in the ileum at colonoscopic examination.

The initial description of most of these diseases began in Chapter 6 and is expanded here. Effort has been made to provide the major presentation of the various diseases in either of the chapters, but they are mentioned in both areas to provide complete coverage.

GENERAL ASPECTS

Examination of the jejunal mucosa was initiated in advance of the development of the fiberoptic endoscopes.[1–4] The biopsies are obtained by the passage of a tube into the beginning of the jejunum, just beyond the ligament of Treitz; its location is confirmed by a radiograph; and suction-type samples of tissue are taken using a capsule with a guillotine apparatus. This provides a biopsy that is larger than those typically taken at endoscopy, which permits better orientation.

Although there are a very large variety of disorders that can affect the jejunum as a part of the small intestine, the mucosal biopsies are mainly obtained to evaluate patients with diarrheal or other malabsorptive disorders and, less often, to detect multifocal lesions such as some of the lymphomas (Table 7-1). This limited use of the biopsy is due to the lack of direct visualization and the need for a lesion that is likely to be diffuse and detected by such a random biopsy. Even with multiple samples, the jejunal mucosal biopsy still has such restricted use. Indeed, this has led to the increased use of direct endoscopy of the duodenum in the evaluation of many of the disorders that had formally been made primarily by jejunal examination.[5–9]

There are efforts to extend the endoscopes to permit direct visualization of inflammatory and tumor lesions of the jejunum.[10–13] These enteroscopes have had only limited use, mainly in the detection of bleeding lesions and in the removal of polyps. The lack of extensive employment of these scopes,

Table 7-1. Major Uses of Jejunal Mucosal Biopsies

Malabsorptive disorders
Infections
Immunologic conditions
Multifocal and diffuse tumors

however, may reflect the small number of disorders that require this instrument.

Normal Structure

The mucosal anatomy is uniform throughout the jejunum and similar to the distal half of the duodenum and to the proximal portion of the ileum.[1,3,14,15] The mucosa is comprised of the epithelium, which is located in the villi and the crypts; of the lamina propria, consisting of loose connective tissue and a large variety of inflammatory cells; and of the muscularis mucosae formed by smooth muscle tissue.

Epithelial Cells

The villi are tall and thin and generally three to five times in height compared to the length of the crypts (Figs. 7-1 and 7-2). Most of the epithelial cells lining the villi are the tall columnar or absorptive type with the prominent brush or striated border (Table 7-2). These are responsible for the absorption of all of the nutrient materials (Fig. 7-3). Scattered along the villi are well formed goblet-type mucous cells that contain weakly acidic mucins[16,17]; these stain poorly with the PAS reaction and strongly with Alcian Blue at pH 2.5. They ordinarily lack sulfated mucins, which are prevalent in the colon. The crypts contain the Paneth cells that are concentrated at the base and filled with large refractile red granules in the cytoplasm[18]; numerous mitotic cells, occupying the lower two-thirds of the crypt; and the less mature forms of the absorptive and mucous cells (see Figs. 6-2 and 6-3).

In addition, there are a variety of neuroendocrine cells located in the crypts and in the lamina propria.[19–21] Those in the crypts tend to be interposed between the other epithelial cells and the basement membrane, have a clear or finely granular and eosinophilic cytoplasm, and express their secretion toward the region of the basement membrane (Fig. 7-4). All of these cells migrate to the tips of the villi where they are shed, with most epithelial cells having a life span of 3 to 4 days.

Inflammatory Cells

The lamina propria consists of a loose framework of fibroblasts, blood and lymphatic vessels, collagen and strands of smooth muscle, together with a variety of inflammatory cells.[22] This compartment makes up the core of the villi and also the space between the crypts. Present are many mononuclear-type inflammatory cells, including macrophages, lymphocytes, and plasma cells, as well as a variable number of eosinophils. Neutrophils are ordinarily not present. Most of the lymphocytes in the lamina propria region are of the B-cell type; there are also a fair number of lymphocytes, mainly of the T-cell class, located within the epithelial layer overlying the villi[23] (Fig. 7-5). In addition, there are scattered lymphoid nodules that extend throughout the full thickness of the mucosa (Fig. 7-6). On the luminal aspect, many of the epithelial cells are flattened, and contained here are also M cells that specialize in antigen collection[24] (see Fig. 8-3). These nodules are normal throughout the small intestine and are more heavily concentrated in the gross Peyer's patches in the ileum. Secreted by the lymphocytes and plasma cells are immunoglobulins of the various classes, including IgG and IgM, which mainly pass into the local lymphatics for systemic distribution; and IgA, which combines with the secretory component made by the epithelial cells and is excreted into the intestinal lumen. These cells

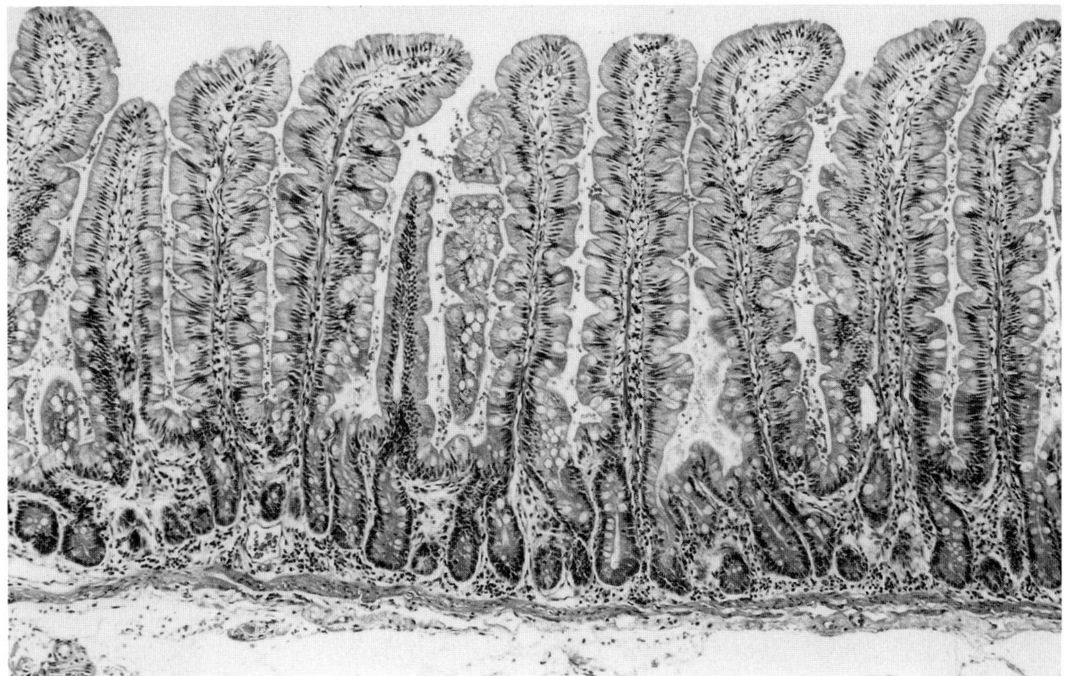

Fig. 7-1. Normal mucosa in the jejunum, showing very tall villi and short crypts, with a ratio of about 4:1. The villi are generally thin, reflecting the presence of only a small amount of inflammatory cells in the lamina propria. The muscularis mucosae and submucosa appear at the bottom (× 105).

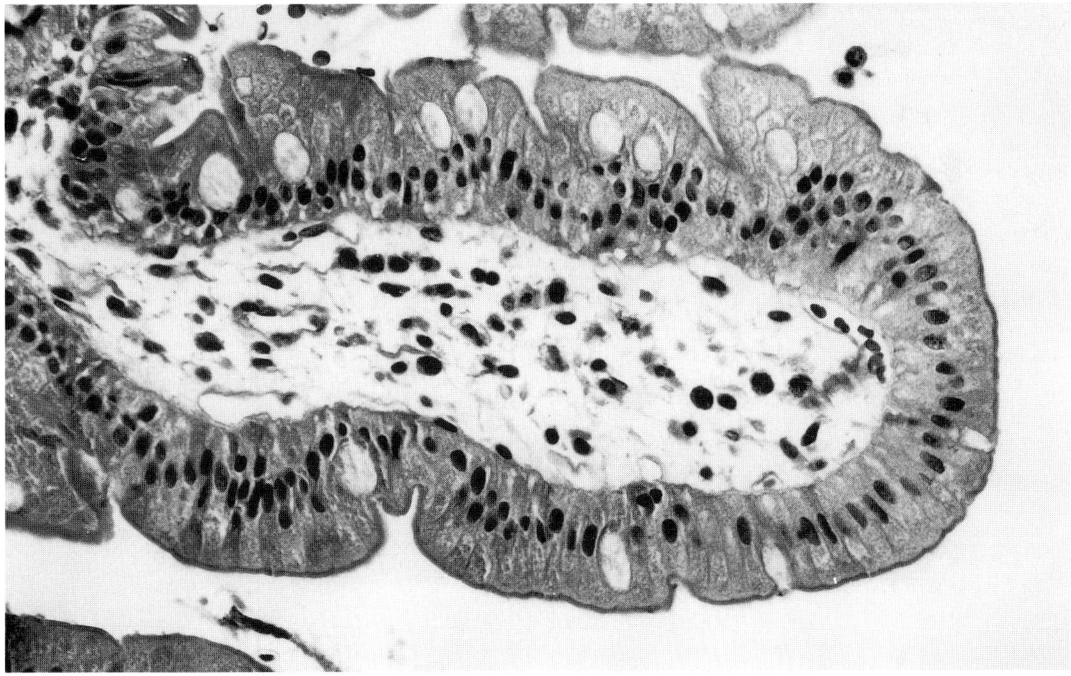

Fig. 7-2. Normal villus in the jejunum, covered by columnar absorptive cells with prominent brush border and by scattered goblet mucous cells. The core of the lamina propria contains few inflammatory cells (× 425).

Table 7-2. Principal Epithelial Cells in Jejunal Mucosa

Villus	
	Absorptive cell
	Goblet mucous cell
Crypt	
	Stem cell
	Less differentiated forms of absorptive and mucous cells
	Paneth cell
	Neuroendocrine cells

are also responsible for the abnormal production of excess IgE that can occur in allergic disorders.

Other Features

It has been suggested that the villous height varies, dependent on age, being somewhat shorter in infants and in older persons, but this has never been absolutely established.[15, 25] There certainly is a great overlap in the histology in all of the age groups, which precludes this use. There probably is some effect from diet, with persons limited to vegetarian meals often showing irregular branching of the villi but no definite change in the epithelial cells. Observer variation has been noted in the assessment of the villous height and particularly in estimating the amount of inflammatory cells in the epithelial layer and lamina propria.[26] This has led to many efforts at quantitation including computer programs,[27–29] but these are not standardized or in current practice.

The renewal of the epithelial cells is derived from the stem cell compartment in the crypts, and there are always several cells in mitoses in each of the crypts. Under normal circumstances, these cells differentiate and extend into the villi, undergo maturation mainly to absorptive and to mucous cells, and migrate to the tips of the villi where they are discarded. The control of the crypt cell growth is largely determined or regulated

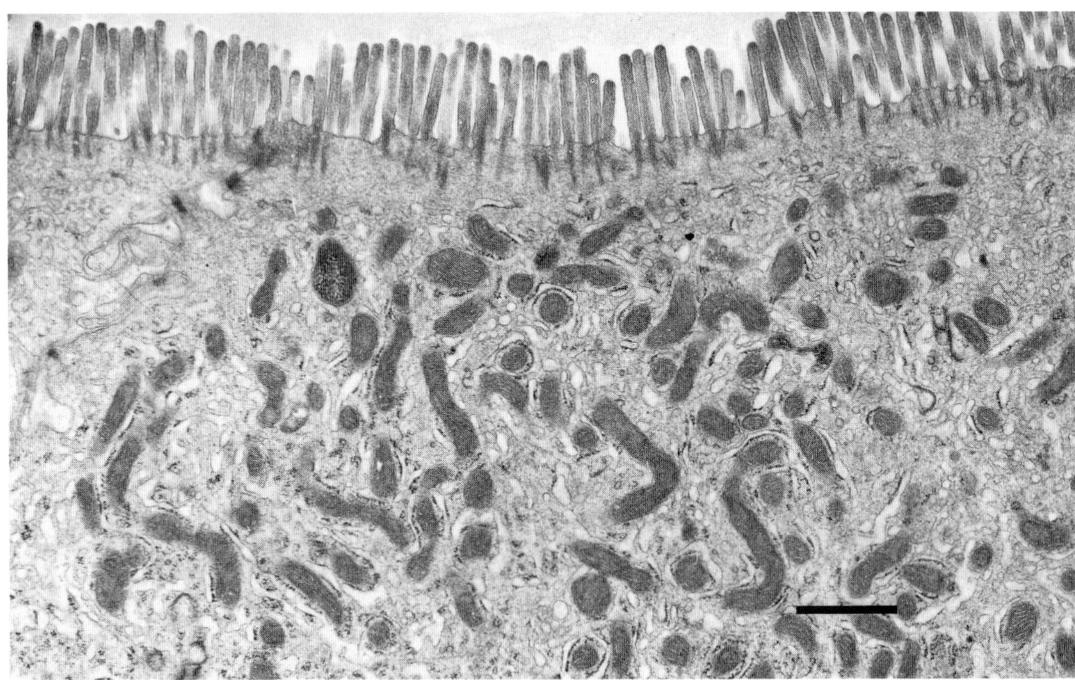

Fig. 7-3. Electron micrograph of absorptive cells in the small intestine. There are closely packed, tall microvilli on the luminal surface, numerous mitochondria, prominent smooth and rough endoplasmic reticulum, and few lysosomes (× 12,500; bar = 1 μm).

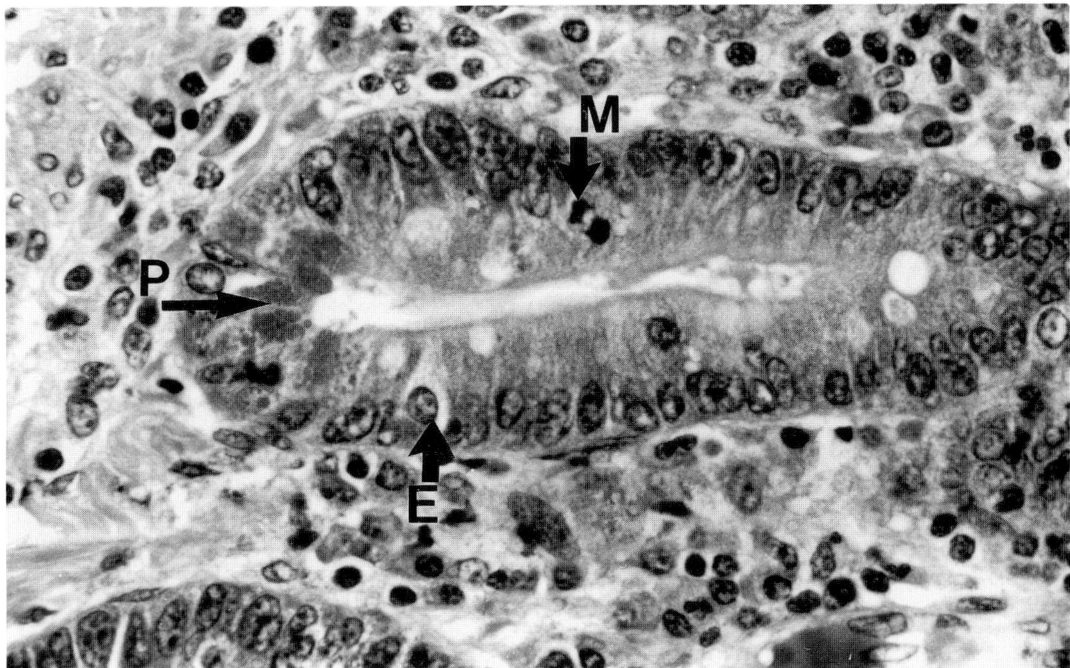

Fig. 7-4. Jejunal crypt, showing Paneth cells (P) with large cytoplasmic granules in the luminal aspect; endocrine cells with fine granules in the basal portion or with clear cytoplasm (E); and mitoses (M) (× 635).

by the villous epithelial cells. When there is damage to these villi, there is a feedback resulting in a hyperplasia of the crypts, unless they also had been damaged. This pattern of injury is highly prevalent and seen in most of the disorders affecting the small intestine. In contrast, when the injury is directed at the crypt area, there can develop poor maturation and shortening of the villi but also a failure to achieve any feedback and to develop a crypt hyperplasia.

Biopsy Material

As mentioned, most of the samples are obtained by blind biopsy and are used to identify disorders that are diffuse or multifocal. The tubes are variable and include those with a single capsule and also ones that have multiple openings or bores to permit obtaining several samples.

Orientation and Fixation

In the evaluation of most of the malabsorptive disorders, it is especially important to achieve excellent orientation of the specimen. This is needed to adequately evaluate the height of the villi and its ratio to the crypts. This orientation can be best achieved by placing the specimens on filter paper, with the mucosal side up; allowing them to stick for about 10 to 15 seconds; and then placing the paper and sample into the bottle or capsule with fixative. This orientation can be facilitated by all workers being adequately familiar with the topography of the specimens; included are the pathologists and residents, as well as the histotechnologist, who are processing the specimens. The choice of fixative is not rigid. The best cytologic detail is achieved by the use of solutions that contain heavy metals such as B5 and Hollande's, but neutral formalin is still extensively used

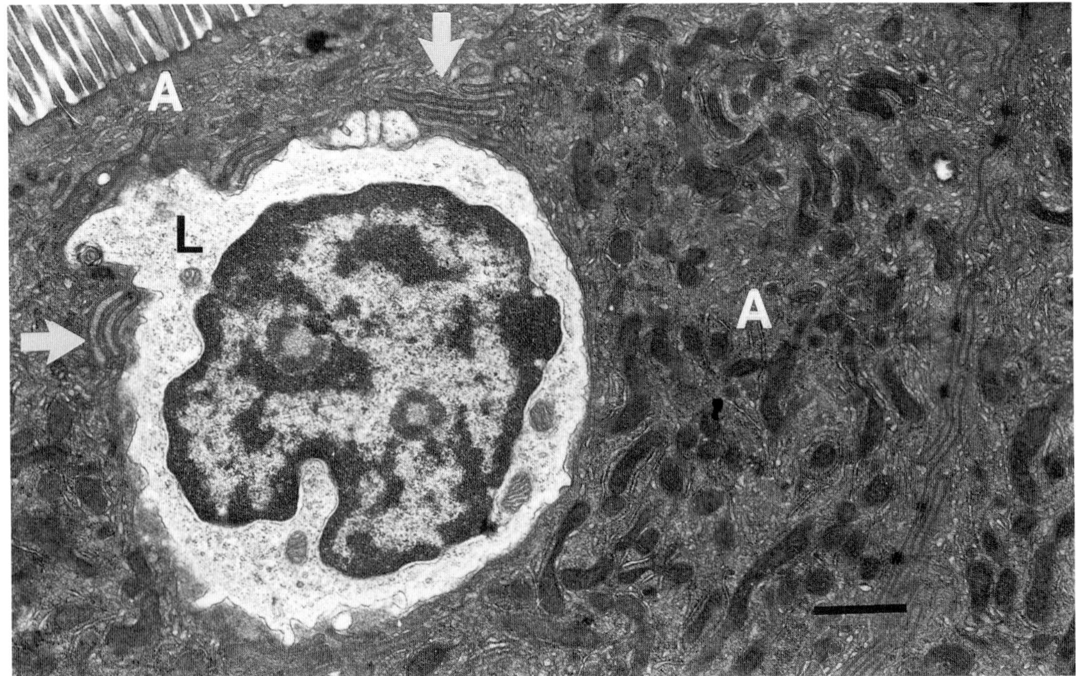

Fig. 7-5. Electron micrograph of intraepithelial lymphocyte (L). The cell is squeezed between the interdigitating lateral plasma membranes (arrow) of the intestinal absorptive cells (A) (× 11,625; bar = 1 μm).

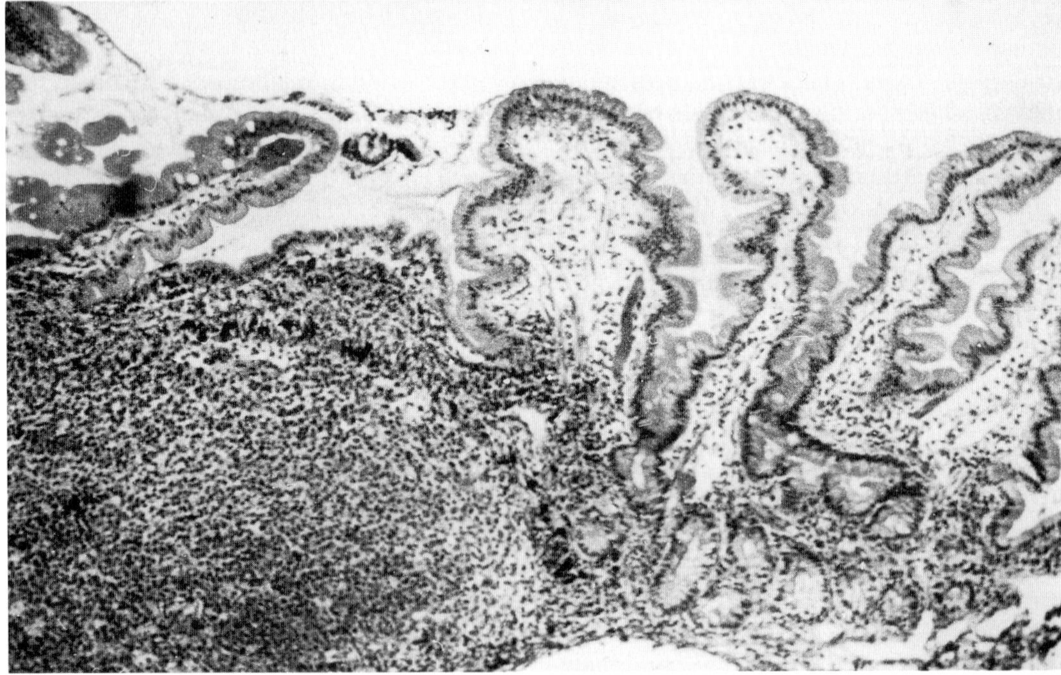

Fig. 7-6. Lymphoid nodule in the normal jejunal mucosa. A well formed nodule with follicle center appears at the left.

biopsies help to distinguish other common malabsorptive disorders such as celiac disease, and diseases with more florid and specific histologic features, as described below.

VASCULAR DISORDERS

Varices and Vascular Malformations

Varices resulting from portal hypertension are typically noted in the esophagus and stomach, but may exceptionally extend into the duodenum and rarely into the jejunum[56] (see Table 4-4). Their presence is probably favored by prior surgery and the appearance of fibrous peritoneal adhesions in the area. They are rarely appreciated by routine studies and are not typically detected by biopsy (see Fig. 4-9). Other vascular lesions of the jejunum are uncommon and include Dieulafoy's type of ulcer with a prominent central artery,[57] telangiectasia,[58] and hemangiomas that may cause problems by bleeding.[59] In such cases, angiographic studies are commonly used in documenting and localizing their presence. There are also recent efforts to use longer enteroscopes to directly capture the lesions, with the potential advantage of applying laser in their local treatment.[11, 13] There is typically no biopsy material from the endoscopic procedure.

Ischemic Lesions

Ischemic injury of the small intestine is commonly observed due to reduced blood flow in the mesenteric circulation from cardiogenic or other forms of shock; to thrombosis and embolism involving the major distributing arteries; and to a variety of small vessel diseases such as vasculitis, amyloid, and atheromatous embolization.[60, 61] The effects on the intestinal wall are highly variable and include no change if there is adequate collaterals, mucosal damage alone in the mildest lesions, and mural or transmural infarction with sustained disease.[62, 63] The mucosal lesions are associated with edema, hemorrhage, and relatively minor necrosis. Cases with persistent ischemia show extension of the infarction into the wall, and this may be associated later with reperfusion and a neutrophilic reaction; alternatively, transmural disease develops if the ischemia is unabated. In all of these situations the diagnosis is largely captured by the clinical information and the radiographic studies. Endoscopic examination is only helpful if the infarction extends to the distal portion of the duodenum or ileum, where it might be seen at endoscopy. The diagnosis is usually not established or monitored by mucosal examination. (See Ch. 9 for further details.)

Small Vessel Diseases

As noted above, small vessel diseases can be involved by direct inflammatory lesions in vasculitis,[64–66] by deposition such as amyloid, and by emboli, particularly atheromatous material.[67, 68] All of these situations can lead to focal areas of vascular compromise, mucosal hemorrhages, and ulcerations. In contrast to the upper and lower portions of the alimentary tract that are readily visualized by endoscopy, the lesions in the jejunum are not easily appreciated and are only rarely detected by multiple biopsies. All types of vasculitis can be involved, and the lesions associated with Henoch-Schönlein syndrome are most distinctive, revealing depositions of IgA not only in the vessels but also in the overlying mucosa.[69]

CHEMICAL AND RADIATION INJURY

All of the chemical and physical effects in the jejunum are the same as those seen in the duodenum but are less easily appreciated by mucosal biopsy because of the lack of direct visualization. More often, the diagnoses are established by the clinical and radiographic findings and are supported by mucosal biopsy of equivalent lesions in the more proximal parts of the alimentary tract such as the duodenum and stomach.

Chemotherapy Effects

Damage to the intestinal mucosa can follow the administration of chemotherapy for a wide variety of systemic tumors.[70, 71] The small intestine is particularly sensitive and is one of the organs that serves to limit the use of these toxic chemicals. The early lesions are associated with crypt injury and erosion or ulceration, together with prominent acute inflammation. Most of these subside without difficulty, but strictures and fistulae can exceptionally develop. Extensive lesions are more likely to occur in patients who are receiving multiple drugs together with radiation. In assessing any lesions, it is important to also consider the potential for secondary infections and for residual or recurrent tumor. To evaluate such cases, biopsies are more often obtained from the duodenal mucosa at upper endoscopy or from the colon. Overall, most of the drugs act on the crypts leading to poor villous development and to a lack of compensatory hyperplasia, referred to as *primary crypt injury,* in contrast to the more common villous injury that is seen in celiac disease and in most infections.[72] This can help in the differential diagnosis. Such crypt injury is seen in ischemic disease, in effects from radiation, in nutritional changes, and in a familial enteropathy known as *microvillous inclusion disease.* (These are described further in the section "Malabsorptive Disorders" below.)

Drug-Induced Enteritis

A wide variety of effects in the intestines are caused by various medications[71, 73–75] (Table 7-4). These include reduction in mucosal defenses by the long-standing use of corticosteroid hormones, anti-inflammatory and immunosuppressive agents; the promotion of altered flora by antibiotics and other antimicrobial drugs: poor motility and pseudo-obstruction by a large number of anticholinergic and antidepressant drugs; hemorrhages from anticoagulants; and ischemic lesions from several drugs used to treat cardiovascular and hypertensive diseases. All of these factors can operate in any part of the alimentary tract, but are especially prominent in the small intestine and in the colon. Contraceptive pills have been associated with various lesions, ranging from focal hemorrhages to intestinal infarctions.[76] Hypersensitivity reactions are also noted to other drugs such as gold salts, which are mainly used for the treatment of rheumatoid disease.[77] This can result in focal ulcers and in larger areas of infarction. The lesions are most common in the colon but can also affect the small intestine and rarely the jejunum.

Table 7-4. Drug Effects in the Intestines

Promotion of infections
Anti-inflammation
Altered flora
Poor motility and pseudo-obstruction
Vascular effects
Hemorrhage
Thrombosis
Vasoconstriction
Hypersensitivity reactions
Direct toxic effects
Ulcer and stricture
Diaphragm

In addition, there are a large number of nonsteroidal, anti-inflammatory drugs (NSAIDs) that are used in the treatment of chronic rheumatoid and other inflammatory disorders. These have largely been developed as alternatives to steroids and to aspirin in efforts to reduce toxicity. Nevertheless, virtually all NSAIDs ultimately cause some damage to the stomach and/or small intestine.[75, 78–81] Most often seen are acute erosions and hemorrhages that rapidly subside after elimination of the medicine. Exceptionally, however, there develops deeper ulceration with stricture formation that can affect any part of the intestinal tract including the jejunum.[82, 83] Also noted is the formation of bands or diaphragms causing more prominent and permanent irregularity of the lumen; these are comprised mainly of a mixture of fibrous and muscle tissue.[84, 85] The diagnoses are often made by radiographic study, with biopsy used to identify equivalent lesions in the upper parts of the small intestine. It is currently estimated that lesions in the small intestine occur in one-quarter to one-third of all patients taking NSAIDs.

One of the more common agents associated with deeper ulcers and strictures is enteric-coated potassium chloride, and the effects appear to be maximal in the jejunum.[86, 87] Because of this complication, this medication is less commonly used at present. (Discussions on drug-induced enteritis are also presented in Chs. 4 and 6.)

Radiation Effects and Injury

Radiation is typically employed for the treatment of lymphomas and other tumors affecting the small intestine and the neighboring retroperitoneum.[88, 89] It also may be used as a conditioning agent in preparation for bone marrow transplants. The small intestinal muscosa is exquisitely sensitive to radiation, with the effects principally occurring at the crypt level, equivalent to the action of many chemotherapeutic agents.[71, 90–95] This leads to arrest of the crypt activity and failure to produce overlying villi, resulting in prompt desquamation and erosion or ulceration (Table 7-5). These changes are seen at the crypt level in a matter of hours and lead to mucosal loss in 1 to 2 days. There is often a marked degree of edema in the submucosa, beyond that amount expected in acute injury. At this time, there are the effects of the ulceration and a mild obstruction of the small intestine. These early changes typically subside over the course of the next few weeks, but there can develop signs of chronic disease in the form of fibrous structures from deeper ulcers, and exceptionally fistulae.[96] These complications are generally kept to a minimum with modern techniques.

Table 7-5. Radiation Effects in the Intestines

Acute Effects
Ulceration
Submucosal edema
Chronic effects
Mucosal atrophy
Telangiectasia
Atypical stromal cells
Fibrosis

Biopsy examination can be helpful in the early stages because the lesion is typically diffuse and involves the distal duodenum, which is obtainable at endoscopy. The study is done not only to confirm the features compatible with radiation but also to exclude secondary infections and tumor. The features seen in biopsy that support chronic changes include persistent atrophy of the mucosa in the form of shortened villi and normal size or reduced length of the crypts; irregularly dilated venules in the lamina propria; fibroblasts and other mesenchymal cells with enlarged and irregular nuclei; and occasional fibrosis (see Fig. 2-22).

INFECTIONS

There are a large variety of infectious disorders that affect the small intestinal mucosa, and many of these were studied in the past in jejunal mucosal biopsies. Currently, more attention is placed on detecting the organisms in the duodenum at upper endoscopy because of the ease of access and the potentially greater yield. This subject was introduced in Chapter 6 and is extended here (see Table 6-5).

General Features

In the jejunum, infection presents an added potential effect on the processes of digestion and absorption, and this is especially prominent in the cases with bacterial proliferation involving the small intestine (see "Malabsorption Disorders" below). Biopsy samples primarily are taken to establish the particular inflammatory condition, but also, and more often, to detect the particular causative microorganism. This applies especially to the opportunistic infections, including the cellular inclusions of herpes and cytomegaloviruses, the atypical mycobacterial and fungal infections, and the many parasitic agents. In addition there are numerous infections, largely of a bacterial nature, that are best detected by cultures. Material is obtained from aspirates of the small intestine and also from colonic sources. These cultures are needed for establishing infections due to species of *Vibrio, Shigella, Salmonella, Campylobacter,* and *Yersinia.* Many of these bacterial infections are also associated with colonic disease. In special instances, material is taken directly from the mucosa to look for viral agents, using in-situ hybridization, ultrastructural study, and special culture techniques. (The major alterations induced by the infectious agents are presented in Chs. 2, 4, and 6.)

Viral Infections

Viral Enteritis

Viral enteritis is the term ordinarily applied to cases that are due to the common pathogenic viruses, including rotavirus, reovirus, adenoviruses, and the Norwalk agent.[97–101] These cases also are commonly referred to as *gastroenteritis,* but this is a probable misnomer since the gastric mucosa is not ordinarily involved. The viruses infest the villous epithelial cells and lead to their rapid destruction. This results in a compensatory hyperplasia of the crypts, and at first glance the mucosa resembles the colon, just like in celiac disease. Indeed, the differential of the sprue syndrome, particularly in children, always includes a viral enteritis. Also seen are degeneration of the surface epithelial cells, an increase of lymphocytes in this layer, and a mild increase of mononuclear inflammatory cells in the lamina propria. Not present are many neutrophils or granulomas. The lesions typically subside over the course of several days, and there is ordinarily complete restoration of the mucosa within a couple of weeks.

The lesions may be focal or diffuse, but the full extent of the small intestinal mucosa in a particular case is rarely established. Considering the limited effects on the patients, it is probable that the damage is restrictive and does not involve the entire small bowel. Biopsies are not typically taken to establish the viral disorder but rather to rule out some other sustained condition. This is especially done in children who present with chronic diarrhea, and the differential largely consists of celiac disease, allergic enteritis, and prolonged viral enteritis.

Opportunistic Viral Infections

The opportunistic viral infections include cases due to the herpes simplex and to cytomegalovirus.[102–106] Typically seen are focal ulcers, with the viral inclusions present in the epithelial cells and in the underlying granulation tissue, particularly in the endothelial cells, macrophages, and fibroblasts (Plates 1A and 1B). The lesions usually involve multiple areas of the small intestine and even the entire alimentary tract. As a result, biopsies are more often taken from other areas, such as the duodenum and colon, to establish the diagnosis. The herpes lesions tend to be more common in areas with squamous epithelium, such as the esophagus and anal areas, whereas CMV can be found anywhere. The yield is considerably greater if biopsies are taken from ulcerated lesions rather than intact mucosa. The features of the inclusions are described in Chapter 2.

Human Immunodeficiency Virus

There are AIDS patients with chronic diarrhea in whom a particular microorganism cannot be identified, and these effects are thought to be due to the primary virus infecting the intestinal cells.[107–112] Electron microscopic studies have demonstrated viral-like particles in the mucosa of the duodenum and jejunum, occasionally present in the epithelial cells, but more prominently appearing within the macrophages and dendritic cells in lymphoid nodules (Fig. 7-7). A clear link to the causation of AIDS or to the clinical symptoms has not been firmly established. It is important to search for opportunistic organisms in these cases, as described in other sections.

Bacterial Infections

Common Agents

There are a multitude of ordinary bacterial infections that can affect the small intestine alone or, more often, in conjunction with colonic disease.[113,114] For most of these disorders, regular culture techniques are employed to look for the particular agent; these include species of *Vibrio, Shigella, Salmonella, Clostridium, Campylobacter, Yersinia,* as well as *Escherichia coli* and other coliforms.[115–120] The effects on the tissue are highly variable and depend on the mode of injury induced by the bacteria (Table 7-6). In *Vibrio* infection resulting in cholera, the total effect is from toxins leading to reduced absorption of sodium and water, and there is no damage to the mucosa. Most of the other bacteria are associated with invasive organisms, leading to ulceration and marked acute inflammation. Some of the cases due to *Salmonella* reveal a prominent mononuclear cell infiltrate, implying sustained immunologic reaction; cases due to *clostridium* are often associated with pronounced degrees of necrosis; and the yersinial infections typically reveal sharply localized microabscesses that must be distinguished from ordinary granulomas[119] (see Ch. 8).

Clostridial Infections

Some of the bacteria cause more distinctive morphologic lesions than others. Cases due to *Clostridium difficile* are typically associated with prominent inflammatory membranes overlying sharply localized ulcerated areas; these have been referred to as the lesions of *pseudomembranous enteritis* and are typically seen in conjunction with equivalent and more common lesions in the large intestine of pseudomembraneous colitis[121,122] (cf. Fig. 9-30). The small bowel lesion is much less common, is usually seen in children, and probably is more frequent in the ileal area. Similarly, patients with leukemia or any other disorder that promotes marked reduction in inflammatory cells can develop a neutropenic ileocolitis, which is typically due to infection by highly toxic clostridial agents such as *C. septicum*[123,124]; these cases show extensive necrosis and bacteria but little inflammation. Despite these useful features, it should be emphasized that these disorders more often involve the distal part of the small intestine and are not typically revealed in aspiration-type jejunal mucosal biopsies. As mentioned, the diagnosis of most bacterial infections involving the small intestine usually depends on culture of fecal material.

Other Bacterial Infections

Infections due to *Mycobacterium tuberculosis* and to *Actinomyces israelii* more often are concentrated in the ileum and colonic regions, showing extensive ulceration and fibrosis.[125,126] More prevalent throughout the jejunal mucosa are the infections due to *Mycobacterium avium intracellulare* and other recently described species.[127–129] These typically present as opportunistic infections in

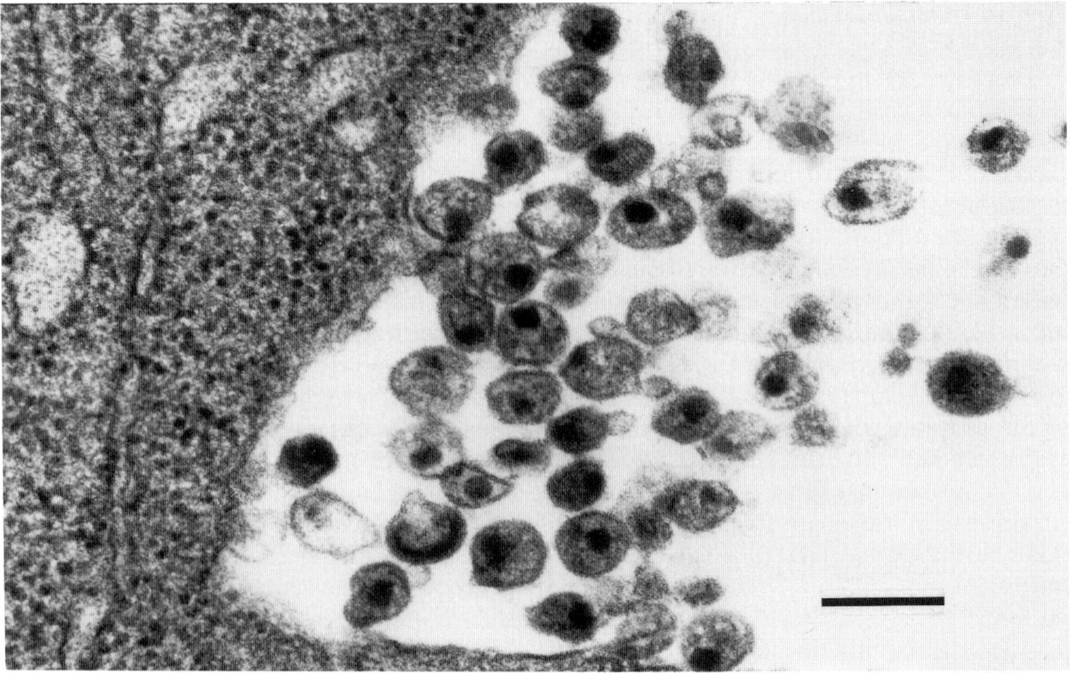

Fig. 7-7. Electron micrograph of HIV on surface of monocyte. The mature viral particle is round, measures on average 100 nm in diameter, and has a very electron-dense eccentric or central core (× 81,000; bar = 0.2 μm).

patients with AIDS or other immunosuppressive disorders. There is marked infiltration of the lamina propria with the organisms, lying free or within macrophages. Lesions range from poor or no granuloma formation to large nodules of macrophages. Biopsies are distinctive, revealing the increased macrophages together with the vast number of organisms seen on acid-fast stain (Figs. 6-12 and 6-13, and Plate 1D). Currently, these infections are more often detected in distal duodenal biopsies at endoscopy. Due to the large growth by the organisms, they also can be readily seen on stool smears by a modified acid-fast stain. Rarer causes of bacterial infection include syphilis, Whipple's disease (which is described below under "Malabsorptive Disorders"), and malakoplakia, which is more frequent in the colon.[130–132]

Table 7-6. Examples of Effects of Bacteria in the Intestines

Bacterial Group	Major Tissue Feature
Vibrio	None
Shigella	Acute inflammation
Salmonella	Chronic inflammation
Clostridium	Pseudomembrane
Yersinia	Microabscess
Mycobacterium	Granuloma

Fungal Infections

Most often seen are the opportunistic fungal infections, complicating cases with necrosis due to the effects of drugs and/or radiation in the treatment of malignant tumors; and occurring in patients who are immunosuppressed due to the large variety of primary and secondary conditions. Infections due to *Candida* are most frequent and involve several species.[133, 134] Much less common are secondary infections associated with *Aspergillus* and with *Phycomyces.*[135–137] Infection with the pathogenic fungi, including *Histoplasma* and *cryptococcus,* also typically occurs in immunocompromised patients.[138–140] Cases with histoplasmosis can reveal granulomas with variable necrosis, and special stains such as methenamine silver are needed to identify the tiny organisms. The other fungi can ordinarily be seen with the H & E and accented by the silver strain or the PAS reaction. The features of the fungal organisms are described in Chapter 2 (Plates 1E–F).

Protozoal Infections

Some protozoal infections, such as with species of *Cryptosporidium,* occur in immunocompetent patients and are ordinarily associated with a short duration, reversible colitis in children.[141, 142] Most of the protozoal infections affect the immunocomprised patients and often determine the clinical complications and survival in these patients.[143] Most commonly seen are infections due to *Giardia*[144–149] (Fig. 6-14 and Plate 2A), *cryptosporidium* and other coccidia[150–156] (see Figs. 6-15 and 6-16, and Plate 4B), and the several species of Microsporidia[157–164] (see Figs. 6-17 and 6-18, and Plate 4C). The latter includes the Enterocytozoan group and *Septata intestinalis,* with newer species being found. Rarer protozoal infections are those due to *Isospora,*[165–167] *Pneumocystis,*[168, 169] *Leishmania,*[170] *Toxoplasma,*[171] and *Cyclospora*[172] (see Color Plate 4D). The characteristics and major locations of the common organisms are presented in Chapter 6.

These agents are detected in biopsies that are largely performed to evaluate patients with immunodeficiency problems. The biopsies may help to establish this disorder but are probably most useful in identifying the particular microorganism, which is more likely responsible for the presenting symptoms. Accordingly, examination and stains are applied to look for viral inclusions, for acid-fast bacilli, for the various opportunistic fungi and protozoa, and for helminthic ova. Routinely performed are H & E, methenamine silver or PAS, acid-fast stain, and modified Gram stain, with optional addition of Giemsa.

Helminthic Infections

Injury to the jejunal mucosa can result from many worms and their ova, and specific diagnoses can be obtained in biopsy samples. Examples include localized inflammatory reactions with prominent eosinophils due to *Strongyloides* (see Fig. 6-19) and granulomas associated with schistosomiasis[173–175] (Fig. 9-23 and Plate 2F). This general topic is discussed in Chapters 6 and 9.

MALABSORPTIVE DISORDERS

The traditional and long-standing use of jejunal mucosal biopsies has been for the evaluation of patients with malabsorptive disorders.[176, 177] The biopsies are taken to confirm that the patient has a malabsorptive condition, to identify the particular disorder or to provide a more restricted differential diagnosis, to monitor the patients following specific therapy, and to detect complications. The jejunal biopsies are most useful in conditions that are diffuse, since a single sample can provide the necessary information. For those disorders that tend to be focal, multiple biopsies are often needed.

Over the past decade, however, there has been extensive use of endoscopic-type biopsies, typically obtained from the duodenum at upper endoscopy.[5–8, 178, 179] These are especially helpful in those conditions that always involve the duodenum, such as the sprue disorders and most infections. The biopsies act as a useful screening tool, since a negative sample serves to eliminate celiac disease. The finding of an abnormal duodenal biopsy is not as specific, since the differential would also include the common disorder of peptic duodenitis. Nevertheless, upper endoscopy, which permits evaluation of the esophagus, stomach, and duodenum, is now being used more extensively in evaluation of patients with small intestinal diseases. The jejunal biopsy is more commonly used in children, and is reserved for providing specificity in the more difficult cases. It also remains essential in those conditions that may be limited to the jejunum, such as a malignant lymphoma.

Clinical Syndromes

Maldigestion

This results from a failure to digest the major nutrients in the foods, including the breakdown of the neutral fats and triglycerides to monoglycerides and free fatty acids, the proteins to the dipeptides and amino acids, and the complex carbohydrates to the disaccharides and monosaccharides. The smaller elements are needed for the final process of absorption by the intestinal mucosa. Failure in the digestive process can result from prior gastric resection, leading to bypass and potential for poor mixing of the contents with the pancreatic and biliary excretions; inadequate digestive enzymes from the pancreas due to tissue destruction or to obstruction of the major duct; and critical reduction in the bile salts, which serve as detergents for optimal digestion of fats (Table 7-7). The bile salt depletion can have multiple causes, including failure of production by the liver, bile duct obstruction, bacterial proliferation causing destruction of the major and most functional bile salts, and lack of reabsorption in the terminal ileum due to disease or bypass.

In all of these situations, there results an inadequate digestion and excess excretion of fats. In addition, the excess fat and altered bile salts can be toxic to the colon, leading to further diarrhea. The small bowel mucosa in all of these conditions is variable, ranging from normal to a patchy but nonspecific and relatively mild villous injury; the latter is probably related to stasis and the local effects of the excess bacteria. The small bowel biopsy in these cases also serves to rule out intrinsic intestinal disease.

Table 7-7. Clinical Syndromes and Causes of Malabsorption

Maldigestion
Prior gastrectomy
Pancreatic insufficiency and ductal obstruction
Bile salt reduction
Malabsorption
Rapid transit
Bypass or loss of intestine
Mucosal diseases
Bacterial proliferation
Multiple diverticula
Strictures and fistulae
Afferent loop syndrome
Protein-losing conditions and lesions
Ménétrier's disease and chronic gastritis
Celiac disease and allergic gastroenteritis
Infections and immunologic deficiencies
Lymphangiectasia
Villous adenoma, carcinoma, and lymphoma

Malabsorption

This results when the patient is capable of digesting the major nutrients but cannot deliver them beyond the mucosal barrier. This can be due to rapid transit or bypass as a result of surgery or fistulae; to loss of intestine; and to a very large number of mucosal disorders.

In these conditions, there is sufficient digestion of the nutrients, but one or more may be inadequately absorbed into the circulation. The deficit can range from a highly specific condition, such as primary lactase deficiency in which the lactose cannot be finely broken down into its components of glucose and galactose, to a condition such as celiac disease in which all of the nutrient elements are inadequately absorbed, resulting in extensive nutritional and metabolic problems in the patients.

Bacterial Proliferation

This has also been referred to as the *bacterial stasis* or *blind loop* syndrome.[180, 181] There are multiple causes, including the presence of diverticula, strictures, fistulae, or other unnatural pockets such as an exaggerated afferent loop following a gastrectomy. In all of these situations, there is stasis and the proliferation of bacteria in the small intestinal lumen, which is ordinarily sterile or nearly so. This also occurs in any condition that interferes with the regular peristalsis and, therefore, can be seen in all of the pseudoobstructive disorders that affect the small intestine (see above under "Motor and Mechanical Disorders").

Stasis and bacterial proliferation can also complicate many of the other maldigestive and malabsorptive disorders, due to the retention in the lumen of large amounts of inadequately processed nutrient elements. The small bowel biopsy features are highly variable. In cases due primarily to stasis, the biopsies range form normal to showing patchy but ordinarily mild villous injury. If more severe and diffuse villous injury is encountered, the possibility of an underlying or coexisting malabsorptive disorder must be considered.

Protein-Losing Enteropathy

Protein-losing enteropathy refers to a lesion or condition that is associated with marked protein loss in the intestinal lumen. It is typically due to the excess production of the protein substance or extensive oozing from an inflamed lesion, and the exuded protein exceeds the capacity for its reabsorption. The same effect can occur with equivalent lesions in other parts of the gut, including the stomach and colon. The result is a decline in the serum proteins, particularly the albumin level, and in the promotion of edema.

Considering the wide range of lesions that can be associated with protein loss, it is clear that some result from discrete lesions or tumors, whereas others are but one feature in a more generalized malabsorptive condition. Exceptionally, just about any condition can be associated with a dominance of this feature. For example, this has been seen in allergic disorders, in granulomatous diseases, in infections, and in hyperplastic conditions.[182–186]

Biopsy Evaluation and Patterns

Biopsy Preparation

It is essential that the biopsy be properly oriented to allow for accurate evaluation of the villous and crypt heights and their ratio.[1, 187] Problems in this assessment can occur with tangential sections, causing the villi to appear shorter than normal. This is usually appreciated by noting cross sections rather than a longitudinal profile of the crypts. The method to achieve optimal orientation is described in the "Normal Structure" section above.

In many instances where the biopsy is not completely well oriented, there still may be adequate villi to determine normality. It should be stressed that tangential cuts cannot result in improvement of the villous height, so their normal appearance can be considered an accurate finding independent of the overall orientation. Also, in most conditions associated with villous shortening and active disease, there is damage to the epithelial cells overlying the villi and often an increase in the inflammatory cells in this region. Again, their absence helps to support a lack of significant disease, even in less than perfectly oriented specimens.

Other difficulties can occur when the biopsies are superficial. There can be distortion from the procedure, leading to edema and hemorrhage within the lamina propria; flattening of surface epithelial cells and discharge of mucus form the goblet cells; and failure to appreciate the characteristics of

Table 7-8. Patterns of Injury Observed by Jejunal Mucosal Biopsy

	Villous Injury	Crypt Injury
Villous shortening	Mild to marked	Mild to moderate
Complete loss of villi	In severe cases	Rare
Increased intraepithelial lymphocytes	Prominent	Uncommon
Crypts	Hyperplasia	Normal or hypoplasia

epithelial cells adjacent to normal lymphoid follicles. The latter may normally appear shortened, lacking any mucus, and are often associated with inflammatory cells.

Biopsy Patterns

There are two major patterns of injury involving the jejunal mucosa, represented by direct effects on the crypts and on the villi (Table 7-8). The damage at the crypt level leads to reduced numbers of cells formed and to shortened villi, and this is associated with a lack of compensatory crypt hyperplasia. The crypts either appear normal or even slightly shortened. This pattern is noted in a variety of conditions, including ischemic disease, some infections and immunologic disorders, effects of many chemicals and of radiation, a severe protein under-nutrition, and the familial disorder of microvillous inclusion disease (Table 7-9). In this pattern of injury, there is usually only a minor degree of degeneration of the surface epithelial cells and no marked increase in inflammatory cells, either in the epithelial area or in the lamina propria.

The more common pattern of injury to the small intestinal mucosa is at the level of the villi. This is the type seen in celiac disease, in allergic disorders, with most infectious agents, in the stasis syndrome, and in most immunologic disorders. There is damage to the epithelial cells, particularly the absorptive cells, leading to their degeneration and to progressive loss of the villi, and this is associated with a compensatory hyperplasia of the crypts, presumably due to a feedback mechanism. It is believed that the mature epithelial cells ordinarily make a chalone-like substance that ordinarily inhibits the crypt growth; when the mature epithelial cells are damaged, there is the lack of this inhibitor, resulting in the stimulation of the crypt stem cells. In general, there is a close correlation between the degree of villous shortening and the level of crypt hyperplasia. This can reach the maximum, as revealed by complete loss of villi and the greatest amount of crypt elongation, which is typically seen in the severe cases of active celiac disease. The disorders associated with villous injury typically show damage of the epithelial cells and considerable increases in inflammatory cells involving the epithelial zone and the lamina propria.

Table 7-9. Causes of Crypt Injury

Chemical injury
Radiation
Ischemia
Protein under-nutrition
Microvillus inclusion disease

General Biopsy Features and Diagnoses

There are five major forms of small bowel mucosal abnormalities that are seen in the malabsorptive cases (Table 7-10). These include cases without structural abnormalities, such as the disaccharidase deficiencies; cases with nonspecific features of enteritis that is always diffuse, as seen in celiac disease; cases with nonspecific enteritis that is more often focal than diffuse, similar to most cases of viral disease and of bacterial proliferation; cases with specific and diagnostic features

Table 7-10. Biopsy Patterns in the Major Causes of Malabsorption

Condition	Usual Biopsy Pattern	
	Diffuse	Focal
Disorders with normal mucosa		
Maldigestive conditions		
Primary disaccharidase deficiencies		
Monosaccharidase deficiencies		
Peptidase deficiences		
Disorders with nonspecific enteritis		
Celiac disease	X	
Allergic enteritis		X
Refractory sprue and collagenous sprue	X	
Tropical sprue	X	
Bacterial proliferation syndrome		X
Viral enteritis		X
Immunodeficiency disorders in children	X	
Disorders with specific features		
Whipple's disease	X	
Immunodeficiency disorders in adults	X	
Infections with recognizable organisms		X
Lymphangiectasia		X
Amyloidosis and Waldenstrom's macroglobulinemia		X
Mastocytosis, granulomatous diseases, and histiocytosis		X
Abetalipoproteinemia, Tangier's disease, and other storage disorders		X

that are almost always diffuse, such as Whipple's disease; and cases with specific features that are more commonly focal than diffuse, such as particular depositions and many of the infections with recognizable microorganisms.

Accordingly, a jejunal mucosal biopsy in a patient with a possible malabsorptive disorder may be normal, show a nonspecific enteritis that is either focal or diffuse, or reveal a specific and diagnostic abnormality. A normal biopsy can be seen as evidence that the patient does not have a malabsorptive condition, but it also would be present in those disorders characterized by focality or without structural abnormality. It is, therefore, important to consider the taking of multiple samples in those diseases that tend to be focal, such as with infections and allergic lesions. The finding of a normal biopsy or of a focal lesion serves to exclude those diseases that are always diffuse, such as celiac disease, and this can be especially helpful as a screening practice. Conversely, biopsies showing diffuse but otherwise nonspecific disease can be seen in a very large variety of conditions, including those that are always diffuse as well as cases that may be focal or diffuse.

Disorders with Normal Mucosa

Most patients with a maldigestive condition have a normal small intestinal mucosa (Table 7-10). In addition, this is seen in cases of the various disaccharidase deficiencies, including primary absences of lactase, sucrase, and isomaltase. The lactase absence is highly prevalent in the non-white populations of the world, presumably related to major evolutionary changes that were associated with switching from hunting to dairy products for survival. The mucosa is completely normal but there is a total lack of the disaccharidase in the brush border. In early studies of these conditions, biopsies were taken for biochemical analyses, but these are no longer done. Rather, the particular deficiency is suggested by the clinical information and specific diagnoses are provided by tolerance tests. The lactose is ordinarily split into galactose and glucose, and these can be measured in the blood and urine following the ingestion of a set quantity of the disaccharide.

The primary deficiencies must be distinguished from the secondary loss of disaccharidases, which can occur in any damage to the villous epithelial cells. The latter are distinguished by the association with malabsorption of other elements besides the specific disaccharide. Other rare causes of malabsorption associated with a normal structure include the primary enzyme deficiencies required for absorption of monosaccharides and of amino acids, and these patients do not ordinarily have biopsy studies.

Celiac Disease

This is a common disorder that is associated with a diffuse but nonspecific enteritis that can involve all age groups.[189–190] Other common terms for this disorder are *non-tropical sprue* and *gluten-sensitive* or *associated enteropathy*. It is especially common in infants and children but the disease can present in adults and in the elderly. It is thought to have an immunologic basis with the patient reacting to gluten and particularly to the gliadin fraction that is contained in many of the wheats.[191] The disease starts in the proximal small intestine, including the duodenum, and spreads over time to involve the entire small bowel if not arrested. As a result, there is malabsorption of virtually all food substances, and this can be associated with significant clinical problems.

Diagnosis and Major Biopsy Features

The diagnosis is suggested by the clinical information and is largely made by the small intestinal mucosal biopsy.[192] Samples of the jejunum reveal, in most cases, a diffuse enteritis with marked to complete loss of the villi together with compensatory hyperplasia of the crypts (Table 7-11). Also present is evidence of damage to the surface epithelial cells with major loss of microvilli, as well as a great increase of inflammatory cells in both the lamina propria and the epithelial layer (Fig. 7-8). The latter is mainly associated with an increase of T-type lymphocytes. The inflammation of the lamina propria consists mostly of B-type lymphocytes and plasma cells with variable amounts of eosinophils and usually inconspicuous neutrophils. The diagnosis of celiac disease is supported by the finding of the diffuse and particularly severe enteritis, but the lesion is not specific. Equivalent lesions can be seen in patients with infections, allergic disorders, and immunological conditions. Accordingly, one must consider the response to a gluten-free diet for additional support of the diagnosis.

In adults, the prompt functional and clinical improvement typically establishes the diagnosis without further biopsy examinations in most cases. In children, in contrast, the differential including allergic and viral disorders is more prevalent, and subsequent biopsies are more regularly employed to confirm the healing and to evaluate the effects of gluten challenge.[193] Repeat biopsies after gluten withdrawal typically reveal the features of a healing enteritis without active disease, as described below. If the second biopsy shows active disease or only partial healing, the possibilities of poor dietary compliance or of other diseases must be considered.

Stages of Disease

The full range of lesions can be present in patients with celiac disease. The mildest form, seen typically in the patients who are

Table 7-11. Biopsy Features in Celiac Disease

Shortening of villi
Degeneration of absorptive cells with reduced number and height of microvilli
Increased intraepithelial lymphocytes
Crypt hyperplasia with increased mitoses and endocrine cells
Increased mononuclear inflammatory cells and eosinophils in lamina propria

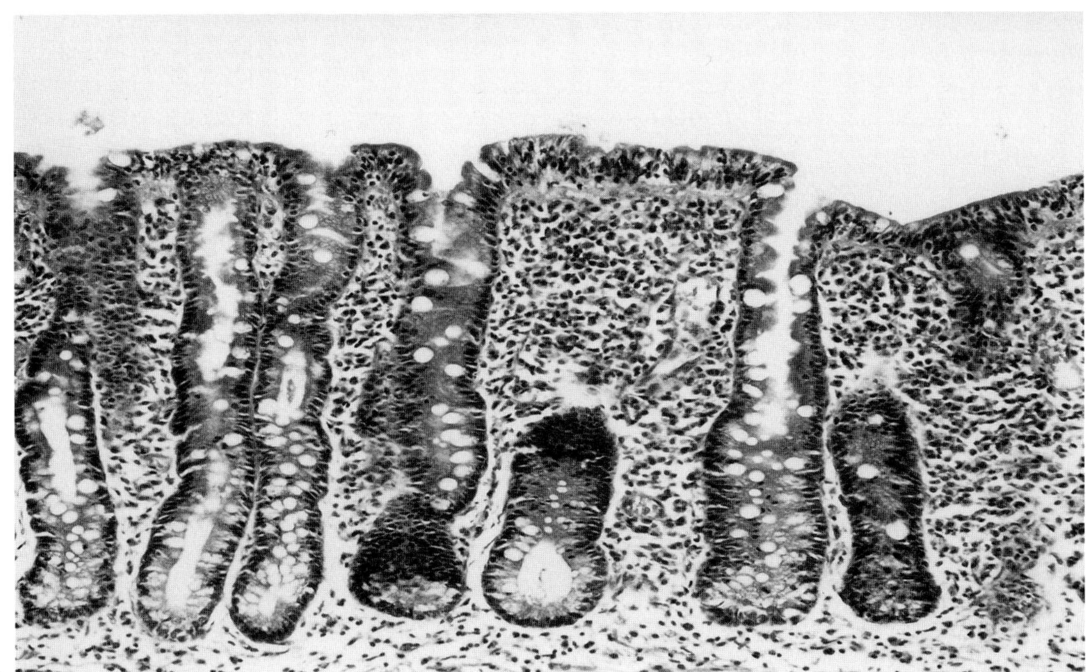

A

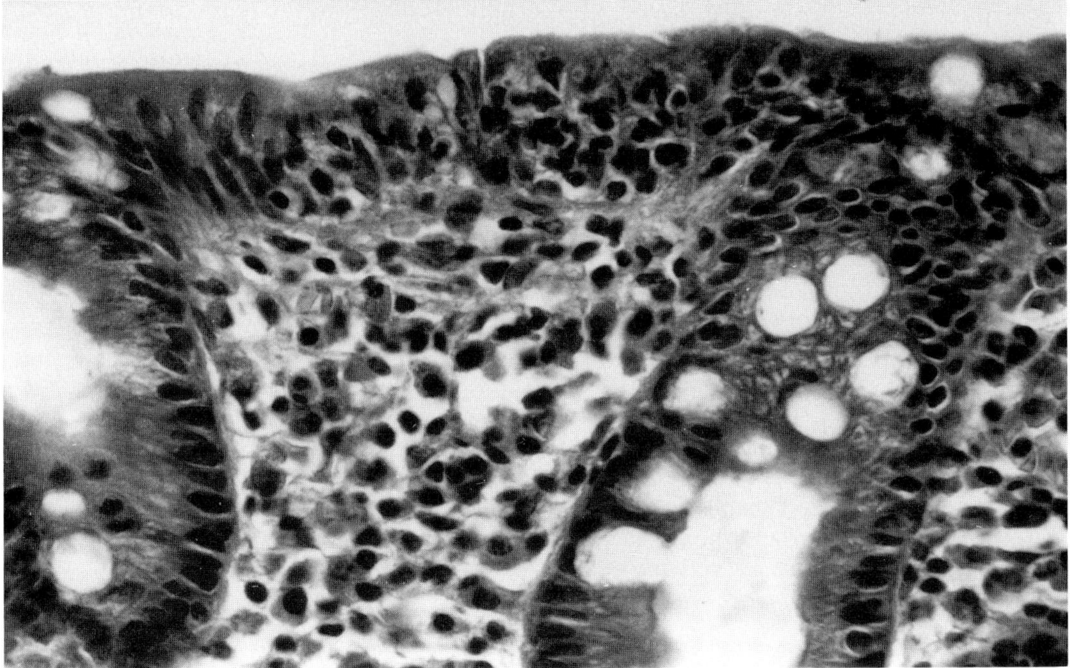

B

Fig. 7-8. Severe example of active celiac disease in the jejunum. **(A)** There is diffuse and total loss of the villi, marked crypt hyperplasia, and increased inflammatory cells in the lamina propria. (× 170). **(B)** Noted is a marked increase of intraepithelial lymphocytes in the surface layer, indicative of active disease (× 635).

receiving gluten challenge, shows only mild shortening of the villi, but distinct damage to the surface epithelial cells with a loss of microvilli and an increase of lymphocytes in the epithelial layer[193, 194] (Fig. 7-9). When this is noted following the reintroduction of gluten, it serves to clinch the diagnosis of celiac disease.

The more severe cases show greater loss or complete absence of the villi, together with more inflammation (Fig. 7-8). The absorptive epithelial cells on the villi show the greatest effects of injury, which are best visualized by ultrastructure.[195, 196] Noted are an overall shortening of the cells, a marked reduction together with blunting of the surface microvilli, and prominent vacuoles, mostly lipid in nature, within the cytoplasm. The amount of crypt hyperplasia is largely proportional to the degree of villous damage and shortening, being maximal when there are no villi. Also noted within the elongated crypts are increased numbers and more irregular locations of Paneth cells and of neuroendocrine cells.[197]

With healing, there is a prompt diminution in the inflammatory reaction and restitution of the columnar epithelial cells and their surface microvilli (Fig. 7-10). This closely correlates with the functional and clinical improvement. The reappearance of villi takes a longer interval, probably on the order of months (Fig. 7-11). Biopsies are occasionally encountered when patients are in this healing phase. At first glance they may appear as evidence of disease, since there are shortened villi and crypt hyperplasia. Lacking, however, are the features of damaged epithelial cells or of increased lymphocytes in the surface epithelial layer, and the diagnosis of a healing rather than of an active enteritis can be made in such instances.

Use of Duodenal Biopsy

As mentioned above, duodenal endoscopy and biopsy are now being extensively substituted in the initial evaluation of patients with celiac disease. This is based on the information that the celiac disease always involves the duodenum, and the biopsies can be employed for screening. If they are completely normal, this serves to exclude a case of untreated celiac disease. Conversely, evidence of villous damage in the duodenum could represent celiac disease, but could also represent other common disorders that affect the duodenum, particularly peptic duodenitis. Accordingly, attempts are made to take biopsies from the more distal region of the duodenum to provide greater specificity. Overall, the finding of a severe enteritis with total loss of the villi in the distal duodenum can probably also be considered as putative evidence of celiac disease, similar to what is done in the jejunum. The endoscopic biopsies are smaller but appear to provide the essential information in most cases. This smallness leads to greater difficulty in orientation, which can be helped by obtaining multiple levels of the tissue samples.

Clinical Associations and Complications

An increase in incidence of celiac disease is noted in many conditions, including patients with diabetes mellitus, selective IgA deficiency, dermatitis herpetiformis, and possibly primary biliary cirrhosis and sarcoidosis.[198–200] The link with the skin disorder seems best established, and it has been shown that the subtype with linear deposition of IgA is particularly prone to be associated with active celiac disease.[201] Most of the patients with dermatitis herpetiformis have a mild degree of enteritis and therapy is probably only needed for those with clinically evident disease[202] (Fig. 7-12). It has been further proposed that treatment with a gluten-free diet may help to resolve some of the skin lesions.

It has been suggested that there is an increase of celiac disease in patients with collagenous and lymphocytic colitis and possi-

A

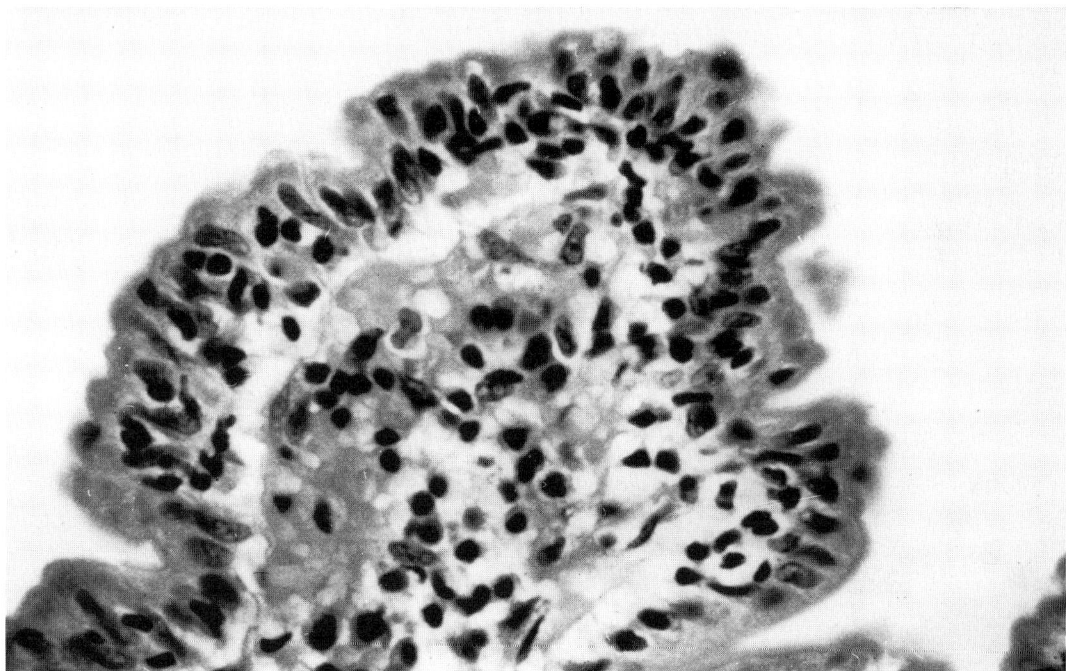

B

Fig. 7-9. Jejunal mucosal biopsy, taken after gluten challenge. **(A)** The villi are only mildly shortened, but there is an increase in inflammatory cells in the lamina propria and villous epithelial layer. **(B)** Surface of villus, showing marked infiltrate of lymphocytes in the surface epithelium together with degeneration of the cells (compare with Fig. 7-2).

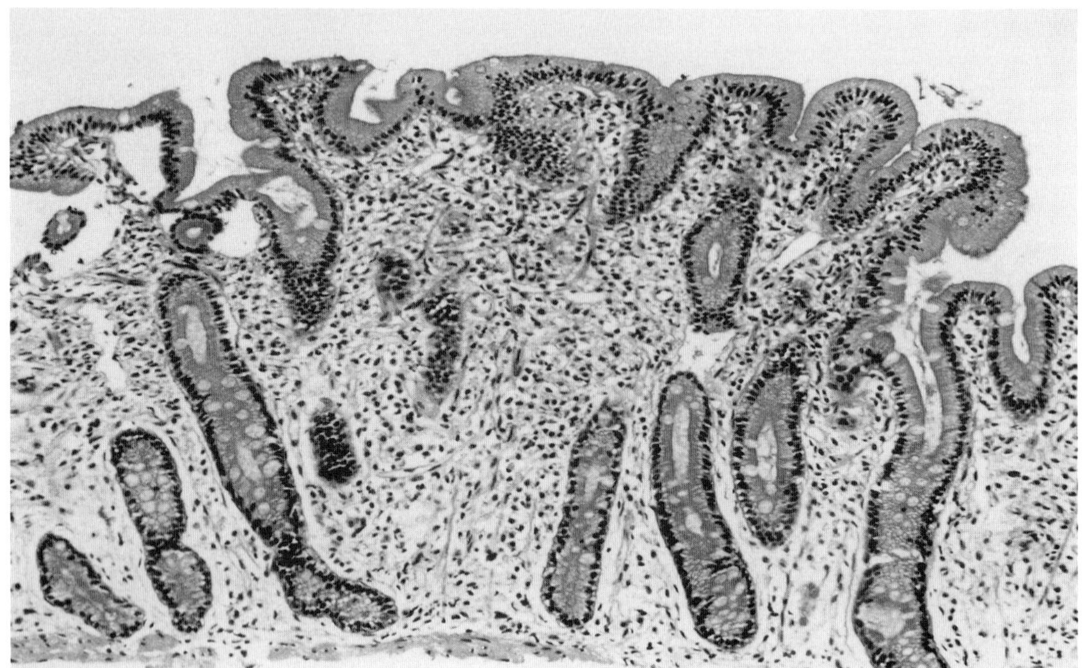

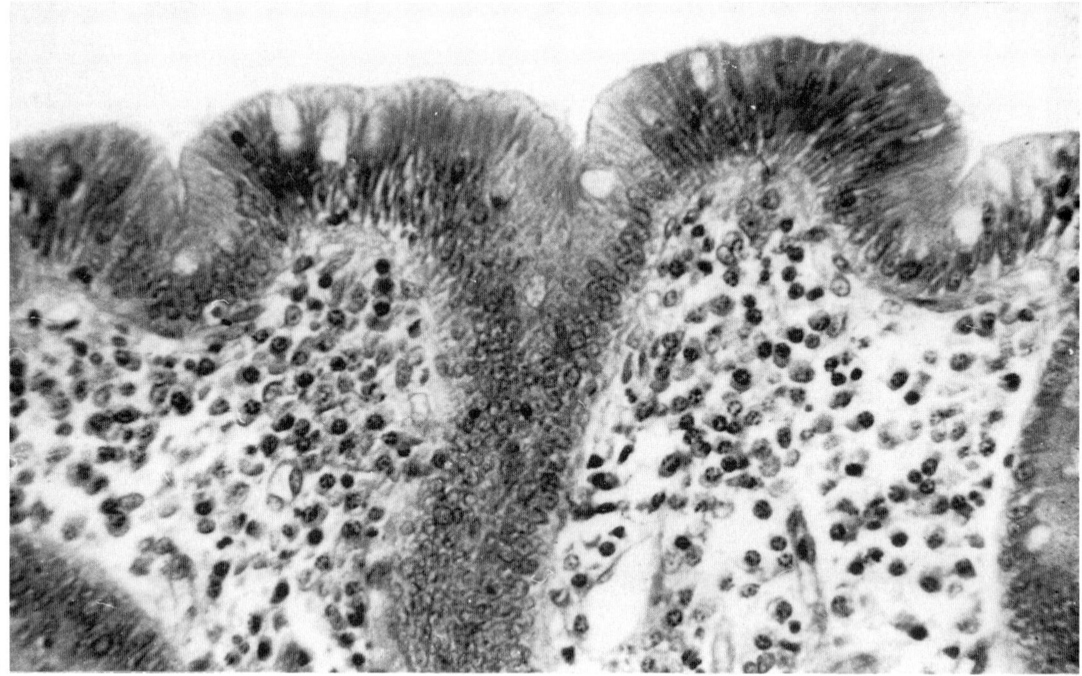

Fig. 7-10. Early healing phase of celiac disease, after gluten withdrawal. **(A)** There is minimal villous formation and persistence of the crypt hyperplasia, but considerable reduction in the inflammation of the lamina propria (compare with Fig. 7-8A) (× 68). **(B)** Surface of jejunal mucosa, showing a marked decrease of intraepithelial lymphocytes and a partial restitution of the epithelial cells (compare with Figs. 7-8B and 7-9B).

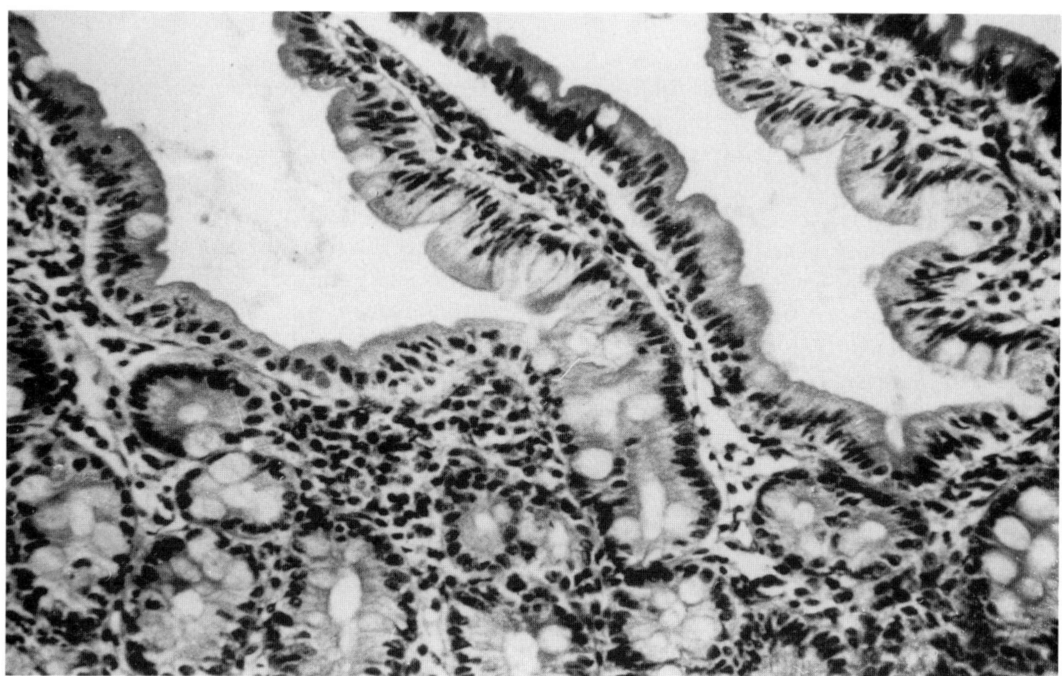

Fig. 7-11. Late healing phase of celiac disease, revealing the return of the villi.

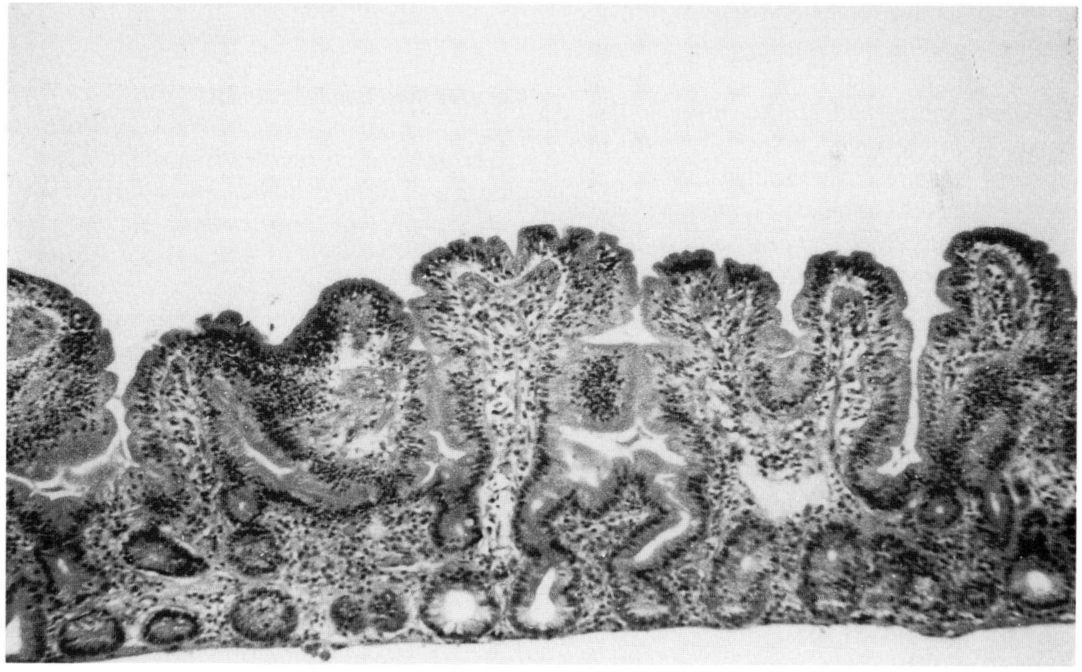

Fig. 7-12. Jejunal mucosal biopsy, in case of dermatitis herpetiformis. Noted are moderate villous shortening, crypt hyperplasia, and increased inflammatory cells. The features are compatible with a mild case of active celiac disease.

bly in those with lymphocytic gastritis, based on finding increased lymphocytes in the surface epithelial layer in colonic and gastric mucosae.[203–206] Alternatively, the finding of the increased intraepithelial lymphocytes in these other gut epithelia may represent a more widespread reaction to the gluten. For example, it has been noted in the gastric antral mucosa in over 60 percent of celiac cases, and the lesion reverses following elimination of dietary gluten[207] (see Fig. 4-18).

Many of the cases of celiac disease appear in adults and in elderly patients,[208] and these are thought to have latent disease in advance of their clinical findings.[209] Some of these cases present following the occurrence of a transient and reversible disorder that calls attention to the problem in the alimentary tract, such as a coincidental infection. It has been suggested that such cases of latent celiac disease may increase the overall diagnosis by 12 percent.[210]

Most patients are able to control their disease throughout their life without further problems. A small percentage become unresponsive to their diet, leading to a recurrence of villous injury and clinical effects. These have been termed cases of *refractory sprue.*[211] It is presently thought that this presages the development of a lymphoproliferative disorder, which may be associated with the formation of ulcers in the small intestine and stomach and ultimately with the development of a malignant lymphoma, largely of the T-cell type.[212–214] The diagnosis of the lymphoma is particularly difficult in the early stages, and is associated with scattered foci of highly atypical lymphoid cells embedded in the lamina propria (Fig. 7-13). In patients with celiac disease who are refractory to diet or who develop ulcers, the clinical suspicion of lymphoma should be enhanced, leading to multiple biopsy samples. Patients with celiac disease are also at an increased risk for the development of epithelial neoplasms, including adenomas, adenocarcinoma, and carcinoid tumors.[215–217]

Allergic Enteritis

Disease Due to a Single Allergen

Allergic enteritis due to a single allergen most commonly develops as an allergic reaction to cow's milk protein or to soy protein, leading to the formation of multiple foci of enteritis and to the potential for bleeding and for malabsorption.[218–223] The lesions tend to be focal in the small intestine, requiring several samples for the diagnosis. The biopsies of the affected areas show partial villous shortening, prominent damage to the surface epithelial cells with many vacuoles in the cytoplasm, and a large increase of eosinophils in the form of aggregates that involve the lamina propria and extend into the surface epithelium (see Fig. 6-20). A change in diet with elimination of the particular offending allergen is typically associated with prompt resolution of the clinical problem and a return of the mucosa to normal. Repeat biopsies are ordinarily not obtained.

Eosinophilic Gastroenteritis

The mucosal form of eosinophilic gastroenteritis is thought to have an allergic basis and to represent those cases in which there are multiple allergens that cannot be fully identified.[224–227] This leads to greater damage of the mucosa with more likelihood of significant bleeding, of protein loss, and of malabsorption. The lesions are similar to those noted with cows milk or soy protein but are usually more prominent. About 10 percent of the cases affecting the small bowel can show a diffuse enteritis with marked to complete loss of the villi, identical in appearance to celiac disease.[228] In most instances, however, multiple samples are needed to document the focal lesions in the small bowel.[229] Furthermore, the presence of eosinophils is not specific, since they can be seen in many other conditions including celiac disease, infections, and granulomatous disorders.[230, 231]

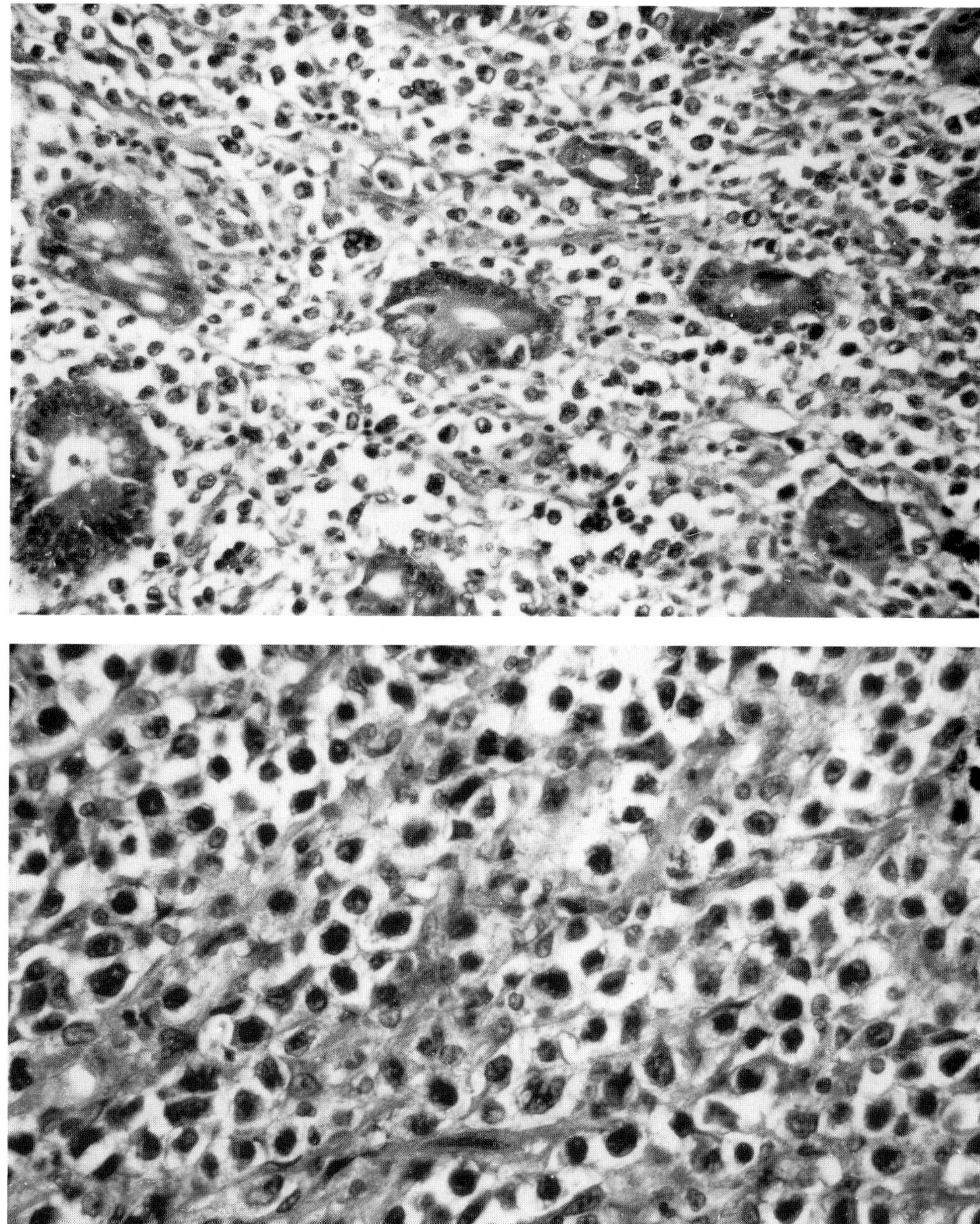

Fig. 7-13. Malignant lymphoma of the jejunum, complicating a case of celiac disease. **(A)** There is a prominent infiltrate of enlarged lymphoid cells in the lamina propria. The crypts are partially destroyed. **(B)** Diffuse infiltrate of enlarged and pleomorphic lymphoid cells. Most cases are composed of T cells.

In contrast, more marked and diffuse lesions are noted in the gastric antrum, which can serve as a more sensitive and specific marker for the diagnosis of allergic or eosinophilic gastroenteritis (see Fig. 4-31 and Table 4-11). Accordingly, biopsies of the small bowel can support the diagnosis of allergic disease, but samples of the gastric antrum are probably more helpful.

Lesions of allergic disease are also commonly noted in the esophagus, whereas they tend to be particularly sparse in the gastric corpus and in the colon in older children.[228] A different form of allergic disease that involves the rectal and colonic mucosa occurs in young infants in reaction to dietary proteins, but this typically resolves without sequellae, and it is not associated with the eosinophilic gastroenteritis that is seen in older children and young adults.

Other Disorders with Nonspecific Enteritis

Refractory Sprue

Refractory sprue represents the cases that resemble celiac disease both clinically and by biopsy but fail to respond to a gluten-free diet.[211] As noted above, it may occur late in the course of a patient with well established celiac disease; in such instances, it is often a sign of impending development of lymphoma. Other cases present at an earlier stage, showing the clinical features of celiac disease and the same biopsy, but fail to respond adequately or at all to a gluten-free diet. These patients frequently require steroids or other immunosuppressive agents for treatment and ultimately develop complications from such prolonged therapy. Biopsies of patients with refractory sprue show a severe and nonspecific enteritis that mimics celiac disease. It has been suggested that there is less perfect development of the crypts, with a relative depletion of goblet mucous cells and a paucity of well formed Paneth cells[232] (Fig. 7-14). These criteria, however, do not appear to be present in most cases. There is also a word of caution about the evaluation of Paneth cells that may fail to show the bright red granules after fixation in heavy metal solutions. In such cases they still should be recognized but as cells with vacuolated cytoplasm.

Collagenous Sprue

The lesion of collagenous sprue shows a marked deposition of collagen within the lamina propria and is now thought to be a variant of long-standing or refractory cases of celiac disease.[233,234] There are rare associations with collagenous colitis but no clear connection between the two disorders.[235]

Tropical Sprue

Tropical sprue represents cases of severe malabsorption and diffuse enteritis that are noted in the tropical regions.[236–240] The cases are thought to be due to chronic infections and are especially associated with reduced absorption of folates. Indeed, treatment with folates alone or together with antibiotics is usually beneficial. The biopsy features are those of a diffuse enteritis, usually with marked shortening but not complete loss of the villi, increased inflammation, and crypt hyperplasia (Fig. 7-15). On an absolute scale, the biopsy features cannot be distinguished from those in celiac disease or from any other nonspecific enteritis. It appears that the lesions are always diffuse. The diagnosis is essentially made by noting the response to the specific therapy.

Ulcerative Jejunoileitis

Ulcerative jejunoileitis was a condition described in patients with ulcers of the jejunum and ileum that could not be ascribed to

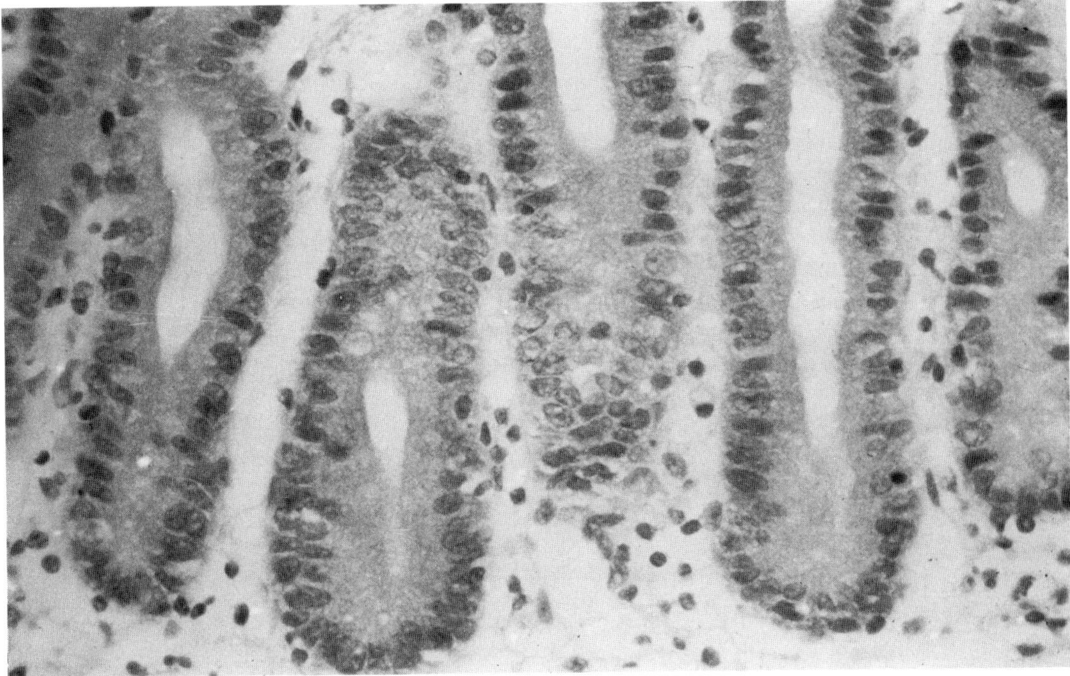

Fig. 7-14. Refractory sprue in the jejunum. Shown are crypts that lack Paneth cells and mature goblet mucous cells (compare with Fig. 7-4).

Crohn's disease.[241, 242] It is now thought, however, to be a feature of long-standing celiac disease and a possible marker of the development of lymphoma.[212] This is no longer considered to be a separate entity.

Effects of Microorganisms

As noted above, the functional effects seen in the bacterial proliferation syndromes are largely due to the depletion of bile salts, but there can be secondary changes in the mucosa.[180, 181] These typically take the appearance of patchy and relatively mild enteritis. Biopsies show the shortened villi, elongated crypts, and increased inflammatory cells. In most instances, the biopsy can readily be distinguished from celiac disease because of the patchy and mild nature.

Infection due to a variety of common viruses can be associated with a focal or diffuse enteritis that can range from mild to severe disease and simulate celiac disease, particularly in children.[98–101] The viruses can be seen with ultrastructural examination but this is ordinarily not done. Following recovery, there is a prompt return of the mucosa to normal. There are exceptional cases of prominent malabsorption that is associated with a generalized fungal or parasitic infection.[243]

Immunodeficiency Disorders in Children

Reversible immunodeficiency conditions have been noted, and include transient hypogammaglobulinemia of infants and nodular lymphoid hyperplasia.[244, 245] The former shows shortened villi and elongated crypts, but typically lacks the reduction in plasma cells that is noted in the same condition in adults. The disorder is made worse by complicating infections, such as *Giardia,* but usually resolves over a short period of time. In

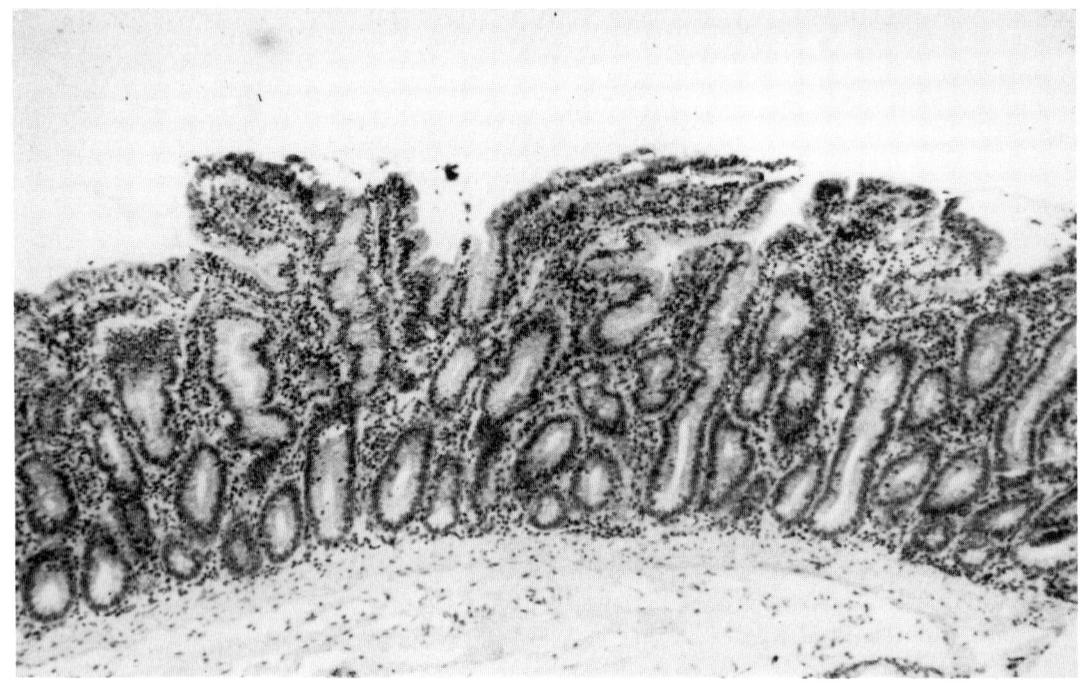

A

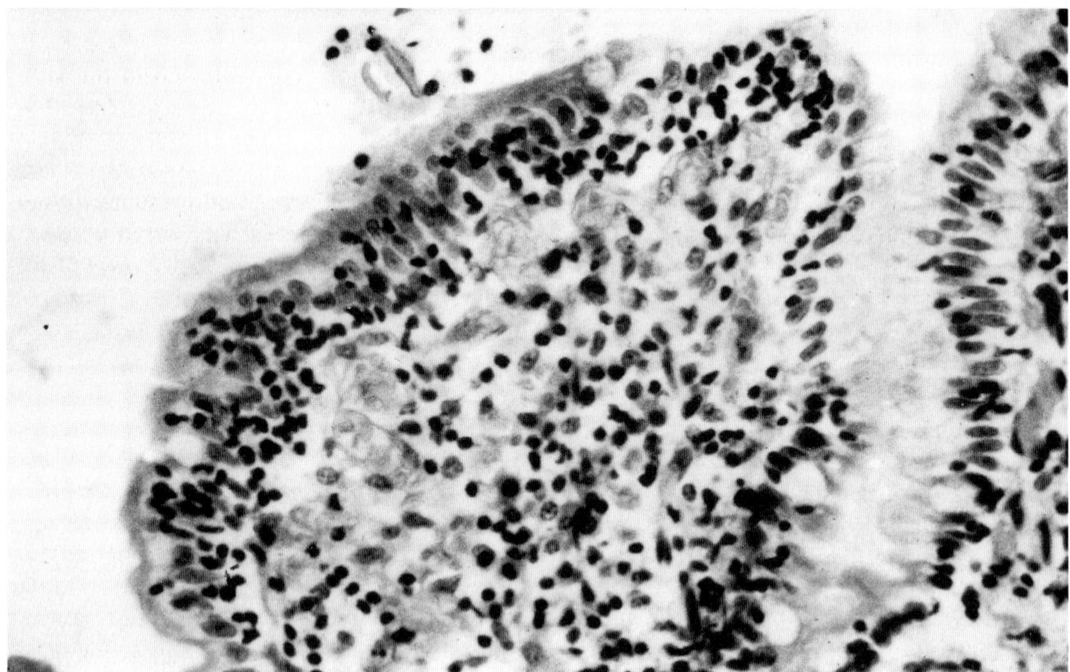

B

Fig. 7-15. Tropical sprue in the jejunum. **(A)** There is diffuse and marked shortening of the villi and crypt hyperplasia, similar to that seen in celiac disease. **(B)** Surface of shortened villus, showing a marked increase of intraepithelial lymphocytes, indicative of an active enteritis.

lymphoid hyperplasia, radiographs note prominent lymphoid nodules throughout the small intestine, and these can be readily appreciated in biopsy samples. There are usually no other problems in the mucosa, which reveals villi of normal height and no other increase in inflammatory cells. Again, the clinical symptoms appear to be related to secondary opportunistic infections, and most of these cases resolve over time. There is no clear relation of nodular lymphoid hyperplasia to the development of lymphoma in children.

Crohn's Disease

Many patients with Crohn's disease affecting typical areas of the ileum and colon develop minor microscopic lesions of the upper and midportions of the gut.[246, 247] Biopsies may reveal a patchy and mild enteritis without granulomas, and the diagnosis requires the finding of the disease in the more typical area. The discovery of the microscopic lesions does not signify certain development of clinical disease in these areas. Accordingly, much less attention has been recently placed on examination of the entire gut in such cases. Rather, the prognosis and treatment is largely determined by the gross appearance of disease.

Whipple's Disease

Whipple's disease is a rare disorder due to the bacterium *Tropheryma whippelii,* which has not yet been cultured.[248–251] There can develop lesions in many organs of the body, with the greatest amount occurring in the small intestine. In this site there is a massive accumulation of macrophages containing the organisms that tend to block the lymphatics, resulting in malabsorption, principally of fats.

The small bowel biopsy is highly distinctive, revealing many macrophages with a finely vacuolated appearance in the lamina propria (Fig. 7-16). These stain intensely with the PAS reaction and represent the coats of the bacteria (Fig. 7-17). The actual bacterial nature is disclosed by ultrastructural examination (Fig. 7-18), and is supported by both molecular and immunocytochemical studies.[249, 252, 258] Utilizing polymerase chain reaction (PCR) technology, the organism has been identified in peripheral blood monocytes and in tissue specimens, both normal and diseased.[254] Also noted in the lamina propria are dilated lymphatics from the obstruction of this circulation. The epithelial cells appear normal by light microscopy but may show minor alterations of the microvilli that are associated with reduced lactose digestion;[255] these revert to normal after treatment.

The lesions are usually diffuse in the jejunum and can extend in a patchy fashion into the duodenum where they may be captured by an endoscopic biopsy.[248, 256] Exceptionally, the disease is concentrated in the submucosa with relative sparing of the mucosa.[257]

Treatment with antibiotics typically results in clinical improvement and ultimate reduction of the bacteria.[258, 259] Biopsies taken during the healing phase still reveal the many macrophages but with less intense PAS staining, as well as the appearance only of coats of organisms by ultrastructure (Fig. 7-19).

The lesions of Whipple's disease can be mimicked by infection due to *Mycobacterium avium intercellularae* (MAI), which is now much more common, with frequent appearance in the AIDS population. In this disorder there are also many macrophages with a prominent cytoplasm. In contrast to Whipple's disease, the cytoplasm in infection due to MAI is more typically granular and the organisms are revealed with the acid-fast stain (see Figs. 6-12 and 6-13). A word of caution is that the mycobacteria can also be stained with the PAS reaction, which can

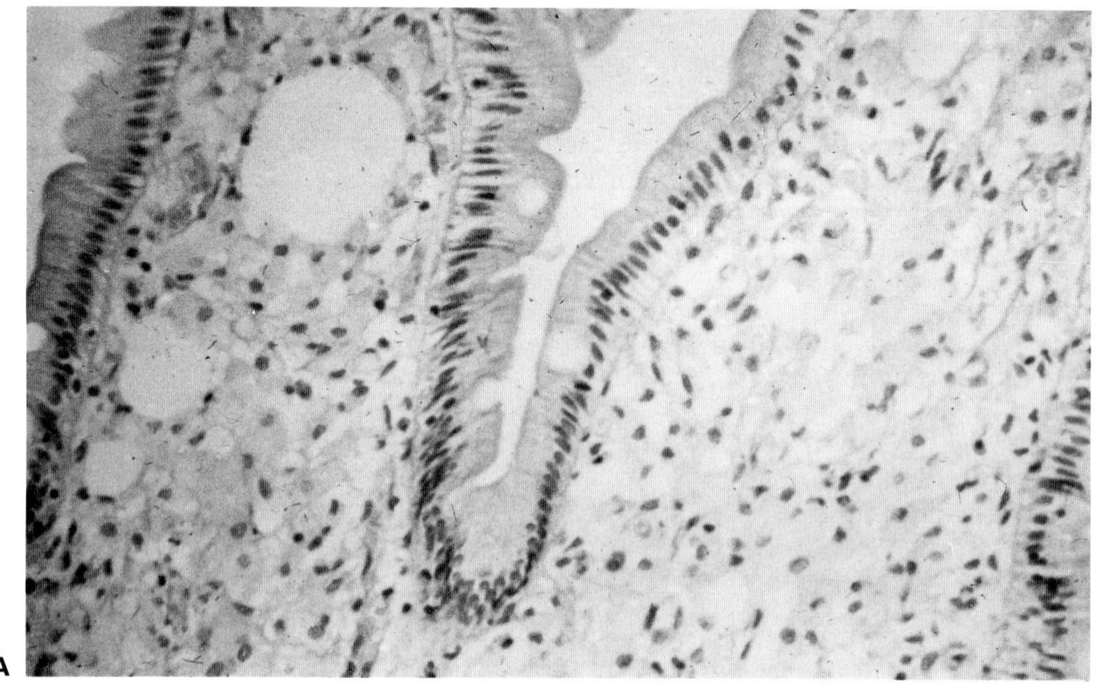

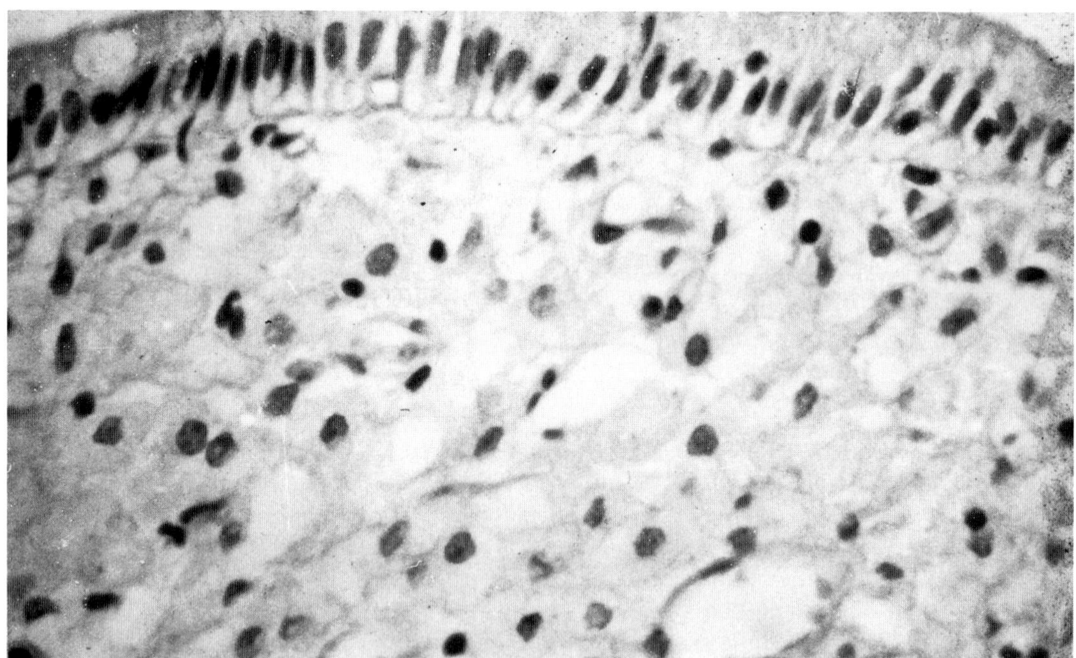

Fig. 7-16. Whipple's disease in the jejunal mucosa. **(A)** There is distention of the lamina propria in the villous cores due to the many enlarged macrophages. Dilated lymphatic lumina are present at the left. **(B)** Villus, showing the many macrophages with finely granular or foamy cytoplasm in the lamina propria. The overlying epithelial cells are normal.

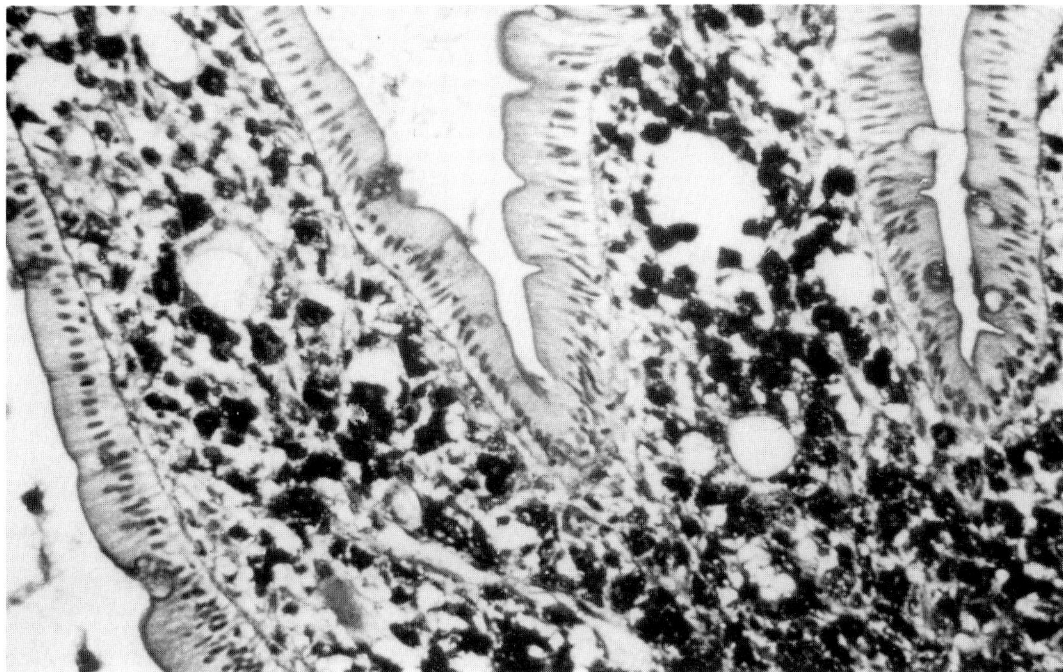

Fig. 7-17. Whipple's disease. Periodic acid-Schiff (PAS) reaction, accenting the macrophages in the lamina propria. The unstained spaces in the villous cores are lymphatics.

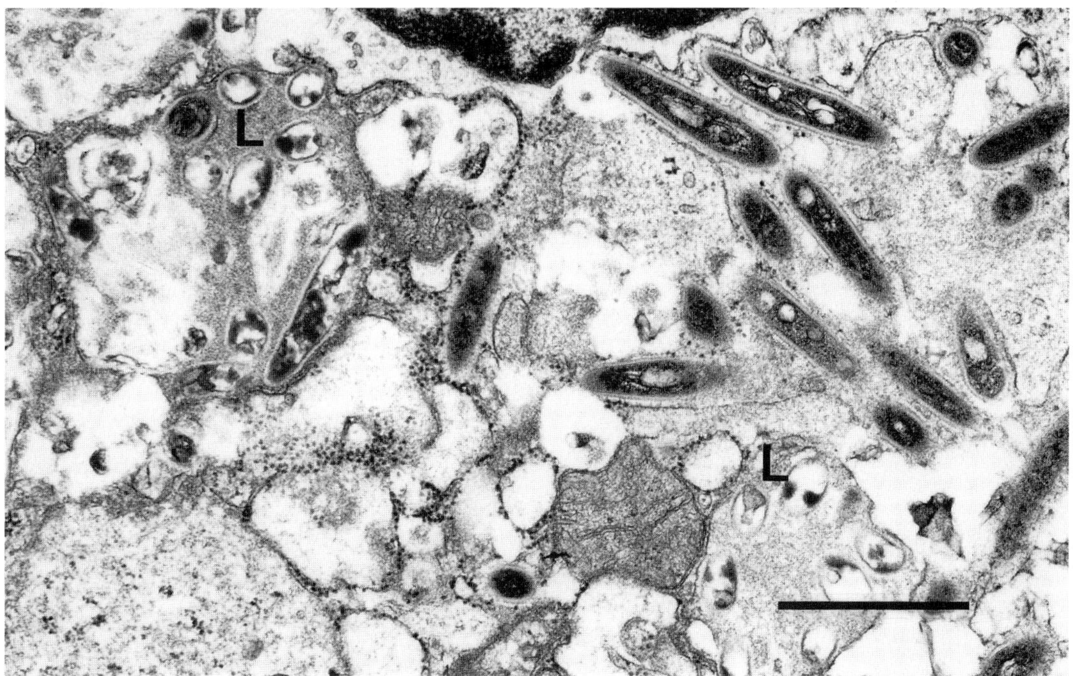

Fig. 7-18. Electron micrograph of bacteria found in Whipple's disease. Intact rod-shaped bacilli are free in the cytoplasm of the macrophages, and secondary lysosomes (L) contain cell wall material and degenerating bacteria (× 25,000; bar = 1 μm).

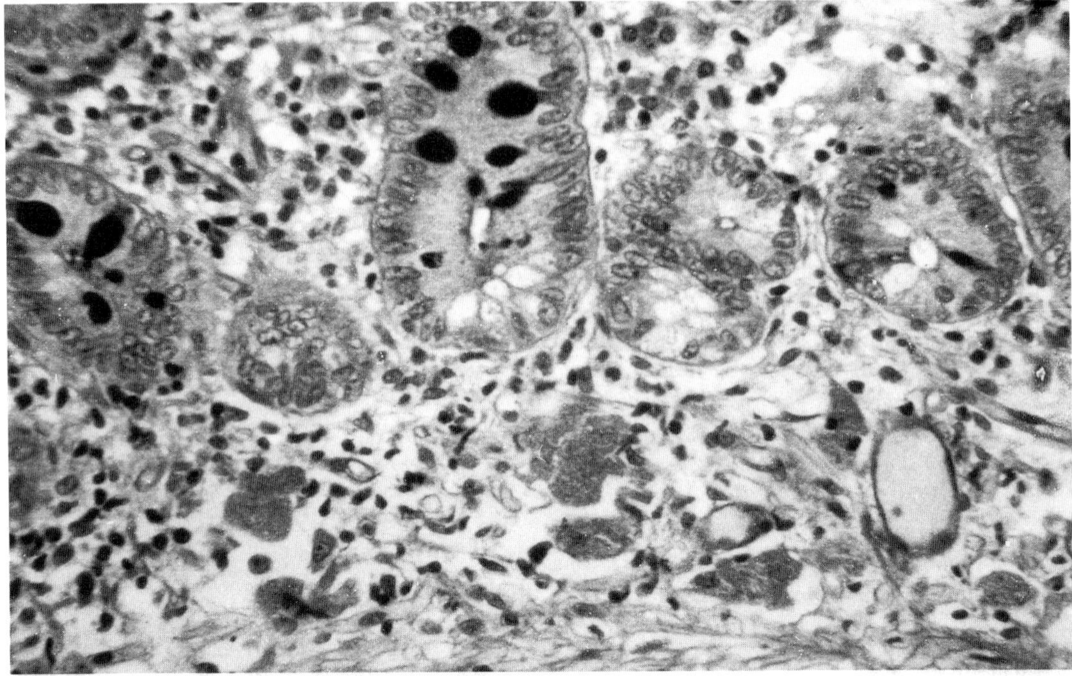

Fig. 7-19. Whipple's disease in the healing phase, after treatment with antibiotics. PAS reaction reveals marked reduction of the macrophages and their staining at the base. The stronger staining is in the goblet mucous cells of the crypts. The muscularis mucosae appear at the bottom.

cause erroneous interpretations. Biopsies are performed in patients with Whipple's disease to render the diagnosis and to follow the case after therapy. Exceptionally noted is a granulomatous reaction that may occur in the mucosa or in the adjoining lymph nodes.[260] The granulomas are of the sarcoid type, with well formed epithelioid cells and giant cells, and lack any significant necrosis.

Immunodeficiency Disorders

As noted above, some of the disorders that affect infants and children lack much in the way of abnormalities, but the patients have clinical problems that appear to be largely related to secondary infections. The disorders in children are mostly reversible. There are other conditions that can affect adults as well that show more distinctive features[261–263] (see Table 6-6).

Agammaglobulinemia

Agammaglobulinemia is an inherited disorder in men in which there is a failure to produce immunoglobulins, but the patients are protected by complete T-cell function. Biopsies reveal normal mucosal structure except for the complete absence of plasma cells. There are usually no major clinical problems in the gastrointestinal tract unless there is an associated disorder in the T cells.

Selective IgA Deficiency

Patients with selective IgA deficiency lack the ability to produce the secretory immunoglobulin, but this is compensated by the increased production of other immunoglobulins, particularly IgM.[264] Accordingly, the biopsy may be completely normal, with a full complement of plasma cells as appreciated by ordinary H & E stain. Immunocytochemical stains show, however, that these are mainly comprised of cells producing IgG and IgM and none revealing stains for IgA. Except for an increased prevalence of celiac disease, these patients ordinarily do not have other gastrointestinal problems.

Hypogammaglobulinemia

Cases of hypogammaglobulinemia in adults may or may not be associated with prominent nodular lymphoid hyperplasia.[265] Compared to the childhood cases, the adult forms more regularly show a considerable depletion in plasma cells within the lamina propria, and there is usually clinical problems related to secondary infections with *Giardia* and other protozoal agents. The disorders tend to be more protracted in adults and are productive of greater complications, including the development of lymphomas and carcinomas. Biopsies typically show marked enteritis with reduced villi and elongated crypts, but a relative lack of inflammation and, particularly, a sparse number of plasma cells (Fig. 7-20). Most symptomatic cases are associated with secondary infections, typically from protozoa.

Acquired Immunodeficiency Syndrome

Cases of AIDS do not show a standard effect in the intestines. Some are associated with focal or diffuse lesions in the small intestine with mild to moderate villous injury, but most cases reveal normal structure. A variety of viral-like particles have been noted in the epithelial cells and macrophages of the small intestine and are thought to be responsible for some of the symptoms, but this is not fully established[107–113] (see Fig. 7-7). In general, the problems are due instead to the numerous opportunistic infections that can occur throughout the alimentary tract. Biopsies are largely done to identify the organisms. Aside from the H & E, stains such as the modified Gram, methenamine silver, PAS, and acid-fast are commonly obtained to look for the microorganisms. (See "Infections" above for further details.)

Other Disorders with Specific Features

There are many other disorders with specific features that can be appreciated in mucosal biopsies of the small intestine, including the jejunum. Some of these are associated with bleeding, excess secretion of proteins, and variable degrees of malabsorption. There also may be involvement of other parts of the gut, particularly the colon and rectum.

Infections

Included are the many diseases with recognizable fungi, protozoa, and ova, which are described above in the section on "Infections."

Depositions

Jejunal mucosal biopsies have been used in the past to detect amyloid material, as well as the macroglobulinemic deposits of Waldenstrom's disease[266, 267] (Fig. 7-21). In these circumstances, the biopsy shows fibrillar eosinophilic material within the lamina propria and involving vessel walls. The amyloid can be accented by the Congo Red stain, yielding green birefringence under polaroid light. The nature of the material is best visualized with electron microscopic examination (see Fig. 4-35 and Plate 4D). At the present time, samples of other parts of the gut are more often used to detect amyloid and other deposits, particularly from the rectum and the stomach (Fig. 9-46).

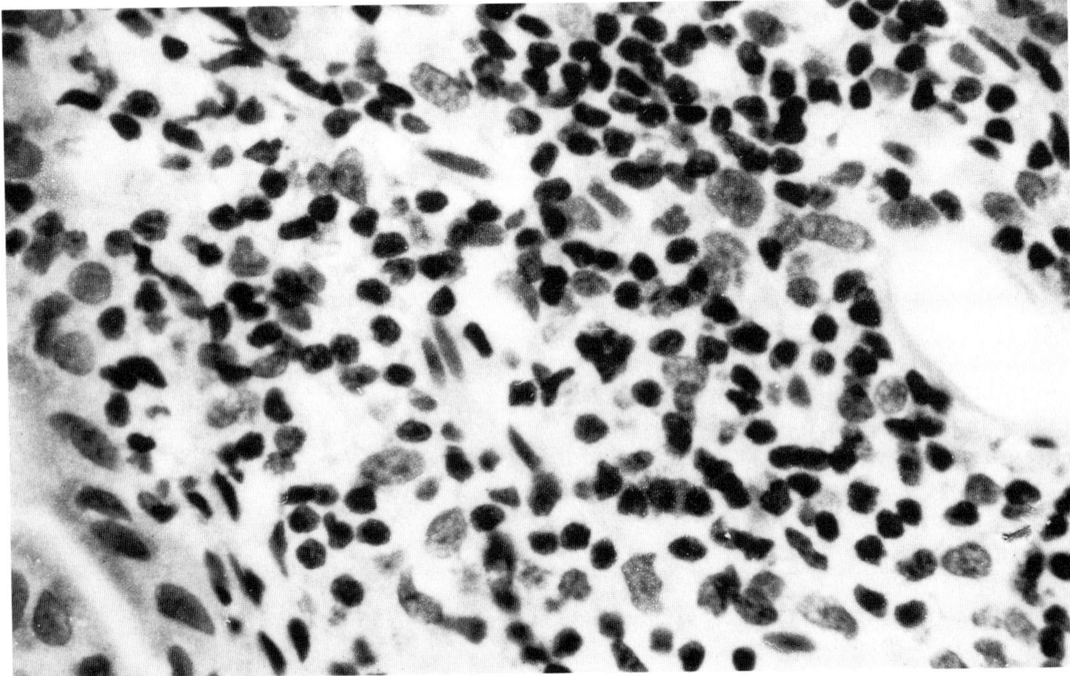

Fig. 7-20. Hypogammaglobulinemic sprue in jejunal mucosa. There is a prominent mononuclear cell infiltrate in the lamina propria, but lacking mature plasma cells.

Mastocytosis

Cases of systemic mastocytosis are associated with the deposition of large quantities of mast cells in many tissues.[268–270] These can be seen in the small intestinal mucosa as clumps of large granulated cells in the lamina propria (Fig. 7-22). They are best visualized with metachromatic stains such as Toluidine Blue, and also contain specific granules as evidenced by ultrastructural examination. There is usually only mild injury in the small intestine in contrast to other organs such as the liver, where there can develop an increased fibrosis.

Granulomatous Diseases

The most common granulomatous disorder is Crohn's disease, which is typically more prevalent in the ileum and colon. Cases can involve any part of the small intestine and the disease can range from microscopic foci to grossly evident ulcers with fistulae and strictures.[271, 272] The diagnosis is largely established by radiographic studies and by biopsies of the upper and lower tract taken at endoscopy or at time of operation. Jejunal mucosal biopsy is usually not obtained but may show features of nonspecific inflammation and, less often, well formed granulomas (see Fig. 4-41). The other granulomatous disorders are discussed in the section "Miscellaneous Conditions" below.

Histiocytosis

Clusters of macrophages are seen in many conditions, including Whipple's disease and mycobacterial infections, storage disorders, and granulomatous diseases. Rare conditions include the dissemination of Langerhan's cells in the entity of histiocytosis.[273, 274] These can occur in any parts of the body including the small intestine, but are not usually detected with random jejunal biopsy.

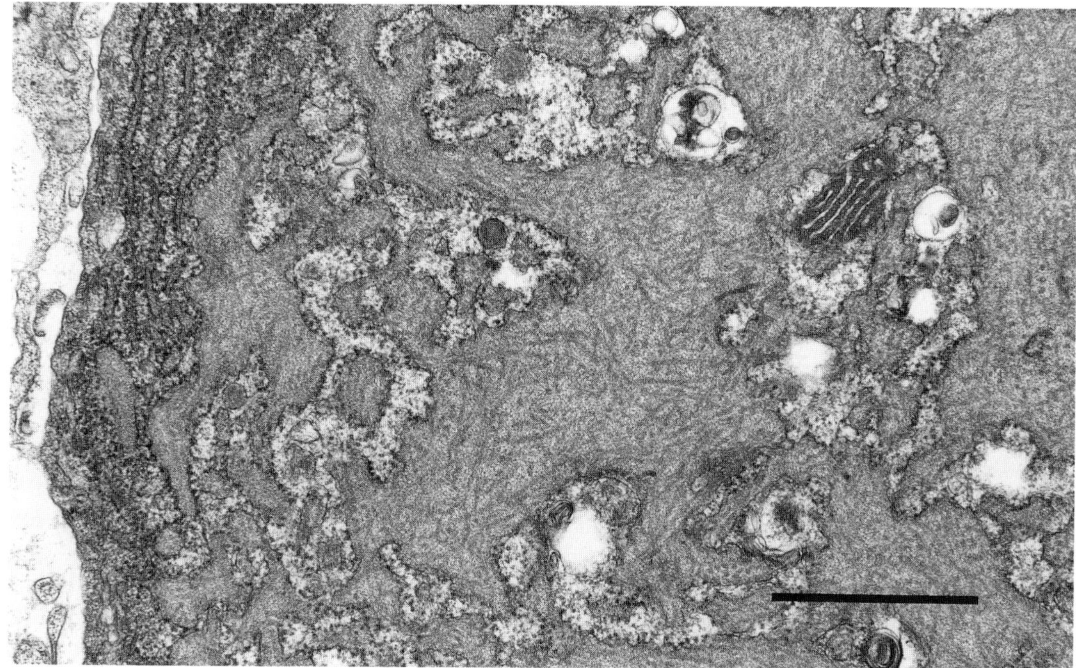

Fig. 7-21. Electron micrograph of plasma cell in Waldenstrom's macroglobulinemia. The rough endoplasmic reticulum has very distended cisternae that contain fibrillary inclusions representing immunoglobulin (× 27,000; bar = 1 μm).

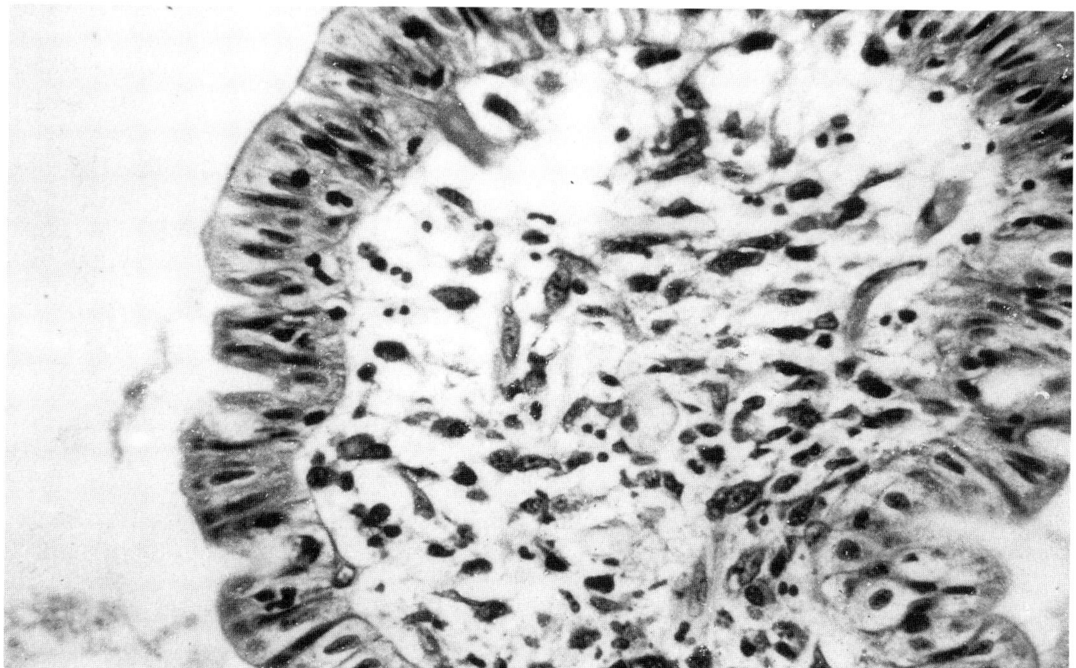

Fig. 7-22. Mastocytosis in the jejunal mucosa. The lamina propria in the villous core contains an increase of mast cells and eosinophils (toluidine blue stain).

Lymphangiectasia

Cases of primary lymphangiectasia are associated with lesions in several organs including the alimentary tract.[275–277] The lesions appear to represent microscopic hamartomas of the lymphatics and are most often present in the small intestine, where the greatest amount of lymphatic tissue ordinarily occurs. The lesions are focal and easily missed by a random single jejunal sample. Accordingly, endoscopic examination with multiple biopsies has proven more useful. The biopsies show the conglomeration of dilated lymphatics in a patchy area of the lamina propria within the biopsy, with the rest of the mucosa appearing normal (Fig. 7-23). Exceptionally, the lesion extends into the submucosa. Patients typically develop problems from the oozing of the leaky lymphatics, resulting in losses of lymphocytes and protein. Additional problems can develop from larger lesions in the skin and soft tissues of the body.

These lesions should be distinguished from secondary lymphangiectasia resulting from the effects of lymphatic obstruction, which may be at the level of the large ducts or even due to constrictive pericarditis.[277] In these secondary cases there is a more generalized dilation of the lymphatics, which are otherwise not abnormal. Biopsy shows prominent dilation of the mucosal lymphatics in practically all villous cores. It is important to distinguish this from exaggerated lacteals in a normal state.

Abetalipoproteinemia

Abetalipoproteinemia represents rare cases in which the patients are able to digest and absorb fats but cannot produce the chylomicrons that are needed to leave the epithelial cells.[278] There results an accumulation of the fats within the absorptive cells and a deficiency in the draining lymphatics. Biopsies show a normal overall structure but a marked increase of triglycerides within the cytoplasm (Fig. 7-24). This is revealed by many vacuoles in H & E processed sections. The lipid nature can be demonstrated with fat stains on tissues that have not been processed in alcohol or by ultrastructural examination. The appearance is identical to the normal mucosa following a fatty meal. The diagnosis is typically made by biochemical studies, and biopsies are not ordinarily obtained.

Tangier Disease

Tangier disease represents patients with abnormal metabolism of the alpha lipoproteins.[279, 280] The cases are associated with prominent hemolytic anemia and with the deposition of macrophages containing lipid vacuoles in many tissues of the body. Most notably involved are the tongue, liver, spleen, and gastrointestinal tract. Any part of the gut can be affected, but the lesions are more commonly seen in the large intestine as yellow to orange nodules and streaks. Biopsy shows the marked infiltrate of the lipid-filled macrophages in the lamina propria and submucosa, and their nature is best appreciated with ultrastructural study[281] (see Fig. 9-49). The diagnosis is typically established by biochemical means, but biopsy may be done to exclude other problems such as infections and tumors.

Microvillous Inclusion Disease

Microvillous inclusion disease is a rare disorder affecting young infants and associated with intractable diarrhea, and is usually familial.[282–285] Biopsies reveal a marked shortening of the villi and usually only modest crypt hyperplasia. The overlying epithelial cells may be only slightly shortened, but reveal a pronounced loss of the microvilli (Fig. 7-25). Compared to other cases of enteritis, there is usually no prominent inflammation.

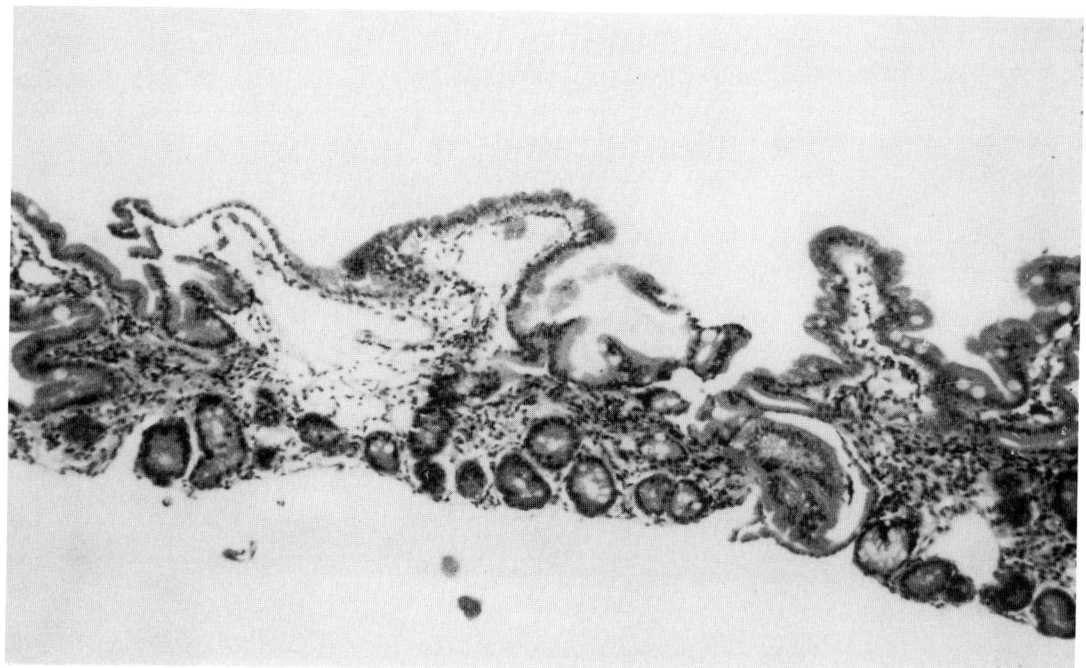

A

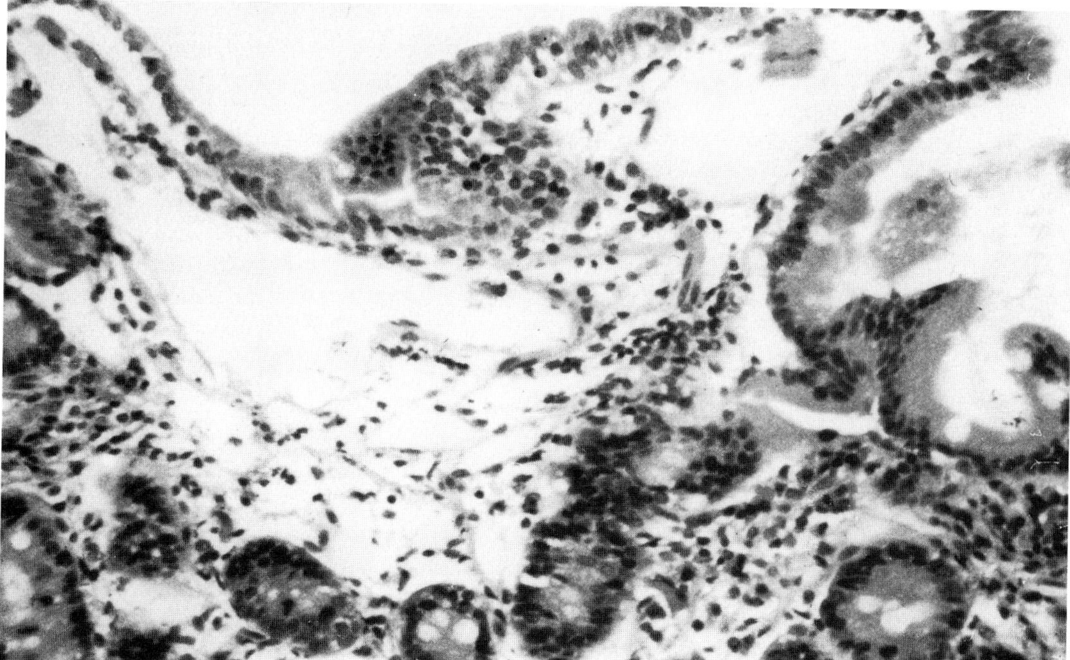

B

Fig. 7-23. Primary lymphangiectasia in the jejunal mucosa, with surface at top. **(A)** There is a focal area in the center with marked and irregular dilation of lymphatics, resulting in distortion and shortening of the overlying villi. **(B)** The lymphatic structure appearing at the left is complex, suggesting that this represents a microhamartoma rather than a simple dilation of normal vessels.

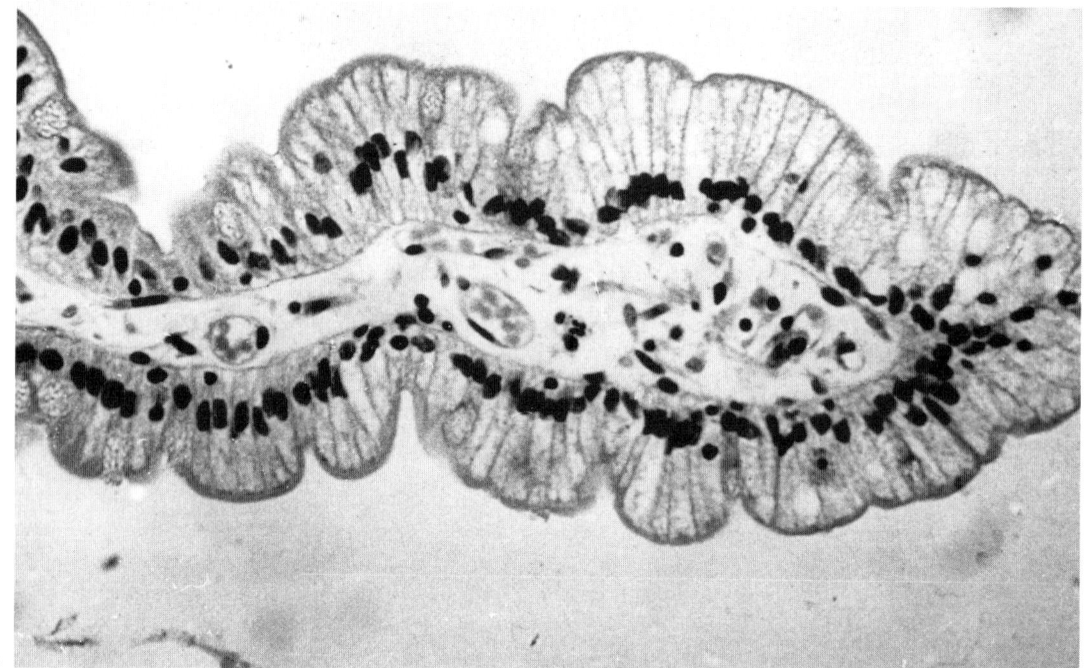

A

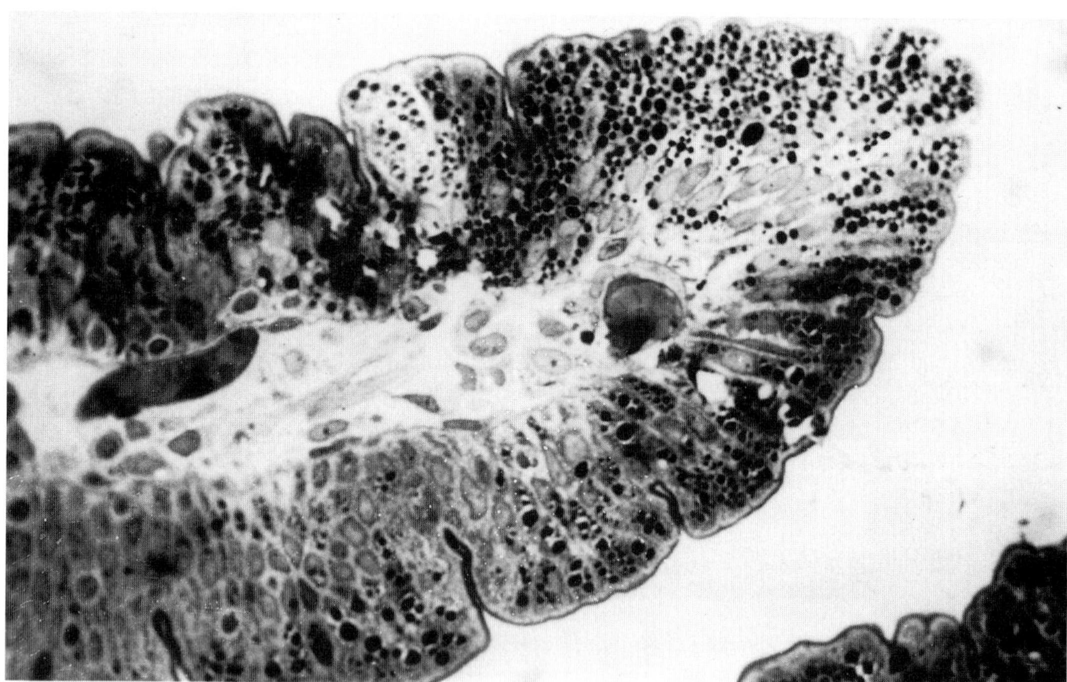

B

Fig. 7-24. Abetalipoproteinemia in the jejunal mucosa. **(A)** Villus of normal dimensions, showing marked vacuolization of the columnar absorptive cells due to retention of cytoplasmic triglycerides. The appearance is similar to a normal villus following a fatty meal. **(B)** One-micrometer-thick plastic section of affected villus, that was fixed in osmium tetraoxide and stained with Toluidine Blue. The triglyceride is preserved and revealed as dark droplets within the cytoplasm.

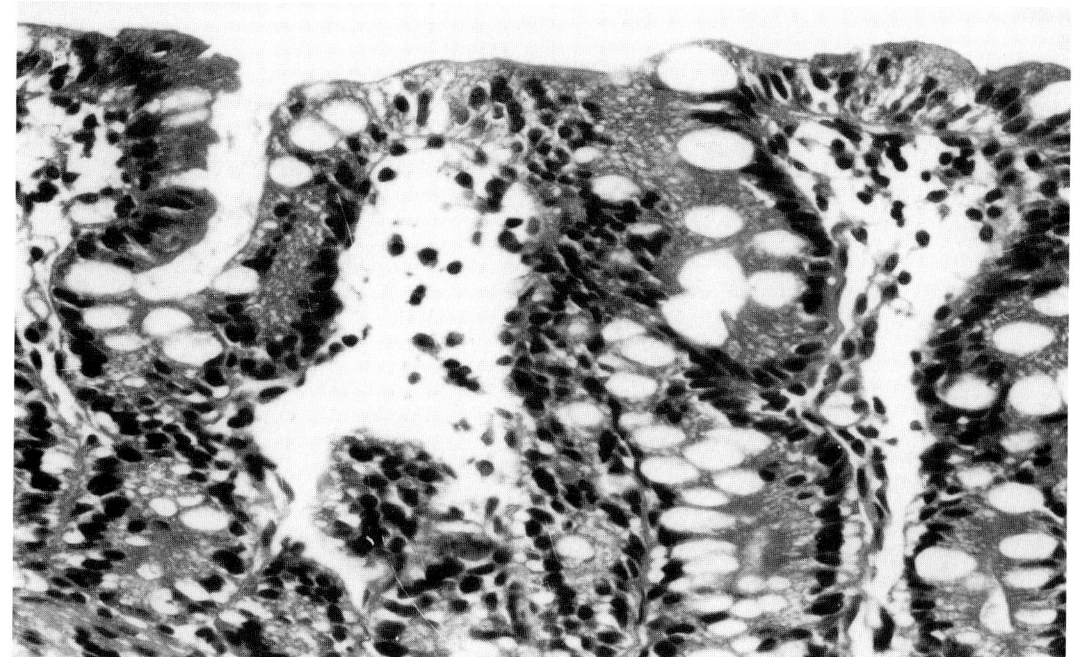

A

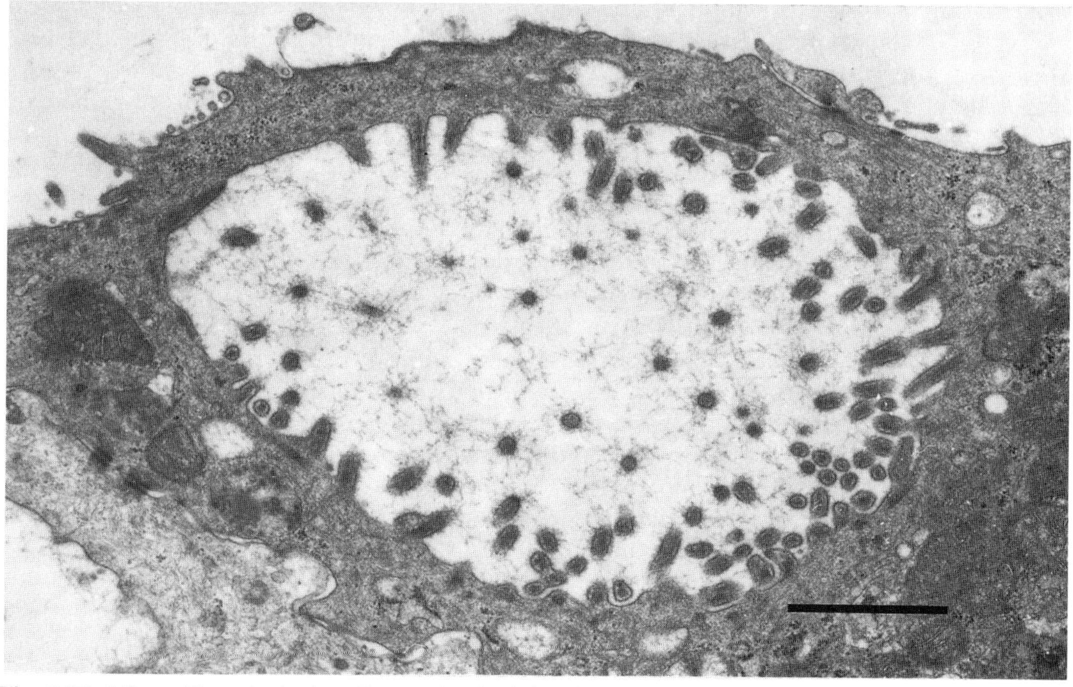

B

Fig. 7-25. Microvillous inclusion disease in the jejunal mucosa. **(A)** Noted are the absence of villi and the appearance of intact crypts. The surface epithelial cells appearing at the top lack a well defined brush border (× 425). **(B)** Electron micrograph of an epithelial cell, showing a well formed intracytoplasmic inclusion lined by microvilli that have filamentous cores, glycocalyx coats, and poorly developed terminal rootlets. The surface of the epithelial cell is almost devoid of microvilli. These are all characteristic features of microvillous inclusion disease (× 20,250; bar = 1 μm). (Courtesy of Dr. Antonio Perez-Atayde, Children's Hospital, Boston, MA.)

The pathognomonic feature is observed with electron microscopy, showing inversion of microvillous structures within the apical portion of the cytoplasm of the absorptive cells.[286, 287] This also can be appreciated by the use of stains that outline the brush border at light microscopy; examples are the PAS reaction and histochemical stains for markers in this structure, such as carcinoembryonic antigen and alkaline phosphatase.[288, 289]

Disorders Associated with Crypt Injury

As described above, some diseases of the small intestinal tract are due to more direct injury of the crypts rather than of the villi (cf. Table 7-9). This leads to reduced formation of the mature cells and to shortened villi, but there is a lack of compensatory hyperplasia of the crypts. Also, compared to the cases with villous injury, those with the crypt injury show less destruction of the surface epithelial cells and an overall reduced degree of inflammation. The expected causes are those that preferentially damage the crypt cells, such as ischemic disease, radiation, and the antimetabolite types of drugs. This also seems to be the preferred site for injury due to a restricted number of infections (such as some species of *Salmonella*), to cases of graft-versus-host disease, and to severe protein under-nutrition in infants.[290]

Biopsy can readily show the crypt type of injury, best appreciated by the lack of proportional crypt hyperplasia and the relative paucity of inflammatory cells. This information can be helpful in restricting the list of potential etiologic agents.

MUCOSAL POLYPS

Overall, polypoid lesions of the jejunum are uncommon and not easily accessed.[291, 292] As a consequence, this is rarely a source for jejunal mucosal biopsy examination. Most tumors are recognized because of the occurrence of clinical symptoms and are demonstrated by radiographic studies. There have been recent attempts with longer scopes, termed *enteroscopes,* to reach and remove some of these lesions, but this is as yet not standard practice.[293, 294] This subject is covered in Chapter 6 and is briefly reviewed here.

Non-Neoplastic Polyps

Various types of polyps can be found throughout the small intestinal mucosa, including the jejunum. These include nodules of heterotopic gastric mucosa, localized inflammatory-type polyps, and isolated hamartomatous lesions. Other polypoid lesions seen in the intestinal tract are cases of localized lymphoid hyperplasia,[245] inflammatory fibroid polyps,[295, 296] and adenomyomas that probably represent variants of pancreatic heterotopia.[297] Multiple inflammatory pseudopolyps can occur in cases of severe chronic inflammatory conditions such as Crohn's disease, but these tend to be more common in the ileal region.[298]

Most of the polypoid lesions are asymptomatic. They can cause problems by bleeding and by obstruction, the latter mainly due to intussusception. The diagnosis is usually established by examination of resected specimens and not by biopsy in the jejunum.

Adenoma

Adenomas are generally uncommon in the jejunum and most go unnoticed[299] (see Fig. 6-22). As in other parts of the gut, adenomas are prone to develop carcinoma, and any larger lesion must be removed. They are increased in the adenomatous polyposis syndromes and, possibly, in cases of chronic enteritis such as celiac disease.

Polyposis Syndromes

Juvenile Polyposis Syndrome

Multiple juvenile polyps are more typically seen in the colon and rectum but there are rare generalized forms with lesions in all parts of the gut, including the stomach and small intestine.[300, 301] The polyps are comprised of hyperplastic glands with prominent cystic change, as well as an edematous and inflamed lamina propria. Dysplasia and carcinoma can develop in these syndromes but are more typical in the colon.[302]

Peutz-Jeghers Syndrome

Hamartomatous polyps occur in the Peutz-Jeghers syndrome with involvement of the small intestine in 90 percent of cases.[303–305] The polyps in this location are highly distinctive, revealing a marked proliferation of hyperplastic and metaplastic small intestinal glands together with prominent wide bands of smooth muscle, representing a harmartoma of the entire mucosa (see Fig. 6-23). The polyps are typically multiple and can cause symptoms by enlargement and intussusception, or by bleeding. It also may be associated with a growth into the wall of the small intestine, representing a localized form of enteritis cystic profunda. It is necessary in such cases to exclude an invasive carcinoma, which is typically done by noting the lack of cytologic atypism or of tumor stroma. Compounding the issue is the recognition that carcinoma can complicate these polyps in any part of the gut.[306–308] Because of the tendency for enlargement and production of symptoms, many of these polyps need removal, but this usually requires surgical operation rather than endoscopic polypectomy in the jejunum.

Cronkhite-Canada Syndrome

Cases of Cronkhite-Canada syndrome also can affect the small intestine.[309–311] These are associated with multiple irregular nodules and foci of atrophy in the mucosa in the formation of small polyps (see Fig. 10-18). The lesions show edema, inflammation, and prominent cystic change. The diagnosis usually requires knowledge of more generalized polyposis and of the extraintestinal manifestations. These are described in Chapter 4.

Adenomatous Polyposis Syndrome

In the adenomatous polyposis syndromes involving the colon, lesions ultimately occur in the upper tract as well, with preference for the stomach and the duodenum.[312–317] There appears to be a slight increase of adenomas as well in the jejunum and ileum.[318, 319] (See discussions of adenomatous polyposis in Chs. 5 and 6).

OTHER TUMORS

Most of the tumors described in the duodenum can involve the jejunum[320] (see Table 6-7). Mucosal biopsy is most useful in those tumors that are very large or multicentric, permiting detection by multiple random samples. This proves to be particularly helpful with the malignant lymphomas. In the rest of the tumors affecting the jejunum, the diagnosis is more often established by operation.

Adenocarcinoma

Most adenocarcinomas of the small intestine occur in the duodenum, and they are especially rare in the jejunum and ileum.[321–324] There is a probable increase in patients with AIDS, celiac disease, and Crohn's disease.[216, 325–328] The latter are more often seen in the ileum, reflecting the greater frequency of Crohn's disease in that area, and may be associated with dysplasia.[329] Adenocarcinomas complicating foci of gastric heterotopia have also been described.[330] As noted above, carcinomas can develop in association with preexisting adenoma.[318, 319]

Jejunal mucosal biopsy is rarely obtained in cases of adenocarcinoma. Most reveal highly atypical glands together with tumor stroma (see Fig. 6-25A); linitis plastica lesions have also been described.[331] The diagnosis of adenocarcinoma of the jejunum is practically always dependent on the examination of a surgical specimen.

Endocrine Tumors

Endocrine tumors include carcinoid tumors[332–334] (see Figs. 6-26 and 8-13), composite tumors composed of a mixture of carcinomatous and endocrine elements[335–337] (see Fig. 10-30), and rare neuroendocrine carcinomas[338, 339] (see Fig. 3-19). All of these tumors are much more common in the duodenum and ileum (see descriptions in Chs. 6 and 8). It is rare to obtain any jejunal mucosal biopsies in these cases.

Lymphoid Tumors

Lymphoid tumors are the most commonly observed tumors in jejunal mucosal biopsies, reflecting their higher incidence in this area and also their involvement of a larger surface area. As a consequence, they can be more readily sampled by blind biopsies. In an effort to enhance their detection, multiple samples are often obtained. The lesions share characteristics with those described in the stomach and duodenum (see Chs. 5 and 6).

Benign Hyperplasia

Focal lymphoid nodules are located throughout the small intestine, and one or two may be included in any jejunal mucosal biopsy. An increase in the size and number of these nodules is often seen in the small intestine, including the jejunal mucosa, and has been termed *nodular lymphoid hyperplasia.* This may be sharply localized, multicentric, or seemingly diffuse. The nodules can be readily appreciated in radiographic studies and followed during the course of the disorders.[340, 341] The lesions are most often seen in children and probably represent a common reaction to a variety of enteric infections and other diseases.

In adults, they tend to be more often associated with symptomatic disease. Patients with lymphoid hyperplasia can develop diarrhea, which is due to a variety of underlying conditions. Particularly important are the presence of immunodeficiency diseases, such as acquired hypogammaglobulinemia. In these conditions, the symptoms appear to be most related to the appearance of secondary infections, particularly by *Giardia* and other protozoal agents.

It is supposed that some cases of lymphoid hyperplasia can persist and proceed into the formation of lymphomas, but this is probably a rare event. Nevertheless, the appearance on radiographs of persistent and enlarging nodules should serve as a marker for suspicious lesions. Multiple samples are typically taken for histology, and marker studies may be added in the difficult cases.[342] The biopsy in hyperplasia shows enlarged but otherwise well formed lymphoid follicles with prominent germinal centers and without any large sheets of monomorphic cells, markedly atypical forms, or prominent necrosis.

Malignant Lymphoma

Malignant lymphoma is the most common malignant tumor involving the jejunum.[343–349] Cases can present that are localized to the small intestinal area, are part of a regional involvement with lesions also noted in the abdominal and retroperitoneal lymph nodes, and as a component of a systemic disease. The lesions in the jejunum are most often multicentric, and their large size can help in providing positive biopsies.

The great majority of the lymphomas occurring in otherwise well patients are of the non-Hodgkin's B-cell type, with all varieties, including follicular and small and large cell forms. The tumors are increased in patients with celiac disease[350, 351] and with prolonged immunologic deficiencies.[352, 353] Of interest, the tumors seen in the celiac patients are almost always of the T-cell class.[354] The Mediterranean form of malignant lymphoma, termed *immunoproliferative small intestinal disease (IPSID),* is associated with a greater amount of plasma cell proliferation.[355–360] In the earlier stages there is a chronic enteritis with benign-appearing plasma cells, similar to that seen in most cases of celiac disease and other malabsorptive disorders. Later lesions develop more prominent masses of plasma cells and ultimately lymphoma formation. It has been suggested that these stages can be monitored and detected by small bowel biopsy (see Ch. 6 for further details). Other types of lymphoma that rarely affect the small intestine include multiple lymphomatous polyposis, Burkitt's disease, histiocytic tumors, Hodgkin's disease, and localized plasmacytomas.[361–366] These are rarely detected by biopsy of the mucosa.

The diagnosis on jejunal mucosal biopsy of malignant lymphoma is usually easier than that occurring in the stomach. This may be due to the samples being taken from larger and possibly more advanced lesions. The biopsies typically reveal broad sheets of tumor cells without follicle formation (Fig. 7-26). There is often a marked infiltration by the tumor cells into any remaining crypt epithelium, and, typically, prominent extension into the region of the muscularis mucosae and the submucosa. The larger lesions can develop secondary ulcers, and acute inflammatory cells are often associated in the superficial regions. In any case of suspected lymphoma, it is best to fix the samples in B5 or other metal-containing solutions, which allows for improved cytologic appearance. The more differentiated tumors are recognized by smaller cell size and less irregularity of the nuclei, and they are distinguished from inflammatory conditions by their monomorphism. Marker studies identifying monotypic growth can be of assistance. The less differentiated lymphomas show more overt tumor with larger and irregular cells. Since carcinoma is so much rarer in this area, immunocytochemical stains to distinguish it from the large cell forms of lymphoma are often not needed.

The greatest difficulty in diagnosing lymphoma occurs in the patients with long-standing celiac disease, since the earlier lesions tend to be very focal and tiny in size.[354] Multiple samples should be examined, looking especially for clusters of atypical cells (Fig. 7-13). Immunocytochemical studies can be of assistance in identifying the clusters of T-cell lineage. Considering the focality, several samples and multiple levels of each sample are often examined to identify or exclude the lesion. As noted above, patients with celiac disease who develop refractory sprue or ulcers are especially at risk for the development or presence of lymphoma and need the extra search for the tumor.

Mesenchymal Tumors

Mesenchymal tumors can affect the jejunum. They are much less likely to be detected in mucosal biopsy samples in this area, however, and practically all diagnoses involve examination of operative specimens. The benign stromal tumors described include leiomyoma and lipoma (see Figs. 3-20 and 10-34); granular cell and other neural tumors (Fig. 3-21); angioma, glomus tumor, and hemangiopericytoma (Fig. 5-28); and lymphangioma.[367–374] The generic or undifferentiated stromal tumors, believed to be of muscle or nervous origin, can involve any part of the small intestine (see Fig. 5-24). They are less common than those seen in the stomach but appear to be more aggressive, with most lesions larger than 5 cm in diameter considered

A

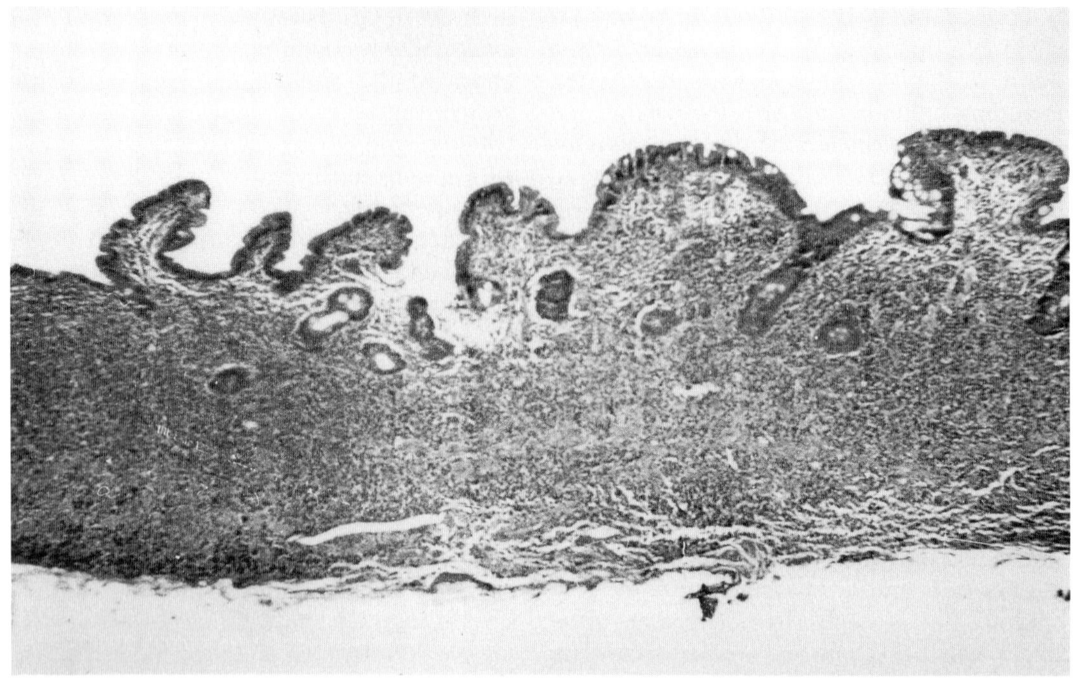

B

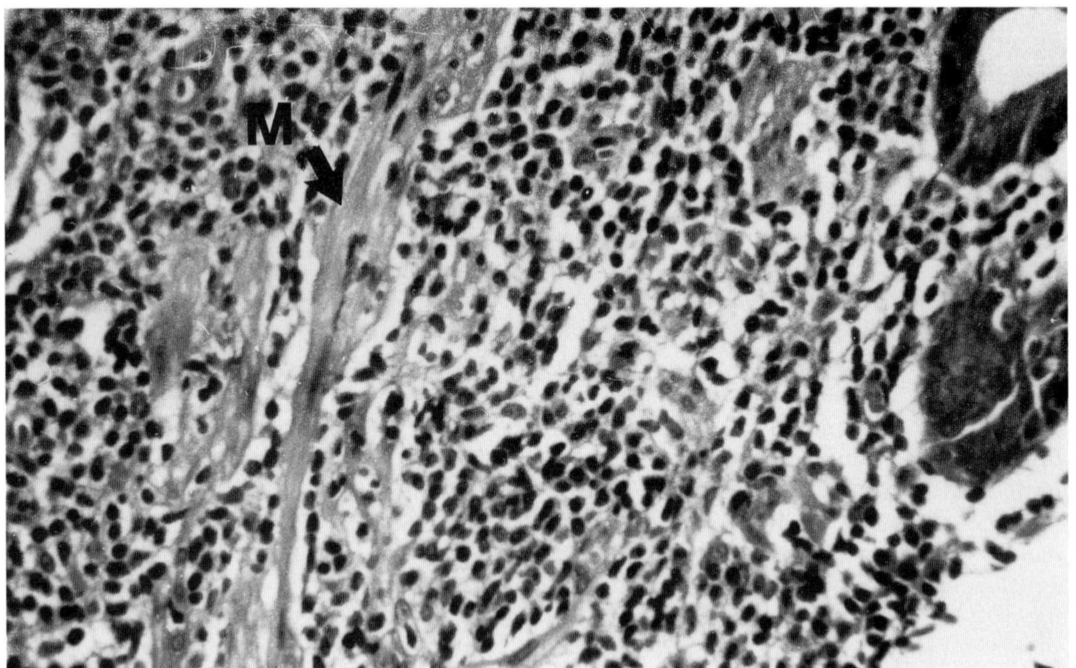

Fig. 7-26. Malignant lymphoma in the jejunal mucosa. **(A)** There is a dense infiltrate of small lymphocytes in the mucosa, resulting in crypt destruction and villous shortening. **(B)** The lymphoma is comprised of small, relatively uniform cells. It is present in both the mucosa (right) and submucosa (left), and there is infiltration and destruction of the muscularis mucosae (M).

potentially malignant.[367] (See Chs. 5 and 6 for more details.)

There are a wide variety of sarcomas noted, including leiomyosarcoma, lipsarcoma, angiosarcoma, and malignant neural lesions.[375–379] Rare instances of rhabdomyosarcoma, malignant mesenchymoma, osteosarcoma, granulocytic sarcoma, and malignant fibrous histiocytoma have also been cited in the small intestine.[380–383] These cases do not typically present in jejunal mucosal biopsies.

Kaposi's sarcoma frequently involves the small intestine in patients with AIDS, and is often associated with multiple opportunistic infections.[384–389] The lesions are best diagnosed by direct inspection such as occurs in the stomach and duodenum, revealing ragged ulcerated areas. Biopsies show the compact spindly cells with hemorrhage and mild atypism, which must be distinguished from ordinary granulation tissue (Fig. 6-28). (See Ch. 6 for further details.)

Other Primary Tumors

There has been rare mention of other primary lesions involving the jejunum, including pleomorphic carcinoma, carcinosarcoma, and choriocarcinoma[390–392] (see Figs. 3-10 and 3-26). These are probably more common in the stomach and duodenum.

Secondary and Metastatic Tumors

Extension of tumors into the jejunal region is generally rare and most often occurs from tumors of lymph nodes or retroperitoneal masses. Metastatic lesions to the jejunum can develop as in any part of the small intestine. Most often seen are nodules of malignant melanoma, leukemia, and lymphoma[393–395] (Fig. 5-31). Of the carcinomas those arising in the lung, breast, and germ cell tumors appear to be the most frequent.[396, 397] All of these lesions are not typically detected in jejunal mucosal biopsies.

MISCELLANEOUS CONDITIONS

There are many other disorders that can affect the small intestine, leading occasionally to their discovery in jejunal mucosal biopsies.

Depositions

Amyloid

The small intestine can be involved in cases of primary or secondary amyloidosis, with deposits noted in the mucosa or in the vessel walls.[398–402] The latter can result in localized areas of ischemic injury leading to focal ulceration and bleeding. Less often noted are infiltrates in the wall, resulting in reduced motility and pseudo-obstruction.[48] As mentioned, most cases are detected instead by biopsies of the stomach and rectum (Fig. 9-46 and Plate 4D). (See section on "Malabsorptive Disorders" above for more details.)

Pigments

Hemosiderin can be found in macrophages within the lamina propria in any case of resolving hemorrhage, and this is increased in patients with hemosiderosis.[403] There is increased iron within the epithelial cells overlying the villi in patients with hemochromatosis, but this is not typically surveyed in these patients. Lipofuscin-type pigments are noted in macrophages in many conditions, including several storage disorders, Langerhans' cell histiocytosis, and chronic granulomatous disease.[404] There is no relation to melanosis coli or to melanosis of the duodenum.

Storage Disorders

There are many diseases associated with the deposition of a wide variety of substances in the body tissues (Table 7-12). These most frequently involve muscles, nerves, and macrophages. At present, most of the diagnoses are established by samples of blood and muscles with appropriate biochemical studies. Traditionally, samples were taken from the mucosa of the gastrointestinal tract, particularly from the rectum and colon, to help in the diagnoses. These lesions can exceptionally also involve the small intestinal mucosa and be detected in mucosal biopsy. It should be stressed that this is now a rare source of positive diagnoses. Included are cases with depositions of lipoproteins seen in abetalipoproteinemia and in Tangier disease[278–281] (see Figs. 7-24 and 9-49); the glycolipids represented by Fabry's disease, deposits of gangliosides, and Niemann-Pick disease[53, 405, 406]; and the lipid pigment disorders of lipofuscinosis (ceroidosis) and the brown bowel syndrome[407, 408] (Plate 4C and Fig. 9-48). Deposits have also rarely been noted in patients with lysosomal storage disorders, cystinosis, cholesterol ester storage diseases, and the mucopolysaccharidoses.[409–412]

Biopsy in all of these deposit disorders reveals the abnormal substance within the macrophages and muscle or nervous tissue elements.[404, 413] Their nature is suggested by their appearance, with vacuoles favoring lipids, granular material associated with carbohydrate substances, and the pigment disorders; these features are accented by ultrastructural study. It is important to distinguish localized inflammatory conditions that can mimic these lesions, particularly granulomas, infections due to *Mycobacterium avium*, and other diseases with macrophage proliferation.

Collagen

An increase in collagen within the lamina propria is noted in some of the late cases of celiac disease and has been termed *collagenous sprue*.[233, 234] This may be seen on mucosal biopsy and must be distinguished from other causes of protein deposits, such as amyloid, and from other cases with extensive fi-

Table 7-12. Depositions in the Intestinal Mucosa

Deposit	Chemical Substance
Protein Deposits	
Amyloid, light chains, and macroglobulins	
Collagenous sprue and collagenous enterocolitis	
Infantile systemic hyalinosis	
Lipoid proteinosis	
Neutral fat and triglycerides	
Xanthoma	
Abetalipoproteinemia	
Tangier disease	
Glycolipids	
Fabry's disease	Ceramide trihexoside
Tay–Sachs and other gangliosidoses	Ganglioside
Nieman–Pick disease	Sphingomyelin
Lipid pigments	
Lipofuscinosis	Lipofuscin
Brown bowel syndrome	Lipofuscin
Other	
Wolman's disease	Cholesterol ester
Cystinosis	Cystine
Mucopolysaccharidoses	Heparin and other sulfates

brosis, such as systemic sclerosis. In the latter, the fibrous tissue is typically deposited in the submucosa and muscle coats rather than in the mucosa. There are rare instances of more superficial collagen deposition beneath the surface epithelium seen in association with cases of collagenous colitis.[235]

Other Depositions

Rarely seen are deposits of lipids within the macrophages, termed *xanthomas,* which are probably related to localized hemorrhages.[44] These are more common in the stomach (Fig. 4-37). Other rare conditions include infantile systemic hyalinosis in which there are deposits of a protein-type material in many tissues of the body, including the small intestinal mucosa and submucosa[415]; and lipoid proteinosis, which reveals deposits in the intestine as well as the skin.[416] Such cases need to be distinguished from other conditions with proteinaceous deposits, particularly amyloidosis.

Granulomatous Diseases

The major granulomatous disorder is Crohn's disease, which is discussed above (see "Malabsorptive Disorder"). Sarcoidosis of the small intestine is rare.[417–419] Seen are multiple granulomas without necrosis, but the diagnosis should be supported by findings in other more typical organs such as the lungs. Other conditions that can be associated with granulomas include reactions to foreign bodies, various infections, and the rare disorders of chronic granulomatous disease and malakoplakia.[131, 420]

Localized collections of Langerhans' cells can be seen in cases of systemic histiocytosis, and these are usually distinguished from other granulomas because of the uniformity of the cells[273, 274]; they also stain positively for S-100 and have distinctive granules on ultrastructure (see Fig. 4-38).

Metabolic Disorders

Cystic Fibrosis

There have been extensive studies of the mucosa throughout the alimentary tract in patients with cystic fibrosis.[421] It was noted both in the small and large intestine that the goblet mucous cells are often larger than those seen in normal persons, but there were no differences in mucosubstances. There was, however, considerable overlap with the findings in normal persons, and this feature has not proven useful in the diagnosis. It is known that patients with cystic fibrosis can develop excess amounts of mucus and that this can cause obstruction in relatively small chambers such as the appendix, bronchi, and pancreatic ducts. It is also thought that the intrauterine form of meconium ileus is the major source for development of jejunal atresias.[32]

Megaloblastic Anemias

In patients with megaloblastic anemia due to any cause, the megaloblastic change can also be appreciated in the epithelium throughout the alimentary tract.[422, 423] This can be seen in mucosal biopsies in patients with severe folate or B12 deficiency, and it is important not to confuse them with tumor cells.

Renal Diseases

The small intestinal mucosa is frequently affected in patients with uremia, revealing foci of congested vessels, hemorrhage, and ulcers, which tend to be more common in the upper portion.[424–426] Because of the immunosuppressive therapies often used in these patients, secondary infections are common and particularly affect the gastrointestinal tract. There are also several diseases that simultaneously involve both areas, such as vasculitis and amyloidosis.

Skin Diseases

Dermatitis Herpetiformis

As noted above, there is a definite genetic link with cases of celiac disease.[199, 200] Most patients with dermatitis herpetiformis have mild changes in the small intestinal mucosa, which are usually not clinically evident. If symptoms develop, biopsy should be performed because of the strong likelihood that it is due to celiac disease. The biopsy features in the mucosa are otherwise identical to those of celiac disease (see Fig. 7-12). The lesions tend to be milder probably because of detection at an ealier stage.

Acrodermatitis Enteropathica

Acrodermatitis enteropathica is a rare inherited skin disorder that is related to zinc deficiency and is associated with alterations of the small intestinal mucosa.[427, 428] Noted are a villous injury and alterations of the Paneth cells, with loss of normal granules and the presence of rod-shaped inclusions. The diarrhea and tissue changes are reversed by zinc therapy.

Other Skin Diseases

The intestinal tract can also be involved in patients with erythema multiforme and with Kohlmeier-Degos disease, but the lesions are more typically found in the large bowel[404, 429] (see Ch. 9).

Soft Tissue Diseases

There are many soft tissue diseases that can be associated with deposition of connective tissue materials or with defects in the composition of the stromal components of the intestinal tract. All of these may lead to abnormal function of the muscular coats and promote pseudo-obstructive disorders; included are the disorders of systemic sclerosis, Fabry's disease, and pseudoxanthoma elasticum. As mentioned above, biopsies are rarely obtained to establish the diagnosis. Rather, these patients can develop pseudo-obstruction, stasis, and bacterial proliferation, leading to patchy foci of active enteritis. They are described in the sections on "Motor and Mechanical Disorders" and "Malabsorptive Disorders".

A prominence of mucosal eosinophils and mast cells has been noted in the small intestinal biopsies obtained from patients with a variety of connective tissue disorders.[430] These include patients with systemic sclerosis, dermatomyositis, and systemic lupus erythematosis. The cellular infiltrate is most pronounced in the basal portion of the mucosa, separating the crypts from the muscularis mucosae (Fig. 7-27).

Tumorlike Conditions

Pneumatosis Intestinalis

Pockets of air or other gases can be present in the mucosa or wall of any part of the gut, including the small intestine.[431–433] There are two principal types. The most common is associated with extension of air from the lungs or a perforated organ, such as from peptic ulcers. These areas are usually unassociated with any prominent inflammation, are mainly comprised of air, and lack foreign body reaction. The second form of pneumatosis is due to localized destruction of tissue, most often ischemic disease, promoting the invasion by gas-forming bacteria. These

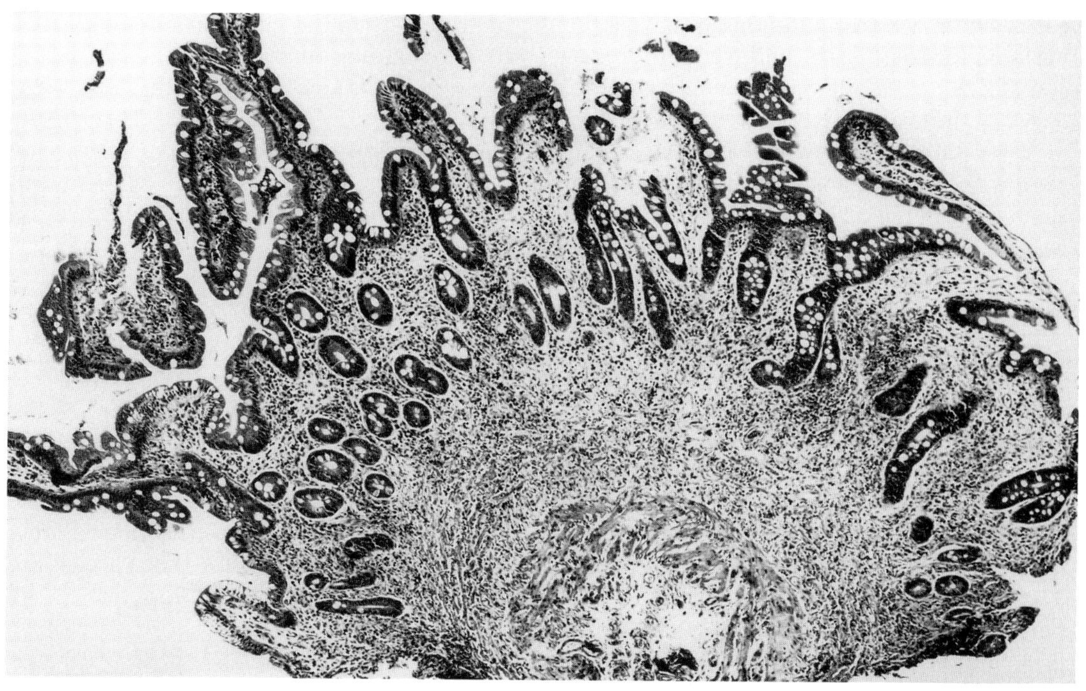

A

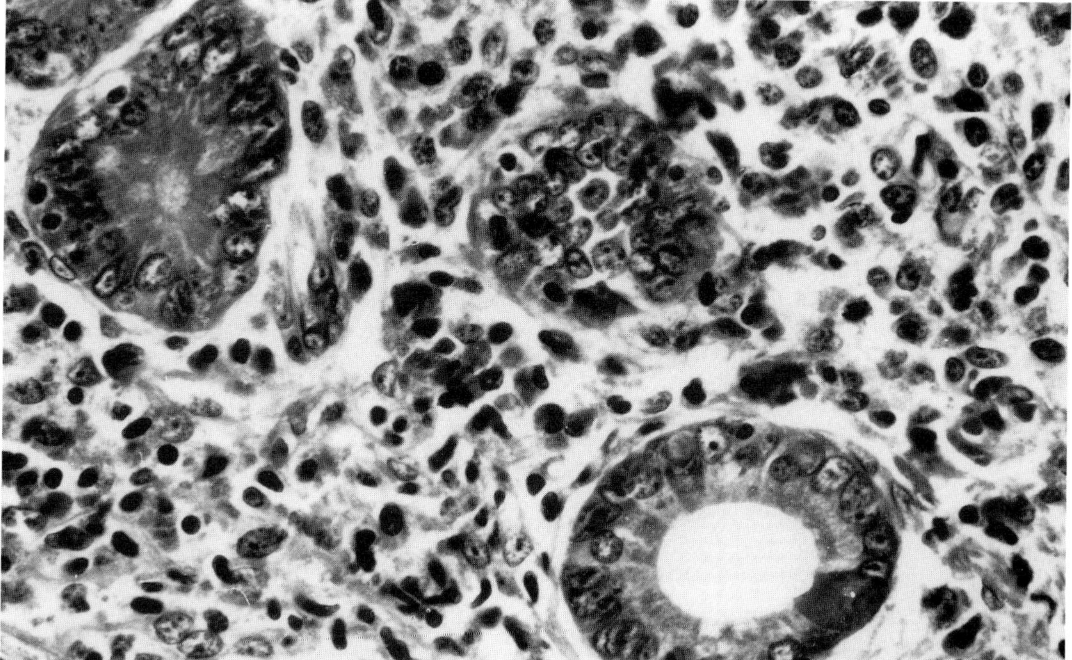

B

Fig. 7-27. Mucosal inflammation of the jejunum, seen in cases of connective tissue disorders. **(A)** There is a marked inflammatory infiltrate in the base of the mucosa separating the crypts and the muscularis mucosae appearing at the bottom. The villi appear normal (× 68). **(B)** Seen is the inflammation in the lamina propria, including many eosinophils (× 635).

cases show greater inflammation, contain variable forms of gases, and frequently show giant cells at the edges.

All of these gaseous lesions are more common in the small intestine and are readily seen with radiographic studies. It is rare for them to be detected in mucosal biopsy examination of the small intestine. Rather, they are best visualized by direct study, particularly in the colon and rectum (Figs. 8-16 and 9-42).

Endometriosis

Endometriosis is a common disorder that frequently involves the intestine, particularly the ileum and the distal part of the colon.[434] The lesions are usually concentrated in the peritoneal aspect and in the muscularis propria, and only rarely extend into the mucosa. Accordingly, it is virtually never seen in a jejunal mucosal biopsy.

Other Tumorlike Conditions

The small bowel occasionally can be involved in cases with myeloid metaplasia, revealing foci of hematopoiesis in any portion, including the mucosa.[435, 436]

Other Inflammatory Disorders

Enteritis Cystica

Enteritis cystica represents a lesion in which mature small intestinal mucosal tissue extends into the submucosa or muscularis propria.[437, 438] It is seen most often in cases with severe chronic inflammatory conditions such as Crohn's disease[439, 440]; and in a localized version underlying hamartomatous Peutz-Jeghers polyps.[441, 442] It is distinguished from carcinoma by noting the lack of any cytologic atypism, and that the stroma more closely resembles normal lamina propria rather than the irregular edematous tissue surrounding tumors.

Ulcerative Jejunoileitis

This is described above in the section on Celiac Disease.

Bypass Enteritis

Jejunoileal bypass has been done in patients with morbid obesity. The bypass area can develop stasis leading to bacterial proliferation and patchy foci of enteritis.[443] Also noted in these segments is an increased prevalence of pneumatosis.[433] The areas are rarely sampled by mucosal biopsy.

Graft-versus-Host Disease

Graft-versus-host disease is seen most often in patients who have had bone marrow or small bowel transplants.[444–446] The initial 2 to 3 weeks are associated with the effects of preparative chemotherapy and radiation, and subside. The later changes in the small intestine are largely due to the effects of the graft. Milder lesions are associated with infiltrates of mononuclear cells, largely directed to the crypt area. This can lead to interference with the growth of the villi and eventually to ulceration in the severe cases. In turn, the ulcers can be complicated by secondary infections, particularly by fungi. The diagnosis is more often established by skin biopsies. Small intestinal biopsies are mainly done to exclude other conditions and, particularly, to identify infections.

Small Bowel Transplant

Limited studies in humans have demonstrated effects involving mononuclear cells and a delayed hypersensitivity type of reaction, similar to that seen in other transplants.[447–449] More severe and rapid findings involve vascular compromise leading to hemorrhagic infarction. Biopsies have been largely obtained from the distal segments at the ileum in these cases (see Fig. 8-15).

MISCELLANEOUS CONDITIONS

Patients with Zollinger-Ellison syndrome can develop peptic lesions, including ulcers, in the distal duodenum and jejunum.[104] These are not typically examined by biopsy.

Nonspecific ulcers can appear in any part of the small intestine, including the jejunum.[450, 451] It is important to rule out the major known etiologies, including effects of drugs and other chemicals, radiation, ischemic lesions, and complications of infections. Those that develop in the jejunum are more often seen following NSAIDs or enteric-coated potassium chloride. After exclusion of all of these cases, there still remain some patients with ulcers; these tend to be more common in children. The diagnosis is typically dependent on the clinical information and on radiographic studies. Biopsies are uncommonly done and serve largely to exclude other more specific causes.

REFERENCES

1. Perera DR, Weinstein WM, Rubin CE: Small intestinal biopsy. Human Pathol 6:157–217, 1975
2. Rubin CE, Robbins WO III: Peroral biopsy of the small intestine. A review of its diagnostic usefulness. Gastroenterology 49:676–697, 1965
3. Dobbins WO III: Small bowel biopsy in malabsorptive states. pp. 137–188. In Norris HT (ed): Pathology of the Colon, Small Intestine, and Anus. 2nd Ed. Churchill Livingstone, New York, 1991
4. Sheahan DG, Rotterdam H: Small intestine. pp. 315–575. In Rotterdam H, Sheahan DG, Sommers SC (eds): Biopsy Diagnosis of the Digestive Tract. 2nd Ed. Raven Press, New York, 1993
5. Scott BB, Jenkins D: Endoscopic small intestinal biopsy. Gastrointest Endosc 27:162–167, 1981
6. Gillberg R, Kastrup W, Mobachen H et al: Endoscopic duodenal biposy compared with biopsy with the Watson capsule from the upper jejunum in patients with dermatitis herpetiformis. Scand J Gastroenterol 17:305–308, 1982
7. Mee AS, Burke M, Vallon AG et al: Small bowel biopsy for malabsorption: comparison of the diagnostic accuracy of endoscopic forceps and capsule biopsy specimens. Br Med J 291:769–772, 1985
8. Achkar E, Carey WD, Petras R et al: Comparison of suction capsule and endoscopic biopsy of small bowel mucosa. Gastrointest Endosc 32:278–281, 1986
9. Holdstock G, Eade OE, Isaacson P, Smith CL: Endoscopic duodenal biopsy in coeliac disease and duodenitis. Scand J Gastroenterol 14:717–720, 1979
10. Iida M, Yamamoto T, Yao T et al: Jejunal endoscopy using a long duodenofiberscope. Gastrointest Endosc 32:233–236, 1986
11. Gastout CG, Schroeder KW, Burton DD: Small bowel enteroscopy: an early experience in gastrointestinal bleeding of unknown origin. Gastrointest Endosc 37:5–8, 1991
12. Lewis BS, Kornbluth A, Waye JD: Small bowel tumors: yield of enteroscopy. Gut 32:763–765, 1991
13. Chong J, Tagle M, Barkin JS et al: Small bowel push-type fiberoptic enteroscopy for patients with occult gastrointestinal bleeding or suspected small bowel pathology. Am J Gastroenterol 89:2143–2146, 1994
14. Burhol PG, Myren T: Jejunal biopsy findings in healthy young men. Scand J Gastroenterol 3:346–350, 1968
15. Variend S, Phillips AD, Walker-Smith JA: The small intestinal mucosal biopsy in childhood. Perspect Pediatr Pathol 1:57–78, 1984
16. Goldman H, Ming S-C: Mucins in normal and metaplastic gastrointestinal epithelium: histochemical distribution. Arch Pathol 85:580–586, 1968
17. Filipe MI: Mucins in the human gastrointestinal epithelium: a review. Invest Cell Pathol 2:195–216, 1979

18. Mathan M, Hughes J, Whitehead R: The morphogenesis of the human Paneth cell. An immunocytochemical ultrastructural study. Histochemistry 87:91–96, 1987
19. Sjolund K, Sanden G, Hakonson R, Sundler F: Endocrine cells in human intestine: an immunocytochemical study. Gastroenterology 85:1120–1130, 1983
20. Lechago J: The endocrine cells of the digestive tract. General concepts and historic perspective. Am J Surg Pathol 11(suppl 1):63–70, 1987
21. Dayal Y: Neuroendocrine cells and their proliferative lesions. pp. 305–365. In Norris HT (ed): Pathology of the Colon, Small Intestine, and Anus. 2nd Ed. Churchill Livingstone, New York, 1991
22. Keren F: Structure and function of the immunologic system of the gastrointestinal tract. pp. 69–80. In Ming S-C, Goldman H (eds): Pathology of the Gastrointestinal Tract. WB Saunders, Philadelphia, 1992
23. Ferguson A: Intraepithelial lymphocytes of the small intestine. Gut 18:921–937, 1977
24. Owen RL, Jones AL: Epithelial cell specialization within human Peyer's patches: an ultrastructural study of intestinal lymphoid follicles. Gastroenterology 66:189, 1974
25. Corazza GR, Franzzoni M, Gatto MRA, Gasbarrini G: Ageing and small bowel mucosa: a morphometric study. Gerontology 32:60–65, 1986
26. Corazza GR, Bonvicini F, Franzzoni M et al: Observer variation in assessment of jejunal biopsy specimens. Gastroenterology 83:1217–1222, 1982
27. Dunnill MS, Whitehead R: A method for the quantitation of small intestinal biopsy specimens. J Clin Pathol 25:243–246, 1972
28. Corazza GR, Franzzoni M, Dixon MF, Gasbarrini G: Quantitative assessment of the mucosal architecture of jejunal biopsy specimens: a comparison between linear measurement, stereology, and computer-aided microscopy. J Clin Pathol 38:765–770, 1985
29. Slavin G, Sowter C, Robertson K et al: Measurement in jejunal biopsies by computer-aided microscopy. J Clin Pathol 33: 254–261, 1980
30. Bower RJ, Sieber WK, Kiesewetter WB: Alimentary tract duplications in children. Ann Surg 188:669–674, 1978
31. Adair HM, Trowell JE: Squamous cell carcinoma arising in a duplication of the small bowel. J Pathol 133:25–31, 1981
32. Carpenter HM: Pathogenesis of congenital jejunal atresia. Arch Pathol 73:390–396, 1962
33. Jeffrey I, Durrans D, Wells M, Fox H: The pathology of meconium ileus equivalent. J Clin Pathol 36:1292–1297, 1983
34. Thoeni RF, Gedgaudas RK: Ectopic pancreas: usual and unusual features. Gastrointest Endosc 5:37–42, 1980
35. Franzin G, Musola R, Negri A et al: Heterotopic gastric (fundic) mucosa in the duodenum. Endoscopy 14:166–167, 1982
36. Vizcarrondo FJ, Wang T-Y, Brady PG: Heterotopic gastric mucosa: presentation as a rugose duodenal mass. Gastrointest Endosc 29:107–111, 1983
37. Tsadilas T: Duodenal polyp composed of ectopic gastric mucosa. Dig Dis Sci 29: 475–477, 1984
38. Tsubone M, Kozura S, Taki T et al: Heterotopic gastric mucosa in the small intestine. Acta Pathol Jpn 34:1425–1431, 1984
39. Jabbori M, Goresky CA, Lough J et al: The inlet patch: heterotopic gastric mucosa in the upper esophagus. Gastroenterology 89:352–356, 1985
40. Shah KK, DeRidder PH, Shah KK: Ectopic gastric mucosa in proximal esophagus. Its clinical significance and hormonal profile. J Clin Gastroenterol 8:509–513, 1986
41. Galligan ML, Uhlich T, Lewin KJ: Heterotopic gastric mucosa in the jejunum causing intussusception. Arch Pathol Lab Med 107:335–336, 1983
42. Caruso ML, Marzullo F: Jejunal adenocarcinoma in congenital heterotopic gastric mucosa. J Clin Gastroenterol 10:92–94, 1988
43. Krishnamurthy S, Kelly MM, Rohrmann CA, Schuffler MD: Jejunal diverticulosis. A heterogeneous disorder caused by a variety of abnormalities of smooth muscle or myenteric plexus. Gastroenterology 85:538–547, 1983
44. Sibile A, Willcox R: Jejunal diverticulitis. Am J Gastroenterol 87:655–658, 1992
45. Friedman LS, Kirkham SE, Thistletwaite JR et al: Jejunal diverticulosis with perforation as a complication of Fabry's disease. Gastroenterology 86:558–563, 1984

46. Anuras S: Intestinal pseudo-obstruction syndrome. Annu Rev Med 39:1–15, 1988
47. Tada S, Iida M, Yao T et al: Intestinal pseudo-obstruction in patients with amyloidosis: clinicopathologic differences between chemical types of amyloid protein. Gut 34:1412–1417, 1993
48. Steen LE, Oberg L: Familial amyloidosis with polyneuropathy: roentgenological and gastroscopic appearance of gastrointestinal involvement. Am J Gastroenterol 78: 417–420, 1980
49. Rothstein RD: Gastrointestinal motility disorders in diabetes mellitus. Am J Gastroenterol 85:782–785, 1990
50. Marshall JB, Kretschmar JM, Gerhardt DC et al: Gastrointestinal manifestations of mixed connective tissue disease. Gastroenterology 98:1232–1238, 1990
51. Mitros FA, Schuffler MD, Teja K, Anuras S: Pathologic features of familial visceral myopathy. Hum Pathol 13:825–833, 1982
52. Krishnamurthy S, Schuffler MD: Pathology of the neuromuscular disorders of the small intestine and colon. Gastroenterology 93: 610–639, 1987
53. Sheth KJ, Werlin SL, Freeman ME, Hodach AE: Gastrointestinal structure and function in Fabry's disease. Am J Gastroenterol 76:246–251, 1981
54. Beighton PH, Murdoch JL, Votteler T: Gastrointestinal complications of the Ehlers-Danlos syndrome. Gut 10:1004–1008, 1969
55. Schuffler MD, Kaplan LR, Johnson L: Small-intestinal mucosa in pseudoobstruction syndrome. Am J Dig Dis 23:821–828, 1978
56. Nagral AS, Joshi AS, Bhatia SJ et al: Congestive jejunopathy in portal hypertension. Gut 34:694–697, 1993
57. Vedlhuyzen van Zanten SJO, Bartelsman JFWM, Schipper MEI, Tytgat GNJ: Recurrent massive hematemesis from Dieulafoy vascular malformations—a review of 101 cases. Gut 27:213–222, 1986
58. Sassaris M, Pang G, Hunter F: Telangiectasias of the gastrointestinal tract. Report of six cases and review. Endoscopy 15:85–88, 1983
59. Eastman J, Nazek M, Mangeis D: Localized arteriovenous malformation of the jejunum. Arch Pathol Lab Med 118:181–183, 1994
60. Williams LF Jr: Vascular insufficiency of the intestines. Gastroenterology 61:757–777, 1971
61. Norris HT: Vascular Disorders. pp. 214–239. In Ming S-C, Goldman H (eds): Pathology of the Gastrointestinal Tract. WB Saunders, Philadelphia, 1992
62. Whitehead R: The pathology of ischemia of the intestines. Pathol Annu 11:1–52, 1976
63. Swerdlow SH, Antonioli DA, Goldman H: Intestinal infarction: a new classification. Arch Pathol Lab Med 105:218, 1981
64. Shepherd HA, Patal C, Bamforth J, Isaacson P: Upper gastrointestinal endoscopy in systemic vasculitis presenting as an acute abdomen. Endoscopy 15:307–311, 1983
65. Camilleri M, Pusey CD, Chadwick VS, Rees AJ: Gastrointestinal manifestations of systemic vasculitis. Q J Med 206:141–149, 1983
66. Burke AP, Sobin LH, Virmani R: Localized vasculitis of the gastrointestinal tract. Am J Surg Pathol 19:338–349, 1995
67. Taylor NS, Gueft B, Lebowich RJ: Atheromatous embolization: a cause of gastric ulcers and small bowel necrosis. Gastroenterology 47:97, 1964
68. Socinski MA, Frankel JP, Morrow PL, Krawitt L: Painless diarrhea secondary to intestinal ischemia: diagnosis of atheromatous emboli by jejunal biopsy. Dig Dis Sci 29:674–677, 1984
69. Morichau-Beauchant M, Touchard G, Maire P et al: Jejunal IgA and C3 deposition in adult Henoch-Schönlein purpura with severe intestinal manifestations. Gastroenterology 82:1438–1442, 1982
70. Cunningham D, Morgan RJ, Mills PR et al: Functional and structural changes of the human proximal small intestine after cytotoxic therapy. J Clin Pathol 38:265–270, 1985
71. Goldman H, Szabo S: Chemical and physical disorders. pp. 141–170. In Ming S-C, Goldman H (eds): Pathology of the Gastrointestinal Tract. WB Saunders, Philadelphia, 1992
72. Trier JS: Morphologic alterations induced by methotrexate in the mucosa of the human proximal intestine. Gastroenterology 42: 295–305, 1962
73. Riddell RH: The gastrointestinal tract. pp. 515–606. In Riddell RH (ed): Pathology of Drug-Induced and Toxic Diseases. Churchill Livingstone, New York, 1982

74. Lewis JH: Gastrointestinal injury due to medicinal agents. Am J Gastroenterol 81: 819–834, 1986
75. Lee FD: Drug-related pathological lesions of the intestinal tract. Histopathology 25:303–308, 1994
76. Hoyle M, Kennedy A, Prior AL et al: Small bowel ischemia and infarction in young women taking oral contraceptives and progestational agents. Br J Surg 64:533–537, 1977
77. Jackson CW, Haboubi NY, Whorwell PJ, Schofield PF: Gold-induced enterocolitis. Gut 27:452–456, 1986
78. Henry D, Dobson A, Turner C: Variability in the risk of major gastrointestinal complications from non-aspirin non-steroidal anti-inflammatory drugs. Gastroenterology 105:1078–1088, 1993
79. Bjornason I, Hayallar J, Macpherson AJ, Russell AS: Side effects of nonsteroidal anti-inflammatory drugs on the small and large intestine in humans. Gastroenterology 104: 1832–1847, 1993
80. Morris AJ, Madhok R, Sturrock RD et al: Enteroscopic diagnosis of small bowel ulceration in patients receiving non-steroidal anti-inflammatory drugs. Lancet 1:520, 1991
81. Lanza FL: Gastrointestinal toxicity of newer NSAIDS. Am J Gastroenterol 88:1318–1323, 1993
82. Matsukashi N, Yamada A, Hiraishi M et al: Multiple strictures of the small intestine after long-term nonsteroidal anti-inflammatory drug therapy. Am J Gastroenterol 87:1183–1186, 1992
83. Bjornson I, Price AB, Zanelli G et al: Clinicopathological features of nonsteroidal anti-inflammatory drug-induced small intestinal strictures. Gastroenterology 94:1070–1074, 1988
84. Lang J, Price AB, Levi AJ et al: Diaphragm disease: pathology of disease of the small intestine induced by non-steroidal anti-inflammatory drugs. J Clin Pathol 41: 516–526, 1988
85. Fellows IW, Clarke JMF, Roberts PF: Non-steroidal anti-inflammatory drug-induced jejunal and colonic diaphragm disease: a report of two cases. Gut 33:1424–1426, 1992
86. Weiss SM, Rutenberg HL, Paskin DL, Zeren HA: Gut lesions due to slow-release KCL tablets. N Engl J Med 296:111–112, 1977
87. Barloon T, Moore SA, Mitros FA: A case of stenotic obstruction of the jejunum secondary to slow-release potassium. Am J Gastroenterol 81:192–194, 1986
88. Berthrong M, Fajardo LF: Radiation injury in surgical pathology. Part II. Alimentary tract. Am J Surg Pathol 5:153–178, 1981
89. Case records of the MGH. Radiation enteritis. N Engl J Med 330:627–632, 1994
90. Trier JS, Browning TH: Morphologic response of the mucosa of human small intestine to x-ray exposure. J Clin Invest 45:194, 1966
91. Novak JM, Collinness JT, Donowitz M et al: Effects of radiation on the human gastrointestinal tract. J Clin Gastroenterol 1:9, 1979
92. Poddar PK, Bauer JJ, Gelerent I et al: Radiation injury to the small intestine. Mt Sinai J Med 49:144–149, 1982
93. Haddad GK, Grodsinsky C, Allen H: The spectrum of radiation enteritis. Dis Colon Rectum 26:590–594, 1983
94. O'Brien PH, Jenette JM, Darvin AJ: Radiation enteritis. Am Surg 53:501–504, 1987
95. Yeoh EK, Horowitz M: Radiation enteritis. Surg Gynecol Obstet 165:373–376, 1987
96. Sher ME, Bauer J: Radiation-induced enteropathy. Am J Gastroenterol 85:121–128, 1990
97. Kapikian AZ: Viral gastroenteritis. JAMA 269:627–630, 1993
98. Schreiber DS, Blacklow NR, Trier JS: The mucosal lesion of the proximal small intestine in acute infectious nonbacterial gastroenteritis. N Engl J Med 288:1318–1323, 1973
99. Shepherd RW, Butler DG, Cutz E et al: The mucosal lesion in viral enteritis. Gastroenterology 76:770–777, 1979
100. Kaplan JE, Goodman RA, Schonberger LB et al: Gastroenteritis due to Norwalk virus: an outbreak associated with a municipal water system. J Infect Dis 146:190–197, 1982
101. Blacklow NR, Greenberg HB: Viral gastroenteritis. N Engl J Med 325:252–264, 1991
102. Hinnant KL, Rotterdam HZ, Bell ET, Tapper ML: Cytomegalovirus infection of the alimentary tract: a clinicopathological correlation. Am J Gastroenterol 81:944–950, 1986
103. Chetty R, Roskell DE: Cytomegalovirus infection in the gastrointestinal tract. J Clin Pathol 47:968–972, 1994

104. Cheung ANY, Ng IOL: Cytomegalovirus infection of the gastrointestinal tract in non-AIDS patients. Am J Gastroenterol 88:1882–1886, 1993
105. Wassalle JA, Sedgwick JH, Dawson PJ, Fabri PJ: Intestinal herpes simplex infection presenting with intestinal perforation. Am J Gastroenterol 87:1475–1477, 1992
106. Wu G-D, Shintaku IP, Chien K, Geller SA: A comparison of routine light microscopy, immunohistochemistry, and in-situ hybridization for the detection of cytomegalovirus in gastrointestinal biopsies. Am J Gastroenterol 84:1517–1520, 1989
107. Ehrenpreis ED, Patterson BK, Brainer JA et al: Histopathologic findings of duodenal biopsy specimens in HIV-infected patients with and without diarrhea and malabsorption. Am J Clin Pathol 97:21–28, 1992
108. Fontana M, Boldorini R, Zulin G et al: Ultrastructural changes in the duodenal mucosa of HIV-infected children. J Ped Gastroenterol Nutr 17:255–260, 1993
109. Ullrich R, Zeitz M, Heise W et al: Small intestinal structure and function in patients infected with human immunodeficiency virus (HIV): evidence for HIV-induced enteropathy. Ann Intern Med 111:15–21, 1989
110. Greenson JK, Belitsos PC, Yardley JH, Bartlett JG: AIDS enteropathy—occult enteric infections and duodenal mucosal alterations in chronic diarrhea. Ann Intern Med 114:366–372, 1991
111. Heise C, Dandekar S, Kumor P et al: Human immunodeficiency virus infection of enterocytes and mononuclear cells in human jejunal mucosa. Gastroenterology 100: 1521–1527, 1991
112. Grohmann GS, Glass RI, Pereira HG et al: Enteric viruses and diarrhea in HIV-infected patients. N Engl J Med 329:14–20, 1993
113. Guerrant RL, Bobak DA: Bacterial and protozoal gastroenteritis. N Engl J Med 325:327–340, 1991
114. Abrams GD: Infectious disorders of the intestine. pp. 621–642. In Ming S-C, Goldman H (eds): Pathology of the Gastrointestinal Tract. WB Saunders, Philadelphia, 1992
115. Rabbani GH: Cholera. Clin Gastroenterol 3:507–528, 1986
116. Nalin DR: Cholera and severe toxigenic diarrhoeas. Gut 35:145–149, 1994
117. Islam MM, Azad AK, Bardhan PK et al: Pathology of shigellosis and its complications. Histopathology 24:65–71, 1994
118. Blaser MJ, Reller LB: Campylobacter enteritis. N Engl J Med 305:1444–1452, 1981
119. El-Maraghi NRH, Mair NS: The histopathology of enteric infection with Yersinia pseudotuberculosis. Am J Clin Pathol 71:631–639, 1979
120. Gleason TH, Patterson SD: The pathology of Yersinia enterocolitica ileocolitis. Am J Surg Pathol 6:347–355, 1982
121. Buts J-P, Weber AM, Morin CL: Pseudomembraneous enterocolitis in childhood. Gastroenterology 73:823–827, 1977
122. Wiesen S, Gregg PA, Kershenobich P et al: Pseudomembranous enteritis: rediscovery of a previously well-described entity? Am J Gastroenterol 87:1631–1633, 1992
123. King A, Rampling A, Wight DGD, Warren RE: Neutropenic enterocolitis due to Clostridium septicum infection. J Clin Pathol 37:335–343, 1984
124. Newbold KM, Lord MG, Baglin TP: Role of clostridial organisms in neutropenic enterocolitis. J Clin Pathol 40:471, 1987
125. Marshall JB: Tuberculosis of the gastrointestinal tract and peritoneum. Am J Gastroenterol 88:989–999, 1993
126. Brown JR: Human actinomycosis: a study of 181 subjects. Hum Pathol 4:319–330, 1973
127. Gray JR, Rabeneck L: Atypical mycobacterial infections of the gastrointestinal tract in AIDS patients. Am J Gastroenterol 84:1521–1524, 1989
128. Maschek H, Georgil A, Schmidt RE et al: Mycobacterium genavense. Autopsy findings in three patients. Am J Clin Pathol 101:95–99, 1994
129. Roth RI, Owen RZ, Keren DF, Volberding PA: Intestinal infection with Mycobacterium avium in acquired immune deficiency syndrome (AIDS): histological and clinical comparison with Whipple's disease. Dig Dis Sci 30:497–504, 1985
130. Schlossberg D, Rudy FR, Jackson FW, Dumalag LB: Syphilitic enteritis. Arch Intern Med 144:811–812, 1984
131. McClure J: Malakoplakia of the gastrointestinal tract. Postgrad Med J 57:95, 1981
132. Volpicelli NA, Salyer WR, Milligan FD et al: The endoscopic appearance of the duode-

num in Whipple's disease. Johns Hopkins Med J 138:19, 1976
133. Eras P, Goldstein MJ, Sherlock P: Candida infection of the gastrointestinal tract. Medicine (Baltimore) 51:367–379, 1972
134. Joshi SN, Garvin PJ, Sunwoo YC: Candidiasis of the duodenum and jejunum. Gastroenterology 89:829–833, 1981
135. Lyon DT, Schubert TT, Mantia AG, Kaplan MH: Phycomycosis of the gastrointestinal tract. Am J Gastroenterol 72:379–394, 1979
136. Young RC, Bennett JE, Vogel CL et al: Aspergillosis: the spectrum of the disease in 98 patients. Medicine (Baltimore) 49:147, 1970
137. Whiteway DE, Virata RL: Mucormycosis. Arch Intern Med 139:944, 1979
138. Cappell MS, Mandell W, Grimes MM, Neu HC: Gastrointestinal histoplasmosis. Dig Dis Sci 33:353–360, 1988
139. Washington K, Gottfried MR, Wilson ML: Gastrointestinal cryptococcosis. Modern Pathol 4:707–711, 1991
140. Miller DP, Everett ED: Gastrointestinal histoplasmosis. J Clin Gastroenterol 1:233, 1979
141. Isaacs D, Hunt GH, Phillips AD et al: Cryptosporidiosis in immunocompetent children. J Clin Pathol 38:76–81, 1985
142. Wolfson JS, Richter JM, Waldron MA et al: Cryptosporidiosis in immunocompetent patients. N Engl J Med 312:1278–1282, 1985
143. Simon D, Brandt LJ: Diarrhea in patients with the acquired immunodeficiency syndrome. Gastroenterology 105:1238–1242, 1993
144. Sun T: The diagnosis of giardiasis. Am J Surg Pathol 4:256–271, 1980
145. Oberhuber G, Stolte M: Giardiasis-analysis of histological changes in biopsy specimens of 80 patients. J Clin Pathol 43:641–643, 1990
146. Thornton SA, West AH, DuPont HL, Pickering LK: Comparison of methods for identification of Giardia lamblia. Am J Clin Pathol 80:858–860, 1983
147. Marshall JB, Kelley DH, Vogele K: Giardiasis: diagnosis by endoscopic brush cytology of the duodenum. Am J Gastroenterol 79:517–519, 1984
148. Lager DJ, Landos SK: Correlative light and scanning electron microscopy of intestinal giardiasis, cryptosporidiosis, and spirochetosis. Ultrastruct Pathol 15:585–592, 1991
149. McHenry R, Bartlett MS, Lehman GA, O'Connor KW: The yield of routine duodenal aspiration for Giardia lamblia during esophagogastroduodenoscopy. Gastrointest Endosc 33:425–426, 1987
150. Guarda LA, Stein SA, Cleary KA, Ordonez NG: Human cryptosporidiosis in the acquired immune deficiency syndrome. Arch Pathol Lab Med 107:562–566, 1983
151. Godwin TA: Cryptosporidiosis in the acquired immunodeficiency syndrome: a study of 15 autopsy cases. Hum Pathol 22:1215–1224, 1991
152. Phillips AD, Thomas AG, Walker-Smith JA: Cryptosporidium, chronic diarrhea and the proximal small intestinal mucosa. Gut 33:1057–1061, 1992
153. Genta RM, Chappell CL, White AC et al: Duodenal morphology and intensity of infection in AIDS-related intestinal cryptosporidiosis. Gastroenterology 105:1769–1775, 1993
154. Lefkowitch JH, Krumholz S, Feng Chen KC et al: Cryptosporidiosis of the human small intestine: a light and electron microscopic study. Hum Pathol 15:746–752, 1984
155. Marcial MA, Madara JL: Cryptosporidium: cellular localization, structural analysis of absorptive cell-parasite membrane-membrane interactions in guinea pigs, and suggestion of protozoan transport by M cells. Gastroenterology 90:83–94, 1986
156. Bird RG, Smith MD: Cryptosporidiosis in man: parasite life cycle and fine structural pathology. J Pathol 132:217–233, 1980
157. Orenstein LM, Chiang J, Steinberg W et al: Intestinal microsporidiosis as a cause of diarrhea in human immunodeficiency virus–infected patients: a report of 20 cases. Hum Pathol 21:475–481, 1990
158. Peacock CS, Blanchard C, Tovey DG et al: Histological diagnosis of intestinal microsporidiosis in patients with AIDS. J Clin Pathol 44:558–563, 1991
159. Shadduck JA, Orenstein JM: Comparative pathology of microsporidiosis. Arch Pathol Lab Med 117:1215–1219, 1993
160. Orenstein JM, Tenner M, Cali A, Kotler DP: A microsporidian previously undescribed in humans, infecting enterocytes and macrophages, and associated with diarrhea in an

acquired immunodeficiency syndrome patient. Hum Pathol 23:722–728, 1992
161. Weber R, Bryan RT, Owen RL et al: Improved light-microscopic detection of microsporidia spores in stool and duodenal aspirates. N Engl J Med 326:161–166, 1992
162. Giang TT, Kotler DP, Garro ML, Orenstein MD: Tissue diagnosis of intestinal microsporidiosis using the chromotrope-2R modified trichrome stain. Arch Pathol Lab Med 117:1149–1251, 1993
163. Vangool T, Snijdoors F, Reiss P et al: Diagnosis of intestinal and disseminated microsporidial infections in patients with HIV by a new rapid fluorescence technique. J Clin Pathol 46:694–700, 1993
164. Orenstein JM: Microsporidiosis in the acquired immunodeficiency syndrome. J Parasitol 77:843–864, 1991
165. Shein R, Gelb A: Isospora belli in a patient with acquired immunodeficiency syndrome. J Clin Gastroenterol 6:525–528, 1984
166. DeHovitz JA, Pape JN, Boncy M, Johnson WD Jr: Clinical manifestations and therapy of Isospora belli infection in patients with the acquired immunodeficiency syndrome. N Engl J Med 315:87–90, 1986
167. Trier JS, Moxey PC, Schimmel EM, Robles E: Chronic intestinal coccidiosis in man: intestinal morphology and response to treatment. Gastroenterology 66:923–935, 1974
168. Carter TR, Cooper PH, Petri WA et al: Pneumocystic carinii infection of the small intestine in a patient with acquired immune deficiency syndrome. Am J Clin Pathol 89:679–683, 1988
169. Chiampi NP, Sundberg RD, Klompus JP, Wilson AJ: Cryptosporidial enteritis and pneumocystic pneumonia in a homosexual man. Hum Pathol 14:734–737, 1983
170. Muigai R, Shaunak S, Gatei DG et al: Jejunal function and pathology in visceral leishmoniasis. Lancet 2:476–479, 1983
171. Stemmermann GN, Hayochi T, Globes GA et al: Cryptosporidiosis: report of a fatal case complicated by disseminated toxoplasmosis. Am J Med 69:637–642, 1980
172. Ortega YR, Sterling CR, Gilman RH et al: Cyclospora species: a new protozoan pathogen of humans. N Engl J Med 328: 1308–1312, 1993
173. Brasitus TA, Gold RP, Kay RH et al: Intestinal stronglyoidiasis. Am J Gastroenterol 73:65–69, 1980
174. Milder JE, Walzer PD, Kilgore G et al: Clinical features of Strongyloides stercoralis infection in an endemic area of the United States. Gastroenterology 80:1481–1488, 1981
175. Strickland GT: Gastrointestinal manifestations of schistosomiasis. Gut 35:1334–1337, 1994
176. Perera DR, Weinstein WM, Rubin CE: Small intestinal biopsy. Human Pathol 6:157–217, 1975
177. Dobbins WO III: Small bowel biopsy in malabsorptive states. pp. 137–188. In Norris HT (ed): Pathology of the Colon, Small Intestine, and Anus. 2nd ed. Churchill Livingstone, New York, 1991
178. Goldman H, Antonioli DA: Mucosal biopsy of the esophagus, stomach and proximal duodenum. Hum Pathol 13:423–448, 1982
179. Holdstock G, Eade OE, Isaacson P, Smith CL: Endoscopic duodenal biopsy in coeliac disease and duodenitis. Scand J Gastroenterol 14:717–720, 1979
180. King CE, Toskes PP: Small intestine bacterial overgrowth. Gastroenterology 76:1035–1055, 1979
181. Sherman P, Lichtman S: Small bowel bacterial overgrowth syndrome. Dig Dis Sci 5:157–171, 1987
182. Waldmann TA: Protein-losing enteropathy. Gastroenterology 50:422–443, 1966
183. Popovic OS, Brkic S, Bojic P et al: Sarcoidosis and protein-losing enteropathy. Gastroenterology 78:119–125, 1980
184. Bank S, Trey C, Gans I et al: Histoplasmosis of the small bowel with "giant" intestinal villi and secondary protein-losing enteropathy. Am J Med 39:492–501, 1965
185. Kure CF, Gwavova N: Protein losing enteropathy: an unusual presentation of intestinal schistosomiasis. Gut 28:616–618, 1987
186. Wolber RA, Owen DA, Anderson FH, Freeman HJ: Lymphocytic gastritis and giant gastric folds associated with gastrointestinal protein loss. Modern Pathol 4:13–15, 1991
187. Yardley JH: Malabsorptive disorders. pp. 725–767. In Ming S-C, Goldman H (eds): Pathology of the Gastrointestinal Tract. WB Saunders, Philadelphia, 1992

188. Yardley JH, Bayless TM, Norton JH et al: Celiac disease: a study of the jejunal epithelium before and after a gluten-free diet. N Engl J Med 267:1173, 1962
189. Falchuk ZM: Update on gluten-sensitive enteropathy. Am J Med 67:50, 1979
190. Trier JS: Celiac sprue. N Engl J Med 325:1709–1719, 1991
191. Kagnoff MF: Immunopathogenesis of celiac disease. Immunol Invest 18:499–508, 1989
192. Katz AJ, Falchuck ZM: Definite diagnosis of gluten-sensitive enteropathy. Gastroenterology 75:695–700, 1978
193. Bramble MG, Zucolato S, Wright NA, Record CC: Acute gluten challenge in treated adult coeliac disease: a morphometric and enzymatic study. Gut 26:169–174, 1985
194. Egan-Mitchell B, Fottrell PF, McNicholl B: Early or precoeliac mucosa: development of gluten enteropathy. Gut 22:65–69, 1981
195. Rubin W, Ross LL, Sleisenger MH, Wesser E: An electron microscopic study of adult celiac disease. Lab Invest 15:1720–1747, 1966
196. Shiner M: Ultrastructural changes suggestive of immune reactions in the jejunal mucosa of coeliac children following gluten challenge. Gut 14:1–12, 1973
197. Pietroletti R, Bishop AE, Carlei F et al: Gut endocrine cell population in coeliac disease estimated by immunocytochemistry using a monoclonal antibody to chromogranin. Gut 27:838–843, 1986
198. Collin P, Reunala T, Pukkala E et al: Coeliac disease–associated disorders and survival. Gut 35:1215–1218, 1994
199. Fry L, Seah PP, Harper PG et al: The small intestine in dermatitis herpetiformis. J Clin Pathol 27:817–824, 1974
200. Gawkrodger DJ, McDonald C, O'Mahoney S, Ferguson A: Small intestinal function and dietary status in dermatitis herpetiformis Gut 32:377–382, 1991
201. de Franchis R, Primignani M, Cipolla M et al: Small-bowel involvement in dermatitis herpetiformis and in linear IgA bullous dermatosis. J Clin Gastroenterol 5:429–436, 1983
202. Leonard J, Haffenden G, Tucker W et al: Gluten challenge in dermatitis herpetiformis. N Engl J Med 308:816–819, 1983
203. Breen EG, Farren C, Connolly CE, McCarthy CF: Collagenous colitis and coeliac disease. Gut 28:364, 1987
204. Yardley JH, Lazenby AJ, Giardiello FM, Bayless TM: Collagenous, "microscopic", lymphocytic, and other gentler and more subtle forms of colitis. Hum Pathol 21:1089–1091, 1990
205. Wolber R, Owen D, Freeman H: Colonic lymphocytosis in patients with celiac sprue. Hum Pathol 21:1092–1096, 1990
206. Wolber R, Owen D, Del Buona L et al: Lymphocytic gastritis in patients with celiac sprue or sprue-like intestinal disease. Gastroenterology 98:310–315, 1990
207. Alsaigh N, Odze R, Antonioli D et al: Gastric and esophageal inflammatory changes in pediatric celiac disease. Modern Pathol 8:57A, 1995
208. Hankey GL, Holmes GKT: Coeliac disease in the elderly. Gut 35:65–67, 1994
209. Weinstein WM: Latent celiac sprue. Gastroenterology 66:489–493, 1974
210. Unsworth DJ, Brown DL: Serological screening suggests that adult coeliac disease is underdiagnosed in the UK and increases the incidence by up to 12%. Gut 35:61–64, 1994
211. Trier JS, Falchuk ZM, Carey MC et al: Celiac sprue and refractory sprue. Gastroenterology 75:307–316, 1978
212. Isaacson P, Wright DH: Malignant histiocytosis of the intestine: its relationship to malabsorption and ulcerative jejunitis. Hum Pathol 9:661–677, 1978
213. Baer AN, Bayless TM, Yardley JH: Intestinal ulceration and malabsorption syndromes. Gastroenterology 79:754–765, 1980
214. Roehrkasse RL, Roberts IM, Wald A et al: Celiac sprue complicated by lymphoma presenting with multiple gastric ulcers. Gastroenterology 91:740–745, 1986
215. Holmes GK, Prior P, Lane MR et al: Malignancy in coeliac disease—effect of a gluten free diet. Gut 30:333–338, 1989
216. Straker PJ, Gunasekaran S, Brady PG: Adenocarcinoma of the jejunum in association with celiac sprue. J Clin Gastroenterol 11:320–323, 1989
217. Gardiner GW, Van Patter T, Murray D: Atypical carcinoid tumor of the small bowel

complicating celiac disease. Cancer 56:2716–2722, 1985

218. Shiner M, Ballard J, Brook CGD et al: Intestinal biopsy in the diagnosis of cow's milk protein intolerance without acute symptoms. Lancet 2:1060–1063, 1975
219. Ament M, Rubin CE: Soy protein—another cause of the flat intestinal lesion. Gastroenterology 62:227–234, 1972
220. Perkkio M, Savilahti E, Kuitunen P: Morphometric and immunohistochemical study of jejunal biopsies from children with intestinal soy allergy. Fin Eur J Pediatr 137:63–69, 1981
221. Rosekrans PCM, Meijer CJIM, Cornelisse CJ et al: Use of morphometry and immunohistochemistry of small intestinal biopsy specimens in the diagnosis of food allergy. J Clin Pathol 33:125–130, 1980
222. Grybowski JD: Gastrointestinal milk allergy in infants. Pediatrics 40:354–360, 1967
223. Walker-Smith JA, Harrison M, Kilby A et al: Cow's milk–sensitive enteropathy. Arch Dis Child 53:375–380, 1978
224. Klein NC, Hargrove RL, Sleisenger MH et al: Eosinophilic gastroenteritis. Medicine (Baltimore) 40:299–319, 1970
225. Talley NJ, Shorter RG, Phillips SF et al: Eosinophilic gastroenteritis: a clinicopathological study of patients with disease of the mucosa, muscle layers and subserosal tissues. Gut 31:54–58, 1990
226. Goldman H: Allergic disorders. pp. 171–187. In Ming S-C, Goldman H (eds): Pathology of the Gastrointestinal Tract. WB Saunders, Philadelphia, 1992
227. Lee C-M, Changchien C-S, Chen P-C et al: Eosinophilic gastroenteritis: 10 years experience. Am J Gastroenterol 88:70–74, 1993
228. Goldman H, Proujansky R: Allergic proctitis and gastroenteritis in children: clinical and mucosal biopsy features in 53 cases. Am J Surg Pathol 10:75–86, 1986
229. Leinbach GE, Rubin CE: Eosinophilic gastroenteritis: a simple reaction to food allergens? Gastroenterology 59:874–889, 1970
230. Blackshaw AJ, Levison DA: Eosinophilic infiltrates of the gastrointestinal tract. J Clin Pathol 39:1–7, 1986
231. Walker NI, Croese J, Clouston AD et al: Eosinophilic enteritis in northeastern Australia. Pathology, association with *Ancylostoma caninum,* and implications. Am J Surg Pathol 19:328–337, 1995
232. Creamer B, Pink IJ: Paneth cell deficiency. Lancet 1:304–306, 1967
233. Weinstein WM, Saunders DR, Tytgat GN, Rubin CE: Collagenous sprue: an unrecognized type of malabsorption. N Engl J Med 283:1297–1301, 1970
234. Zeman RK, Toffler RB: Collagenous sprue. Am J Gastroenterol 70:541–544, 1978
235. Eckstein RP, Dowsett JF, Riley JW: Collagenous enterocolitis: a case of collagenous colitis with involvement of the small intestine. Am J Gastroenterol 83:767–771, 1988
236. Schenk EA, Samloff IM, Klipstein FA: Morphologic characteristics of jejunal biopsy in celiac disease and tropical sprue. Am J Pathol 47:765–781, 1965
237. Cook GC: Aetiology and pathogenesis of postinfective tropical malabsorption (tropical sprue). Lancet 1:721–723, 1984
238. Swanson VL, Thomasson RW: Pathology of the jejunal mucosa in tropical sprue. Am J Pathol 46:511–551, 1965
239. Lindenbaum J: Tropical enteropathy. Gastroenterology 64:637–652, 1973
240. Mathan M, Mathan VI, Baker SJ: An electron microscopic study of jejunal mucosal morphology in control subjects and in patients with tropical sprue in Southern India. Gastroenterology 68:17–32, 1975
241. Jeffries GH, Steinberg H, Sleisenger MH: Chronic ulcerative (nongranulomatous) jejunitis. Am J Med 44:47–59, 1968
242. Modigliani R, Poitras P, Galian A et al: Chronic non-specific ulcerative duodenojejunoileitis: report of four cases. Gut 20:318–328, 1979
243. Orchard JL, Luparello F, Bruskill D: Malabsorption syndrome occurring in the course of disseminated histoplasmosis. Am J Med 66:331–335, 1979
244. Perlmutter PH, Leichtner AM, Goldman H, Winter HS: Chronic diarrhea associated with hypogammaglobulinemia and enteropathy in infants and children. Dig Dis Sci 30:1149–1155, 1985
245. Atwell JD, Burge D, Wright D: Nodular lymphoid hyperplasia of the intestinal tract in infancy and childhood. J Ped Surg 20:25–29, 1985

246. Tanaka M, Kimura K, Sakai H et al: Long-term follow-up for minute gastroduodenal lesions in Crohn's disease. Gastrointest Endosc 32:206–209, 1986
247. Schuffler MD, Chaffee RE: Small intestinal biopsy in a patient with Crohn's disease of the duodenum. (The spectrum of abnormal findings in the absence of granulomas.) Gastroenterology 76:1009–1014, 1979
248. Comer GM, Brandt LJ, Abissi CJ: Whipple's disease: a review. Am J Gastroenterol 78:107–114, 1983
249. Relman DA, Schnidt TM, MacDermott RP, Falkow S: Identification of the uncultured bacillus of Whipple's disease. N Engl J Med 327:193–301, 1992
250. Yardley JH, Hendrix TR: Combined electron and light microscopy in Whipple's disease: demonstration of "bacillary bodies" in the intestine. Bull Johns Hopkins Hosp 109:80–95, 1961
251. Dobbins WO III, Kawanishi H: Bacillary characteristics in Whipple's disease: an electron microscopic study. Gastroenterology 80:1468–1475, 1981
252. Keren DF, Weisburger WR, Yardley JH et al: Whipple's disease: demonstration by immunoflorescence of similar bacterial antigens in macrophages from three cases. Johns Hopkins Med J 139:51–59, 1976
253. Du Boulay CE: An immunohistochemical study of Whipple's disease using the immunoperoxidase technique. Hum Pathol 13:925–929, 1982
254. Richman LS, Freeman WR, Green WR et al: Uveitis caused by Tropheryma whippelii (Whipple's bacillus). N Engl J Med 352:363–366, 1995
255. Ectors NL, Geboes KJ, De Vos RM et al: Whipple's disease: a histological, immunocytochemical, and electron microscopic study of the small intestinal epithelium. J Pathol 172:73–79, 1994
256. Volpicelli NA, Salyer WR, Milligan FD et al: The endoscopic appearance of the duodenum in Whipple's disease. Johns Hopkins Med J 138:19, 1976
257. Kuhajda FP, Belitsos NJ, Keren DF, Hutchins GM: A submucosal variant of Whipple's disease. Gastroenterology 82:46–50, 1982
258. Denholm RB, Mills PR, More IAR: Electron microscopy in the long-term follow-up of Whipple's disease. Am J Surg Pathol 5:507–516, 1981
259. Fleming JL, Wiesner RG, Shorter RG: Whipple's disease: clinical, biochemical and histopathologic features and assessment of treatment of 29 patients. Mayo Clin Proc 63:539–551, 1988
260. Cho C, Linscheer WG, Hirschkorn MA, Askutosh K: Sarcoid-like granulomas as an early manifestation of Whipple's disease. Gastroenterology 87:941–947, 1984
261. Rosen FS, Cooper MD, Wedgewood RJP: The primary immunodeficiencies. N Engl J Med 311:235–242, 300–310, 1984
262. Ament ME: Immunodeficiency syndromes of the gut. Scand J Gastroenterol 20(suppl 114):127–135, 1985
263. Gillin JS, Shike M, Alcock N et al: Malabsorption and mucosal abnormalities of the small intestine in the acquired immunodeficiency syndrome. Ann Intern Med 102:619–622, 1985
264. Cunningham-Rundles C: Selective IgA deficiency. J Pediatr Gastroenterol Nutr 7:482–484, 1988
265. Webster ADB, Kenwright S, Ballard J et al: Nodular lymphoid hyperplasia of the bowel in primary hypogammaglobulinaemia: study of in vivo and in vitro lymphocyte function. Gut 18:364–372, 1977
266. Bedine MS, Yardley JH, Elliott HL et al: Intestinal involvement in Waldenstrom's macroglobulinemia. Gastroenterology 65:308–315, 1973
267. Brandt LJ, Davidoff A, Bernstein LH et al: Small intestinal involvement in Waldenstrom's macroglobulinemia: case report and review of the literature. Dig Dis Sci 26:174–180, 1981
268. Ammann RW, Vetter D, Deyhle P et al: Gastrointestinal involvement in systemic mastocytosis. Gut 17:107–112, 1976
269. Braverman DZ, Dollberg L, Shiner M: Clinical, histological and electron microscopic study of mast cell disease of the small bowel. Am J Gastroenterol 80:30–37, 1985
270. Fishman RS, Fleming CR, Li CY: Systemic mastocytosis with review of gastrointestinal manifestations. Mayo Clin Proc 54:51–54, 1979
271. Haggitt RC, Meissner WA: Crohn's disease of the upper gastrointestinal tract. Am J Clin Pathol 59:613–622, 1973

272. Lescut D, Vanco D, Bonniere P et al: Perioperative endoscopy of the whole small bowel in Crohn's disease. Gut 34:647–649, 1993
273. Lee RG, Braziel RM, Stenzel P: Gastrointestinal involvement in Langerhans cell histiocytosis (Histiocytosis X): diagnosis by rectal biopsy. Modern Pathol 3:154–157, 1990
274. Yu RCH, Attra A, Quinn CM et al: Multisystem Langerhans' cell histiocytosis with pancreatic involvement. Gut 34:570–572, 1993
275. Dobbins WO III: Electron microscopic study of the intestinal mucosa in intestinal lymphangiectasia. Gastroenterology 51:1004–1017, 1966
276. Strober W, Wochner RD, Carbone PP, Waldmann TA: Intestinal lymphangiectasia: a protein-losing enteropathy with hypogammaglobulinemia, lymphocytopenia and impaired homograft rejection. J Clin Invest 46:1643–1656, 1967
277. Asakura H, Miur S, Morishita T et al: Endoscopic and histopathological study on primary and secondary intestinal lymphangiectasia. Dig Dis Sci 26:312–320, 1981
278. Greenwood N: The jejunal mucosa in two cases of A-beta-lipoproteinemia. Am J Gastroenterol 65:160–162, 1976
279. Ferrans VJ, Fredrickson DS: The pathology of Tangier disease: a light and electron microscopic study. Am J Pathol 78:101, 1975
280. Herbert PN, Forte T, Heinen RJ, Fredrickson DS: Tangier disease. N Engl J Med 299:519–521, 1978
281. Dechelotte P, Kantelip B, de Laguillaumie BC et al: Tangier disease. A histological and ultrastructural study. Pathol Res Pract 180:424–430, 1985
282. Phillips AD, Jenkins P, Rafat F, Walker-Smith JA: Congenital microvillus atrophy: specific diagnostic features. Arch Dis Child 60:135–140, 1985
283. Schofield DE, Agostini RM, Yunis EJ: Gastrointestinal microvillus inclusion disease. Am J Clin Pathol 98:119–124, 1992
284. Davidson GP, Cutz E, Hamilton JR, Gall DG: Familial enteropathy: a syndrome of protracted diarrhea from birth, failure to thrive, and hypoplastic villus atrophy. Gastroenterology 75:783–790, 1978
285. Cutz E, Rhoads JM, Drumm B et al: Microvillus inclusion disease: an inherited defect of brush-border assembly and differentiation. N Engl J Med 320:646–651, 1989
286. Bell SW, Kerner JA Jr, Sibley RK: Microvillous inclusion disease. The importance of electron microscopy for diagnosis. Am J Surg Pathol 15:1157–1164, 1991
287. Rhoads JM, Vogler RC, Lacey SR et al: Microvillus inclusion disease: in vitro jejunal electrolyte transport. Gastroenterology 100:811–817, 1991
288. Groisman GM, Ben-Izhak O, Schwersenz A et al: The value of polyclonal carcinoembryonic antigen immunostaining in the diagnosis of microvillous inclusion disease. Hum Pathol 24:1232–1237, 1993
289. Lake BD: Microvillus inclusion disease: specific diagnostic features shown by alkaline phosphatase histochemistry. J Clin Pathol 41:880–882, 1988
290. Stanfield JP, Hutt MSR, Tunnicliffe R: Intestinal biopsy in kwashiorkor. Lancet 2:519–523, 1965
291. Ashley SW, Ells SA: Tumors of the small intestine. Semin Oncol 15:116–128, 1988
292. Cooper HS: Benign polyps of the intestines. pp. 786–815. In Ming S-C, Goldman H (eds): Pathology of the Gastrointestinal Tract. WB Saunders, Philadelphia, 1992
293. Lewis BS, Kornbluth A, Waye JD: Small bowel tumors: yield of enteroscopy. Gut 32:763–765, 1991
294. Chong J, Tagle M, Barkin JS et al: Small bowel push-type fiberoptic enteroscopy for patients with occult gastrointestinal bleeding or suspected small bowel pathology. Am J Gastroenterol 89:2143–2146, 1994
295. LiVolsi VA, Perzin KH: Inflammatory pseudotumors (inflammatory fibrous polyps) of the small intestine. Am J Dig Dis 20:325–326, 1975
296. Navas-Palacios JJ, Colima-Ruizdelgado F, Sanchez-Larrea, Cortes-Consino J: Inflammatory fibroid polyps of the gastrointestinal tract. An immunohistochemical and electron microscopic study. Cancer 51:1682–1690, 1983
297. Gal R, Rathwolfson L, Ginzburg M, Kessler E: Adenomyomas of the small intestine. Histopathology 18:369–371, 1991
298. Kahn E, Daum F: Pseudopolyposis of the small intestine in Crohn's disease. Hum Pathol 15:84–86, 1984

299. Perzin KH, Bridge MF: Adenomas of the small intestine: a clinicopathologic review of 51 cases and a study of their relationship to carcinoma. Cancer 48:799, 1981
300. Roth SI, Helwig EB: Juvenile polyps of the colon and rectum. Cancer 16:468–479, 1963
301. Sachatello CR, Pickren JW, Grace JT: Generalized juvenile gastrointestinal polyposis. Gastroenterology 58:669, 1970
302. Stemper TJ, Kent TH, Summers RW: Juvenile polyposis and gastrointestinal carcinoma: a study of a kindred. Ann Intern Med 83:639–646, 1975
303. Williams GT, Bussey HJR, Morson BC: Hamartomatous polyps in Peutz-Jeghers syndrome. N Engl J Med 299:101, 1978
304. Foley TR, McGarrity TJ, Abt AB: Peutz-Jeghers syndrome: a clinicopathologic survey of the "Harrisburg Family" with a 49-year follow-up. Gastroenterology 95: 1535–1540, 1988
305. Burdick D, Prior JT: Peutz-Jeghers syndrome. A clinicopathologic study of a large family with a 27 year follow-up. Cancer 50:2139–2146, 1982
306. Dodds WJ, Schulte WJ, Hensley GT, Hogan WJ: Peutz-Jeghers syndrome and gastrointestinal malignancy. AJR 115:374–377, 1972
307. Giardiello FM, Welsh SB, Hamilton SR et al: Increased risk of cancer in the Peutz-Jeghers syndrome. N Engl J Med 316:1511–1514, 1987
308. Perzin KH, Bridge MF: Adenomatous and carcinomatous changes in hamartomatous polyps of the small intestine (Peutz-Jeghers syndrome). Cancer 49:971–983, 1982
309. Ali M, Weinstein J, Biempica J et al: Cronkhite-Canada syndrome: report of a case with bacteriologic, immunologic, and electron microscopic studies. Gastroenterology 79:731, 1980
310. Daniel ES, Ludwig SL, Lewin KJ et al: The Cronkhite-Canada syndrome. An analysis of clinical and pathologic features and therapy in 55 patients. Medicine 61:293–309, 1982
311. Burke AP, Sobin LH: The pathology of Cronkhite-Canada polyps: a comparison to juvenile polyposis. Am J Surg Pathol 13:940–946, 1989
312. Jarvinen H, Nyberg M, Peltokallio P: Upper gastrointestinal tract polyps in familial adenomatous coli. Gut 24:333–339, 1983
313. Sarre RG, Frost AG, Jagelman DG et al: Gastric and duodenal polyps and familial adenomatous polyposis: a prospective study of the nature and prevalence of upper gastrointestinal polyps. Gut 28:306–314, 1987
314. Domizio P, Talbort IC, Spigelman AD et al: Upper gastrointestinal pathology in familial adenomatous polyposis—results from a prospective study of 102 patients. J Clin Pathol 43:738–743, 1990
315. Odze R, Gallinger S, So K, Antonioli D: Duodenal adenomas in familial adenomatous polyposis: relation of cell differentation and mucin histochemical features to growth pattern. Modern Pathol 7:376–384, 1994
316. Burt RW, Berenson MM, Lee RG et al: Upper gastrointestinal polyps in Gardners syndrome. Gastroenterology 86:295–301, 1984
317. Shemesk E, Bat L: A prospective evaluation of the upper gastrointestinal tract and periampullary region in patients with Gardner syndrome. Am J Gastroenterol 80:825–827, 1985
318. Ross JE, Mara JE: Small bowel polyps and carcinoma in multiple intestinal polyposis. Arch Surg 108:736–738, 1974
319. Phillips LG Jr: Polyposis and carcinoma of the small bowel and familial colonic polyposis. Dis Colon Rectum 24:478–481, 1981
320. Fenoglio-Preiser CM, Pascal RR, Perzin KH: Tumors of the intestines. Atlas of Tumor Pathology, second series, fascicle 27. Armed Forces Institute of Pathology, Washington DC, 1990
321. Bridge MF, Perzin KH: Primary adenocarcinoma of the jejunum and ileum. A clinicopathologic study. Cancer 36:1876–1887, 1975
322. Arthaud JB, Guinee VF: Jejunal and ileal adenocarcinoma. Am J Gastroenterol 72:638–646, 1979
323. Live TF, Biggart JD: Primary adenocarcinoma of the jejunum and ileum—clinicopathological review of 25 cases. J Clin Pathol 43:533–536, 1990
324. Ming S-C: Adenocarcinoma and other malignant epithelial tumors of the intestines. pp. 816–857. In Ming S-C, Goldman H (eds): Pathology of the Gastrointestinal Tract. WB Saunders, Philadelphia, 1992
325. Danzig JB, Brandt LJ, Reinus JF, Klein RS: Gastrointestinal malignancy in patients with AIDS. Am J Gastroenterol 86:715–718, 1991

326. Greenstein AJ, Sachar DB, Smith H et al: Patterns of neoplasia in Crohn's disease and ulcerative colitis. Cancer 40:403–407, 1980
327. Gyde SN, Prior P, Macartney JC et al: Malignancy in Crohn's disease. Gut 21: 1024–1029, 1980
328. Lashner BA: Risk factors for small bowel cancer in Crohn's disease. Dig Dis Sci 37:1179–1184, 1992
329. Simpson S, Traube J, Riddell RH: The histological appearance of dysplasia (precarcinomatous change) in Crohn's disease of the small and large intestine. Gastroenterology 81:492–501, 1981
330. Caruso ML, Marzullo F: Jejunal adenocarcinoma in congenital heterotopic gastric mucosa. J Clin Gastroenterol 10:92–94, 1988
331. Andrup H, Ajode P: Primary linitis plastica of the small bowel. Case report. Acta Chir Scand 154:319–321, 1988
332. Sanders RJ, Axtell HK: Carcinoids of the gastrointestinal tract. Surg Gynecol Obstet 119:369–380, 1984
333. Moryana TN, Satkunam N: A comparative immunohistochemical study of jejunoileal and appendiceal carcinoids. Implications for histogenesis and pathogenesis. Cancer 70:1081–1088, 1992
334. Lechago J: Gastrointestinal neuroendocrine cell proliferations. Hum Pathol 25:1114–1122, 1994
335. Kubo T, Watanabe H: Neoplastic argentaffin cells in gastric and intestinal carcinomas. Cancer 27:447–454, 1971
336. Klappenbach RS, Kurman RJ, Sinclair CF, James LP: Composite carcinoma—carcinoid tumors of the gastrointestinal tract. A morphologic, histochemical and immunocytochemical study. Am J Clin Pathol 84:137–143, 1985
337. Lewin K: Carcinoid tumors and the mixed (composite) glandular-endocrine cell carcinomas. Am J Surg Pathol 11(suppl 1):71–86, 1987
338. Gould Ve, Valaitis J, Trujillo Y et al: Neuroendocrinoma of the jejunum: electron microscopic and biochemical analysis. Cancer 46:713–717, 1980
339. Alpers CE, Beckstead JH: Malignant neuroendocrine tumor of jejunum with osteoclast-like giant cells. Enzyme histochemistry distinguishes tumor cells from giant cells. Am J Surg Pathol 9:57–64, 1985
340. McDonald GB, Schuffler MD, Kadin ME, Tytgat GNJ: Intestinal pseudoobstruction caused by diffuse lymphoid infiltration of the small intestine. Gastroenterology 89:882–889, 1985
341. Gudjonsson H, Jones M, Krawitt EL, Kaye MD: Pseudolymphoma of the jejunum. Dig Dis Sci 32:1314–1318, 1987
342. Mir R, Kahn LB, Selzer G: Immunohistochemistry of primary gastrointestinal lymphomas: a study of 76 cases. Histopathology 10:391–403, 1986
343. Dragosics B, Bauer P, Radaszkiewicz T: Primary gastrointestinal non-Hodgkin's lymphoma. A retrospective clinicopathologic study of 150 cases. Cancer 55:1060–1073, 1985
344. Appelman HD, Hirsch SD, Schnitzer B, Coon WW: Clinicopathologic overview of gastrointestinal lymphomas. Am J Surg Pathol 9(3)(suppl):71–83, 1985
345. Netto D, Nowak JA, Balaban EP, Demian SDE: Primary lymphoma of the duodenum. Surg Pathol 4:57–67, 1991
346. Isaacson PG: Gastrointestinal lymphoma. Hum Pathol 25:1020–1029, 1994
347. Lewin KJ, Ranchod M, Dorfman RF: Lymphoms of the gastrointestinal tract: a study of 117 cases presenting with gastrointestinal disease. Cancer 42:693, 1978
348. Weingrad DN, DeCosse JJ, Sherlock P et al: Primary gastrointestinal lymphoma: a 30-year review. Cancer 49:1258–1265, 1982
349. Filippa DA, Lieberman PH, Weingrad DN et al: Primary lymphoma of the gastrointestinal tract. Analysis of prognostic factors with emphasis on histological type. Am J Surg Pathol 7:363–372, 1983
350. Cooper BT, Holmes GK, Ferguson R, Cooke WT: Celiac disease and malignancy. Medicine (Baltimore) 59:249–261, 1980
351. Swinson CM, Slavin G, Coles EC, Booth CC: Celiac disease and malignancy. Lancet 1:111–115, 1983
352. Matuchansky C, Touchard G, Lemaire M et al: Malignant lymphoma of the small bowel associated with diffuse nodular lymphoid hyperplasia. N Engl J Med 313:166–172, 1985
353. Steinberg JJ, Bridges N, Feiner HD, Valensi Q: Small intestinal lymphoma in three pa-

tients with acquired immune deficiency syndrome. Am J Gastroenterol 8:21–26, 1985
354. Isaacson PG, Spencer J, Connolly CE et al: Malignant histiocytosis of the intestine: a T-cell lymphoma. Lancet 2:688–691, 1985
355. Al-Bahrani ZR, Al-Mondhiry H, Bakir F, Al-Saleem T: Clinical and pathologic subtypes of primary intestinal lymphoma. Experience with 132 patients over a 14-year period. Cancer 52:1666–1672, 1983
356. Khojasteh A, Haghehenass M, Haghighi P: Immunoproliferative small intestinal disease. A "third-world lesion". N Engl J Med 308:1401–1405, 1983
357. Tabbone F, Mourali N, Cammoun M, Najjar T: Results of laparotomy in immunoproliferative small intestinal disease. Cancer 61:1699–1706, 1988
358. Price SK: Immunoproliferative small intestine disease: a study of 13 cases with alpha heavy-chain disease. Histopathology 17:7–18, 1990
359. Commoun M, Jaofowa H, Tabbone F et al: Immunoproliferative small intestinal disease without X-chain disease. A pathological study. Gastroenterology 96:750–763, 1989
360. Isaacson PG, Dogan A, Price SK, Spencer J: Immunoproliferative small intestinal disease. An immunohistochemical study. Am J Surg Pathol 13:1023–1033, 1989
361. Fernandes BJ, Amato D, Goldfinger M: Diffuse lymphomatous polyposis of the gastrointestinal tract. A case report with immunohistochemical studies. Gastroenterology 88:1267–1270, 1985
362. Stessens L, Van Den Oord JJ, Geboes K et al: Gastrointestinal lymphomatous polyposis. Gastroenterology 90:2041–2042, 1986
363. Milchgrub S, Kamel OW, Wiley E et al: Malignant histiocytic neoplasms of the small intestine. Am J Surg Pathol 16:11–20, 1992
364. Miettinen M, Fletcher CDM, Lasota J: True histiocytic lymphoma of the small intestine. Analysis of two S-10 protein-positive cases with features of interdigitating reticulum cell sarcoma. Am J Clin Pathol 100:285–292, 1993
365. Devaney K, Jaffe ES: The surgical pathology of gastrointestinal Hodgkin's disease. Am J Clin Pathol 95:794–801, 1991
367. Appelman HD: Mesenchymal tumors of the gastrointestinal tract. pp. 310–350. In Ming S-C, Goldman H (eds): Pathology of the Gastrointestinal Tract. WB Saunders, Philadelphia, 1992
368. Khansur T, Balducci L, Tavassoli M: Granular cell tumor. Cancer 60:220–222, 1987
369. Boyle L, Lack EE: Solitary cavernous hemangioma of small intestine. Case report and literature review. Arch Pathol Lab Med 117:939–941, 1993
370. Johnston J, Helwig EB: Granular cell tumors of the gastrointestinal tract and perianal region. A study of 74 cases. Dig Dis Sci 26:807–816, 1981
371. Daimaru Y, Kido H, Hashimoto H, Enjoji M: Benign schwannoma of the gastrointestinal tract: a clinicopathologic and immunohistochemical study. Hum Pathol 19:257–264, 1988
372. Fuller CE, Williams GT: Gastrointestinal manifestations of type-1 neurofibromatosis (von Recklinghausen's disease). Histopathology 19:1–12, 1991
373. Hamilton WH, Shelburne JD, Bossen EH, Lowe JE: A glomus tumor of the jejunum masquerading as a carcinoid tumor. Hum Pathol 13:859–861, 1982
374. Olsen EGJ, Wellwood JM: Hemangiopericytoma of the small intestine. A report of three cases. Br J Surg 57:66–69, 1970
375. Ranchod M, Kempson RL: Smooth muscle tumors of the gastrointestinal tract and retroperitoneum: a pathologic analysis of 100 cases. Cancer 39:255, 1977
376. Evans HL: Smooth muscle tumors of the gastrointestinal tract. A study of 56 cases followed for a minimum of 10 years. Cancer 56:2242–2250, 1985
377. Chiotasso PJ, Fazio VW: Prognostic factors of 28 leiomyosarcomas of the small intestine. Surg Gynecol Obstet 155:197–202, 1982
378. Atik M, Whittlesey RH: Liposarcoma of the jejunum. Ann Surg 146:837–842, 1957
379. Taxy JB, Battifora H: Angiosarcoma of the gastrointestinal tract. A report of three cases. Cancer 62:210–216, 1988
380. Sato N, Zaloudek C, Geelhoed GW, Orenstein JM: Malignant mesenchymoma of the small intestine. Arch Pathol Lab Med 108:164–167, 1984
381. Nojima T, Gebhardt MC, Mankin HJ, Schiller AL: Extraosseous osteosarcoma presenting with intestinal hemorrhage: case report

and literature review. Hum Pathol 17:85–87, 1986

382. Miliauskas JR, Crowley KS: Granulocytic sarcoma (chloroma) of the small intestine with associated megakaryocytes. Pathology 17:559, 661–662, 1985
383. Fu Y-S, Gabbiani G, Kaye GI, Lattes R: Malignant soft tissue tumors of probable histiocytic origin (malignant fibrous histiocytomas): general considerations and electron microscopic and tissue culture studies. Cancer 35:176–198, 1975
384. Saltz RK, Kurtz RC, Lightdale CJ et al: Kaposi's sarcoma. Gastrointestinal involvement and correlation with skin findings and immunologic function. Dig Dis Sci 29:817–823, 1984
385. Bernal A, del Junco GW, Gibson SR: Endoscopic and pathologic features of gastrointestinal Kaposi's sarcoma: a report of four cases in patients with the acquired immune deficiency syndrome. Gastrointest Endosc 31:74–77, 1985
386. Freedman SL, Wright TL, Altman DF: Gastrointestinal Kaposi's sarcoma in patients with acquired immunodeficiency syndrome. Endoscopic and autopsy findings. Gastroenterology 89:102–108, 1985
387. Parente F, Cernushi M, Orlando G et al: Kaposi's sarcoma and AIDS-frequency of gastrointestinal involvement and its effect on survival—a prospective study in a heterogeneous population. Scand J Gastroenterol 26:1007–1012, 1991
388. Rose HS, Balthazar EJ, Megibow AJ et al: Alimentary tract involvement in Kaposi's sarcoma: radiographic and endoscopic findings in 25 homosexual men. Am J Radiol 39:661–666, 1982
389. Templeton AC: Kaposi's sarcoma. Pathol Annu 16:315–336, 1981
390. Bak M, Teglbjaerg PS: Pleomorphic (giant cell) carcinoma of the intestine. An immunohistochemical and electron microscopic study. Cancer 64:2557–2564, 1989
391. Radi MF, Gray GF, Scott HW: Carcinosarcoma of ileum in regional enteritis. Hum Pathol 15:385–387, 1984
392. Harada N, Misawa T, Chijijwa Y et al: A case of extragenital choriocarcinoma in the jejunum. Am J Gastroenterol 86:1077–1079, 1991
393. Raijman I: Duodenal metastases from lung cancer. Endoscopy 26:752–753, 1994
394. Goodman PL, Karakousis CP: Symptomatic gastrointestinal metastases from malignant melanoma. Cancer 48:1058–1059, 1981
395. Geboes K, DeJaeger E, Rutgierts P, Vantrappen G: Symptomatic gastrointestinal metastases from malignant melanoma. A clinical study. J Clin Gastroenterol 10:64–70, 1988
396. Regan JR, Gibbons RB: Adenocarcinoma of the lung presenting as hematemesis secondary to jejunal metastasis: a case report and review of the literature. Mil Med 153:30–32, 1988
397. Sweetenham JW, Whitehouse JM, Williams CJ, Mead GM: Involvement of the gastrointestinal tract by metastases from germ cell tumor of the testes. Cancer 61:2566–2570, 1988
398. Rocken C, Saeger W, Linke RP: Gastrointestinal amyloid deposits in old age—report on 110 consecutive autopsical patients and 98 retrospective bioptic specimens. Pathol Res Pract 190:641–649, 1994
399. Gilat T, Spiro HM: Amyloidosis and the gut. Am J Dig Dis 13:619–633, 1968
400. Shousha S, Lowdell CP, Bull TB, Parkins RA: Secondary amyloidosis of the gastrointestinal tract: an electron microscopic study. Hum Pathol 16:596–601, 1985
401. Shimizu S, Yoshinaka M, Tada M et al: A case of primary amyloidosis confined to the small intestine. Gastroenterol Jpn 21:513–517, 1986
402. Coughlin GP, Remer RG, Grant AK: Endoscopic diagnosis of amyloidosis. Gastrointest Endosc 26:154, 1980
403. Astaldi G, Meardi G, Lisino T: The iron content of jejunal mucosa obtained by Crosby's biopsy in haemochromatosis and haemosiderosis. Blood 28:70–82, 1966
404. Goldman H: Systemic and miscellaneous disorders. pp. 351–380. In Ming S-C, Goldman H (eds): Pathology of the Gastrointestinal Tract. WB Saunders, Philadelphia, 1992
405. Schneck L, Volk BW, Saifer A: The gangliosidoses. Am J Med 46:245–263, 1969
406. Dinari G, Rosenbach Y, Grunebaum M et al: Gastrointestinal manifestation of Niemann-Pick disease. Enzyme 25:407–412, 1980

407. Fox B: Lipofuscinosis of the gastrointestinal tract in man. J Clin Pathol 20:806–813, 1967
408. Horn T, Svendsen LB, Johansen A, Backer O: Brown bowel syndrome. Ultrastruct Pathol 8:357–361, 1985
409. Glew RH, Basu A, Prence EM, Remaley AT: Lysosomal storage diseases. Lab Invest 53:250–269, 1985
410. Morecki R, Paunier L, Hamilton JR: Intestinal mucosa in cystinosis. Arch Pathol 86:297–307, 1968
411. Partin JC, Schubert WK: Small intestinal mucosa in cholesterol ester storage disease: a light and electron microscope study. Gastroenterology 57:542–558, 1969
412. Dorfman A, Matalon R: The mucopolysaccharidoses: a review. Proc Natl Acad Sci USA 73:630–637, 1976
413. Lake BD: Storage disorders involving the alimentary tract. pp. 269–276. In Whitehead R (ed): Gastrointestinal and Oesophageal Pathology. Churchill Livingstone, New York, 1989
414. Coletta U, Sturgill BC: Isolated xanthomatosis of the small bowel. Hum Pathol 16:422–424, 1985
415. Landing BH, Nadorra R: Infantile systemic hyalinosis. Pediatr Pathol 6:55–79, 1986
416. Caccamo D, Jaen A, Telenta M et al: Lipoid proteinosis of the small bowel. Arch Pathol Lab Med 118:572–574, 1994
417. Rauf A, Davis P, Levendoglu H: Sarcoidosis of the small intestine. Am J Gastroenterol 83:187–189, 1988
418. MacFarlane DA: Intestinal sarcoidosis. Br J Surg 4:639–642, 1955
419. Sprague R, Harper P, McClain S et al: Disseminated gastrointestinal sarcoidosis: case report and review of the literature. Gastroenterology 87:421–425, 1984
420. Ament ME, Ochs HD: Gastrointestinal manifestations of chronic granulomatous disease. N Engl J Med 288:382–387, 1973
421. Park RW, Grand RJ: Gastrointestinal manifestations of cystic fibrosis: a review. Gastroenterology 81:1143–1161, 1981
422. Graham RM, Rheault MH: Characteristic cellular changes in epithelial cells in pernicious anemia. J Lab Clin Med 43:235–245, 1954
423. Foroozan P, Trier JS: Mucosa of the small intestine in pernicious anaemia. N Engl J Med 277:553–559, 1967
424. Gupta S, Walker DL, Keshavarzian A, Hodgson HJF: Upper endoscopy for occult bleeding in renal failure. J Clin Gastroenterol 9:43–45, 1987
425. Franzin G, Musola R, Mencarelli R: Morphological changes of the gastroduodenal mucosa in regular dialysis in uremic patients. Histopathology 6:429–437, 1982
426. Musola R, Franzin G, Mora R, Manfrini C: Prevalence of gastroduodenal lesions in uremic patients undergoing dialysis and after renal transplantation. Gastrointest Endosc 30:343–346, 1984
427. Prasad AS: The role of zinc in gastrointestinal and liver disease. Clin Gastroenterol 12:713–741, 1983
428. Mack D, Koletzko B, Cunnane S et al: Acrodermatitis enteropathica with normal serum zinc levels: diagnostic value of small bowel biopsy and essential fatty acid determination. Gut 30:1426–1429, 1989
429. Casparie MK, Moyer JWR, Vanhuyster BJW et al: Endoscopic and histopathologic feature of Dego's disease. Endoscopy 23:231–234, 1991
430. DeSchryver-Keiskemeti K, Clouse RE: A previously unrecognized subgroup of "eosinophilic gastroenteritis": association with connective tissue diseases. Am J Surg Pathol 8:171, 1984
431. Smith BH, Welter LH: Pneumatosis intestinalis. Am J Clin Pathol 48:455–465, 1967
432. Yale CE, Balish E: Pneumatosis cystoides intestinalis. Dis Colon Rectum 19:107–111, 1976
433. Doolas A, Breyer RH, Franklin JL: Pneumatosis cystoides intestinalis following jejunoileal by-pass. Am J Gastroenterol 72:271–275, 1979
434. Stahl C, Grimes EM: Endometriosis of the small bowel. Case reports and review of the literature. Obstet Gynecol Surv 42:131–136, 1987
435. Sharma BK, Pounder RE, Cruse JP et al: Extramedullary haemopoiesis of the small bowel. Gut 27:873–875, 1986
436. Schreibman D, Brenner B, Jacobs R et al: Small intestinal myeloid metaplasia. JAMA 259:2580–2582, 1988
437. Kyriakos M, Condon SC: Enteritis cystica profunda. Am J Clin Pathol 69:77–85, 1978

438. Saul SH, Wong lK, Zinsser KR: Enteritis cystica profunda: association with Crohn's disease. Hum Pathol 17:600–603, 1986
439. Aftalion B, Lipper S: Enteritis cystica profunda associated with Crohn's disease. Arch Pathol Lab Med 108:532–533, 1984
440. Alexis J, Lubin J, Wallach M: Enteritis cystica profunda in a patient with Crohn's disease. Arch Pathol Lab Med 113:947–949, 1989
441. Shepherd NA, Bussey HJR, Jass JR: Epithelial misplacement in Peutz-Jeghers polyps; a diagnostic pitfall. Am J Surg Pathol 11:743–749, 1987
442. Spjut HJ, Helgason AG, Trabanino JG: Jejunitis cystica profunda in a hamartomatous polyp. Am J Surg Pathol 11:328–332, 1987
443. Goldman H: Other inflammatory disorders of the intestines. pp. 689–696. In Ming S-C, Goldman H (eds): Pathology of the Gastrointestinal Tract. WB Saunders, Philadelphia, 1992
444. Snover DC, Weisdorf SA, Vercolotti GM et al: A histopathologic study of gastric and small intestinal graft-versus-host disease following allogeneic bone marrow transplantation. Hum Pathol 16:387–392, 1985
445. Spencer GD, Shulman HM, Mayerson D et al: Diffuse intestinal ulceration after marrow transplantation: a clinicopathologic study of 13 patients. Hum Pathol 17:621–633, 1986
446. Schraut WH, Lee KKW, Dawson PJ, Hurst RD: Graft-versus-host disease induced by small bowel allografts: clinical course and pathology. Transplantation 41:286–290, 1986
447. Cohen Z, Silverman RE, Wassef R, Levy GA et al: Small intestinal transplantation using Cyclosporine. Transplantation 42:613–621, 1986
448. Grant D: Intestinal transplantation: current status. Transplant Proc 21:2869–2871, 1989
449. Hurlbut D, Ohene-Fianko D, Grant D, Garcia B: Histopathologic diagnosis of intestinal rejection following clinical small bowel transplantation. Modern Pathol 5:43A, 1992
450. Boydstan JS Jr, Gaffey TA, Bartholomew LG: Clinicopathologic study of non-specific ulcers of the small intestine. Dig Dis Sci 26:911–916, 1981
451. Thomas WEG, Williamson RCN: Nonspecific small bowel ulceration. Postgrad Med J 61:587–591, 1985

8

Disorders of the Ileum

This chapter concentrates on diseases that primarily involve or present in the ileum, either in its normal position or as part of a stoma or anastomotic procedure.[1-3] Many other conditions can affect the ileum as a part of the small intestine, and these are generally presented in Chapters 6 and 7; they are briefly mentioned here for completeness. Similarly, disorders that occur in the colon can also involve the ileum, and the principal presentation, when the effects are more prominent in the large intestine, is given in Chapters 9 and 10.

GENERAL ASPECTS

As endoscopes were developed for examination of the lower part of the gastrointestinal tract, most attention was directed toward extending the study from the rectum and sigmoid colon to the rest of the large intestine. For a considerable time, there appeared to be little interest in the visualization of the terminal ileum as a general or common procedure. It has been subsequently realized, however, that with a little extra effort and skill, this can be accomplished in the large majority of cases. It is estimated that useful information can be obtained by the examination of the ileum in almost one-third of the cases. This is particularly indicated for disorders that commonly affect the area or in which there is radiographic evidence of disease in that region (Table 8-1). As noted below, examination of the ileal segment is also commonly obtained following anastomotic and stomal procedures.

NORMAL STRUCTURE

The ileal mucosa shares the overall common structure with the rest of the small intestine, consisting of villi and crypts covered by epithelial cells; a lamina propria with a variety of inflammatory cells; and a muscularis mucosae comprised of two layers of smooth muscle tissue.[1, 3]

Epithelium

The villi are generally three to four times as tall as the crypts, similar to other parts of the small bowel (Fig. 8-1). There are a greater number of goblet mucous cells along the villi; these comprise about one-half of

Table 8-1. Uses of Ileal Mucosal Biopsies

Presence of ileitis
Crohn's disease versus other ileitis
Evaluation of stomas and anastomoses
Detection of tumors

the epithelial cells lining the villi, in contrast to the proximal portions where they are only the small minority. The mucin is otherwise similar to the rest of the small intestine, consisting mainly of the non-sulfated, less acidic type that stains well with Alcian Blue at pH 2.5.[4, 5] The crypts contain the stem and dividing cells, Paneth cells at the base, and endocrine cells largely interspersed between the other epithelial cells and the basement membrane[6] (see Fig. 6-2). (See Chs. 6 and 7 for further details regarding the features of the epithelial cells in the small intestine.)

Lamina Propria

The distal ileal region normally has the greatest amount of lymphoid tissue, which is concentrated in the mucosa and submucosa.[7] This is appreciated grossly as Peyer's patches, and there are also more isolated lymphoid nodules in the intervening mucosa, compared to other parts of the small intestine[8] (Fig. 8-2). All of these structures are comprised of well formed lymphoid nodules with prominent germinal centers, and they present as areas of granularity or nodularity on endoscopic visualization. Overlying the nodules in the surface epithelium are the specialized M cells that assist in the antigen trapping[9] (Fig. 8-3). The intervening lamina propria contains all forms of mononuclear inflammatory cells including lymphocytes, plasma cells and macrophages as well as eosinophils, whereas neutrophils are ordinarily not present.

Effects of Operations

The ileal mucosal structure becomes modified at sites of anastomosis and stomas. At a minimum, there is an atrophy of the mucosal

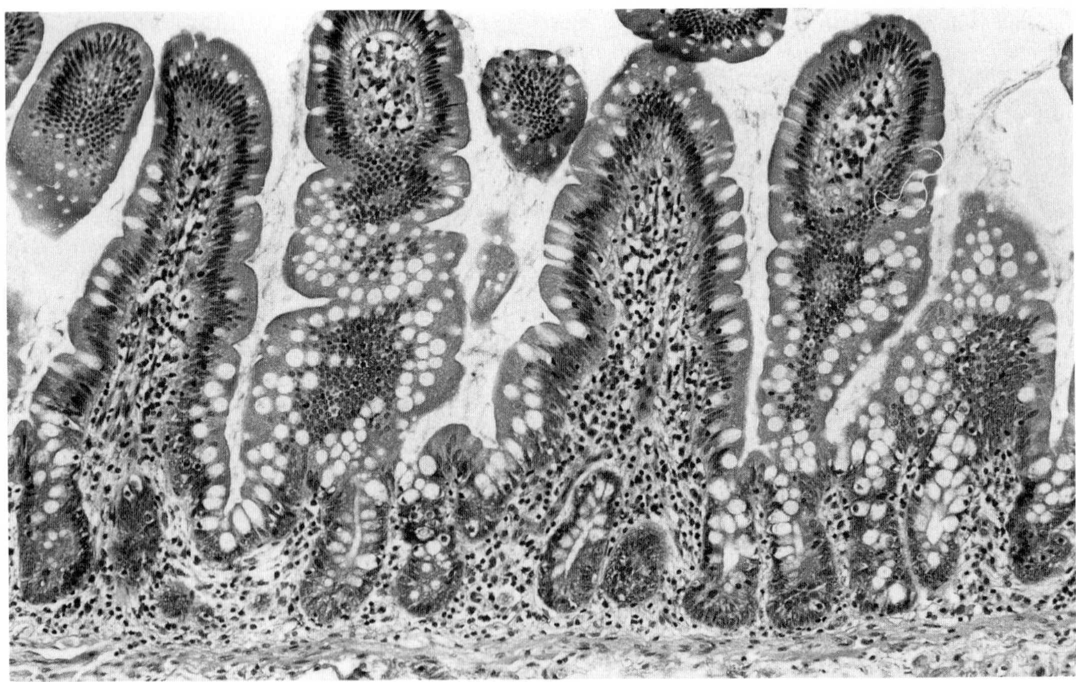

Fig. 8-1. Normal ileum. As in other parts of the small intestine, there are tall tapered villi and short crypts, but there are more goblet mucous cells on the villous surface. Noted are a moderate amount of inflammatory cells in the lamina propria and the muscularis mucosae (bottom) (× 140).

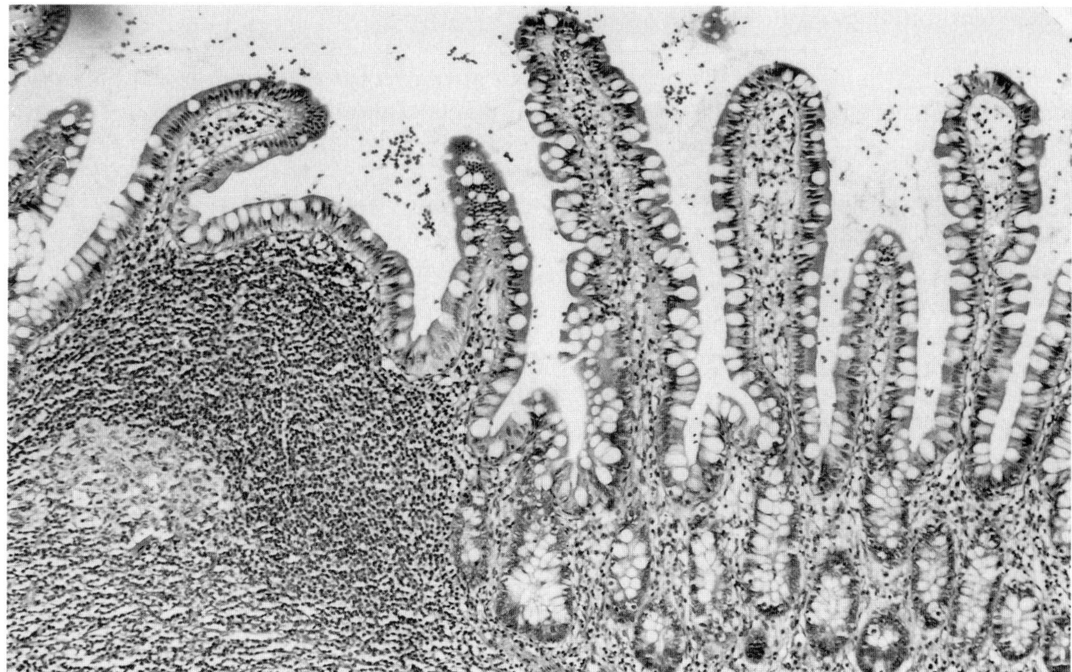

Fig. 8-2. Peyer's patch of the normal ileum. The edge is present on the left, comprised of large lymphoid nodules with prominent follicle centers. The villi overlying the lymphoid tissue are shortened and distorted (× 105).

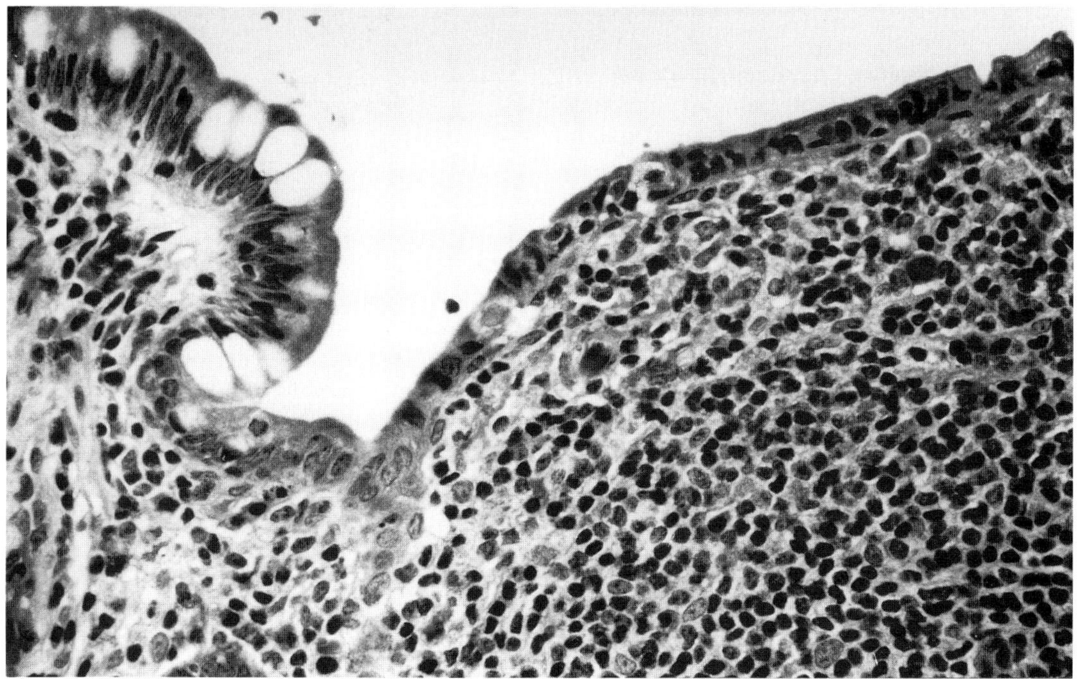

Fig. 8-3. Microfold (M) cells in the ileal mucosa. They are typically located overlying a lymhoid nodule, as seen at the right. The cells are cuboidal or flattened, lack cytoplasmic mucin, and are frequently admixed with inflammatory cells. Compare with absorptive and mucous cells at the left (× 425).

structures, and these must be discounted before considering significant disease. These are described below in the section on "Ileal Procedures" under "Idiopathic Inflammatory Bowel Disease".

Biopsy Material

Intact Ileum

Inspection of the distal 5 to 10 cm of the terminal ileum can be readily obtained at the time of colonoscopy.[10–12] It is ordinarily only done in cases in which the appearance or biopsies of the ileum might relate to presenting symptoms or to associated diseases of the colon. More common indications are patients with idiopathic inflammatory bowel disease, particularly Crohn's disease, and those with apparent masses or other gross lesions in the ileum as evidenced by radiographic examination. There are wide estimates that probably reflect differences in skills, with most suggesting that the ileum can be adequately examined in 75 percent of the cases. At present, the instruments do not permit evaluation of the more proximal portions of the intact ileum. More extensive endoscopic studies can be performed at the time of operation.[13]

Stomas and Anastomoses

Examination of the ileal mucosa is routinely considered following surgical procedures. These include the stoma and contiguous ileum at sites of ileostomy, both of the regular and Kock's continent types; the ileum proximal to ileo–colic anastomoses; and the ileal pouches, formed as reservoirs and connected with the anal musoca.[14–16]. There is now a strong tendency for performance of operations that conserve the anal sphincter, resulting in the need for much greater evaluations of ileal pouches. Following any of these surgical procedures there can develop an atrophy of the ileal mucosa, which does not reflect any clinical symptoms or recurrence of original disease. This is described further in the section on "Idiopathic Inflammatory Bowel Disease" below.

Special Studies

The large majority of diagnoses are rendered by routine H & E study. As in other parts of the gut, special chemical and immunocytochemical stains are employed to help in the identification of special disorders, principally in realizing the nature of particular tumors or of microorganisms (see Table 5-2).

DEVELOPMENTAL AND MECHANICAL DISORDERS

Cysts, stenoses, and diverticula can affect the ileum as in other parts of the small intestine; these are described in Chapters 6 and 7.

Meckel's Diverticulum

This is the most common diverticulum noted in the ileum, and it can be involved in many disease processes leading to significant clinical symptoms.[17, 18] Most commonly noted are areas of gastric heterotopia, which tissue can function, leading to localized ulceration in the adjacent mucosa.[19, 20] The acid-peptic effect is almost always in the small intestinal–type mucosa that is immediately adjacent to the gastric tissue, and this may be in the diverticulum itself or in the regular ileal mucosa if the entire diverticulum is transformed into gastric tissue. In these situations, there can develop an ulcer with bleeding, and this is one of the more common sources of acute bleeding or anemia in children. The diagnosis is typically obtained by scans. The diverticulum can also be the source of prominent inflammation, due either to localized perforation or to the intrusion of the diverticulum into the ileal lumen. The latter can lead to an intussusception and localized area of obstruction with secondary ischemic damage and inflammation. Meckel's diverticula can also be affected by endometriosis, various hamartomas, and tumors of all types.[21, 22] In all of these situations the diagnosis is largely suggested by the features of small bowel obstruction, and the particular cause is determined at surgical examination. Endoscopic examination and mucosal biopsy are not obtained.

Obstruction and Pseudo-Obstruction

The several conditions that lead to mechanical obstruction or to pseudo-obstruction involving the small intestine are detailed in Chapters 6 and 7[23] (cf. Table 7-3). Most commonly noted in the ileum are intussusceptions. These are more typically due to simple hypermotility in infants and young children, whereas there is almost always a mucosal tumor identified in adult patients. The lead points for the intussusception may be any mobile mucosal or submucosal nodule; more commonly seen are adenoma, lipoma, carcinoid tumor, and inflammatory fibroid polyp. Any of these tumors can affect the more distal parts of the ileum and the intussusception can extend into the cecal and ascending colon region. In such cases, they may be visualized by endoscopy but biopsies are not typically obtained. Rather, the diagnosis almost always requires surgical examination. This is discussed further in the section on "Tumors" below.

VASCULAR DISORDERS

Varices and Vascular Malformations

Ileal varices can develop in patients with portal hypertension, particularly if there have been surgical procedures in this area leading to localized fibrous peritoneal adhesions.[24] This is most often seen following operations in the right lower portion of the abdomen, particularly following appendectomy. All other forms of vascular malformations that occur in the small intestine can also involve the ileum[25] (see Table 4-4). Mucosal examination and sampling is not ordinarily obtained from these vascular lesions.

Ischemic Disorders

The ileum is commonly affected by ischemic disease, usually in conjunction with contiguous colonic involvement.[26] Major causes are reduced splancnic blood flow due to shock, thrombosis or embolism of large vessels, and vasculitis. These result in varying degrees of infarction, ranging from mucosal to transmural disease.[27–29] When the ischemic disease is concentrated in the terminal ileum, it can closely resemble and be confused with Crohn's disease.[30] Endoscopic examination and biopsy is usually not performed in the ileum with ischemic lesions but rather in the associated colonic areas; this topic is discussed in Chapter 9.

Localized areas of ischemic damage can occur in the ileum at sites of anastomosis and at stomas. These are readily appreciated by the characteristic features of hemorrhage and necrosis of the mucosa with minimal inflammatory reaction during the most acute stage. With time and reperfusion, there develops ulceration and marked neutrophilic reaction, simulating other forms of enteritis. As in other parts of the gut, the ischemic lesions when reversible tend to be more superficial. Biopsies may be obtained in such cases and they help to exclude other causes, particularly recurrent Crohn's disease.

Small Vessel Diseases

The ileal segment can be involved with amyloid, with atheromatous emboli, and with vasculitis, as in other parts of the small intestine.[31] All of these conditions favor localized areas of ischemic damage and hemorrhage. Mucosal biopsy of the ileum is ordinarily not obtained in these conditions. (See Chs. 6 and 7 for details.)

IDIOPATHIC INFLAMMATORY BOWEL DISEASE

General Uses and Features

Examination and biopsy of the ileal mucosa is most commonly performed in patients with ulcerative colitis and Crohn's disease.[32] Included are studies of the terminal ileum and of the mucosa proximal to anastomoses and stomas.[14, 33–35] The studies are done to identify or confirm an inflammatory condition, to distinguish idiopathic inflammatory bowel disease (IBD) from other forms of ileitis, and to recognize any complications (Table 8-1). The indications vary somewhat dependent on the particular site of the ileum, whether in its normal anatomical position or following a surgical procedure.

In studying mucosal biopsies certain features, such as depth of ulceration or inflammation and the presence of deep fissures, cannot be considered. Overall, biopsy of the ileal mucosa can demonstrate the presence of an ileitis, indicate whether the lesions are focal or diffuse, and show special features such as granulomas. Since ulcerative colitis does not involve the ileum, the biopsy examination is largely performed to identify Crohn's disease and to distinguish it from other potential causes of ileitis, particularly following surgical procedures. (The general features of ulcerative colitis and of Crohn's disease are provided in Chapter 9.)

Ulcerative Colitis

Of patients with extensive colitis who have involvement of the ascending colon or cecum, about 10 percent develop a dilation of the terminal ileum called *backwash ileitis.* This had been thought to be due to reflux of colonic inflammation into the ileum, but it may instead represent obstruction and stasis of the ileum. In either case, there develops a dilation of the terminal ileum, most prominent in the distal most 5 to 10 cm, and this can be appreciated by radiographic or gross endoscopic study. However, there are no gross ulcerations.

Biopsy Features

Mucosal biopsy may be performed to distinguish backwash ileitis from an ulcerating disorder of the ileum, particularly in making the distinction between ulcerative colitis and Crohn's disease. Biopsy in such cases reveals intact epithelium and a possible increase of mononuclear inflammatory cells and of lymphoid nodules in the mucosal area (Fig. 8-4). There is, however, no evidence of erosion or ulceration, or of a neutrophilic infiltrate. The appearance of ulcers with or without granulomas in the intact distal ileum would provide potential evidence that the patient does not have ulcerative colitis, and would lead to consideration of Crohn's disease and of other disorders that might be associated with ileitis, particularly infections and ischemic disease.

Following surgical treatment for ulcerative colitis, patients may have an ileostomy or an ileal pouch, and these are described in the section on "Ileal Procedures" below.

Crohn's Disease

Crohn's disease commonly involves the terminal ileum, either alone or in conjunction with disease that affects more of the small intestine or of the colon. The lesions in the ileum are usually diffuse and often, but not always, extend to the ileocecal valve. Accordingly, in most instances endoscopy and biopsy can be expected to detect ileal

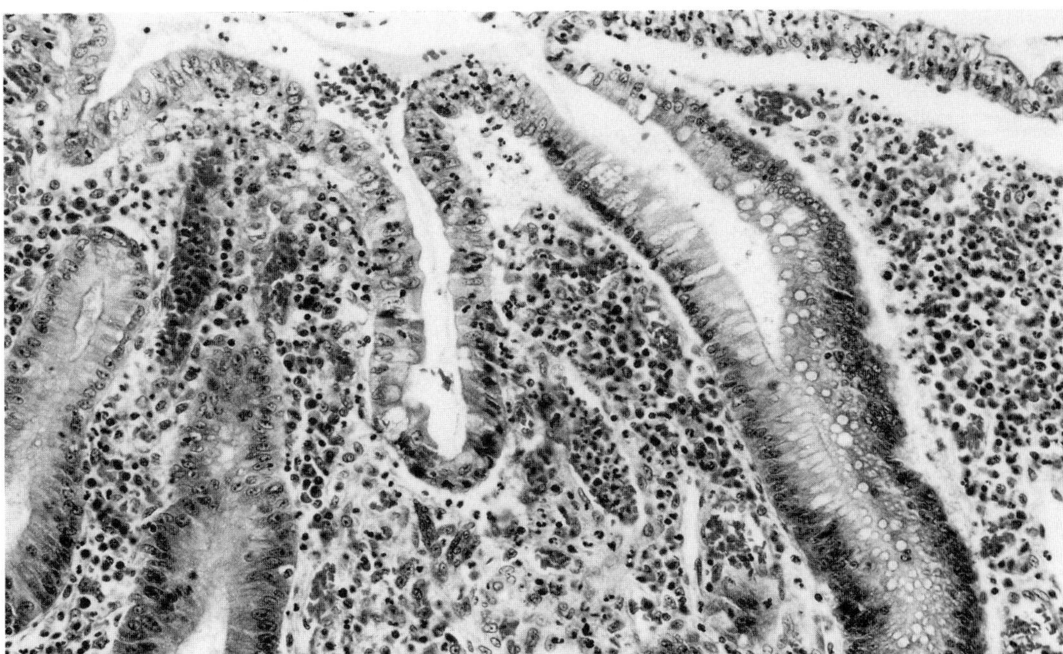

Fig. 8-4. Backwash ileitis in a case of ulcerative colitis. There is flattening of the villi, crypt hyperplasia, and marked increase of inflammatory cells, mainly mononuclear cell type, in the lamina propria. Some of the inflammation extends into the surface epithelium, but there is no ulceration (× 210).

involvement in Crohn's disease when present. Often, however, the appearance of small bowel disease is first appreciated by radiographic examination, and if apparently confined to this area, endoscopy may not be initially performed. Conversely, if the lesions are not certain, and, particularly, if there is associated colonic disease, endoscopy is commonly obtained, and it is in these cases where biopsy of the distal ileum can be particularly helpful in establishing the disease. If ulcerating disease is demonstrated in the ileum it serves to clinch that the patient does not have ulcerative colitis.

Biopsy Features

Mucosal biopsy can identify acute and chronic lesions as well as granulomas in about one-quarter of the cases (Table 8-2). The chronic effects include villous shortening or absence with commensurate crypt hyperplasia, increase of mononuclear inflammatory cells and of eosinophils in the lamina propria, presence of Paneth cells throughout the crypts rather than just in the basal portion, pyloric gland metaplasia, and hypertrophy of the mucosa in the form of an inflammatory pseudopolyp (Fig. 8-5). The pyloric

Table 8-2. Mucosal Biopsy Features in Crohn's Disease

Acute or active disease
Erosions and ulcers
Neutrophilic reaction
Glandular regeneration
Chronic disease
Villous shortening and crypt hyperplasia
Increase of mononuclear inflammatory cells and of eosinophils
Prominent lymphoid nodules
Presence of Paneth cells throughout crypt length
Pyloric gland metaplasia
Inflammatory pseudopolyps
Granulomas

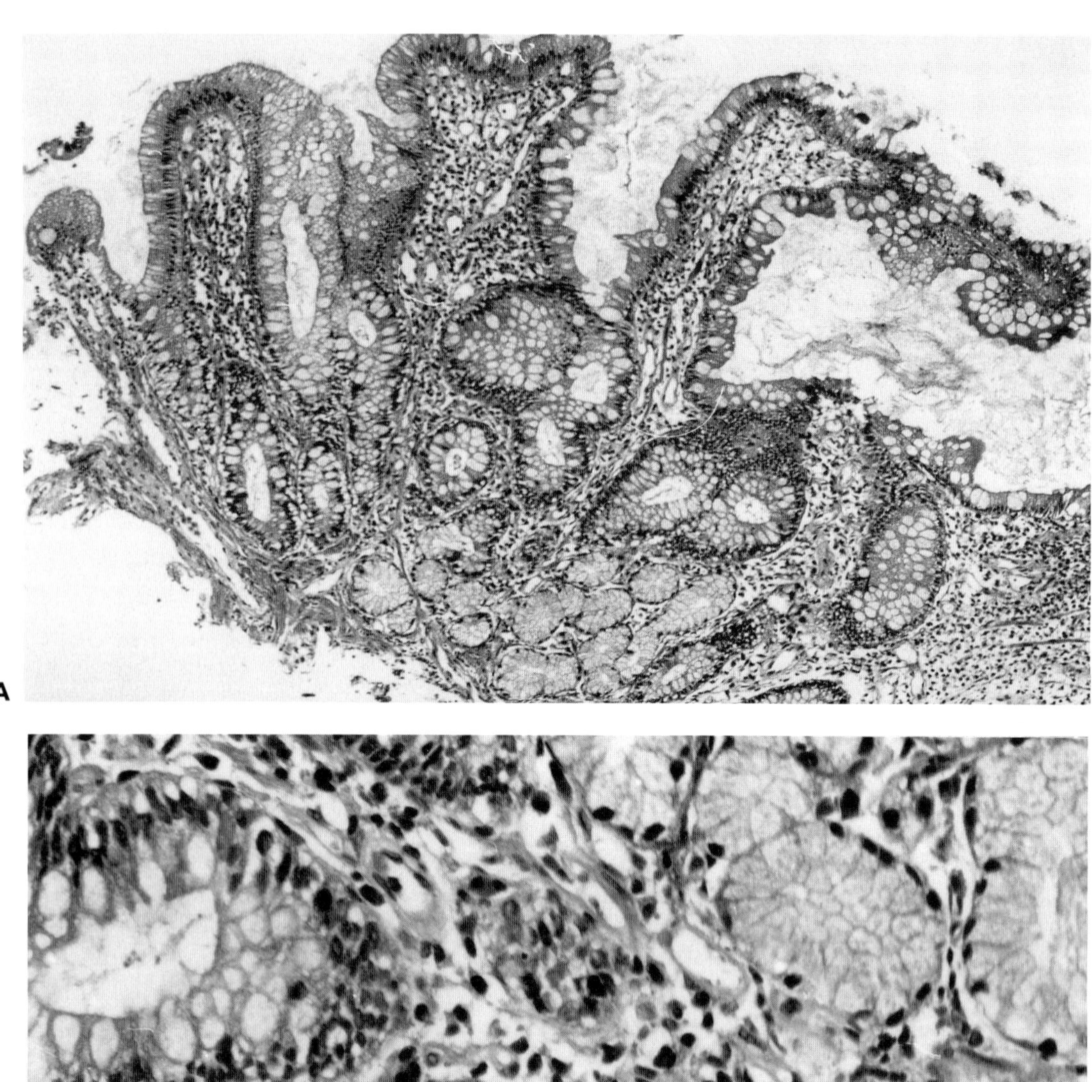

Fig. 8-5. Crohn's disease of the ileum. **(A)** Noted are focal villous loss (upper left) and pyloric gland metaplasia (bottom center), indicative of chronic disease (× 105). **(B)** Closer view of the pyloric glands on the right, showing cytoplasm filled with mucus and flattened nuclei. Compare with cross section of normal crypts at the left (× 425).

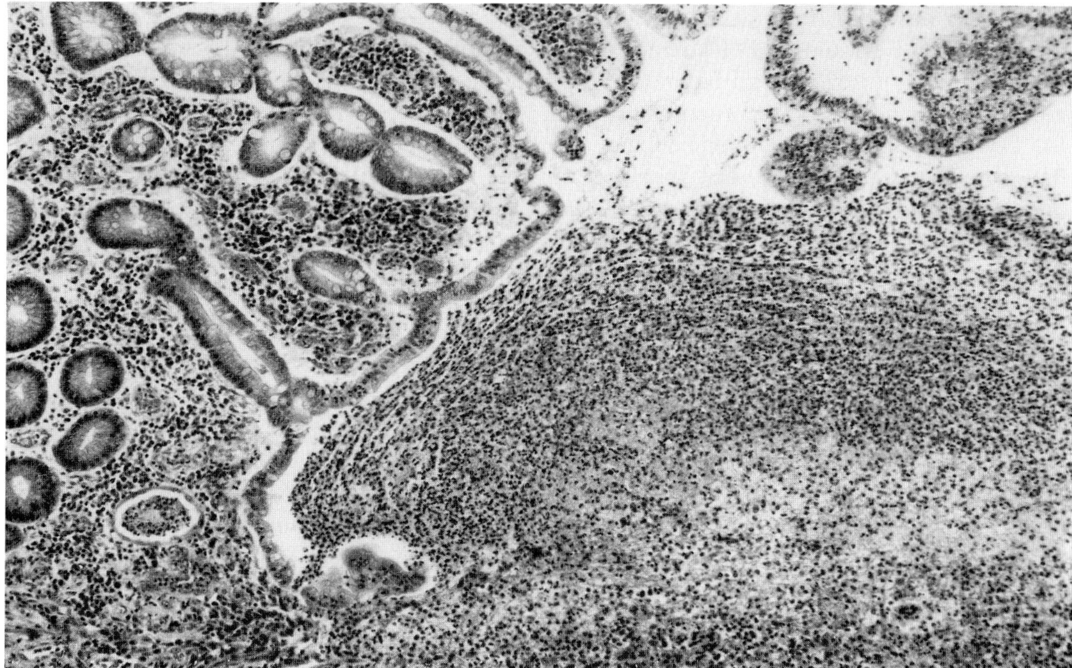

Fig. 8-6. Active Crohn's disease of the ileum. Noted is an ulcer with marked acute inflammation (right) (× 105). Contrast with Figure 8-4 of backwash ileitis in ulcerative colitis, which has inflammation but lacks ulceration.

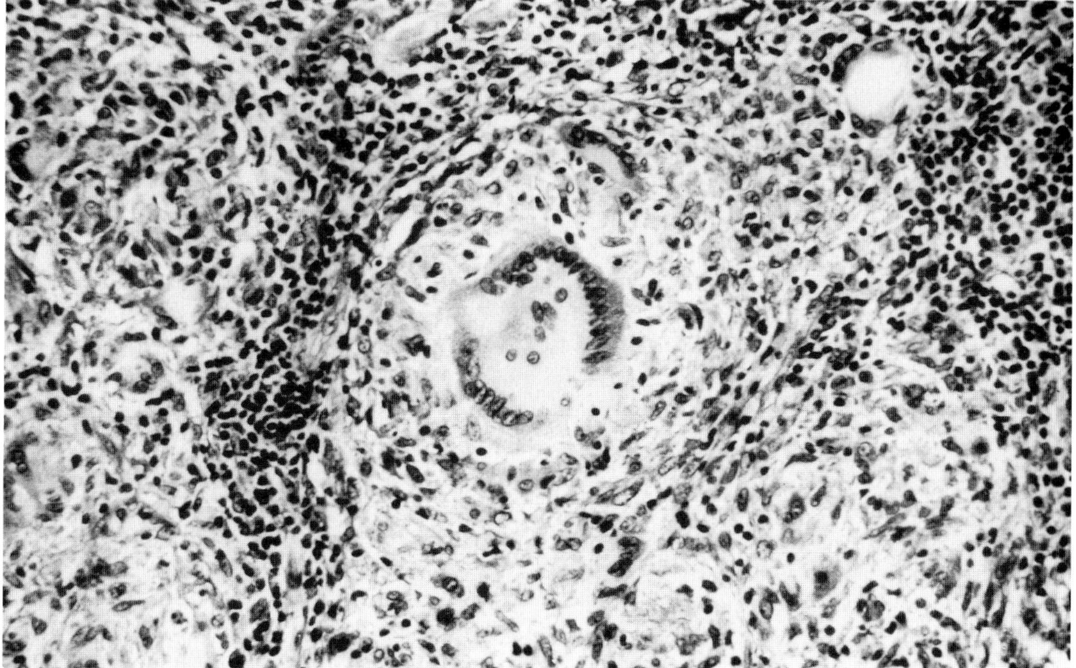

Fig. 8-7. Granuloma in Crohn's disease. There are several well formed granulomas with prominent giant cells and no necrosis.

metaplasia may be pronounced, resulting in grossly evident nodules.[36] Features of acute disease include erosions and ulcerations together with a neutrophilic reaction (Fig. 8-6). The granulomas are well formed and lack necrosis; they may be present in areas of inflammation or in mucosa that is not otherwise involved[37] (Fig. 8-7). In most cases the biopsy acts to identify that the patient has an ileitis, and thus is determining the extent of disease rather than the specific form. It should be remembered that the diagnosis of an inflammatory bowel disease that is idiopathic first requires the exclusion of other specific cases. The finding of ileitis serves to exclude an ulcerative colitis, but it may be necessary to rule out other conditions that can affect the terminal ileum. Included in the latter would be ischemic disease that shows hemorrhagic necrosis or superficial ulceration with marked neutrophilic reaction[30]; specific infections, such as tuberculosis, which reveal characteristic granulomas with necrosis or recognizible microorganisms[38]; and effects of drugs, which might show focal ulcers with acute inflammation only or fibrous strictures.[32]

Examination of the ileum following anastomosis or ileostomy is described in the section on "Ileal Procedures" below. In such cases, it is important to appreciate that the ileal mucosa can be affected by other factors such as mechanical, vascular, or infectious processes (Table 8-3). Accordingly, stringent criteria are needed to accept the presence of recurrent Crohn's disease.[34, 35, 39–41]

Ileal Procedures

Bypass

Bypass of either a portion of the ileum or the entire segment can occur as the result of a fistula or be constructed in the treatment of morbid obesity. The bypassed ileal segment undergoes a moderate atrophy, which may proceed to shortening and irregular folds.[42] Inflammatory changes and lesions of pneumatosis have also been described.[43, 44] Most of these alterations are reversed once continuity is reestablished.

Following ileostomy the distal ileal segment and colon can develop mild inflammatory changes, which simulate inflammatory bowel disease. These are usually more striking in the colon where they have been termed *diversion-related colitis.*[45–47] The lesions are largely eliminated by restoration of intestinal continuity. (This disorder is discussed in Ch. 9.)

Surgical bypass of diseased segments of small intestine, including the ileum, was formerly done for patients with Crohn's disease based on the assumption that resection should not be performed in such cases. The segments typically revealed continuing disease with progressive fibrosis and were particularly likely to develop carcinoma. This procedure is no longer employed.

Mucosal biopsy is ordinarily not obtained in the conditions with bypass of the ileum, except occasionally following an ileostomy. The features of diversion-related inflammation are ordinarily nonspecific, and the diagnosis requires the historical information and is assured by improvement after reunion of the intestinal segments.

Ileostomy

Included are the regular ileostomies and the Kock's continent type, which are performed for a large variety of conditions.[14–16] This may be needed for patients without idiopathic IBD who require extensive colonic resection and temporary or permanent ileostomy; it is most often done in patients with marked neuromuscular abnormalities, widespread ischemic disease, and intestinal polyposis syndromes. In the cases of idiopathic IBD, the ileostomy may be performed in patients with Crohn's disease who require a total colectomy, and also in those with ulcerative colitis in whom the ileo–anal pouch cannot be achieved.

The ileum at the site of the stoma is subject to prolapse, and this can result in foci of hemorrhagic necrosis as well as erosions with acute and chronic inflammation[48, 49] (Table 8-3). The frequency is increased in patients with the continent type of ileostomy.[50, 51] There is also marked fibrosis in the underlying tissue with scattered giant cells presumably reacting to suture material in most instances. All of these features are nonspecific and are not related to the original disorder. Also noted in a small percentage of cases is a condition termed *prestomal ileitis,* in which the ileum for several centimeters reveals scattered ulcers.[52] These are superficial and are unassociated with any sinus tracts or granulomas. Their exact cause is not known but the condition appears to be declining. It is usually associated with dilation of the ileal segment in contrast to recurrent Crohn's disease, which more often shows stenosis as well as deep sinus tracts away from the stroma.

Most often noted in the ileum proximal to the stoma is an atrophy of the mucosa that is probably present to some degree in all patients. This is characterized by shortening of the villi and reactive crypt hyperplasia, with the villous : crypt ratio approaching 2 : 1 or 1 : 1 in most cases (Fig. 8-8). Exceptionally, there may be complete absence of the villi in patchy areas together with even greater crypt hyperplasia. The Paneth cells are seen throughout the crypts and are not limited to their normal basal portion. There is no associated damage to the epithelium nor acute inflammation, which serves to rule out any active ileitis. Mucosal biopsies are commonly obtained to exclude any significant disorder, particularly recurrence of Crohn's disease that shows focal ulcers, pyloric metaplasia, and both acute and chronic inflammation.[53] Granulomas can also be found, but only if they were present in previously resected segments.

Table 8-3. Conditions in Ileal Stomas and Anastomoses

Nonspecific mucosal atrophy
Vascular, mechanical, and infectious lesions
Prestomal ileitis
Pouchitis: acute and chronic
Recurrent Crohn's disease
Tumors: adenoma and adenocarcinoma

Ileocolic Anastomosis

Ileocolic anastomosis is typically performed in patients who have segmental involvement of the ileum and colon, and is most often done for patients with Crohn's disease or with an ischemic disorder. Since the distal colon and rectum are always involved in ulcerative colitis, this procedure is ordinarily not available in that condition.

As with patients who have ileostomies, the ileum immediately adjacent to the anastomosis may reveal nonspecific effects of vascular damage or suture reaction and, occasionally, results of prolapse or wound infection. All of these show relatively nonspecific features. Otherwise, the ileal mucosa routinely shows evidence of atrophy that is usually mild (as described above in the section on "Ileostomy"). In both areas, biopsy evidence of Crohn's disease is in the form of deeper ulcers; certain features of chronic disease, such as marked increases of mononuclear inflammatory cells and eosinophils, and pyloric gland metaplasia; and the appearance of granulomas that are not related to crypt rupture or to foreign body material. In the assessment one should also consider other features that cannot be appreciated in the biopsy examination, such as strictures or deep sinus tracts; these can be realized by radiographic study.

In the various procedures of bypass, stoma, or anastomosis, it is important to distinguish the expected effects of the surgery in the form of mucosal atrophy without active ileitis; any changes that might be due to vascular, mechanical, or infectious complications; and the presence of true recurrence of

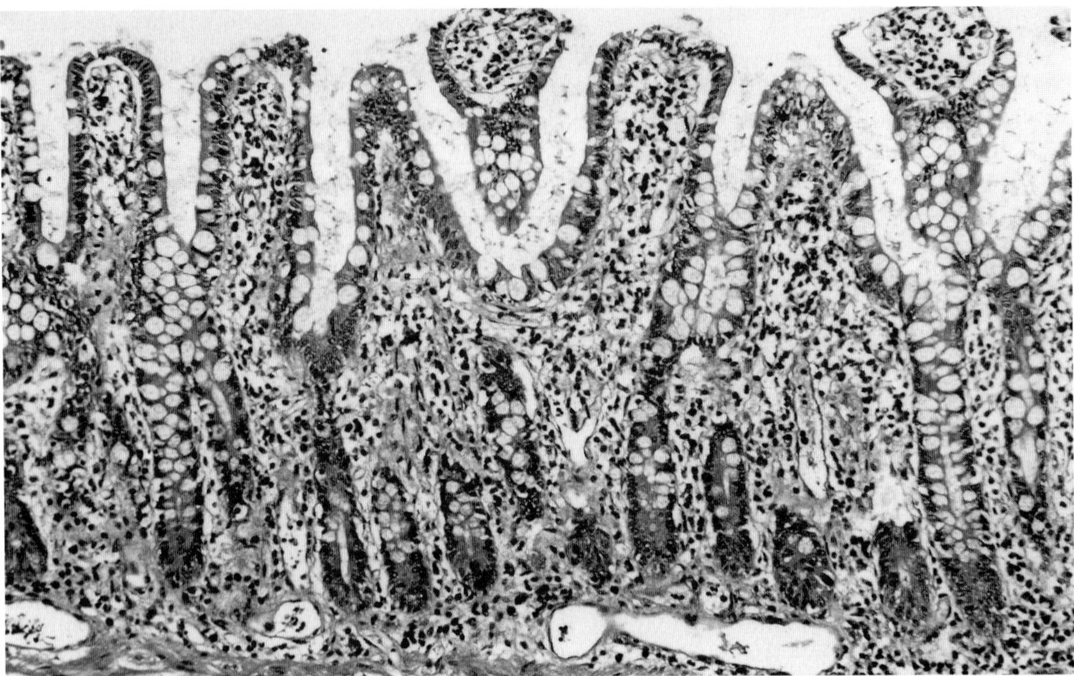

Fig. 8-8. Mucosal atrophy of the ileum, proximal to an ileostomy stoma. Noted are shortening of the villi and crypt hyperplasia, resulting in a ratio of 1:1. There is a slight increase of mononuclear inflammatory cells in the lamina propria but no ulceration or neutrophils (× 140).

disease, particularly of Crohn's disease (Table 8-3).

Ileal Pouch

The creation of an ileal reservoir, or pouch, and its anastomosis to the anal mucosa is now commonly performed for many patients who require a total colectomy and who otherwise have a normal ileum and anal sphincter. This is particularly suited for patients with familial colonic polyposis and for many patients with ulcerative colitis. Because of the potential for small bowel disease, it is not ordinarily performed in those with Crohn's disease. This has led to substantial improvement in patient well being since they have preserved anal function instead of an ileostomy.

About 20 to 25 percent of the patients with a well formed pouch develop inflammation in the form of focal areas of friability or ulceration.[54–58] Most of these respond to one or two trials of metronidazole or other antibiotics and eventually do very well. Biopsy in such cases shows relatively superficial erosion or ulceration with neutrophilic reaction, as well as the expected mild to moderate ileal mucosal atrophy (Fig. 8-9). There are no granulomas, and the features are entirely nonspecific. Exceptionally, biopsy reveals other changes in the form of hemorrhagic necrosis as evidence of prolapse or other ischemic damage, suture abscesses, or deeper ulcers due to fungal or other infections; these are present in only a few percent of the cases and must be distinguished from the usual case of nonspecific pouchitis.[32, 59]

A smaller group of the patients, probably on the order of 5 percent, develop persistent or recurrent ulcers or general inflammation of the pouch that requires more sustained therapy.[16, 60–62] Of importance, the pouch is

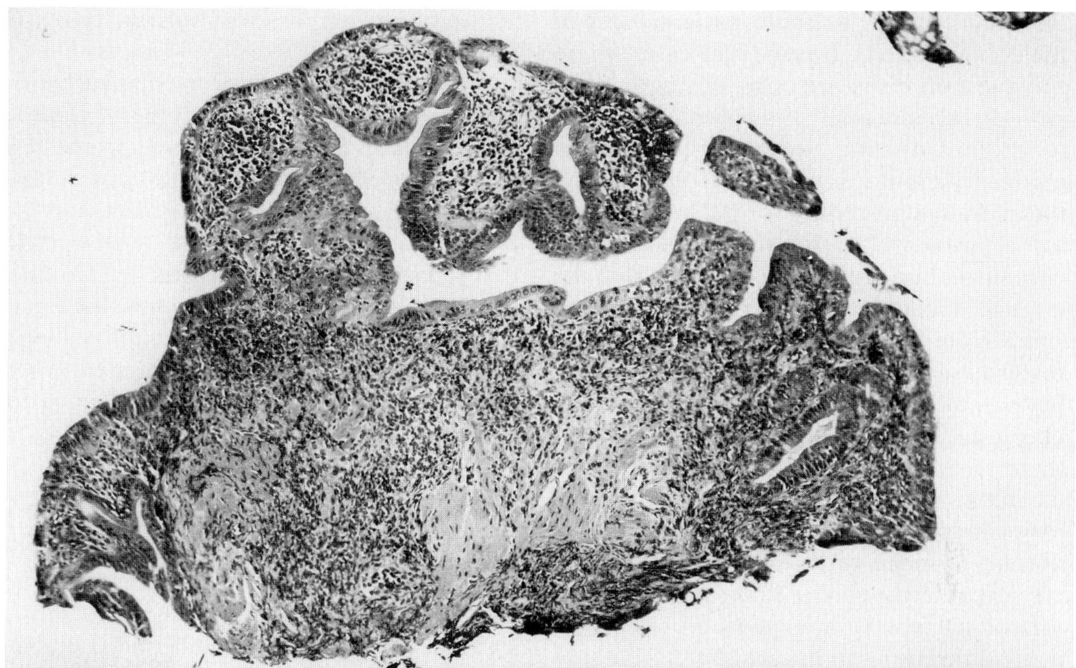

A

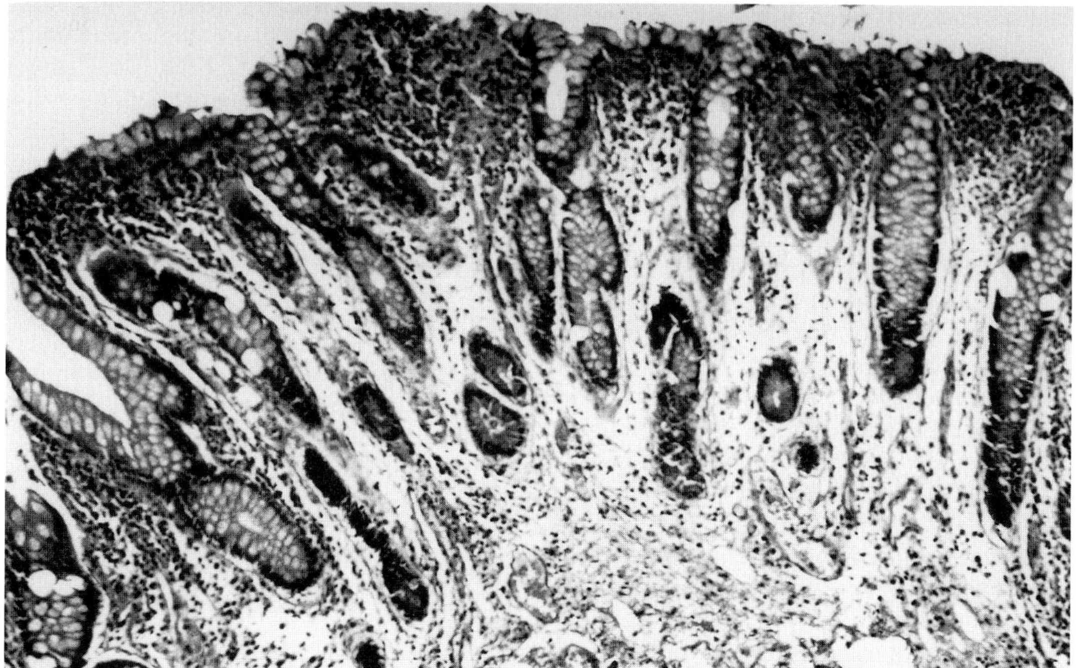

B

Fig. 8-9. Ileal pouchitis. **(A)** Noted in the active phase are shortening and irregularity of the villi, degeneration of the surface epithelial cells with loss of goblet mucous cells and crypts, and considerable inflammation in the stroma that extends into the muscularis mucosae appearing at the bottom. There are no granulomas (× 105). **(B)** Chronic effect of pouchitis. The mucosa is flat and resembles the colon, due to loss of villi and marked crypt hyperplasia. The crypts contain many mucous cells, and there is relatively little inflammation in the lamina propria (× 105).

typically retained in these patients despite the chronic effects. It is in these cases where the question often arises as to whether the patient truly had ulcerative colitis as opposed to Crohn's disease, because the lesions of chronicity are more common in those having the operative procedure for IBD rather than for polyposis.[63–66] The mere presence of chronic disease should not be a sign that the original diagnosis was in error. Rather, the slides from the initial resection should be reviewed and the diagnosis based on those findings alone. In patients with an incorrect diagnosis who develop Crohn's disease, there is a greater amount of, and deeper, ulceration with sinus tract formation and occasional appearance of granulomas. It is important to make certain that these changes are supported by similar findings in the original colonic resection. Equivalent cases with deep ulceration or granulomatous inflammation can be seen in patients with an original diagnosis of ulcerative colitis who then develop infections or foreign body reactions. To emphasize again, the diagnosis of ulcerative colitis or Crohn's disease should be primarily based on the original colonic resection and not simply on the findings of chronic ulceration in the pouch.

In the patients with chronic pouchitis, there develops a progressive atrophy of the ileal mucosa so that it resembles colonic tissue, in the form of total loss of villi and the presence only of crypts.[55, 60, 65] There is not only a histologic resemblance but also the adoption of other features of colonic mucosa, including the presence of sulfated mucins in the goblet cells and ultrastructural features supportive of colonic tissue. This is seen more commonly in the patients who had the pouch following resection for ulcerative colitis rather than those with polyposis. It has led to the supposition that the pouchitis in these cases may be a consequence of conversion of the mucosa to a colonic type, and a recurrence of the ulcerative colitis. This is not proven but there remains concern that over the long term the mucosa may be subject to other complications such as dysplasia and carcinoma.

Overall, biopsy in patients with ileal reservoir pouches are commonly done to identify a pouchitis and to exclude other specific vascular or infectious causes. In the more severe and chronic cases, it may be necessary to review the original resection to be certain that it was ulcerative colitis and not Crohn's disease. Long-term changes of the ileal mucosa indicate a conversion to colonic-type tissue, and further studies are needed to see whether additional complications, such as neoplasia, will develop in the pouches.

Complications

As noted above, the ileal mucosa at the site of a stoma or anastomosis often shows signs of atrophy. This is usually mild but may be more pronounced, particularly in cases with chronic pouchitis. Biopsies are occasionally done to identify or confirm an ileitis, and it is important to rule out other causes due to vascular, mechanical, or infectious processes.

Enteritis Cystica Profunda

Patients with severe Crohn's disease and deep ulcerations can develop the misplacement of epithelium into the wall.[67–69] There results a suspicious mass with extension into the wall that resembles invasive carcinoma, but biopsies reveal the inflammatory nature of the epithelium and the lack of any dysplastic change involving the nuclei. These lesions can occur in any part of the small bowel including the ileum. They are most often identified in surgical specimens.

Dysplasia and Carcinoma

Patients with Crohn's disease are at an increased risk for the development of invasive adenocarcinomas.[70–73] This is most often detected in the colon but is also noted in the small intestine and, apparently more likely, in bypass segments.[74, 75] The lesions typically present with strictures or complex fissures and the diagnosis is readily established by histologic examination that reveals the dysplastic epithelium and the invasive tumor.[76–81] Screening of the ileal or other small intestinal mucosa is not done because of the difficulty in surveying such a large area, and because of the low yield. Cases of longstanding chronic colitis are more apt to have screening procedures, and these are discussed in Chapter 10.[82, 83] Other tumors involving the small bowel have been noted in patients with Crohn's disease, including endocrine lesions and malignant lymphoma. Again, these are not typically detected by mucosal biopsy of the ileum.

CHEMICAL AND RADIATION INJURY

Chemotherapy and Drug Effects

The changes in the ileum due to chemotherapy and the many drugs currently employed are the same as those in the rest of the small intestine, and these are primarily described in Chapters 6 and 7[84–89] (see Table 7-4). It has been suggested that some of the strictures and muscular diaphragms that occur in patients taking nonsteroidal anti-inflammatory drugs (NSAIDs) are more often seen in the ileum.[90–93] The diagnosis is still largely by radiographic examination and study of surgical specimens, and these are not detected by mucosal biopsy. Reactions to gold salts, typically used in the treatment of chronic rheumatoid arthritis, more often affect the ileum as well as the colon.[94, 95] These cases can show injury ranging from focal small ulcers to more extensive enteritis and colitis that resemble ischemic disease. The diagnosis is mainly made by the colonic findings together with the historical information.

Radiation Effects and Injury

The changes in the ileum due to radiation are generally the same as those seen in the rest of the small intestine,[96–100] and they are covered in Chapters 6 and 7 (see Table 7-5). In brief, the acute changes include ulceration and marked edema; and the chronic effects reveal fibrosis with stricture, vascular dilation and thickenings; and atypical-appearing mesenchymal cells. Because of the natural narrowing of the ileocecal area, the effects from radiation are sometimes maximal in this region, and lead to stricture. Exceptionally, there can be sinus tracts and perforations.

INFECTIONS

General Features

Most of the infections occurring in the duodenum and jejunum also involve the ileum, but mucosal biopsy of this area is rarely used in their detection (see Chs. 6 and 7, and Table 6-5 for details). The characteristics of many of the microorganisms are described more fully in Chapter 2.

Some of the infections are more florid or concentrated in the ileum, either alone or in conjunction with colonic disease (Table 8-4). These are mentioned in this section.

Viral Infections

Infections due to adenovirus appear to be more common in the ileum and are associated with a increased likelihood of intussus-

Table 8-4. Infections of the Ileum[a]

Adenovirus
Necrotizing enterocolitis
Neutropenic enterocolitis
Pseudomembranous enterocolitis
Yersinial infection
Tuberculosis
Anisakiasis

[a] List of infectious disorders that are more commonly seen in the ileum than in other parts of the small intestine. They are often associated with colonic involvement.

ception.[101] In some cases there is the formation of an inflammatory or fibroblastic polyp that serves as a lead point, but this is not always present. Patients may present with intestinal obstruction either at the small intestinal or proximal colonic level. The diagnosis is usually dependent on study of the operative specimen and not typically made by mucosal biopsy.

The reader should refer to Chapters 6 and 7 for details related to the common forms of viral enteritis, HIV infection, and opportunistic lesions of the small intestine. All of these can involve the ileum and are exceptionally sampled by mucosal biopsy at time of colonoscopy.[102]

Bacterial Infections

Bacterial infections are generally described in Chapters 6 and 7 (see Table 7-6). There are certain bacterial infections that more commonly involve the ileum, usually together with disease of the right side of the colon. These include necrotizing enterocolitis, which is seen typically in infants and is thought to be due to a combination of poor blood flow and secondary infection[103, 104]; neutropenic enterocolitis due to highly destructive bacteria such as *Clostridium septicum,* in which there is extensive ischemic necrosis and many bacteria but minimal inflammatory reaction[105, 106]; and pseudomembranes enterocolitis due to *C. difficile,* which presents with inflammatory membranes and is most characteristic in the colon.[107, 108] Although the ileum can be involved in most of these disorders, the mucosal biopsies are almost always from the colon only (see Ch. 9).

Similarly, infections due to *Yersinia,* to *M. tuberculosis,* and to *Actinomyces* are more typical for this area. The yersinial infections are associated with marked lymphoid hyperplasia and with microabscesses,[109, 110] whereas tuberculosis in this region typically reveals prominent granulomas with necrosis[38, 111] (see Chs. 6 and 7 for more details). Biopsy of the ileum is rarely obtained but can be helpful because of the characteristic histologic features.[112]

Fungal and Parasitic Infections

These are mostly a consequence of fungal and other opportunistic infections and are described in the other chapters.[113] Anisakiasis due to the ingestion of raw fish typically involves the ileocecal area and can be associated with a transmural inflammatory disorder characterized by sinus tract formation that mimics Crohn's disease.[114–116] The diagnosis is established by identifying the worm fragments in the mural abscesses. Ileal mucosal biopsy can occasionally reveal the various fungal and parasitic infections with the recognizible organisms. (The reader should refer to Ch. 2 for descriptions of the organisms and Chs. 6 and 7 for the effects on the small intestine.)

TUMORS

The ileum can be involved by all of the tumors affecting the small intestine, as portrayed in Chapters 6 and 7[117–119] (see Table 6-7). It is uncommon for these to be observed at endoscopy of the intact ileum. More often, they are detected in ileal segments proximal to stomas and anastomoses.

Mucosal Polyps

Non-Neoplastic Polyps

Inflammatory pseudopolyps are commonly seen in cases of chronic enteritis, including Crohn's and ischemic diseases[120, 121]

(Table 8-5). Juvenile and hamartomatous polyps also occur, either isolated or as part of a polyposis syndrome[122–128] (see Chs. 6 and 7 for further details). More frequently observed in the ileum are nodules of lymphoid hyperplasia, related to the increased amount of this tissue in the area.[129, 130] These typically present as nodules, and mucosal biopsies reveal well-formed lymphoid tissue with enlarged lymphoid follicles. They are possibly increased in patients with the adenomatous polyposis syndromes.[131, 132]

Often noted is a prominence of the ileocecal valve, which is due to an exaggerated amount of adipose tissue and has been termed *lipomatosis* or *lipohyperplasia.*[133] Biopsy reveals the mature adipose tissue with relatively atrophic mucosa overlying it (Fig. 8-10). Also more common in this area is the inflammatory fibroid polyp, which is thought to represent a fibrous or muscular tumor that undergoes extensive inflammation[134–136] (Fig. 8-11). This typically projects into the lumen and may be the source of an intussusception, extending through the ileocecal valve into the right colon. A variant of this tumor with more evident muscular elements, termed an *inflammatory myoglandular tumor,* can also present with intussusception.[137] The diagnosis is usually obtained by the obstruction and examination of the mass, and biopsy is not ordinarily involved.

Adenomas

Adenomas are typically found in patients with familial adenomatous polyposis coli[138, 139] (Fig. 8-12). Most of the lesions were formerly seen in ileostomy stomas, before the alternative use of ileoanal anastomosis.[140–142] Both pure adenomas and those associated with invasive adenocarcinoma are now appearing in the ileal pouches, and some screening system will be needed to detect them and to prevent the development of carcinoma.

Table 8-5. Mucosal Polyps of the Ileum

Inflammatory pseudopolyp
Hamartomatous polyps
Lymphoid hyperplasia
Lipomatosis of ileocecal valve
Inflammatory fibroid polyp
Inflammatory myoglandular polyp
Adenoma

Adenocarcinoma

Primary adenocarcinomas of the jejunum and ileum are generally rare and present as advanced tumors with obstruction[143–146] (see Fig. 6-25A). They are increased in patients with celiac disease,[147, 148] with immunodeficiency conditions,[149] and particularly in cases of Crohn's disease.[70–75] Since most of the latter lesions involve the ileum, the related cancers are also in this area. These typically present with the delayed finding of a stricture. They are largely not accessible by routine endoscopic examination of the distal ileum.

An increased frequency of adenocarcinoma is also seen in ileostomy segments and in ileal pouches[150–161]; included are all forms of operations and subsets of patients. The tumors have been noted in patients who had colectomy for polyposis, for ulcerative colitis, and for Crohn's disease. It is probable that most of the cancers are preceded by benign adenomas or dysplastic lesions and that a screening program would be beneficial. Endoscopy and mucosal biopsy could be readily obtained from the ileum at sites of stomas and pouches, to look for benign neoplastic epithelium.

Rarely noted in the ileum are variants of carcinoma, including adenosquamous carcinoma, pure squamous cell carcinoma, and carcinosarcoma[162–164] (see Figs. 3-10 and 3-17). As with the other malignant tumors, these are ordinarily not detected by mucosal biopsy of the ileum.

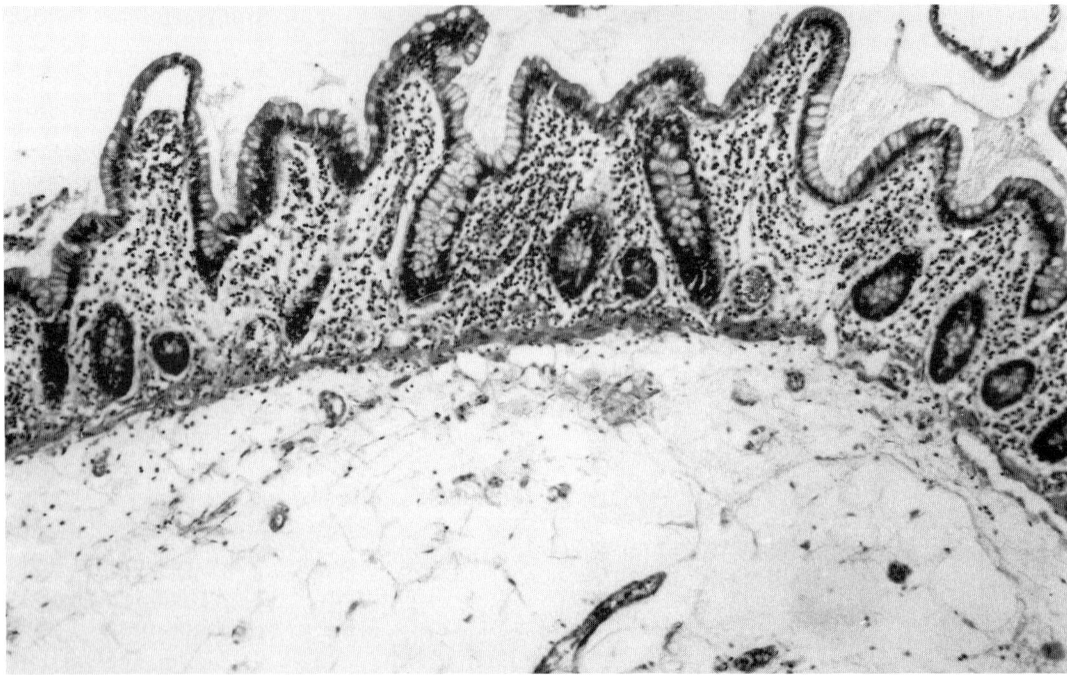

Fig. 8-10. Lipomatosis of the ileocecal valve. Appearing at the bottom is abundant and mature adipose tissue. The overlying mucosa appearing at the the top is compressed and atrophic (× 105).

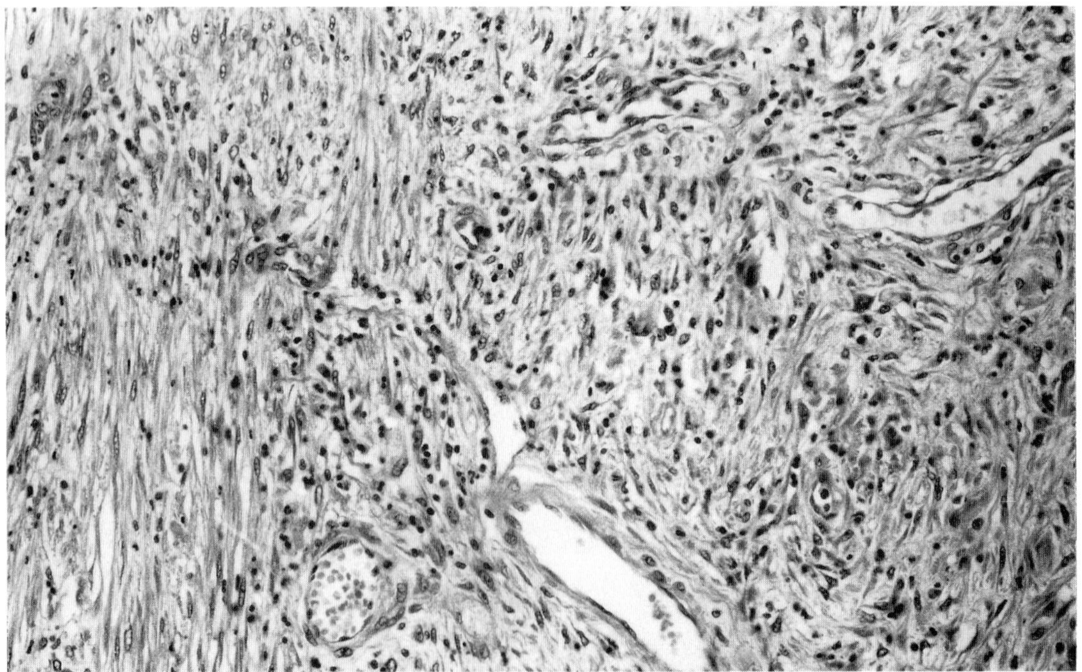

Fig. 8-11. Inflammatory fibroid polyp. The tumor is mainly comprised of spindle cells that lack atypism, edema, and scattered inflammatory cells including many eosinophils (× 210).

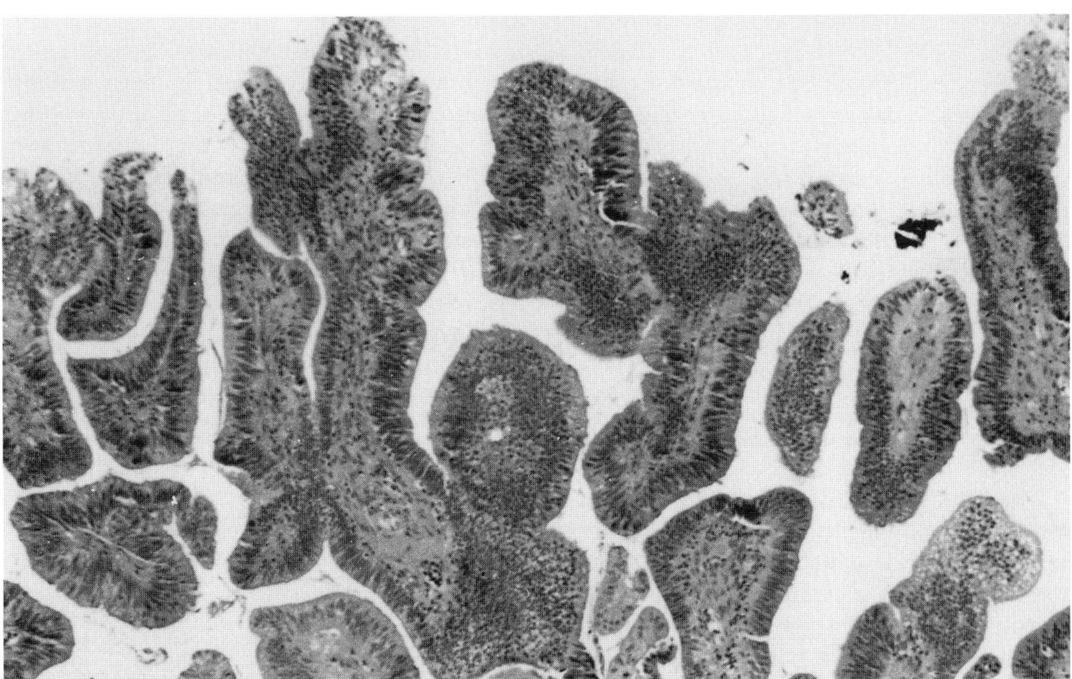

Fig. 8-12. Adenoma of the ileum, in a case of Gardner's syndrome. Villous fronds of the tumor are seen, covered by dysplastic epithelium (× 105).

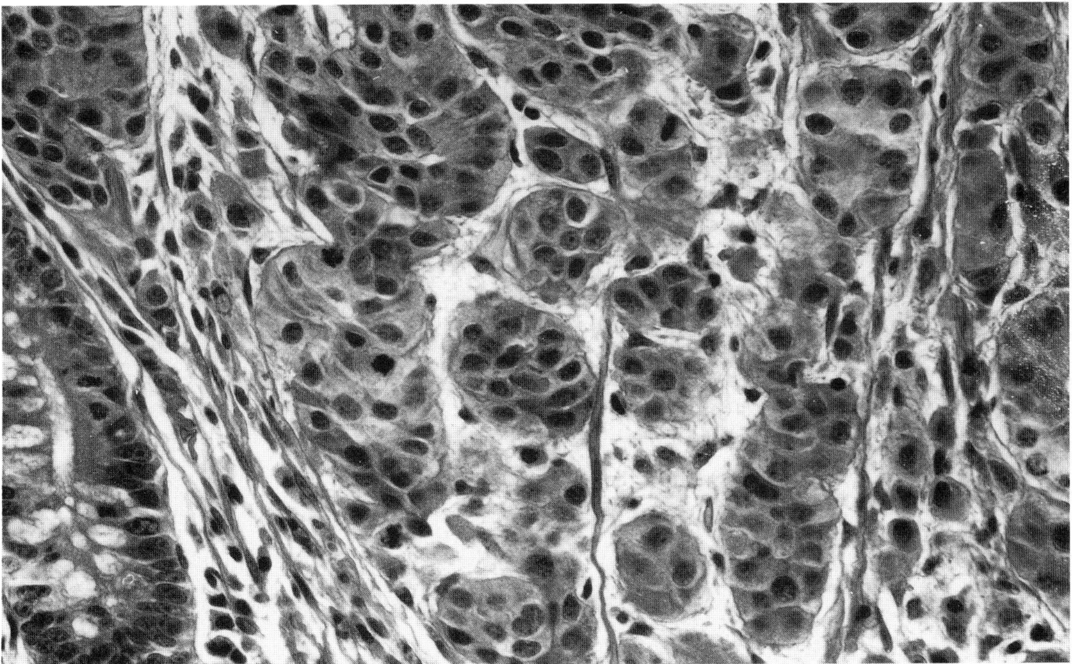

Fig. 8-13. Carcinoid tumor of the ileum. Noted are cords of highly regular cells with central nuclei and prominent cytoplasm. A fragment of a normal crypt appears at the bottom left (× 425).

Endocrine Tumors

The distal ileum is one of the more common sites for the presence of carcinoid tumors.[165, 166] These are located at the base of the mucosa and extend into the submucosa; they appear as flat polyps or plaques and may rarely be detected by endoscopy and mucosal biopsy (Fig. 8-13). As in other parts of the small intestine, there can also be mixtures of carcinomas and endocrine cells and less differentiated malignant forms.[167–169]

Lymphoid Tumors

The benign lymphoid polyps are described above in the section on "Mucosal Polyps".[129–132] Malignant lymphomas occur in the ileum, and it is estimated that this might be the most common site in patients without any preexisting factor, such as celiac disease or other chronic enteritis.[170–172] In the latter the lesions are more common in the duodenum and jejunum. As in other parts of the small intestine, most of the lymphomas are of the non-Hodgkin's B-cell type (Fig. 8-14). They are typically found by radiographic examination and the diagnosis is provided by examination of surgical specimens. To date, endoscopy and biopsy has only rarely been used to detect ileal lymphomas[173] (see Chs. 6 and 7 for more details).

Mesenchymal, Secondary, and Metastatic Tumors

Mesenchymal, secondary, and metastatic tumors are generally the same in the ileum as in other areas of the small intestine.[174] See Chapters 6 and 7 for details.

MISCELLANEOUS CONDITIONS

Malabsorptive Disorders

Many of the conditions affecting the small intestine that are associated with malabsorption or a protein-losing syndrome can also affect the ileum.[175] In celiac disease the involvement in this location is thought to be a sign of late and advanced disease. In many other disorders, such as allergic enteritis, the full extent of ileal involvement is not known because of inadequate sampling.

There are two major substances that are maximally absorbed in the ileal region: vitamin B_{12} and bile salts. Accordingly, loss of ileum by disease or surgery can result in megaloblastic anemia and in maldigestion of fats. The principal disorder in this area that can be associated with these deficiencies is Crohn's disease. It is estimated that patients who have lost or bypassed the distal 100 cm of ileum eventually develop fat malabsorption. In addition, the nonabsorbed bile salts pass into the colon where they are irritable and productive of diarrhea.

Documentation of ileal involvement is typically obtained by radiographic and functional studies. Biopsy is ordinarily not obtained.

Granulomatous Diseases

Aside from Crohn's disease, the causes of granulomas in the ileum are few, and include infections and foreign body reactions.[176, 177] This subject is covered in Chapters 6 and 7.

Depositions

The ileum can be involved with the same deposits that occur in other parts of the small bowel. These include amyloid, xanthomas, and the many storage diseases,[177–179] but they are not accessed by ileal mucosal biopsy. Exogenous pigments are commonly noted in the lymphoid tissue of the Peyer's patches, mainly consisting of carbon and other ingested elements.[180, 181]

Reactive Arthritis

Patients with nonspecific arthritis, including those with the spondylitis form, often have focal lesions of the ileal mucosa.[182, 183]

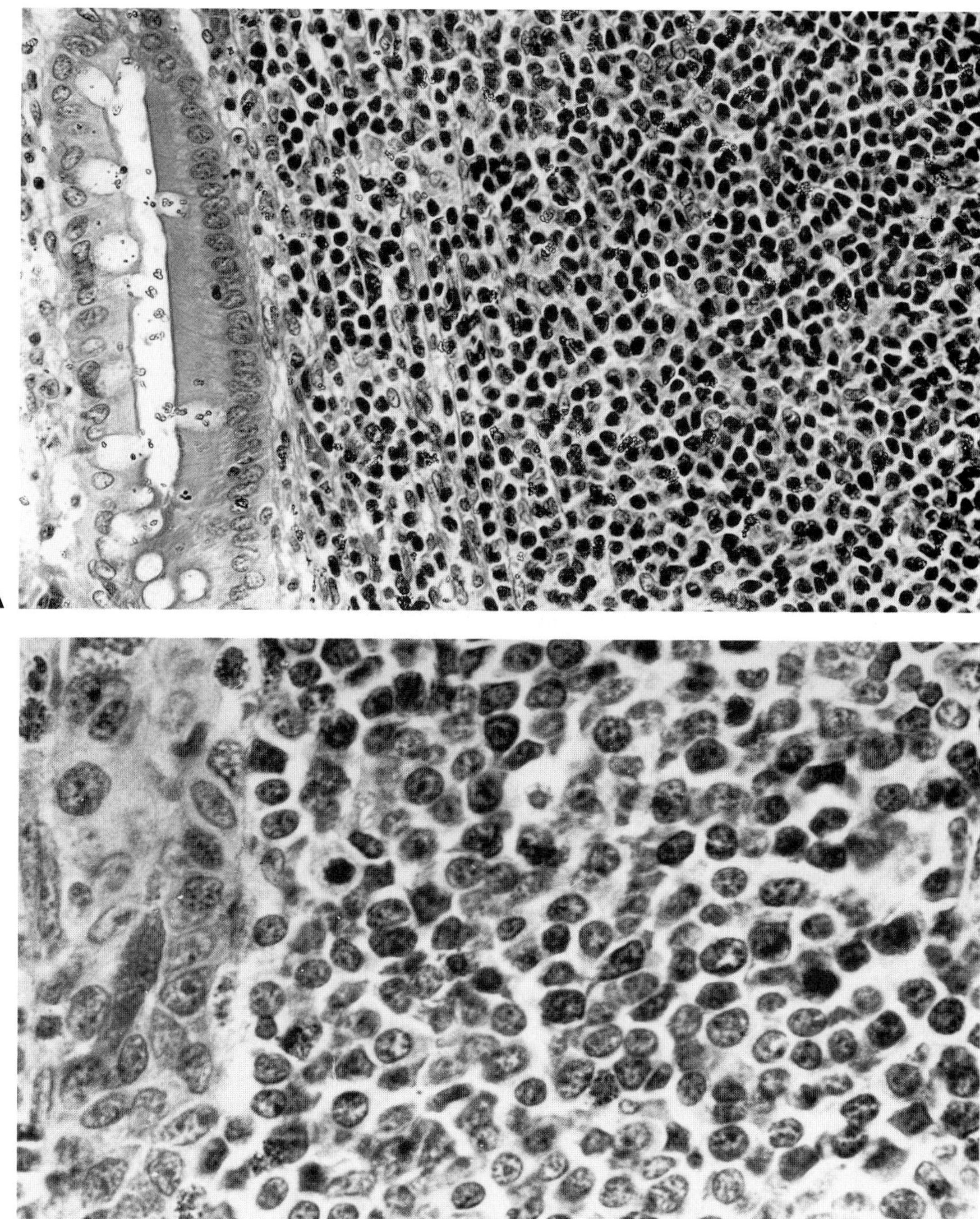

Fig. 8-14. Malignant lymphoma of the ileum. **(A)** There is a diffuse infiltrate of enlarged lymphoid cells in the mucosa. Lacking are mature plasma cells. An unaffected crypt appears at the left (× 425). **(B)** Closer view, showing the enlarged and slightly irregular and hyperchromatic nuclei of the lymphoma cells. A crypt appears at the left (× 680).

Endoscopic studies have revealed superficial ulcers with acute and chronic inflammation and no granulomas. The mucosal biopsy features are entirely nonspecific, and the lesions are not directly related to any drug therapy. Although their distribution is similar to Crohn's disease, the more distinctive chronic changes are lacking, and most of the patients are asymptomatic. Despite the possible association, endoscopy of the ileum is ordinarily not performed in these cases unless the patient has prominent symptoms.

Immunologic Disorders

It is not known whether the principal allergic conditions, such as those involving the upper gut or the colorectum, affect the ileum.[184] Whatever the case, this area is not sampled. The condition of eosinophilic gastroenteritis can occur in the ileum but this is usually the nonallergic, mural form in which there are no mucosal lesions.

The reader should refer to Chapters 6 and 7 for details regarding the major immunodeficiency disorders and for graft-versus-host reactions[185, 186] (see Table 6-7). In limited studies involving small bowel transplants, biopsies are mostly taken from the ileum at the site of an ileostomy[187–189] (Fig. 8-15). The features observed include mononuclear infiltrates as a sign of acute and chronic rejection; these are initially focal and concentrated in the crypt epithelial area, but later extend to involve large parts of the mucosa and submucosa. The hyperacute cases are due to vascular compromise and reveal extensive hemorrhagic necrosis.

Tumorlike Conditions

Endometriosis typically affects the distal part of the small intestine, but usually the peritoneal surface and muscularis propria.[190, 191] Involvement of the mucosa is rare and biopsies are not obtained. As noted above, pneumatosis intestinalis can be seen in any part of the intestine and appears to be more common in bypassed segments[44] (Fig. 8-16). Endoscopic survey and biopsy are rarely obtained in these conditions.

Other Inflammatory Disorders

The reader should refer to Chapters 6 and 7 for the changes seen in metabolic disorders, for the lesions associated with skin diseases, and for the effects of soft tissue abnormalities. The changes noted in bypass of the ileum and in the condition of enteritis cystica profunda are described in the section above on "Idiopathic Inflammatory Bowel Disease".

Chronic Jejuno-Ileitis

This nonspecific condition was described to portray patients with multiple ulcers of unknown etiology involving the jejunum and ileum, which did not correspond to ordinary Crohn's disease.[192, 193] It was later realized that most if not all of these cases probably represented complications of celiac disease associated with the refractory form, the development of ulcers, and the later formation of lymphomas. This is no longer considered to be an accepted entity.

Behçet's Disease

Behçet's disease is an uncommon condition that is characterized by acute ulcers of the skin, oral cavity, and intestinal tract.[194, 195] Multiple lesions may occur in the distal ileum and colon and resemble Crohn's disease. Ileal mucosal biopsies are rarely obtained and reveal the ulcers together with nonspecific inflammation and the absence of granulomas (Fig. 8-17). The diagnosis depends on noting the full distribution of le-

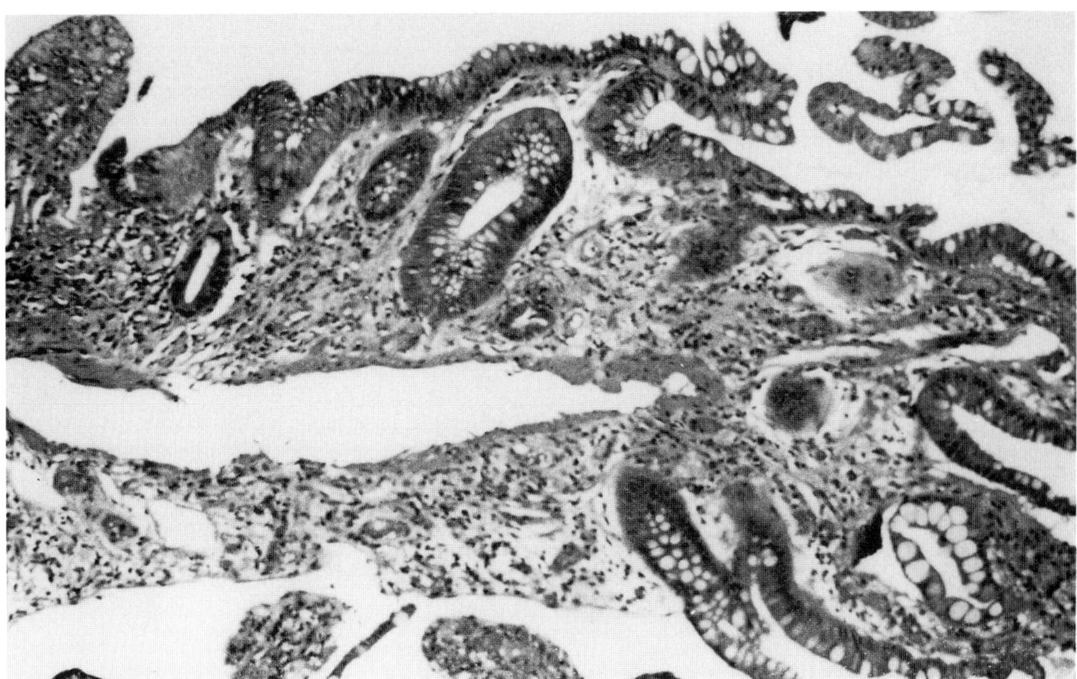

Fig. 8-15. Ileal mucosa in a patient with a small bowel transplant. The biopsy was taken two months after the transplant. There is almost total loss of the villi and a reactive crypt hyperplasia.

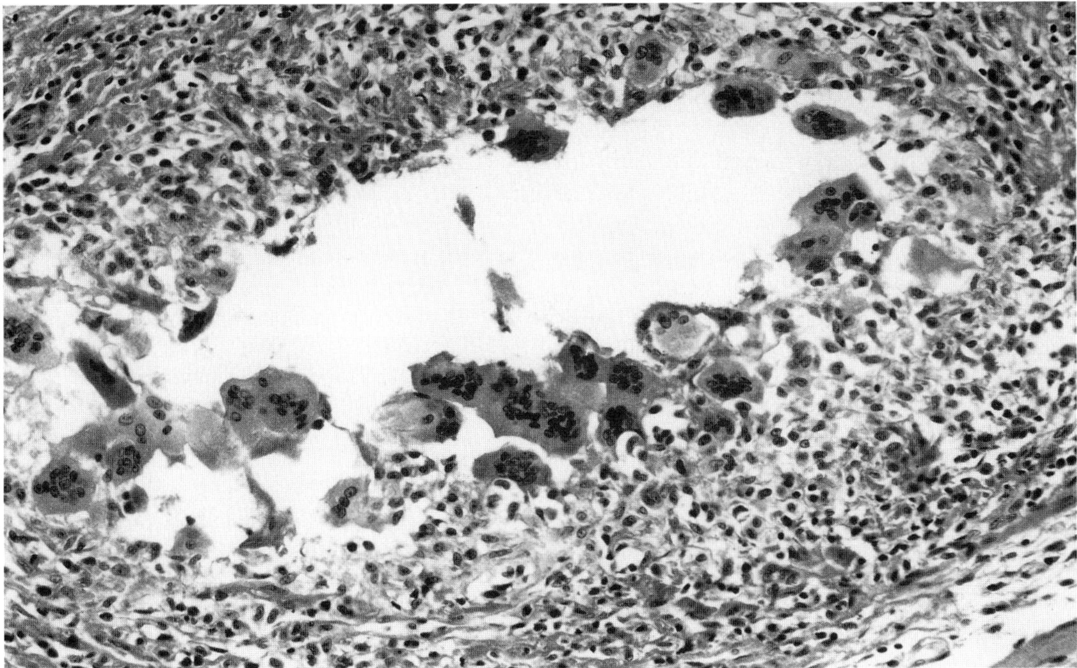

Fig. 8-16. Pneumatosis in the ileum. There is a gas-filled space surrounded by many multinucleated macrophages and other inflammatory cells (× 210).

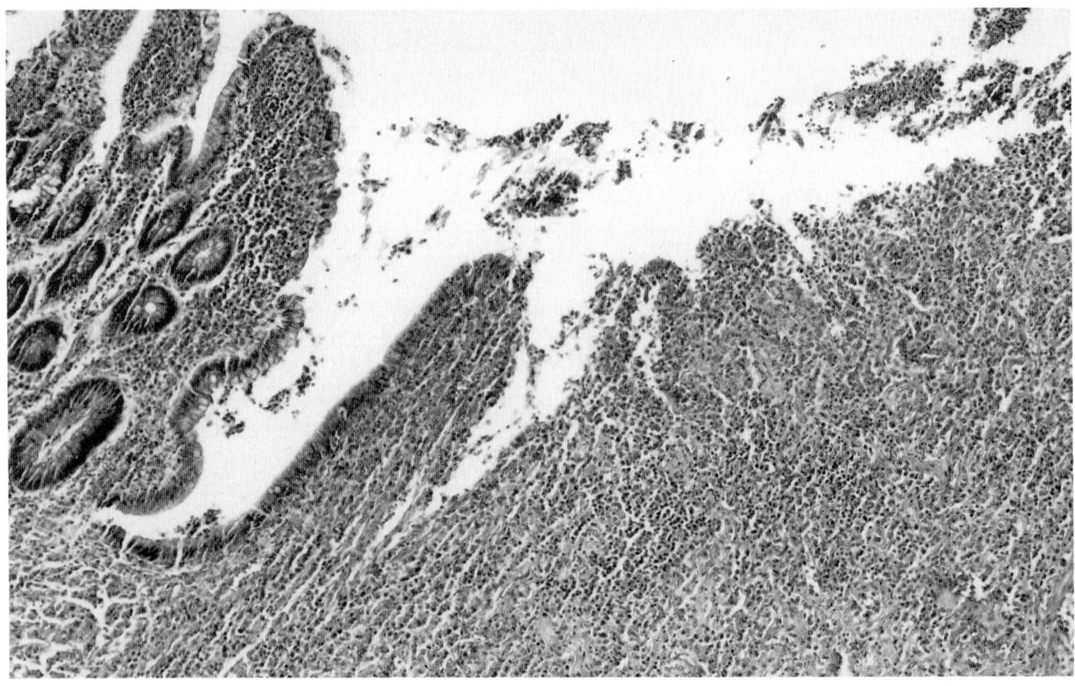

Fig. 8-17. Behçet's disease in the ileum. Present is an ulcer with marked inflammation and granulation tissue. The features are nonspecific. A fragment of inflamed mucosa appears at the left (× 105).

sions, including the presence of the oral and cutaneous ulcers.

REFERENCES

1. Goldman H, Antonioli DA: Mucosal biopsy of the rectum, colon and distal ileum. Human Pathol 13:981–1012, 1982
2. Whitehead R: Mucosal Biopsy of the Gastrointestinal Tract. 4th Ed. pp. 161–282. WB Saunders, Philadelphia, 1990
3. Sheahan DG, Rotterdam H: Small intestine. pp. 315–575. In Rotterdam H, Sheahan DG, Sommers SC (eds): Biopsy Diagnosis of the Digestive Tract. 2nd Ed. Raven Press, New York, 1993
4. Goldman H, Ming S-C: Mucins in normal and metaplastic gastrointestinal epithelium: histochemical distribution. Arch Pathol 85:580, 1968
5. Filipe MI: Mucins in the human gastrointestinal epithelium: a review. Invest Cell Pathol 2:195–216, 1979
6. Lechago J: The endocrine cells of the digestive tract. General concepts and historic perspective. Am J Surg Pathol 11(suppl 1): 63–70, 1987
7. Keren F: Structure and function of the immunologic system of the gastrointestinal tract. pp. 69–80. In Ming S-C, Goldman H (eds): Pathology of the Gastrointestinal Tract. WB Saunders, Philadelphia, 1992
8. Spencer J, Finn T, Isaacson PG: Human Peyer's patches: an immunohistochemical study. Gut 27:405–410, 1986
9. Jacob E, Baker SJ, Swaminathan SP: "M" cells in the follicle-associated epithelium of the human colon. Histopathology 11:941–952, 1987
10. Coremans G, Rutgeerts P, Geboes K et al: The value of ileoscopy with biopsy in the diagnosis of intestinal Crohn's disease. Gastrointest Endosc 30:167–172, 1984
11. Goldin E, Rachmilewitz D: Ileoscopic diagnosis of terminal ileitis. Gastrointest Endosc 30:11–14, 1984
12. Borsch G, Schmidt G: Endoscopy of the terminal ileum. Diagnostic yield in 400 consecu-

tive specimens. Dis Colon Rectum 28: 499–501, 1985
13. Lescut D, Vanco D, Bonniere P et al: Perioperative endoscopy of the whole small bowel in Crohn's disease. Gut 34:647–649, 1993
14. Goldblatt MS, Corman ML, Haggitt RC et al: Ileostomy complications requiring revision: Lahey Clinic experience, 1964–1973. Dis Colon Rectum 20:209–214, 1977
15. Cranley B: The Kock reservoir ileostomy: a review of its development, problems, and role in modern surgical practice. Br J Surg 70:94–99, 1983
16. Svaninger G, Nordgren S, Oresland T, Hulten L: Incidence and characteristics of pouchitis in the Koch continent ileostomy and the pelvic pouch. Scand J Gastroenterol 28:695–701, 1993
17. Seagram CG, Louch RE, Stephens CA, Wentworth P: Meckel's diverticulum: a 10-year review of 218 cases. Can J Surg 11:369–373, 1968
18. Meguid M, Erakis AJ: Complications of Meckel's diverticulum in infants. Surg Gynecol Obstet 139:541–544, 1974
19. Goldman H: Other inflammatory disorders of the intestines. pp. 689–696. In Ming S-C, Goldman H (eds): Pathology of the Gastrointestinal Tract. WB Saunders, Philadelphia, 1992
20. Tsubone M, Kozura S, Taki T et al: Heterotopic gastric mucosa in the small intestine. Acta Pathol Jpn 34:1425–1431, 1984
21. Yamaguchi K, Maeda S, Kitamura K: Adenocarcinoma in Meckel's diverticulum: case report and literature review. Aust NZ J Surg 59:811–813, 1989
22. Kusumoto H, Yoshitake H, Mochida K et al: Adenocarcinoma in Meckel's diverticulum: report of a case and review of 30 cases in the English and Japanese literature. Am J Gastroenterol 87:910–913, 1992
23. Krishnamurthy S, Schuffler MD; Pathology of the neuromuscular disorders of the small intestine and colon. Gastroenterology 93:610–639, 1987
24. Norris HT: Vascular Disorders. pp. 214–239. In Ming S-C, Goldman H (eds): Pathology of the Gastrointestinal Tract. WB Saunders, Philadelphia, 1992
25. Meyer CI, Troncale FJ, Galloway S, Sheahan DG: Arteriovenous malformations of the bowel: an analysis of 22 cases and a review of the literature. Medicine (Baltimore) 60:36–48, 1981
26. Brandt LJ, Boley SJ: Ischemic intestinal syndromes. Adv Surg 15:1–45, 1981
27. Haglund U, Hulten L, Ahren O, Lundgren O: Mucosal lesions in the human small intestine in shock. Gut 16:976–984, 1975
28. Whitehead R: The pathology of ischemia of the intestines. Pathol Annu 11:1–52, 1976
29. Swerdlow SH, Antonioli DA, Goldman H: Intestinal infarction: a new classification. Arch Pathol Lab Med 105:218, 1981
30. Brophy CM, Frederick WG, Scklessel R, Barwick KW: Focal segmental ischemia of the terminal ileum mimicking Crohn's disease. J Clin Gastroenterol 10:343–347, 1988
31. Camilleri M, Pusey CD, Chadwick VS, Rees AJ: Gastrointestinal manifestations of systemic vasculitis. Q J Med 206:141–149, 1983
32. Goldman H: Ulcerative colitis and Crohn's disease. pp. 643–688. In Ming S-C, Goldman H (eds): Pathology of the Gastrointestinal Tract. WB Saunders, Philadelphia, 1992
33. Rhodes JB, Kirsner JB: The early and late course of patients with ulcerative colitis after ileostomy and colectomy. Surg Gynecol Obstet 121:1303, 1965
34. Fawaz KA, Glotzer DJ, Goldman H et al: Ulcerative colitis and Crohn's disease of the colon: a comparison of the long-term postoperative courses. Gastroenterology 71:372–378, 1976
35. Vender RJ, Rickert RR, Spiro HM: The outlook after total colectomy in patients with Crohn's colitis and ulcerative colitis. J Clin Gastroenterol 1:209, 1979
36. Ming S-C, Simon M, Tandar BN: Gross gastric metaplasia of ileum after regional enteritis. Gastroenterology 44:63–68, 1963
37. Kuramoto S, Oohara T, Ihara O et al: Granulomas of the gut in Crohn's disease. A step sectioning study. Dis Colon Rectum 30:6–11, 1987
38. Tandon HD, Prakash A: Pathology of intestinal tuberculosis and its distinction from Crohn's disease. Gut 13:260–269, 1972
39. Greenstein AJ, Sachar DB, Pasternack BS: Reoperation and recurrence in Crohn's colitis and ileocolitis. N Engl J Med 293:685, 1975

40. Rutgeerts P, Geboes K, Vantrappen G et al: Natural history of Crohn's disease at the ileocolonic anastomosis after curative surgery. Gut 25:665–672, 1984
41. Sachar DB, Wolfson DM, Greenstein AJ et al: Risk factors for postoperative recurrence of Crohn's disease. Gastroenterology 85:917–921, 1983
42. Passaro E Jr, Drenick E, Wilson SE: Bypass enteritis: a new complication of jejunoileal bypass for obestiy. Am J Surg 131:169–174, 1976
43. Causey JQ; Granulomatous colitis and ileitis complicating jejunoileal bypass. Arch Intern Med 138:1727, 1978
44. Doolas A, Breyer RH, Franklin JL: Pneumatosis cystoides intestinalis following jejunoileal bypass. Am J Gastroenterol 72:271–275, 1979
45. Glotzer DJ, Glick ME, Goldman H: Proctitis and colitis following diversion of the fecal stream. Gastroenterology 80:438–441, 1981
46. Ma CK, Gottlieb C, Haas PA: Diversion colitis: a clinicopathologic study of 21 cases. Hum Pathol 21:429–436, 1990
47. Komorowski RA: Histologic spectrum of diversion colitis. Am J Surg Pathol 14:548–554, 1990
48. Turnbull RB Jr, Weakley FL, Farmer RG: Ileitis after colectomy and ileostomy for nonspecific ulcerative colitis. Dis Colon Rectum 7:427–435, 1964
49. Bechi P, Romagnoli P, Cortesini C: Ileal mucosal morphology after total cholectomy in man. Histopathology 5:667, 1981
50. Bonello JC, Thow GB, Manson RR: Mucosal enteritis: a complication of the continent ileostomy. Dis Colon Rectum 24:37–41, 1981
51. Go PM, Lens J, Bosman FT: Mucosal alterations in the reservoir of patients with Koch's continent ileostomy. Scand J Gastroenterol 22:1076–1080, 1987
52. Knill-Jones RP, Morson BC, Williams R: Prestomal ileitis: clinical and pathological findings in five cases. Q J Med 39:287, 1970
53. Church JM, Fazio VW, Lavery IC: The role of fiberoptic endoscopy in the management of the continent ileostomy. Gastrointest Endosc 33:203–209, 1987
54. Madden MV, Farthing MJG, Nicholls RJ: Inflammation of ileal reservoirs: "pouchitis". Gut 31:247–249, 1990
55. deSilva HJ, Millard PR, Kettlewell M et al: Mucosal characteristics of pelvic ileal pouches. Gut 32:61–65, 1991
56. Salemans JM, Nogengast FM, Lubbers EJ, Kuijper SJ: Postoperative and long-term results of ileal pouch and anastomosis for ulcerative colitis and familial polyposis coli. Dig Dis Sci 37:1882–1889, 1992
57. Apel R, Cohen Z, Andrews CW Jr et al: Prospective evaluation of early morphological changes in pelvic ileal pouches. Gastroenterology 107:435–443, 1994
58. Sandborn WJ: Pouchitis following ileal pouch–anal anastomosis: definition, pathogenesis, and treatment. Gastroenterology 107:1856–1860, 1994
59. Blazeby JM, Durdey P, Warren BF: Polypoid mucosal prolapse in a pelvic ileal reservoir. Gut 35:1668–1669, 1994
60. Helander KG, Ahren C, Philipson BM et al: Structure of mucosa in continent ileal reservoirs 15 to 19 years after construction. Hum Pathol 21:1235–1238, 1990
61. Santos MC, Thompson JS: Late complications of the ileal pouch–anal anastomosis. Am J Gastroenterol 88:3–10, 1993
62. Carraro PS, Talbot IC, Nicholls RJ: Long-term appraisal of the histological appearances of the ileal reservoir mucosa after restorative proctocolectomy for ulcerative colitis. Gut 35:1721–1727, 1994
63. Subramani K, Harpaz N, Bilotta C et al: Refractory proctitis: does it reflect underlying Crohn's disease? Gut 34:1539–1542, 1993
64. Knober H, Ligumsky M, Ohon E et al: Pouch ileitis—recurrence of the inflammatory bowel disease in the ileal reservoir. Am J Gastroenterol 81:199–220, 1986
65. Berman JJ, Ullah A: Colonic metaplasia of ileostomies: biological significance for ulcerative colitis patients following total colectomy. Am J Surg Pathol 13:955–960, 1989
66. Luukkonen P, Jarvinen H, Tanskanen M, Kahri A: Pouchitis—recurrence of the inflammatory bowel disease? Gut 35:243–246, 1994
67. Aftalion B, Lipper S: Enteritis cystica profunda associated with Crohn's disease. Arch Pathol Lab Med 108:532–533, 1984
68. Saul SH, Wong LK, Zinsser KR: Enteritis cystica profunda: association with Crohn's disease. Hum Pathol 17:600–603, 1986

69. Alexis J, Lubin J, Wallach M: Enteritis cystica profunda in a patient with Crohn's disease. Arch Pathol Lab Med 113:947–949, 1989
70. Weedon DD, Shorter RG, Ilstrup DM et al: Crohn's disease and cancer. N Engl J Med 289:1099–1103, 1973
71. Lightdale CJ, Sternberg SS, Posner G et al: Carcinoma complicating Crohn's disease. Am J Med 59:262–268, 1975
72. Gyde SN, Prior P, Macartney JC et al: Malignancy in Crohn's disease. Gut 21:1024–1029, 1980
73. Choi PM, Zelig MP: Similarity of colorectal cancer in Crohn's disease and ulcerative colitis: implications for carcinogenesis and prevention. Gut 35:950–954, 1994
74. Senay E, Sachar DB, Keokane M, Greenstein AJ: Small bowel carcinoma in Crohn's disease. Distinguishing features and risk factors. Cancer 63:360–363, 1989
75. Lashner BA: Risk factors for small bowel cancer in Crohn's disease. Dig Dis Sci 37:1179–1184, 1992
76. Simpson S, Traube J, Riddell RH: The histological appearance of dysplasia (precarcinomatous change) in Crohn's disease of the small and large intestine. Gastroenterology 81:492–501, 1981
77. Fresko D, Lazarus SS, Doton J, Reingold M: Early representation of carcinoma of the small bowel in Crohn's disease ("Crohn's carcinoma"). Case reports and review of the literature. Gastroenterology 82:783–789, 1982
78. Collier PE, Turowski P, Diamond DL: Small intestinal adenocarcinoma complicating regional enteritis. Cancer 55:516–521, 1985
79. Warren R, Barwick KW: Crohn's colitis with carcinoma and dysplasia. Report of a case and review of 100 small and large bowel resections for Crohn's disease to detect incidence of dysplasia. Am J Surg Pathol 7:151–159, 1983
80. Petras RE, Mir-Madjlessi SH, Farmer RG: Crohn's disease and intestinal carcinoma. A report of 11 cases with emphasis on associated epithelial dysplasia. Gastroenterology 93:1307–1314, 1987
81. Cuvelier C, Bekaert E, De Potter C et al: Crohn's disease with adenocarcinoma and dysplasia. Macroscopical, histological, and immunohistochemical aspects of two cases. Am J Surg Pathol 13:187–196, 1989
82. Riddell RH, Goldman H, Ransohoff DF et al: Dysplasia in inflammatory bowel disease: standardized classification with provisional clinical applications. Hum Pathol 14:931–968, 1983
83. Eklom A, Helmick C, Zack M, Adami H-O: Ulcerative colitis and colorectal cancer: a population-based study. N Engl J Med 323:1228–1233, 1990
84. Riddell RH: The gastrointestinal tract. pp. 515–606. In Riddell RH (ed): Pathology of the Drug-Induced and Toxic Diseases. Churchill Livingstone, New York, 1982
85. Lewis JH: Gastrointestinal injury due to medicinal agents. Am J Gastroenterol 81:819–834, 1986
86. Goldman H, Szabo S: Chemical and physical disorders. pp. 141–170. In Ming S-C, Goldman H (eds): Pathology of the Gastrointestinal Tract. WB Saunders, Philadelphia, 1992
87. Allison MC, Howatson AG, Torrance CJ et al: Gastrointestinal damage associated with the use of nonsteroidal anti-inflammatory drugs. N Engl J Med 327:749–754, 1992
88. Bjornason I, Hayllar J, Macpherson AJ, Russell AS: Side effects of nonsteroidal anti-inflammatory drugs on the small and large intestine in humans. Gastroenterology 104:1832–1847, 1993
89. Lee FD: Drug-related pathological lesions of the intestinal tract. Histopathology 25:303–308, 1994
90. Bjornson I, Price AB, Zanelli G et al: Clinicopathological features of nonsteroidal anti-inflammatory drug-induced small intestinal strictures. Gastroenterology 94:1070–1074, 1988
91. Lang J, Price AB, Levi AJ et al: Diaphragm disease: pathology of disease of the small intestine induced by non-steroidal anti-inflammatory drugs. J Clin Pathol 41:516–526, 1988
92. Matsukashi N, Yamada A, Hiraishi M et al: Multiple strictures of the small intestine after long-term nonsteroidal anti-inflammatory drug therapy. Am J Gastroenterol 87:1183–1186, 1992
93. Monihan JM, Hensley SD, Sobin LH: Nonsteroidal anti-inflammatory drug-induced diaphragm disease arising in a bypassed ileal

segment. Am J Gastroenterol 89:610–612, 1994
94. Jackson CW, Haboubi NY, Whorwell RJ, Schofield PF: Gold-induced enterocolitis. Gut 27:452–456, 1986
95. Geltner D, Sternfeld M, Becker SA, Kori M: Gold-induced ileitis. J Clin Gastroenterol 8:184–186, 1986
96. Berthrong M, Fajardo LF; Radiation injury in surgical pathology. Part II. Alimentary tract. Am J Surg Pathol 5:153–178, 1981
97. Poddar PK, Bauer JJ, Gelerent I et al: Radiation injury to the small intestine. Mt Sinai J Med 49:144–149, 1982
98. Galland RB, Spencer J: The natural history of clinically established radiation enteritis. Lancet 1:1257–1258, 1985
99. Sher ME, Bauer J: Radiation-induced enteropathy. Am J Gastroenterol 85:121–128, 1990
100. Gase records of the Massachusetts General Hospital. Radiation enteritis. N Engl J Med 330:627–632, 1994
101. Montgomery EA, Popek EJ: Intussusception, adenovirus, and children: a brief reaffirmation. Hum Pathol 25:169–174, 1994
102. Lepinski SM, Hamilton JW: Isolated cytomegalovirus ileitis detected by colonoscopy. Gastroenterology 98:1704–1706, 1990
103. Kliegman RM, Fanaroff AA: Necrotizing enterocolitis. N Engl J Med 310: 1093–1103, 1984
104. Cheromcha DP, Hyman PE: Neonatal necrotizing enterocolitis. Inflammatory bowel disease of the newborn. Dig Dis Sci 33(March suppl):78S–84S, 1988
105. Newbold KM, Lord MG, Baglin TP: Role of clostridial organisms in neutropenic enterocolitis. J Clin Pathol 40:471, 1987
106. Wade DS, Nava HR, Douglas HO Jr: Neutropenic enterocolitis. Clinical diagnosis and treatment. Cancer 69:17–23, 1992
107. Buts J-P, Weber AM, Morin CL: Pseudomembraneous entercolitis in childhood: Gastroenterology 73:823–827, 1977
108. Wiesen S, Gregg PA, Kershenobich P et al: Pseudomembraneous enteritis: rediscovery of a previously well-described entity? Am J Gastroenterol 87:1631–1633, 1992
109. El-Maraghi NRH, Mair NS: The histopathology of enteric infection with Yersinia pseudotuberculosis. Am J Clin Pathol 71:631–639, 1979
110. Simmonds SD, Noble MA, Freeman JH: Gastrointestinal features of culture-positive Yersinia enterocolitica infection. Gastroenterology 92:112–117, 1987
111. Palmer KR, Patil DH, Basran GS et al: Abdominal tuberculosis in urban Britain—a common disease. Gut 26:1296–1305, 1985
112. Bhargava DK, Tandon HD: Ileocoecal tuberculosis diagnosed by colonoscopy and biopsy. Aust N Z J Surg 50:583–585, 1980
113. Prescott RJ, Harris M, Banerjee SS: Fungal infections of the small and large intestines. J Clin Pathol 45:806–811, 1992
114. Pinkus GS, Coolidge C, Little MD: Intestinal anisakiasis: first case report from North America. Am J Med 59:114–120, 1975
115. Watt IA, McLean NR, Girdwood RWA et al: Eosinophilic gastroenteritis associated with a larval anisakine nematode. Lancet 2:893–894, 1979
116. McKerrow JH, Sakanari J, Deerdorff TL: Anisakiasis: revenge of the sushi parasites. N Engl J Med 319:1228–1229, 1988
117. Fenoglio-Preiser CM, Pascal RR, Perzin KH: Tumors of the intestines. Atlas of Tumor Pathology, second series, fascicle 27. Armed Forces Institute of Pathology, Washington DC, 1990
118. Cooper HS: Benign polyps of the intestines. pp. 786–815. In Ming S-C, Goldman H (eds): Pathology of the Gastrointestinal Tract. WB Saunders, Philadelphia, 1992
119. Ming S-C: Adenocarcinoma and other malignant epithelial tumors of the intestines. pp. 816–857. In Ming S-C, Goldman H (eds): Pathology of the Gastrointestinal Tract. WB Saunders, Philadelphia, 1992
120. Woelfel GF, Campbell DN, Penn I et al: Inflammatory polyposis in an ileal blind loop. Gastroenterology 84:1020–1024, 1983
121. Kahn E, Daum F: Pseudopolyposis of the small intestine in Crohn's disease. Hum Pathol 15:84–86, 1984
122. Haggitt RC, Reid BJ: Hereditary gastrointestinal polyposis syndromes. Am J Surg Pathol 10:871–877, 1986
123. Listron MB, Fenoglio-Preiser C: Short course. Gastrointestinal polyps. Modern Pathol 2:161–181, 1989

124. Sachatello CR, Pickren JW, Grace JT: Generalized juvenile gastrointestinal polyposis. Gastroenterology 58:669, 1970
125. Williams GT, Bussey HJR, Morson BC: Hamartomatous polyps in Peutz-Jeghers syndrome. N Engl J Med 299:101, 1978
126. Estrada R, Spjut HJ: Hamartomatous polyps in Peutz-Jeghers syndrome. A light-, histochemical and electron-microscopic study. Am J Surg Pathol 7:747–754, 1983
127. Giardiello FM, Welsh SB, Hamilton SR et al: Increased risk of cancer in the Peutz-Jeghers syndrome. N Engl J Med 316: 1511–1514, 1987
128. Burke AP, Sobin LH: The pathology of Cronkhite-Canada polyps: a comparison to juvenile polyposis. Am J Surg Pathol 13:940–946, 1989
129. Atwell JD, Burge D, Wright D: Nodular lymphoid hyperplasia of the intestinal tract in infancy and childhood. J Ped Surg 20:25–29, 1985
130. Rubin A, Isaacson PG: Florid reactive lymphoid hyerplasia of the terminal ileum in adults: a condition bearing a close resemblance to low-grade malignant lymphoma. Histopathology 17:19–26, 1990
131. Thomford NR, Greenberger NJ: Lymphoid polyps of the ileum associated with Gardner's syndrome. Arch Surg 96:289–291, 1968
132. Dorazio RA, Whelan TJ Jr: Lymphoid hyperplasia of the terminal ileum associated with familial polyposis coli. Ann Surg 171:300–302, 1970
133. Tawfik OW, McGregor DH: Lipohyperplasia of the ileocecal valve. Am J Gastroenterol 87:82–87, 1992
134. Benjamin SP, Hawk WA, Turnbull RB: Fibrous inflammatory polyps of the ileum and cecum: review of five cases with emphasis on differentiation from mesenchymal neoplasms. Cancer 39:1300–1305, 1977
135. Shimer GR, Helwig EB: Inflammatory fibroid polyps of the intestine. Am J Clin Pathol 81:708–714, 1984
136. Kim YI, Kim WH: Inflammatory fibroid polyps of gastrointestinal tract. Am J Clin Pathol 89:721–727, 1988
137. Griffiths AP, Hopkinson JP, Dixon MF: Inflammatory myoglandular polyp causing ileoileal intussusception. Histopathology 23: 596–598, 1993
138. Heimann TM, Cohen LB, Bolnick, K, Szporn AH: Villous polyposis of the ileum: report of a case. Am J Gastroenterol 80:983–985, 1985
139. Jass JR, Stewart SM, Officer NMF: Villous adenoma of ileum in Lynch II syndrome. Histopathology 22:186–187, 1993
140. Hamilton SR, Bussey HJR, Mendelsohn G et al: Ileal adenomas after colectomy in nine patients with adenomatous polyposis coli/ Gardner's syndrome. Gastroenterology 77: 1252, 1979
141. Beart RW, Fleming CR, Banks PM: Tubulovillous adenomas in a continent ileostomy after proctocolectomy for familial polyposis. Dig Dis Sci 27:553–556, 1982
142. Nakahara S, Itoh H, Iida M et al: Ileal adenomas in familial polyposis coli. Differences before and after colectomy. Dis Colon Rectum 28:875–877, 1985
143. Bridge MF, Perzin KH: Primary adenocarcinoma of the jejunum and ileum. A clinicopathologic study. Cancer 36:1876–1887, 1975
144. Arthaud JB, Guinee VF: Jejunal and ileal adenocarcinoma. Am J Gastroenterol 72: 638–646, 1979
145. Live TF, Biggart JD: Primary adenocarcinoma of the jejunum and ileum—clinicopathological review of 25 cases. J Clin Pathol 43:533–536, 1990
146. Sellner F: Investigations on the significance of the adenoma-carcinoma sequence in the small bowel. Cancer 66:702–715, 1990
147. Cooper BT, Holmes GK, Ferguson R, Cooke WT: Celiac disease and malignancy. Medicine (Baltimore) 59:249–261, 1980
148. Swinson CM, Slavin G, Coles EC, Booth CC: Celiac disease and malignancy. Lancet 1:111–115, 1983
149. Danzig JB, Brandt LJ, Reinus JF, Klein RS: Gastrointestinal malignancy in patients with AIDS. Am J Gastroenterol 86:715–718, 1991
150. Strykes SJ: Primary stomal adenocarcinoma. An unusual complication of ileostomy. Dis Colon Rectum 26:47–49, 1983
151. Smart PJ, Sastry S, Wells S: Primary mucinous adenocarcinoma developing in an ileostomy stoma. Gut 29:1607–1612, 1988
152. Gadacz TR, McFadden DW, Gabrielson EW et al: Adenocarcinoma of the ileostomy: the latent risk of cancer after colectomy for

ulcerative colitis and familial polyposis. Surgery 107:698–703, 1990
153. Vasilevsky CA, Gordon PH: Adenocarcinoma arising at the ileocutaneous junction occuring after protocolectomy for ulcerative colitis. Br J Surg 73:378, 1986
154. Bedetti CD, De Risio VJ: Primary adenocarcinoma arising at an ileostomy site. An unusual complication after colectomy for ulcerative colitis. Dis Colon Rectum 29:572–575, 1986
155. Primrose JN, Quirke P, Johnston D: Carcinoma of the ileostomy in a patient with familial adenomatous polyposis. Br J Surg 75:384, 1988
156. Johnson JA, Talton DS, Poole GV: Adenocarcinoma of a Brooke ileostomy for adenomatous polyposis coli. Am J Gastroenterol 88:1122–1124, 1993
157. Suarez V, Alexander-Williams J, O'Connor HJ et al: Carcinoma developing in ileostomies after 25 or more years. Gastroenterology 95:205–208, 1988
158. Carter D, Choi H, Otterson M, Felford GL: Primary adenocarcinoma of the ileostomy after colectomy for ulcerative colitis. Dig Dis Sci 33:509–512, 1988
159. Sherlock DJ, Suarez V, Gray JG: Stomal adenocarcinoma in Crohn's disease. Gut 31:1329–1332, 1990
160. Taylor BA, Wolff BG, Dozois RR et al: Ileal pouch–anal anastomosis for chronic ulcerative colitis and familial polyposis coli complicated by adenocarcinoma. Dis Colon Rectum 31:358–362, 1988
161. Stern H, Wolfisch S, Mullen B: Cancer in an ileoanal reservoir: a new late complication? Gut 31:473–475, 1990
162. Griesser GH, Schumacher U, Eifeldt R, Horney H-P: Adenosquamous carcinoma of the ileum. Report of a case and review of the literature. Virchows Arch A Pathol Anat Histopathol 406:483–487, 1985
163. Platt CC, Haboubi NY, Schofield PF: Primary squamous cell carcinoma of terminal ileum. J Clin Pathol 44:253–254, 1991
164. Radi MF, Gray GF, Scott HW: Carcinosarcoma of ileum in regional enteritis. Hum Pathol 15:385–387, 1984
165. Sanders RJ, Axtell HK: Carcinoids of the gastrointestinal tract. Surg Gynecol Obstet 119:369–380, 1984
166. Moryana TN, Satkunam N: A comparative immunohistochemical study of jejunoileal and appendiceal carcinoids. Implications for histogenesis and pathogenesis. Cancer 70: 1081–1088, 1992
167. Iwafuchi M, Watanabe H, Iishihara N et al: Neoplastic endocrine cells in carcinomas of the small intestine: histochemical and immunohistochemical studies of 24 tumors. Hum Pathol 18:185–194, 1987
168. Klappenbach RS, Kurman RJ, Sinclair CF, James LP: Composite carcinoma–carcinoid tumors of the gastrointestinal tract. A morphologic, histochemical and immunocytochemical study. Am J Clin Pathol 84:137–143, 1985
169. Toker C: Oat cell carcinoma of the small bowel. Am J Gastroenterol 61:481–483, 1976
170. Lewin KJ, Ranchod M, Dorfman RF: Lymphomas of the gastrointestinal tract: a study of 117 cases presenting with gastrointestinal disease. Cancer 42:693, 1978
171. Weingrad DN, DeCosse JJ, Sherlock P et al: Primary gastrointestinal lymphoma: a 30-year review. Cancer 49:1258–1265, 1982
172. Appelman HD, Hirsch SD, Schnitzer B, Coon WW: Clinicopathologic overview of gastrointestinal lymphomas. Am J Surg Pathol 9(3)(suppl):71–83, 1985
173. Estrin HM, Farhi DC, Ament AA, Yang P: Ileoscopic diagnosis of malignant lymphoma of the small bowel in acquired immunodeficiency syndrome. Gastrointest Endosc 33: 390–391, 1987
174. Appelman HD: Mesenchymal tumors of the gastrointestinal tract. pp. 310–350. In Ming S-C, Goldman H (eds): Pathology of the Gastrointestinal Tract. WB Saunders, Philadelphia, 1992
175. Yardley JH: Malabsorptive disorders. pp. 725–767. In Ming S-C, Goldman H (eds): Pathology of the Gastrointestinal Tract. WB Saunders, Philadelphia, 1992
176. Haggitt RC: Granulomatous disease of the gastrointestinal tract. pp. 257–305. In Ioachim HL (ed): Pathology of Granulomas. Raven Press, New York, 1983
177. Goldman H: Systemic and miscellaneous disorders. pp. 351–380. In Ming S-C, Goldman H (eds): Pathology of the Gastrointestinal Tract. WB Saunders, Philadelphia, 1992

178. Coletta U, Sturgill BC: Isolated xanthomatosis of the small bowel. Hum Pathol 16:422–424, 1985
179. Lake BD: Storage disorders involving the alimentary tract. pp. 269–276. In Whitehead R (ed): Gastrointestinal and Oesophageal Pathology. Churchill Livingstone, New York, 1989
180. Shephard NA, Crocker PR, Smith AP, Levison DA: Exogenous pigment in Peyer's patches. Hum Pathol 18:50–54, 1987
181. Urbanski SJ, Arsenault L, Green FHY, Haber G: Pigment resembling atmospheric dust in Peyer's patches. Modern Pathol 2:222–226, 1989
182. Cuvelier C, Barbatis C, Mielants H et al: Histopathology of intestinal inflammation related to reactive arthritis. Gut 28:394–401, 1987
183. DeVos M, Cuvelier C, Mielants N et al: Ileocolonoscopy in seronegative spondylarthropathy. Gastroenterology 96:339–344, 1989
184. Goldman H: Allergic disorders. pp. 171–187. In Ming S-C, Goldman H (eds): Pathology of the Gastrointestinal Tract. WB Saunders, Philadelphia, 1992
185. Ament ME: Immunodeficiency syndromes of the gut. Scand J Gastroenterol 20(suppl 114):127–135, 1985
186. Snover DC, Weisdorf SA, Vercolotti GM et al: A histopathologic study of gastric and small intestinal graft-versus-host disease following allogeneic bone marrow transplantation. Hum Pathol 16:387–392, 1985
187. Jaffe R, Trager JD, Zeevi A et al: Multivisceral intestinal transplantation: surgical pathology. Pediatr Pathol 9:633–654, 1989
188. Hurlbut D, Garcia B, Ohene-Bianco D et al: Immunohistochemical assessment of mucosal biopsies following human intestinal transplantation. Transplant Proc 24:1195–1196, 1992
189. Oliva MM, Perman JA, Saavedra JM et al: Successful intestinal transplantation for microvillus inclusion disease. Gastroenterology 106:771–774, 1994
190. Parr NJ, Murphy C, Holt S et al: Endometriosis and the gut. Gut 29:1112–1115, 1988
191. Cappell MS, Friedman D, Mikhail N: Endometriosis of the terminal ileum simulating the clinical, roentgenographic, and surgical findings in Crohn's disease. Am J Gastroenterol 86:1057–1062, 1991
192. Jeffries GH, Steinberg H, Sleisenger MH: Chronic ulcerative (nongranulomatous) jejunitis. Am J Med 44:47–59, 1968
193. Modigliani R, Poitras P, Galian A et al: Chronic non-specific ulcerative duodenojejunoileitis: report of four cases. Gut 20: 318–328, 1979
194. Baba S, Maruta M, Ando K et al: Intestinal Behçet's disease: report of five cases. Dis Colon Rectum 19:428–440, 1976
195. Lee RG: The colitis of Behçet's syndrome. Am J Surg Pathol 10:888–893, 1986

9

Inflammatory Disorders of the Colon and Rectum

The inflammatory lesions of the colon and rectum are presented in this chapter, and the tumors of the colon and rectum are presented in Chapter 10.

GENERAL ASPECTS

Examination of the rectum and sigmoid colon by rigid endoscopes has long been possible. Study of the entire colon was largely hampered, however, by the limitation of the rigid endoscopes to this distal region and by the preferential use of biopsies for only grossly evident inflammatory or tumor lesions. The appearance of flexible endoscopes resulted in a dramatic increase in the number of examinations and allowed for complete evaluation of the colon.[1–4] It soon became evident that the procedure was useful in a wide variety of conditions, not only to establish the diagnosis but also to provide information on the natural history and complications of many lesions[5–7] (Table 9-1). It also was realized that biopsy was needed in many situations where the mucosa appeared to be grossly normal, since it could provide more sensitive information regarding inflammatory lesions in the tissue sample. Sigmoidoscopy and colonoscopy utilizing flexible endoscopes are now commonly employed for multiple reasons, including diagnosis, determining extent and severity of lesions, assessment of the disorders following therapy, and surveying for complications. The choice of sigmoidoscopy or colonoscopy is essentially determined by the symptoms and the probability of location of the lesions.

Most of the disorders affect both the rectum and the colon; these are described together, with notation when there are peculiarities in distribution. In many of the conditions, the rectum and sigmoid are highly representative and can be readily accessed by sigmoidoscopy. The lesions may be just as prominent in the more proximal parts of the colon but are more easily obtained by examination of the lower portion.

Table 9-1. Inflammatory Disorders of the Colon and Rectum

Effects of motor and mechanical disorders
Ischemic disease and vasculitis
Infections
Idiopathic inflammatory bowel disease
Ulcerative colitis
Crohn's disease
Chemical and drug injury
Radiation injury
Allergic and immunologic disorders
Miscellaneous conditions
Collagenous and lymphocytic colitis
Diversion colitis
Solitary rectal ulcer syndrome
Granulomatous diseases
Skin diseases

Normal Structure

Except for the distal few centimeters of the rectum, the mucosal structure throughout the large intestine is generally similar. As in other parts of the gut, there are the three major compartments of the epithelium, the lamina propria, and the muscularis mucosae[8–10] (Table 9-2).

Epithelium

The epithelium forms long and closely packed crypts that extend from the surface to the muscularis mucosae (Fig. 9-1). Throughout the colon there are occasional separations of the crypts into two or more branches just beneath the surface. This should be distinguished from the more prominent budding in the mid- or lower portion of the crypts that represents chronic disease. The crypts are largely composed of goblet-type mucous cells that are rich in sialylmucin and sulfomucins[11, 12] (Fig. 9-2). The mucin stains strongly with Alcian Blue at both pH 2.5 and 1.0, as well as with the high-iron diamine reaction. There is typically only mild staining with the PAS reaction for the neutral mucins. Mitoses are normally present in the basal one-third of the crypts and extend to higher regions in reparative and neoplastic disorders. The surface of the mucosa is covered in part by the mucous cells and also with columnar cells that are involved in absorption of water and electrolytes (Fig. 9-3). The goblet mucous cells are similar to those in the small intestine, displaying basal and often flattened-appearing nuclei and a cytoplasm that is distended with the mucus granules. The absorptive cells on the surface show a basal but more elongated nucleus together with a granular-type cytoplasm.

Table 9-2. Normal Components of the Colonic Mucosa

Epithelium
Goblet mucous cells
Absorptive cells
Microfold (M) cells
Paneth cells
Endocrine cells
Lamina propria
Lymphocytes and plasma cells
Macrophages and eosinophils
Lymphoid nodules
Vessels and ganglia
No lymphatics
Muscularis mucosae
Smooth muscle layers

Paneth cells are typically restricted to the cecum and the beginning of the ascending colon. They are concentrated in the base of the crypts, revealing the large red refractile granules in the cytoplasm (see Fig. 6-2). Their presence in the upper portions of the crypts and in the more distal portions of the colon are a sign of repair and typically correlate with chronic disease. There are a modest number of endocrine cells that are located in the lower portion of the crypts and are interspersed between the mucous cells and the basement membrane[13–15] (see Fig. 7-4). They are well defined by the presence of fine eosinophilic granules in the cytoplasm and rounded or flattened nuclei, with the apex of the cells directed toward the basement membrane.

Lamina Propria

Just beneath the basement membrane is a thin collagen layer. This is very slender, measuring 2 to 3 μm in thickness in the right

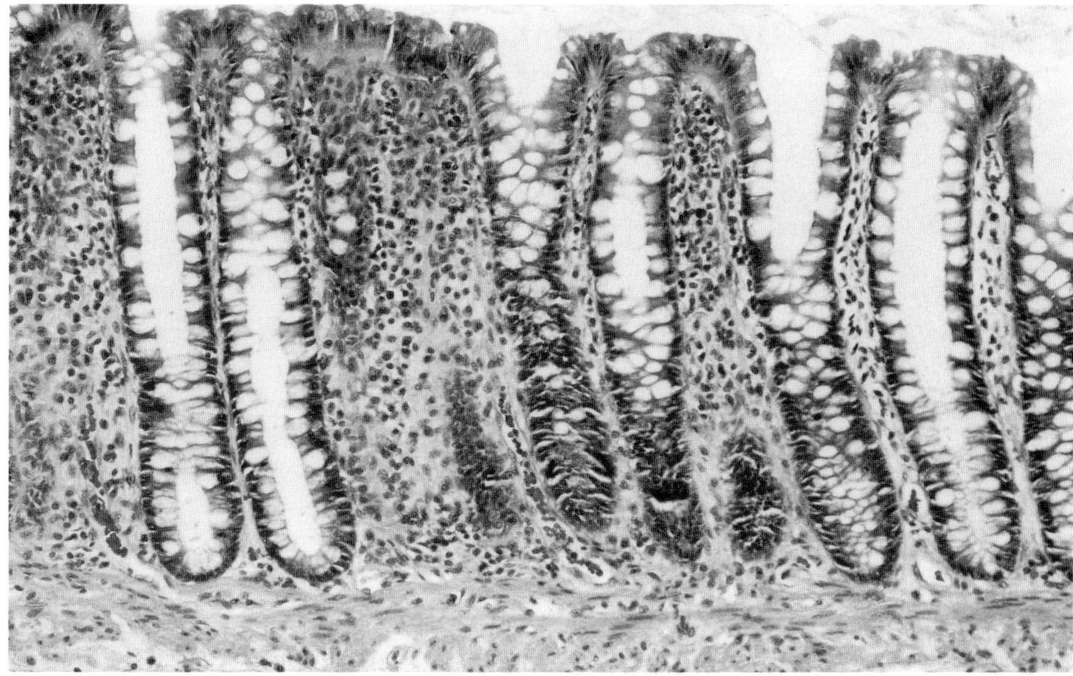

Fig. 9-1. Normal colon. Shown are straight crypts extending from the mucosal surface to the muscularis mucosae appearing at the bottom. The crypts mainly contain goblet mucous cells. There is a moderate amount of mononuclear inflammatory cells in the lamina propria between the crypts (× 170).

side of the colon and increasing to 3 to 4 μm in the left portion. The layer is best seen below the surface epithelium but is generally inconspicuous and merges with the rest of the lamina propria. Throughout the lamina propria are inflammatory cells of most types, including macrophages, lymphocytes, plasma cells, eosinophils, and a rare neutrophil.

Scattered throughout the colon and rectum are lymphoid nodules that extend from the surface to the upper portion of the submucosa, breaking the muscularis mucosae in these areas[16, 17] (Fig. 9-4). A section directly through the nodule reveals a well formed follicle center, surrounded by mature lymphocytes that extend into the epithelial region. These are important structures to appreciate because the tissues immediately adjacent to the follicles may show alterations that simulate inflammatory disorders, but which simply represent variations of normal. Thus the crypts just next to the lymphoid nodules typically show depletion of mucus granules, and the epithelia overlying the nodules are flattened or cuboidal and include the microfold or M cells that are involved in antigen trapping and transfer[18] (see Fig. 8-3). There are also an increased number of inflammatory cells in the epithelial region adjacent to the lymphoid nodules, particularly on the surface, which consist of lymphocytes and a few neutrophils. Such lymphoid nodules are commonly seen in mucosal biopsies. There are usually one or two present; when more are noted, it should be indicated in the diagnosis and may correlate with a reparative feature, especially in children. The lymphoid nodules are more often noted in the rectum and also tend to develop greater hyperplasia in this region.

Also commonly present in the lamina propria are clusters of macrophages with foamy cytoplasm, which usually stain positive for

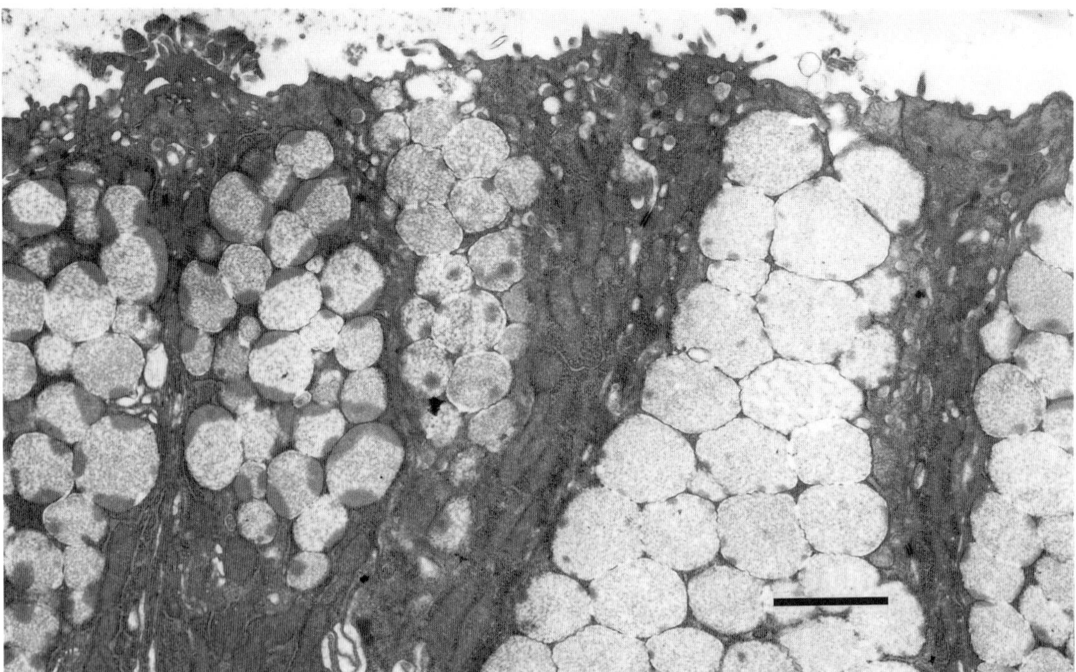

Fig. 9-2. Electron micrograph of normal goblet mucous cells in the colonic crypt. The goblet cells contain numerous mucin granules, and the apical microvilli are short and irregular (× 7500; bar = 2μm).

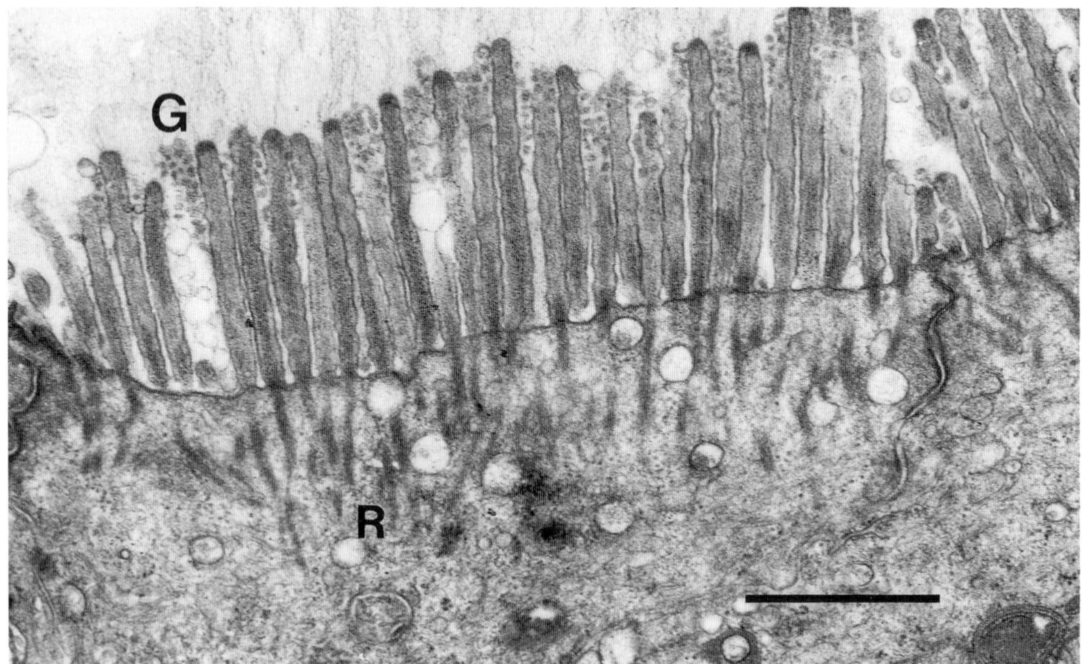

Fig. 9-3. Electron micrograph of absorptive cells from the surface colon epithelium. The rigid microvilli have a core of microfilaments that extend into the apical cytoplasm to form "rootlets" (R), and have a coat of glycocalyx with associated glycocalyceal bodies (G). Such microvilli are primarily found on the apical surface of gastrointestinal tract mucosal absorptive cells (× 25,000; bar = 1 μm).

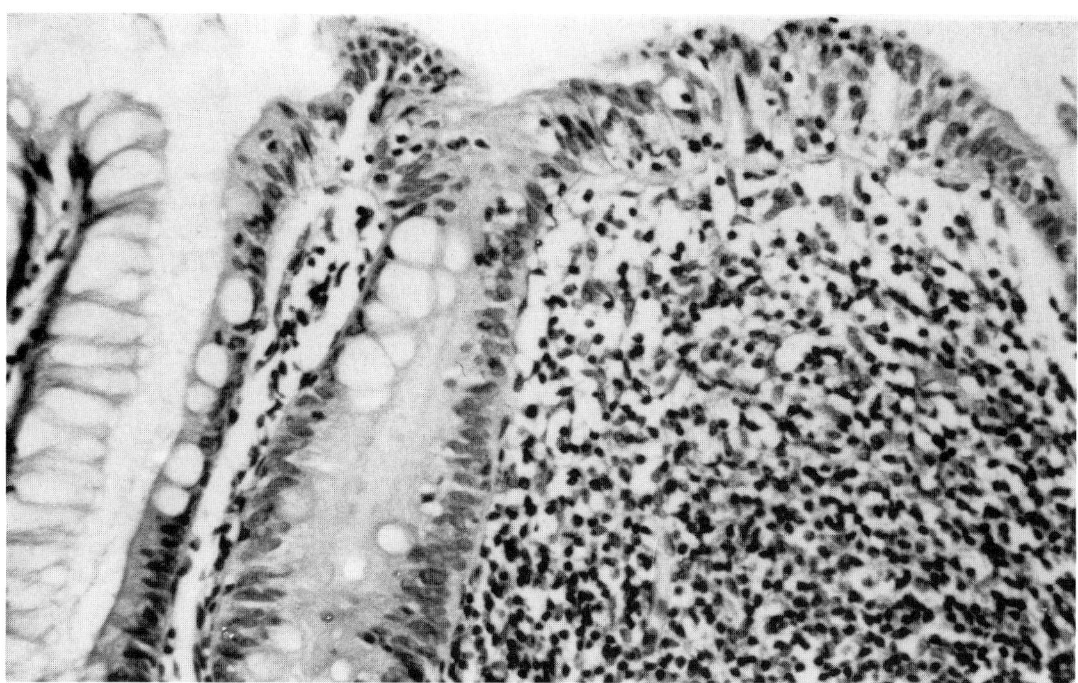

Fig. 9-4. Lymphoid nodule in the normal colonic mucosa. The lymphoid tissue appears at the right. The adjacent crypt shows a loss of mucus from the epithelial cells, and the surface epithelial layer is infiltrated by inflammatory cells.

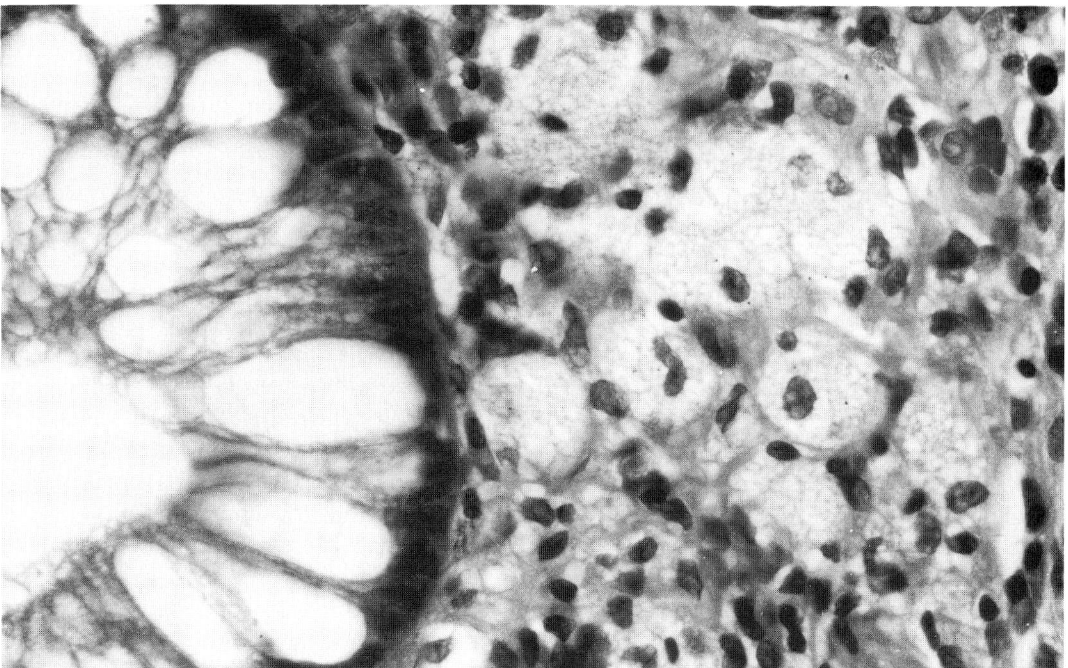

Fig. 9-5. Muciphages in the normal colonic mucosa. Present in the lamina propria appearing at the right is a cluster of macrophages with irregular vacuoles in their cytoplasm. The mucinous nature can be determined by positive stains for PAS, Alcian Blue, and mucicarmine. A crypt appears at the left (× 635).

mucins[19] (Fig. 9-5). These were once considered to be the effect of excess laxative use but are now thought to represent a normal finding. They are usually in the superficial region of the mucosa but can extend to the basal part. It is important to recognize this normal cell to avoid confusion with storage disorders and granulomatous lesions. The lamina propria also contains a small amount of fibrous and muscle tissue, venules and capillaries, and rare ganglia. In contrast to the small intestine, the lymphatics are limited to the submucosa and the region of the muscularis mucosae, and they do not extend higher in the lamina propria in the normal state.[20]

Muscularis Mucosae and Submucosa

The muscularis mucosae is made up of a double layer of smooth muscle (Fig. 9-6). This is typically thickened in many inflammatory disorders. Only minimal amounts of superficial submucosa are present in most endoscopic biopsies. whereas larger quantities are represented in the aspiration-type biopsies. The submucosa is mainly composed of adipose tissue and contains larger arteries and veins, lymphatics, strands of fibrous tissue, discrete ganglia, and scattered nerves. There may also be small lymphoid aggregates but usually no other inflammatory cells.

Lower Rectum

In the lower rectum the mucosa shows features that are indistinguishable from those seen in chronic colitis (Fig. 9-7). There is marked shortening and branching of the crypts and their separation from a thickened muscularis mucosae. There is also usually an increase in the amount of lymphoid nodules in this region. If biopsies are taken from the rectum without exact notation of their location, the report must indicate that such features of atrophy would be compatible with normal in the lower rectum whereas they would be indicative of disease if higher in the gut.

Biopsy Material

Most of the biopsies are obtained at the time of endoscopy. These tend to be small and prone to the traumatic effects of the procedure. Typically, they mainly consist of the mucosa with only scant submucosal tissue. When a larger sample including the submucosa is needed, aspiration-type biopsies can be obtained. These are ordinarily taken from the rectum and are needed to examine the submucosa for ganglia, for vasculitis, or for the presence of amyloid and other infiltrative disorders.

The large majority of the diagnoses are readily established by routine H & E sections. Special stains are employed to identify microorganisms, and immunocytochemical stains may be helpful in establishing the presence and types of tumors. Electron microscopy is an important adjunct that can help in the precise identification of a particular microorganisms or storage condition.

Effects of Procedures

The effects of preparatory enemas and of the procedures must be recognized and discounted before considering abnormalities in the mucosa (Table 9-3). Earlier use of irritating enemas resulted in a mild colitis, which is described in the section on "Chemical Injury" below. Currently, there is the ready use of osmotic solutions that invariably produce an edema of the lamina propria[21] (Fig. 9-8). This results in a separation of the crypts from themselves and from the muscularis mucosae, but is distinguished from atrophy by the otherwise uniform appearance of the crypts. The endoscopic procedure can result in mild trauma that leads to patches of hemorrhage within the lamina propria.[22] Also

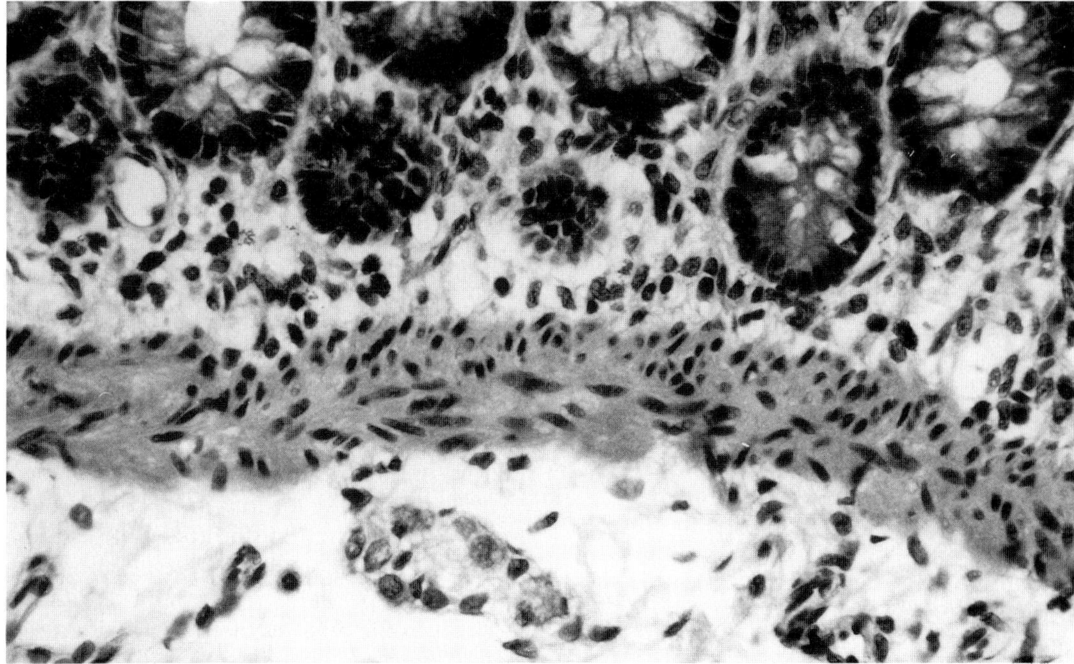

Fig. 9-6. Normal colon, showing base of crypts (top), the muscularis mucosae, and the superficial part of the submucosa, which contains normal ganglion cells (bottom center) (× 425).

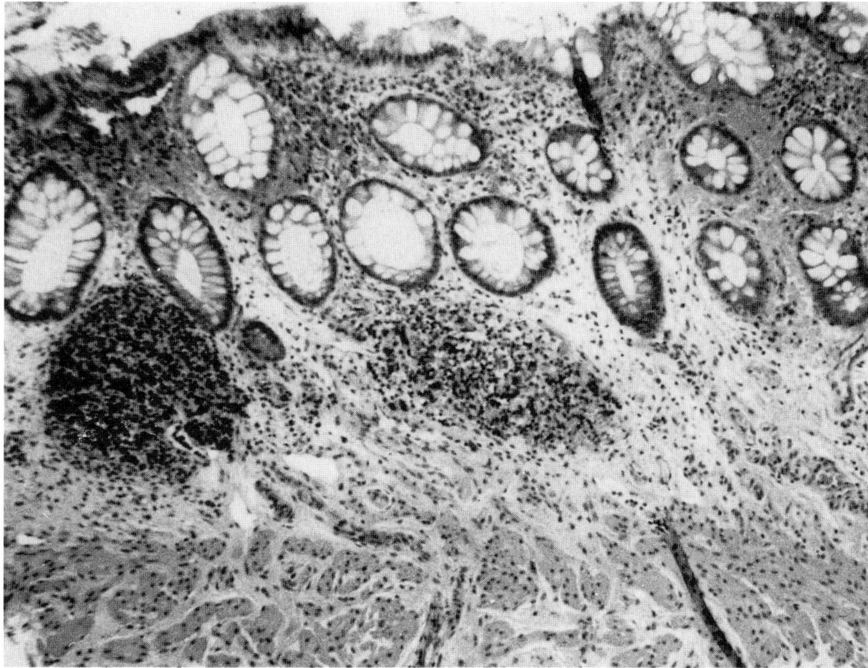

Fig. 9-7. Normal mucosa in the lower part of the rectum. Compared to the rest of the large intestine (see Fig. 9-1), there are crypt shortening with separation from the muscularis, numerous small lymphoid aggregates at the base, and a thickened muscle layer. In the more proximal parts of the rectum and colon, the presence of these features would signify a chronic colitis.

Table 9-3. Effects of Preparatory Solutions and Procedures on the Mucosa

Flattening of surface epithelium
Loss of mucus granules from goblet cells
Edema and hemorrhage in lamina propria
Rare neutrophil

noted are a variable loss of mucus granules from the epithelial cells and an occasional flattening of the surface epithelium. All of these features are distinguished from actual inflammatory disorders by the absence of degeneration of the epithelium and of a neutrophilic reaction. The edema in the lamina propria can also cause a variable shifting of the mononuclear cells in this compartment, suggesting the appearance of increases of the cells; the absence of other features of chronic disease helps to exclude this diagnosis.

General Pathologic Features

Inflammatory lesions of the colon and rectum are seen as a direct consequence of a large variety of lesions, such as infections and immunologic disorders, and also occur as a secondary consequence to other conditions, such as ischemia and mechanical disorders (Table 9-1). As noted above, it is essential that the normal structure and any variations, as well as the effects of preparatory enemas and biopsy procedures, be well appreciated before rendering a diagnosis of acute colitis or proctitis.

Acute Colitis

The features of acute or active disease include actual degeneration of the surface or crypt epithelium in conjunction with the presence of numerous neutrophils in the epithelial area and in the lamina propria (Table 9-4). At the extreme, there can occur erosions and ulcers (Fig. 9-9). Features of repair include regeneration of the crypts and surface epithelium and the potential for the development of an inflammatory pseudopolyp. Depending on the particular etiology, there also may be increases in other inflammatory cells including eosinophils, macrophages, and lymphocytes. The general architecture of the straight crypts without extensive branching is typically retained in an acute colitis.

Chronic Colitis

There are many features of chronic colitis or proctitis[22] (Fig. 9-10). Least helpful is the simple appearance of mononuclear inflammatory cells in the lamina propria, since these are normally located in this region and may appear increased due to small samples or the effects of enema-induced edema. This feature is only useful when there is a great increase in the amount of cells, usually associated with an increase in the number of eosinophils as well. Other more certain findings of chronic disease include complex branching of the crypts, their separation from the muscularis mucosae, a villiform surface, and the presence of Paneth cells in regions beyond the most proximal part of the colon. Less often seen are pyloric metaplasia, a great increase in the endocrine cells, and fibrosis within the lamina propria. These various features have been best cataloged in cases of chronic idiopathic inflammatory bowel disease, but would apply for any chronic disorder. When documented, they serve to exclude an acute lesion.

Stages of Colitis

All of the inflammatory disorders can be categorized into the stages of acute colitis or proctitis, of chronic inactive (quiescent) colitis corresponding to a remission, and of chronic active colitis at times of clinical relapse. It is typically possible by biopsy to indicate the major stage but not the exact

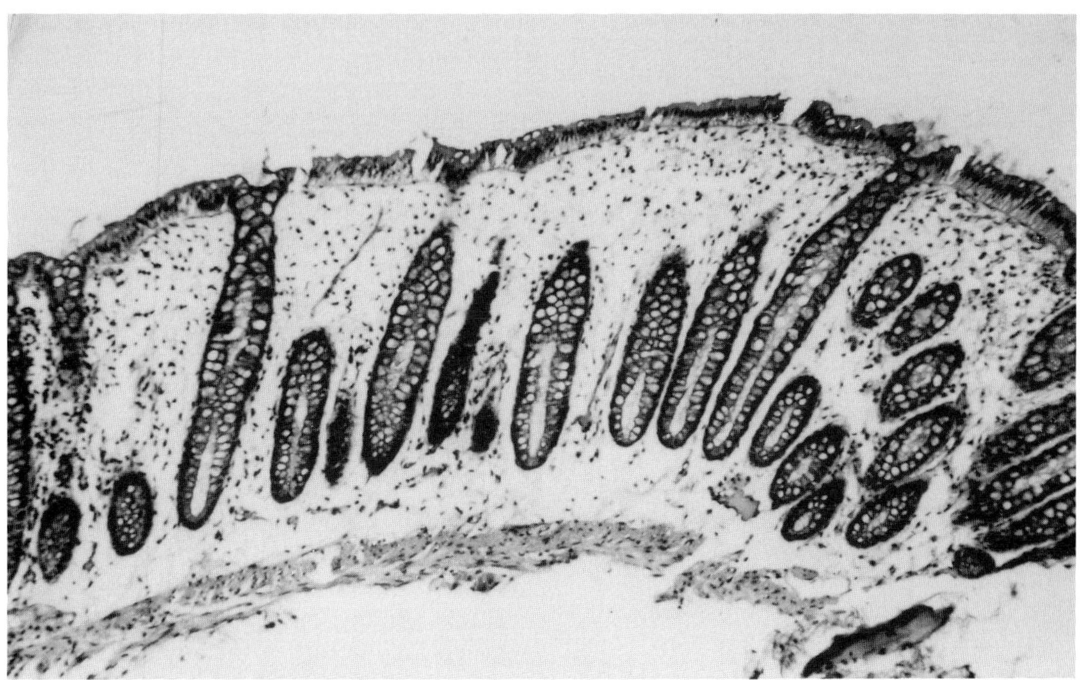

Fig. 9-8. Effect on the colonic mucosa of oral solutions used to prepare for colonoscopy. There is marked edema of the lamina propria, causing separation of the crypts, without any increase of inflammatory cells or damage of the epithelium.

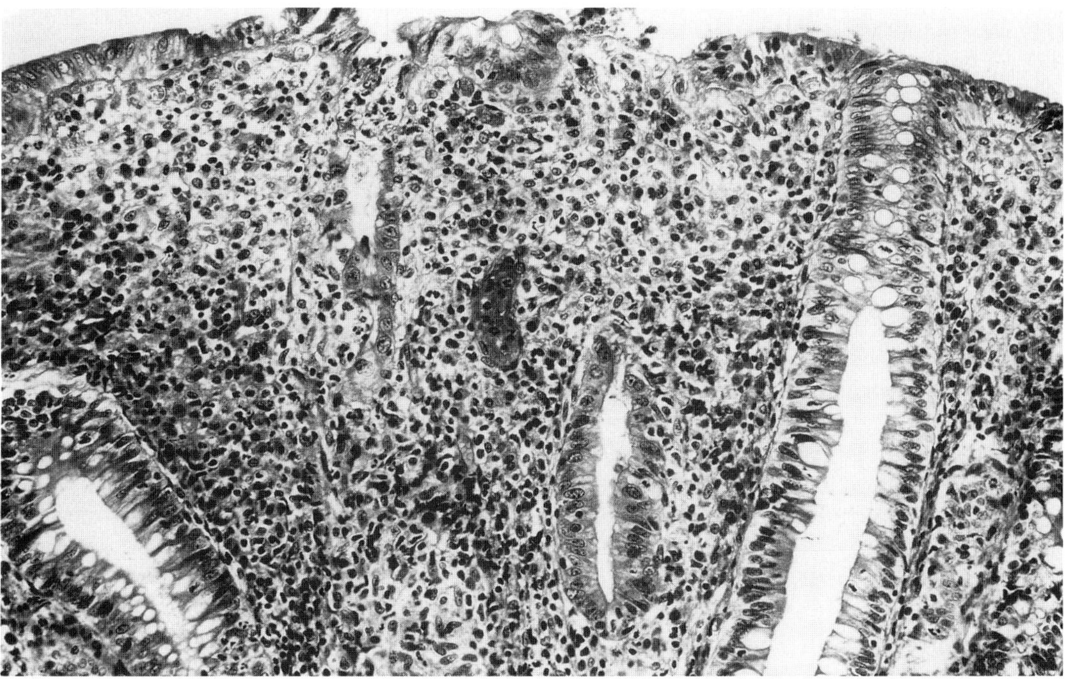

Fig. 9-9. Acute colitis due to a bacterial infection. Noted is a marked increase of neutrophils in the lamina propria, with focal extension into the surface and crypt epithelia. The normal crypt architecture is maintained (× 210).

Table 9-4. Biopsy Features of Colitis

Acute or active colitis
Degeneration of surface and crypt epithelium
Neutrophilic infiltrate in crypts and lamina propria
Ulceration and granulation tissue
Chronic colitis
Crypt irregularity due to budding and shortening
Villiform surface
Paneth cell metaplasia
Large increase in mononuclear inflammatory cells and eosinophils
Small lymphoid nodules and plasma cells beneath the base of crypts
Variable features: increased endocrine cells, pyloric gland metaplasia, fibrosis

etiology. Thus the finding of an acute colitis could represent an infectious disorder or the early stage of an idiopathic inflammatory bowel disease; similarly, the finding of a chronic active colitis may signify ulcerative colitis, ischemic disease, or any other chronic condition.

DEVELOPMENTAL DISORDERS

Developmental disorders of the colon and rectum are more often identified in younger patients and are typically seen in pediatric pathology services.

Cysts and Stenoses

A variety of retention and of duplication cysts can occur in the colon and rectum. These are usually located in the wall but may cause mucosal problems by bulges and by rare ulceration. Endoscopic biopsies are rarely obtained. Exceptionally, tumors can develop in duplication cysts, showing a variety of cell types including squamous differentiation.

Atresia and congenital stenoses are much less common than in the small bowel.[23] These typically present with obstructive effects, leading to secondary inflammatory lesions that may be assessed by biopsies (described below in the section on "Mechanical Obstruction").

Heterotopic Tissues

Heterotopic tissues are generally rare in the large intestine.

Stomach Tissue

Foci of gastric corpus tissue occur in the rectum[24, 25] (see Table 2-5). The gastric corpus tissue is well formed and can function, leading to production of acid and pepsins.[26] Because of the normal stasis in this region, the acid production can lead to ulceration that typically occurs in the adjacent colonic mucosa, which is otherwise unprotected from the acid.[27–29] It is common to see deep ulcerations and fistulae in this region.[30] These lesions are most often noted in children. Biopsies are done to establish the ulceration and to exclude other causes, such as infections or tumors. The finding of intact gastric corpus mucosa is needed to secure the diagnosis, but this is usually not obtained until there is a resection of the area. Occasionally noted on the surface of the epithelium are adherent *Helicobacter pylori,* but these do not appear to contribute to the inflammation.[31] As described in other chapters, heterotopic gastric mucosa is more commonly seen in the duodenum and in the upper part of the esophagus[32, 33] (see Fig. 6-7).

Other Tissues

Rarely noted in the large intestine are foci of pancreatic tissue and of salivary gland remnants[34, 35] (see Fig. 4-8A). These do not ordinarily cause clinical problems and are not usually detected by biopsy.

AGANGLIONOSIS

Hirschsprung's Disease

The most common form of aganglionosis is Hirschsprung's disease, in which there is a short segment of lower sigmoid or rectum devoid of ganglia.[36–38] This area becomes constricted and the proximal part of the colon shows the effects of obstruction, leading to dilation and secondary inflammatory damage of the mucosa. This typically appears in young infants, and biopsies are commonly employed together with manometry to make the diagnosis.[39, 40]

Biopsy Features

Since the ganglia are concentrated in the submucosa, a deeper, aspiration-like biopsy is often needed. Indeed, some have formally recommended that there be a transmural biopsy. Nevertheless, as an initial screening procedure, the more superficial type with submucosa is usually sufficient. Sought are well formed ganglia in the submucosa (Fig. 9-6). They also may be rarely noted within the lamina propria. There are many stains that can be used to accent the ganglia and nerves, including those for acetyl cholinesterase, for neuron-specific enolase, and for nitric oxide synthetase.[41–45] In cases of Hirschsprung's disease, there is typically a proliferation of nerves in addition to the loss of the ganglia (Fig. 9-11). There also are variations of the disorder in which occasional ganglia are found together with prominent nerve proliferation.[46] On study of the biopsies, multiple levels should be examined, looking for the presence of ganglia and for any alteration of the nerves. Their definite finding serves to exclude the diagnosis. If no ganglia are seen, deeper transmural biopsies or manometry may be needed to establish the diagnosis.

As a result of the obstruction and stasis, an inflammation can be noted in the mucosa proximal to the obstruction.[47] Biopsies reveal nonspecific, acute colitis that must be distinguished from infections and allergic disease.

Other Types

There are rare forms of aganglionosis in which the segment of colon without ganglia is much longer. This can be limited to the left colon, show segmental distribution, or involve the entire colon. Biopsy in such cases is largely used to determine the extent of the disease and is more often obtained from colostomy sites or from the edges of surgical resections.

MOTOR AND MECHANICAL DISORDERS

There are many obstructive conditions, either of a mechanical or motor nature, which can lead to secondary damage of the mucosa and an inflammatory lesion. It is thought that this is due to increased pressure, secondary ischemic damage, and resultant inflammatory changes.

MECHANICAL OBSTRUCTION

Causes and Location

There are several causes of mechanical obstruction, including atresia and aganglionic segments in infants and children, volvulus and hernias, inflammatory strictures, and tumors. Whatever the cause, the proximal colon can become dilated and develop secondary pressure-induced ischemic damage.[48–50] This can lead to hemorrhage and necrosis, ulceration and fibrosis. The location of the obstructive effects is highly variable and not necessarily just next to the narrowed portion of the colon. Indeed, the lesions can skip several centimeters and even be distantly lo-

A

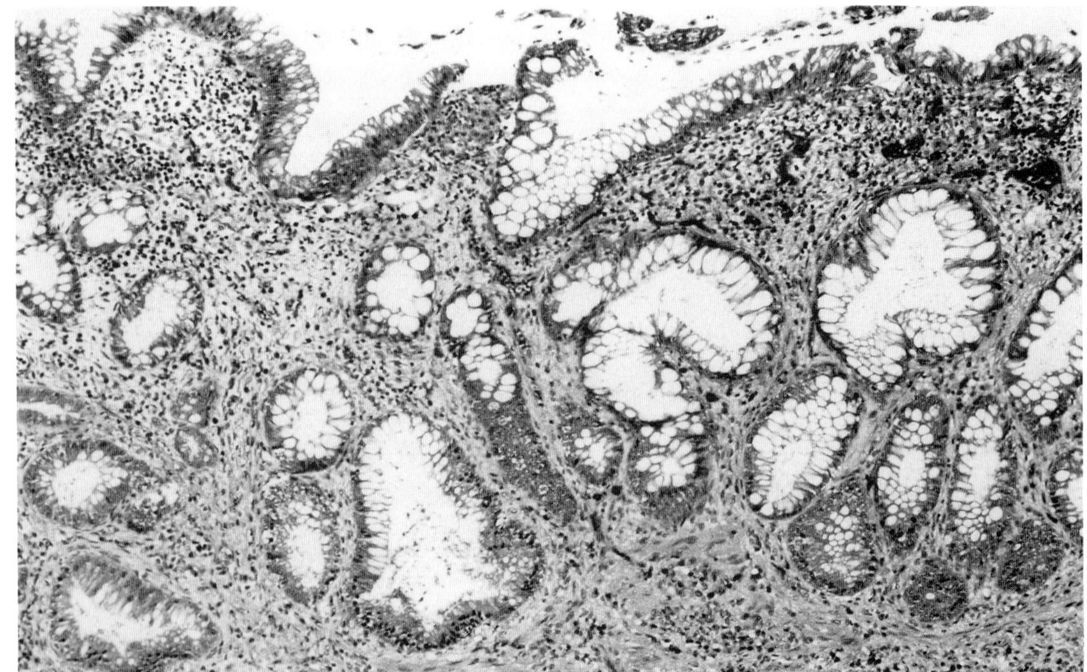

B

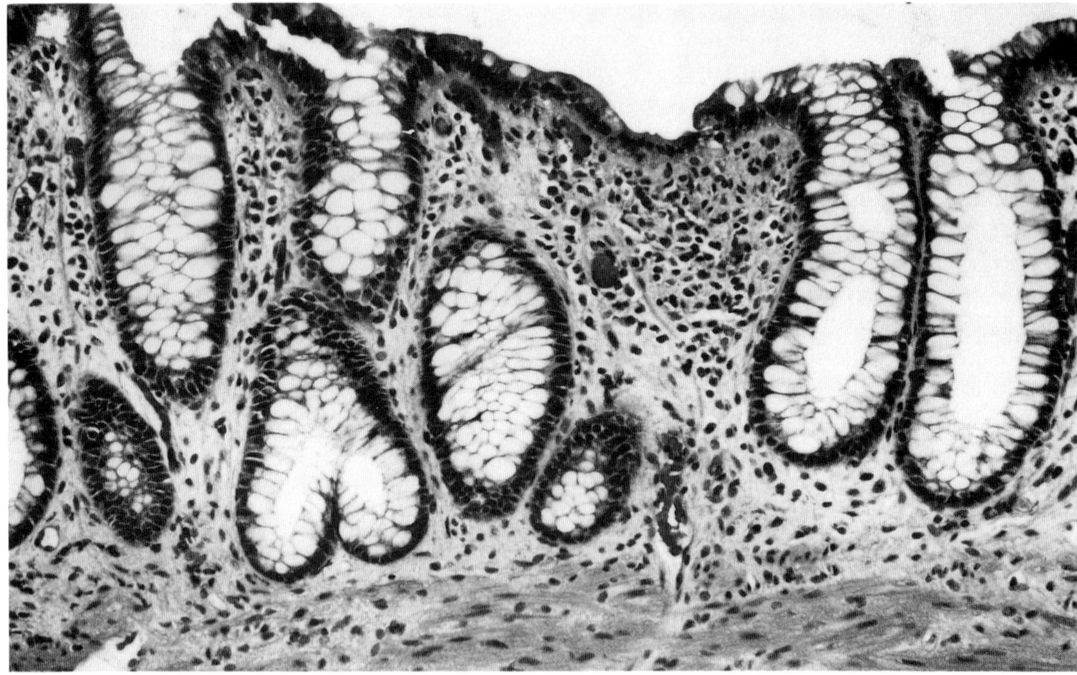

Fig. 9-10. Examples of mucosal changes in chronic colitis. **(A)** Irregular architecture, due to a marked branching of the crypts. The surface appears at the top (×105). **(B)** Atrophy of the mucosa, showing shortened crypts (right) and branching (left). There is no active inflammation (× 210). (*Figure continues.*)

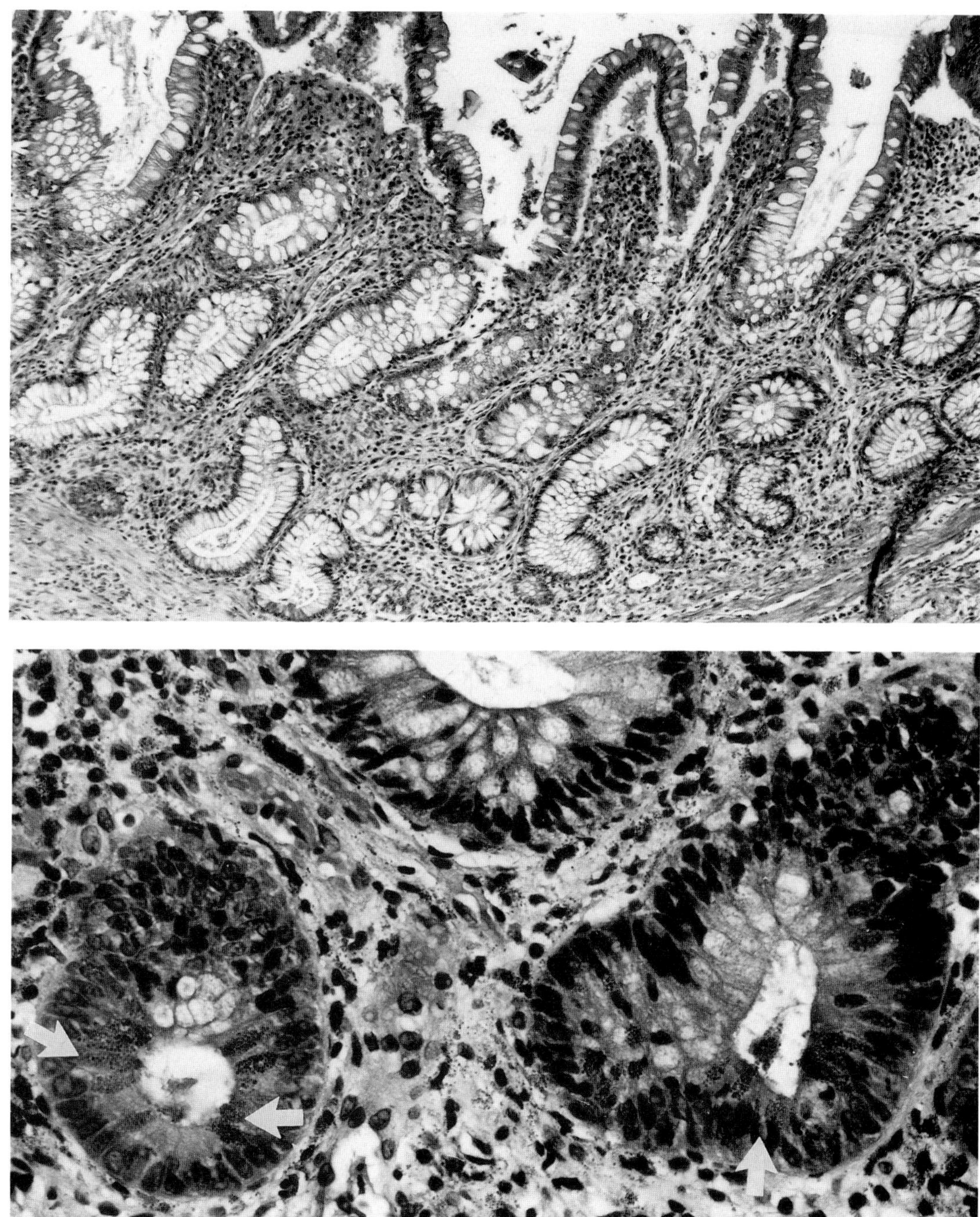

Fig. 9-10 (*Continued*). **(C)** Villiform surface (top), resulting from increased edema and inflammation in the lamina propria (×105). **(D)** Paneth cell metaplasia, present in the crypts (arrows). There also are many eosinophils in the lamina propria, seen as finely granulated cells (× 425).

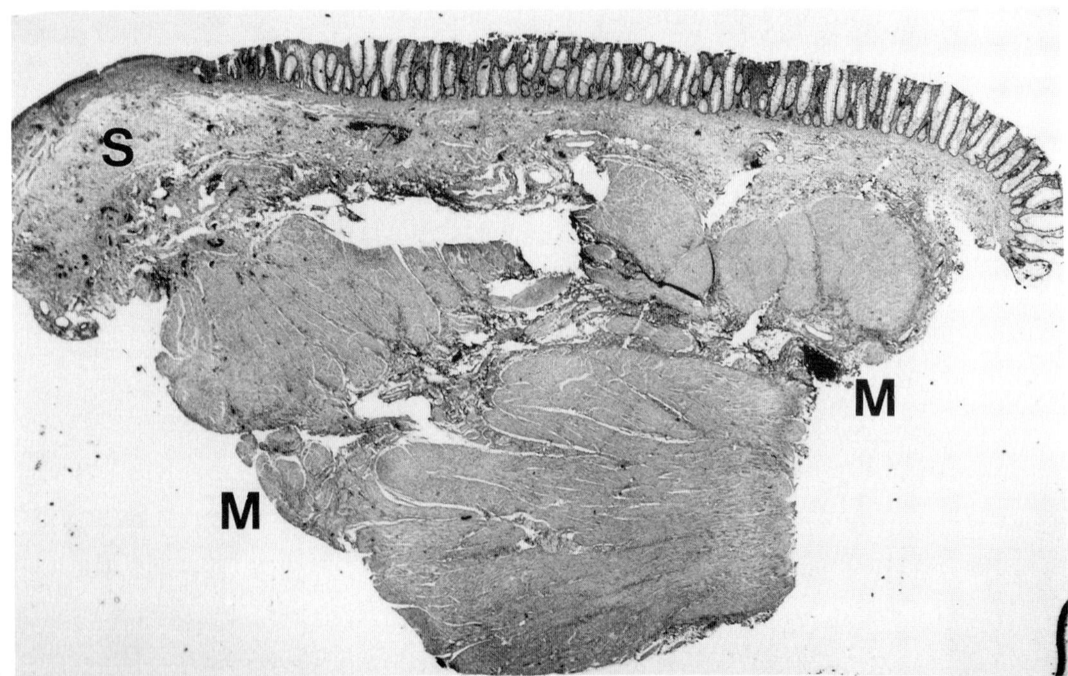

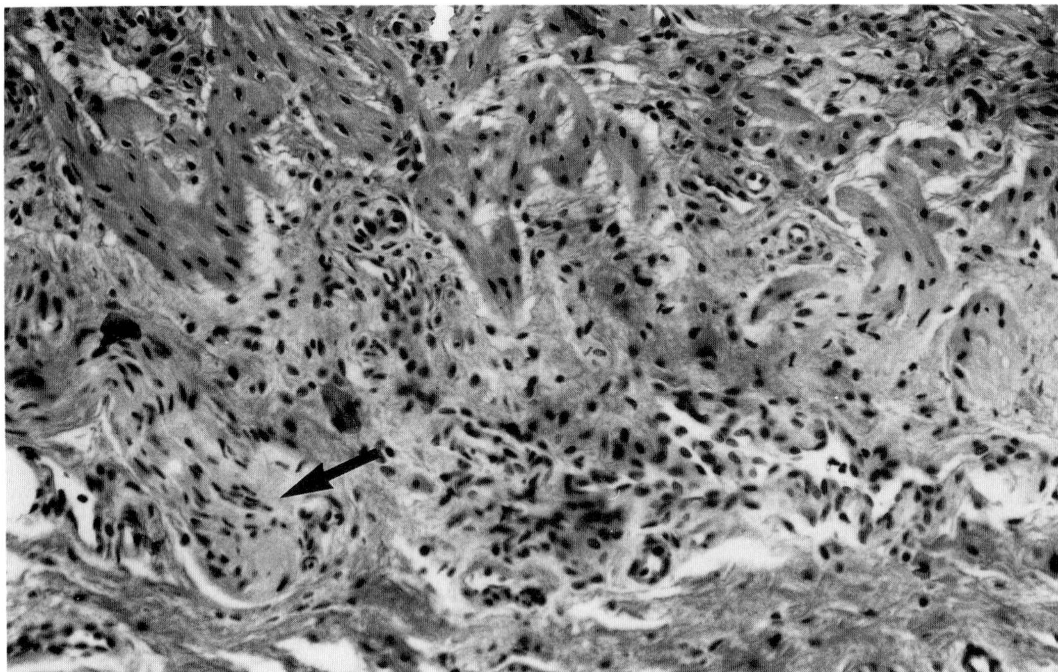

Fig. 9-11. Hirschsprung's disease of the colon. **(A)** Transmural biopsy, with mucosal surface appearing at the top. Such samples are needed to confirm the absence of ganglia in the submucosal (S) and myenteric (M) regions (× 14). **(B)** Submucosa, showing increased nerves (arrow) but no ganglia. A portion of the muscularis mucosae appears at the top (× 210). Compare with Figure 9-6 of normal colon. (*Figure continues.*)

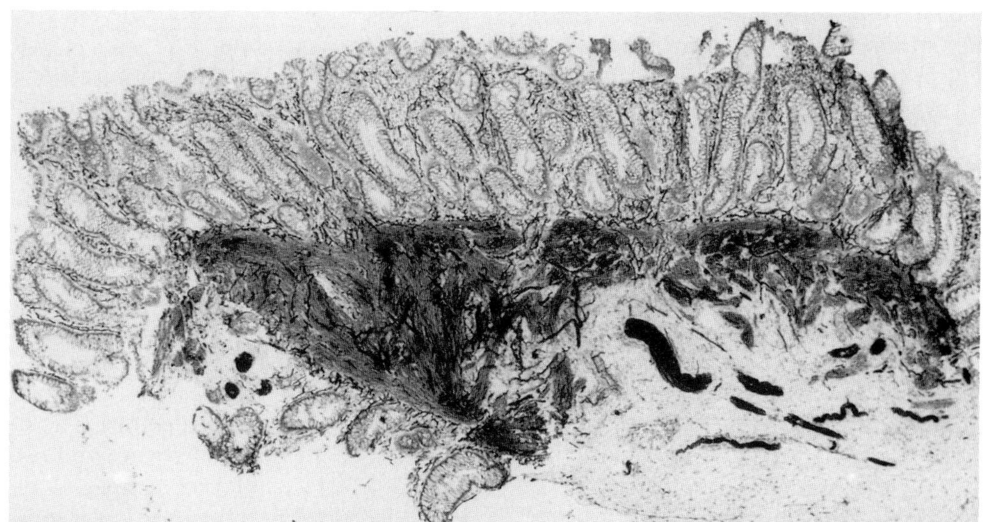

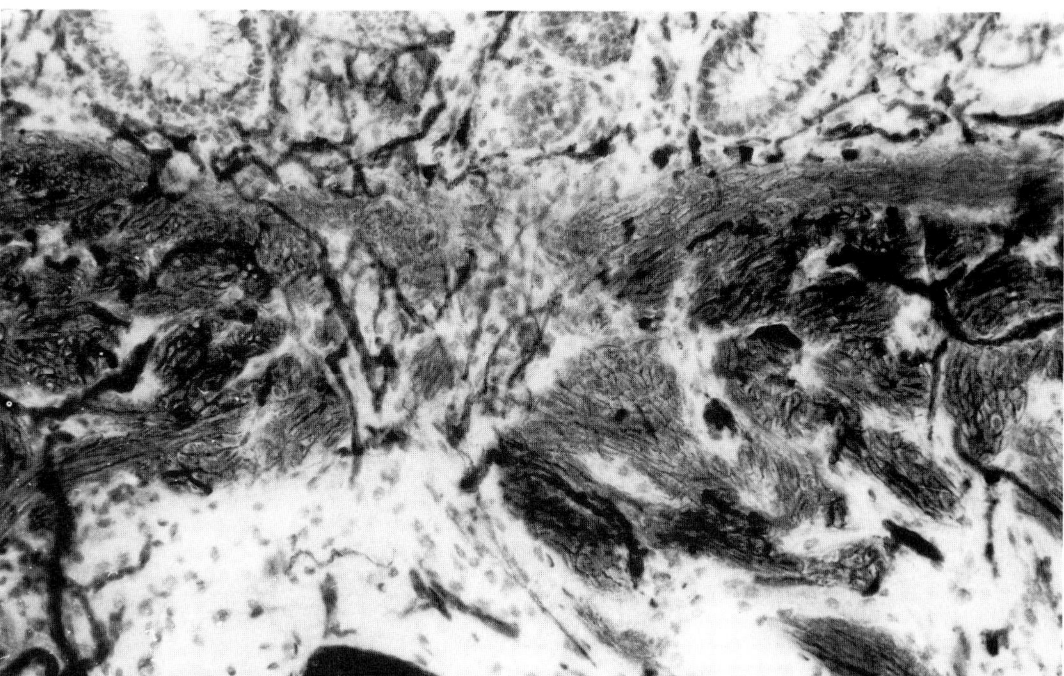

Fig. 9-11 (*Continued*). **(C)** Biopsy stained for acetylcholinesterase, demonstrating the enhanced staining of the hyperplastic nerves in the submucosa. The mucosa appears at the top (× 42). **(D)** Closer view of the hyperplastic nerves, stained for acetylcholinesterase. There are no ganglia (× 210).

cated in the cecum and ascending colon. The site is probably determined by local vasculature and other physical parameters, such as the natural diameter of an area; the effects of pressure may be greater in regions with greater diameter, such as the cecum.

Biopsy Features

Biopsies are usually obtained of the more distal obstructive lesion. Occasionally, they are also taken from the more proximal region, and it is important to distinguish this secondary obstructive lesion from a primary inflammatory condition in which stenosis then develops. Most helpful is the finding of no inflammatory lesion distal to the obstruction. The biopsy features of the obstructive colitis are entirely nonspecific, revealing acute or chronic colitis with prominent ulceration and variable fibrosis. The lesions usually extend only into the submucosa but can exceptionally spread through the full wall with the development of fissures or fistulae, simulating Crohn's disease.[51] The precise diagnosis requires the delineation of an obstructive lesion.

Pseudo-Obstruction

Causes

In cases of pseudo-obstruction, there is obstruction to flow but the absence of an actual mechanical disorder. This is due to a variety of disorders affecting the nerves or muscles of the bowel wall, which may be primary and familial or of a secondary nature[52–54] (see Table 7-3). This condition can be seen in several endocrine disorders and as a consequence of drugs.[55] It is also observed when there is significant loss of the musculature due to systemic sclerosis, to the deposition of amyloid material, or the presence of other abnormal connective tissue substances.[56–59] Whatever the particular cause, there results a marked dilation of the colon leading to secondary ischemic and inflammatory changes in the mucosa.

Biopsy Features

Biopsies may be obtained and are usually nonspecific. The effects are usually milder than in obstructive colitis, showing increased inflammatory cells in the lamina propria and uncommon erosions or ulcers of the mucosa. The diagnosis is typically dependent on the clinical information or examination of the surgical specimen. Exceptionally, deeper biopsies of the intestinal wall may reveal the characteristic lesion of a myopathy or infiltrative disorder.[60] Frequently, patients with these disorders also have similar effects in the small intestine and, occasionally, in the esophagus.

Diverticular Disease

Common Features

Diverticular disease is a common acquired condition of the colon characterized by outpouchings, which tend to increase with age and to be more heavily concentrated in the left portion.[61] They are thought to result from the effects of increased intraluminal pressure and possibly accentuated by the increasing constipation associated with older patients.[62, 63] Nevertheless, diverticula can also be seen in younger patients, where they are more often on the right side. A major problem is the potential for perforation of the diverticula, leading to foci of peridiverticulitis or of larger abscesses. In such cases, the patients typically present with a localized area of colonic narrowing and irritation, and the differential diagnosis is that of a focal or segmental colitis; included are diverticular disease, Crohn's disease, and ischemic lesions. Endoscopy can be of particular help in distinguishing these conditions, since both Crohn's and ischemic disease are associated with intrinsic involvement of the mucosa whereas diverticular disease more often shows a normal mucosa or at most a focal crypt abscess.

Uncommon Features

The edges of the diverticula may be slightly raised, simulating small polyps. This may become exaggerated due to further inversion of the diverticula or prolapse of the mucosal folds.[64, 65] Uncommonly, a case of diverticular disease may show more numerous patches of inflammation, simulating segmental colitis, and it is not clear whether this is a variant of idiopathic inflammatory bowel disease in conjunction with the diverticular disease.[66] The diverticula can also be associated with a massive bleed, and these are more often seen in lesions involving the right side of the colon.[67, 68] The diagnosis is typically established by the clinical and angiographic information, and biopsies are not obtained.

VASCULAR DISORDERS

VARICES AND VASCULAR MALFORMATIONS

Varices

Hemorrhoidal varices are very common and present with pain or acute bleeding.[69] The varices are typically located at the junction of the anal and rectal mucosa and appear as protruded veins with secondary erosions and thromboses. Biopsies are not ordinarily obtained. An enhancement of these varices and their location in other parts of the colon can be seen in patients with portal hypertension. Their presence in the other sites is accentuated if the patient had previous surgery and the development of fibrous adhesions.[70] Biopsies may reveal more widespread venular dilation in the lamina propria, which has been called a *vascular* or *portal colopathy*[71, 72] (Fig. 9-12). These effects of portal hypertension are much more commonly seen in the esophagus, stomach, and small bowel.

Vascular Ectasia

An important cause of hemorrhage, particularly in older patients, is vascular ectasia, or angiodysplasia.[73–77] This is typically present in the cecum or ascending colon and is thought to be due to localized pressure that leads to dilated veins and to secondary arteriovenous channels. The patients present with spontaneous massive hemorrhage, and the diagnosis was formerly largely established by angiography or by examination of surgical specimens. However, at the time of the acute hemorrhage, or within a few days, endoscopy is increasingly being performed to localize such lesions and to eliminate them by cautery. This has resulted in a substantial reduction in the number of needed resections.[76] Such lesions should be sought in any older patient who presents with major hemorrhage and lacks an obvious tumor or history of inflammatory bowel disease. Biopsies are uncommonly taken, and reveal localized foci of marked dilation of venules in the lamina propria and, variably, associated clot on the surface (Fig. 9-13).

Vascular ectasias in other parts of the large bowel are uncommon.[78] They can be seen in patients with generalized telangiectatic disorders, but the lesions tend to be more prominent in the proximal and midportion of the gut. The diagnoses are generally secured by the history and the endoscopic appearance and biopsies are not obtained.

Vascular Tumors

There are many vascular tumors that can affect the large bowel, as in other parts of the gut. These include hemangiomas, Kaposi's sarcoma, angiosarcoma, and lymphangiomas. More often seen and biopsied at endoscopy are patients with Kaposi's sarcoma, which can occur in any part of the gut. The biopsy is highly characteristic, revealing closely packed spindle cells with nuclear atypism and evidence of fresh and old hemorrhage. The lesions tend to be deep and may show only a small fragment on the biopsy (see Ch. 10 for further details).

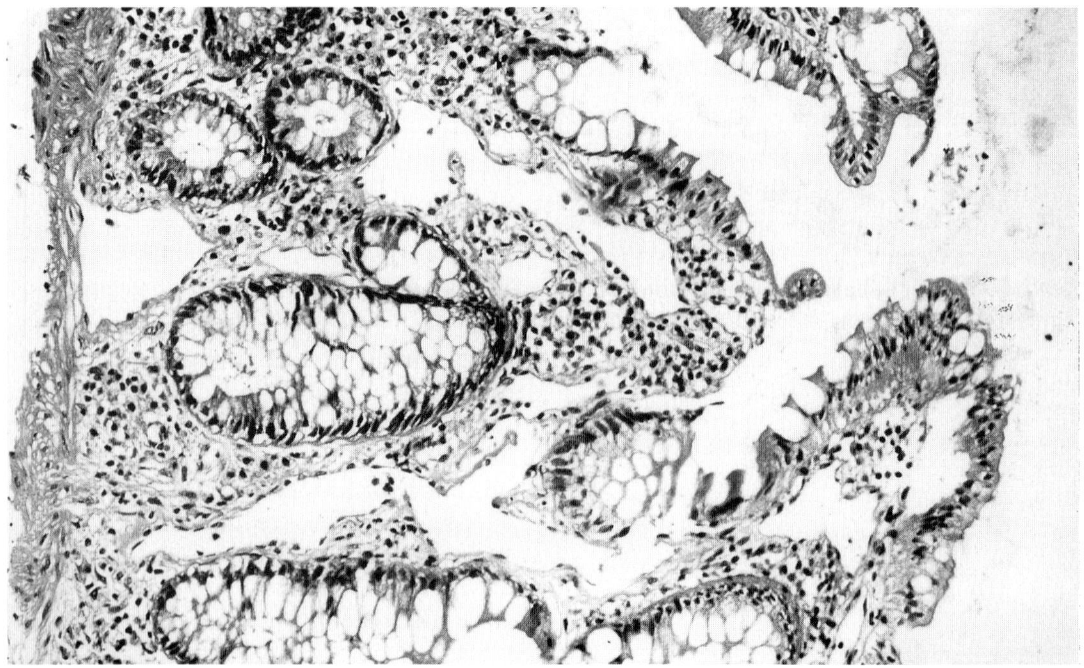

Fig. 9-12. Congestive colopathy. Noted are marked dilation of the venules in the lamina propria. The muscularis appears at the left (× 210).

Small Vessel Diseases

Vasculitis

As in other parts of the gut, the vessels of the large intestine can be affected by vasculitis that is caused by a variety of diseases[69, 79, 80] (Table 9-5). This can result in localized or more extensive areas of ischemic damage of the overlying mucosa as represented by hemorrhages, ulcers, and infarcts, and these lesions are readily detected by endoscopic biopsy (Fig. 9-14). The diagnosis of the vascular lesion by biopsy requires a deeper type of sample to include the submucosa where the major vessels that can be affected are present. These are best obtained by aspiration-type biopsies of the rectum. Often, the diagnosis is identified by the clinical information and the biopsy of other sites, such as the skin. Nevertheless, the lesions are present in the colon and could probably be readily accessed, if needed.

The conditions that are most often associated with a generalized vasculitis that includes involvement of the gut are systemic lupus erythematosis and rheumatoid arthritis.[81–83] Indeed, it has been suggested that patients with rheumatoid disease may show vasculitis in up to 10 to 15 percent of cases. Other causes that less commonly or rarely affect the colon include polyarteritis nodosa, allergic vasculitis, Henoch-Schönlein's disease and Wegener's granulomatosis.[84–87] In the hemolytic-uremic syndrome, which is more often seen in children, the cases may present with marked edema and hemorrhage of the colonic mucosa.[88, 89] The diagnosis is usually established by the general clinical findings and surgical inspection rather than by biopsy.

Other Vessel Diseases

Vascular changes that are probably of a secondary nature are also seen in many other inflammatory diseases, and are especially prominent in Crohn's disease.[90] These are ordinarily present in the deeper parts of the

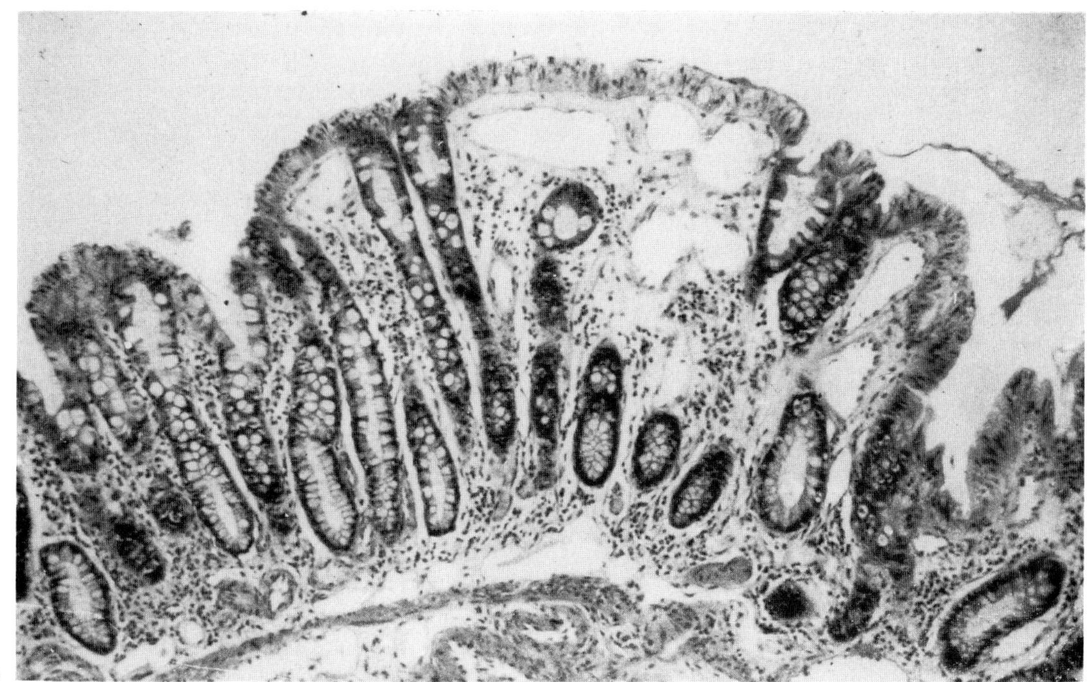

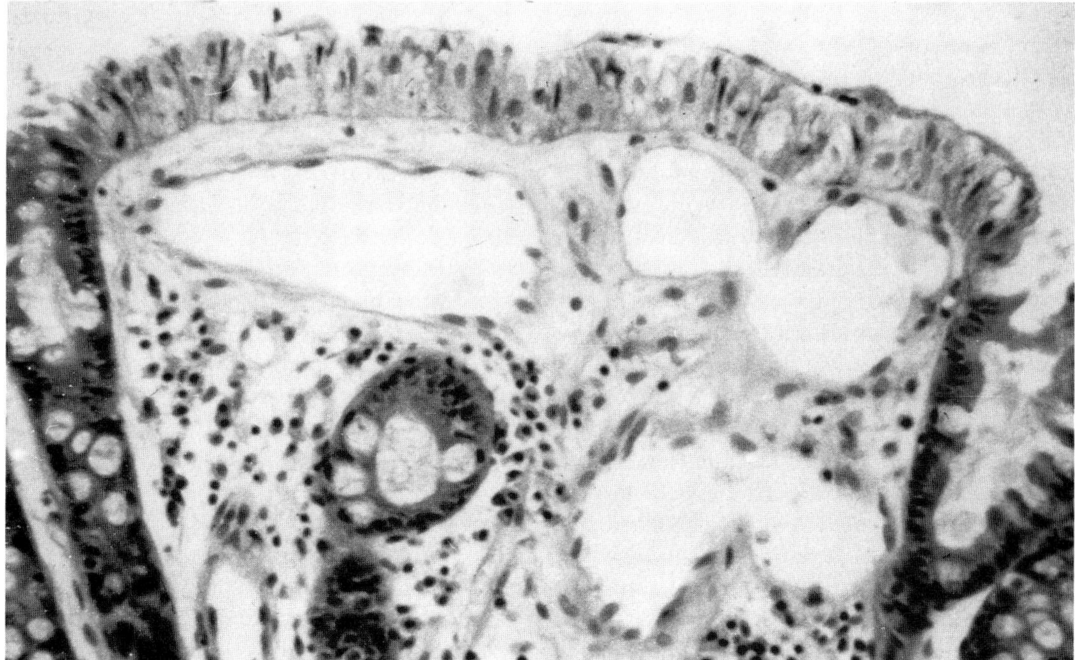

Fig. 9-13. Vascular ectasia (angiodysplasia) of the colon. **(A)** There is a localized area of dilated vessels in the mucosa. The submucosa appears at the bottom. **(B)** Closer view, showing the dilated venules.

Table 9-5. Causes of Intestinal Vasculitis

Systemic lupus erythematosus
Rheumatoid arthritis
Polyarteritis nodosa
Henoch-Schönlein's disease
Hemolytic-uremic syndrome
Churg-Strauss vasculitis
Wegener's granulomatosis

wall and are not seen by biopsy. The small vessels can also be affected by infiltration of substances such as amyloid (see "Depositions" under "Miscellaneous Conditions") and by atheromatous emboli[91–94] (Fig. 9-15). The emboli lead to localized areas of ischemia, resulting in ulcers and inflammatory polyps.

Ischemic Disease

Causes and General Effects

Ischemia of the large bowel can have many causes, including a general reduction of blood flow due to shock, development of thromboses or emboli in the arterial system, or the presence of venous compression as a consequence of hernias and other mechanical conditions[95–97] (Table 9-6). Rare causes include trauma, infections, and vasculitis affecting the principal arteries. Whatever the cause, the effects are generally stereotyped, resulting in a progressive damage of the bowel wall that begins in the mucosa.[98, 99] The mildest lesion affects the mucosa only and is initially associated with necrosis and hemorrhage.[100] Following reflow there is superficial ulceration of the mucosa together with a marked neutrophilic reaction. By the time most biopsies are secured, the examples reveal this inflammatory lesion that has been termed *ischemic colitis.* These lesions, when limited to the mucosa, are reversible but may recur. With more prolonged ischemia the ulcers extend into the submucosa and deeper parts of the wall, and are associated with persistence and with the development of fibrosis and the potential for inflammatory strictures. The most severe cases show transmural infarction that may perforate. These various lesions can be categorized as *mucosal infarcts,* as *mural infarcts,* and as *transmural infarcts.*[99]

Location of Disease

The location of the lesion is highly variable, and often localized or segmental. The presence of a dual circulation from the superior and inferior mesenteric vessels favors that there be a greater number of lesions in the splenic flexure region, which is a watershed area of the two circulations. Also, the lower sigmoid and the rectum ordinarily have a dual vascular supply. Nevertheless, probably due to local small vessel disease, ischemic lesions have now been seen in practically all locations of the colon including the rectum, and the diagnosis cannot be discounted simply because of multiple circulations.[101, 102]

Biopsy Features

Biopsy features are generally nonspecific. In the earliest mucosal lesions, they reveal the characteristic necrosis and hemorrhage with minimal inflammation, but biopsies are rarely obtained at such an early time (Fig. 9-16). More often, they show erosions and acute inflammation. The findings are very similar to the lesions seen in antibiotic-associated colitis due to *Clostridium difficile.* They can be separated from chronic idiopathic inflammatory bowel disease in the early stage because of the lack of complex branching. However, when the lesions extend into the wall there is the propensity for chronic colitis, and the features can no longer be easily distinguished from IBD. Biopsy in these more severe cases shows irregular glands, occasional inflammatory pseudopolyps, and fibrosis.

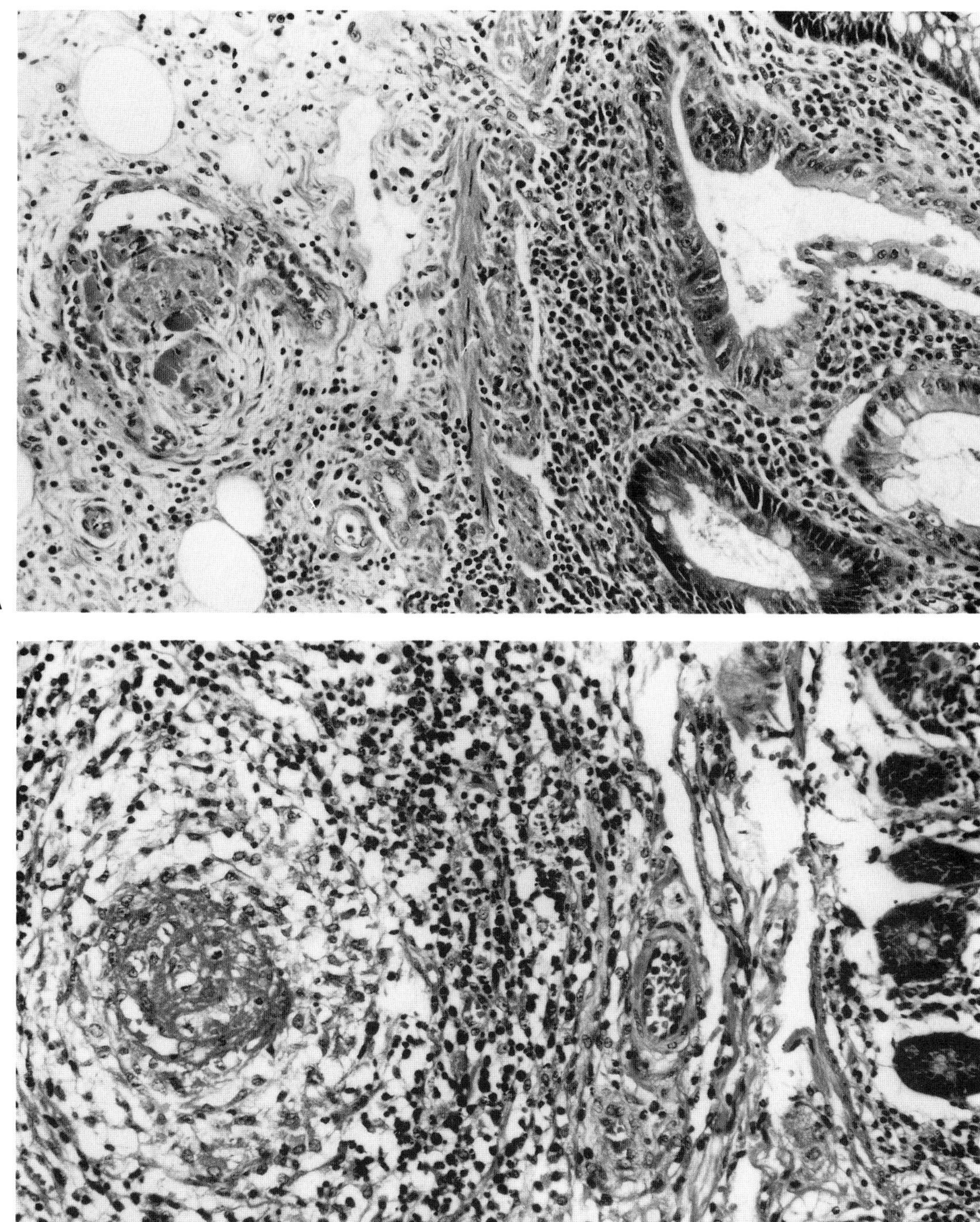

Fig. 9-14. Examples of vasculitis. **(A)** The submucosal vein (left) shows a damaged wall and contains an organizing thrombus. There appears surrounding inflammation in the submucosa and mucosa (right) (× 210). **(B)** In the submucosa (left) is a necrotic artery with marked inflammation. The base of the mucosa appears at the right (× 210).

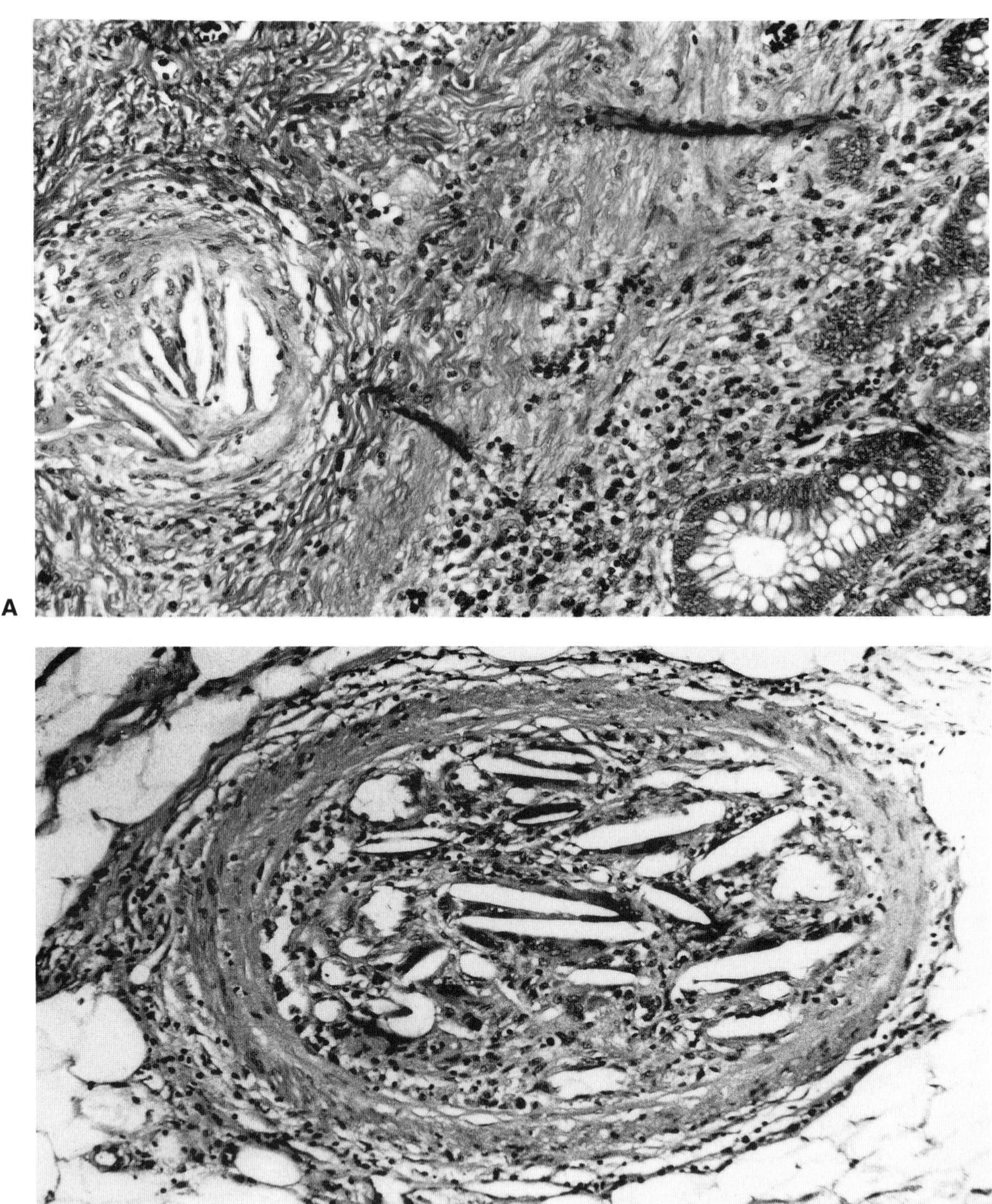

Fig. 9-15. Atherosclerotic embolus. **(A)** The submucosal artery (left) is filled with slit-shaped spaces that represent cholesterol material. The bottom of the mucosa appears at the right (× 210). **(B)** Closer view of a submucosal artery, showing the atheromatous material filling the lumen.

Table 9-6. Ischemic Disease of the Colon and Rectum

Causes
Low arterial blood flow
Arterial atherosclerosis, thrombi, and emboli
Venous thrombi and compression
Vasculitis and trauma
Effects
Mucosal infarct
Mural infarct
Transmural infarct
Complications
Reversible but recurrent
Persistence and stricture
Perforation

Related Conditions

There are many other conditions that are thought to have an ischemic basis as either the sole or the contributing factor in their development. These include necrotizing enterocolitis seen in young infants, the effects of sickle cell disease, pseudomembraneous colitis due to *C. difficile,* and the results of some other infections and of radiation.[69, 103–106] In all of these diseases there is constriction or narrowing of vessels leading to the ischemic effects. The cases are associated with prominent hemorrhage, necrosis, and fibrosis. Biopsies are entirely nonspecific, showing the inflammatory features, and the exact diagnosis requires the full clinical information.

INFECTIONS

There are a wide variety of infections that involve the colon and rectum, and these are largely diagnosed by smears and cultures of stool specimens (Table 9-7).

General features

The general and specific effects of the various infectious agents are described in detail in Chapter 2, and the major features are summarized here. The effects are highly dependent on the type of action of the organisms, whether they induce necrosis and a chemotactic reaction, are associated with an immunologic response, or depend on toxin production.[107] These variations are best demonstrated in the bacterial infections (see Table 7-6). Otherwise, the inflammatory reactions are of a general nature and similar to those seen in other conditions in the colon.

Diagnosis

The diagnosis is dependent on the finding of the particular microorganism, in either smears or cultures of stool specimens, or within biopsy material. The biopsies are generally obtained to document the presence of a colitis and to identify or exclude an infection.[108, 109] Endoscopy reveals a focal colitis in the early stages and more diffuse lesions later in the course. The biopsies in the early stages of most bacterial infections show prominent cryptitis and neutrophilic infiltrate that is concentrated in the superficial portion of the mucosa.

Some of the agents can be readily seen on H & E preparations, including the viral inclusions, fungal and most protozoal organisms, and helminthic ova. The special stains that are of particular help are Gram stain for the identification of Microsporidia and several bacteria, the PAS reaction or methenamine silver stain for most fungi, and the acid-fast stain for tubercle bacilli and *Mycobacterium avium* complex. Electron microscopy is especially helpful in detection and delineation of the various protozoa.

Cases with Increased Frequency

Homosexual males have an increased prevalence of numerous microorganisms in the colon, associated with increased episodes of diarrhea and dysentery.[110, 111] Most of the lesions noted are not unique but simply represent an increased frequency, such as examples of bacterial and amoebic infections. Also noted are more venereal infections in-

A

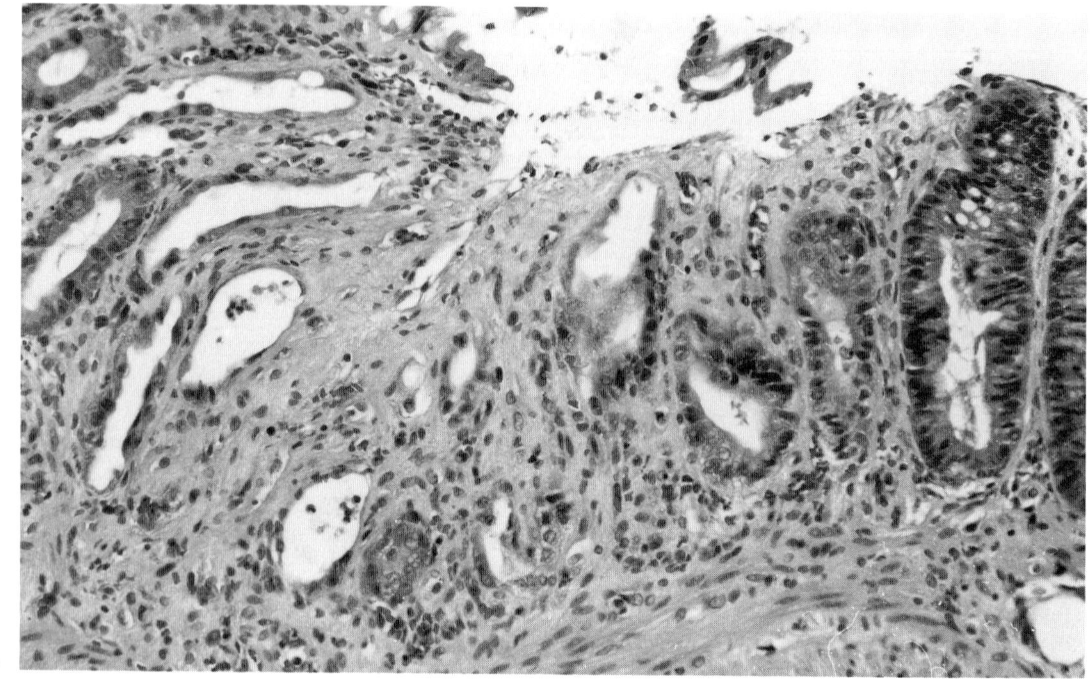

B

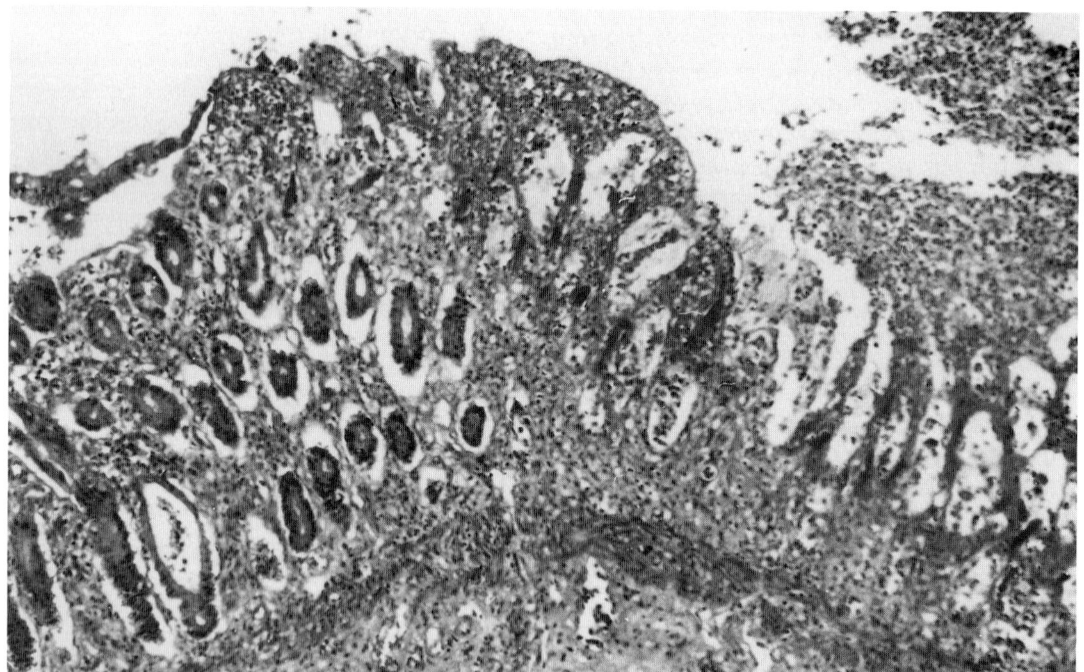

Fig. 9-16. Ischemic colitis. **(A)** Early lesion, showing dropout of crypts and spotty hemorrhage in the lamina propria without acute inflammation (× 210). **(B)** Later lesion. Revealed are more prominent necrosis, hemorrhage in the lamina propria, and focal inflammatory exudate (right) resembling pseudomembranous colitis (× 105).

Table 9-7. Infections of the Colon and Rectum

Viral	Fungal
Herpes simplex	*Candida*
Cytomegalovirus	*Phycomyces*
Adenovirus	*Aspergillus*
	Histoplasma
Chlamydial	*Blastomyces*
Chlamydia trachomatis	*Cryptococcus*
Other agents	
	Protozoal
Bacterial	*Entamoeba*
Shigella	*Cryptosporidium*
Salmonella	Microsporidia
Campylobacter	*Balantidium*
Escherichia coli	*Leishmania*
Yersinia	*Toxoplasma*
Mycobacterium tuberculosis	
Mycobacterium avium	Helminthic
Actinomyces	*Schistosoma*
Clostridium	*Strongyloides*
	Anisakis

volving the anorectal area, including syphilis and gonorrhea.

In the AIDS and other immunocompromised patients, endoscopy and biopsy are often performed to look for opportunistic infections. Particularly sought are cytomegalovirus, *Mycobacterium avium,* fungi, Microsporidia, and *Cryptosporidium.* Electron microscopy of rectal biopsy in AIDS patients has shown viral-like particles in the crypt epithelial and mesenchymal cells, but the results have not been constant.[112, 113] In addition, biopsies are needed in these patients to look for tumors, especially Kaposi's sarcoma and malignant lymphoma.[114]

Viral Infections

The several agents that induce diarrhea by causing a viral enteritis do not ordinarily affect the colon mucosa.[115] Lesions are more often seen in immunocompromised patients, and biopsies are performed to identify or confirm that there is a colitis and to secure the diagnosis by noting the particular viral inclusion.

Herpes Simplex

The herpes infections are more typically found in the squamous epithelium of the anal region but can exceptionally involve the colonic crypts in the lower colon and rectum.[116, 117] Biopsy reveals the rounded nuclear inclusions that are usually surrounded by a halo (Plate 1A). The viral bodies can be noted alone or together with variable degrees of necrosis and acute inflammation. Herpes infection has also been observed in patients with chronic colitis who have received corticosteroid therapy.

Cytomegalovirus

More common are infections caused by cytomegalovirus.[118, 119] These are usually seen in immunocompromised patients but can also occur as a self-limited disorder in immunocompetent persons.[120, 121] The location of the inclusion is dependent on whether there is associated necrosis. They are typically found in the absorptive cells within the crypts as an isolated lesion, and in the endothelial cells and other mesenchymal elements in areas of ulceration and granulation tissue (Fig. 9-17). It is still not established whether one should treat based on the simple finding of the organism, or require the presence of an inflammatory lesion.

Biopsies are taken from areas of ulceration and also from random areas of normal mucosa.[122] Both the nuclear and cytoplasmic inclusions can be seen, and these are described in Chapter 2 (Plate 1B). The endothelial cell nuclei in granulation tissue are often enlarged and somewhat smudgy, causing occasional difficulty in distinguishing them from CMV inclusions. In such cases, immunocytochemical stain for the viral antigens can provide specificity.[123] It has also been suggested that a greater frequency of inclusions can be detected by in-situ hybridization techniques.

Cytomegalovirus infection may also complicate cases of severe ulcerative colitis or

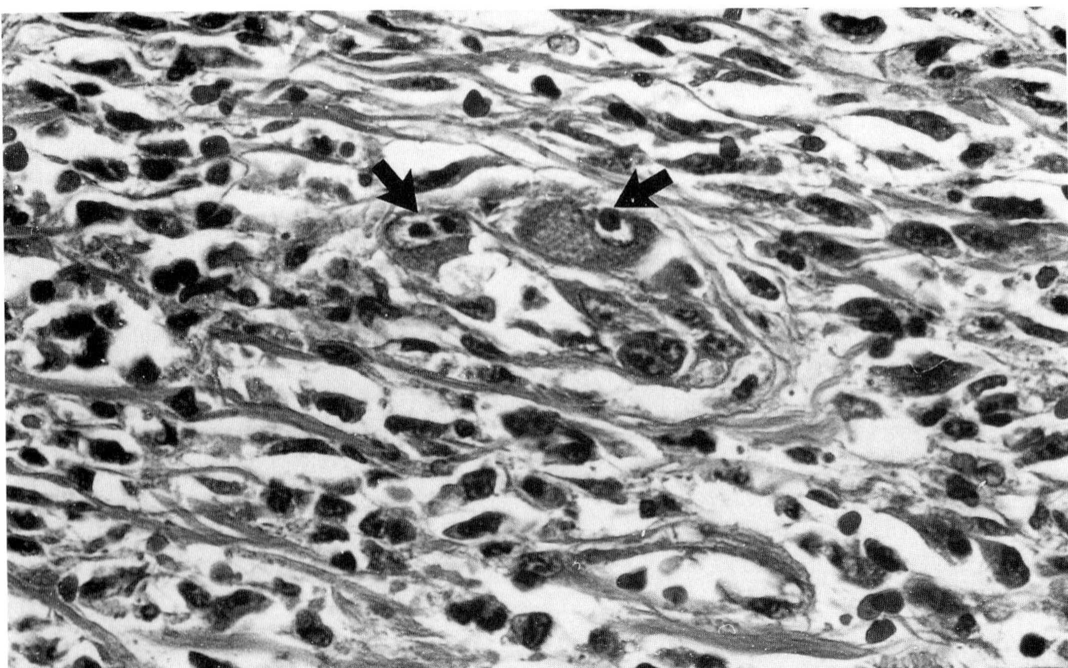

Fig. 9-17. Cytomegalovirus infection of the colon. Shown is the granulation tissue at the base of an ulcer. Both intranuclear and intracytoplasmic inclusions are seen in the endothelial cells appearing in the center (arrows) (× 635).

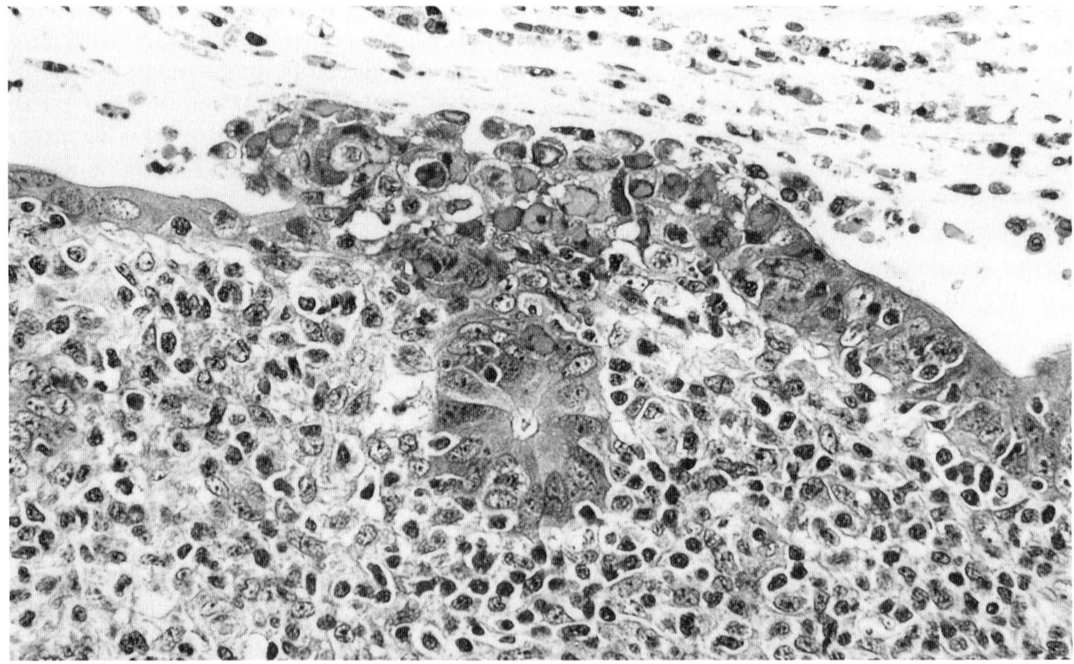

Fig. 9-18. Adenovirus infection of the colon. There is a clump of infected cells on the mucosal surface. The shed cells contain nuclei with large ground glass inclusions (× 425).

Crohn's disease where the patients have been immunocompromised.[124] The presence of CMV is associated with greater necrosis and the potential for perforation and spread to internal organs such as the liver.

Adenovirus

The adenoviruses are also associated with colitis and are probably more common in immunodepressed patients.[125, 126] Most commonly affected are the goblet mucous cells in the upper portions of the colonic crypts and on the surface epithelium. Noted are a very prominent enlargement of the nuclei and a shaggy cell border (Fig. 9-18). There tends to be a clumping of these cells and tiny erosions on the surface of the colonic mucosa. Similar lesions are seen in the appendix.

Chlamydial Infections

Chlamydia represent a less common cause of infectious colitis.[127–129] The lesions tend to be concentrated in the distal colon and rectum and to be associated with a marked lymphocytic reaction. The best documented lesions are those due to *Chlamydia trachomatis* as seen in lymphogranuloma venereum, in which there is a pronounced proliferation of lymphoid tissue with poorly formed granulomas.[129, 130] It is usually associated with superficial ulceration. Several chlamydial agents can cause lesions, and the diagnosis is ordinarily established by serologic examination.

Biopsies reveal the colitis or proctitis and can suggest the particular cause by noting the pronounced lymphoid reaction. It is important in such cases to exclude idiopathic IBD, typically by the lack of a history of chronic disease. The chlamydial infections also may uncommonly be associated with prominent hemorrhage in the mucosa, resembling the lesions seen in ischemic disease.[131]

Bacterial Infections

There are a very large number of bacteria that can act on the colon[107] (Table 9-7). The pathologic features are highly variable, ranging from effects due to toxin production to highly destructive lesions with extensive ulcerations; lesions that can involve any part of the colon to those that are concentrated in one region, such as the cecum or rectum; and conditions that are associated with prominent necrosis and neutrophilic reaction in contrast to others that have an immunologic reaction with profound mononuclear cell proliferation (see Table 7-6).

Acute Bacterial Dysentery

Acute colitis with necrosis and a neutrophilic reaction is commonly due to species of *Shigella, Salmonella,* invasive *Escherichia coli, Yersinia,* and *Campylobacter*.[132–136] Less often, cases of acute colitis result from streptococcal and staphylococcal organisms. The lesions may be focal or diffuse, involving any part of the rectum and colon, and are associated with a marked neutrophilic reaction in the mucosa together with progressive destruction of the crypts that begins from the luminal surface. The most severe cases show focal ulceration. The patients present with cloudy or bloody diarrhea, and the diagnosis is typically established by bacterial culture.

Biopsy is obtained in uncertain cases and shows a severe, acute colitis that is otherwise nonspecific (Fig. 9-9). The major features are a cryptitis and a neutrophilic infiltrate that usually affects the upper one-half to two-thirds of the mucosa. The normal architecture of straight crypts is preserved in the acute phase. With healing, there is loss of the neutrophils and complete restitution of the crypts, without any persistent abnormality. Exceptionally a prolonged infection, usually due to *Shigella,* develops; this can show features of chronic colitis in the form of crypt budding and atrophy, similar to that seen in chronic IBD.

Acute Self-Limited Colitis

Some of the cases with typical clinical and pathologic features of acute colitis initially fail to reveal a causative agent, and these have been termed *acute self-limited colitis.*[109] Ultimately an etiologic agent, usually a less commonly sought bacterium, is found in 30 to 40 percent of cases. These examples of acute colitis must be distinguished from the acute phase of ulcerative colitis. (See the section on "Other Inflammatory Disorders" for details.)

Salmonella Infections

Salmonella infections of the colon present varied effects dependent on the particular species involved.[137–139] Some cases reveal an acute necrotizing colitis, as described above. Other species are associated with less necrosis and more immunologic reaction. Biopsies mainly show an increase in lymphocytes within the epithelial layer and surrounding the crypts.

Typhoid fever, representing infection with *Salmonella typhi,* more commonly involves the small bowel but may extend into the large intestine. It is characterized by very marked proliferation of macrophages and of lymphoid nodules. The diagnosis requires culture.

Escherichia coli Infections

There are several effects due to *E. coli* in the colon, dependent on theparticular species and the pathologic action (Fig. 9-19): some grow within the lumen and cause disease by the production of a toxin that acts on the absorptive cells and is productive of a watery diarrhea similar to that seen in cholera (toxogenic); organisms that selectively adhere to the surface of the crypt epithelial cells and are more commonly seen in AIDS patients (enteroadherent); strains that release toxins causing marked hemorrhage of the mucosa and simulating ischemic disease (enterohemorrhagic); and species that can release strong enzymes that lead to invasion of the organisms and extensive necrosis productive of an acute dysentery (enteropathogenic or invasive). The diagnosis in practically all of these cases is established by culture of stool specimens.

Biopsies are obtained in selected cases and show the findings to match each of the major types of *E. coli.* Accordingly, there is a normal mucosa with the toxogenic strains, the finding of clumps of bacteria on the surface columnar cells with the adherent type, an acute colitis with erosions associated with the invasive form, and pronounced hemorrhage with the vascular toxin species.[140]

Mycobacterial Infections

Most cases of colonic tuberculosis are localized in the cecal and proximal colon region.[141–143] Noted are large areas of ulcerations and granulomas with prominent caseation (Fig. 9-20). This disorder is very uncommon in most of the developed countries but is increased in AIDS patients. Biopsies reveal the necrosis and occasionally the granulomas.[144] The diagnosis is dependent on the finding of organisms by acid-fast stain or by their culture.

Also noted in immunocompromised patients are infections due to *Mycobacterium avium* complex, which typically reveal much less necrosis and poor granuloma formation[145–147] (Fig. 6-12 and Plate 1D). Indeed, any patient with AIDS probably needs an

A
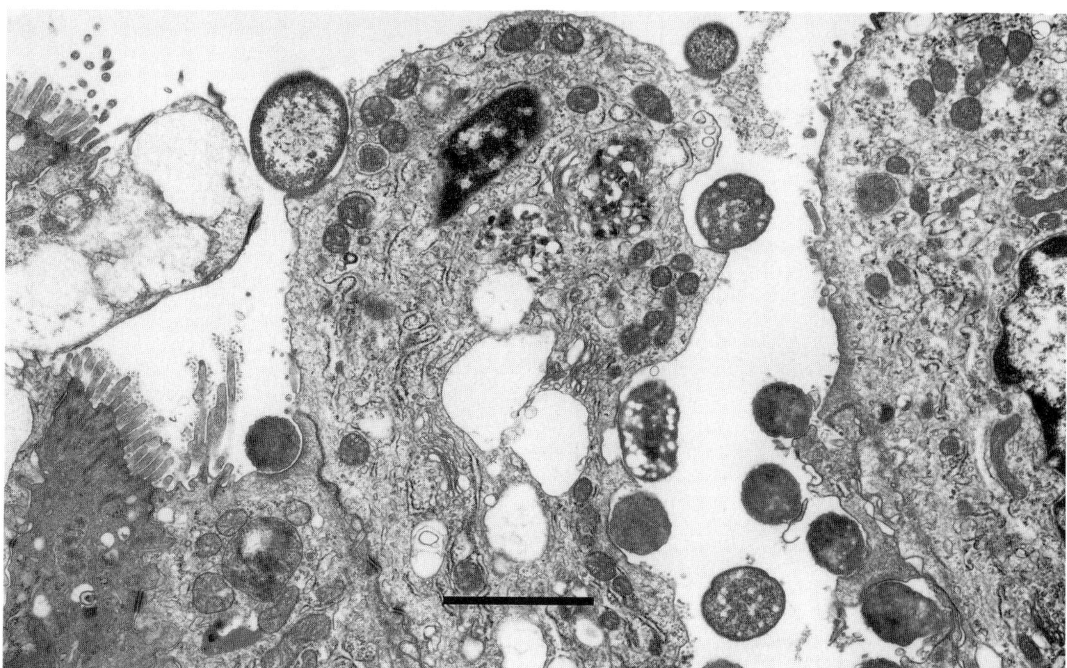

B
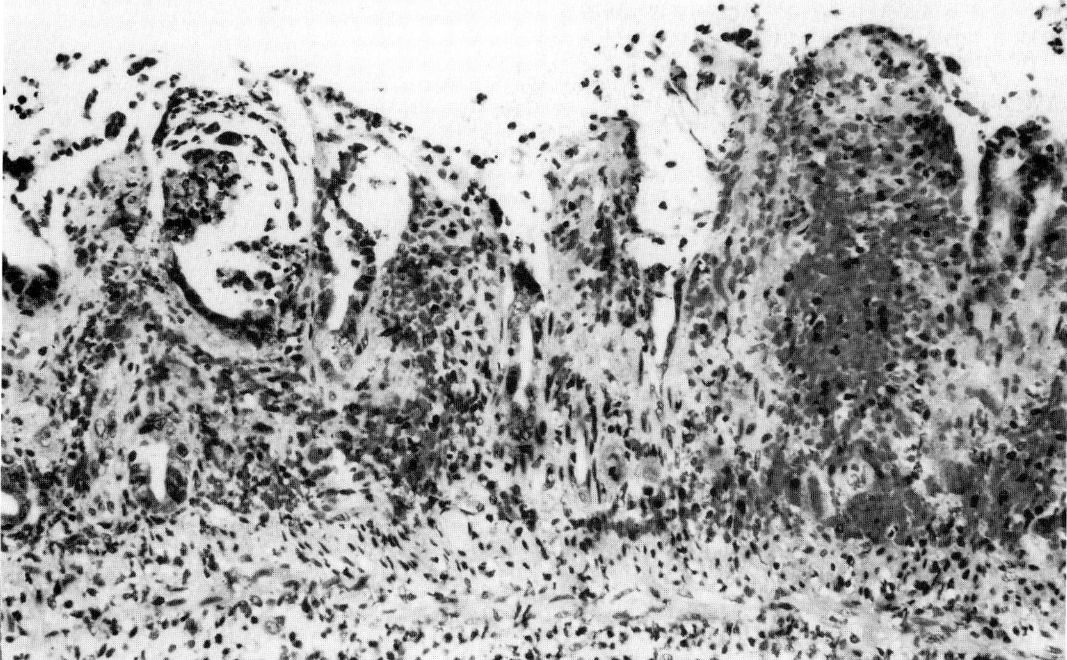

Fig. 9-19. **(A)** Electron micrograph of bacteria adhering to the surface of absorptive cells of the colon epithelium. The epithelial cells that are attacked by the bacteria have lost their normal microvilli, as seen on the left. Note that in this case, the bacteria are intimiately associated with the cell membrane, which appears to surround them, but do not invade the cells (× 9400; bar = 2 μm). **(B)** Hemorrhagic colitis due to *E. coli.* There is diffuse hemorrhage in the lamina propria together with crypt destruction. The muscularis mucosae appears at the bottom (× 210).

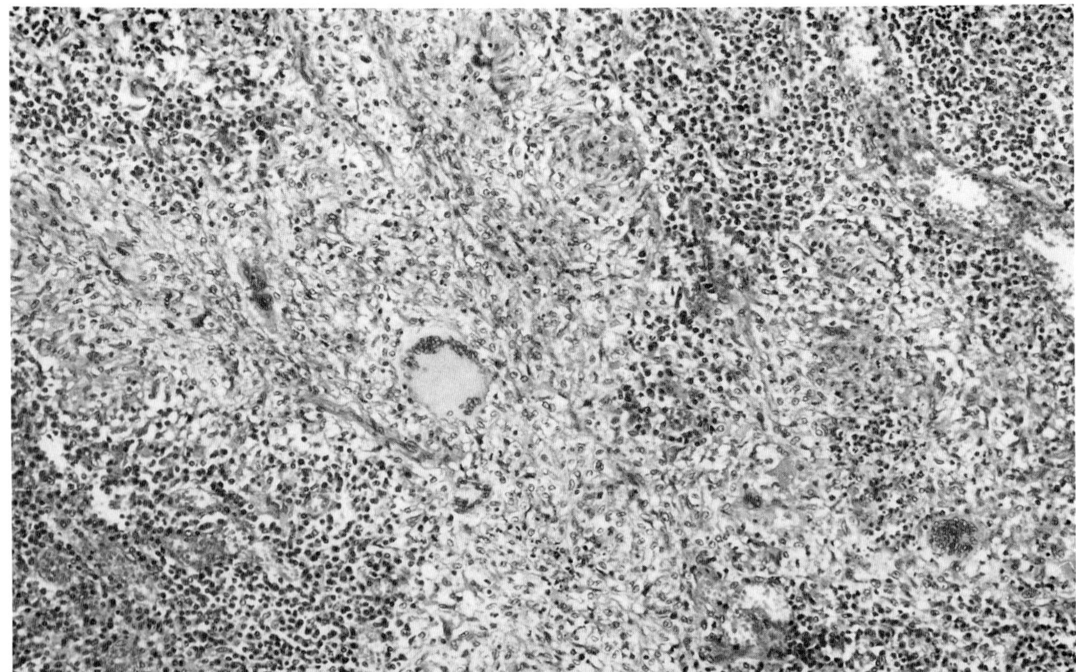

Fig. 9-20. Tuberculosis of the colon. There are granulomas with prominent giant cells and extensive necrosis (× 140).

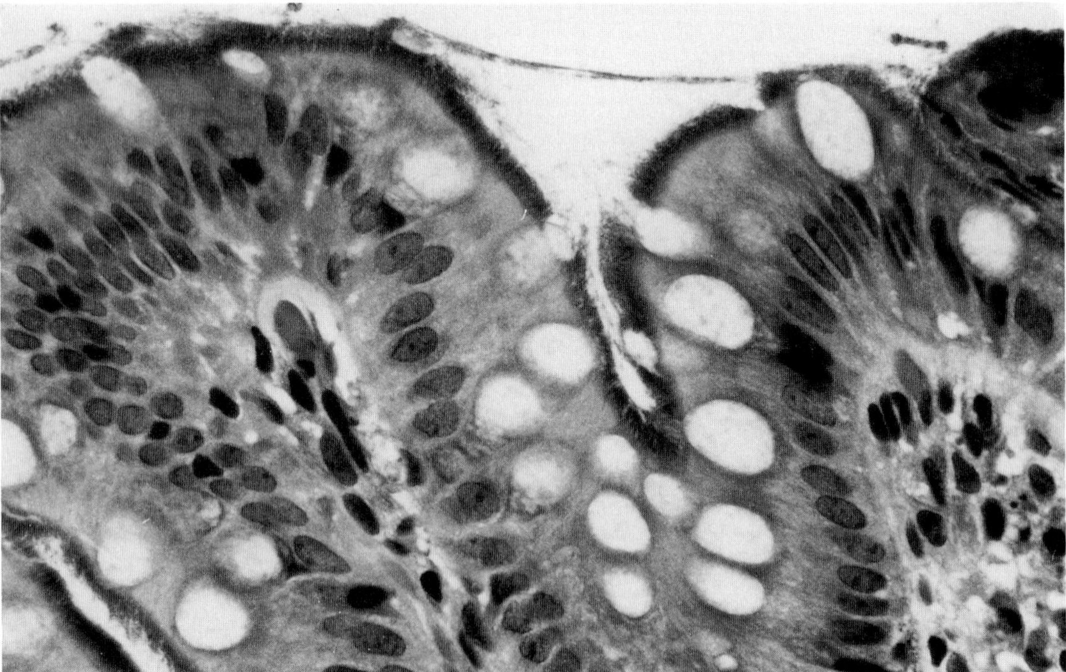

Fig. 9-21. Spirochetosis of the colon. Overlying the surface and the crypt epithelial cells are closely packed spiral-shaped bacteria, resulting in the appearance of a dark and fuzzy coat (Dieterle's silver stain, × 635).

acid-fast stain to exclude the presence of the organisms, which are typically congregated in the lamina propria. The infection is probably less common in the colon than in the small intestine and the upper part of the gut.

Spirochetosis

Spirochetosis of the rectum or colon is a condition characterized by the presence of a large number of spirochetes on the surface of the columnar epithelial cells in these regions.[148–150] There results an apparent thickening of the surface membrane, which resembles a brush border (Fig. 9-21). The spirochetes can be identified by Gram, Giemsa, or silver stains as well as by electron microscopy. The lesion appears to be more common in homosexual patients. Some studies have suggested mild clinical problems, whereas others indicate no definite functional problems. The lesions are not seen by endoscopy, and biopsies are often taken in the evaluation of some other disorder. At present, the finding of spirochetosis has no definite clinical significance.

Other Bacterial Infections

Infection due to yersinial agents can either be associated with a common acute dysentery and colitis or reveal small microabscesses.[151] The lesions are more common in the distal ileum and appendix and are not ordinarily revealed on biopsy. Actinomycosis is usually seen in debilitated patients; it is also concentrated in the distal ileum and proximal colonic region and associated with extensive necrosis with potential for fistula formation.[152] The diagnosis is typically established by finding the sulfur granules in resected specimens. Syphilis is rare in the colon, whereas gonococcal infection tends to be more concentrated in the anal region.[153] Other rare examples of colitis include *Legionella* infection, which can cause a severe inflammation that simulates ulcerative colitis.[154]

There are other disorders in which bacteria participate in the pathogenesis, including necrotizing enterocolitis and neutropenic enterocolitis, and these are described in the section on "Other Inflammatory Disorders." The antibiotic-associated, pseudomembraneous colitis due to *C. difficile* is presented in the section on "Chemical Injury".[106]

Fungal Infections

Fungal infections are described in earlier chapters and are briefly summarized here. The general characteristics of the lesions and descriptions of the organisms are largely contained in Chapter 2 (Plates 1E & F). Infection in the colon has been seen with practically all fungal agents and is most often noted in immunocompromised patients.[155] They are usually due to *Candida* and less often to *Phycomyces* and *Aspergillus.*[156–158] There commonly is extensive necrosis and acute inflammation, and biopsies are obtained to idenfity the organisms and to exclude other causes, particularly recurrent tumor. Infections can also be seen with the pathogenic types of fungi, and cases of colitis have been noted with *Histoplasma, Blastomyces,* and *Cryptococcus.*[159–162] These cases may show giant cell and granuloma formation, and the organisms are best visualized with methenamine silver stains. Overall, such fungal infections are uncommon in the colon.

Protozoal Infections

Amoebiasis

The most common protozoal infection is amoebic dysentery due to *Entamoeba histolyticum,* which is associated with a widespread colitis.[163, 164] The diagnosis is best made by identifying the organisms in either smears of the stool or smears made directly from ulcerated lesions. Biopsy may be done to establish the colitis and to obtain material for diagnosis (Fig. 9-22 and Plate 2E). The organisms are highly characteristic, measuring about 30 to 40 μm in diameter, and contain prominent nuclei and ingested material, such as well-formed red blood cells. They are about twice the size of macrophages and can be readily seen in H & E preparations. It has been suggested that they can be accentuated in iron hematoxylin stains. The organisms can be found in any part of the bowel wall but tend to be highly concentrated over areas of ulcerations.

Giardia Infestation

Giardia lamblia may be found in stools but is usually not associated with a colitis. Rather, the organisms tend to proliferate in the small bowel mucosa and to be associated with a malabsorptive disorder (Fig. 6-14 and Plate 2A).

Coccidial Infections

Cryptosporidium are a common cause of a reversible colitis in children who are immunocompetent.[165, 166] The diagnosis is typically established by identifying the organism on smears by use of a modified acid-fast stain. In immunodepressed patients, the cryptosporidial organisms tend to be more prominent in the small bowel and are associated with a profound diarrhea.[167, 168] They also may proliferate in other parts of the gut, including the stomach and the colon. The organisms are easy to recognize as 3- to 5-μm spherical agents that are on the top of the surface and crypt epithelium (Fig. 6-15 and Plate 2B). They can easily be seen by the H & E and be accented by Giemsa and many other stains. There is usually no invasion by the organisms or any associated necrosis.

Recently, cases of Microsporidia infection have been noted in the colon.[169–171] These are much more common in the small intestine but may exceptionally involve the colonic epithelial cells. The diagnosis is established by noting the agent in the cytoplasm of the crypt and surface epithelial cells, best visualized with Gram stains (see Fig. 6-17 and Color Plate 4C). (See Chapters 6 and 7 for further descriptions of cryptosporidial and microsporidial organisms.)

Other Protozoal Infections

Other uncommon-to-rare causes of colitis from protozoal agents include *Balantidium* and other *Amoeba, Leishmania, Trypanosoma,* and *Toxoplasma.*[172–174] In all of these cases, the diagnosis requires the identification of the particular agent. Eletron microscopic examination can be of considerable assistance in the detection and precise identification of the particular protozoal organism (see Figs. 6-16 and 6-18).

Helminthic Infections

The diagnosis of helminthic infection is established by detection of the ova in the stools or in biopsy specimens.

Schistosomiasis

Lesions can develop in the colon due to infection with *Schistosoma japonicum* and *S. mansoni.*[175, 176] In the early stages, before there is an immunologic reaction, there is the presence of a marked number of ova within the mucosa and minimal inflammation. More typical, however, is the finding of a colitis at the time of a profound immunologic reaction to the eggs (Fig. 9-23 and Plate 2F). Noted are large nodules in the submucosa and mucosa, in which one can find the ova, and these are surrounded by a marked

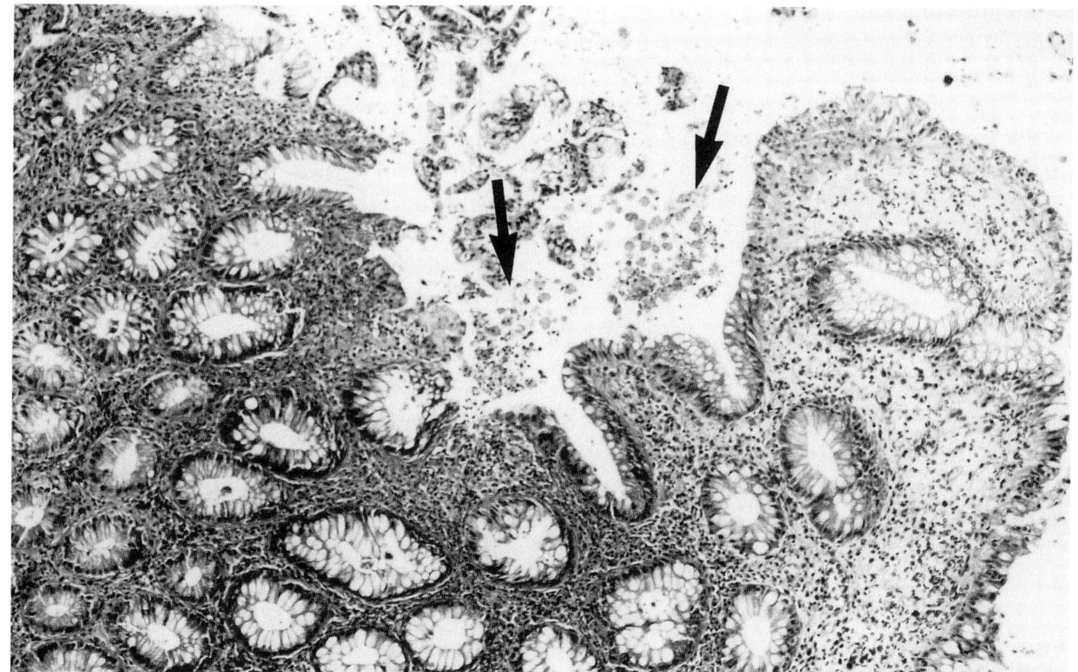

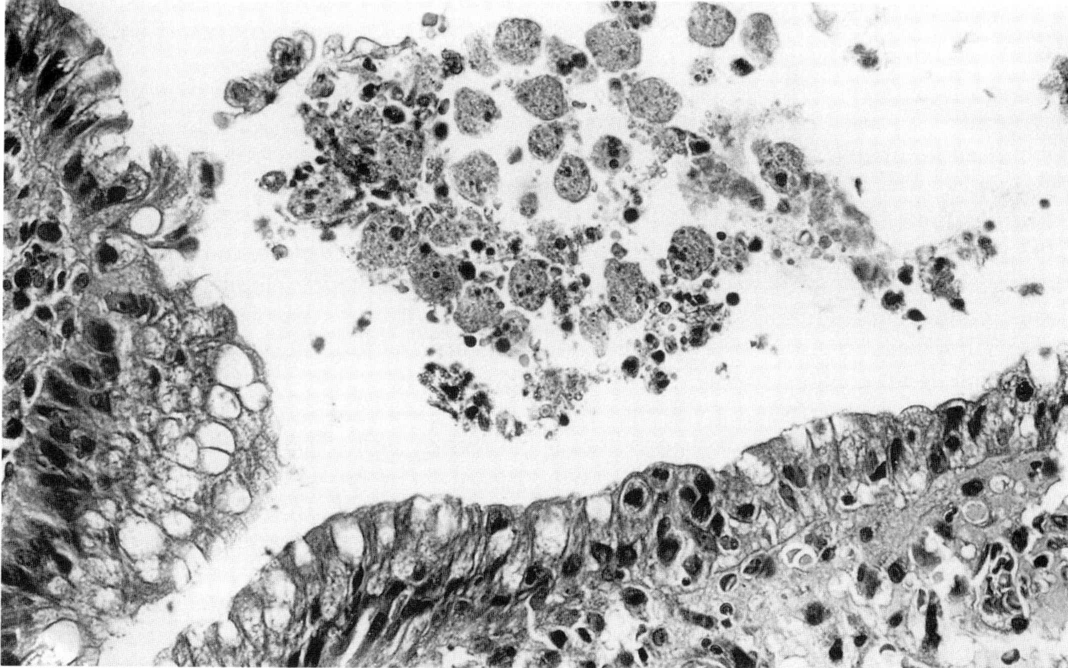

Fig. 9-22. Amoebiasis of the colon. **(A)** Colonic biopsy with small erosion (top center). Numerous amoebae are in the adjacent lumen (arrows) (× 105). **(B)** Closer view of amoebae in the lumen (× 425).

inflammatory and fibrotic reaction. Eosinophils are particularly conspicuous. The prominant granulomatous reaction can result in the formation of inflammatory polyps in the colon and rectum, which may be single or multiple.[177] In the healing phase there is progressive resolution of the inflammation, and only rare eggs and scattered pigment are seen.

Strongyloides

Infection by *Strongyloides stercoralis* is almost exclusively seen in immunocompromised patients, revealing ulcers and fragments of the worms or ova.[178, 179] They can be found in any part of the gut but are probably more common in the upper and midportions (see Fig. 6-19).

Other Helminthic Infections

Anisakis marina more typically affects the ileum and stomach but may rarely involve the colon.[180, 181] There is a marked inflammatory reaction that resides in the wall, and biopsies do not readily capture the lesion. There are other common worms in the colon and appendix, including *Enterobius* and *Trichuris,* but these do not usually cause a prominent colitis that leads to biopsy.

IDIOPATHIC INFLAMMATORY BOWEL DISEASE

Biopsy of patients with idiopathic inflammatory bowel disease (IBD) accounts for the majority of specimens in the evaluation of inflammatory conditions of the colon and rectum. These include the cases of ulcerative colitis (UC) and of Crohn's disease (CD).[22, 182–185]

General Aspects

Lacking knowledge of the specific etiology or pathogenesis of these inflammatory conditions, the diagnosis is dependent on a constellation of clinical, radiographic and endoscopic findings, and histologic features.[186–190] In this setting, the biopsy should be considered as an important but not exclusive tool in generating the diagosis. Some of the potential discriminating features, such as transmural inflammation and deep fissures or fistulae, are not available in the assessment of the biopsy. It is important to link the histologic information with the gross findings that are obtained by endoscopy and full radiographic examination. The potential findings available in a mucosal biopsy are a normal mucosa as evidence of a normal rectum or skip area, a diffuse colitis involving the entire specimen and multiple samples, a focal colitis, and granulomas that may occur together with or independent of a colitis. These are further discussed under "Biopsy Uses" below.

Ulcerative Colitis

Ulcerative colitis (UC) is a chronic disorder that can affect children and acults of all ages. There is one major peak incidence occurring in the early 20s and a smaller rise occurring in the mid-50s.

Etiology and Clinical Course

The cause of ulcerative colitis is unknown, but thought to represent an autoimmune disorder with the colonic and rectal mucosa serving as the target tissue. The primary action is in the mucosal layer and may proceed to ulceration and deeper involvement due to secondary pressure effects. The disease is characterized by periodic relapses and remissions, with a highly variable degree of severity ranging from minimal symptoms

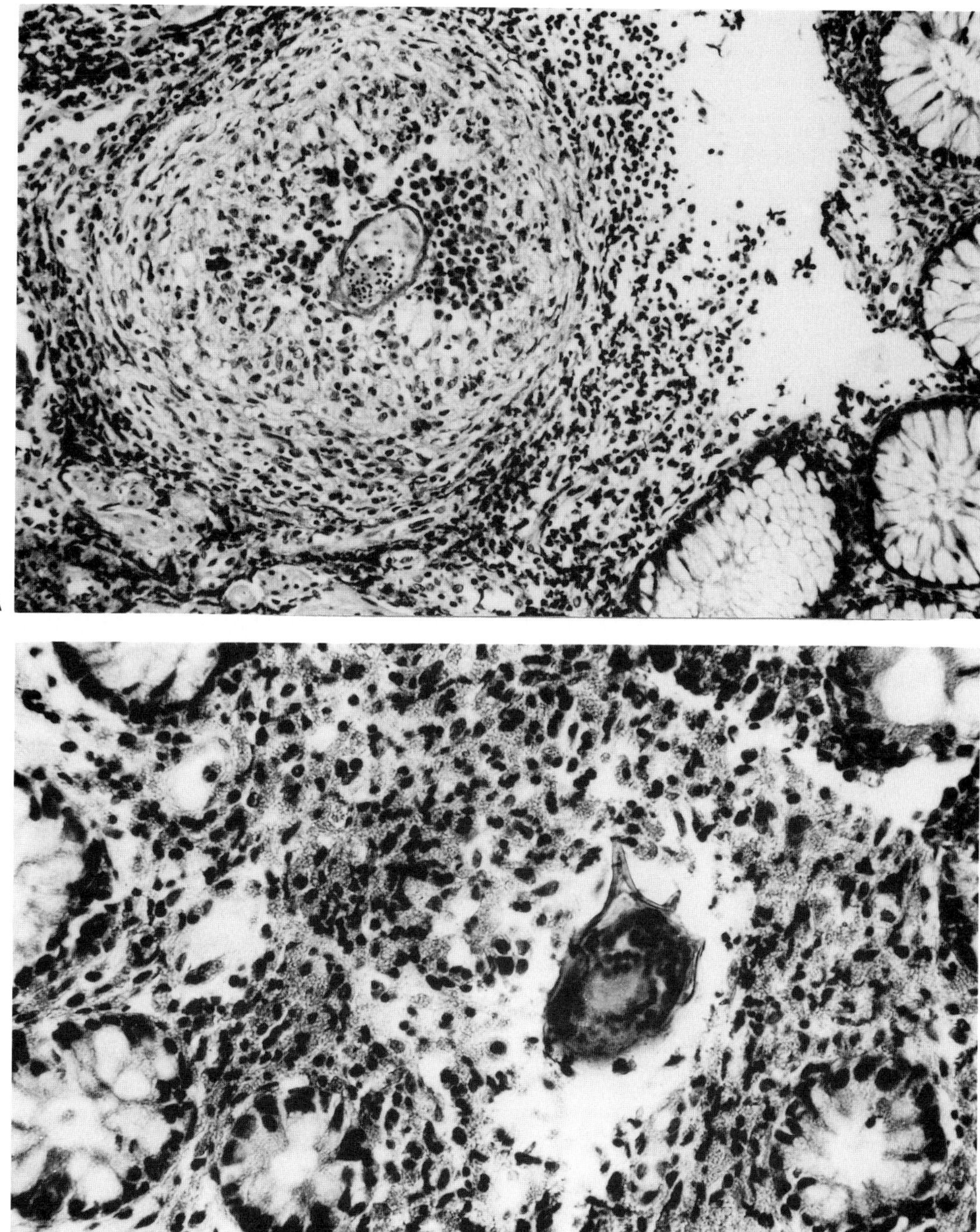

Fig. 9-23. Schistosomiasis of the colon. **(A)** There is a well formed granuloma in the submucosa (left). This is associated with several eosinophils and an egg (center). Some crypts appear at the right. **(B)** Ovum of *Schistosoma mansoni* with lateral spine together with an eosinophilic reaction in the mucosa.

to extensive disease that requires significant therapy.

Distribution of Disease

The disease always affects the rectum and may extend in a diffuse fashion to involve the more proximal parts of the colon. It is estimated that the lesions are limited to the rectum and distal colon in one-third of cases, extend to the midportion in another one-third, and ultimately involve the entire large bowel in the remaining one-third of cases. The ulcerative disorder is limited to the large bowel and appendix. In the very severe cases, there can occur a dilation and inflammation of the terminal ileum unassociated with ulceration, and known as *backwash ileitis;* this is thought to be due to either reflux through an incompetent ileocecal valve or, more likely, to a static segment of ileum in cases with generalized colitis. In contrast to Crohn's disease, there is no evidence that the ulcerative disorder can affect the ileum or any other part of the gut.

Diagnosis

The diagnosis of ulcerative colitis first requires complete exclusion of other possible causes, particularly infections, ischemic disease, and mechanical disorders. Lacking any specific feature, the diagnosis is dependent on the demonstration of rectal involvement; diffuse disease of any other portion of the colon that may extend to the cecum; the lack of any skip areas except for lesions in the cecum or appendix; disease that is largely limited to the mucosa and submucosa, except when there is severe involvement and secondary pressure changes; the absence of any discrete fissures or fistulae; and a completely nonspecific histology without any granulomas, except those of a foreign body type.

Pathologic Features

There is diffuse involvement of the mucosa with acute and chronic inflammation, ulcers, and inflammatory pseudopolyps (Fig. 9-24A). The ulcers frequently extend into the superficial submucosa and are associated with prominent inflammation in that area.[189] In about one-third of resected cases, there is more severe involvement with ulcers extending into the muscularis propria; in such instances, inflammation can be found in the serosal area.[190] There are no discrete fissures or fistulae. Poorly formed granulomas can be found in the mucosa next to ruptured crypts, presumably reacting to exuded mucus. There are no well formed, sarcoid-type granulomas in this or any other part of the bowel wall. The disease is limited to the rectum and colon, and there is no evidence of ulcerating disease in other parts of the tract. The only exceptions to the absence of skip lesions is the area of cecum and appendix, which may be involved even in cases with less than total colitis.[191, 192]

Biopsy Features

There are several reasons for endoscopy and biopsy of the rectum and colon in patients with ulcerative colitis. The biopsies serve to identify that the patient has colitis, that there is chronic disease, and to distinguish active and inactive forms.[182–184, 193, 194] The biopsies of affected areas always show diffuse abnormalities, with alterations seen in all portions of a biopsy and in all the samples. In contrast, biopsies from the area proximal to the overt disease may be completely normal.

The pathologic features in the mucosa depend on the stage of the disease (Table 9-4). Initially there is pronounced acute inflammation with cryptitis that cannot be distinguished from other types of acute colitis of an infectious or other etiology. With time there develop many features to signify the chronic disease, including alteration of the architecture due to multiple branching of the crypts, crypt atrophy with separation of their bases from the muscularis mucosae, a chronic inflammatory infiltrate in the basal part of the lamina propria, a villiform surface, and Paneth cell metaplasia[195–198] (Figs. 9-10 and 9-24B). Also noted are an increase in the number of endocrine cells and the appearance of many lymphoid nodules[199–201] (Fig. 9-24C). The latter can be especially pronounced in retained distal segments following subtotal colectomy, and has been called *follicular proctitis and colitis.*

There also can be persistence of inflammatory pseudopolyps, including giant and papillary forms.[202, 203] These may occur in the absence of active disease, and small biopsies may simply reveal normal or mildly atrophic mucosa. In such cases the gross findings are needed to establish the existence of the polyps (see Ch. 10).

Table 9-8. Complications of Ulcerative Colitis

Toxic megacolon
Secondary infections
Drug effects
Colitis cystica profunda
Dysplasia and adenocarcinoma

Complications

The complications of ulcerative colitis are listed in Table 9-8, and are discussed below. The ileal abnormalities that are noted following colonic surgery are described in Chapter 8.

Toxic Megacolon. In the severe cases of ulcerative colitis, there is marked production of blood and fluid that extends into the lumen and causes secondary distention of the colon. This is associated with ischemic damage of the wall leading to marked congestion and the potential for multiple fissures and perforation. These cases are ordinarily evident by their severe symptomatology and radiographic study that shows the dilated bowel. Biopsy is contraindicated in such cases to avoid perforation.

Secondary Infections. Cases of ulcerative colitis can develop secondary infections that lead to the return of symptoms. This has been noted with many organisms, particularly *Campylobacter, Salmonella* and *C. difficile.*[204] Biopsies are indistinguishable from ordinary relapses of chronic ulcerative colitis, and the diagnosis is totally dependent on cultures of the stools.

In immunocompromised patients, there can develop secondary infections with herpes or with cytomegalovirus, and these can be associated with greater necrosis and the threat of perforation.[124] The diagnosis is secured by identifying the specific inclusions in the biopsy material, and this can be confirmed by specific immunocytochemical stains. The herpes inclusions are more often seen in the crypt epithelial cells, whereas the CMV inclusions can be found both in epithelial cells and in the mesenchymal elements, particularly endothelial and fibroblastic cells.

Drug Effects. Some patients with IBD react poorly to salicylates that are used in their treatment.[205] The drug can cause a worsening or reactivation of symptoms, presumably as a result of an allergic reaction. Biopsies simply show the active IBD. Such patients also usually respond poorly when given NSAID for other reasons.[206]

Colitis Cystica. In severe cases of chronic colitis, there can be an extension of the glands into the submucosa and deeper parts of the wall, termed *colitis cystica profunda.*[207] It is important in these cases to distinguish this inflammatory effect from the development of a well differentiated carcinoma. The epithelial cells in the misplaced glands are normal or show regeneration in contrast to the dysplastic effects in carcinoma cells.

Neoplasia. Patients with long-standing and extensive ulcerative colitis are particularly prone to the development of dysplasia and carcinoma of the colon.[208, 209] This subject is covered in Chapter 10.

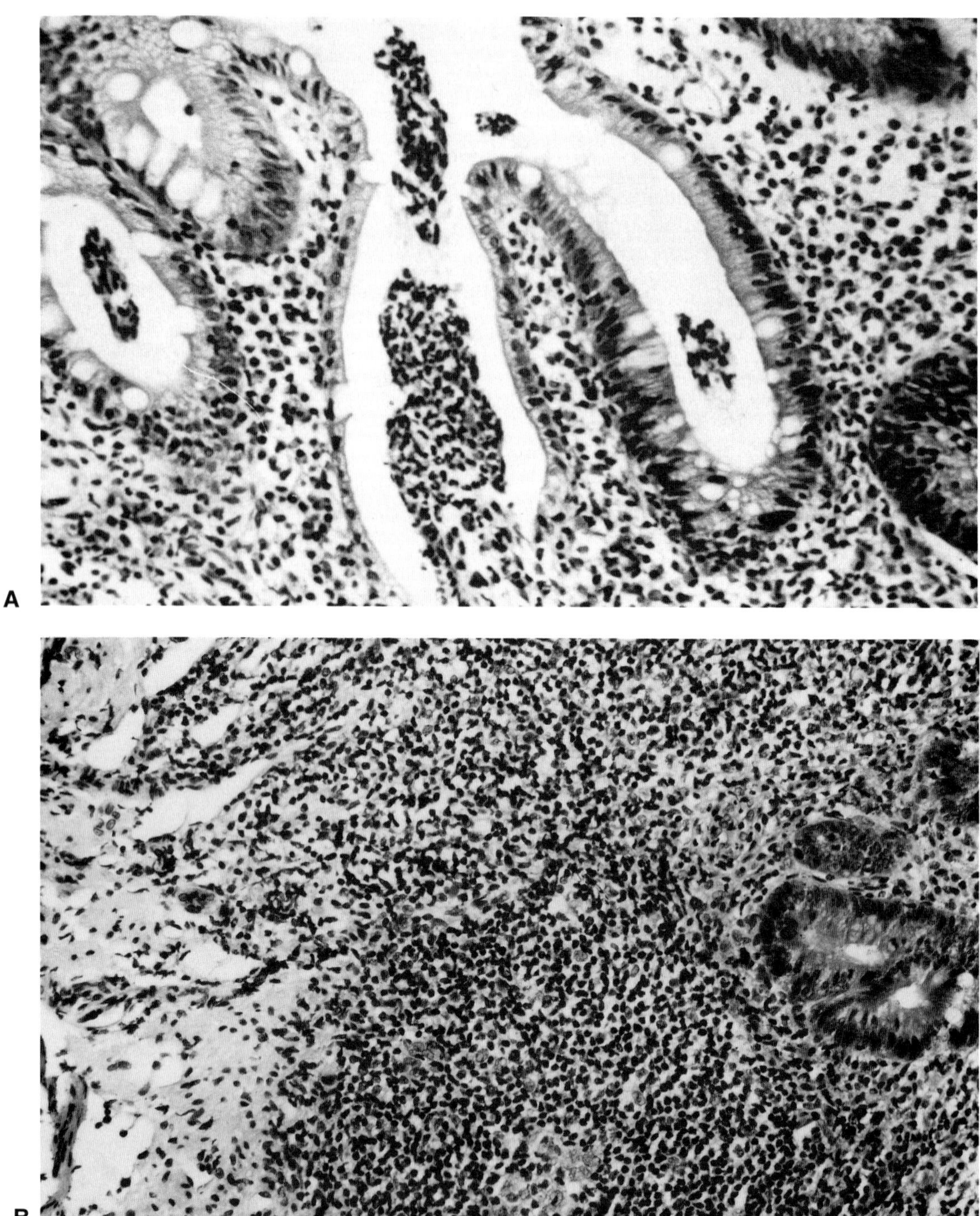

Fig. 9-24. Ulcerative colitis. **(A)** Active disease, indicated by crypt abscesses. **(B)** There is a marked infiltrate of mononuclear inflammatory cells in the base of the lamina propria, separating the crypts (right) and the muscularis (left) (× 210). (*Figure continues.*)

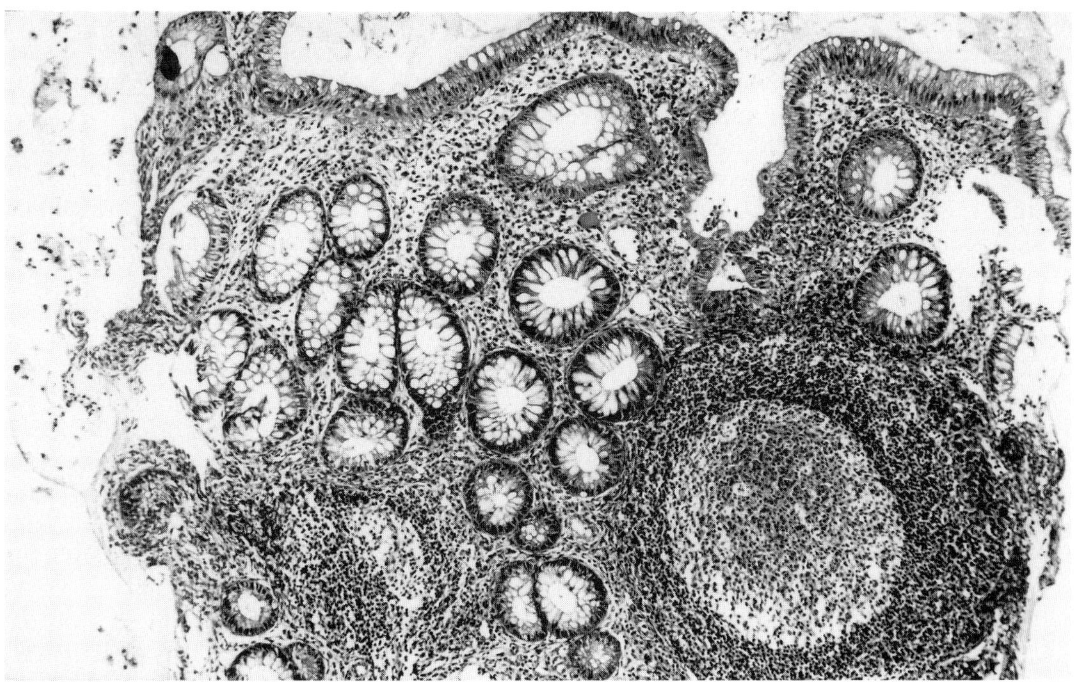

Fig. 9-24 (*Continued*). **(C)** Follicular inflammation. Noted are the irregular surface and crypts of chronic disease as well as a large lymphoid follicle in the lower right (× 105).

Crohn's Disease

Etiology and Clinical Course

Crohn's disease (CD) is a chronic disorder of the gastrointestinal tract of unknown etiology. It is thought to represent a peculiar reaction to some infectious agent but the particular organism has not been established. Potential candidates have been various mycobacteria, cell-deficient bacteria, and viruses. Recently, it has been suggested that the disease might be mediated by a granulomatous vasculitis leading to secondary ischemic lesions.[210]

The disorder can affect persons of all ages, including children and the elderly. It is characterized by repeated relapses of increasing severity, often requiring surgery.

Distribution of Disease

In contrast to ulcerative colitis, Crohn's disease can involve any part of the gastrointestinal tract. Most commonly affected are the distal ileum in 50 percent of cases, the ileum and colon in 35 percent of cases, and the colon alone in 10 percent of cases. The disease tends to be focal or segmental, resulting in skip areas. This is particularly evident in the colon, with rectal sparing in 50 percent of cases and the frequent appearance of a localized Crohn's disease involving any portion of the large intestine. Disease is less often noted in the upper parts of the gut, the rest of the small intestine, the appendix, and the anal region.

Diagnosis

Since Crohn's disease is an idiopathic disorder, it is necessary to first exclude any other specific causes of enteritis or colitis. This typically means infection or unusual diffuse tumors like lymphomas in the small bowel; and other forms of segmental colitis such as diverticular disease or ischemic disease in the colon. It is also important in the colon to differentiate ulcerative colitis and

Crohn's disease. There is no single feature that is present in every case of Crohn's disease. Hence, the diagnosis is dependent on the finding of any one or more of the several distinctive features: focal or segmental disease in the colon, including rectal sparing or other skip areas, seen in 90 percent of cases; the appearance of discrete fissures extending into the muscularis propria or fistulae, noted grossly in one-third and microscopically in two-thirds of cases; and the presence of granulomas that are not of the mucus or other foreign body type, seen in 50 percent of overall cases.[22] Many of these features depend on other examinations such as radiographic, gross endoscopic, or study of surgical specimens. Accordingly, this information should be available in the proper assessment of mucosal biopsies.

Pathologic Features

The lesions may be diffuse or focal within a given segment of disease.[22,189] Characteristically seen are deep ulcers, inflammation that usually involves all portions of the wall, a tendency for the development of early strictures due to fibrosis, the appearance of fissures and fistulae, and the variable presence of granulomas. Prominently noted in the submucosa are lymphoid nodules, fibrosis, dilation of lymphatics, and proliferation of nerves. About 5 to 10 percent of CD cases show more superficial disease with shallow ulcers and less fibrosis. These can usually be distinguished from UC by the tendency for focal lesions and for more prominent serosal inflammation, even in areas of superficial ulceration.

Biopsy Features

Endoscopic examination and biopsy are performed for multiple reasons in patients with Crohn's disease. These include the identification of involvement of the colon in patients with Crohn's disease in another area; the distinction from ulcerative colitis; determination of the full extent of the disease, especially in anticipation of surgery; and the detection of any complications.

The biopsies more often show focal disease, represented by involvement of only a part of a biopsy or of the multiple samples, with the remaining portions appearing totally normal[183, 193] (Fig. 9-25). Features are highly variable, typically showing some evidence of chronic disease with or without active areas. Granulomas can be seen independent of other involvement of the colon; they are noted both in inflamed and otherwise normal areas. The chance of detecting granulomas is dependent on the extent of colonic involvement, occuring in 5 percent or less of patients with gross disease limited to the small intestine and right colon, and extending up to 15 to 25 percent in patients with overt left-sided disease. The prevalence of granulomas can be enhanced by examination of en face sections and also by multiple levels.[211–213] Occasionally, the granulomas are very small and fragmented (termed *microgranulomas*), and these must be distinguished from a normal loose collection of macrophages.[214] It is important to rule out granulomas due to other specific causes, most often to ruptured crypts where poorly formed granulomas can occur secondary to the mucus extrusion into the lamina propria (Fig. 9-26). When in doubt, multiple sections can be obtained to look for the remnants of the crypts. Such mucus-related granulomas are nonspecific and can be seen in ulcerative colitis as well as any other colitis.

Complications

The development of a toxic megacolon, of secondary infections, and of colitis cystica are much less common than in patients with ulcerative colitis, but they can occur (see discussion above, under "Ulcerative Colitis"). The effects on the ileum following surgery are described in Chapter 8; and the complica-

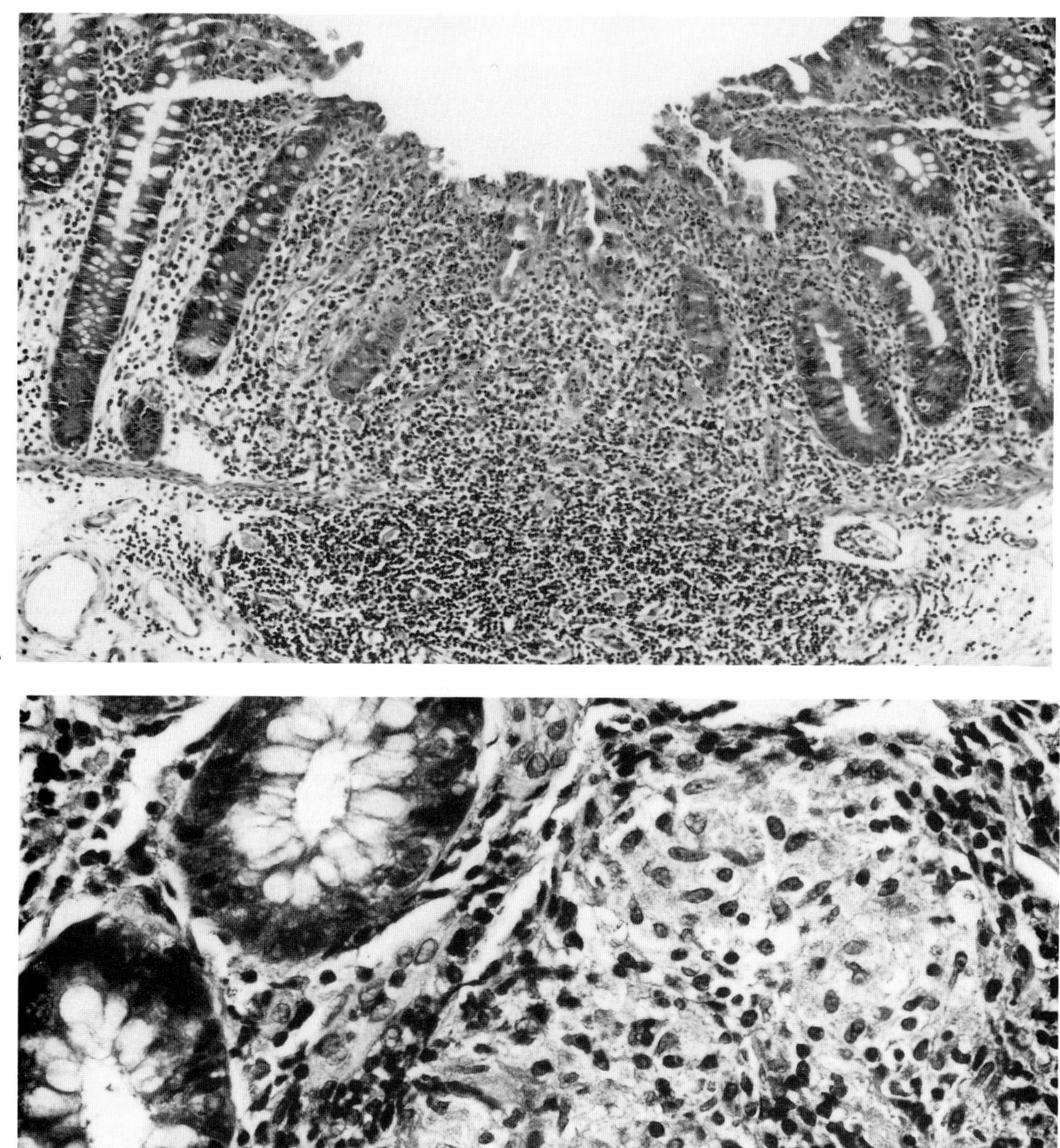

Fig. 9-25. Crohn's disease. **(A)** Focal acute erosion of the colon (top center). The earliest lesions are often noted over the lymphoid nodules; the lymphoid tissue in the subjacent submucosa appearing at the bottom is part of the normal lymphoid nodule. The mucosa appearing at the right is inflamed, whereas the part appearing at the left is normal (× 140). **(B)** There is a granuloma in the mucosa, next to crypts (left). The granulomas in Crohn's disease lack necrosis, and may occur in both normal and diseased areas of the mucosa (× 425).

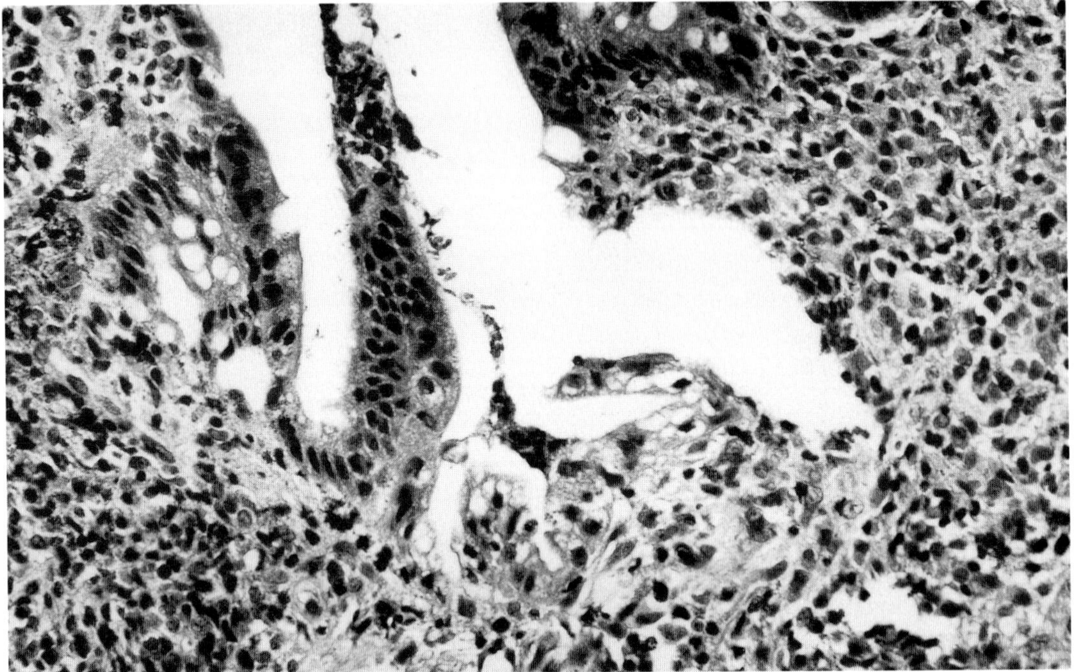

Fig. 9-26. Crypt granuloma. Noted in the center is a ruptured crypt; a poorly formed granuloma appears at the bottom (× 340).

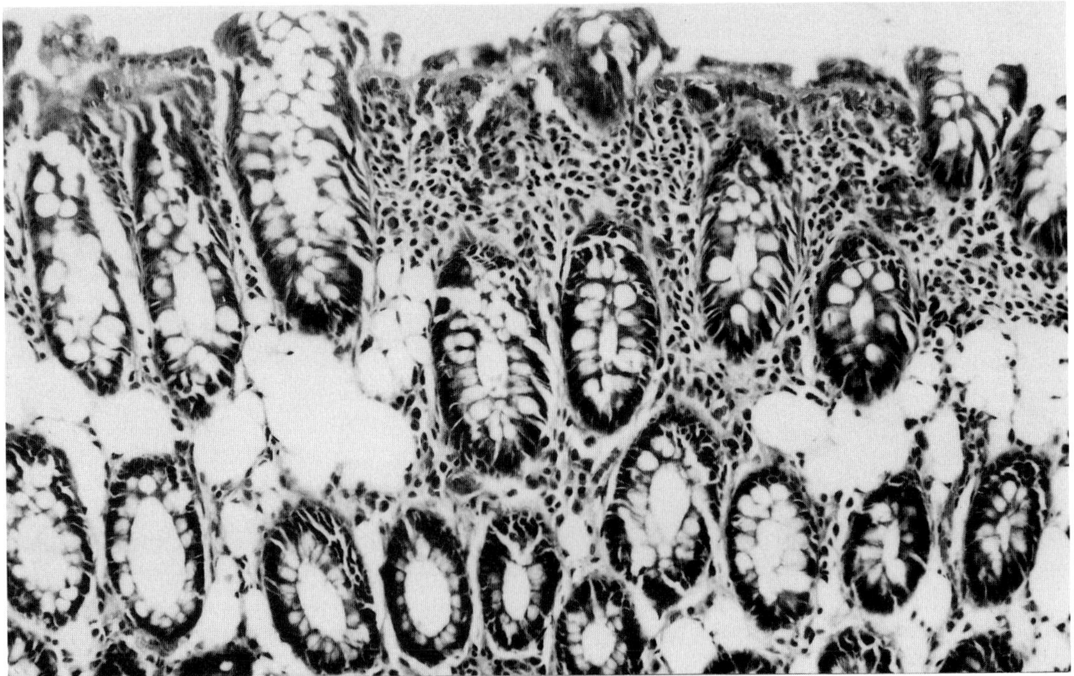

Fig. 9-27. Pseudolipomatosis in the colon. Noted are apparent spaces in the lamina propria. Although they resemble adipose cells, ultrastructural study reveals only artifactual spaces due to shrinkage from fixation (× 210).

tions of dysplasia and carcinoma are contained in Chapter 10.[215, 216]

Biopsy Uses

There are multiple reasons for examination of the rectum and colon in patients with IBD[7, 183, 217] (Table 9-9). Included are the exclusion of other specific causes of colitis, the identification or verification of a colitis or proctitis, the differentiation of acute versus chronic colitis, the distinction between UC and CD, the determination of the extent and severity of the disease, the assessment following therapy, and the detection of complications including dysplasia and carcinoma. It is especially helpful for the essential information and particular reason for the endoscopy to be provided on the requisition slip. Also useful are the gross findings, and modern technology permits sending a copy of the endoscopic appearance together with the requisition form.

Exclusion of Other Specific Causes

Uncommonly, the biopsy is obtained to rule out some other form of colitis that has a specific histology. Thus, early ischemic disease shows necrosis and hemorrhage with minimal inflammation, and antibiotic-associated colitis may reveal highly discrete membranes with sharply demarcated crypt inflammation. In addition, specific microorganisms, such as *Amoeba* or viral inclusions, may be realized. Overall, the appearance of such specific lesions in the assessment of patients for ulcerative colitis is uncommon.

Table 9-9. Mucosal Biopsy in Inflammatory Bowel Disease

Exclusion of other specific diseases
Identification of colitis and proctitis
Differentiation of acute versus chronic colitis
Distinction between UC and CD
Determination of disease extent, severity, and response to therapy
Detection of neoplasia

Identification of Colitis and Proctitis

A very common request for endoscopy and biopsy is to establish that the patient has a proctitis or colitis. Biopsies are routinely recommended whatever the findings are at the gross level. It is now evident that the gross evaluation may not be precise except in instances with marked inflammation or overt ulceration. Thus, although the mucosa may appear grossly normal, microscopic evidence of disease can be appreciated in the biopsy. This is particularly so in the case of determining chronic features and relatively mild active disease. Conversely, some of the cases with grossly evident abnormalities of a mild or uncertain nature, such as simple erythema, may reveal a normal histology, suggesting that the effects may be due to the endoscopic procedure. Whatever the case, biopsy examination is essential to establish or to confirm that the patient has a proctitis or colitis. The microscopic slide also offers a permanent record of this finding. In determining that the patient has a colitis, evidence is sought of chronic and/or active disease and not necessarily any specific feature.

Differentiation of Acute Versus Chronic Colitis

In the initial presentation of a case of proctitis or colitis, an effort may be made to distinguish IBD from an episode of an acute self-limited colitis that is most often due to infections[195–197] (Table 9-4). The acute cases show overall preservation of crypt architecture and cryptitis that is typically more marked in the superficial portion of the mucosa (Fig. 9-9). In contrast, cases of chronic colitis reveal some combination of crypt irregularity due to budding of the glands; crypt atrophy displayed as shortened crypts that are irregularly separated from the muscularis mucosae; a villiform surface; Paneth cell metaplasia; a large increase of mononuclear inflammatory cells; the presence of small lymphoid nodules; and the appearance of lymphocytes and plasma cells at the base of the mucosa beneath the crypts (Figs. 9-10 and 9-24). It has been estimated that one or more of these features of chronic disease can be seen in over 70 percent of cases of IBD within the first few weeks of the disease presentation.

More variable features of chronic disease are an increase in the number of endocrine cells, pyloric gland metaplasia, and the presence of fibrosis in the mucosa. In the biopsy showing chronic colitis, there is often an artifactual separation of the mucosal elements due to the variable location of the inflammatory cells[218] (Fig. 9-27). This was previously thought to represent adipose tissue and to be a sign of prior ulceration with extension of the material from the submucosa. It has now been demonstrated to represent just tissue separation from the fixation.

In the early cases that lack definite features of chronic disease, the differentiation of acute versus chronic colitis is dependent on the subsequent clinical course. Endoscopy and biopsy performed after a few months of therapy may be helpful, revealing complete restitution of normal mucosa in the cases of acute self-limited colitis and the presence of chronic features in most cases of IBD. The detection of chronic disease may be limited by the small biopsies taken and by the effects of therapeutic enemas.[219] Normal biopsies were observed in almost 30 percent of UC patients who received drug enemas. Accordingly, the finding of normal mucosa in a single biopsy, especially in the distal colon, does not completely rule out a chronic disease. Multiple samples may be needed to establish the chronicity.

Distinction between Ulcerative Colitis and Crohn's Disease

As noted previously, the differential between these two entities depends on the considering of a combination of features both of a gross and microscopic type. It is, therefore, essential to have information pertaining to the gross endoscopic and radiographic findings available at the time of biopsy examination. Given a biopsy sample, certain features are not available, such as the presence of fissures or sinus tracts and the notation of mural and transmural inflammation. Thus, although Crohn's disease may reveal very prominent lymphatic dilation and nerve proliferation in the submucosa, this cannot be appreciated in mucosal samples.

The potential findings on biopsy are a normal specimen, indicative of a spared area; the presence of a diffuse colitis, meaning that the entire specimen and all samples are affected; the finding of a focal colitis, represented in single or multiple samples; and the detection of a granuloma, independent of the feature of colitis.[7, 193] The findings of a normal biopsy to support that the rectum is not involved nor any other skip area, a focal colitis, or a granuloma all serve to identify that the patient has Crohn's disease, since these features are not seen in ulcerative colitis (Fig. 9-25). They may, however, occur in infections that must be excluded whenever one encounters a focal colitis with or without granulomas. Conversely, the finding of a diffuse colitis would support a diagnosis of ulcerative colitis but would not be specific, since it also can occur in a random area in a case of Crohn's disease. Accordingly, the diagnosis of ulcerative colitis remains the ultimate one of exclusion.

Determination of Disease Severity and Response to Therapy

Independent of the particular diagnosis, the biopsies may be obtained to determine the degree of severity of the disease, particularly whether active or inactive, and the response to therapy.[220] For the assessment of active disease, particularly important are the degree of cryptitis, ulceration, and neutrophilic reaction. Cases showing only scant cryptitis with relatively rare neutrophils typically correlate with clinically inactive disease.

Extent of Disease

Endoscopic examination and biopsy may be employed to determine the extent of disease, whichever the primary diagnosis. For example, in patients with long-standing ulcerative colitis in whom there has been evident gross disease as demonstrated by radiograph and sigmoidoscopy limited to the left colon, complete coloscopic examination may be warranted to determine the full extent of the disease. This is based on the impression that patients with more extensive colitis have a greater chance for the complications of dysplasia and carcinoma. In such examinations, biopsies should be obtained because the areas of inactive disease may be grossly normal. Any abnormalities in the form of chronic or active colitis are sought.

Another example would be patients with established Crohn's disease involving the ileum and colon or colon alone, for whom there is planned a segmental resection with anastomosis. The best time to determine the full extent of the disease is by endoscopy prior to the operation. In such cases the gross appearance is particularly important in assessing the extent of surgery, and biopsies are added for confirmation in any uncertain cases. In all of these examples, the particular diagnosis is not in question but rather the extent of the disease. Accordingly, evidence of chronic or active colitis without any distinguishing features is sought in the biopsy.

Detection of Neoplasia

Patients with long-standing idiopathic inflammatory bowel disease have an increased risk for the development of epithelial dysplasia and adenocarcinoma.[208, 209] At any time, endoscopy and biopsy may be needed to evaluate a mass lesion, remembering that most prove to be inflammatory pseudopolyps. Great caution is needed in the evaluation of these biopsies, since the polyps may be associated with marked epithelial alterations due to the inflammation and repair. In general, the inflammatory pseudopolyps reveal considerable stroma with edema and inflammation and show great variation in the appearance of the epithelia, including many normal or mildly damaged areas. In contrast, areas of polypoid dysplasia show denser glands and more uniform abnormalities in the epithelium.

Because of the considerable risk for the development of carcinoma, patients with long-standing IBD ultimately need surveillance to look for dysplasia or cancer.[221–223] This topic is covered in Chapter 10.

Tumor should also be suspected in patients with long-standing colitis who have persistent strictures or fistulae. Patients with Crohn's disease can develop these strictures as a consequence of inflammation early in the course of the disease, but their finding later may be more ominous. It may be difficult to access these regions, particularly strictures, and brush cytology might be tried similar to what is done in the upper gut.

Indeterminate Colitis

The term *indeterminate colitis* has been used for cases with ambiguous features that prevent the clear delineation between ulcerative colitis and Crohn's disease.[187, 224, 225] It is probably best to retain this term only for instances in which there is incomplete information regarding the distribution of the disease or incomplete examination of its full features. Accordingly, this term might be used at times of early biopsy examination prior to more extensive endoscopic, radiographic, and surgical examination.

Cases with Overlap of Features

Indeterminate colitis has unfortunately also been used to describe cases with shared features, but this is probably not helpful. For example, patients with diffuse colitis simulating ulcerative colitis may exceptionally show microscopic fissures extending into the muscularis propria and granulomas, and such cases should more appropriately be categorized as Crohn's disease. Conversely, there may be cases that appear to be focal based on the gross examination but this is due to uneven severity, and microscopic examination reveals a diffuse disorder[224]; it would be best to regard such cases as ulcerative colitis. Many other microscopic features have been heralded as more prominent in one or the other form of colitis but are not specific; these include inflammatory pseudopolyps, lymphoid nodules, lymphatic dilation, fibrosis, and proliferation of nerves. These features may be more common in UC or CD but can occur in either form.

Cases of Ulcerative Colitis

Ulcerative colitis is typically diffuse but may show uneven involvement simulating skip areas, and it has now been established that the right side of the colon can be skipped in the face of cecal and appendiceal lesions.[191, 192] Also, it is important to distinguish so-called backwash ileitis from actual ulcerative involvement of the ileum, with the latter favoring Crohn's disease. Although ulcerative colitis dominantly affects the mucosa and submucosa, about one-third of the surgically treated cases reveal extension of ulceration into the muscularis propria, and these are associated with patchy serosal or transmural inflammation.[190]

Cases of Crohn's Disease

Although Crohn's disease usually is protrayed as a segmental and transmural condition, there are exceptions, with superficial or diffuse disease noted in 5 to 10 percent of the cases.[190, 226] Similarly, the rectum can be involved in half of the cases, and any one of the distinctive features, such as fissures or granulomas, may be absent. Indeed, grossly evident sinus tracts are seen in only one-third of the cases, and granulomas in only 25 percent of the biopsies. In all of these situations, there can be overlap and confusion in the distinction between ulcerative colitis and Crohn's disease.

Summary

There are no special features of indeterminate colitis. Indeed, the author believes that it would be better to describe the variable features and to note the degrees of uncertainty with regard to the precise diagnosis at the time of early biopsy rather than use this diagnostic term. In this regard, it is exceedingly important to remember that the diagnostic distinction of ulcerative colitis and Crohn's disease is based on a combination of gross and microscopic features.

CHEMICAL AND DRUG INJURY

The colonic and rectal mucosa is readily injured by a large array of chemicals and drugs that are applied at a local or systemic level[227, 228] (Table 9-10).

Chemotherapy Effects

The various chemotherapeutic agents used as adjuncts in the treatment of cancers can easily damage the colonic mucosa since it is

Table 9-10. Chemical and Drug Injury in the Colon

- Chemotherapy
- Enemas and cathartics
- Antibiotic-associated colitis
- Other drugs
  - NSAIDs
  - Hormones
  - Anticholinergic- and antidepressant-induced pseudo-obstruction
  - Gold-induced colitis
  - Miscellaneous effects

constantly replicating. The effects are usually not as advanced as in the small intestine. Nevertheless, there can occur edema and ulceration, usually limited to the superficial region, with only rare examples of sinus tracts or perforation. Colonic carcinomas are common and may require chemotherapy, but the agent usually used, 5-fluorouracil, is not especially toxic.[229]

Biopsy Features

Biopsy in these cases reveals nonspecific features, in the form of cryptitis, ulcers, acute and chronic inflammation, and variable granulation tissue. The studies are usually performed not only to look for effects of therapy but also to rule out other problems in such patients, notably recurrence of tumor and the appearance of opportunistic infections.

Enemas and Cathartics

Many of these lesions have been eliminated or lessened due to more judicious use of the various solutions.

Enema Effects

Bland solutions such as saline may cause slight edema of the lamina propria but no other signs of injury. Earlier use of more caustic substances was associated with occasional development of a mild acute colitis, characterized by damage to the epithelial cells on the surface, and in the upper portions of the crypt associated with edema and congestion of the lamina propria together with a rare neutrophil[230] (Fig. 9-28). In biopsy evaluation of such cases the absence of regeneration was usually a sign that this was a very recent event and did not correlate with the clinical history of a longer duration.[231] The present use of oral hypertonic solutions results in prominent edema but usually no damage to the epithelial cells of inflammation[21] (Fig. 9-8). In these cases, it is important to rule out the potential for enema effect before considering the diagnosis of a more important colitis.

More marked necrosis has been occasionally noted with some of the stronger hypertonic solutions such as Kayexalate, and crystals may be seen in the biopsies[232] (Fig. 9-29). Examples of enemas containing soap solutions and accidental inclusions of alcohol or hydrogen peroxide were associated with extensive necrosis and shedding of the mucosa.[233, 234] The diagnosis in such cases is established by the clinical information and does not usually require biopsy.

Laxative Effects

It has been suggested that the entity of melanosis coli is related to excess use of certain laxatives.[235] In such cases there is the appearance of increased lipofuscin within the macrophages in the lamina propria. Extensive and continued use of laxatives can lead to atrophy and shortening of the gut, affecting both the terminal parts of the small intestine and the colon. The diagnosis is typically established by the clinical and radiographic findings. With laxative abuse, the patients present with diarrhea lacking a specific cause, and the ultimate diagnosis is dependent on obtaining the appropriate history.[236] In these examples with excess laxatives, there are no specific features in the biopsies.

Antibiotic-Associated Pseudomembranous Colitis

Etiology and Pathogenesis

This is a relatively common form of acute colitis, due to the ingestion of a large variety of antibiotics or other substances that can alter the bowel flora in the large intestine.[106, 237] It has been demonstrated that the

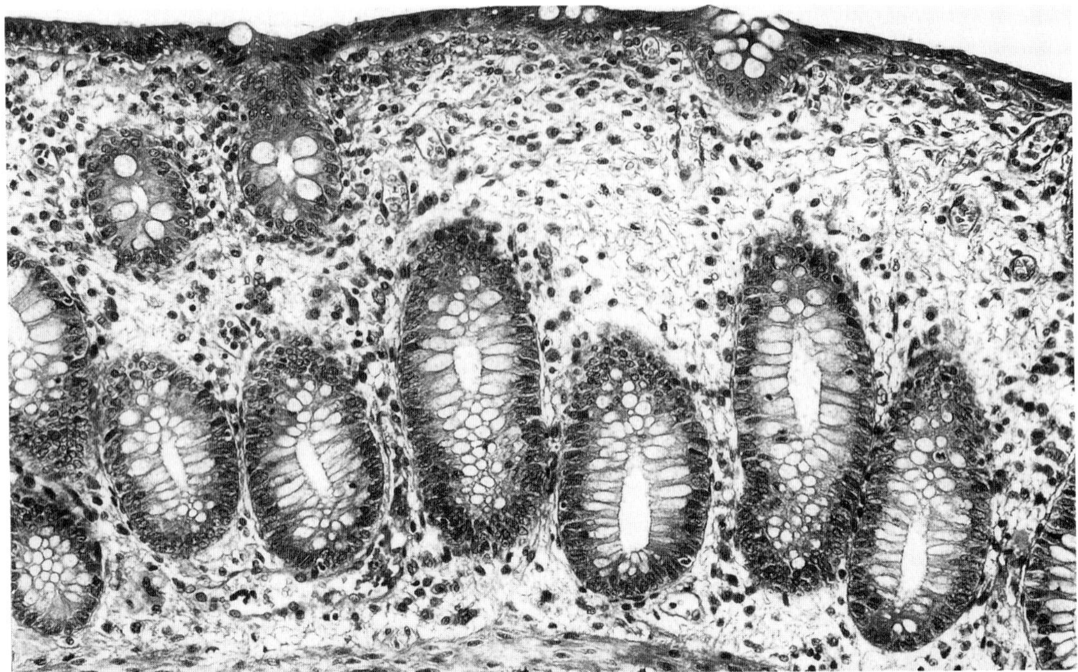

Fig. 9-28. Mild injury due to enema. There is edema of the lamina propria, flattening of the surface epithelium, and dilated capillaries. Some cases show rare neutrophils, but there are no mitoses. The muscularis appears at the bottom (× 210).

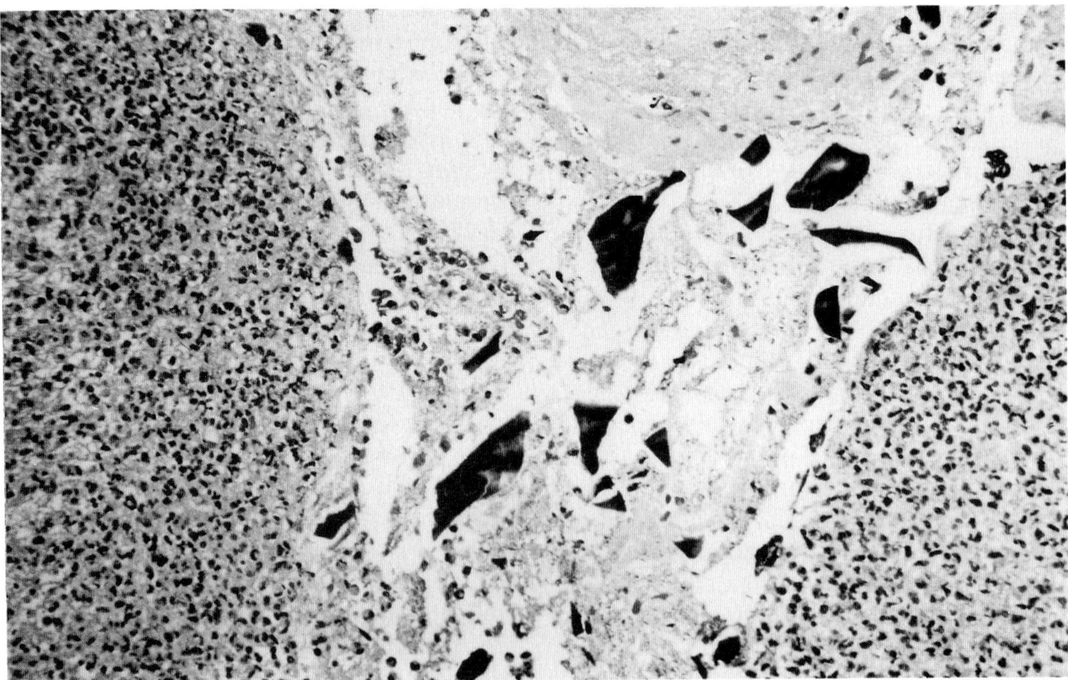

Fig. 9-29. Acute colitis due to Kayexalate enema. Noted are ulceration with marked acute inflammation and densely basophilic, irregularly shaped crystals.

cases are due to a selective overgrowth of *Clostridium difficile,* which in turn releases two important toxins. One of these acts on the local vasculature leading to an ischemic-type lesion that results in a florid form of acute colitis.

Endoscopic Features

There is marked variation in clinical presentation from relatively mild diarrhea to severe dysentery. Endoscopy may show patchy or more confluent lesions involving any part of the colon. In the earlier stages the characteristic sharply circumscribed and small, yellow, slightly raised membranes, or *pseudomembranes,* can be seen. In more advanced cases, there can develop an extreme edema of the mucosa and wall with the threat of perforation.

Biopsy Features

The diagnosis is typically made by a biologic assay of the stool for the bacterial toxin. Endoscopic examination is often done to look for the pseudomembranes, helping to establish the diagnosis, and to rule out other causes.[238] Biopsies taken from the early lesions, particularly at the edge of the membranes, reveal a part that is completely normal and adjacent to crypts that have exploded and are covered by a mass of fibrin and neutrophils (Fig. 9-30). In later stages, there is more extensive destruction and edema and the biopsies greatly resemble ischemic bowel disease. Biopsies in such cases show greater edema and necrosis, but there is still a marked predilection for the upper part of the mucosa and there is an overlying heavy membrane.[239] In practice, when on encounters such inflammatory pseudomembranes, it is best to share the possibilities of either a *C. difficile* infection, usually related to antibiotic use, and ischemic bowel disease.

As the disease recedes, the bowel typically returns to normal. In patients with preexisting IBD who develop secondary infections with *C. difficile,* the typical pseudomembranes are absent and the biopsies are indistinguishable from ordinary chronic active colitis.[204]

Other Drugs

There are a multitude of drugs that can affect any part of the intestinal tract by highly varied mechanisms. Some act on both the small and large bowel and others show greater preference for the colon.[240] This subject is extensively covered in reviews and in textbooks, and the major findings at biopsy are presented here.

Nonsteroidal Anti-Inflammatory Drugs

Whereas NSAIDs commonly cause lesions in the stomach and upper small bowel, lesions in the colon are rare.[241, 242] Biopsies are usually nonspecific, showing focal erosions. Rarely, the NSAIDs can lead to more extensive mucosal damage in the colon, usually the proximal portion, resulting in the development of strictures and of mucosal bridges or diaphragms.[243, 244] These drugs may also result in activation of IBD in patients who have proven to be allergic to salicylates.[206] It has also been suggested that they may promote the development of some cases of collagenous colitis.[245]

More extensive disease has also been noted with the use of salicylates and indomethacin in suppositories, resulting in greater cryptitis and necrosis.[246] The diagnosis is usually evident and biopsies are not needed.

Hormones

As in other parts of the gut, corticosteroid treatment can lead to the promotion of opportunistic infections. The estrogenic hor-

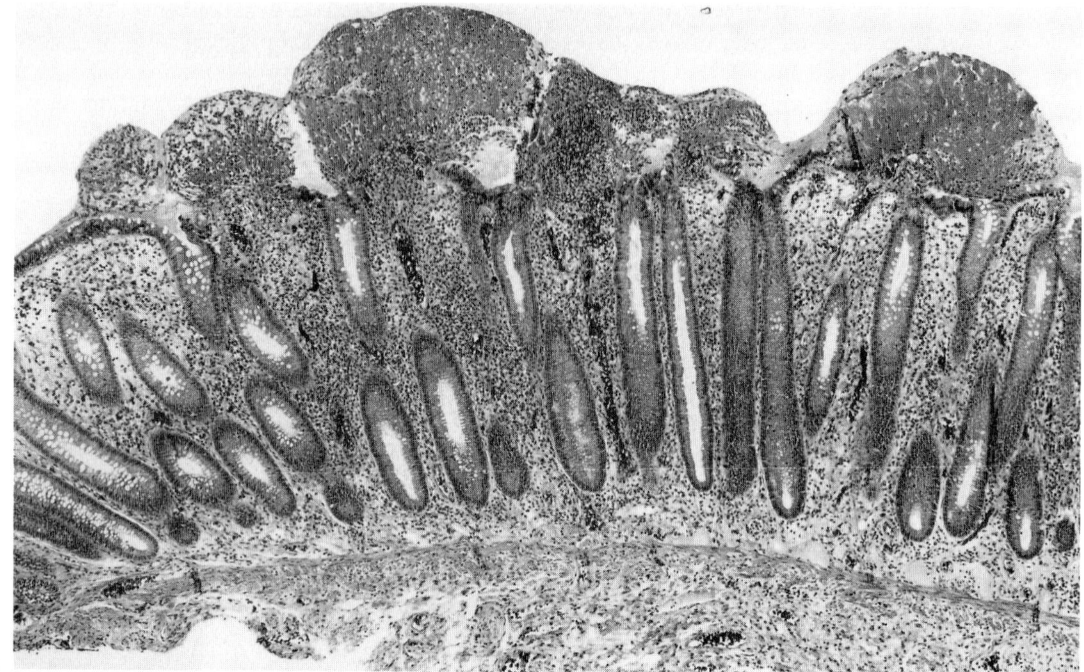
A

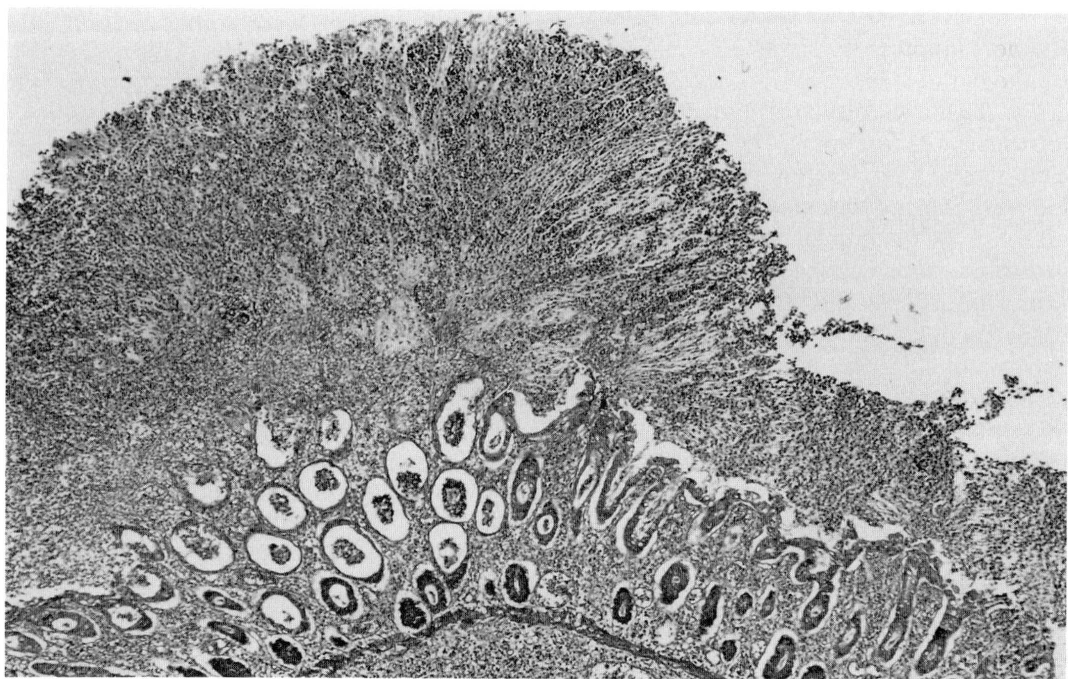
B

Fig. 9-30. Pseudomembranous colitis. **(A)** There are superficial erosions and patches of prominent inflammatory exudate, representing the membranes, on the mucosal surface appearing at the top. Muscularis and submucosa appear at the bottom (× 210). **(B)** More advanced lesion, showing greater necrosis and inflammatory membrane (left). More normal mucosa is seen at the lower right (× 42).

mones, including the oral contraceptive pill, may be associated with the development of thrombi leading to hemorrhages and ischemic lesions in the small or large intestine.[247, 248] These are visualized by radiographic and endoscopic studies, and biopsies reveal mucosal necrosis and regeneration.

Pseudo-Obstruction

Many drugs, including particularly anticholinergic and antidepressant agents, can lead to poor bowel motility favoring pseudo-obstruction that may be manifest in the small or large intestine.[53, 55] This can lead to late effects of ischemic damage. The diagnosis is typically established by the clinical information.

Gold-Induced Colitis

Rheumatoid arthritis patients who are taking gold salts may develop an enteritis or colitis that is not directly related to the total dosage, suggesting an allergic reaction.[249, 250] There develops a focal or more extensive but usually segmental colitis that leads to ulceration and simulates IBD. Biopsies reveal the necrosis and inflammation but are otherwise nonspecific. The lesions typically regress following withdrawal of the drug.

Miscellaneous Drug Effects

Many other lesions have been noted, including hemorrhage from anticoagulants; ischemic lesions from the use of numerous vasoconstrictive drugs; a localized proctitis due to ergot suppositories; and the appearance of pneumatosis from occasional agents.[228, 251, 252] The diagnosis is typically established by the clinical history and biopsy is largely used to rule out other disorders. Additional examples include reactions to the cleaning solutions that were not adequately removed from the endoscopes[253, 254]; colitis presumably of an allergic nature due to isotretinoin and to acyclovir[255, 256]; a toxic megacolon from methotrexate[257]; and ischemic lesions following cocaine abuse.[258]

PHYSICAL INJURY

Radiation Injury

General Effects

The large intestine is relatively resistant to radiation, but can be damaged by the very high radiation doses that are used in the treatment of tumors of some of the adjacent organs, particularly the uterine cervix and the prostate.[259–262] Regularly seen are the acute effects, consisting of prominent edema of the submucosa with variable ulceration, and these usually subside promptly after the treatments[263–265] (see Table 7-5). Chronic effects are common but usually mild, consisting of variable atrophy of the mucosa associated with prominent vascular ectasia and with thickening of the collagen layer beneath the surface and crypt epithelium.[266] This thickening can simulate and be confused with that seen in cases of collagenous colitis. More extensive effects of radiation are seen in a small portion of cases and are probably due to alterations in the larger arteries, leading to narrowing of these arteries and secondary ischemic damage of the bowel.

Biopsy Features

Biopsy is often done in patients not only to find and to establish the effects of radiation but also to exclude other problems in these patients, such as the appearance of recurrent tumor or of opportunistic infections. The biopsy features are generally nonspecific, showing edema and ulcers with acute and chronic inflammation (Fig. 9-31). Suggestive features of radiation effects include

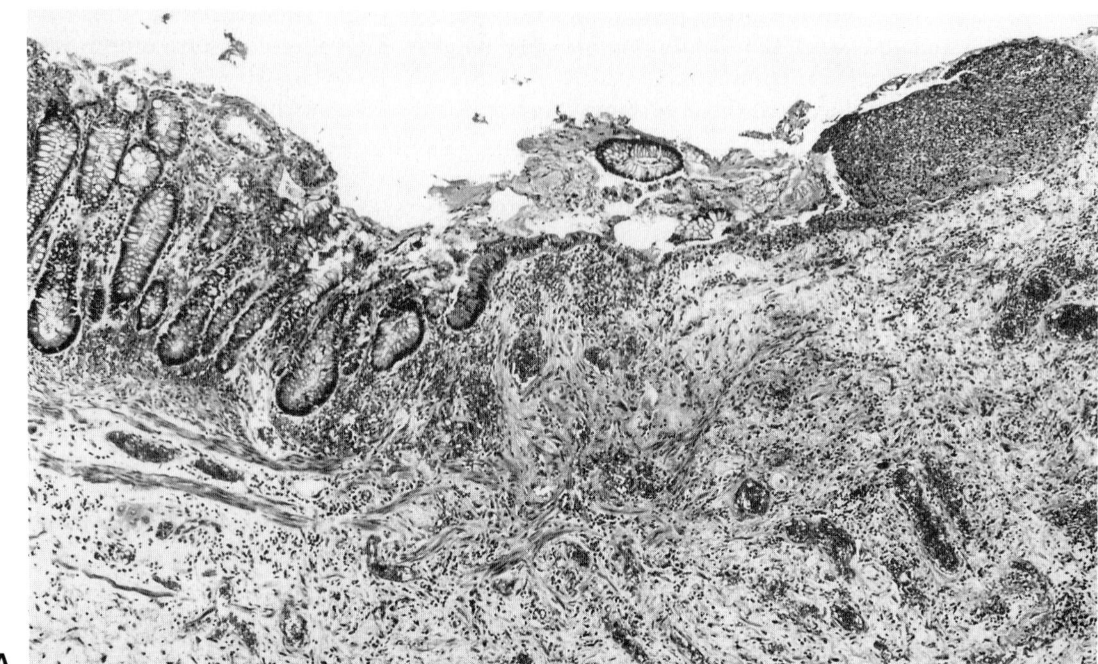

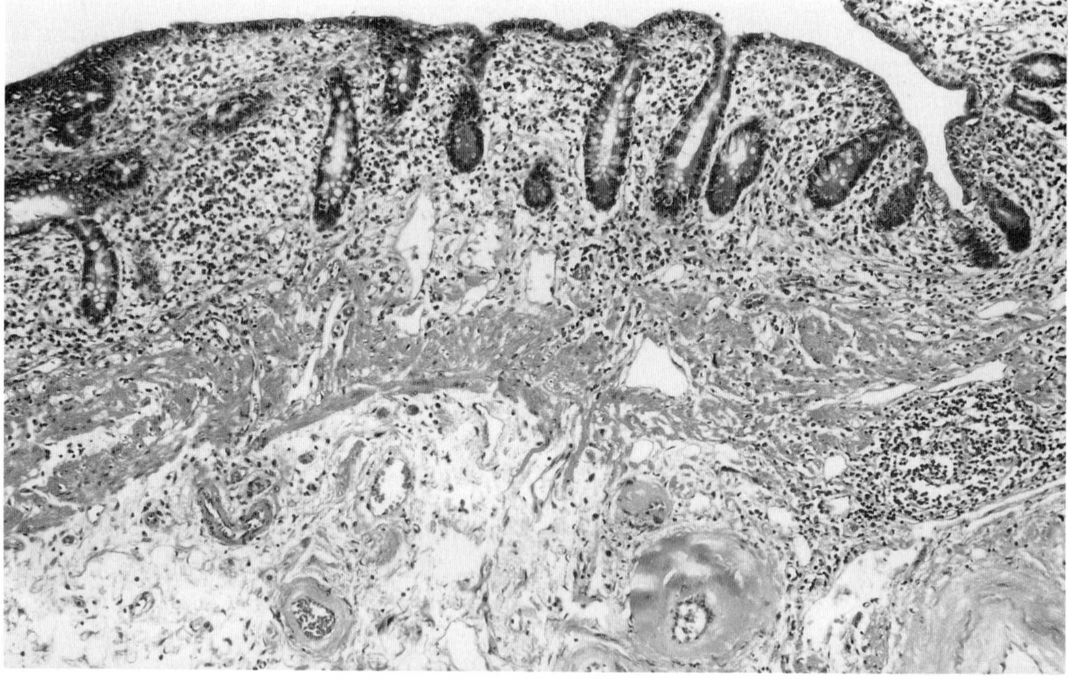

Fig. 9-31. Examples of radiation injury in the colon. **(A)** Acute ulceration with underlying granulation tissue (right). Normal mucosa appears at the left (× 68). **(B)** Chronic radiation effects, showing mucosal atrophy in the form of shortened crypts, thickened muscularis mucosae, and marked hyalinization of the submucosal vessels (× 105). (*Figure continues.*)

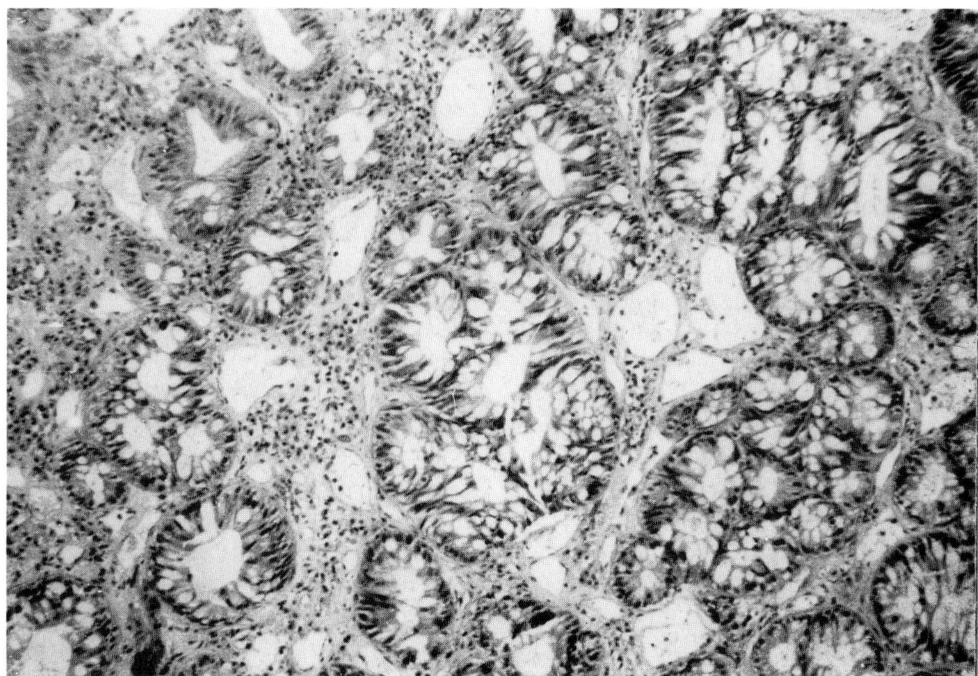

Fig. 9-31 (*Continued*). **(C)** Clumping of the crypts that may be mistaken for dysplasia. These changes occur early after radiation exposure and typically disappear.

prominent telangiectasia, the collagen thickening in the mucosa, and the appearance of enlarged nuclei in the mesenchymal cells underlying areas of ulceration (see Fig. 2-22). The changes in the larger vessels are not seen in the mucosal biopsies.

Complications

Rarely noted are examples of colitis cystica profunds developing in an inflammatory stricture that is associated with radiation.[267] There is probably also a slight increase in tumor formation in the colon as a result of radiation.[268] These effects are seen after many years and are more concentrated in the lower colon and rectum, reflecting the areas receiving the highest dose from treatment of tumors in adjacent organs. A link to radiation has been well established with adenocarcinoma and, possibly, with lymphoma of the colon. It has been suggested that in high-risk groups, surveillance endoscopy and biopsy should be done to look for dysplasia. However, the findings of dysplastic epithelium protrayed in the literature have not been totally convincing. Early after radiation treatment, within the first or second year, there can develop a considerable proliferation of the glands and a mild atypism that simulates dysplasia, but this recedes (Fig. 9-31C). It is probable that the overall risk is insufficient to justify any surveillance program to look particularly for dysplasia.

Foreign Body Effects

Foreign body granulomas readily occur secondary to suture and to mucus from ruptured crypts. These must be appreciated and distinguished from the well formed granulomas that are seen in Crohn's disease.

Barium Granuloma

At the time of radiographic examination, barium may extend into the submucosa and deeper wall, probably through areas of ulceration.[269–271] This can produce small nodules and is most often encountered in the rectum. The biopsy shows a large mass of macrophages containing the finely granular barium material that is refractile but not doubly refractile (Fig. 9-32). There is usually no prominent giant cell formation or fibrosis.

Oleogranuloma

Oleogranulomas represent reactions to oils that are inserted into the rectum, largely for the treatment of hemorrhoids or constipation.[272–274] Some of these are irritating and can evoke marked inflammation and fibrosis. The biopsies show the nodular areas containing multiple irregular spaces, which represent oils that are dissolved in preparation (Fig. 9-33).

IMMUNOLOGIC DISORDERS

Allergic Proctitis and Colitis

Allergic proctitis and colitis occurs almost exclusively in newborns and young infants and represents an anaphylactic reaction to a dietary protein, typically cow's milk or soy bean protein.[275–278] It has also been observed in infants receiving breast milk and is presumably due to the transfer of foreign proteins into that substance.[279] Patients typically present with rectal bleeding or bloody diarrhea in the first 2 weeks, which subsides after a change in the formula. Most studies have concentrated on examination and biopsy of the rectum but it is thought that the lesion probably involves a larger segment of the colon.

Biopsy Features

Biopsies taken at the time of the bleeding reveal an increase of eosinophils within the lamina propria and a focal extension into the epithelium lining the surface and crypts[280] (Fig. 9-34). This can be very focal, and multiple sections are needed to show the lesion.[281] The number of eosinophils in the normal lamina propria is highly variable and appears to be related to the geographic region, being much less in the northern cities and higher in the southern cities of the United States.[282] The severe cases show eosinophils extending into the muscularis mucosae as well. There are typically no changes of a chronic colitis in the form of altered architecture, and the alterations disappear following a change in the dietary protein.[283]

With aging, the allergy is lost due to the development of IgG-type antibodies that prevent the anaphylactic reaction. This disorder appears to differ from allergic or eosinophilic gastroenteritis, which ordinarily affects older children and adults and is associated with lesions dominantly in the upper and mid-intestinal tract.[280, 284] (See Chs. 4 and 6 for further details regarding allergic gastroenteritis.)

Immunologic Deficiencies

Immunologic deficiencies are largely described in Chapters 6 and 7 (see Table 6-6). The principal effects in the large intestine are those of opportunistic infections and an increase in certain tumors.

Primary Immunodeficiency Disorders

The primary immunodeficiency disorders include selective IgA deficiency, hypogammaglobulinemia, agammaglobulinemia, T-cell deficiencies, and other rarer disorders.[285] The more severe cases are seen when there are combined B-cell and T-cell deficiencies.

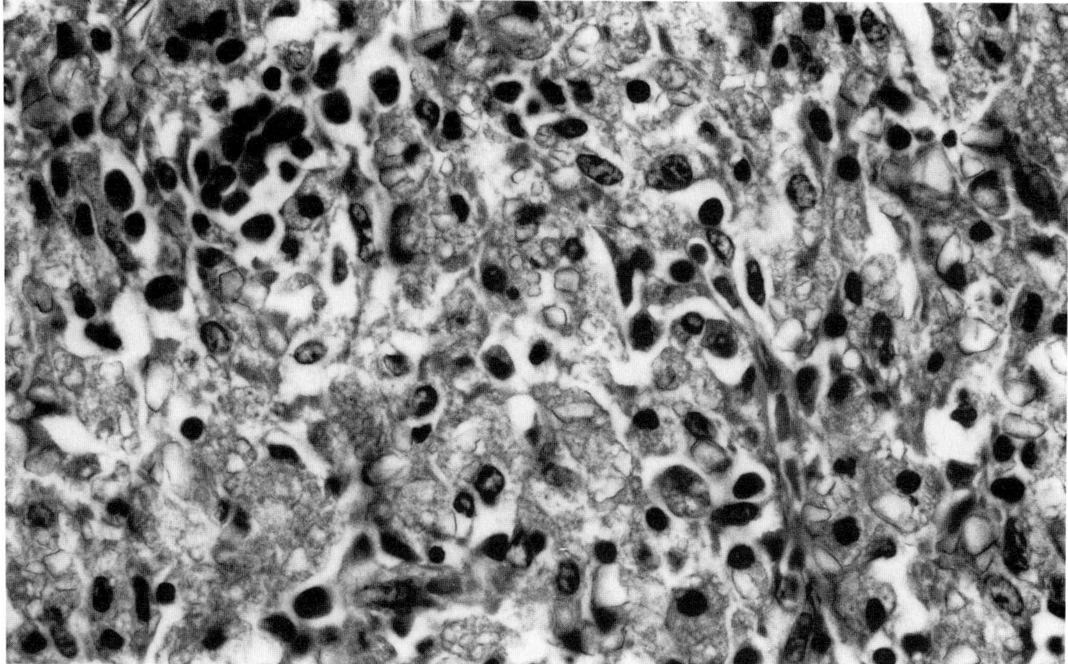

Fig. 9-32. Barium granuloma in the rectum. There is a diffuse infiltrate of macrophages in the submucosa. Noted in the cytoplasm are the tan, refractile granules of barium (× 635).

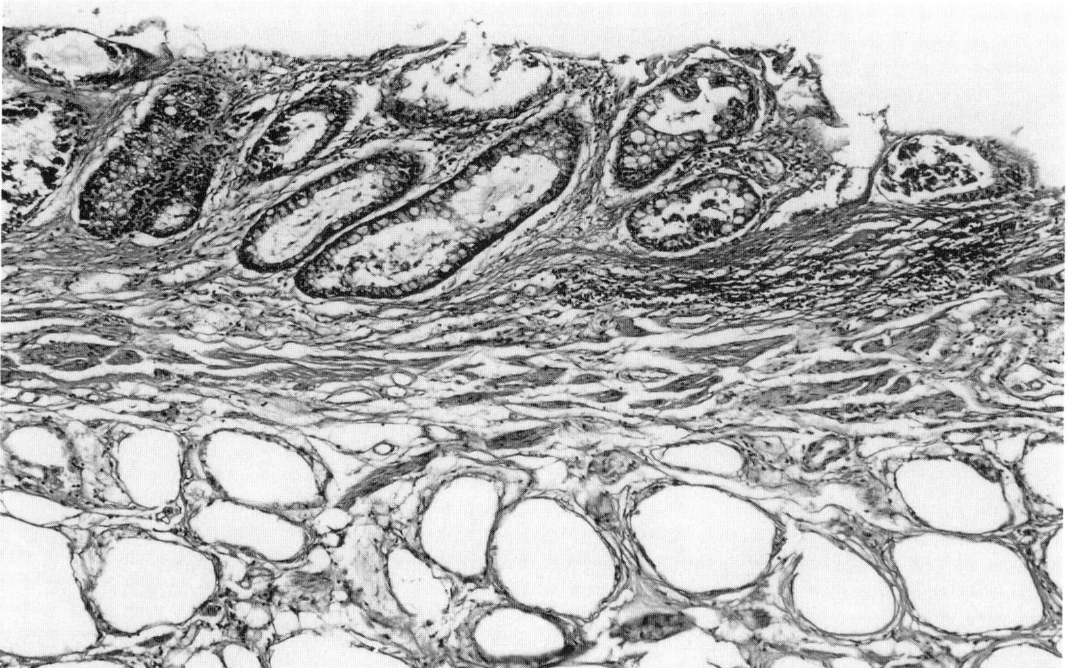

Fig. 9-33. Oil granuloma (oleogranuloma) in the colon. Noted are numerous spaces in the submucosa (bottom) corresponding to the oil substances. There is mild reaction in this case, but other examples show marked fibrosis. The compressed mucosa appears at the top (× 105).

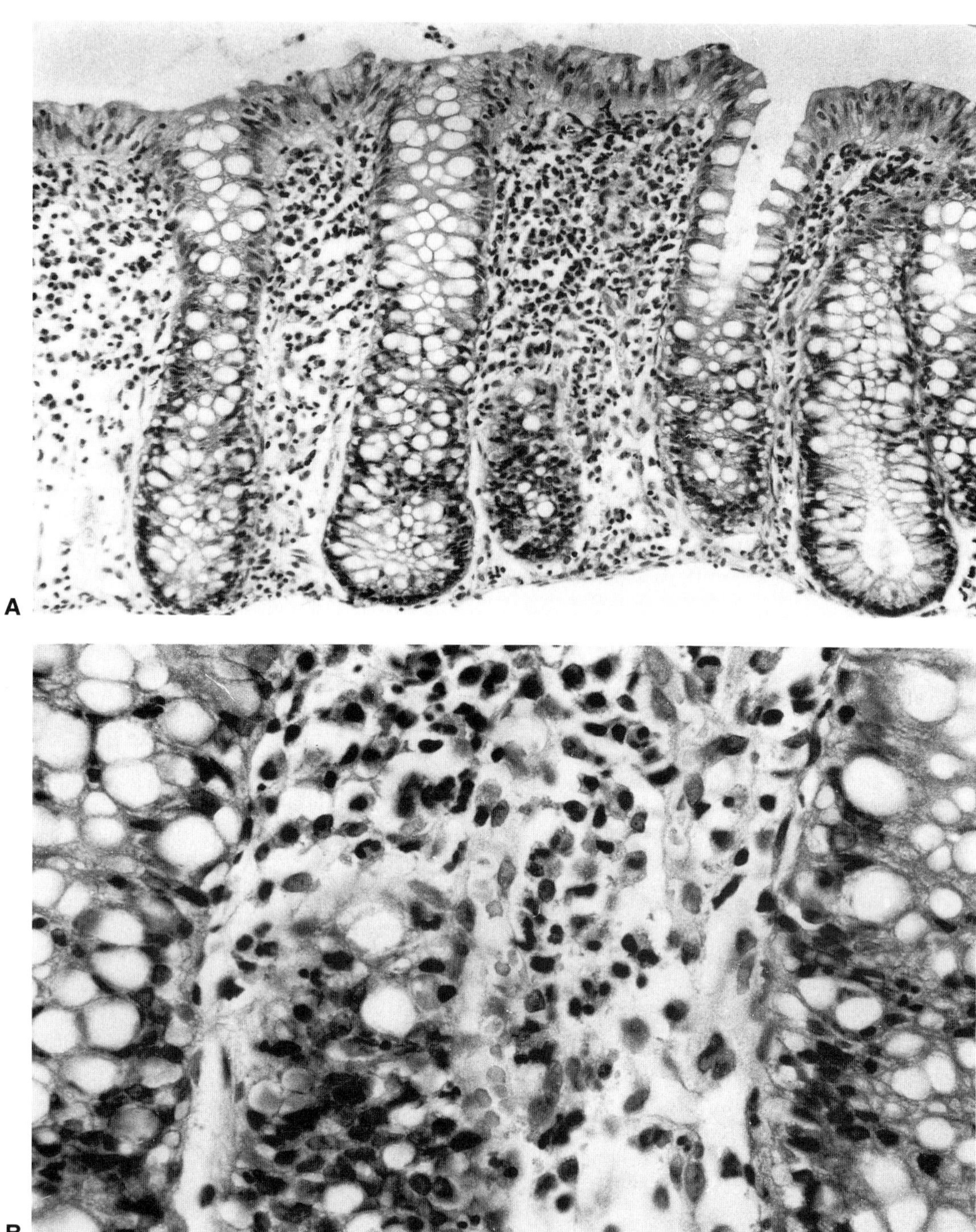

Fig. 9-34. Allergic proctitis. **(A)** The overall crypt architecture is normal. Noted is an increase of inflammatory cells in the upper portion of the lamina propria (× 210). **(B)** Closer view, revealing the many eosinophils in the lamina propria with focal extension into the crypt epithelial layer (× 635).

A variety of opportunistic infections can occur in the large intestine, and these are outlined in Chapter 7.

Acquired Disorders

Acquired disorders are represented by cases of AIDS and patients with various transplants. All of these cases are at risk for infections due to a variety of opportunistic agents, notably to herpes and cytomegalovirus, to *Mycobacterium avium,* to *Candida* and other fungi, and to *Cryptosporidium* and Microsporidia.[114, 286–288] There also is a definite increase in Kaposi's tumors and probably an enhanced degree of lymphoma. Biopsy is largely done to identify the various infections and tumors.

Graft-versus-Host Disease

Graft-versus-host disease can develop following bone marrow and other transplants and is due to a lymphocytic reaction by the graft tissue.[289] Lesions of the intestine, including the colon and rectum, regularly occur.

Biopsy Features

Biopsy of early lesions shows focal lymphocytic infiltrate around and into the crypt epithelium, which is associated with prominent apoptosis[290] (Fig. 9-35). The lesions can be very focal and can require multiple sections for identification. They are not totally specific, as similar lesions can be seen in some infections such as salmonellosis. More severe reactions are associated with erosions and ulcers and prominent acute inflammation, findings that are also entirely nonspecific.[291] The skin appears to be the preferred site for documentation of this disorder, and intestinal biopsies are now less often obtained.

OTHER INFLAMMATORY DISORDERS

Collagenous Colitis

Collagenous colitis is an uncommon condition that almost always involves middle-aged and older women.[292, 293] The patients present with prolonged watery diarrhea, and radiographic and colonoscopic examinations are normal. The etiology is not known, and there is irregular response to anti-inflammatory agents. Although the disease is thought to primarily affect the colon, there are examples of synchronous involvement of the small bowel and suggestions that the disorder may be seen more often in patients with celiac disease and with other autoimmune disorders.[294, 295] It also has been observed in some patients receiving NSAIDs.[245]

Biopsy Features

The biopsy features are distinctive, revealing a thickening of the collagen layer beneath the basement membrane of the surface epithelium[296–304] (Fig. 9-36). It is restricted to this region and does not extend down along the crypts. The lesion is often continuous but also may be patchy, particularly in the earlier and in the resolving phases of the disease[305, 306] (Fig. 9-37). The change is typically more marked in the proximal colon, whereas the distal part and, particularly, the rectum may be spared. Accordingly, a negative rectal biopsy does not exclude this condition.

The normal collagen layer in this region ranges from 2 to 3μm on average, whereas the lesion in collagenous colitis is usually 10 μm or greater in thickness. Similar thickenings can be seen, however, in other conditions, especially in idiopathic IBD, radiation damage, and other colitides.[302, 304] Therefore, the simple finding of the collagen thickening is not sufficient. There must also be the appropriate clinical syndrome.

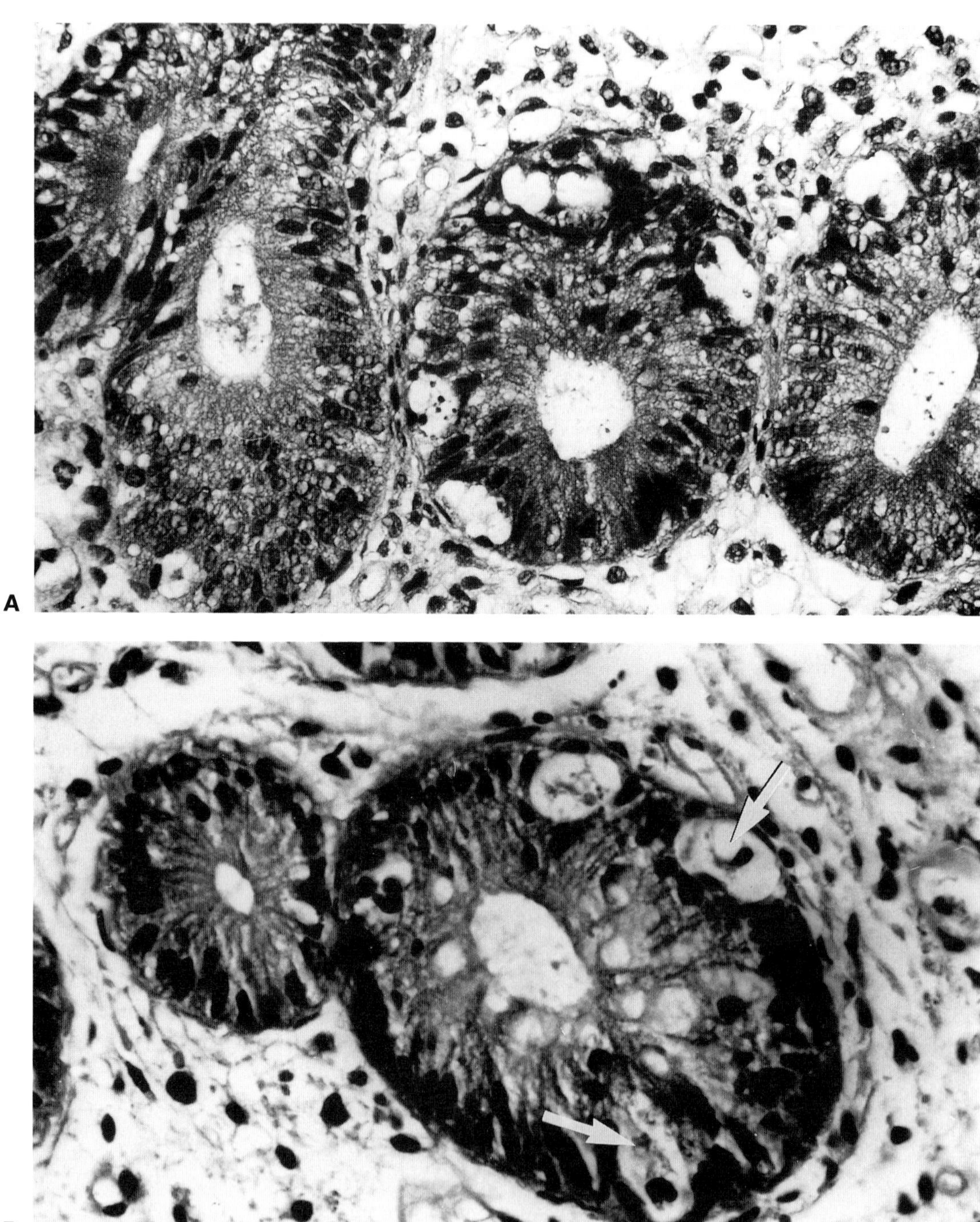

Fig. 9-35. Graft-versus-host disease in the colon. **(A)** Base of the crypts, revealing focal infiltrate of lymphocytes into the epithelial layer (× 425). **(B)** Closer view of the crypts to show the increase in apoptotic cells (arrows) (× 635).

It has also been noted that many cases reveal an increase in the amount of lymphocytes within the surface epithelium, similar to that seen in the small bowel in celiac sprue.[292] It is possible that the combination of the collagen thickening and the increased inflammation of the surface epithelium will prove to be the best marker of collagenous colitis. Of interest, despite the prolonged course, there are typically no other changes of chronic disease in the form of crypt budding or atrophy. It has been suggested that there may be focal increase of mononuclear inflammatory cells in the lamina propria, but this is difficult to document.

With regression of the disease, the collagen layer becomes patchy and finally disappears. There are typically no recurrences. Biopsy is largely performed to document the disease and to exclude other inflammatory conditions.

Lymphocytic Colitis

Lymphocytic colitis was previously termed *microscopic* colitis. The patients present with prolonged watery diarrhea, but unlike those with collagenous colitis, the condition affects either gender and adults of all ages.[292, 293, 307] The etiology is not known. Recent studies suggest a close association of celiac disease and lymphocytic colitis as well as an association with some patients of lymphocytic gastritis.[295] It is possible that some of the examples of lymphocytic colitis that have been noted reflect ongoing inflammation in patients with active celiac disease, but this needs to be substantiated. A case resembling lymphocytic colitis has also been noted in a patient receiving a tonic drug, cyto-3-fort,[308] suggesting that lymphocytic colitis is a response to many disorders including drug reactions.

Biopsy Features

There is typically no colonoscopic or radiographic abnormalities in the large intestine. Biopsy reveals a marked increase of lymphocytes in the surface epithelium, but the absence of a thickened collagen layer[307] (Fig. 9-38). This lymphocytic infiltrate can extend into the upper regions of the crypts. There have been many reports indicating variable increases of chronic and acute inflammatory cells in the lamina propria, but this is not a constant feature. Not much is known of the natural history except that the lesions eventually regress. Biopsy is done to establish the lesion of lymphocytic colitis and to rule out other forms of inflammatory disease.

Diversion Colitis

Patients who have a colostomy for any reason may develop inflammatory changes in the diverted segment of colon and rectum.[309–321] When initially reviewed by endoscopy early after the procedure, the gross endoscopic features resemble a mild ulcerative colitis, but the patients lack any history of lesions in the colon proximal to the stoma. The cause of the inflammatory lesion is not known, but is presumably an effect of the stasis leading to production of excess bacteria or other metabolic substances. Of interest, it has been noted that the installation of fatty acids can cause regression of symptoms in patients who have not had a reanastomosis.[322]

Biopsy Features

Biopsy is entirely nonspecific, initially revealing focal crypt abscesses, superficial erosions, and prominent lymphoid hyperplasia[309, 318] (Fig. 9-39). More long-standing cases may show ulcerations, inflammatory pseudopolyps, and rarely granulomas.[311–321] The diagnosis is absolutely dependent on a combination of the clinical information and the pathologic material. It is ultimately determined by the response to reanastomosis, since the lesions disappear.

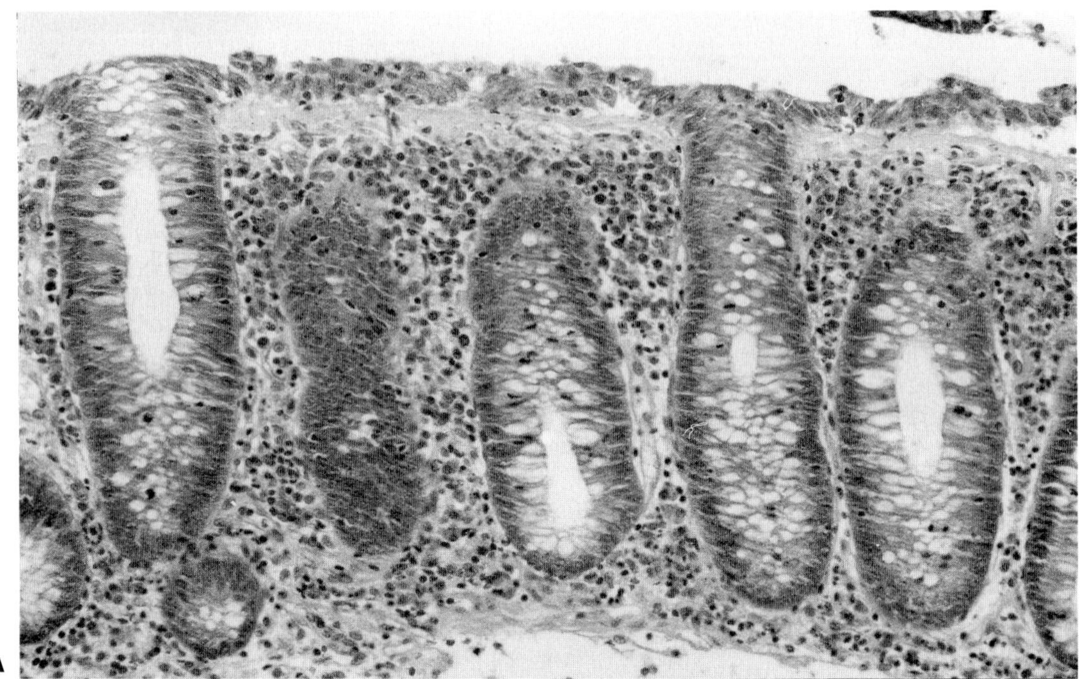

A

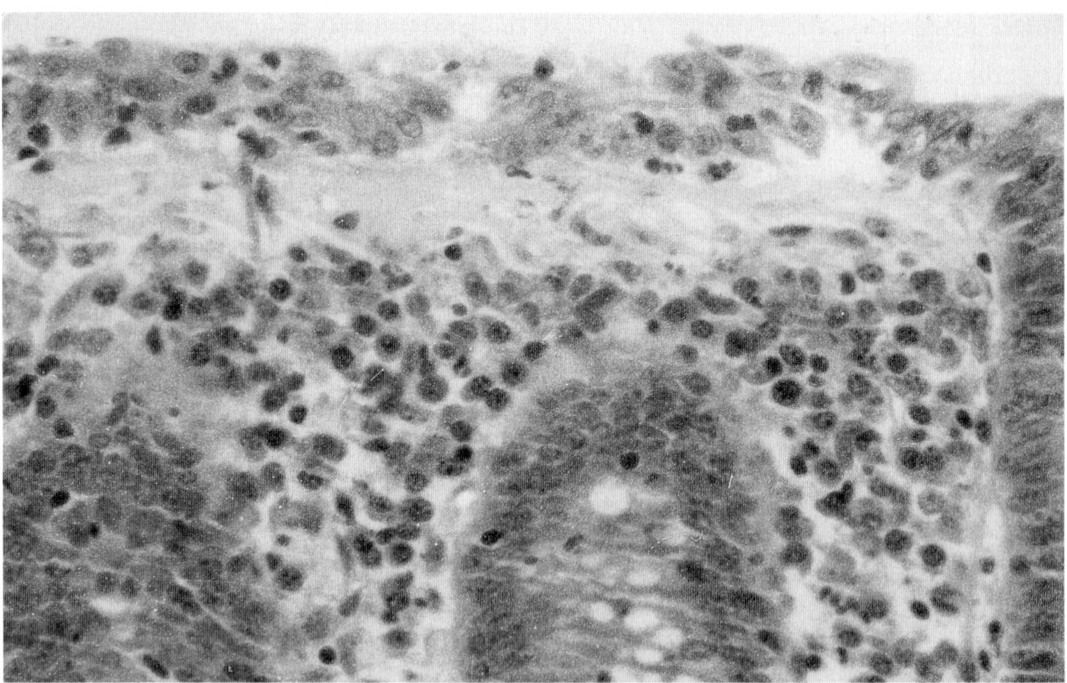

B

Fig. 9-36. Collagenous colitis. **(A)** There is a diffuse thickening of the collagen layer beneath the surface epithelium (top). It does not extend down along the crypts (× 210). **(B)** Closer view of the surface, showing the expanded collagen layer and also increased inflammatory cells in the surface epithelial layer (top) (× 535).

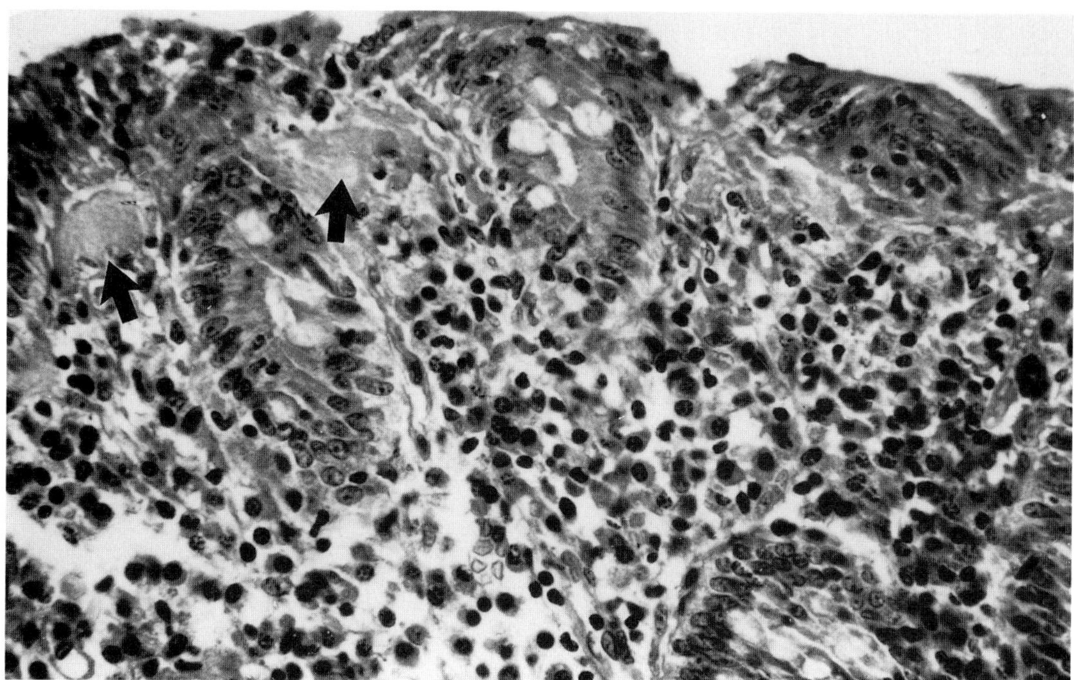

Fig. 9-37. Focal changes in collagenous colitis. The thickening of the collagen layer beneath the surface epithelium is patchy, as seen in the upper left (arrows).

Clinical Aspects

When the colostomy is done in a patient without established IBD, such as for diverticular disease, the appearance of the inflammation in the distal segment can quickly be construed as due to the diverting procedure. In contrast, if the colostomy occurs in a patient with Crohn's disease, the problem arises as to whether the changes in the distal segment represent those of diversion or of early recurrence of the Crohn's disease. It is helpful in such situations to check previous biopsies of the distal area before the colostomy procedure, and there probably should be more extensive involvement with sinus tracts to accept a diagnosis of Crohn's disease in such a situation. If there is any doubt, reanastomosis should settle the issue, leading to resolution of the lesion if it had been due to diversion.[310]

Acute Self-Limited Colitis

Acute self-limited colitis is the term used for patients who present with an acute colitis that eventually resolves over the course of a few months without an established cause.[109, 195–197] Most of these cases are thought to be due to infections but lack culture diagnoses. The importance of the condition is in its distinction from the early phase of chronic inflammatory bowel disease.

Biopsy Features

Biopsies of the acute disorder reveal preservation of the elongated and straight crypts, but the presence of neutrophilic infiltrate in the lamina propria and in the upper portion of the crypts. There are no other features of chronic disease, such as a great increase of

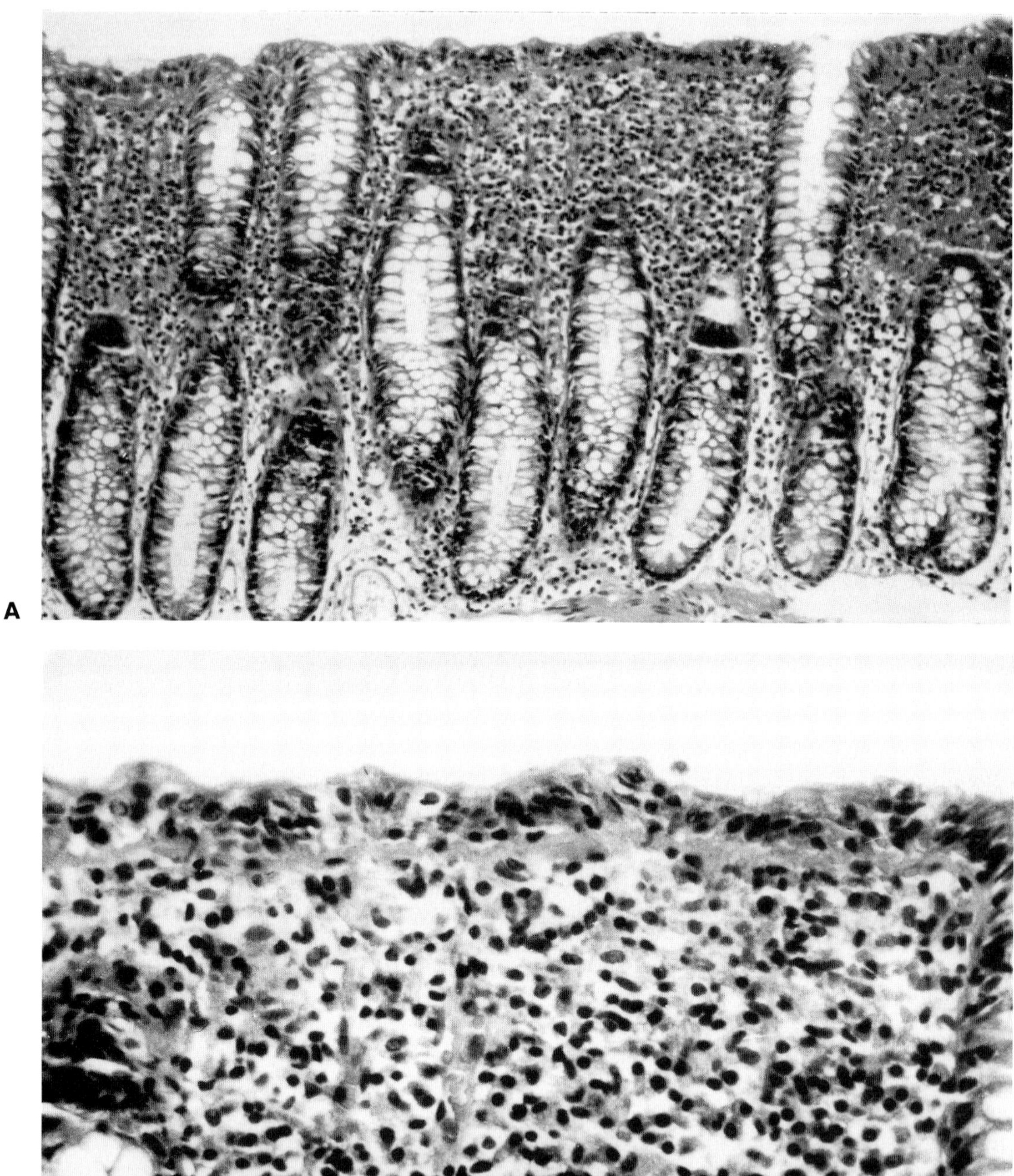

Fig. 9-38. Lymphocytic colitis. **(A)** The mucosa is normal except for an increased amount of inflammation in the superficial part of the mucosa (top). **(B)** Closer view of the surface showing increased inflammatory cells in the surface epithelial layer and adjacent lamina propria. Compared to Fig. 9-36B, there is no increase of the collagen layer.

mononuclear inflammatory cells, crypt budding or atrophy, villifom surface, or Paneth cell metaplasia. It has been estimated that of patients with chronic IBD, features of chronicity may be lacking in 20 to 30 percent of cases at the time of initial biopsy.[197] In these cases the distinction from acute self-limited colitis can only be established by follow up. Biopsy at a later time will show complete resolution of the mucosa in a case of acute colitis, whereas there will usually be some evidence of chronic disease in a patient with IBD. (See above section on "Idiopathic Inflammatory Bowel Disease" for further details.)

Miscellaneous Conditions

Necrotizing Enterocolitis

Necrotizing enterocolitis is a condition that occurs in infants and is associated with extensive ulceration and infarction of the small and large intestine[103, 104] (Fig. 9-40). It is more common in premature infants and is thought to be related to a combination of ischemic bowel disease and secondary infections. The diagnosis is made by clinical and radiographic studies, and biopsies are usually not performed.

Neutropenic Enterocolitis

Neutropenic enterocolitis occurs in patients who have a profound reduction in their leukocyte count due to tumor or to drug therapy.[323–326] The patients present with extensive necrosis of the distal ileum, cecum, and proximal colon. The lesion is due to a secondary infection with *Clostridium septicum* or other highly virulent bacterium. Histology reveals extensive necrosis and marked proliferation of the bacteria without much inflammation. Biopsies are not typically obtained.

Follicular Proctitis and Colitis

Follicular proctitis and colitis is not a special entity but rather a descriptive term, corresponding to a case of chronic colitis with marked proliferation of lymphoid nodules[200] (Fig. 9-24C). It may occur in any case of long-standing chronic inflammatory disease, but is most often noted in patients with ulcerative colitis, and is especially enhanced following a subtotal colectomy.[201, 317] Biopsies simply show the many lymphoid follicles together with the other evidence of chronic colitis. The epithelial cells overlying the lymphoid follicles can show very marked degenerative changes, and biopsies of these areas must be distinguished from epithelial dysplasia.

Behçet's Disease

Behçet's disease is an uncommon disorder that is characterized by ulcerations occurring in the skin, genital region, and variably in the intestinal tract.[327, 328] It may affect the esophagus, stomach, distal small intestine, or colon. The lesions are nonspecific, revealing focal ulcerations and inflammation, and it has been suggested that this may be due to a localized vasculitis, but necrotizing lesions are usually not found[329–332] (see Fig. 8-17). Severe cases may show more extensive necrosis and the potential for perforation. There are typically no granulomas. It must be distinguished from Crohn's disease, which is usually based on the finding of more significant chronic inflammation, granulomas, and sinus tracts. Biopsies of Behçet's disease show nonspecific features and are not diagnostic.

Stercoral Ulcer

Stercoral ulcer represents an ulcer that develops as a result of the pressure effect by impacted feces or foreign bodies on the mucosa.[333] The biopsy is completely nonspecific

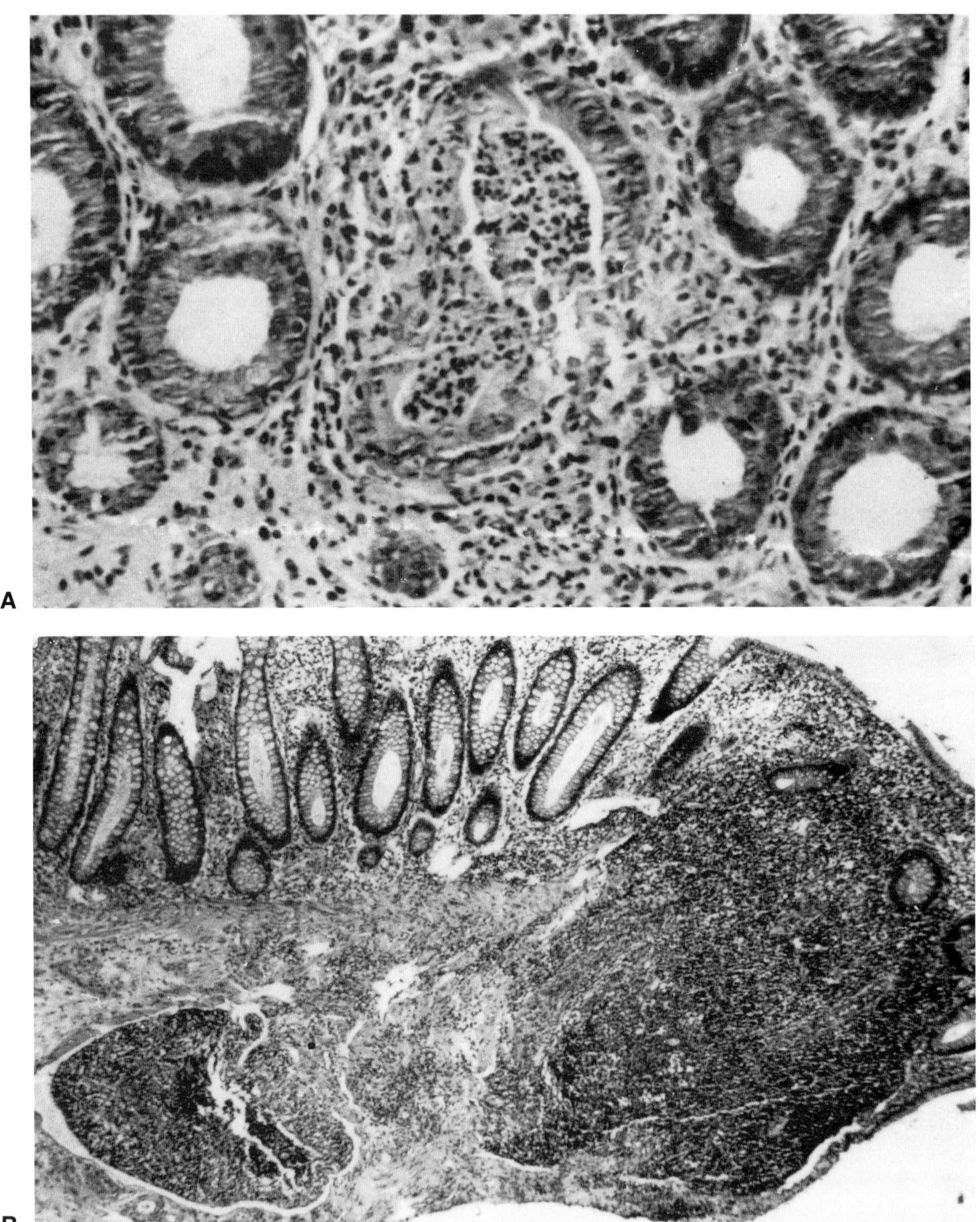

Fig. 9-39. Diversion colitis, showing examples of lesions. **(A)** Focal crypt abscess (center). **(B)** Increased number and size of lymphoid nodules, seen in most cases. (*Figure continues.*)

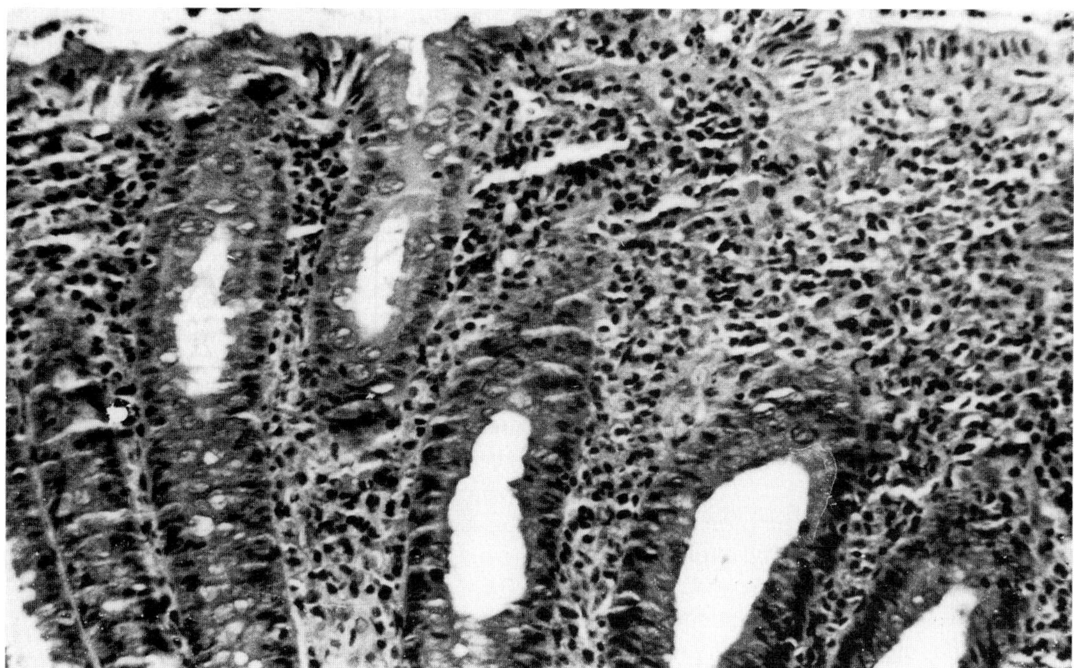

Fig. 9-39 (*Continued*). **(C)** Superficial erosion (upper right). More severe cases show deeper ulcers.

and reveals ulceration, together with acute and chronic inflammation and variable granulation tissue or fibrosis, depending on the age of the lesion. There may also be giant cells and granulomas reacting to foreign elements within the fecal material. Biopsies are uncommonly obtained and largely performed to rule out other ulcerating disorders.

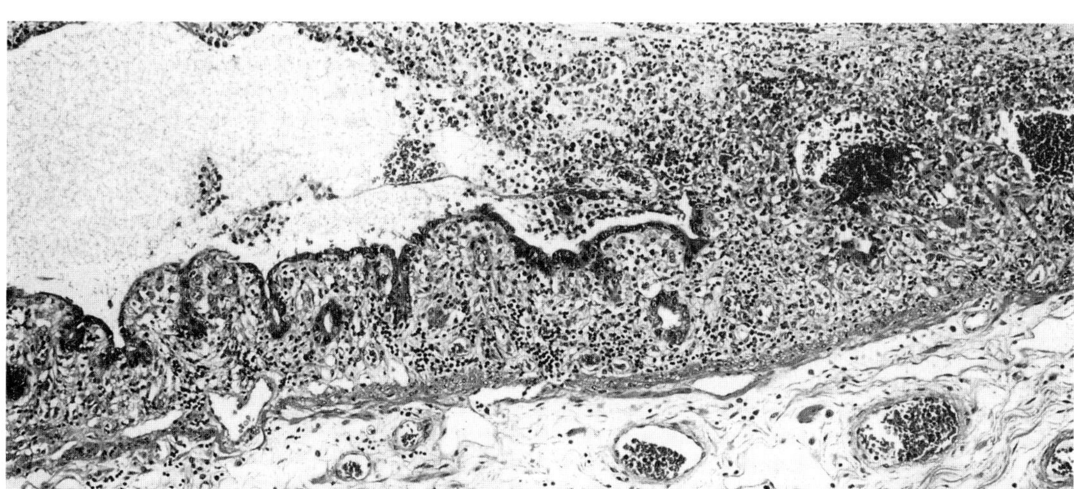

Fig. 9-40. Necrotizing colitis. There is diffuse hemorrhage and necrosis of the mucosa, resembling ischemic disease, together with a focal ulcer and acute inflammatory membrane (right). More advanced lesions show greater necrosis extending into the bowel wall (× 105).

IRRITABLE BOWEL SYNDROME

Irritable bowel syndrome is a common condition that is associated with intermittent watery and mucus-filled diarrhea.[334, 335] There is usually no blood or purulent material. The exact etiology is not established, and treatment is largely of a supportive nature. Endoscopic and biopsy examinations are completely normal.

TUMORLIKE DISORDERS

ENDOMETRIOSIS

Endometriosis is a common condition in which there are endometrial explants outside of the uterine corpus region.[336, 337] The tissue frequently is present in the peritoneum and may extend into the muscularis propria, most often noted in the distal colon. In this region it may be productive of pain, and lead to muscle hypertrophy or to fibrosis.

Biopsy Features

Endometrial tissue is uncommonly located in the mucosa, where it may be associated with cyclic bleeding.[338, 339] Endoscopy reveals nodules of hemorrhagic lesions, and biopsy is diagnostic (Fig. 9-41). Noted are the glands and stroma of the endometrial tissue, which must be distinguished from the native glands as well as from regeneration and tumor. The endometrial glands reveal non-mucous epithelial cells with elongated nuclei, and frequently have a ciliated surface border. Extremely helpful is the recognition of the associated endometrial stroma with the dense cells containing elongated and slightly rounded nuclei. There may be associated hemorrhage in the biopsy as well. Exceptionally, carcinomas can develop in such ectopic foci of the endometrium.[340] The biopsy diagnosis can be suspected by the lack of mucin production and ciliated surface in the tumor cells, but probably needs support from the finding of benign endometrial tissue in adjacent areas.

PNEUMATOSIS

Pneumatosis is a lesion characterized by the presence of gas-filled spaces in the bowel wall.[341, 342] It is most commonly noted as a consequence of emphysema or ruptured peptic ulcer disease in which air extends along the vascular tracts into the small and large intestine. Changes are evident on radiographic examination, and there is usually no major extension into the mucosa requiring biopsy study.

Biopsy Features

Another form of pneumatosis is due to a prior damage to the mucosa, leading to the invasion of gas-forming bacteria.[343] This may be associated with any form of colitis, but is particularly common following ischemic disease. Noted at endoscopy are slightly raised, distensible areas.[344] Biopsy shows the gaseous spaces with variable mononuclear inflammatory cells around the edge (Fig. 9-42; see Fig. 8-16). Frequently noted are giant cells presumably responding to fecal elements. The lesions are commonly seen in the upper submucosa but may also involve the mucosal area. Spaces are readily distinguished from glandular tissue by the lack of any lining epithelial cells, and mucin stains are negative. Oleogranulomas may show multiple clear spaces, but they lack the giant cells and are usually associated with more fibrosis.

Rare Causes

Pneumatosis is noted rarely following colonoscopy, presumably due to small tears in the mucosa, but this is readily reversible.[345]

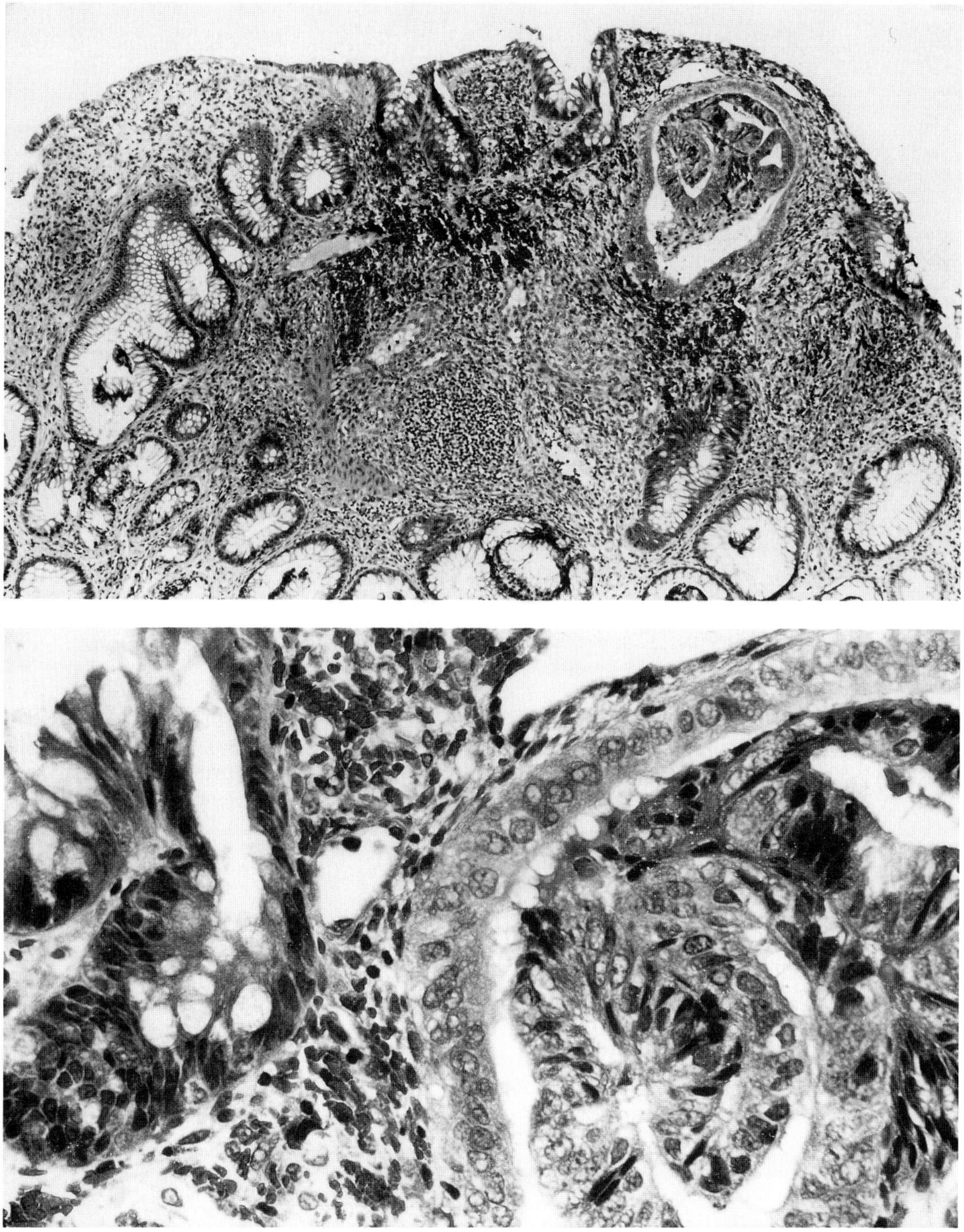

A

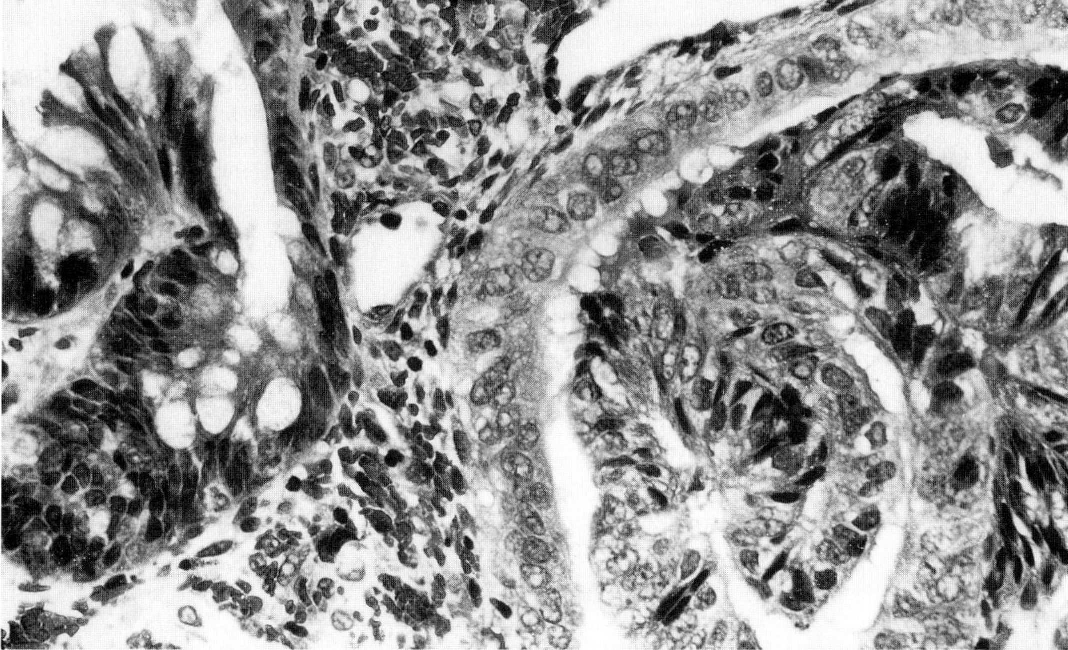

B

Fig. 9-41. Endometriosis in the colon. **(A)** Section of colonic mucosa, revealing focus of endometrial tissue (upper right) (× 85). **(B)** Closer view of mature endometrial glands (right). Compare with the colonic crypts (left) (× 425).

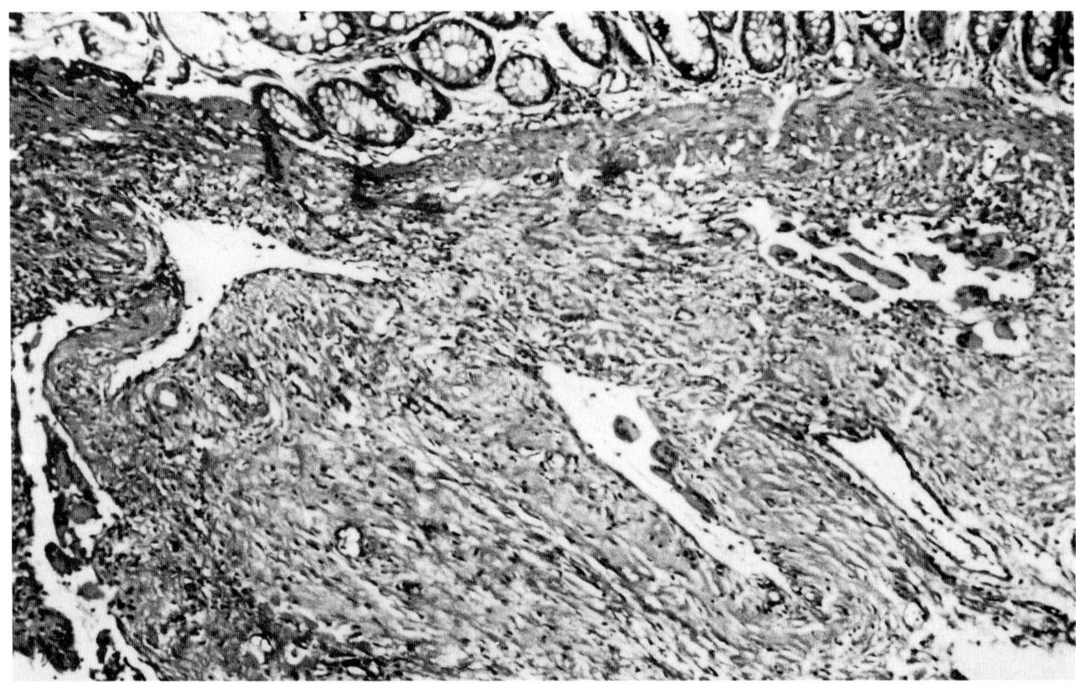

Fig. 9-42. Pneumatosis of the colon. There are numerous gas-filled spaces in the submucosa, surrounded by inflammatory tissue. A portion of the mucosa appears at the top. For a closer view of the pneumatosis and inflammatory reaction, see Figure 8-16.

The lesions also are seen uncommonly with reaction to some drugs and in patients who have had bypass procedures.[336, 346]

Colitis Cystica

Colitis cystica is a condition that is associated with the extension of mature glandular tissue into the submucosa and deeper parts of the bowel wall.[207, 347] It typically develops as a consequence of a chronic inflammatory condition and is most often associated with chronic ulcerative colitis. The lesions also have been seen in patients with other causes of chronic colitis, such as radiation or schistosomiasis. A more localized form is seen in the rectum together with the solitary rectal ulcer syndrome, as described below.[348]

Biopsy Features

Biopsies reveal mature glands extending into the submucosa, and these must be distinguished from neoplasms. The epithelial cells are either completely normal or show only mild regenerative changes, and the stroma resembles lamina propria. In contrast, neoplasms show dysplastic epithelium together with a tumor stroma.

Solitary Rectal Ulcer Syndrome

In the solitary rectal ulcer syndrome there is an initial development of an ulcer in the rectal area. Its pathogenesis is probably variable and related to the age of the patient. One well-studied group are young patients, more often women, with a long history of straining; these patients are thought to have excess constriction of their internal anal sphincter.[349–351] Over time there occurs prolapse with an ulcer and later, by regeneration, the development of a polypoid lesion. The lesions are more often noted on the anterior wall, are almost always single, and are usually in the lower part but may extend several centimeters up the rectum.

Similar lesions are noted in older patients and may be related to incompetent sphincters that lead to prolonged mucosal prolapse.[352, 353] Indeed, it has been suggested that this entity might be termed *mucosal prolapse syndrome.*

Biopsy Features

Biopsy of the early ulcer lesion is entirely nonspecific, revealing necrosis and inflammation. More often obtained are biopsies of the polypoid phase, with an impression that the sample might represent a neoplasm.[349, 354–357] The biopsy features are highly characteristic, revealing a hyperplastic and serrated type of epithelium together with a pronounced increase of fibrous and muscle tissue in the lamina propria (Fig. 9-43). There is no dysplasia of the epithelium in the form of elongated, atypical, or hyperchromatic nuclei. It is, therefore, possible to make this diagnosis or at least to indicate that it is inflammatory, in contrast to an adenoma.

In the later lesions there may be extension of mature tissue into the submucosa, representing a localized example of proctitis cystica, and the surface may develop a villiform arrangement, all features suggestive of neoplasm[348] (Fig. 9-44). However, the epithelial cells show no dysplasia either at the surface or within the submucosal region. They are readily distinguished from invasive carcinoma by the lack of nuclear atypism or tumor stroma. Advanced lesions may also be associated with very large masses, termed *inflammatory cloacogenic polyps.*[358, 359] These remain inflammatory or hyperplastic in nature and are not neoplastic.

MISCELLANEOUS CONDITIONS

Metabolic Disorders

Uremia

Patients with renal failure develop many lesions throughout all portions of the gut.[360, 361] In the colon there can be found areas of hemorrhage, ulcers, or infarcts. Biopsy of any of these lesions is entirely nonspecific.

Cystic Fibrosis

Cases of cystic fibrosis tend to have excess mucus production in multiple organs, including the intestinal tract.[362] Studies have shown an increase in the number of goblet cells and in the size of the mucous part of the cytoplasm in the crypt epithelial cells, but there is considerable overlap with the normal patients and with other inflammatory conditions.[363] Accordingly, colonic or rectal biopsy is ordinarily not obtained in these patients.

Depositions

There are many types of substances that can be deposited within the colonic mucosa (Table 9-11). Fragments of mucus are commonly noted in the colonic lamina propria, resulting from ruptured crypts in cases of active colitis and from previous biopsy sites. These can be associated with poorly formed granulomas. Macrophages that contain mucinous material or small amounts of lipofuscin are normally located in the lamina propria. An increase in foamy macrophages filled with fatty substances has been seen in cases with disordered motor activity[364] (Fig. 9-45).

Amyloid

Amyloid deposits occur in patients with primary or secondary amyloidosis of a systemic nature.[365] Of interest, there does not appear to be an example of localized amyloidosis in the intestinal tract. The amyloid may involve any compartment, but most often is noted in the walls of small arteries, which can be readily accessed by aspiration-type biopsies of the rectum.[366, 367] Indeed, it is a common choice to look for amyloid in

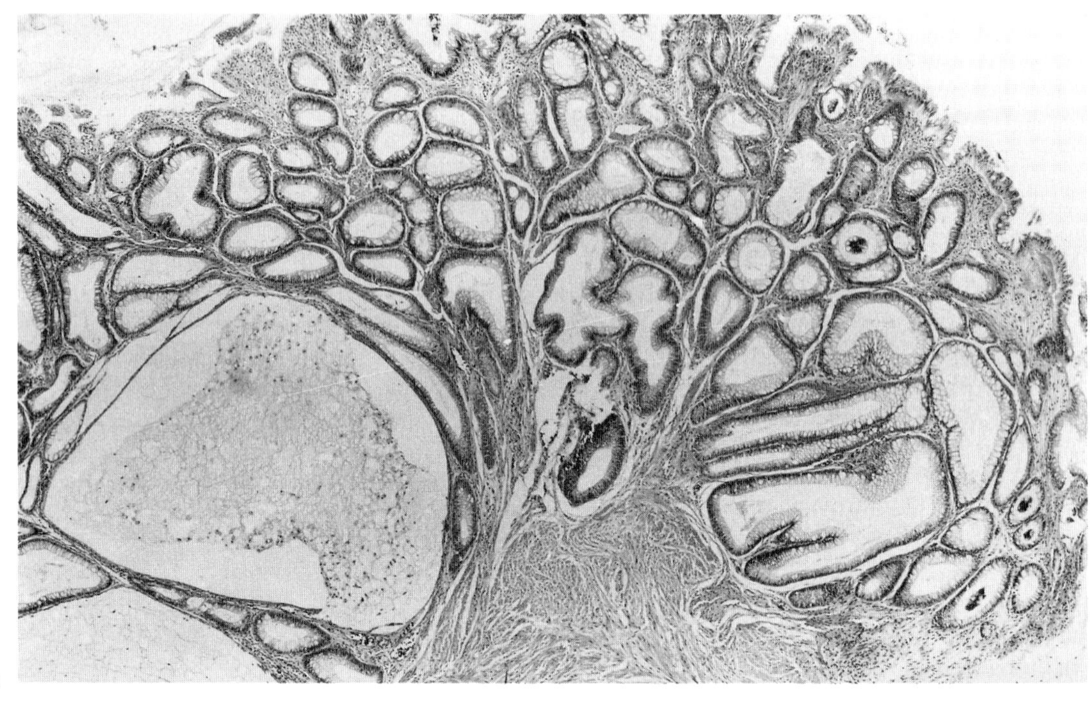

A

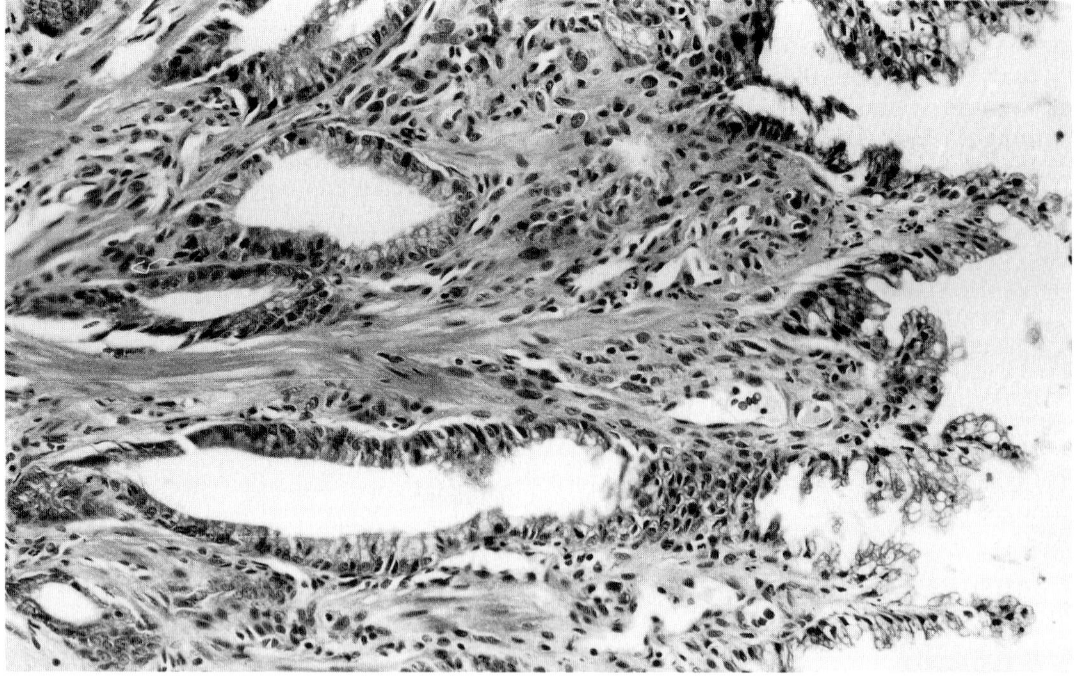

B

Fig. 9-43. Solitary ulcer syndrome of the rectum. **(A)** Polypoid phase, showing irregular glands with cystic change and a prominent fibromuscular stroma (× 42). **(B)** Closer view of the polyp. Noted are the muscle in the lamina propria and the irregular glands with less well formed goblet mucous cells. Near the surface at the right, the crypts appear serrated (× 210).

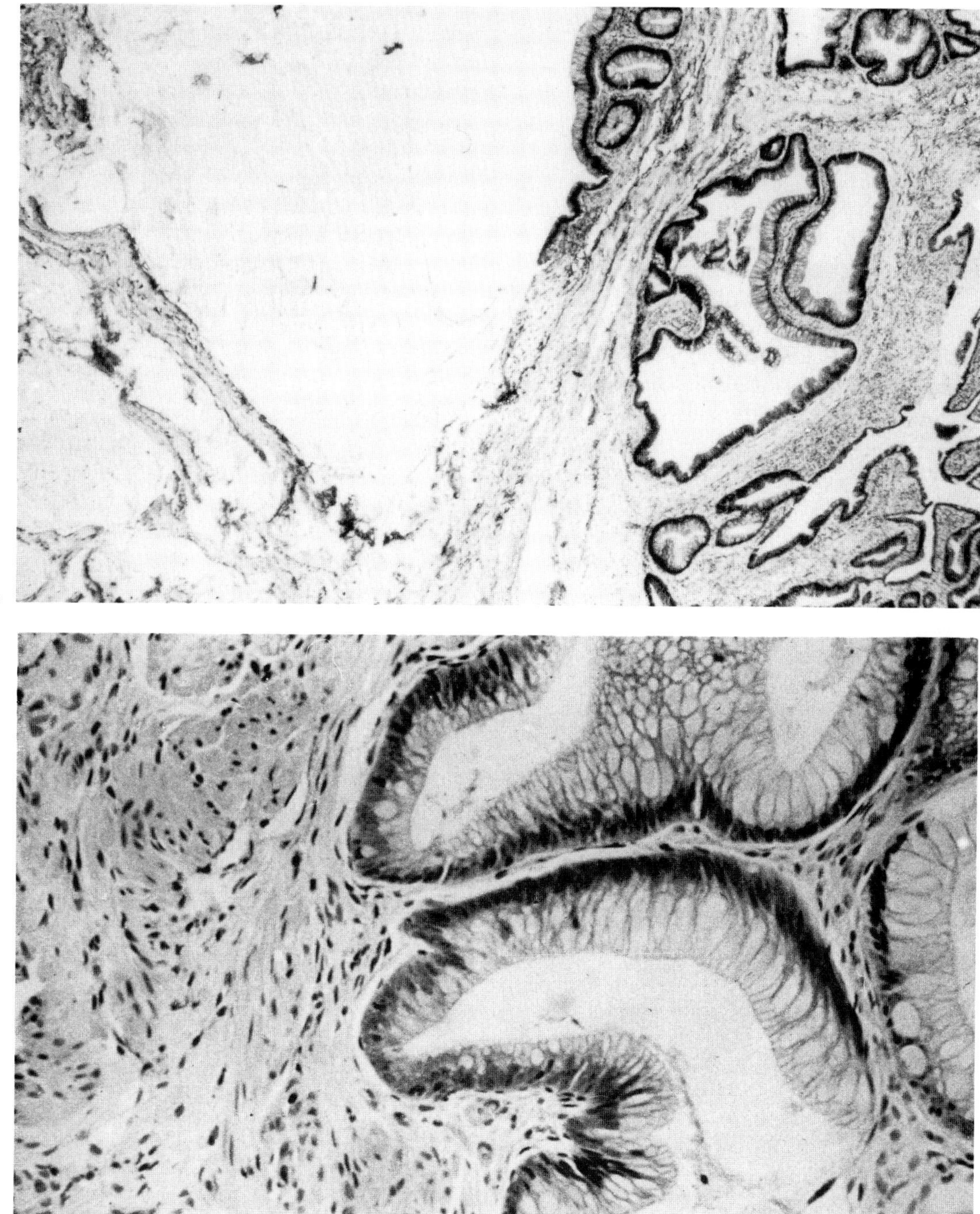

Fig. 9-44. Colitis cystica profunda. (**A**) Polypoid lesion of solitary ulcer syndrome appears at the right. The cystic glands extend into the submucosa (left) (**B**) Closer view of glands in the submucosa, showing mature mucous epithelial cells without atypism.

Table 9-11. Depositions in the Colon and Rectum

Mucin (free and in macrophages)
Amyloidosis
Melanosis coli
Storage diseases
Brown bowel syndrome
Tangier disease
Lipofuscinosis
Other conditions

patients with suspected disease in other organs such as the heart, liver, and kidney.

Biopsies show amyloid concentrated in the vessel walls (Fig. 9-46) and Plate 4D). The material appears as a hyalin type with fracture slits. Less often, the amyloid material is noted in the stromal area of the submucosa or mucosa. Special stains are needed for verification. Crystal Violet and other metachromatic stains are particularly sensitive, but most often used is Congo Red and visualization with polarized light to reveal the specific green birefringence. Electron microscopy can also identify the precise amyloid material[367] (see Fig. 4-35). The amount of amyloid may be very scant; accordingly, even if it is not evident in the routine H & E section, special stains should be employed.

Amyloid can also infiltrate the musculature, leading to a state of poor motility and productive of a pseudo-obstruction.[57, 58] In such cases, the amyloid may not extend into the superficial compartments and may not be seen on endoscopic biopsy.

Melanosis Coli

Melanosis coli is a common condition characterized by the presence of many macrophages that contain lipofuscin within the lamina propria of the rectum and colonic mucosa.[235, 368, 369] It is thought to be related to excess laxative use, but may also be an aging phenomenon. Of interest, the lesion is limited to the large intestine and appendix and does not extend into the small bowel.

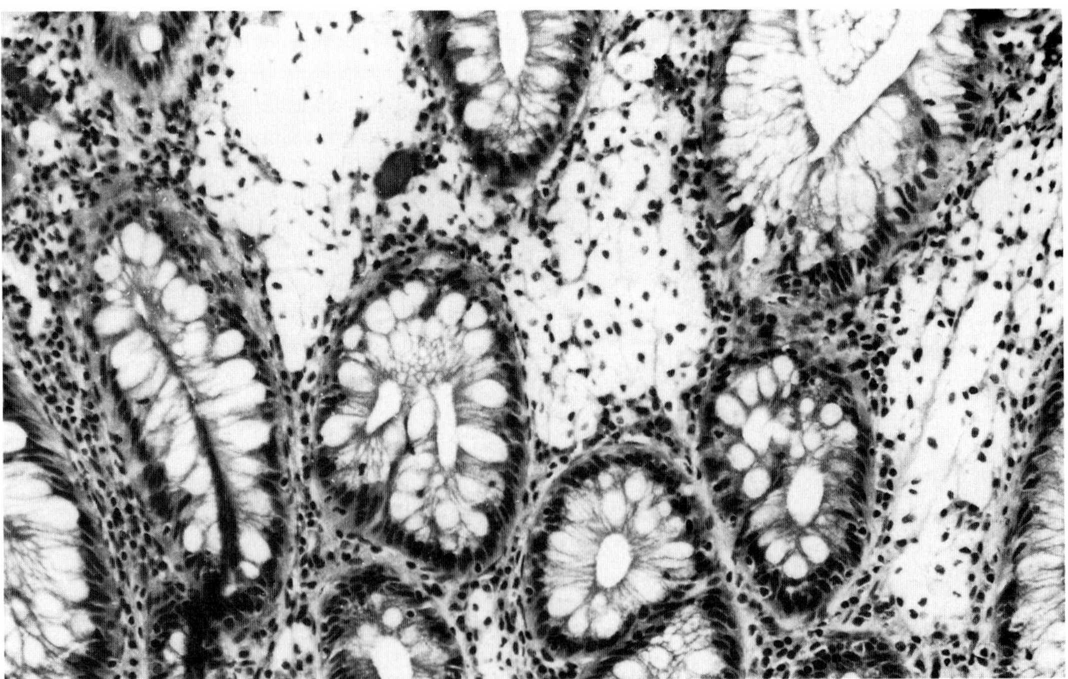

Fig. 9-45. Xanthoma of the colon. The lesion is comprised of macrophages in the lamina propria, which have finely vacuolated cytoplasm and small central nuclei. Stains for mucin are negative (× 210).

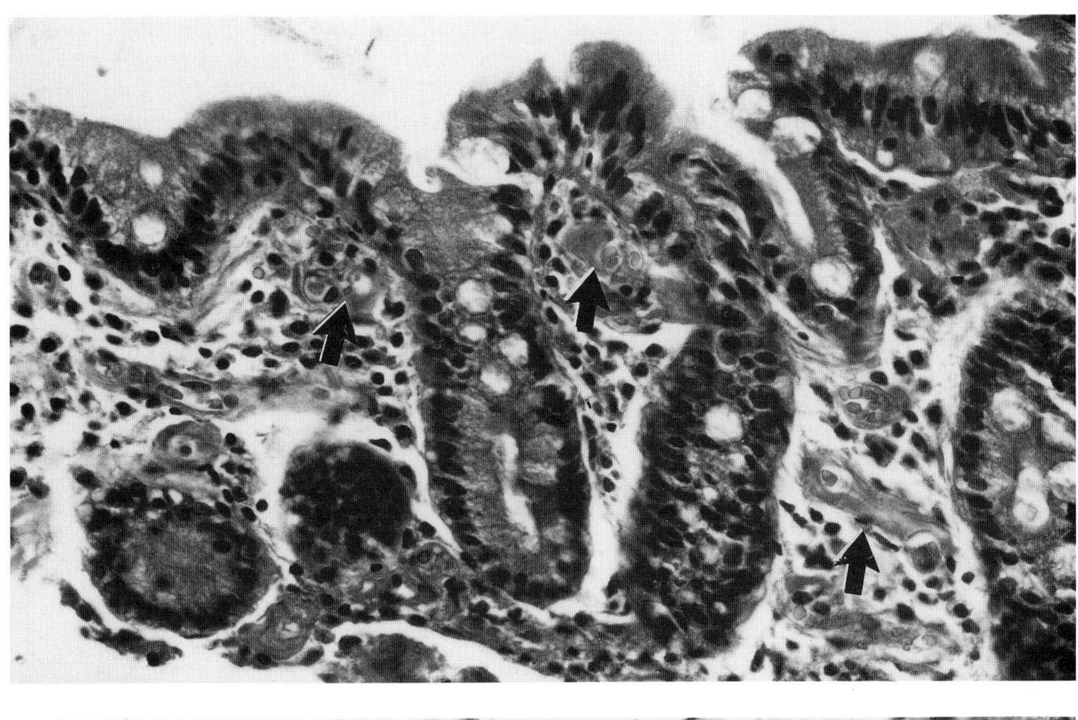

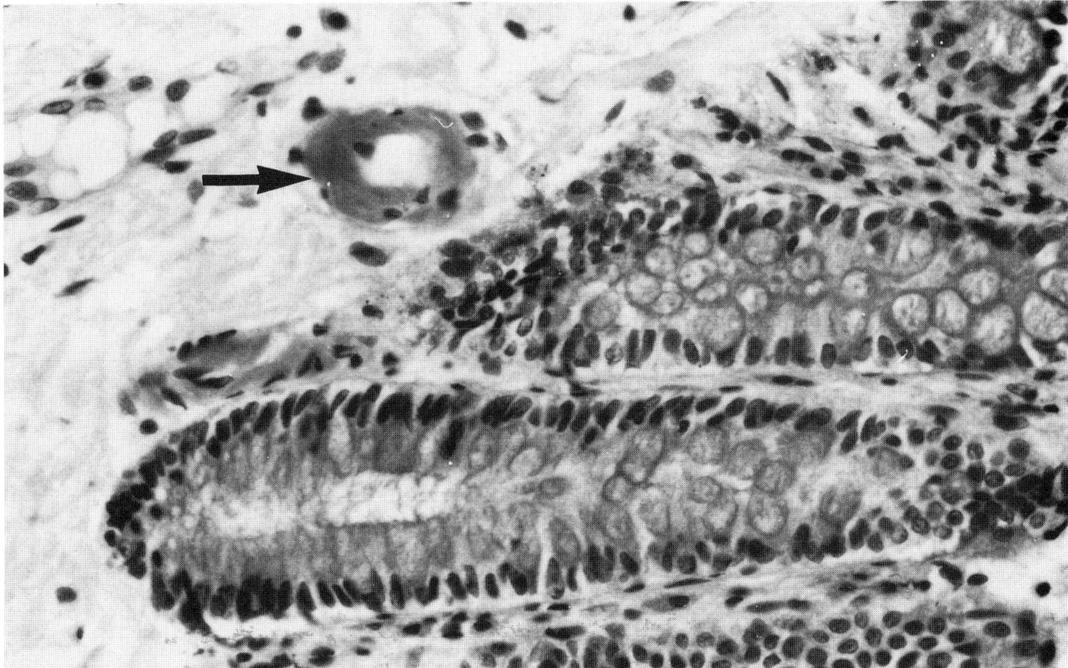

Fig. 9-46. Amyloidosis in the colon. **(A)** Deposits are noted in most of the small vessel walls within the mucosa (arrows). Such lesions are uncommon (× 425). **(B)** More characteristic localization of amyloid in a small artery within the submucosa (arrow). The muscularis is thinned out in this section, and the mucosa appears at the right (× 425).

Biopsies are diagnostic, revealing the macrophages with the fine refractile and colored material (Fig. 9-47). It should be distinguished from hemosiderin, which typically appears as larger, more refractile and shiny granules, and iron stain can be employed in uncertain cases. Other conditions may be associated with macrophages that contain lipofuscin material, including several storage diseases, Langerhans' cell histiocytosis, and chronic granulomatous disease. In these conditions, the macrophages are typically arranged in prominent nodules.

Storage Diseases

There is a large variety of storage diseases that can affect the intestinal tract, and these are described more fully in Chapter 7[370, 371] (see Table 7-12). In the brown bowel syndrome, there is a massive increase of lipofuscin in all parts of the bowel wall, particularly in the muscle coats[372] (Fig. 9-48 and Plate 4C). This may exceptionally extend to the mucosal region, making it difficult to distinguish from ordinary melanosis coli. Other examples of substances that are occasionally seen in the colon include Tangier disease, in which there are large clusters of foamy macrophages in the mucosa and submucosa (Figs. 9-49 and 9-50); and ceroid lipofuscinosis, showing macrophages that contain large amounts of lipochrome pigment, similar to the brown bowel syndrome.[373, 374] Most of the storage diseases are currently diagnosed by examination of other tissues, particularly blood and muscle. Accordingly, biopsy of the intestinal mucosa is now only rarely obtained for these disorders.[375]

Granulomatous Diseases

There are many causes of granulomas that involve any part of the gut, including the large bowel[376] (Table 9-12). These can be seen in connection with various infections, in Crohn's disease, and in reactions to barium, oil, suture, and mucin material (see Figs. 9-20, 9-26, 9-27, 9-32, and 9-33). Rare causes in the gut include sarcoidosis, malakoplakia, histiocytosis, and chronic granulomatous disease. Exceptionally, granulomas have also been noted in cases with vasculitis and tumor. Many of the conditions are discussed in other parts of the chapter; presented in this section are only the rarer lesions.

In the evaluation of tissue for granulomas, it is important to exclude lesions that can resemble them. In particular, it is necessary to delineate germinal centers of lymphoid follicles, ganglia or fragments of nerves, fibrous sheaths around crypts, and bits of smooth muscle tissue. Also commonly seen in the mucosa are clusters of macrophages that contain mucin or fat, scattered giant cells without full granuloma formation, and aggregates of lymphoid tissue, all of which may mimic the appearance of granulomas.

Sarcoidosis

Sarcoidosis rarely affects the gastrointestinal tract, and the diagnosis is dependent on the presence of lesions in some other more distinctive area, such as the respiratory system or liver.[377, 378] The lesions reveal well formed granulomas without necrosis, and there is usually no prominent ulceration or fibrosis (see Fig. 4-42).

Malakoplakia

Malakoplakia more commonly involves the urinary tract but may affect the gut.[379–381] It is seen in children and adults, with most lesions in the large bowel. Noted are large plaques with central ulcers that may extend deeply into the bowel wall. The lesions are thought to be of an infectious nature due to a defect in the ability of leukocytes to eliminate the organisms.[382] However, the ex-

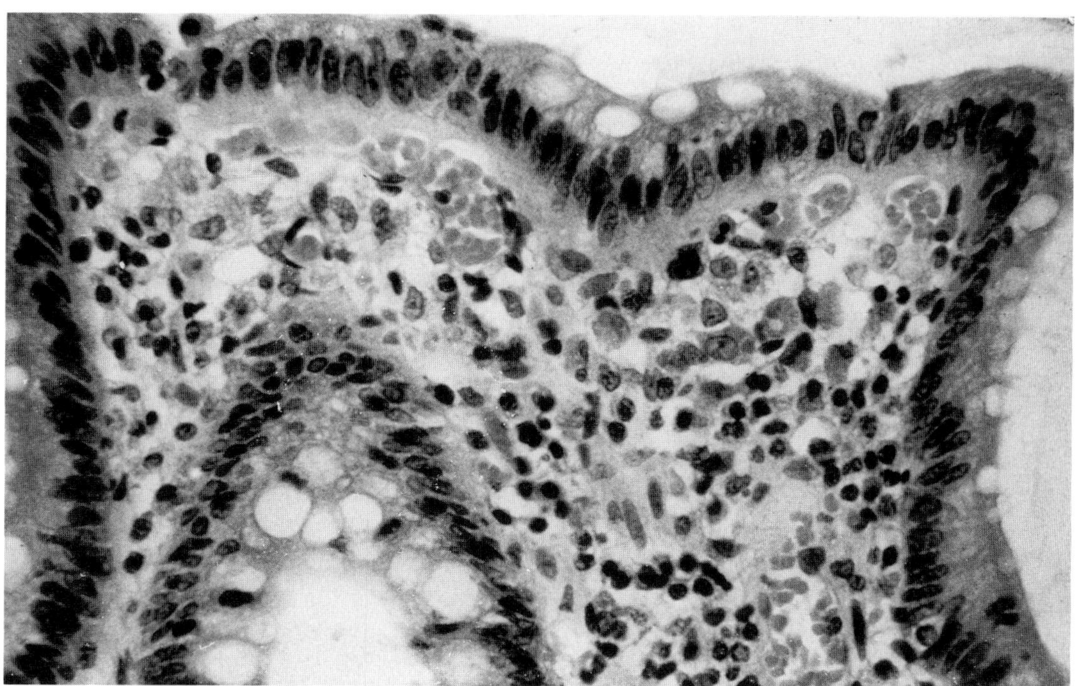

Fig. 9-47. Melanosis coli. Present in the lamina propria are several macrophages that contain the fine lipofuscin pigment.

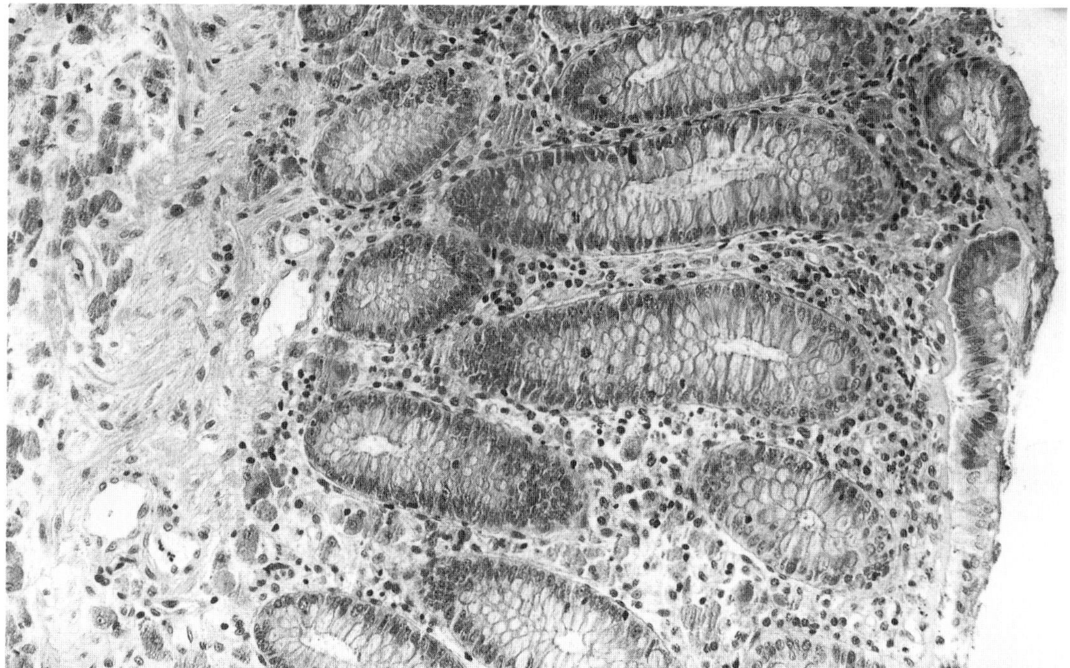

Fig. 9-48. Brown bowel syndrome in the colon. Noted is a greater degree of macrophages with lipofuscin extending into the muscularis mucosae and submucosa (left) (× 210).

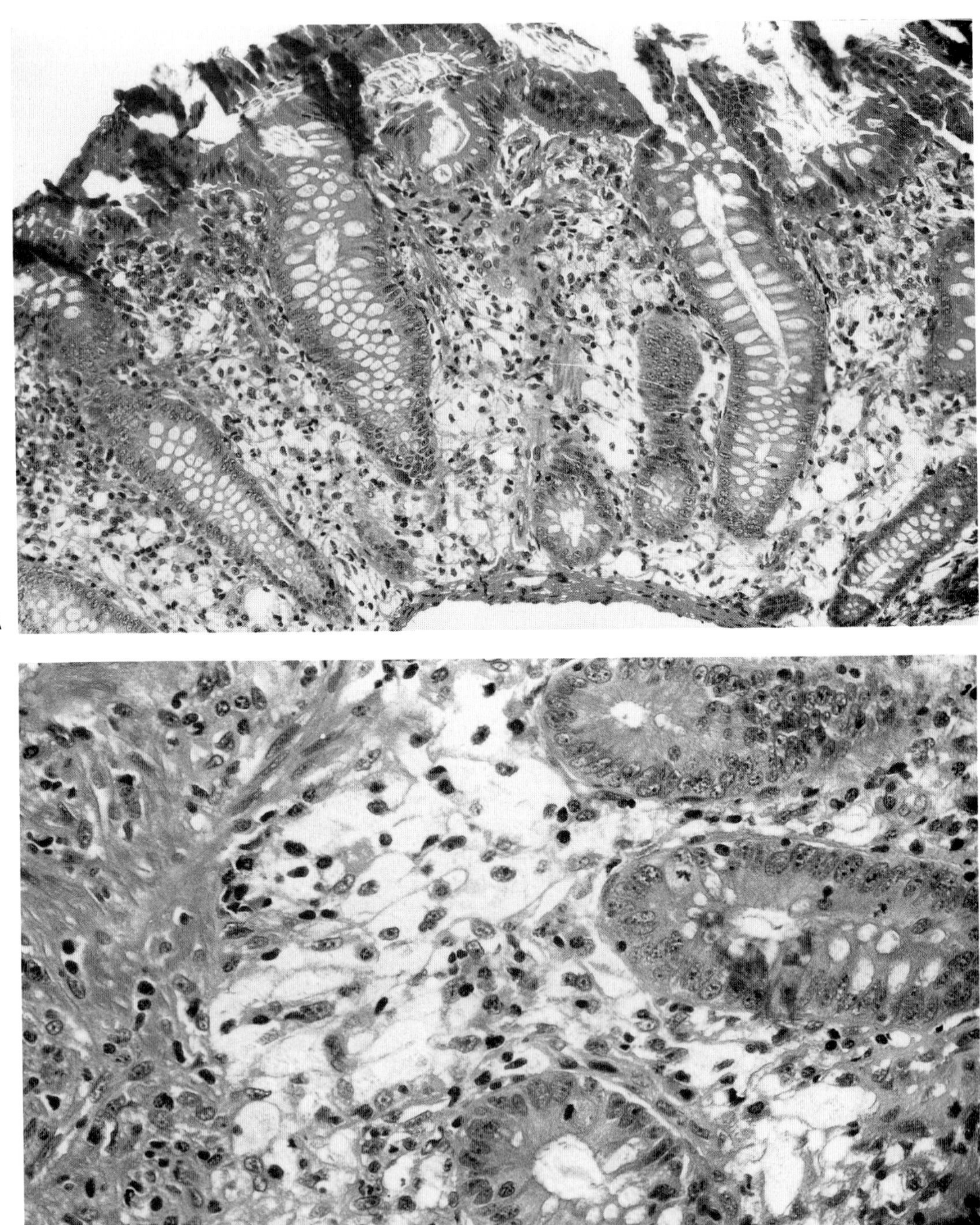

Fig. 9-49. Tangier disease in the colon. **(A)** There is a diffuse infiltrate of vacuolated macrophages in the lamina propria. The mucosal surface appears at the top (× 210). **(B)** Closer view of the clear macrophages that are filled with lipids. The muscularis mucosae appears at the left (× 425).

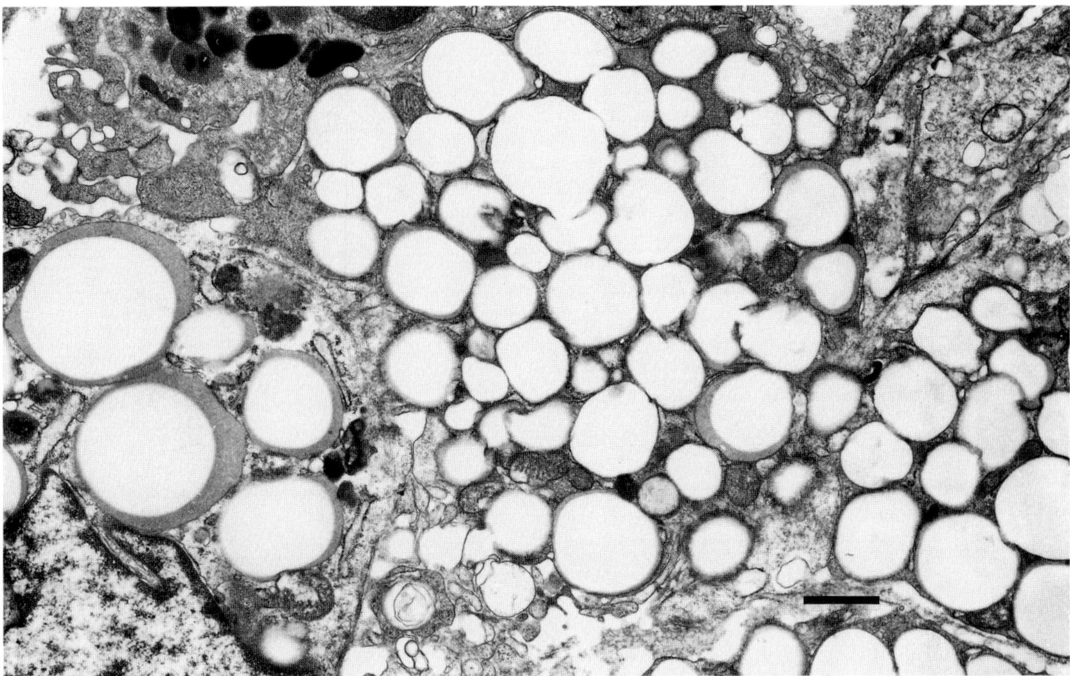

Fig. 9-50. Electron micrograph of macrophages from the colon biopsy of a patient with Tangier disease. The cells are packed with lipid droplets (× 10,000; bar = 1μm).

act etiology and pathogenesis are not established.

Biopsy reveals masses of well formed macrophages with a prominent granular cytoplasm and with striking small, oval Michaelis-Gutmann inclusions (Figs. 9-51 and 9-52). The cytoplasm can be stained with the PAS reaction, which highlights the numerous enlarged lysosomes, and the inclusions are accented by mineral stains such as for iron and calcium (Plate 4B). There appears to be an increased association of malakoplakia with colonic adenomas and carcinomas, and biopsy may also be used to identify or exclude such lesions.[383, 384]

Table 9-12. Causes of Granulomas in the Colon and Rectum

Infections
Crohn's disease
Reactions to barium, oil, suture, and mucin
Rare
Sarcoidosis
Malakoplakia
Langerhans cell histiocytosis
Chronic granulomatous disease

Langerhans' Cell Histiocytosis

Langerhans' cell histiocytosis, the diffuse and severe form of histiocytosis X, uncommonly involves the gastrointestinal tract and is associated with infiltrates of macrophage-like cells in the lamina propria.[385–387] These are arranged in clusters and often contain small amounts of lipofuscin pigment. They represent dendritic cells and can be identified either by electron microscopy, showing the characteristic Birbeck granules, or by stains for S-100 (see Fig. 4-38).

Infiltrates in the gut are uncommon, and biopsy is only performed if there are symptoms or unusual nodules.

Chronic Granulomatous Disease

Chronic granulomatous disease is more common in children and is due to the failure of the macrophages to properly lyse bacterial agents.[388] The patients frequently have se-

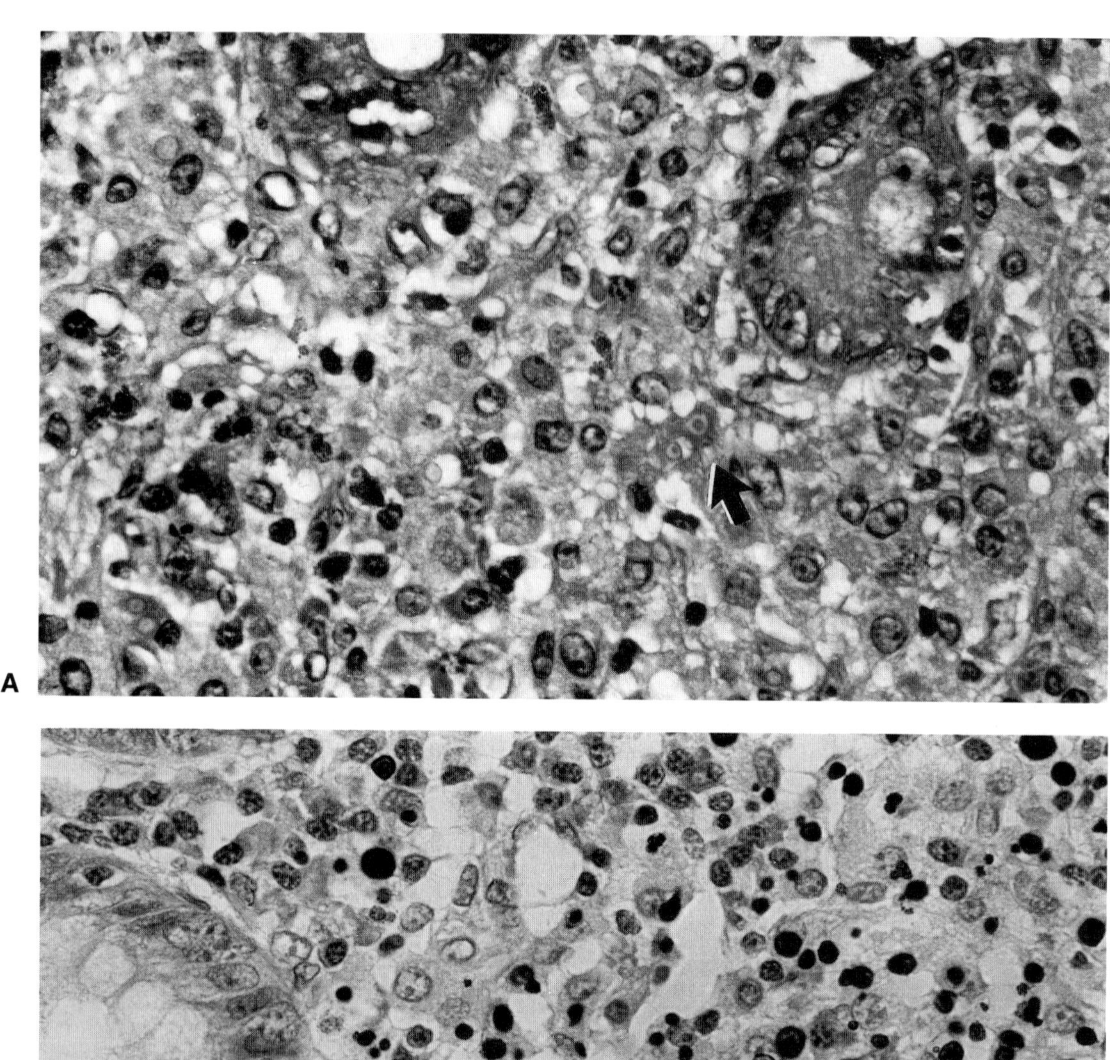

Fig. 9-51. Malakoplakia of the colon. **(A)** There is a dense infiltrate of macrophages in the lamina propria. The cells have a granular cytoplasm due to the presence of many lysosomes and contain the characteristic Michaelis-Gutmann bodies (arrow) (× 635). **(B)** The inclusions are accented by the use of stains for iron and calcium, showing the many densely stained bodies (Von Kossa stain for calcium; × 635).

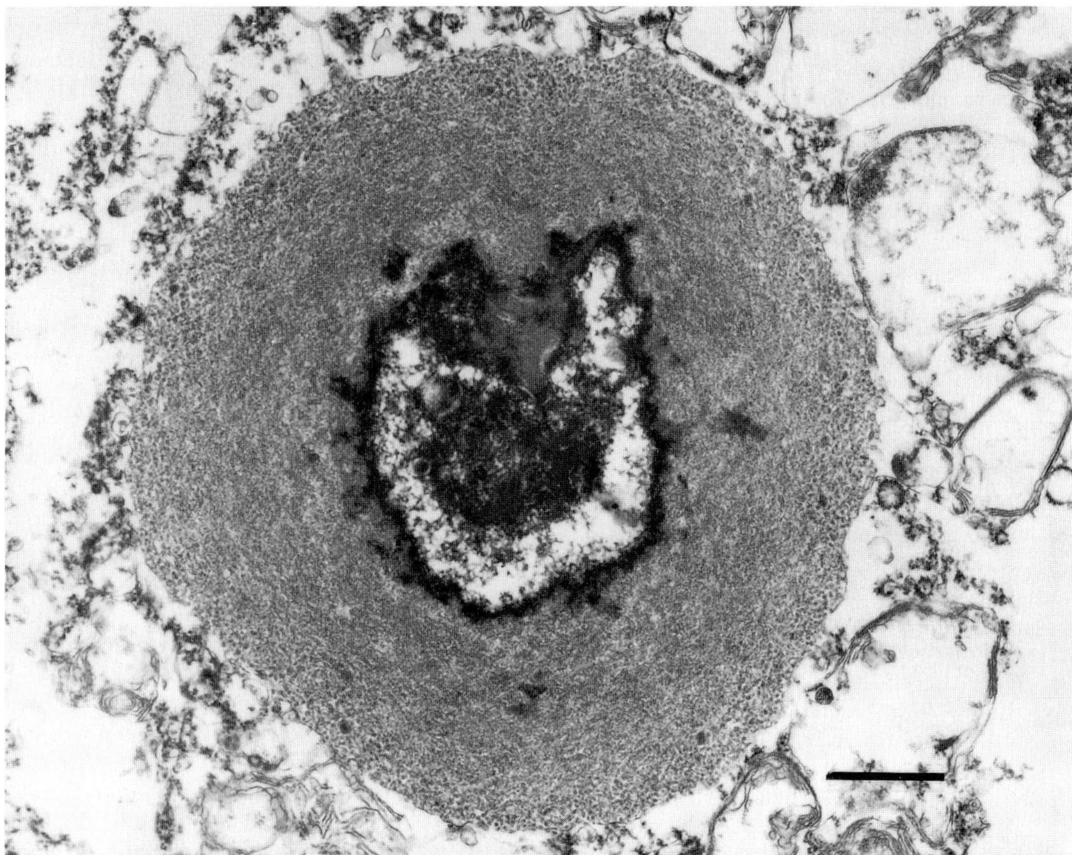

Fig. 9-52. Electron micrograph of a Michaelis-Gutmann body from a case of malakoplakia. The characteristic lamellar (or targetoid) lysosomes are most likely calcified remnants of phagocytized bacteria, and are seen centrally in this example (× 15,000; bar = 1 μm).

vere infections of the skin, and bronchial and pulmonary tissues. There also can develop a marked narrowing of the lower portion of the stomach and occasional ulcers of the large bowel.[389] Biopsies reveal necrosis and inflammation, as well as clusters of macrophages rich in lipofuscin pigment. The diagnosis is dependent on the finding of characteristic lesions in other tissues as well.

Skin Diseases

The colon is rarely involved with cutaneous disorders. Focal areas of hemorrhage, inflammation, and erosion can be seen in cases of erythema multiforme,[390] and more extensive ulcers with the threat of mural necrosis and perforation in Kohlmeier-Degos disease.[391, 392]

Appendiceal Diseases

The lumen and proximal edge of the appendix can often be visualized at endoscopy of the cecum, and there is occasional protrusion of the tissue into the large intestinal lumen. Rare biopsies reveal acute inflammation, the effects of intussusception, and tumors affecting the mucosa of the appendix.[393, 394]

REFERENCES

1. Teague RH, Salmon PR, Read AE: Fiberoptic examination of the colon: a review of 255 cases. Gut 14:139, 1973
2. Haber GB: Role of endoscopy in inflammatory bowel disease. Dig Dis Sci 32:165–255, 1987
3. Morrissey JF, Reichelderfer M: Gastrointestinal endoscopy N Engl J Med 325:1142–1149, 1214–1222, 1991
4. Hirschowitz BI: Development and application of endoscopy. Gastroenterology 104: 337–342, 1993
5. Goldman H, Antonioli DA: Mucosal biopsy of the rectum, colon and distal ileum. Human Pathol 13:981–1012, 1982
6. Haggitt RC: Differential diagnosis of colitis. pp. 325–355. In Goldman H, Appelman HD, Kaufman N (eds): Gastrointestinal Pathology. Williams & Wilkins, Baltimore, 1990
7. Goldman H: Interpretation of large intestinal mucosal biopsies. Hum Pathol 25:1150–1159, 1994
8. Eidelman S, Lagunoff D: The morphology of the normal human rectal biopsy. Hum Pathol 3:389, 1972
9. Shamsuddin AM, Phelps PC, Trump BF: Human large intestinal epithelium: light microscopy, histochemistry and ultrastructure. Hum Pathol 13:790–803, 1982
10. Levine DS, Haggitt RC: Normal histology of the colon. Am J Surg Pathol 13:966–984, 1989
11. Goldman H, Ming S-C: Mucins in normal and metaplastic gastrointestinal epithelium: histochemical distribution. Arch Pathol 85:580, 1968
12. Filipe MI: Mucins in the human gastrointestinal epithelium: a review. Invest Cell Pathol 2:195–216, 1979
13. Sjolund K, Sanden G, Hakonson R, Sundler F: Endocrine cells in human intestine: an immunocytochemical study. Gastroenterology 85:1120–1130, 1983
14. Lechago J: The endocrine cells of the digestive tract. General concepts and historic perspective. Am J Surg Pathol 11(suppl 1): 63–70, 1987
15. Dayal Y: Neuroendocrine cells and their proliferative lesions. pp. 305–365. In Norris HT (ed): Pathology of the Colon, Small Intestine, and Anus. 2nd Ed. Churchill Livingstone, New York, 1991
16. O'Leary AD, Sweeney EC: Lymphoglandular complexes of the colon. Histopathology 10:267–283, 1986
17. Keren F: Structure and function of the immunologic system of the gastrointestinal tract. pp. 69–80. In Ming S-C, Goldman H (eds): Pathology of the Gastrointestinal Tract. WB Saunders, Philadelphia, 1992
18. Jacob E, Baker SJ, Swaminathan SP: "M" cells in the follicle-associated epithelium of the human colon. Histopathology 11:941–952, 1987
19. Azzopardi JG, Evans DJ: Muciprotein-containing histiocytes (muciphages) in the rectum. J Clin Pathol 19:368, 1966
20. Fenoglio CM, Kaye GI, Lane N: Distribution of human colonic lymphatics in normal, hyperplastic, and adenomatous tissue. Gastroenterology 64:51, 1973
21. Pockros RJ, Foroozan P: Golytely lavage versus a standard colonoscopy preparation: effect on normal colonic mucosal histology. Gastroenterology 88:545–548, 1985
22. Goldman H: Ulcerative colitis and Crohn's disease. pp. 643–688. In Ming S-C, Goldman H (eds): Pathology of the Gastrointestinal Tract. WB Saunders, Philadelphia, 1992
23. Schiller AI, Freund H: Congenital colonic atresia and stenosis. Am J Surg 138:721–724, 1979
24. Wolff M: Heterotopic gastric epithelium in the rectum: a report of three new cases with a review of 87 cases of gastric heterotopia in the alimentary canal. Am J Clin Pathol 55:604–616, 1971
25. Yokoyama I, Kozuka S, Ito K et al: Gastric gland metaplasia in the small and large intestine. Gut 18:214–218, 1977
26. Debas HT, Chaun H, Thomson FB et al: Functioning heterotopic oxyntic mucosa in the rectum. Gastroenterology 79:1300, 1980
27. Edouard J, Jouannelle A, Amor A et al: Ulcerated heterotopic gastric mucosa located in the rectum. Gastroenterol Clin Biol 7:39–42, 1983
28. Pistoia MA, Guadagni S, Tisiano D et al: Ulcerated ectopic gastric mucosa of the rectum. Gastrointest Endosc 33:41–43, 1987
29. Murray FE, Lombard M, Dervan P et al: Bleeding from multifocal heterotopic gastric

mucosa in the colon controlled by an H_2-antagonist. Gut 29:848–851, 1988
30. Kaloni BP, Vaezzadeh K, Sieber WK: Gastric heterotopia in rectum complicated by rectovesical fistula. Dig Dis Sci 28:378–380, 1983
31. Dye KR, Marshall BJ, Frierson HF et al: Campylobacter pylori colonizing heterotopic gastric tissue in the rectum. Am J Clin Pathol 93:144–147, 1990
32. Franzin G, Musola R, Negri A et al: Heterotopic gastric (fundic) mucosa in the duodenum. Endoscopy 14:166–167, 1982
33. Jabbori M, Goresky CA, Lough J et al: The inlet patch: heterotopic gastric mucosa in the upper esophagus. Gastroenterology 89:352–356, 1985
34. Duphare H, Nijkawon S, Rana S, Bhargova DK: Heterotopic gastric and pancreatic tissue in large bowel. Am J Gastroenterol 85:68–71, 1990
35. Weitzner S: Ectopic salivary gland tissue in submucosa of rectum. Dis Colon Rectum 26:814–815, 1983
36. Barnes PRH, Lennard-Jones JE, Todd IP: Hirschsprung's disease and idiopathic megacolon in adults and adolescents. Gut 27:534–541, 1986
37. Blisard KS, Kleinman R: Hirschsprung's disease: a clinical and pathologic overview. Hum Pathol 17:1189–1191, 1986
38. Qualman SJ, Murray R: Aganglionosis and related disorders. Hum Pathol 25:1141–1149, 1994
39. Andrany RJ, Isaacs H, Weitzman JJ: Rectal suction biopsy for the diagnosis of Hirschsprung's disease. Ann Surg 193:419–424, 1981
40. Ariel I, Vinograd I, Lernau OZ et al: Rectal mucosal biopsy in aganglionosis and allied conditions. Hum Pathol 14:991–995, 1983
41. Hamoudi AB, Reiner CB, Boles ET et al: Acetylcholinesterase staining activity of rectal mucosa. Its use in the diagnosis of Hirschsprung's disease. Arch Pathol Lab Med 106:670–672, 1982
42. Challa VR, Moran JR, Turner CS, Lyerly AD: Histologic diagnosis of Hirschsprung's disease. The value of concurrent hematoxylin and eosins and cholinesterase staining of rectal biopsies. Am J Clin Pathol 88:324–328, 1987
43. Robey SS, Kukajda FP, Yardley JH: Immunoperoxidase stains of ganglion cells and abnormal mucosal nerve proliferations in Hirschsprung's disease. Hum Pathol 19:432–437, 1988
44. Vinores SA, May E: Neuron-specific enolase as an immunohistochemical tool for the diagnosis of Hirschsprung's disease. Am J Surg Pathol 9:281–285, 1985
45. Vanderwinden J-M, DeLaet M-H, Schiffman SN et al: Nitric acid synthase distribution in the enteric nervous system of Hirschsprung's disease. Gastroenterology 105:969–973, 1993
46. Hall CL, Lampert PW: Immunohistochemistry as an aid in the diagnosis of Hirschsprung's disease. Am J Clin Pathol 83:177–181, 1985
47. Bill AH, Chapman ND: The enterocolitis of Hirschsprung's disease: its natural history and treatment. Am J Surg 103:70, 1962
48. Saegesser F, Sandblom P: Ischemic lesions of the distended colon: a complication of obstructive colorectal cancer. Am J Surg 129:309–315, 1975
49. Nishida T, Iida M, Chijiwa K et al: Obstructive colitis: endoscopic diagnosis using a pediatric colonofiberscope. Gastrointest Endosc 34:140–142, 1988
50. Toner M, Condell D, O'Briain DS: Obstructive colitis. Ulceroinflammatory lesions occurring proximal to colonic obstruction. Am J Surg Pathol 14:719–728, 1990
51. Levine TS, Price AB: Obstructive enterocolitis: a clinico-pathological discussion. Histopathology 25:57–64, 1994
52. Mitros FA, Schuffler MD, Teja K, Anuras S: Pathologic features of familial visceral myopathy. Hum Pathol 13:825–833, 1982
53. Anuras S, Shirazi SS: Colonic pseudo-obstruction. Am J Gastroenterol 79:525–532, 1984
54. Krishamurthy S, Schuffler MD: Pathology of the neuromuscular disorders of the small intestine and colon. Gastroenterology 93:610–639, 1987
55. Evans DL, Rogers JF, Peiper SC: Intestinal dilatation associated with phenothiazine therapy: a case report and literature review. Am J Psychiatry 136:970–972, 1979
56. Schuffler MD, Rohrmann CA, Chaffee RG: Chronic intestinal pseudoobstruction. Medicine 60:173–196, 1981

57. Wald A, Kichler J, Mendelow H: Amyloidosis and chronic intestinal pseudo-obstruction. Dig Dis Sci 26:462–465, 1981
58. Tada S, Iida M, Yao T et al: Intestinal pseudo-obstruction in patients with amyloidosis: clinicopathologic differences between chemical types of amyloid protein. Gut 34:1412–1417, 1993
59. Ferrari BT, Ray JE, Robertson HD et al: Colonic manifestations of collagen vascular diseases. Dis Colon Rectum 23:473, 1980
60. Leon SH, Schuffler MD: Visceral myopathy of the colon mimicking Hirschsprung's disease. Diagnosis by deep rectal biopsy. Dig Dis Sci 31:1381–1386, 1986
61. Almy TP, Howell DA: Diverticular disease of the colon. N Engl J Med 302:324, 1980
62. Ming SC, Fleischner F: Diverticulitis of the sigmoid colon: reappraisal of the pathology and pathogenesis. Surgery 58:627, 1965
63. Morson BC: Pathology of the diverticular disease of the colon. Clin Gastroenterol 4:37, 1975
64. Shah AN, Mazza BR: The detection of an inverted diverticulum by colonoscopy. Gastrointest Endosc 28:188–189, 1982
65. Kelly JK: Plypoid prolapsing mucosal folds in diverticular disease. Am J Surg Pathol 15:871–878, 1991
66. Cawthorn SJ, Gibbs NM, Marks CG: Segmental colitis: a new complication of diverticular disease. Gut 24:500, 1983
67. Casarella WJ, Kanter IE, Seaman WB: Right-sided colonic diverticula as a cause of acute rectal hemorrhage. N Engl J Med 286:450–453, 1972
68. Meyers MA, Alonson DR, Baer JW: Pathogenesis of massively bleeding colonic diverticulosis: new observations. AJR 127:901, 1976
69. Norris HT: Vascular disorders. pp. 214–239. In Ming S-C, Goldman H (eds): Pathology of the Gastrointestinal Tract. WB Saunders, Philadelphia, 1992
70. Moncure AC, Waltman AC, Vandersalm TJ et al: Gastrointestinal hemorrhage from adhesion-related mesenteric varices. Ann Surg 18:24, 1976
71. Kozarek RA, Botoman VA, Bredfeldt JE et al: Portal colopathy: prospective study of colonoscopy in patients with portal hypertension. Gastroenterology 101:1192–1197, 1991
72. Iredale JP, Ridings P, McGinn FP, Arthur MJP: Familial and idiopathic colonic varices: an unusual cause of lower gastrointestinal hemorrhage. Gut 33:1285–1288, 1992
73. Mitsudo SM, Boley SJ, Brandt LJ et al: Vascular ectasias of the right colon in the elderly: a distinct pathologic entity. Hum Pathol 10:585, 1979
74. Pounder DJ, Rowland R, Pieterse AS et al: Angiodysplasia of the colon. J Clin Pathol 35:824–829, 1982
75. Howard CM, Buchanan JD, Hunt RG: Angiodysplasia of the colon. Experience of 26 cases. Lancet 2:16–19, 1982
76. Richter JM, Hedberg SE, Athanasoulis A, Schapiro RH: Angiodysplasia: clinical presentation and colonoscopic diagnosis. Dig Dis Sci 29:481–485, 1984
77. Boley SJ, Brandt LJ: Vascular ectasias of the colon—1986. Dig Dis Sci 31:26S–42S, 1986
78. Meyer CI, Troncale FJ, Galloway S, Sheahan DG: Arteriovenous malformations of the bowel: an analysis of 22 cases and a review of the literature. Medicine (Baltimore) 60:36–48, 1981
79. Camilleri M, Pusey CD, Chadwick VS, Rees AJ: Gastrointestinal manifestations of systemic vasculitis. Q J Med 206:141–149, 1983
80. Burke AP, Sobin LH, Virmani R: Localized vasculitis of the gastrointestinal tract. Am J Surg Pathol 19:338–349, 1995
81. Hoffman BI, Katz WA: The gastrointestinal manifestations of systemic lupus erythematosus: a review of the literature. Semin Arthritis Rheum 9:237–247, 1980
82. Tribe CR, Scott DGI, Bacon PA; Rectal biopsy in the diagnosis of systemic vasculitis. J Clin Pathol 34:843–850, 1981
83. McCurley TL, Collins RD: Intestinal infarction in rheumatoid arthritis. Arch Pathol Lab Med 108:125–128, 1984
84. Shimamoto C, Hirata I, Okshiba S et al: Churg-Strauss syndrome (allergic granulomatous angiitis) with peculiar multiple colonic ulcers. Am J Gastroenterol 85:316–319, 1990
85. Goldman LP, Lindenberg RL: Henoch-Schoenlein purpura: gastrointestinal manifestations with endoscopic correlation. Am J Gastroenterol 75:357–360, 1981

86. Cappell MS, Gupta AM: Colonic lesions associated with Henoch-Schönlein purpura. Am J Gastroenterol 85:1186–1188, 1990
87. Haworth SJ, Pusey CD: Severe intestinal involvement in Wegener's granulomatosis. Gut 25:1296–1300, 1984
88. Whitington PF, Friedman AL, Chesney RW: Gastrointestinal disease in the hemolytic-uremic syndrome. Gastroenterology 76:728–733, 1979
89. Yates RS, Osterholm RK: Hemolytic-uremic syndrome colitis. J Clin Gastroenterol 2:359, 1980
90. Geller SA, Cohen A: Arterial inflammatory-cell infiltration in Crohn's disease. Arch Pathol Lab Med 107:473–475, 1983
91. Romano TJ, Graham SM, Chuong J et al: Bleeding colonic ulcers secondary to atheromatous micoemboli after left heart catheterization. J Clin Gastroenterol 10:693–698, 1988
92. O'Briain DS, Jeffers M, Jay EW, Hourihane DOB: Bleeding due to colorectal atheroembolism. Diagnosis by biopsy of adenomatous polyps or of ischemic ulcer. Am J Surg Pathol 15:1078–1082, 1991
93. Gramlich TL, Hunter SB: Focal polypoid ischemia of the colon: atheroemboli presenting as a colonic polyp. Arch Path Lab Med 118:308–309, 1994
94. Cheville JC, Mitros FA, Vanderzalm G, Platz CE: Atheroemboli-associated polyps of the sigmoid colon. Am J Surg Pathol 17:1054–1057, 1993
95. Williams LF Jr: Vascular insufficiency of the intestines. Gastroenterology 61:757–777, 1971
96. Alschibaja T, Morson BC: Ischemic bowel disease. J Clin Pathol 11:68, 1977
97. Brandt LJ, Boley SJ: Ischemic intestinal syndromes. Adv Surg 15:1–45, 1981
98. Whitehead R: The pathology of ischemia of the intestines. Pathol Annu 11:1–52, 1976
99. Swerdlow SH, Antonioli DA, Goldman H: Intestinal infarction: a new classification. Arch Pathol Lab Med 105:218, 1981
100. Ming SC: Hemorrhagic necrosis of the gastrointestinal tract and its relation to cardiovascular status. Circulation 32:332, 1965
101. Kilpatrick ZM, Farman J, Yasner R et al: Ischemic proctitis. JAMA 205:75, 1968
102. Devroede G, Wobecky S, Masse S et al: Ischemic fecal incontinence and rectal angina. Gastroenterology 83:970–980, 1983
103. Kliegman RM, Fanaroff AA: Necrotizing enterocolitis. N Engl J Med 310:1093–1103, 1984
104. Cheromcha DP, Hyman PE: Neonatal necrotizing enterocolitis. Inflammatory bowel disease of the newborn. Dig Dis Sci 33 (March suppl):78S–84S, 1988
105. Gage TP, Gagnier JM: Ischemic colitis complicating sickle cell crisis. Gastroenterology 84:171–174, 1983
106. Bartlett JG: Antiobiotic-associated colitis. Clin Gastroenterol 8:783, 1979
107. Abrams GD: Infectious disorders of the intestine. pp. 621–642. In Ming S-C, Goldman H (eds): Pathology of the Gastrointestinal Tract. WB Saunders, Philadelphia, 1992
108. Price AB, Jewkes J, Sanderson RJ: Acute diarrhea: Campylobacter colitis and the role of rectal biopsy. J Clin Pathol 32:990–997, 1979
109. Kumar NB, Nostrant TT, Appelman HD: The histopathologic spectrum of acute self-limited colitis (acute infectious colitis). Am J Surg Pathol 6:523–529, 1982
110. Quinn TC, Corey L, Chaffee RG: The etiology of anorectal infections in homosexual men. Am J Med 71:395, 1981
111. Surawicz CM, Goodell SE, Quinn TC et al: Spectrum of rectal biopsy abnormalities in homosexual men with intestinal symptoms. Gastroenterology 91:651–659, 1986
112. Dobbins WO, Weinstein WM: Electron microscopy of the intestine and rectum in acquired immunodeficiency syndrome. Gastroenterology 88:738–749, 1985
113. Blanshard C, Ellis DS, Tovey G, Gazzard BG: Electron microscopy of rectal biopsies in HIV-positive individuals. J Pathol 169: 79–87, 1993
114. Rotterdam H, Tsang P: Gastrointestinal disease in the immunocompromised patient. Hum Pathol 25:1123–1140, 1994
115. Blacklow NR, Greenberg HB: Viral gastroenteritis. N Engl J Med 325:252–264, 1991
116. Goodell SE, Quinn TC, Mertichinian E et al: Herpes simplex virus proctitis in homosexual men. Clinical, sigmoidoscopic and histopathological features. N Engl J Med 308:868–871, 1983

117. Wassalle JA, Sedgwick JH, Dawson PJ, Fabri PJ: Intestinal herpes simplex infection presenting with intestinal perforation. Am J Gastroenterol 87:1475–1477, 1992
118. Hinnant KL, Rotterdam HZ, Bell ET, Tapper ML: Cytomegalovirus infection of the alimentary tract: a clinicopathological correlation. Am J Gastroenterol 81:944–950, 1986
119. Chetty R, Roskell DE: Cytomegalovirus infection in the gastrointestinal tract. J Clin Pathol 47:968–972, 1994
120. Surawicz CM, Myerson D: Self-limited cytomegalovirus colitis in immunocompetent individuals. Gastroenterology 94:194–199, 1988
121. Cheung ANY, Ng IOL: Cytomegalovirus infection of the gastrointestinal tract in non-AIDS patients. Am J Gastroenterol 88: 1882–1886, 1993
122. Goodgame RW, Genta RM, Estrada R et al: Frequency of positive tests for cytomegalovirus in AIDS patients: endoscopic lesions compared with normal mucosa. Am J Gastroenterol 88:338–342, 1993
123. Wu G-D, Shintaku IP, Chien K, Geller SA: A comparison of routine light microscopy, immunohistochemistry, and in-situ hybridization for the detection of cytomegalovirus in gastrointestinal biopsies. Am J Gastroenterol 84:1517–1520, 1989
124. Cooper HS, Roffensperger EC, Jonal L: Cytomegalovirus inclusions in patients with ulcerative colitis and toxic dilatation requiring colonic resection. Gastroenterology 72: 1253, 1977
125. Janoff EN, Orenstein JM, Manischewitz JF, Smith PD: Adenovirus colitis in the acquired immunodeficiency syndrome. Gastroenterology 100:976–979, 1991
126. Maddox A, Francis N, Moss J et al: Adenovirus infection of the large bowel in HIV positive patients. J Clin Pathol 45:684–688, 1992
127. Geller SA, Zimmerman MJ, Cohen A: Rectal biopsy in early lymphogranuloma venereum proctitis. Am J Gastroenterol 74:433, 1980
128. Levine JS, Smith PD, Brugge WR: Chronic proctitis in male homosexuals due to lymphogranuloma venereum. Gastroenterology 79:563, 1980
129. Quinn TC, Goodell SE, Mhrtichian PAC et al: Chlamydia trachomatic proctitis. N Engl J Med 305:195, 1981
130. de la Monte SM, Hutchins GM: Follicular proctocolitis and neuromatous hyperplasia with lymphogranuloma venereum. Hum Pathol 16:1025–1032, 1985
131. Klotz SA, Dautz DJ, Tam MR, Reed KH: Hemorrhagic proctitis due to lymphogranuloma venereum serogroup 12. N Engl J Med 308:1563–1565, 1983
132. Dickinson RJ, Gilmour HM, McClelland DBL et al: Rectal biopsy in patients presenting to an infectious disease unit with diarrheal disease. Gut 20:141–148, 1979
133. Anand BS, Malhotra V, Bhattacharya SK et al: Rectal histology in acute bacillary dysentery. Gastroenterology 90:654–960, 1986.
134. Islam MM, Azad AK, Bardhan PK et al: Pathology of shigellosis and its complications. Histopathology 24:65–71, 1994
135. Colgan T, Lambert JR, Newman A, Luk SC: Campylobacter jejunienterocolitis. Arch Pathol Lab Med 104:571–574, 1980
136. Van Spreauwel JP, Duiersma GC, Meijer CJ et al: Campylobacter colitis: histological, immunohistochemical and ultrastructural findings. Gut 26:945–951, 1985
137. Day DW, Mandal BK, Morson BC: The rectal biopsy appearances in salmonella colitis. Histopathology 2:117, 1978
138. McGovern VJ, Slarutin LJ: Pathology of salmonella colitis. Am J Surg Pathol 3:483, 1979
139. Boyd JF: Pathology of the alimentary tract in Salmonella typhimurium food poisoning. Gut 26:935–944, 1985
140. Kelly J, Oryshak A, Wenetsak M et al: The colonic pathology of Escherichia coli 0157:H7 infection. Am J Surg Pathol 14:87–92, 1990
141. Bhargava DK, Tandon HD: Ileocoecal tuberculosis diagnosed by colonoscopy and biopsy. Aust N Z J Surg 50:583–585, 1980
142. Shah S, Thomas V, Matkan M et al: Colonoscopic study of 50 patients with colonic tuberculosis. Gut 33:347–351, 1992
143. Marshall JB: Tuberculosis of the gastrointestinal tract and peritoneum. Am J Gastroenterol 88:989–999, 1993
144. Malik AK, Bhasin DK, Roy P et al: Demonstration of mycobacterium tuberculosis in colonoscopic biopsies. Histopathology 23: 199–200, 1993
145. Gillin JS, Urmacher C, West R, Shuke M: Disseminated Mycobacterium avium-

intracellulare infection in acquired immunodeficiency syndrome mimicking Whipple's disease. Gastroenterology 85:1187–1191, 1983
146. Roth RI, Owen RZ, Keren DF, Volberding PA: Intestinal infection with Mycobacterium avium in acquired immune deficiency syndrome (AIDS): histological and clinical comparison with Whipple's disease. Dig Dis Sci 30:497–504, 1985
147. Gray JR, Rabeneck L: Atypical mycobacterial infections of the gastrointestinal tract in AIDS patients. Am J Gastroenterol 84: 1521–1524, 1989
148. Nielsen RH, Orholm M, Pederson JO et al: Colorectal spirochetosis: clinical significance of the infection. Gastroenterology 85:62–67, 1983
149. Surawicz CM, Roberts PL, Rompalo A et al: Intestinal spirochetosis in homosexual men. Am J Med 82:587–592, 1987
150. Ferreira RMCD, Phillips AD, Stevens CR et al: Intestinal spirochetosis in children. J Ped Gastroenterol Nutr 17:333–337, 1993
151. Simmonds SD, Noble MA, Freeman JH: Gastrointestinal features of culture-positive Yersinia enterocolitica infection. Gastroenterology 92:112–117, 1987
152. Brown JR: Human actinomycosis: a study of 181 subjects. Hum Pathol 4:319–330, 1973
153. Kilpatrick ZM: Gonorrheal proctitis. N Engl J Med 287:967, 1972
154. Schmidt T, Pfeiffer A, Ehret W et al: Legionella infection of the colon presenting as acute attack of ulcerative colitis. Gastroenterology 97:751–755, 1989
155. Prescott RJ, Harris M, Banerjee SS: Fungal infections of the small and large intestines. J Clin Pathol 45:806–811, 1992
156. Eras P, Goldstein MJ, Sherlock P: Candida infection of the gastrointestinal tract. Medicine (Baltimore) 51:367–379, 1972
157. Lyon DT, Schubert TT, Mantia AG, Kaplan MH: Phycomycosis of the gastrointestinal tract. Am J Gastroenterol 72:379–394, 1979
158. Young RC, Bennett JE, Vogel CL et al: Aspergillosis: the spectrum of the disease in 98 patients. Medicine (Baltimore) 49:147, 1970
159. Cappell MS, Mandell W, Grimes MM, Neu HC: Gastrointestinal histoplasmosis. Dig Dis Sci 33:353–360, 1988
160. Clarkston WK, Bonacini M, Peterson I: Colitis due to Histoplasma capsulation in the acquired immune deficiency syndrome. Am J Gastroenterol 86:913–916, 1991
161. Cimponeriu D, LoPresti P, Lavelanet M et al: Gastrointestinal histoplasmosis in HIV infection: two cases of colonic pseudocancer and review of the literature. Am J Gastroenterol 89:129–131, 1994
162. Washington K, Gottfried MR, Wilson ML: Gastrointestinal cryptococcosis. Modern Pathol 4:707–711, 1991
163. Blumeniranz H, Kasen L, Romen J et al: The role of endoscopy in suspected amebiasis. Am J Gastroenterol 78:15–18, 1983
164. Gonzalez-Ruiz A, Haque R, Aguirre A et al: Value of microscopy in the diagnosis of dysentery associated with invasive Entamoeba histolytica. J Clin Pathol 47:236–240, 1994
165. Isaacs D, Hunt GH, Phillips AD et al: Cryptosporidiosis in immunocompetent children. J Clin Pathol 38:76–81, 1985
166. Wolfson JS, Richter JM, Waldron MA et al: Cryptosporidiosis in immunocompetent patients. N Engl J Med 312:1278–1282, 1985
167. Godwin TA: Cryptosporidiosis in the acquired immunodeficiency syndrome: a study of 15 autopsy cases. Hum Pathol 22:1215–1224, 1991
168. Clayton F, Heller T, Kotler DP: Variation in the enteric distribution of cryptosporidia in acquired immunodeficiency syndrome. Am J Clin Pathol 102:420–425, 1994
169. Orenstein JM: Microsporidiosis in the acquired immunodeficiency syndrome. J Parasitol 77:843–864, 1991
170. Peacock CS, Blanchard C, Tovey DG et al: Histological diagnosis of intestinal microsporidiosis in patients with AIDS. J Clin Pathol 44:558–563, 1991
171. Shadduck JA, Orenstein JM: Comparative pathology of microsporidiosis. Arch Pathol Lab Med 117:1215–1219, 1993
172. Kamberoglou D, Savva S, Adraskelos N et al: Balantidiosis complicating a case of ulcerative colitis. Am J Gastroenterol 85:765–766, 1990
173. Idoate MA, Vazquez JJ, Civeira P: Rectal biopsy as a diagnostic procedure of chronic visceral leishmaniasis. Histopathology 22:589–590, 1993

174. Pauwels A, Merjohas MC, Elioszewicz M et al: Toxoplasma colitis in the acquired immunodeficiency syndrome. Am J Gastroenterol 87:518–519, 1992
175. Gambescia RA, Kaufman B, Noy J et al: Schistosoma mansoni infection of the colon: a case report and review of the late colonic manifestations. Am J Dig Dis 21:988, 1976
176. Mohamed AR, Karawi MA, Yasawy MI: Schistosomal colonic disease. Gut 31:439–442, 1990
177. Dimmette RM, Sproat HF: Rectosigmoid polyps in schistosomiasis. Am J Trop Med Hyg 4:1057–1067, 1955
178. Brasitus TA, Gold RP, Kay RH et al: Intestinal stronglyoidiasis. Am J Gastroenterol 73:65–69, 1980
179. Grove DI: Strongyloidiasis: a conundrum for gastroenterologists. Gut 35:437–440, 1994
180. McKerrow JH, Sakanari J, Deerdorff TL: Anisakiasis: revenge of the sushi parasites. N Engl J Med 319:1228–1229, 1988
181. Minamoto T, Sawaquchi K, Ogino T, Mai M: Anisakiasis of the colon. Report of two cases with emphasis in the diagnostic and therapeutic value of colonoscopy. Endoscopy 23:50–52, 1991
182. Malatjalion DA: Pathology of inflammatory bowel disease in colorectal musocal biopsies. Dig Dis Sci 32:150–155, 1987
183. Goldman H: Colonic mucosal biopsy in inflammatory bowel disease. Surg Pathol 4:3–24, 1991
184. Seldenrijk CA, Morson BC, Meuwissen SGM et al: Histopathological evaluation of colonic mucosal biopsy specimens in chronic inflammatory bowel disease: diagnostic implications. Gut 32:1514–1520, 1991
185. Chong SKF, Blackshaw AJ, Boyle S et al: Histological diagnosis of chronic inflammatory bowel disease in childhood. Gut 26:55–59, 1985
186. Lennard-Jones JE, Lockhart-Mummery HE, Morson BC: Clinical and pathological differentiation of Crohn's disease and proctocolitis. Gastroenterology 54:1162, 1968
187. Glotzer DJ, Gardner RC, Goldman H et al: Comparative features and course of ulcerative and granulomatous colitis. N Engl J Med 282:582–589, 1970
188. Cook MG, Dixon MF: An analysis of the reliability of detection and diagnostic value of various pathologic features in Crohn's disease and ulcerative colitis. Gut 14:255, 1973
189. Price AB, Morson BC: Inflammatory bowel disease: the surgical pathology of Crohn's disease and ulcerative colitis. Hum Pathol 6:7, 1975
190. Fawaz KA, Glotzer DJ, Goldman H et al: Ulcerative colitis and Crohn's disease of the colon: a comparison of the long-term postoperative courses. Gastroenterology 71:372–378, 1976
191. Groisman GM, George J, Harpaz N: Ulcerative appendicitis in universal and nonuniversal ulcerative colitis. Modern Pathol 7:322–325, 1994
192. Kroft SH, Stryker SJ, Rao MS: Appendiceal involvement as a skip lesion in ulcerative colitis. Modern Pathol 7:912–914, 1994
193. Yardley JH, Donowitz M: Colo-rectal biopsy in inflammatory bowel disease. pp. 50–94. In Yardley JH, Morson BC, Abell MR (eds): The Gastrointestinal Tract. Williams & Wilkins, Baltimore, 1977
194. Delpre G, Cevidor I, Steinherz R et al: Ultrastructural abnormalities in endoscopically and histologically normal and involved colon in ulcerative colitis. Am J Gastroenterol 84:1038–1046, 1989
195. Nostrant TT, Kumar NB, Appelman HD: Histopathology differentiates acute self-limited colitis from ulcerative colitis. Gastroenterology 92:318–328, 1987
196. Allison MC, Hamilton-Dutoit SJ, Dhillon AP, Pounder RE: The value of rectal biopsy in distinguishing self-limited colitis from early inflammatory bowel disease. Q J Med 65:985–995, 1987
197. Surawicz CM, Haggitt RC, Husseman M, McFarland LV: Mucosal biopsy diagnosis of colitis: acute self-limited colitis and idiopathic inflammatory bowel disease. Gastroenterology 107:755–763, 1994
198. Symonds DA: Paneth cell metaplasia in diseases of the colon and rectum. Arch Pathol 97:343, 1974
199. Skinner JM, Whitehead R, Piris J: Argentaffin cells in ulcerative colitis. Gut 12:636, 1971
200. Flejou JF, Potet F, Bogomoletz WV et al: Lymphoid follicular proctitis. A condition different from ulcerative proctitis? Dig Dis Sci 33:314–320, 1988

201. Warren BF, Shepherd NA, Bartolo DCC, Bradfield JWB: Pathology of the defunctioned rectum in ulcerative colitis. Gut 34:514–516, 1993
202. Kelly JK, Langevin JM, Price IM et al: Giant and symptomatic inflammatory polyps of the colon in idiopathic inflammatory bowel disease. Am J Surg Pathol 10:420–428, 1986
203. Brozna JP, Fisher RL, Barwick KW: Filiform polyposis: an unusual complication of inflammatory bowel disease. J Clin Gastroenterol 7:451–458, 1985
204. LaMont JT, Trnka YM: Therapeutic implications of Clostridium difficile toxin during relapse of chronic inflammatory bowel disease. Lancet 1:381–384, 1980
205. Chakraborty TK, Bhatia D, Heading RC, Ford MJ: Salicylate induced exacerbations of ulcerative colitis. Gut 28:613–615, 1987
206. Kaufmann HJ, Taubin HL: Nonsteroidal anti-inflammatory drugs activate quiescent inflammatory bowel disease. Ann Intern Med 107:513–516, 1987
207. Herman AH, Nabseth DC: Colitis cystica profunda: localized, segmental, and diffuse. Arch Surg 106:337, 1973
208. Greenstein AJ, Sacher DB, Smith H et al: Cancer in universal and left-sided ulcerative colitis: factors determining risk. Gastroenterology 89:290–294, 1979
209. Gyde SN, Prior P, Allan RN et al: Colorectal cancer in ulcerative colitis: a cohort study of primary referrals from three centers. Gut 29:206–217, 1988
210. Wakefield AJ, Ekbom A, Dhillon AP et al: Crohn's disease: pathogenesis and persistent measles virus infection. Gastroenterology 108:911–916, 1995
211. Hamilton SR, Bussey H Jr, Morson BC: En face histologic technique to demonstrate mucosal inflammatory lesions in macroscopically uninvolved colon of Crohn's disease resection specimens. Lab Invest 42:121, 1980
212. Surawicz CM, Meisel JL, Ylvisaker T et al: Rectal biopsy in the diagnosis of Crohn's disease: value of multiple biopsies and serial sectioning. Gastroenterology 81:66–71, 1981
213. Kuramoto S, Oohara T, Ihara O et al: Granulomas of the gut in Crohn's disease. A step sectioning study. Dis Colon Rectum 30:6–11, 1987
214. Rotterdam H, Korelitz BI, Sommers SC: Microgranulomas in grossly normal rectal mucosa in Crohn's disease. Am J Clin Pathol 67:550, 1977
215. Hamilton SR: Colorectal carcinoma in patients with Crohn's disease. Gastroenterology 89:398–407, 1985
216. Petras RE, Mir-Madjlessi SH, Farmer RG: Crohn's disease and intestinal carcinoma. A report of 11 cases with emphasis on associated epithelial dysplasia. Gastroenterology 93:1307–1314, 1987
217. Holdstock G, DuBoulay CE, Smith CL: Survey of the use of colonoscopy in inflammatory bowel disease. Dig Dis Sci 29:731–734, 1984
218. Snover DC, Sandstad J, Hutton S: Mucosal pseudolipomatosis of the colon. Am J Clin Pathol 84:575–580, 1985
219. Odze R, Antonioli D, Peppercorn M, Goldman H: Effect of topical 5-aminosalicylic acid (5-ASA) therapy on rectal mucosal biopsy morphology in chronic ulcerative colitis. Am J Surg Pathol 17:869–875, 1993
220. Korelitz BI, Sommers SC: Responses to drug therapy in ulcerative colitis. Am J Dig Dis 21:441, 1976
221. Lennard-Jones JE, Melville DM, Morson BC et al: Pre-cancer and cancer in extensive ulcerative colitis; findings among 401 patients over 22 years. Gut 31:800–806, 1990
222. Nugent FW, Haggitt RC, Gilpin PA: Cancer surveillance in ulcerative colitis. Gastroenterology 100:1241–1248, 1991
223. Riddell RH, Goldman H, Ransohoff DF et al: Dysplasia in inflammatory bowel disease: standardized classification with provisional clinical applications. Hum Pathol 14:931–968, 1983
224. Price B: Overlap in the spectrum of nonspecific inflammatory bowel disease: colitis indeterminate. J Clin Pathol 31:567–577, 1978
225. Lee KS, Medline A, Shockey S: Indeterminate colitis in the spectrum of inflammatory bowel disease. Arch Pathol Lab Med 103:173, 1979
226. McQuillan AC, Appelman HD: Superficial Crohn's disease: a study of 10 patients. Surg Pathol 2:231–239, 1989
227. Riddell RH: The gastrointestinal tract. pp. 515–606. In Riddell RH (ed): Pathology of

the Drug-Induced and Toxic Diseases. Churchill Livingstone, New York, 1982

228. Goldman H, Szabo S: Chemical and physical disorders. pp. 141–170. In Ming S-C, Goldman H (eds): Pathology of the Gastrointestinal Tract. WB Saunders, Philadelphia, 1992
229. Miller SS, Muggia AL, Spiro HM: Colonic histologic changes induced by 5-fluorouracil. Gastroenterology 43:391, 1962
230. Meisel JL, Bergman D, Graney D et al: Human rectal mucosa: proctoscopic and morphological changes caused by laxatives. Gastroenterology 72:1274–1279, 1977
231. Leriche M, Devroede G, Sanchez G et al: Changes in the rectal mucosa induced by hypertonic enemas. Dis Colon Rectum 21:227, 1978
232. Scott TR, Graham SM, Schweitzer EJ, Bartlett ST: Colonic necrosis following sodium polystyrene sulfonate (Kayexalate)-sorbitol enema in a renal transplant patient. Dis Colon Rectum 36:607–609, 1993
233. Herreiras JM, Muniain MA, Sanchez S, Garrido M: Alcohol-induced colitis. Endoscopy 15:121–122, 1983
234. Meyer CT, Brand M, DeLuca Va, Spriro HM: Hydrogen peroxide colitis: a report of three patients. J Clin Gastroenterol 3:31–35, 1981
235. Smith B: Pathologic changes in the colon produced by anthraquinone purgatives. Dis Colon Rectum 16:455–458, 1973
236. Oster JR, Materson BJ, Rogers AI: Laxative abuse syndrome. Am J Gastroenterol 74:451, 1980
237. Kelly CP, Pothoulakis C, LaMont JT: Clostridium difficile colitis. N Engl J Med 330:257–262, 1994
238. Price AB, Davies DR: Pseudomembranous colitis. J Clin Path, 30:1–12, 1977
239. Schnitt SJ, Antonioli DA, Goldman H: Massive mural edema in severe pseudomembranous colitis. Arch Pathol Lab Med 107:211–213, 1983
240. Fortson WC, Tedesco FJ: Drug-induced colitis: a review. Am J Gastroenterol 79:878–883, 1984
241. Bjornason I, Hayllar J, Macpherson AJ, Russell AS: Side effects of nonsteroidal anti-inflammatory drugs on the small and large intestine in humans. Gastroenterology 104:1832–1847, 1993
242. Stamm C, Burkhalter E, Pearce W et al: Benign colonic ulcers associated with nonsteroidal anti-inflammatory drug ingestion. Am M Gastroenterol 89:2230–2233, 1994
243. Huber T, Ruchti C, Halter F: Nonsteroidal anti-inflammatory drug-induced colonic strictures: a case report. Gastroenterology 100:1119–1122, 1991
244. Fellows IW, Clarke JMF, Roberts PF: Nonsteroidal anti-inflammatory drug-induced jejunal and colonic diaphragm disease: a report of two cases. Gut 33:1424–1426, 1992
245. Riddell RH, Tonaka M, Mazzoleni G: Nonsteroidal anti-inflammatory drugs as a possible cause of collagenous colitis: a case-control study. Gut 33:683–686, 1992
246. Ueda D, Azuma H, Sakata Y et al: Aminophylline suppository-induced acute proctitis. Am J Gastroenterol 87:889–890, 1992
247. Bernardino ME, Lawson TL: Discrete colonic ulcers associated with oral contraceptives. Dig Dis Sci 21:503–506, 1976
248. Deana DG, Dean RJ: Reversible ischemic colitis in young women. Association with oral contraceptive use. Am J Surg Pathol 19:454–462, 1995
249. Reinhart WH, Kapeller M, Halter F: Severe pseudomembranous and ulcerative colitis during gold therapy. Endoscopy 15:70–72, 1983
250. Jackson CW, Haboubi NY, Whorwell PJ, Schofield PF: Gold-induced enterocolitis. Gut 27:452–456, 1986
251. Worminn B, Hochter W, Seib H-J, Ottenjonn R: Ergotamine-induced colitis. Endoscopy 17:165–166, 1985
252. Eckardt VF, Kanzler G, Remmele W: Anorectal ergotism: another cause of solitary rectal ulcer. Gastroenterology 91:1123–1127, 1986
253. Jonas G, Mahoney A, Murray J, Gertler S: Chemical colitis due to endoscopic cleaning solutions: a mimic of pseudomembranous colitis. Gastroenterology 95:1403–1408, 1988
254. Levine DS: Proctitis following colonoscopy. Gastrointest Endosc 34:269–272, 1988
255. Martin P, Manley PN, Depew WT, Blakeman JM: Isotretinoin-associated proctosigmoiditis. Gastroenterology 93:606, 1987
256. Moshkowitz M, Konikoff FM, Arber N et al: Acyclovir-associated colitis. Am J Gastroenterol 83:2110–2111, 1993

257. Atherton LD, Leib ES, Kaye MD: Toxic megacolon associated with methotrexate therapy. Gastroenterology 86:1583–1588, 1984
258. Brown DN, Rosenholtz MJ, Marshall JB: Ischemic colitis related to cocaine abuse. Am J Gastroenterol 89:1558–1561, 1994
259. May J, Lowenthal J: Irradiation injury to the colon. Gut 6:444–447, 1965
260. Weisbrodt IM, Liber AF, Gordon BS: The effects of therapeutic radiation on colonic mucosa. Cancer 36:931–940, 1975
261. Gilensky NH, Burns DG, Barbezat GO et al: The natural history of radiation-induced proctosigmoiditis: an analysis of 88 patients. Q J Med 202:40–53, 1983
262. Habonbi NY, Schofield PF, Rowland PI: The light and electron microscopic features of early and late phase radiation-induced proctitis. Am J Gastroenterol 83:1140–1144, 1988
263. Warren S, Friedman B: Pathology and pathologic diagnosis of radiation lesions in the gastrointestinal tract. Am J Pathol 18:499–507, 1942
264. Novak JM, Collinness JT, Donowitz M et al: Effects of radiation on the human gastrointestinal tract. J Clin Gastroenterol 1:9, 1979
265. Berthrong M, Fajardo LF; Radiation injury in surgical pathology. Part II. Alimentary tract. Am J Surg Pathol 5:153–178, 1981
266. Hasleton PS, Carr N, Schofield PF: Vascular changes in radiation bowel disease. Histopathology 9:517, 1985
267. Gardiner GW, McAuliffe N, Murray D: Colitis cystica profunda occurring in a radiation-induced colonic stricture. Hum Pathol 15:295–298, 1984
268. Qizilbash AH: Radiation-induced carcinoma of the rectum: a late complication of pelvic irradiation. Arch Pathol 98:118–121, 1974
269. Carney JA, Stephens DH: Intramural barium (barium granuloma) of colon and rectum. Gastroenterology 65:316, 1973
270. Lewis JW, Kerstein MD, Koss N: Barium granuloma of the rectum: an uncommon complication of barium enema. Ann Surg 81:418–423, 1980
271. Phelps JE, Sanowski RA, Kozarek RA: Intramural extravasation of barium simulating carcinoma of the rectum. Dis Colon Rectum 24:388, 1981
272. Hernandez V, Hernandez IA, Berthrong M: Oleogranuloma simulating carcinoma of the rectum. Dis Colon Rectum 10:205–209, 1967
273. Greaney MG, Jackson PR: Oleogranuloma of the rectum produced by Lasonil ointment. Br Med J 2:997–998, 1977
274. Mazier WP, Sun KM, Robertson WG: Oil-induced granuloma (oleoma) of the rectum. Dis Colon Rectum 21:292–294, 1978
275. Jenkins HR, Pincott JR, Soothill JF et al: Food allergy: the major cause of infantile colitis. Arch Dis Child 59:326–329, 1984
276. Dahms BB: Allergic proctitis. Pediatr Pathol 8:429–435, 1988
277. Hill SM, Milla PJ: Colitis caused by food allergy in infants. Arch Dis Child 65:132–133, 1990
278. Goldman H: Allergic disorders. pp. 171–187. In Ming S-C, Goldman H (eds): Pathology of the Gastrointestinal Tract. WB Saunders, Philadelphia, 1992
279. Lake AM, Whitington PF, Hamilton SR: Dietary protein-induced colitis in breast-fed infants. J Pediatr 101:906–910, 1982
280. Goldman H, Proujansky R: Allergic proctitis and gastroenteritis in children: clinical and mucosal biopsy features in 53 cases. Am J Surg Pathol 10:75–86, 1986
281. Winter HS, Antonioli DA, Fukagawa N et al: Allergy-related proctocolitis in infants: diagnostic usefulness of rectal biopsy. Modern Pathol 3:5–10, 1990
282. Pascal RR, Gramlich TL: Geographic variations of eosinophil concentration in normal colonic mucosa. Modern Pathol 6:51A, 1993
283. Odze RD, Bines J, Leichtner AM et al: Allergic protocolitis in infants: a prospective clinicopathologic biopsy study. Hum Pathol 24:668–674, 1993
284. Klein NC, Hargrove RL, Sleisenger MH et al: Eosinophilic gastroenteritis. Medicine (Baltimore) 40:299–319, 1970
285. Ament ME; Immunodeficiency syndromes of the gut. Scand J Gastroenterol 20(suppl 114):127–135, 1985
286. Dworkin B, Wormser GP, Rosenthal WS et al: Gastrointestinal manifestations of the acquired immunodeficiency syndrome: a review of 22 cases. Am J Gastroenterol 80:774–778, 1985
287. Weber JR Jr, Dobbins WO: The intestinal and rectal epithelial lymphocyte in AIDS.

An electron-microscopic study. Am J Surg Pathol 10:627–639, 1986

288. Simon D, Brandt LJ: Diarrhea in patients with the acquired immunodeficiency syndrome. Gastroenterology 105:1238–1242, 1993
289. Ferrara JLM, Deeg HJ: Graft-versus-host disease. N Engl J Med 324:667–674, 1991
290. Sale GE, Shulman HM, McDonald JB et al: Gastrointestinal graft-versus-host disease in man: a clinicopathologic study of the rectal biopsy. Am J Surg Pathol 3:291, 1979
291. Spencer GD, Shulman HM, Mayerson D et al: Diffuse intestinal ulceration after marrow transplantation: a clinicopathologic study of 13 patients. Hum Pathol 17:621–633, 1986
292. Yardley JH, Lazenby AJ, Giardiello FM, Bayless TM: Collagenous, "microscopic", lymphocytic, and other gentler and more subtle forms of colitis. Hum Pathol 21:1089–1091, 1990
293. Saul SH: The watery diarrhea-colitis syndrome. A review of collagenous and microscopic/lymphocytic colitis. Int J Surg Pathol 1:65–82, 1993
294. Eckstein RP, Dowsett JF, Riley JW: Collagenous enterocolitis: a case of collagenous colitis with involvement of the small intestine. Am J Gastroenterol 83:767–771, 1988
295. Wolber R, Owen D, Freeman H: Colonic lymphocytosis in patients with celiac sprue. Hum Pathol 21:1092–1096, 1990
296. Lindstrom CG: "Collagenous colitis" with watery diarrhea: a new entity? Pathol Eur 11:87, 1976
297. Nielsen VT, Vetner M, Harslof E: Collagenous colitis. Histopathology 4:83, 1980
298. Bogomoletz WV, Adnet JJ, Birembault P et al: Collagenous colitis: an unrecognized entity. Gut 21:164, 1980
299. Teglbjaerg PS, Thaysen EH, Jansen HH: Development of collaenous colitis in sequential biopsy specimens. Gastroenterology 87:703–709, 1984
300. Kingham JGC, Levison DA, Morson BC, Dawson AM: Collaenous colitis. Gut 27:570, 1986
301. Flejou JF, Grimaud JA, Molas G: Collagenous colitis. Ultrastructural study and collagen immunotyping of four cases. Arch Pathol Lab Med 198:977–982, 1984
302. Gledhill A, Cole FM: Significance of basement membrane thickening in the human colon. Gut 25:1085–1088, 1984
303. Jesserun J, Yardley JH, Giardiello FM et al: Chronic colitis with thickening of the subepithelial collagen layer (collagenous colitis): histopathologic findings in 15 patients. Hum Pathol 18:839–848, 1987
304. Wang HH, Owings DV, Antonioli DA, Goldman H: Increased subepithelial collagen deposition is not specific for collagenous colitis. Modern Pathol 1:329–335, 1988
305. Carpenter HA, Tremaine WJ, Batts KP et al: Sequential histologic evaluations in collagenous colitis. Dig Dis Sci 37:1903–1909, 1993
306. Tanaka M, Mazzoleni G, Riddell RH: Distribution of collagenous colitis: utility of flexible sigmoidoscopy. Gut 33:65–70, 1992
307. Lazenby AJ, Yardley JH, Giardiello FM et al: Lymphocytic ("microscopic") colitis: a comparative histopathologic study with particular reference to collagenous colitis. Hum Pathol 20:18–28, 1989
308. Beaugerie L, Luboinski J, Brousse N et al: Drug induced lymphocytic colitis. Gut 35:426–428, 1994
309. Glotzer DJ, Glick ME, Goldman H: Proctitis and colitis following diversion of the fecal stream. Gastroenterology 80:438–441, 1981
310. Korelitz BI, Cheskin LJ, Sohn N, Summers SC: Proctitis after fecal diversion in Crohn's disease and its elimination with reanastomosis: implications for surgical management. Report of four cases. Gastroenterology 87:710–713, 1984
311. Lush LB, Reichen J, Levine JS: Aphthous ulceration in diversion colitis: clinical applications. Gastroenterology 87:1171–1173, 1984
312. Bosshardt RT, Abel ME: Proctitis following fecal diversion. Dis Colon Rectum 27:605–607, 1984
313. Ona FV, Bogar JN: Rectal bleeding due to diversion colitis. Am Gastroenterol 80:40–41, 1985
314. Murray FE, O'Brien MJ, Birkett DH et al: Diversion colitis. Pathologic findings in a resected sigmoid colon and rectum. Gastroenterology 93:1404–1408, 1987
315. Ma CK, Gottlieb C, Haas PA: Diversion colitis: a clinicopathologic study of 21 cases. Hum Pathol 21:429–436, 1990

316. Komorowski RA: Histologic spectrum of diversion colitis. Am J Surg Pathol 14:548–554, 1990
317. Geraghty JM, Talbort IC: Diversion colitis: histological features in the colon and rectum after defunctioning colostomy. Gut 32:1020–1023, 1991
318. Yeong ML, Bethwaite PB, Prasad J, Isbister WH: Lymphoid follicular hyerplasia—a distinctive feature of diversion colitis. Histopathology 19:55–61, 1991
319. Haque S, Eisen RN, West AB: The morphologic features of diversion colitis: studies of a pediatric population with no other disease of the intestinal mucosa. Hum Pathol 24:211–219, 1993
320. Roe AM, Warren BF, Brodribb AJM, Brown C: Diversion colitis and involution of the defunctioned anorectum. Gut 34:382–385, 1993
321. Geraghty JM, Charles AK: Aphthoid ulceration in diversion colitis. Histopathology 24:395–397, 1994
322. Harig JM, Soergel KH, Komorowski RA, Wood CM: Treatment of diversion colitis with short chain–fatty acid irrigation. N Engl J Med 320:23–28, 1989
323. Kies MS, Luedke DW, Boyd JF, McCue MJ: Neutropenic enterocolitis. Cancer 43:730–734, 1979
324. King A, Rampling A, Wight DGD, Warren RE: Neutropenic enterocolitis due to Clostridium septicum infection. J Clin Pathol 37:335–343, 1984
325. Newbold KM, Lord MG, Baglin TP: Role of clostridial organisms in neutropenic enterocolitis. J Clin Pathol 40:471, 1987
326. Wade DS, Nava HR, Douglas HO Jr: Neutropenic enterocolitis. Clinical diagnosis and treatment. Cancer 69:17–23, 1992
327. Chajek T, Fainaru M: Behçet's disease: report of 41 cases. Medicine (Baltimore) 54:179, 1975
328. Goldman H: Other inflammatory disorders of the intestine. pp. 697–724. In Ming S-C, Goldman H (eds): Pathology of the Gastrointestinal Tract. WB Saunders Co, Philadelphia, 1992
329. Baba S, Maruta M, Ando K et al: Intestinal Behçet's disease: report of five cases. Dis Colon Rectum 19:428–440, 1976
330. Lee RG: The colitis of Behçet's syndrome. Am J Surg Pathol 10:888–893, 1986
331. Johnson DA, Everhort CW: Colitis in Behçet's syndrome. Gastrointest Endosc 32:58–59, 1986
332. Lakhanpal S, Tani K, Lie JT et al: Pathologic features of Behçet's syndrome: a review of Japanese autopsy registry data. Hum Pathol 16:790–795, 1985
333. Gekas P, Schuster MM: Stercoral perforation of the colon: case report and review of the literature. Gastroenterology 80:1054–1058, 1981
334. Lennard-Jones JE: Functional gastrointestinal disorders. N Engl J Med 308:431–435, 1983
335. Lynn RB, Friedman RS: Irritable bowel syndrome. N Engl J Med 329:1940–1945, 1993
336. Goldman H: Systemic and miscellaneous disorders. pp. 351–380. In Ming S-C, Goldman H (eds): Pathology of the Gastrointestinal Tract. WB Saunders, Philadelphia, 1992
337. Parr NJ, Murphy C, Holt S et al: Endometriosis and the gut. Gut 29:1112–1115, 1988
338. Caccese WJ, McKinley MJ, Bronzo RL, Bronson R: Endoscopic confirmation of colonic endometriosis. Gastrointest Endosc 30:191–193, 1984
339. Langlois NEI, Park KGM, Keenan RA: Mucosal changes in the large bowel with endometriosis: a possible cause of misdiagnosis of colitis? Hum Pathol 25:1030–1034, 1994
340. Amano S, Yamado N: Endometroid carcinoma arising from endometriosis of the sigmoid colon: a case report. Hum Pathol 12:845–849, 1981
341. Yale CE, Balish E: Pneumatosis cystoides intestinalis. Dis Colon Rectum 19:107–111, 1976
342. Galondiuk S, Fazio VW: Pneumatosis cystoides intestinalis: a review of the literature. Dis Colon Rectum 29:358–363, 1986
343. Pieterse AS, Leong AS, Rowland R: The mucosal changes and pathogenesis of pneumatosis cystoides intestinalis. Hum Pathol 16:683–688, 1985
344. Pemberton HW, Smith WG, Holman CB: Pneumatosis cystoides intestinalis diagnosed sigmoidoscopically. Am J Surg 94:472–477, 1957
345. Heer M, Altorfer J, Pirovino M, Schmid M: Pneumatosis cystoides coli: a rare complica-

tion of colonoscopy. Endoscopy 15:119–120, 1983
346. Doolas A, Breyer RH, Franklin JL: Pneumatosis cystoides intestinalis following jejunoileal bypass. Am J Gastroenterol 72:271–275, 1979
347. Wayte DM, Helwig EB: Colitis cystica profunda. Am J Clin Pathol 48:159–169, 1966
348. Stuart M: Proctitis cystica profunda. Incidence, etiology, and treatment. Dis Colon Rectum 27:153–156, 1984
349. Rutter K, Riddell RH: The solitary ulcer syndrome of the rectum. Clin Gastroenterol 4:505–530, 1975
350. Ford MJ, Anderson JR, Gilmour HM et al: Clinical spectrum of "solitary ulcer" of the rectum. Gastroenterology 84:1533–1540, 1983
351. Tjandra JJ, Fazio VW, Church JM et al: Clinical concepts of solitary rectal ulcer. Dis Colon Rectum 25:227–234, 1992
352. DuBoulay CE, Fairbrother J, Isaacson PG: Mucosal prolapse syndrome—a unifying concept for solitary ulcer syndrome and related disorders. J Clin Pathol 36:1264–1268, 1983
353. Womach NR, Williams NS, Holmfield HJM, Morrison JFB: Pressure and prolapse—the cause of solitary rectal ulceration. Gut 28:1228–1233, 1987
354. Bogomoletz W, Fenzy A: Histopathological features of the solitary ulcer syndrome of the rectum. Arch Anat Cytol Pathol 28:329, 1980
355. Saul SH, Sollenberger LC: Solitary rectal ulcer syndrome. Its clinical and pathological underdiagnosis. Am J Surg Pathol 9:411–421, 1985
356. Niv Y, Bat L: Solitary rectal ulcer syndrome—clinical, endoscopic, and histological spectrum. Am J Gastroenterol 81:486–491, 1986
357. Levine DS: "Solitary" rectal ulcer syndrome. Are "solitary" rectal ulcer syndrome and "localized" colitis cystica profunda analogous syndromes caused by rectal prolapse? Gastroenterology 92:243–253, 1987
358. Lobert PF, Appelman HD: Inflammatory colacogenic polyp: a unique inflammatory lesion of the anal transitional zone. Am J Surg Pathol 5:761, 1981
359. Saul SH: Inflammatory cloacogenic polyp: relationship to solitary rectal ulcer syndrome/mucosal prolapse and other bowel disorders. Hum Pathol 18:1120, 1987
360. Mason EE: Gastrointestinal lesions occurring in uremia. Ann Intern Med 37:96, 1952
361. Komorowski RA, Cohen EB, Kauffman HM, Adams MB: Gastrointestinal complications in renal transplant recipients. Am J Clin Pathol 86:161–167, 1986
362. Park RW, Grand RJ: Gastrointestinal manifestations of cystic fibrosis: a review. Gastroenterology 81:1143–1161, 1981
363. Neutra MR, Trier JS: Rectal mucosa in cystic fibrosis: morphological features before and after short-term organ culture. Gastroenterology 75:701, 1978
364. Scheiman J, Elta G, Colturi T, Nostrant T: Colonic xanthomatosis. Relationship to disordered mobility and review of the literature. Dig Dis Sci 33:1491–1494, 1988
365. Rocken C, Saeger W, Linke RP: Gastrointestinal amyloid deposits in old age—report on 110 consecutive autopsical patients and 98 retrospective bioptic specimens. Pathol Res Pract 190:641–649, 1994
366. Kumar SS, Appavu SS, Abcarion H, Barreta T: Amyloidosis of the colon: report of a case and review of the literature. Dis Colon Rectum 26:541–544, 1983
367. Shousha S, Lowdell CP, Bull TB, Parkins RA: Secondary amyloidosis of the gastrointestinal tract: an electron microscopic study. Hum Pathol 16:596–601, 1985
368. Walker NI, Smith MM, Smithers BM: Ultrastructure of human melanosis coli with reference to its pathogenesis. Pathology 25:120–124, 1993
369. Ghadially FN, Walley VM: Melanoses of the gastrointestinal tract. Histopathology 25: 197–207, 1994
370. Brett EM, Lake BD: Reassessment of rectal approach to neuropathology in childhood: review of 307 biopsies over 11 years. Arch Dis Child 50:753, 1975
371. Lake BD: Storage disorders involving the alimentary tract. pp. 269–276. In Whitehead R (ed): Gastrointestinal and Oesophageal Pathology. Churchill Livingstone, New York, 1989
372. Horn T, Svendsen LB, Johansen A, Backer O: Brown bowel syndrome. Ultrastruct Pathol 8:357–361, 1985

373. Ferrans VJ, Fredrickson DS: The pathology of Tangier disease: a light and electron microscopic study. Am J Pathol 78:101, 1975
374. Rapola J, Santavuori P, Savilahti E: Suction biopsy of rectal mucosa in the diagnosis of infantile and juvenile types of neuronal ceroid lipofuscinoses. Hum Pathol 15:352–360, 1984
375. Yamano T, Shimada M, Okada S et al: Ultrastructural study of biopsy specimens of rectal mucosa. Its use in neuronal storage diseases. Arch Pathol Lab Med 106:673–677, 1982
376. Haggitt RC: Granulomatous disease of the gastrointestinal tract. pp. 257–305. *In* Ioachim HL (ed): Pathology of Granulomas. Raven Press, New York, 1983
377. Konda J, Ruth M, Sassaris M et al: Sarcoidosis of the stomach and rectum. Am J Gastroenterol 73:516, 1980
378. Tobi M, Kobrin I, Ariel I: Rectal involvement in sarcoidosis. Dis Colon Rectum 25:491–493, 1982
379. Ranchod M, Kahn LB: Malakoplakia of the gastrointestinal tract. Arch Pathol 94:90, 1972
380. Gonzalez-Angulo A, Corral E, Garcia-Torres R et al: Malakoplakia of the colon. Gastroenterology 48:383, 1965
381. Yunis EJ, Estevez JM, Pinson GJ et al: Malakoplakia: discussion of pathogenesis and report of three cases including one of fatal gastric and colonic involvemet. Arch Pathol 83:180, 1967
382. Abdou NI, NaPombejara C, Sagawa A et al: Malakoplakia: evidence for monocyte lysosomal abnormality correctable by cholinergic agonist in vitro and in vivo. N Engl J Med 297:1413, 1977
383. Robert J, Lagace R, Delage C: Malakoplakia of the colon associated with a villous adenoma. Dis Colon Rectum 17:688–671, 1974
384. Moron CA, West B, Schwartz IS: Malakoplakia of the colon in association with colonic adenocarcinoma. Am J Gastroenterol 84:1580–1582, 1989
385. Oberman HA: Idiopathic histiocytosis: a clinicopathologic study of 49 cases and review of the literature. Pediatrics 28:307–327, 1981
386. Hyams JS, Hoswell JE, Gerber MA, Berman MM: Colonic ulceration in histiocytosis X. J Pediatr Gastroenterol Nutr 4:286–289, 1985
387. Lee RG, Braziel RM, Stenzel P: Gastrointestinal involvement in Langerhans cell histiocytosis (Histiocytosis X): diagnosis by rectal biopsy. Modern Pathol 3:154–157, 1990
388. Ament ME, Ochs HD: Gastrointestinal manifestations of chronic granulomatous disease. N Engl J Med 288:382–387, 1973
389. Werlin SL, Chusid MJ, Caya J et al: Colitis in chronic granulomatous disease. Gastroenterology 82:328–331, 1982
390. Zweiban B, Cohen H, Chandrasoma P: Gastrointestinal involvement complicating Stevens-Johnson syndrome. Gastroenterology 91:469–474, 1986
391. Sidi E, Reinberg A, Spinasse JB, Hinchy M: Lethal cutaneous and gastrointestinal arteriolar thrombosis (malignant atrophying papulosis of Degos). JAMA 174:1170–1173, 1960
392. Casparie MK, Moyer JWR, Vanhuyster BJW et al: Endoscopic and histopathologic feature of Degos disease. Endoscopy 23:231–234, 1991
393. Fazio RA, Wickremesinghe PC, Arsusa EL et al: Endoscopic removal of an intussuscepted mimicking a polyp—an endoscopic hazard. Am J Gastroenterol 77:556–558, 1982
394. Jevon GP, Daya D, Qizilbash AH: Intussusception of the appendix. A report of four cases and review of the literature. Arch Pathol Lab Med 116:960–964, 1992

10

Tumors of the Colon and Rectum

GENERAL ASPECTS

Primary tumors of the colon and rectum, particularly adenocarcinoma, represent one of the largest groups of malignant neoplasms seen in both men and women.[1–3] There are estimates of 150,000 new cases per year in the United States, with expected fatality in one-third of these. It is now appreciated that many of these carcinomas are preceded by benign polyps that can readily be detected and removed at the time of endoscopy.[4, 5] Accordingly, there has been a great surge in endoscopic activity to search for and eliminate the earlier, precancerous lesions.

There also has been considerable work done in identifying patients with preneoplastic conditions of an inflammatory nature, and in defining by epidemiologic and genetic studies large populations with predispositions to colonic and rectal tumors.

Biopsy Material

Biopsy Types

The samples obtained at endoscopy are largely of two types. They include removal of polyps and mucosal biopsies of larger masses, as well as biopsies of suspicious inflammatory, ulcerative, and stricture lesions. In the case of polyps, routine attempts are made to completely excise the smaller lesions, both the sessile and pedunculated forms. Even bigger polyps are commonly removed by the ability to cause their fragmentation, especially if they have a stalk. Also performed are screening and surveillance of chronic inflammatory disorders such as ulcerative colitis, which are prone to the development of dysplasia and carcinoma.

Larger and deeper biopsies can be obtained by the use of the aspiration technique. These provide a bigger sample of the submucosa in addition to the mucosa. They are most commonly taken from the rectal area and are used to look for disorders that are preferentially located in the submucosa, such as vasculitis, amyloid deposition, and ganglionic disorders.

Cytology

Also available for the diagnosis of malignant tumors is cytologic examination.[6, 7] This has not been used as extensively in the colon and rectum as in the upper portions of the gut, presumably because of contamination from fecal material. Nevertheless, there are now methods for improving the quality of such specimens, and it is expected that this will become an important adjunct.[8–11] This may prove to be especially useful in cases with strictures that cannot readily be biopsied. Such areas can be accessed by brushes to provide cytologic specimens. More recent studies have utilized lavage preparation for the detection of dysplasia and carcinoma in patients with ulcerative colitis.[12] Also employed for tumors, especially those extending into the submucosa, is fine-needle aspiration obtained by endoscopy.[13]

The cytologic specimens are most often evaluated for evidence of abnormalities in the epithelial cells (Plates 3E–H). Enlargement of the nuclei, with elongation and overlapping and only minor alterations in chromatin distribution, serve to identify the benign neoplastic cells that are found in adenomas and in areas of dysplasia. The malignant epithelial cells show greater variation in size and shape of the nuclei, more prominent nuclear chromatin with irregular clumping, and enlarged nucleoli. Cytologic preparations may also assist in the identification of unusual tumors, such as squamous carcinoma, melanomas, and sarcomas.

Special Studies

As with most disorders in the gut, the diagnosis of the large majority of tumors can be rendered in the routine H & E sections. Multiple levels might be required to determine whether polyps are completely removed and to detect any degree of invasive tumor (Table 10-1).

Cytochemical Stains

A battery of special immunocytochemical stains is available to help in the major differentiation of epithelial, mesenchymal, and hematopoietic tumors. Most commonly employed are cytokeratins and carcinoembryonic antigen for the delineation of epithelial neoplasms, leukocyte common antigen and other more specific B-cell and T-cell markers for lymphoid tumors, and vimentin together with other stromal markers for the mesenchymal lesions.

Table 10-1. Special Studies of Colonic Tumors

Cytologic smears and brushings
Immunocytochemical stains
Electron microscopy
Flow cytometry
Oncogenes and tumor suppressor genes
Cellular growth stains

Electron Microscopy

Electromicroscopy also can be used in selected cases to help in the distinction of carcinomas from other types of tumors by the finding of prominent cell junctions; of endocrine tumors, by noting the neurosecretory granules; and of other specific features in support of metastatic tumors, such as melanoma. The primary colonic adenocarcinomas reveal prominent glands with microvilli and rootlets, and these features can serve to distinguish them from other secondary or metastatic tumors in the area[14] (Fig. 10-1).

Flow Cytometry

The flow cytometry technique has been extensively used in the study of colonic tumors and their precursors, to search for nondiploid fractions.[15–20] Alterations, including the finding of aneuploidy, are commonly seen in adenomas and carcinomas but are rarely noted in normal or simple inflammatory lesions. Accordingly, this technique can help in selected cases to provide specificity of a neoplastic lesion. As yet, they are not totally reliable in distinguishing the benign neoplastic and malignant proliferations.

Molecular Studies

There has been a recent, enormous surge in studies related to the molecular aspects of tumors of the colon and rectum.[21, 22] Both activated oncogenes and elimination of tumor suppressor genes have been identified

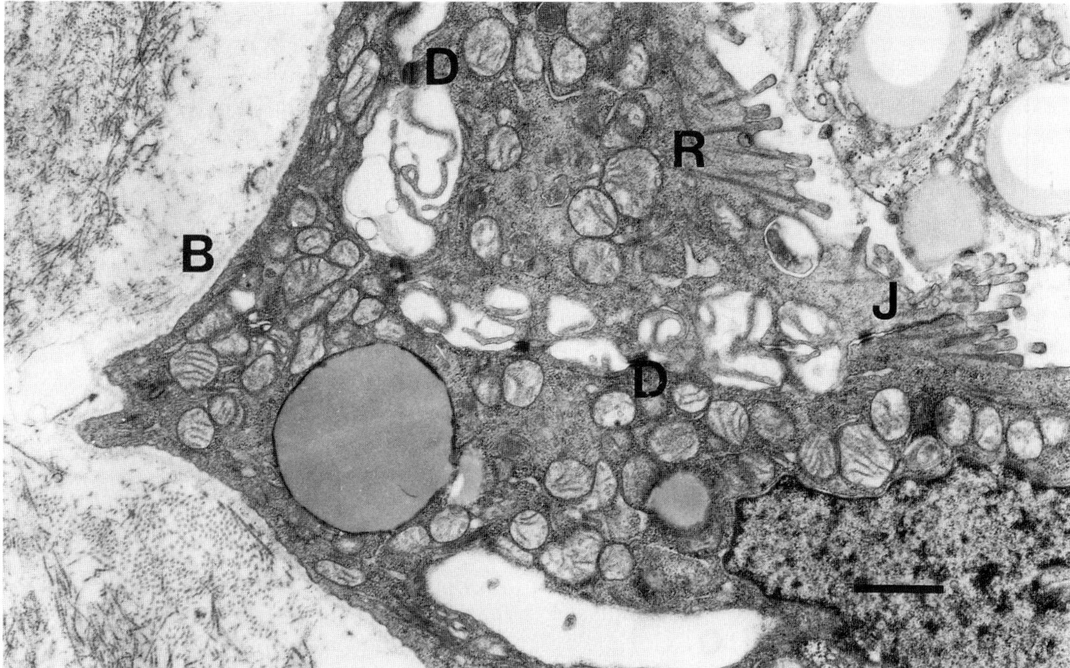

Fig. 10-1. Electron micrograph of an adenocarcinoma with characteristic features of a primary intestinal tumor. The apical luminal surface of the epithelial cells has intestinal-type microvilli with core microfilaments and rootlets (R). A junctional complex (J), desmosome (D), and basal lamina (B) are also seen ($\times$ 11,250; bar = 1 μm).

in the formation of many of the tumors, most notably in the evoluation of benign adenomas to adenocarcinomas. The familial adenomatous polyposis gene has been localized to the 5q21 area, and it is thought that this gene may also be implicated in isolated tumors.[23–25] It has been illustrated that larger adenomas with greater dysplasia frequently show alterations in the oncogenes such as the *ras* group, whereas the later transformation to carcinoma is more correlated with the loss of the normal p53 tumor suppressor gene.

Mutation and altered expression of p53 is seen in dysplasia and adenomas and is especially prominent in adenocarcinomas.[26–28] It is interesting that in the chronic inflammatory disorders that are prone to the development of carcinoma, such as ulcerative colitis, this abnormality in mutant p53 overexpression is seen at an earlier stage before the appearance of overt malignancy.

Immunocytochemical stains and other molecular techniques are now available for the identification of the various genetic alterations. Recently noted have been the finding of alterations in ras, jun, and fos oncoprotein expressions; loss of alleles in chromosomes 17p, 18q, and 22q; and other replication errors.[28–33] These are helping to define the disorders, to evaluate behavior, and to designate patients who are at increased risk for the development of polyps and carcinomas. This possibly can lead to improved selection of populations for endoscopic screening.

Other Growth Studies

Many of the colonic tumors have been studied for their growth potential and activity, utilizing Ki-67 and proliferating cell nuclear antigen (PCNA).[34–37] In general, these correlate with the more aggressive tumors at a greater stage. At the biopsy level, the stains are also being employed to try to help in the pathologic distinction between normal and inflammatory conditions versus adenomas or dysplasia, as well as in separating benign neoplasia from adenocarcinoma.[38, 39]

POLYPS

Polyps of the colon and rectum are very common and probably account for the greatest utilization of endoscopy and biopsy in the lower gut.[5] This is based on the recognition that the large majority of the colorectal carcinomas are probably preceded by an adenoma, which could be systemically sought and eliminated.[40, 41] Since polyps of the colon and rectum are so common, however, there is a need for find populations that would be at greater risk. Part of this is accomplished by identifying patients who have chronic inflammatory conditions or polyposis syndromes. It is hoped that genetic studies will ultimately identify the subsets of the population who are especially at risk for the development of adenoma and carcinoma.

Most of the polypoid lesions discussed herein primarily involve the mucosa (Table 10-2). Lesions in the bowel wall can secondarily project into the lumen, resulting in polypoid stromal tumors such as lipomas.

Inflammatory Polyps

Inflammatory polyps represent nodules of mucosa that have undergone marked inflammation and regeneration. At one time, some were designated as *pseudopolyps,* implying that the mucosa was elevated relative to an adjacent ulceration. It is now clear that the mucosa is usually expanded by the inflammatory tissue, particularly by edema, in all instances. These inflammatory polyps can occur as isolated lesions, presumably developing in areas of localized trauma or erosions. More commonly, they are seen in conjunction with a case of chronic colitis, including expecially ulcerative colitis, Crohn's disease, and ischemic colitis.[42] The polyps in these conditions can vary greatly in number from a few to a massive amount.

Table 10-2. Classification of Major Forms of Colonic Mucosal Polyps

Inflammatory polyps
Pseudopolyps in chronic colitis
Isolated
Lymphoid polyps
Juvenile (retention) polyps
Hamartomatous polyps
Peutz-Jegher
Cronkhite-Canada
Cowden
Hyperplastic (metaplastic) polyps
Neoplastic polyps (adenomas)

Gross Forms

Inflammatory polyps will differ in size, ranging from a few millimeters to giant forms.[43, 44] The highly active examples show prominent bridging of the mucosa due to associated ulceration.[45] Later lesions reveal less active inflammation but persistence of fibromuscular cores together with a papillary or filiform gross configuration.[46] It is necessary to distinguish the larger polyps from neoplasms that also can develop in such patients with chronic inflammatory disorders.

Biopsy Features

The histologic features of inflammatory polyps are variable, dependent on the degrees of activity and healing in the lesions. Potentially noted are mucosa with all features of active and chronic colitis; those mainly consisting of granulation tissue and variable fibrosis; and examples with minimal mucosal changes overlying the fibrous stalks in the larger filiform polyps (Figs. 10-2 and 10-3). Areas with very cellular vascular and fibrous tissue formation resembling stromal neoplasms can be seen.[47] In the actively inflamed areas, there can develop considerable regeneration with marked clustering of glands and piling up of nuclei, and these must

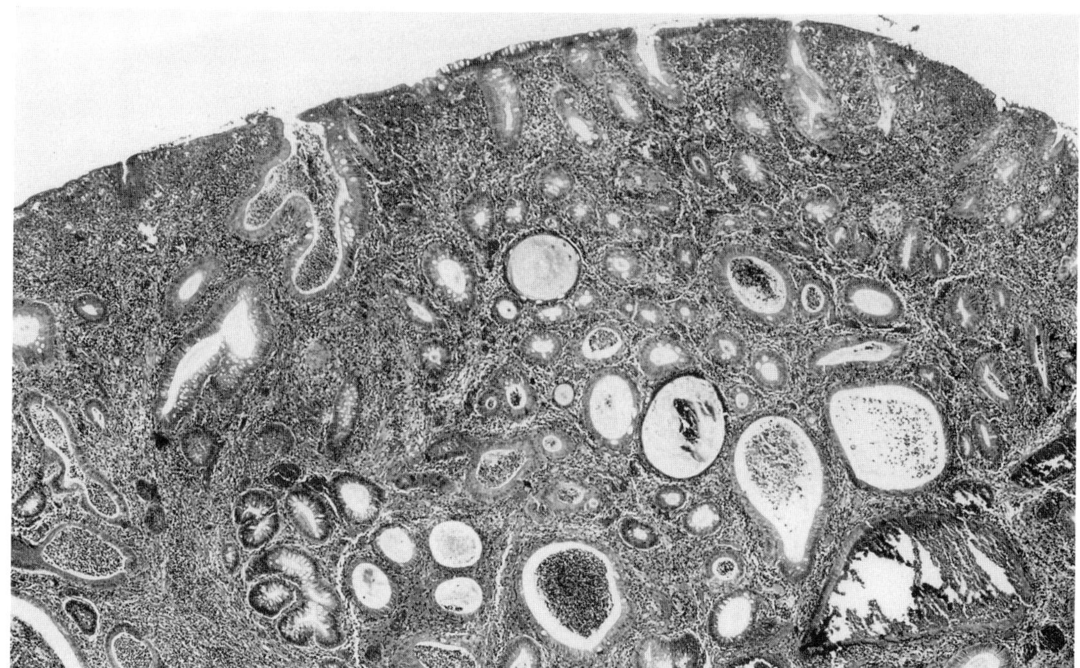

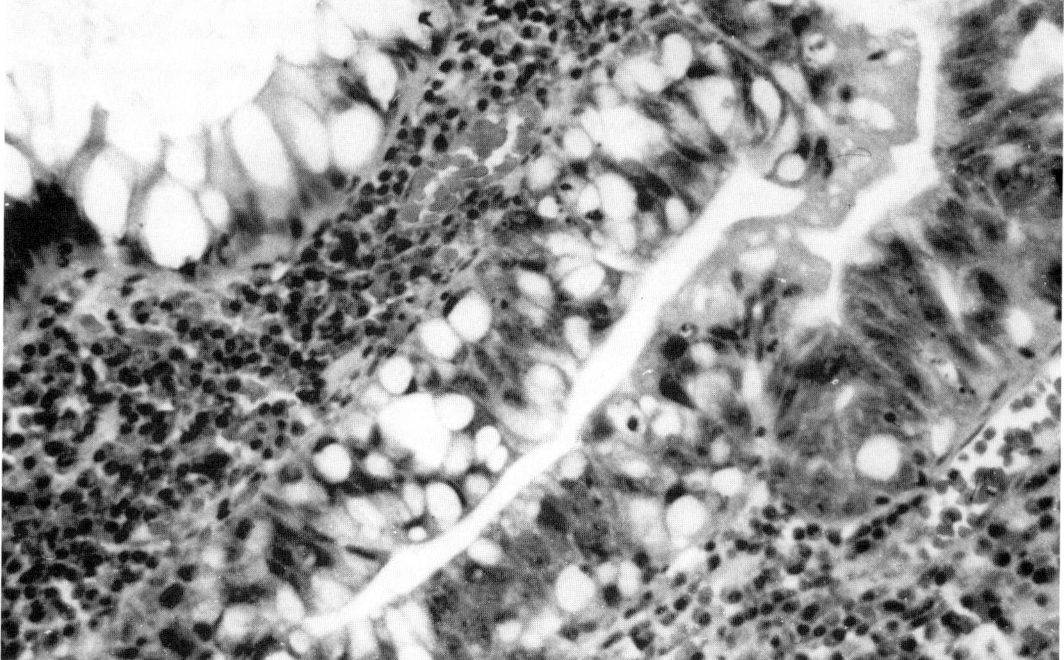

Fig. 10-2. Inflammatory polyp of the colon. **(A)** The polyp is composed of glands with variable cystic change and prominent inflammatory tissue in the stroma. Numerous crypt abscesses are present, and there is no epithelial dysplasia (× 42). **(B)** Focal area of gland with marked cellular proliferation and irregular goblet mucous cells. Such areas must be distinguished from epithelial dysplasia. Portion of normal crypt appears at upper left.

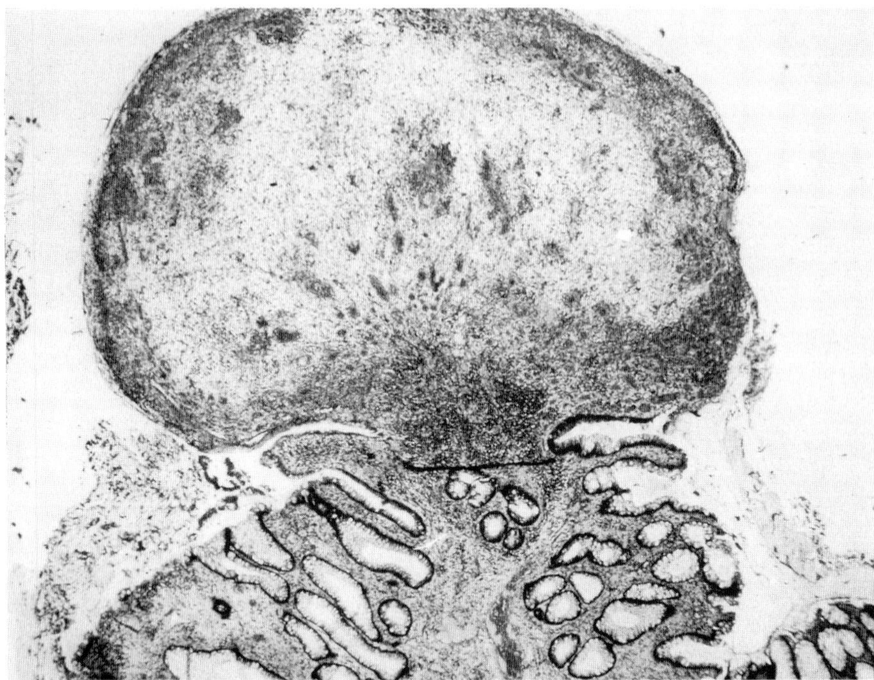

Fig. 10-3. Polypoid nodule of granulation tissue in the rectum. Attached to the mucosa is a mass of granulation tissue. The adjacent mucosa is mildly inflamed.

be distinguished from true dysplasia (Fig. 10-2B). Absent are significant hyperchromasia and abnormal mitoses. Furthermore, polypoid areas of dysplasia typically show more diffuse lesions together with less inflamed stroma.

Juvenile Polyp

The juvenile polyp is considered to be a hamartomatous lesion of the mucosa associated with irregular proliferation of cystic glands and a large quantity of edematous and inflamed stroma.[48] The lesions are most often seen in young children, hence its name, and usually present as a single or a few lesions, which bleed and may recur. They are less commonly noted in older persons and have also been called *retention,* or *hamartomatous polyps.* The diagnosis is secured by removal and examination of the polyp.

Most patients have no problems after the development of one or a few polyps.[49] There are uncommon syndromes associated with a larger number of juvenile polyps that affect the colon alone or the entire gastrointestinal tract, and these are discussed below in the section on "Juvenile Polyposis."

Gross and Biopsy Features

The smaller lesions are sessile and the larger typically have a short stalk. Their surface is smooth in contrast to the convulated and papillary arrangement of adenomas. Histologic features are largely nonspecific and very similar to those seen in inflammatory polyps. There is a mixture of normal, inflamed, and regenerative glands, the latter most often noted near surface erosions (Fig. 10-4). As the lesions enlarge there typically develops a twisting of the stalk and ulcer-

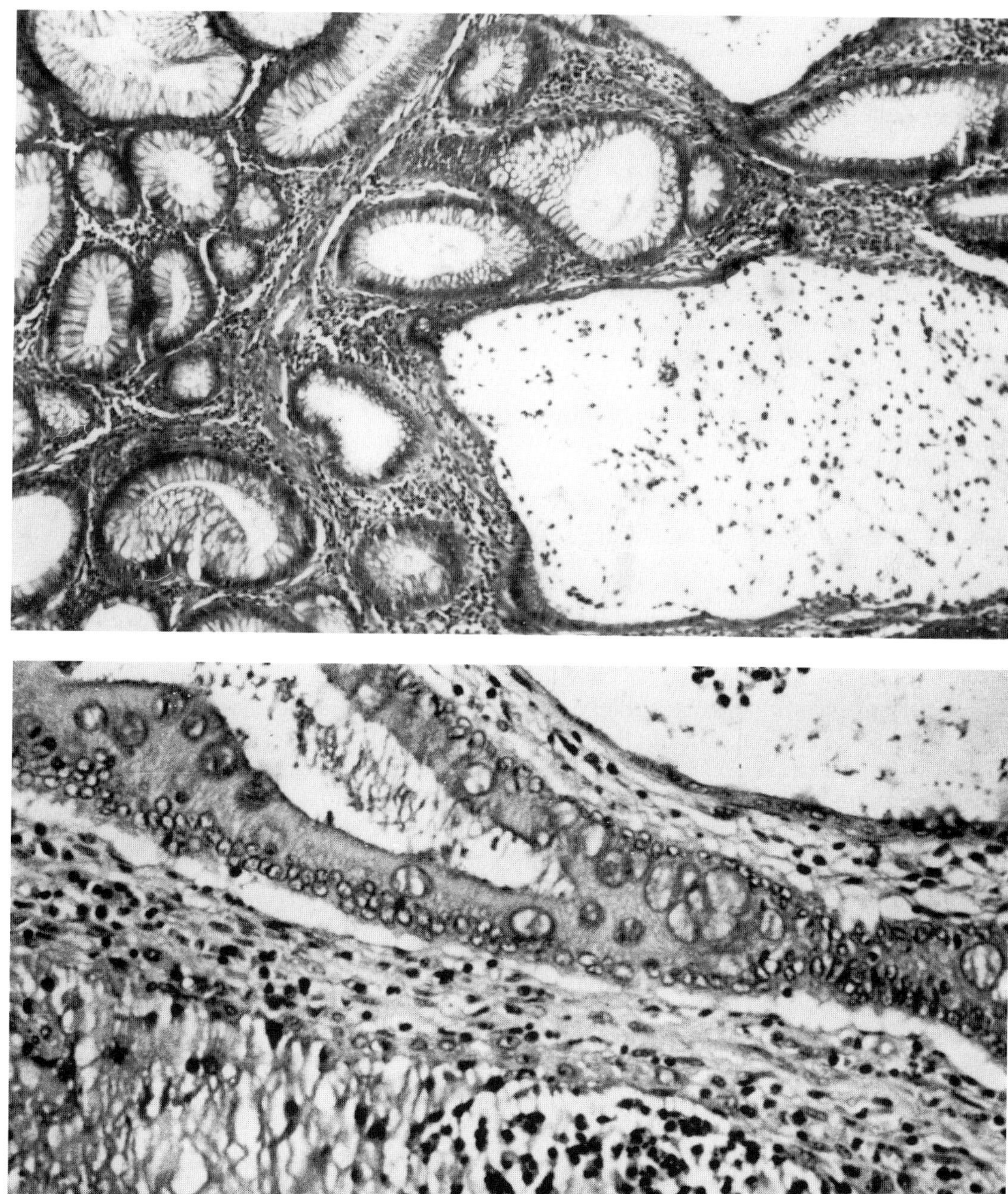

Fig. 10-4. Juvenile (retention) polyp of the colon. **(A)** Noted are mature glands with prominent cystic change and variable amounts of inflammation. There is no epithelial dysplasia. **(B)** Part of polyp near a surface erosion, showing greater inflammation (bottom) and regenerative glands.

ation of the surface, which accounts for the bleeding. The histologic features of such areas reveal mucosal necrosis together with variable amounts of granulation tissue.

Hyperplastic Polyps

Hyperplastic polyps are the most common polyps encountered in the large intestine and have also been called *metaplastic polyps.*[50–53] There are typically no symptoms, and the polyps are noted as incidental findings at the time of endoscopy or examination of surgical specimens. There have been a few reports of cases with multiple hyperplastic polyps that suggest a polyposis syndrome, but this has not been completely accepted.[54]

Gross and Biopsy Features

Practically all of the lesions are less than 1 cm in diameter, with most less than 5 mm. They are sessile and have a smooth surface. The histologic features are characteristic, revealing prominent papillary infoldings of the epithelial cells in the crypts, which present a serrated appearance (Fig. 10-5). Nuclei remain small and basal, and there is highly variable mucus production but it is usually preserved. The polyps are thought to develop as a result of an incomplete maturation or differentiation of the epithelial cells, leading to their persistence rather than loss from the surface.[55]

Inverted Polyp

Occasionally noted is extension of the basal portion of the crypts through the muscularis mucosae into the upper part of the submucosa.[56, 57] This may be particularly prominent and lead to the appearance of an inverted polyp, with most of the glandular proliferation noted in the bottom of the mucosa and in the upper portion of the submucosa. The hyperplastic nature is appreciated by the serrated appearance of the glands, and it can be readily distinguished from invasive carcinoma by the total lack of any dysplasia in the epithelial cells.

Mixed Polyp

Occasionally seen are larger polyps with a prominent papillary or serrated appearance that also show typical nuclear features of dysplasia in the form of elongation, palisading, and variable hyperchromasia[51, 58, 59] (Fig. 10-6). Such lesions have been termed *serrated adenomas* or *mixed hyperplastic polyp and adenoma,* and they have the potential for malignant transformation like other adenomas.[60, 61]

In biopsies that reveal hyperplastic polyps, it is important to correlate this with the size of the lesions. If a polyp is thought to be larger than 1 cm, the finding in a biopsy of a hyperplastic area should not be regarded as absolute evidence that it is typical of the entire lesion. Rather, the whole lesion must be removed to exclude the possibility of a serrated adenoma or of a carcinoma next to a small area of hyperplasia.

Other Non-Neoplastic Polyps

Various other non-neoplastic polyps that occur in the colonic mucosa are listed in Table 10-3 and are discussed below.

Inflammatory Fibroid Polyps

Inflammatory fibroid polyps are more commonly noted in the stomach and ileum but can occur in the colon.[62, 63] They appear as single, usually large lesions with markedly edematous stroma that contains many spindle cells and variable amounts of inflammatory cells, frequently with many eosinophils (Fig. 10-7). The lesions are thought to de-

A

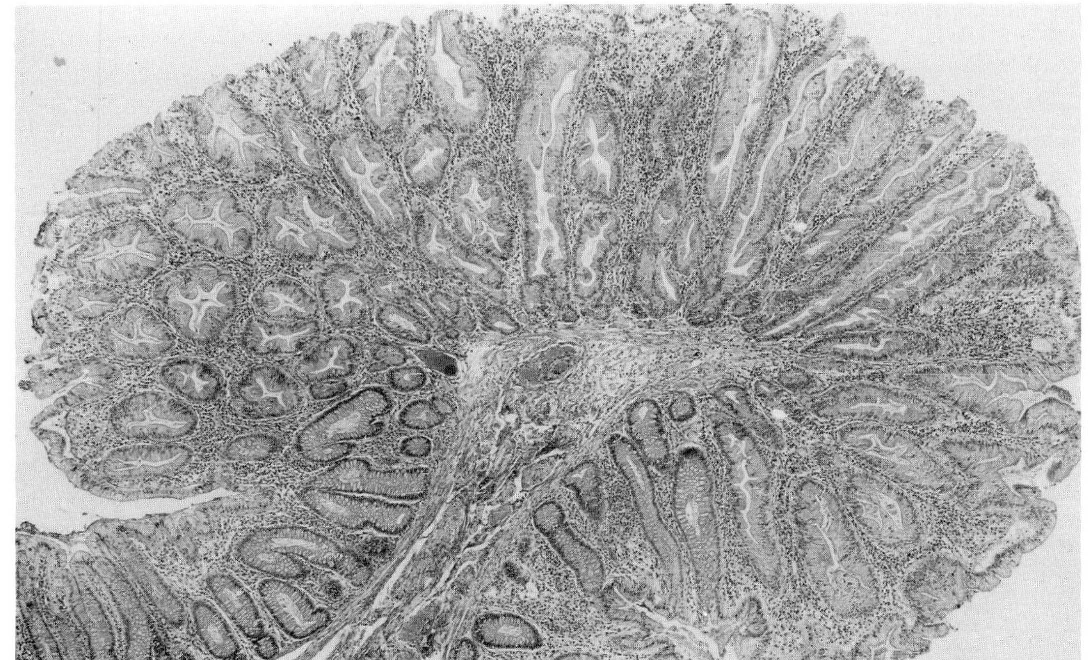

B

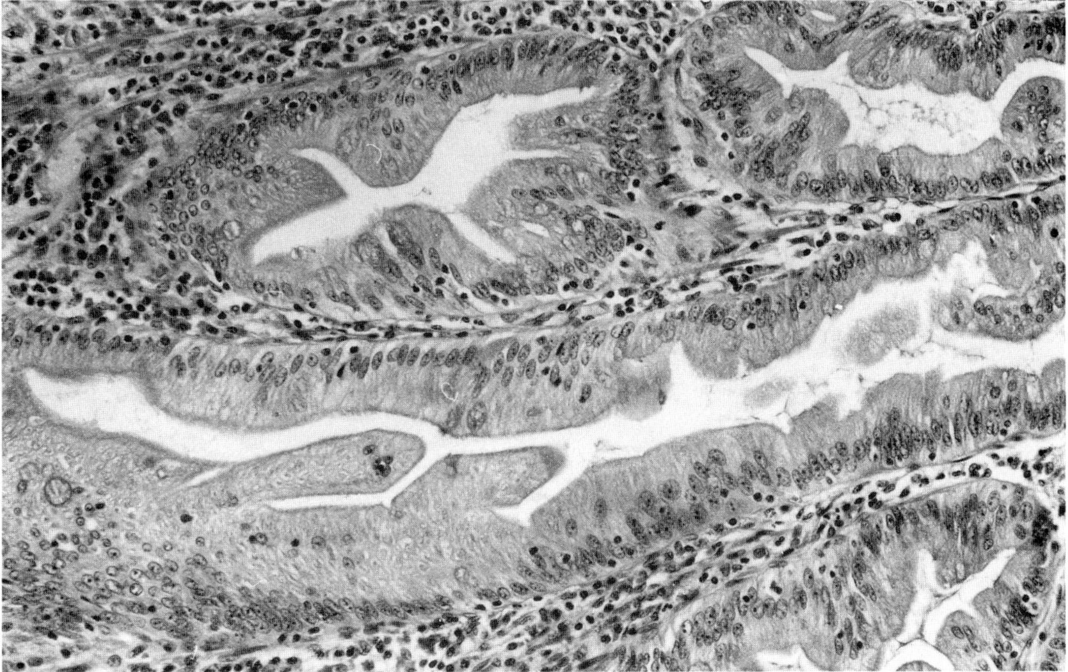

Fig. 10-5. Hyperplastic polyp of the colon. **(A)** The polyp is composed of elongated crypts with prominent papillary infoldings of the epithelial cells. There is no cystic change and relatively little inflammation (× 42). **(B)** Closer view of the hyperplastic crypts, showing the serrated appearance. The epithelial nuclei are mainly basal and lack the features of dysplasia. Cytoplasmic mucin is reduced in this example but can be prominent in other cases (× 210).

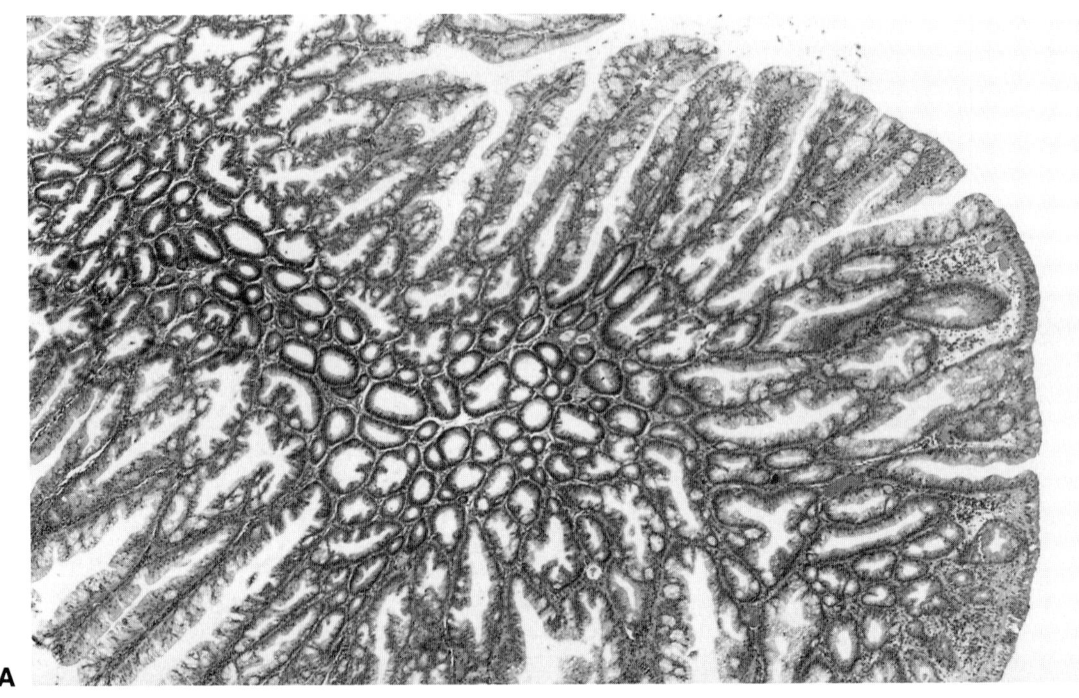

A

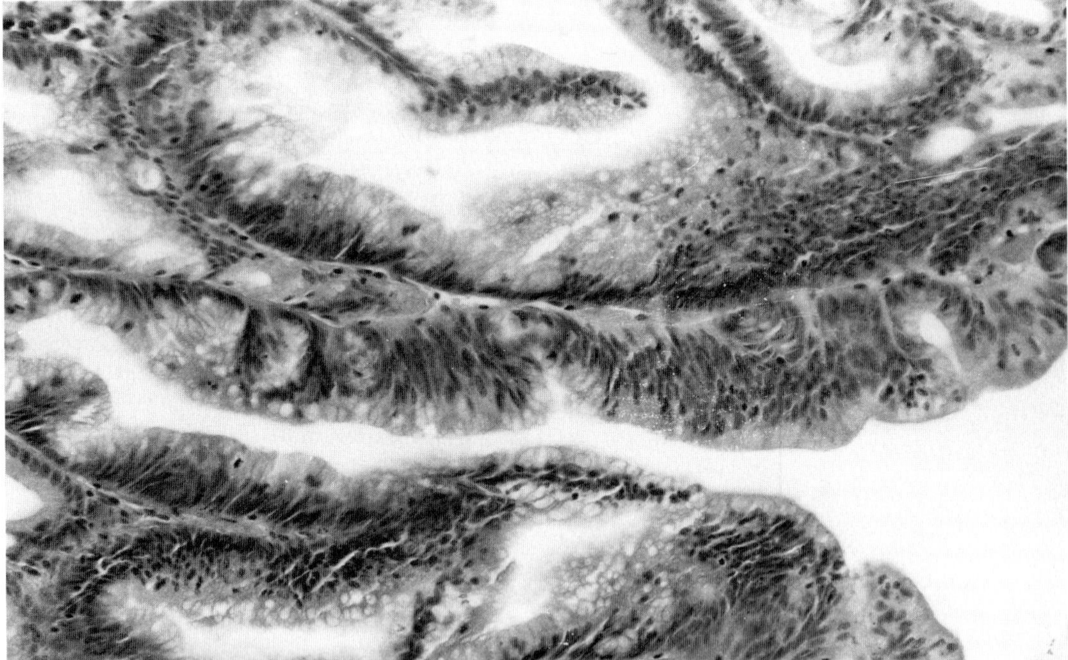

B

Fig. 10-6. Serrated adenoma of the colon. **(A)** Compared to the hyperplastic polyp (Fig. 10-5A), this polyp also shows elongated crypts with characteristic papillary infoldings, but the lesions are typically much larger (× 42). **(B)** The adenomatous nature is based on the finding of the dysplastic nuclei, showing elongation and palisading (× 210). Compare with Figure 10-5B.

Table 10-3. Miscellaneous Polyps in the Colonic Mucosa

Inflammatory fibroid polyp
Inflammatory myoglandular polyp
Non-glandular polyps
Benign lymphoid polyp
Polypoid carcinoid tumor
Mucosal neuroma and ganglioneuroma
Vascular and inflammatory lesions
Polyp due to cholesterol embolus
Mucosal bridge due to drugs
Chronic infections
Tumorlike nodules
Polyp in solitary ulcer syndrome
Endometriosis
Pneumatosis
Mechanical lesions
Intussuception of appendix
Edge or prolapse of diverticulum
Retained stalk after a polypectomy

velop from protrusion of stromal lesions into the luminal area. Biopsies show the inflamed edematous stroma that would be compatible with any inflammatory-type polyp.

Inflammatory Myoglandular Polyps

Recently described is a polyp that is characterized by a prominent admixture of smooth muscle and glandular elements together with inflammatory tissue.[64] The epithelium shows no dysplasia. This may represent a variant of a juvenile or other inflammatory polyp.

Non-Glandular Polyps

Polyps of the colon can also be seen in association with growths of other mucosal elements. Examples are lymphoid polyps due to hyperplasia[65, 66]; nodules of endocrine cells that represent small polypoid carcinoid tumors[67]; and proliferation of ganglia and nerves that can occur in the multiple endocrine neoplasia syndromes, termed *ganglioneuromatosis* or *mucosal neuromas.*[68] These

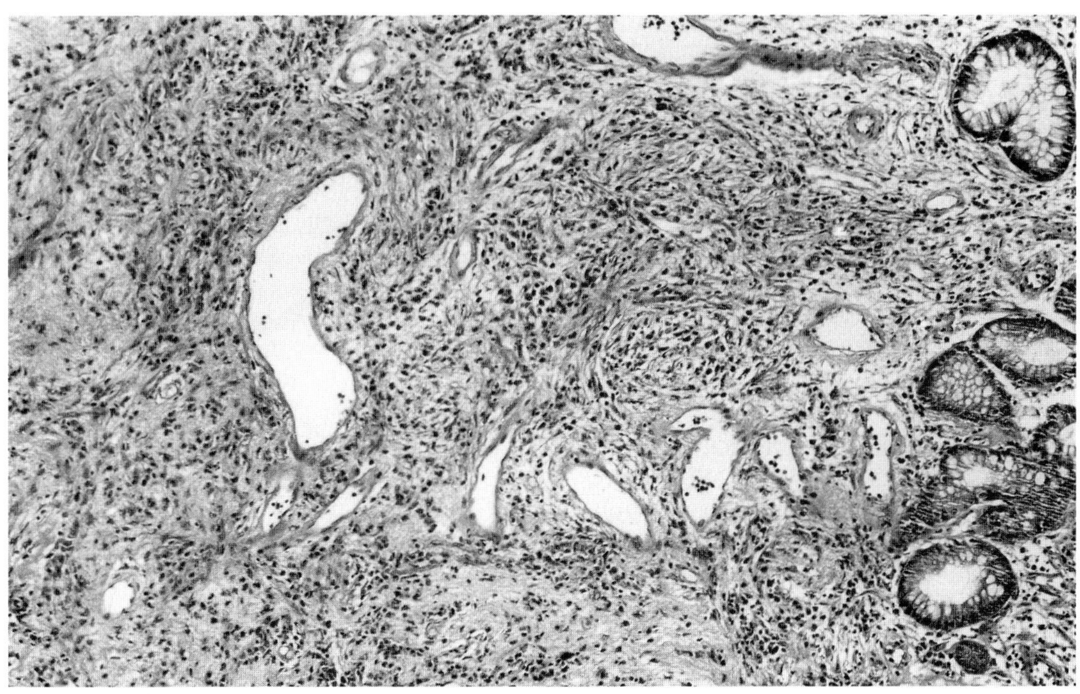

Fig. 10-7. Inflammatory fibroid polyp of the colon. The polyp consists of spindle-shaped cells, variable edema, and prominent inflammation, including many eosinophils. Some colonic crypts appear at the right (× 105). See Figure 8-11 for another example in the ileum.

are discussed below in the section on "Other Tumors."

Miscellaneous Polyps

Projections from the mucosal surface that stimulate inflammatory polyps can be caused by many other conditions, including excess inflammation in areas of ischemic damage secondary to atherosclerotic emboli[69, 70]; mucosal bridges that rarely develop following the ingestion of NSAID[71]; polypoid regions of colitis cystica profunda[72]; and nodular lesions of endometriosis and raised areas of pneumatosis.[73, 74] Mucosal polyps may also be due to intussusception of portions of the appendix into the cecum,[75,76] the edge or prolapse of diverticula into the colonic lumen,[77–79] and the persistence of a large stalk from a polyp that was previously removed.[80] (All of these conditions are described in Ch. 9.).

In addition, inflammatory-type polyps may be encountered in chronic infections such as schistosomiasis,[81] and are regularly seen in the solitary ulcer and mucosal prolapse syndromes [82–84] (cf. Fig. 9-43). The latter can be associated with exceptionally large polyps termed *inflammatory cloacogenic polyps.*[85–87] The polyps in the ulcer syndrome have a characteristic appearance, showing serrated-type glands and a prominent fibromuscular stroma. (See Ch. 9 for further details.)

Adenomas

Adenomas are the most important polyps in the colon and rectum because they are considered to be the major precursor of adenocarcinoma in this area.[88–90] The adenomas are present in about one-quarter of adult patients, and they may be single or multiple. The polyps vary greatly in size, probably dependent on their age; they begin as small sessile lesions, and most develop a stalk as they enlarge.

Morphologic Types

Overall, the adenomas have been divided into the categories of *tubular type,* formerly called adenomatous polyp, based on a relatively smooth or convoluted surface together with elongated glands extending into the polyp; and *villous type,* which is associated with a papillary surface covering at least one-half of the lesion and corresponding to elongated villous-like structures on histology[40, 41] (Table 10-4) and Fig. 10-8. Actually, there appears to be a full morphologic spectrum ranging from tubular, to *mixed* (or *tubulovillous*), to *villous* adenomas, with a rough correlation to size of the lesions.[91, 92]

Biopsy Features

The adenoma is ultimately defined by the histologic presence of benign neoplastic or dysplastic epithelium lining the glands[1, 3, 90, 93] (Fig. 10-9). This may be of a relatively low grade or mild degree in the form of elongated and slightly pallisading nuclei, filling only a portion of the cell, and showing no hyperchromasia. These cells usually show good

Table 10-4. Characteristic of Colonic Adenoma

Types
Tubular
Mixed
Villous
Grades
Low- and high-grade dysplasia
Carcinoma
In-situ
Intramucosal
Invasive
Other elements
Endocrine and Paneth cells
Squamous and osseous metaplasia
Variants
Serrated adenoma
Flat adenoma

mucin production. More marked degrees of dysplasia, termed high grade, reveal greater nuclear palisading and irregularity, more occupation of the total cell together with less mucin production, and variable hyperchromasia and loss of polarity of the cells. There is probably a full range of dysplastic features ranging from the low grade to high grade. Previous studies had tried to separate these into more categories, such as mild, moderate, and severe, but this has no special utility.

Frequently seen in adenomas are other elements, including an increase in endocrine cells and the appearance of Paneth cells[94–96] (Fig. 10-9C). These are also seen in carcinomas, and are not associated with any functional activity. Less common are foci of squamous metaplasia, and rarely noted are areas of osseous metaplasia.[97, 98] These probably reflect signs of chronic irritation and do not impart any special significance to the adenomas. The features are not unique to adenomas and can be seen in other polyps. In particular, Paneth cells are often noted in hamartomatous polyps, and their presence in a polypoid lesion should not exclude the possibility of a neoplasm. Adenomas also may contain variable amounts of smooth muscle; these are typically in fine strands in contrast to the broad bands noted in hamartomatous polyps.[99]

Shortly after biopsies of an adenoma, there may be misplacement of the benign glands into the upper regions of the submucosa.[100] This is recognized by either a lack of any greater dysplasia in the epithelial cells or of the appearance of a desmoplastic stroma, which help to distinguish the adenoma from invasive carcinoma. Rarely observed is the presence of a well differentiated squamous cell carcinoma that is intimately related to a large adenoma.[101] It is supposed that this might develop from areas of squamous metaplasia, but precise documentation is lacking. Also reported is the rare presence of malakoplakia in close association with a colonic adenoma[102] (see Fig. 9-51).

Associated Carcinoma

Once a polyp is identified to be an adenoma, it may be of interest to determine whether it is tubular, mixed, or villous, and to indicate the range of dysplasia; but it is most important to look for associated carcinoma. This is an area that has been extensively investigated, and it has been suggested that the carcinoma can appear in three stages within a polyp: *in-situ carcinoma, intramucosal carcinoma,* and *invasive carcinoma.*[103–105] The in-situ carcinoma is represented by highly dysplastic glands together with a cribiform arrangement, but no transgression by the cells through the basement membrane into the lamina propria (Fig. 10-10). Since such cases are never associated with metastatic disease, many investigators prefer to term such lesions as simply the end of the spectrum of high-grade dysplasia rather than using the term carcinoma.

Cases of intramucosal carcinoma show greater irregularity of glands together with apparent invasion of the lamina propria, but no extension into the muscularis mucosae or submucosa (Fig. 10-11). Again, there appears to be very little chance of deeper spread or metastases, since the colonic mucosa ordinarily lacks lymphatics.[106] It is probably still important to identify this lesion so that additional sections may be sought to look for more significant invasion.

Finally, the term invasive carcinoma is used when there is a definite extension of the carcinoma into and through the muscularis mucosae, showing tumor in the submucosa or stalk region (Fig. 10-12).

The presence of infiltrative or invasive carcinoma is typically associated with a tumor type of stroma that consists of loose mesenchymal tissue with variable inflammation and fibrosis. The submucosal tissue is best identified by noting structures that are peculiar to this area, particularly large amounts of adipose tissue, nerves, lymphatics, and medium-sized blood vessels. Invasive carcinoma in the submucosa or stalk of a polyp

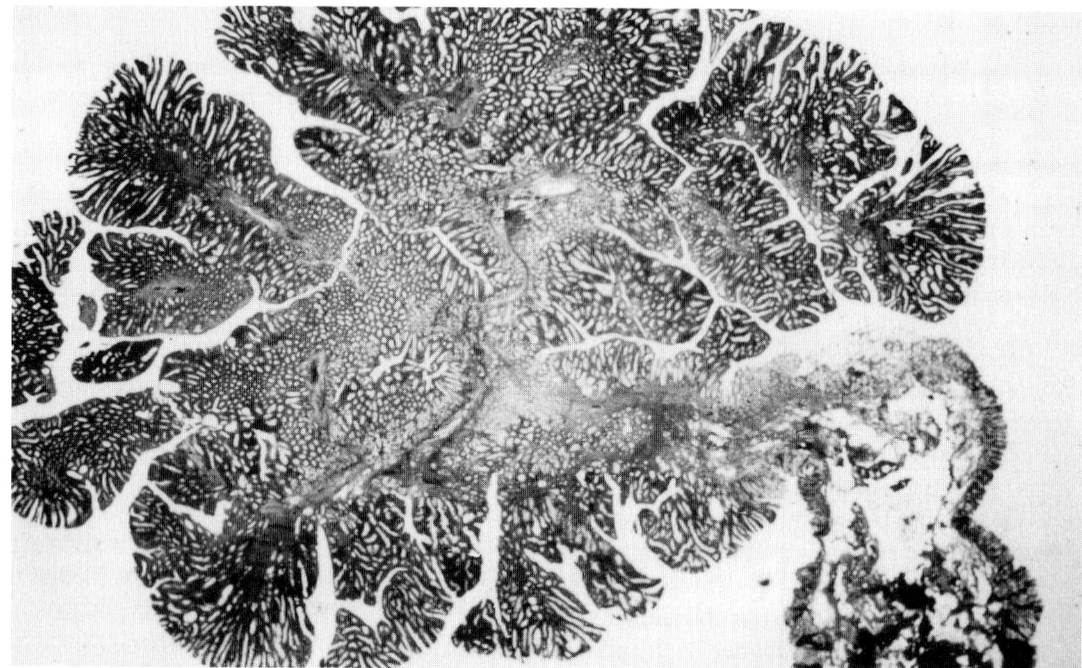

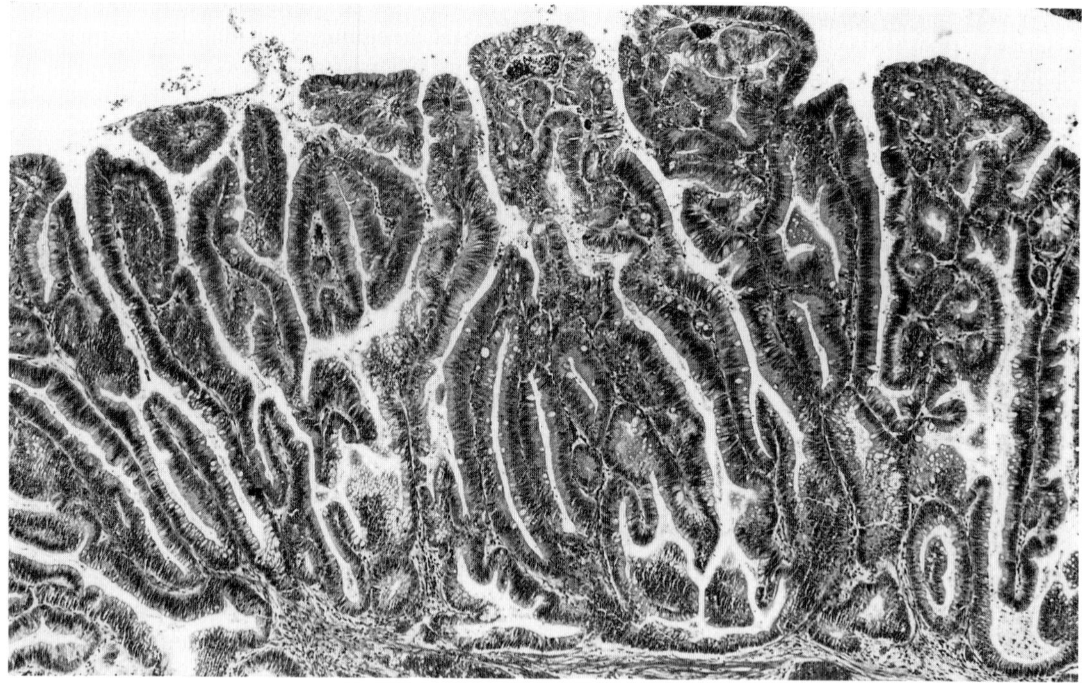

Fig. 10-8. Adenoma of the colon. Examples of the major morphologic forms are shown. **(A)** Adenoma with stalk, predominantly tubular. The surface of the adenoma is lobulated, and the stalk appearing at the lower right is covered by normal mucosa. **(B)** Sessile adenoma, mainly villous. The polyp is composed of fine fronds, imparting a papillary configuration (× 56). *(Figure continues.)*

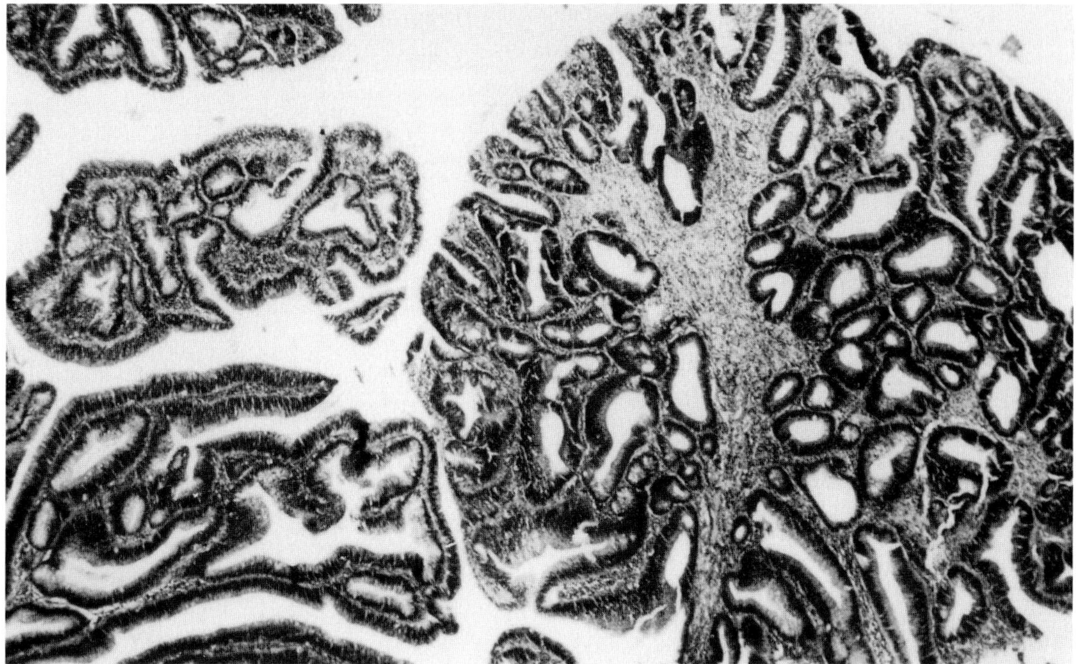

Fig. 10-8 *(Continued).* **(C)** Tubulovillous adenoma. Noted on the surface are distinct areas of villous shape (left) and tubular shape (right). Many adenomas larger than 1 cm are of this type.

must be distinguished from misplacement of benign epithelium[107–110] (Table 10-5). The latter is more often seen in large adenomas and is thought to be due to a twisting of the polyp with breakdown of the underlying muscularis mucosa and extension of the adenoma into the submucosa (Fig. 10-13). Such areas of misplaced epithelium are distinguished from carcinoma by noting that the epithelial cells show the same degree of dysplasia throughout the adenoma, and that the stroma still resembles the components of the lamina propria. In addition, there is often a prominent degree of hemosiderin surrounding such lesions.

Serrated Adenoma

A variant of the adenoma is the serrated adenoma, or mixed hyperplastic polyp-adenoma.[58, 59] These are lesions that have crypts with prominent papillary infoldings of the epithelial cells resembling hyperplastic polyps, but with the typical dysplastic epithelium of adenomas (Fig. 10-6). They are also larger and more papillary in appearance. It is not completely established whether they arise from the conversion of a hyperplastic polyp into an adenoma or simply have shared features. Nevertheless, they behave like adenomas, including having the propensity for carcinoma.[58, 60] It has been estimated that they represent just a few percent of all of the adenomas. The importance in biopsies is that the investigator not be fooled by the serrated appearance, which suggests a hyperplastic polyp, but to provide the exact diagnosis based on the nuclear characteristics of an adenoma.

Flat Adenoma

A minority of the colonic adenomas remain relatively flat as they enlarge, and may develop a central depression.[111–113] It has

A

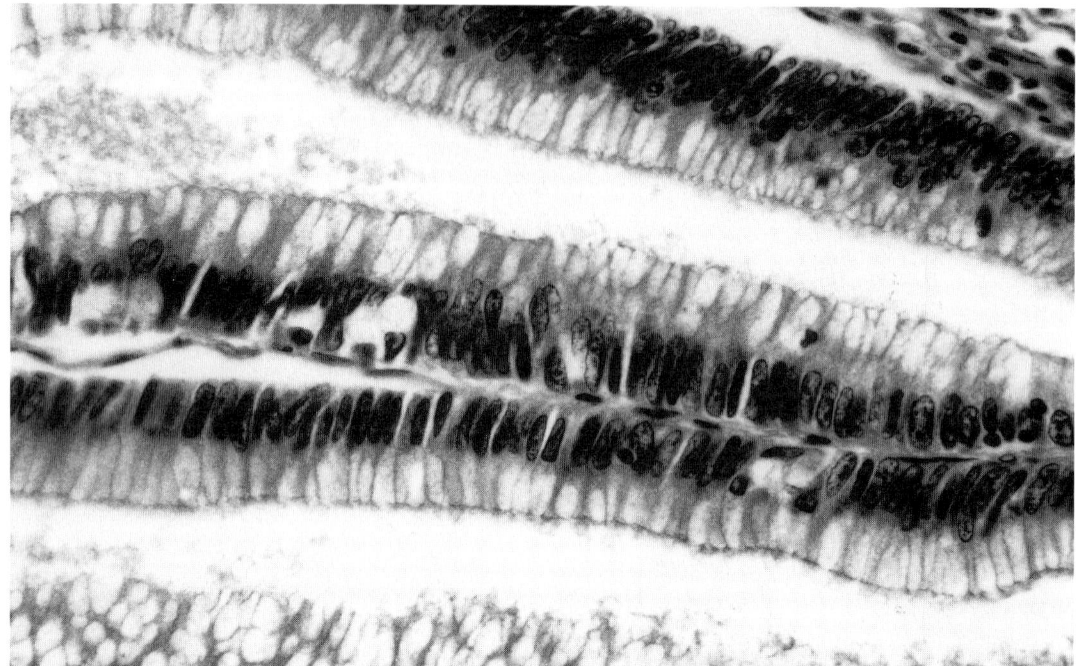

B

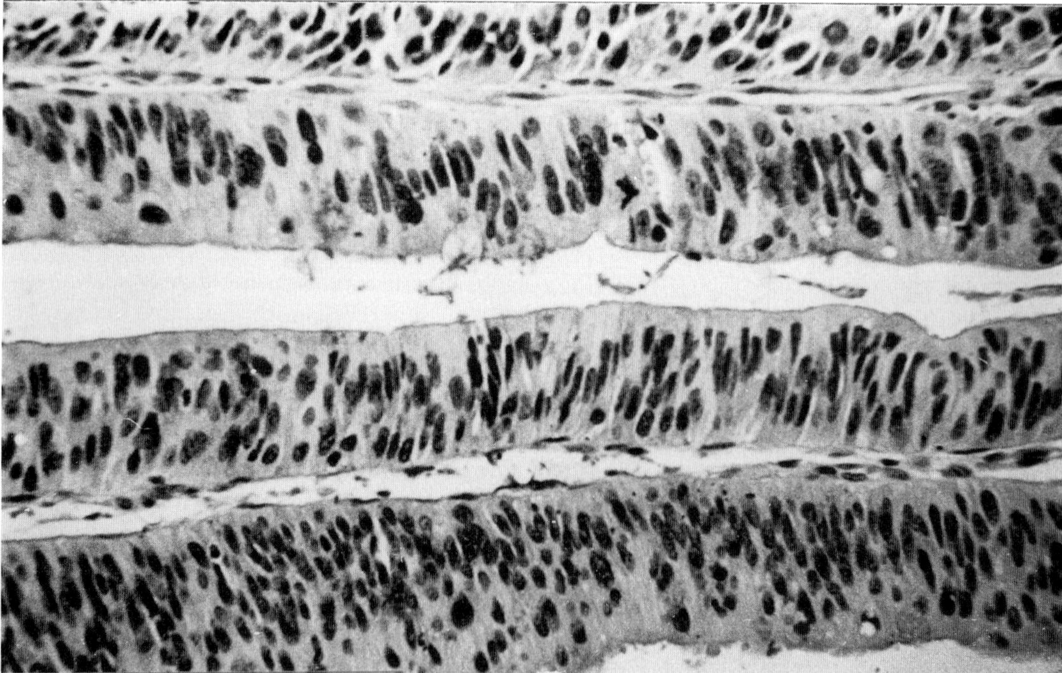

Fig. 10-9. Adenoma of the colon, showing histologic features. **(A)** Adenoma with low-grade dysplasia. Shown are two crypts with relatively slight nuclear alterations. There is nuclear elongation limited to the basal half of the cells and no hyperchromasia (× 425). **(B)** Adenoma with high-grade dysplasia. There is marked variation in the size and shape of the epithelial nuclei, and they are present throughout the cell length. *(Figure continues.)*

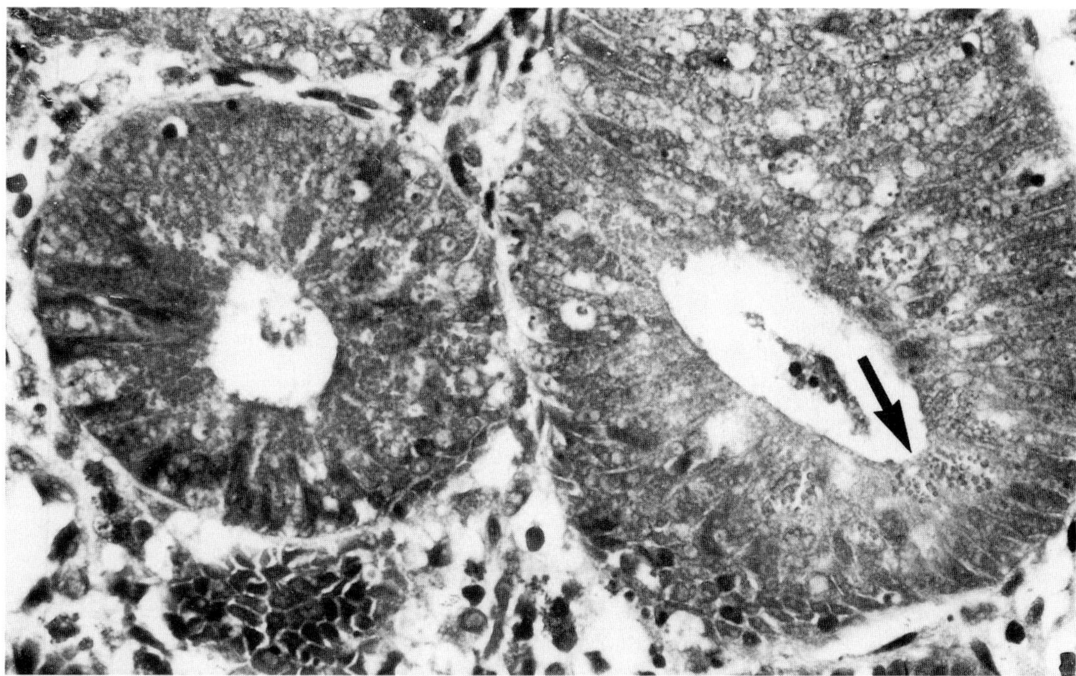

Fig. 10-9 *(Continued).* **(C)** Paneth cells in an adenoma. Shown are two adenomatous glands that contain abundant Paneth cell granules (arrow). The granules are large, highly refractile, and are located in the cytoplasm next to the glandular lumen (× 635).

been suggested that these lesions may be particularly aggressive and undergo malignant change at a more rapid pace. There are hereditary disorders associated with an increase in the appearance of flat adenomas, these either limited to the large intestine or associated with similar lesions in the stomach and duodenum.

Management of Polyps

Both sigmoidoscopy and colonoscopy are commonly employed for the detection and removal of polyps, and it is most important to distinguish the adenoma from the other non-neoplastic lesions.[114] The latter are largely separated by their histologic features or history and are typically not related to carcinoma, with the exception of the uncommon polyposis syndromes. In contrast, once an adenoma is identified, evidence is sought of carcinoma and, particularly, invasive tumor extending into the stalk or submucosa of a sessile lesion[115–123] (Fig. 10-14). Additional data regarding the carcinoma are its degree of differentiation, and whether there is evidence of any extension into vascular spaces in the stalk region. Based on many studies, it is felt that total polypectomy by endoscopy is sufficient not only for pure adenomas but also for those that contain carcinoma, provided the tumor is well or moderately differentiated, does not extend into vascular spaces, and may invade the stalk but has not reached the cauterized margin of excision (Table 10-6).

Conversely, because of the greater potential for residual carcinoma and its spread, colectomy is more commonly recommended for polypoid adenomas having carcinoma that is either poorly differentiated, shows apparent invasion of lymphatics or blood vessels, or extends to the stalk base. In addition,

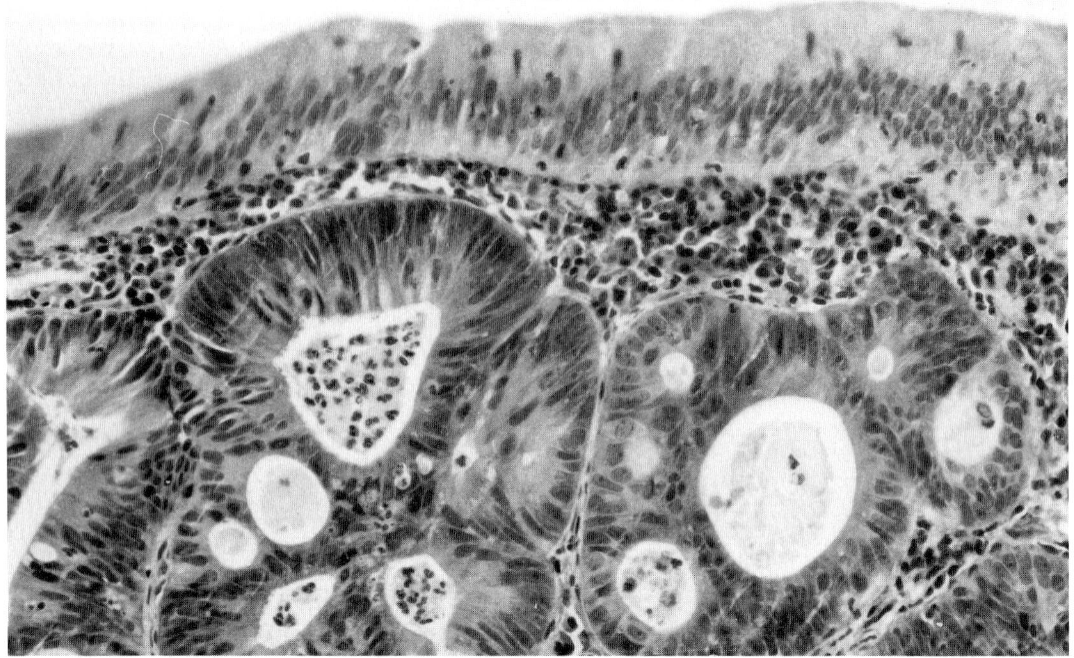

Fig. 10-10. Adenoma of the colon with carcinoma in-situ. Noted are glands with marked nuclear dysplasia and a prominent cribiform arrangement. The glands still have intact basement membranes and are surrounded by lamina propria, signifying that there is no invasion. Many prefer to designate this lesion as the upper limit of high-grade dysplasia (× 340).

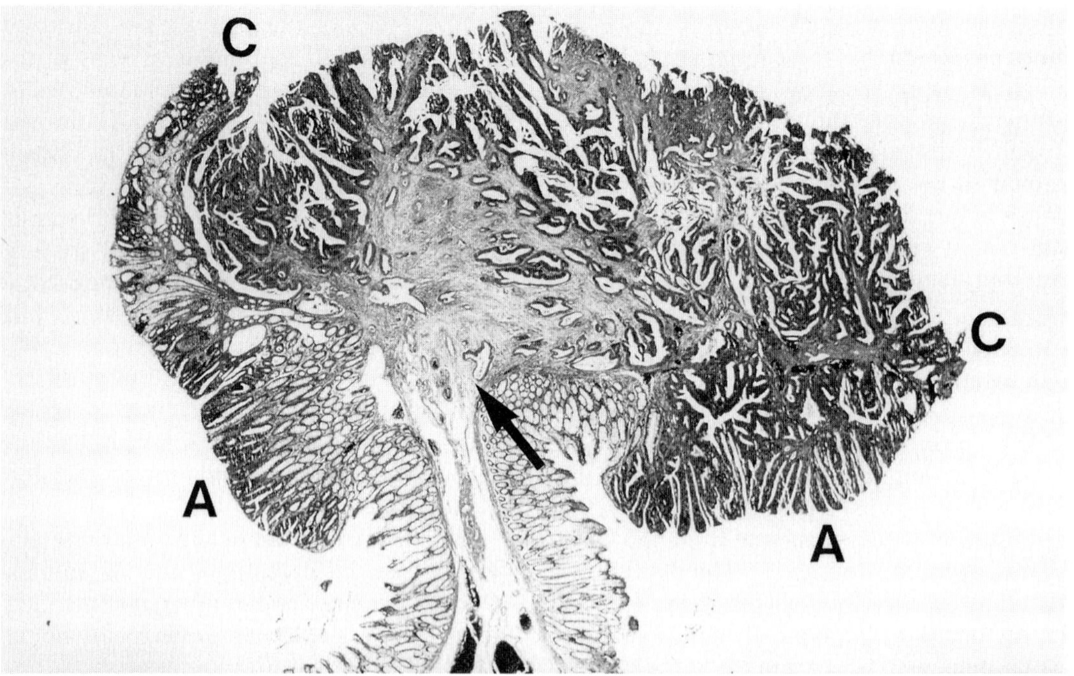

Fig. 10-11. Adenoma of the colon with adenocarcinoma. Shown is a stalked adenoma (A) with an area of adenocarcinoma (C) that is predominantly in the head of the polyp. The carcinoma extends into the lamina propria (mainly intramucosal) but also invades the submucosa in the upper part of the stalk (arrow). The rest of the stalk is free of tumor and is covered by normal colonic mucosa. Such lesions are ordinarily treated by polypectomy (see text) (× 105).

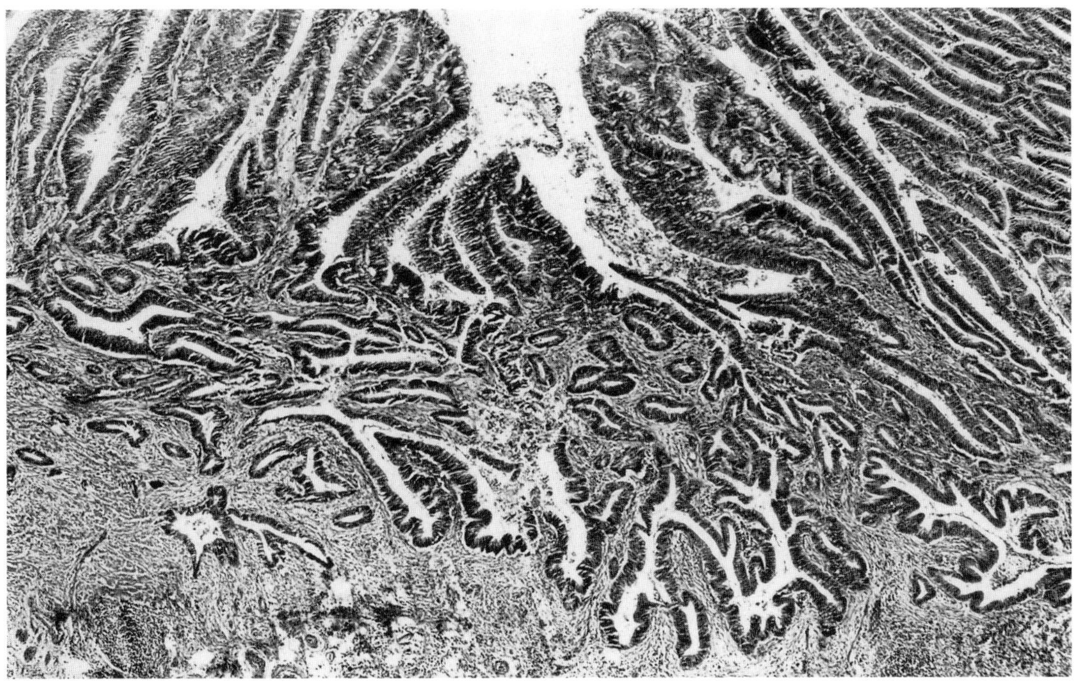

Fig. 10-12. Adenoma of the colon with invasive adenocarcinoma. This is a sessile villous adenoma (upper left and upper right), with a central area of invasive adenocarcinoma. The tumor extends into the submucosa (bottom). These tumors usually require a colectomy (see text) (× 440).

because of the inability to totally judge the degree of invasion, probably all sessile adenomas containing invasive carcinoma need a resection.

Polyposis Syndromes

A variety of syndromes, largely hereditary, are associated with the development of multiple polyps in the colon and rectum[40, 41, 124, 125] (Table 10-7). These vary in their nature and in association with carcinoma. Accordingly, it is most important that biopsies be obtained to provide specific diagnoses that will help in decisions on therapy regarding the entire colon. Only the cases of adenomatous polyposis and its variants are associated with a great increase of carcinoma development that requires prophylactic colectomy. The other syndromes show more variable development of carcinoma and can usually be managed more conservatively in the initial stages.

Adenomatous Polyposis Coli

Adenomatous polyposis coli is a hereditary syndrome in which massive numbers of adenomas begin to develop in the mid-teen

Table 10-5. Misplaced Epithelium versus Invasive Carcinoma

Feature	Misplaced	Carcinoma
Degree of dysplasia	Same as rest of adenoma	Often of higher degree
Stroma	Lamina propria	Loose mesenchyme
Edge of tissue in submucosa	Rounded	Irregular
Hemosiderin	Prominent	Sparse or absent

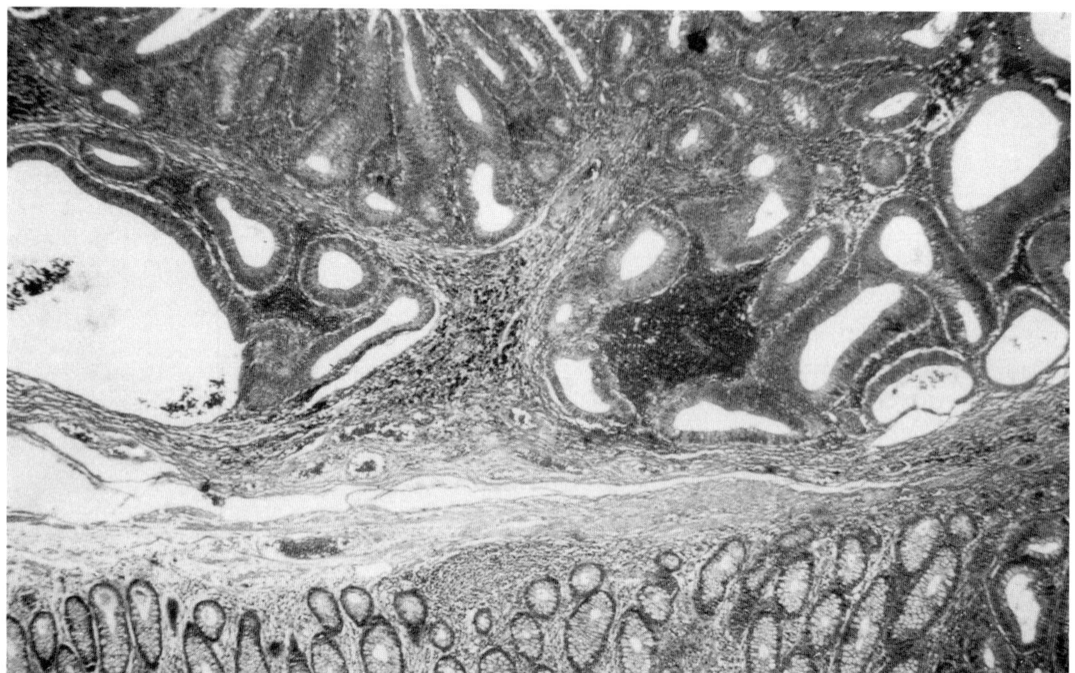

A

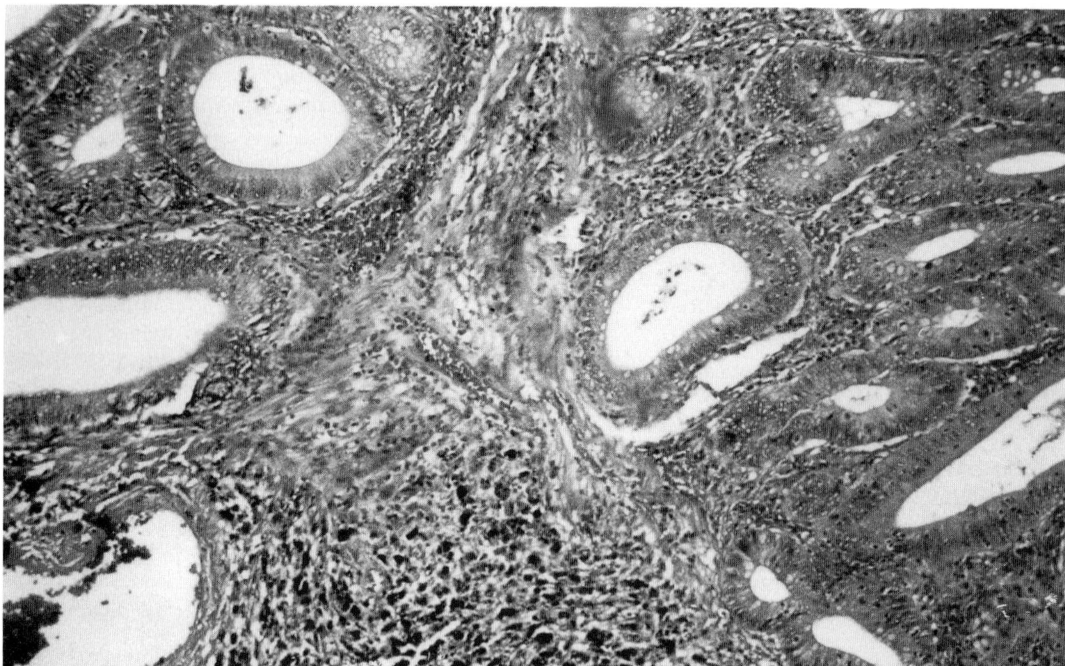

B

Fig. 10-13. Adenoma of the colon with misplaced epithelium. **(A)** Shown is the stalk with a covering of normal mucosa at the bottom. The submucosal core of the stalk contains a circumscribed nodule of adenoma that is surrounded by fibrous tissue and hemosiderin deposits. **(B)** Closer view of misplaced adenoma. The stroma between the glands has the features of normal lamina propria, and a focus of hemosiderin appears at the bottom.

years, and there is a projected chance of carcinoma in virtually all cases.[126] Extensive molecular studies have been conducted, and the gene alteration responsible for the syndrome is present in the 5q21 region.[21–25] There is a variant termed *Gardner syndrome* in which there are associated extraintestinal lesions, including desmoid tumors and various hamartomatous lesions of the bones and jaw.[127] Recently noted is the presence of a nasopharyngeal angiofibroma in some cases.[128] It has also been suggested that Gardner syndrome can show a lesser number of adenomas in the colon, but there is probably considerable overlap between this variant and the full syndrome. In addition, the patients are prone to the development of adenomas and carcinomas in other parts of the gut, particularly the stomach and the duodenum.[129–131] They also appear in ileostomy stomas and ileal pouches following total colectomy.[132–136] (See Chs. 5, 6, and 8 for further details.)

All morphologic forms of adenomas are present in adenomatous polyposis coli, including pedunculated, sessile, flat, and depressed types.[126, 136] Biopsy of the polyps reveals adenomas with varying degrees of dysplasia ranging from low to high grade. In addition, since the propensity for neoplasia is so great, biopsy even of flat areas between the polypoid lesions usually reveals microscopic foci of adenomas (Fig. 10-15) This can be particularly helpful in distinguishing a polyposis syndrome from a case of multiple but not diffuse polyps, since microscopic adenomas in patients without the syndrome are rare.[137] Confirmation of the adenomatous process in the polyps and in the flat mucosa is sought at endoscopy. The chance of carcinoma greatly increases with age. In patients in their teens or twenties, the colectomy specimen typically shows only the adenomas.

Prophylactic colectomy is ordinarily done once the patient is sufficiently mature and capable of handling this procedure.[138] This formerly required a permanent ileostomy, but has now been greatly supplanted by ileo–anal anastomosis with pouch formation. Because of the likelihood of early colectomy before the development of carcinoma or its deep invasion, the overall prognosis is generally good in these patients.

Juvenile Polyposis

Juvenile polyposis is a less common, usually familial disorder in which multiple juvenile-type polyps are seen in the colon and rectum.[139–141] The patients present with multiple bleeding episodes, and require polypectomy or even partial resections of the colon. In contrast to adenomatous polyposis, there are usually fewer polyps in the juvenile cases and there is less likelihood for early carcinoma development. Accordingly, a prophylatic colectomy is ordinarily not recommended in the cases that lack dysplasia.

Examination of the excised polyps reveals the typical juvenile type, with prominent cystic glands, epithelium that is normal or regenerative but not dysplastic, and considerable edema and inflammation in the stroma.[142] Samples of the intervening mucosa not involved with the polyps frequently show slightly irregular glands and edema, supportive that there is a more generalized lesion[143] (Fig. 10-16A). With increasing age there is a small potential for the development of adenomas and carcinomas.[144–147] It has been suggested, therefore, that surveillance with removal of polyps be done to look for dysplastic epithelium. This can vary considerably from juvenile polyps with small foci of dysplasia to lesions that have been totally transformed into adenomas (Fig. 10-16B). If such dysplastic lesions persist or recur, consideration should be given to colonic resection.

Exceptionally, the juvenile polyps are present throughout the intestinal tract and even in the stomach.[148] In the latter location, they are indistinguishable from the ordinary inflammatory and hyperplastic polyps in that region.

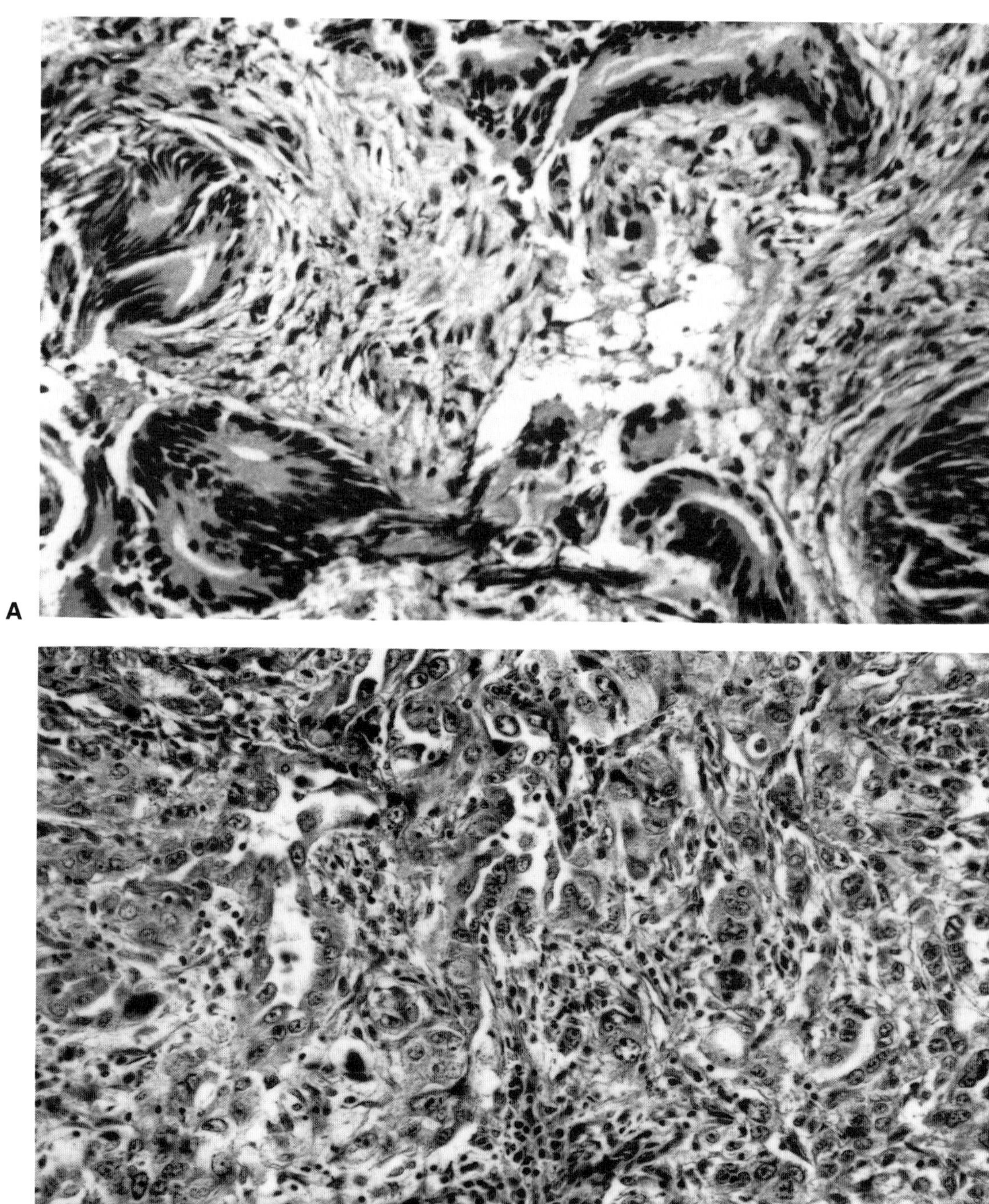

Fig. 10-14. Adenocarcinoma in adenoma of the colon. Examples of features that usually dictate the need for a colectomy: **(A)** Base of stalk, revealing malignant glands and marked cautery effect. **(B)** Poorly differentiated adenocarcinoma. Noted is a sheet of malignant cells with occasional small gland formation (× 210). *(Figure continues.)*

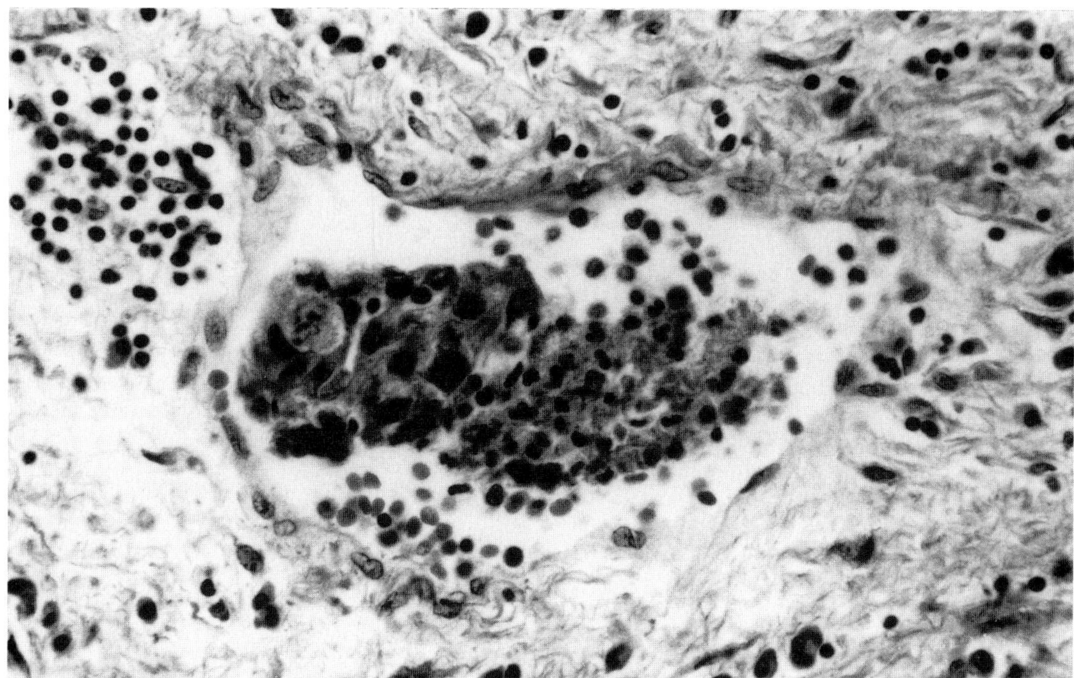

C

Fig. 10-14 *(Continued).* **(C)** Vascular invasion. A clump of tumor cells is seen in the lumen of the vein (× 425).

Table 10-6. Management of Colonic Adenomas with Carcinoma

Polypectomy usually sufficient for:
In-situ or intramucosal carcinoma
Invasive carcinoma into stalk submucosa
Well or moderately differentiated
No vascular invasion
No extension to base of stalk
Colectomy considered for:
Invasive carcinoma into stalk submucosa
Poorly differentiated
Vascular invasion
Extension to base of stalk
Invasive carcinoma into submucosa of sessile lesion

Table 10-7. Colonic Polyposis Syndromes

Adenomatous polyposis coli
Juvenile polyposis
Peutz-Jeghers syndrome
Cronkhite-Canada syndrome
Turcot syndrome
Cowden syndrome
Flat adenoma syndrome

Peutz-Jeghers Syndrome

Peutz-Jeghers syndrome is an uncommon hereditary disorder in which there are multiple polyps in all portions of the gut, being particularly pronounced in the small intestine.[149, 150] The lesions in that site are highly characteristic, revealing a hamartomatous proliferation of the mucosa in the form of complex glands, and broad bands of well formed smooth muscle (see Fig. 6-23). Both normal and regenerative glands are present, and there are abundant goblet mucous cells and Paneth cells. The polyps in the colon vary in appearance, with some showing the typical features, and others resembling the juvenile-type polyps with the prominent edema and dilated glands (Fig. 10-17).

There is a slight increase of cancer development in patients with this syndrome, in all parts of the gastrointestinal tract and in other tissues including the breast, pancreas, uterus, and ovary.[151, 152] Areas of adenomatous epithelium and of carcinoma can be seen in the

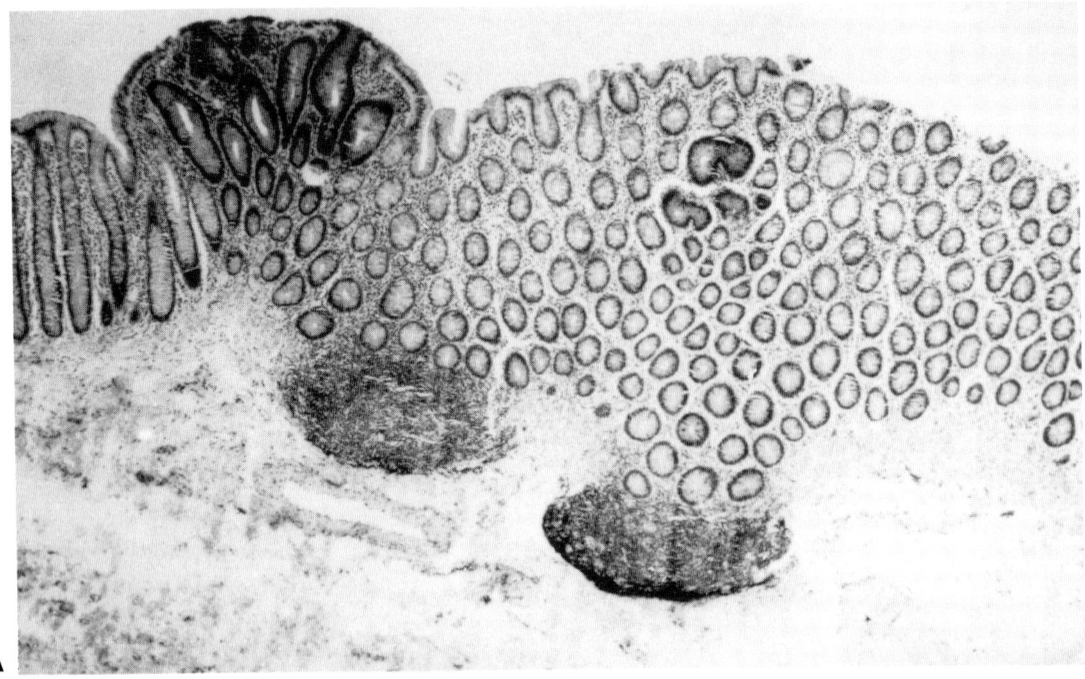

A

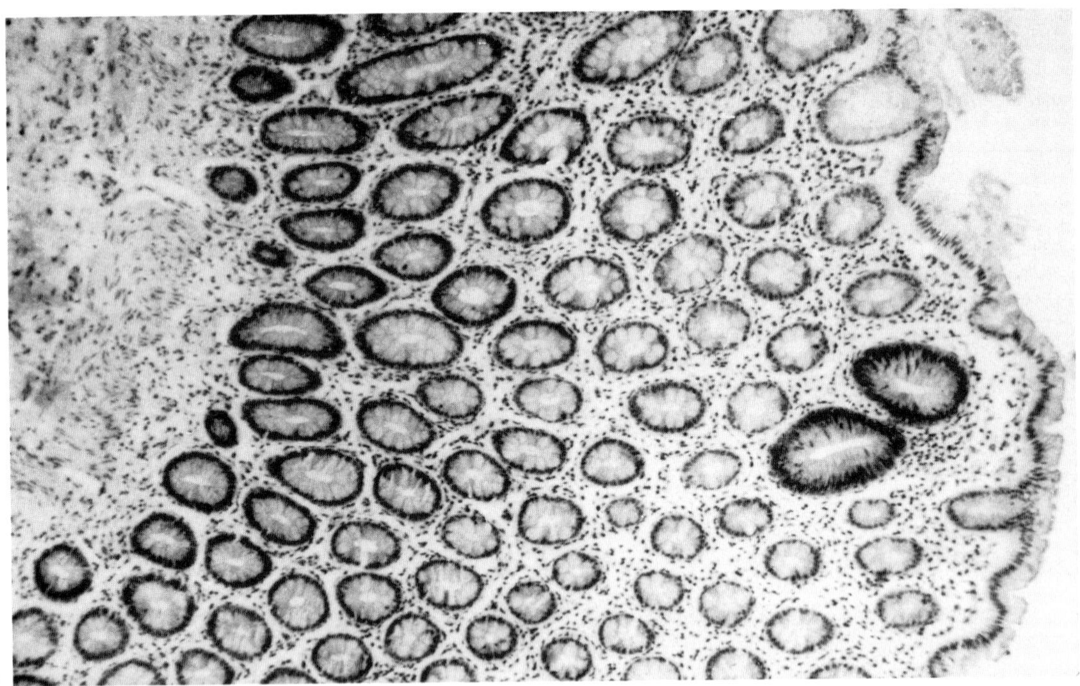

B

Fig. 10-15. Adenomatous polyposis in the colon. **(A)** Section of colonic mucosa and submucosa, revealing a small adenoma (left) and microscopic foci of adenomatous change (right). There are also prominent lymphoid nodules appearing in the lower part. **(B)** Closer view of flat mucosa with a tiny area of adenomatous glands appearing at the right. The submucosa appears at the left.

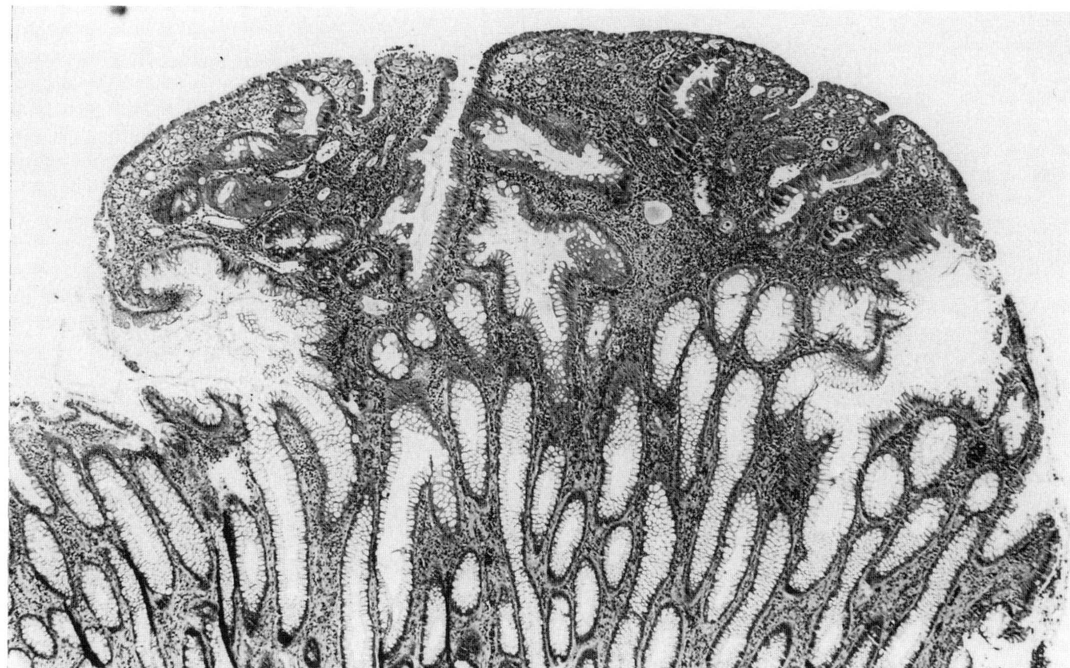

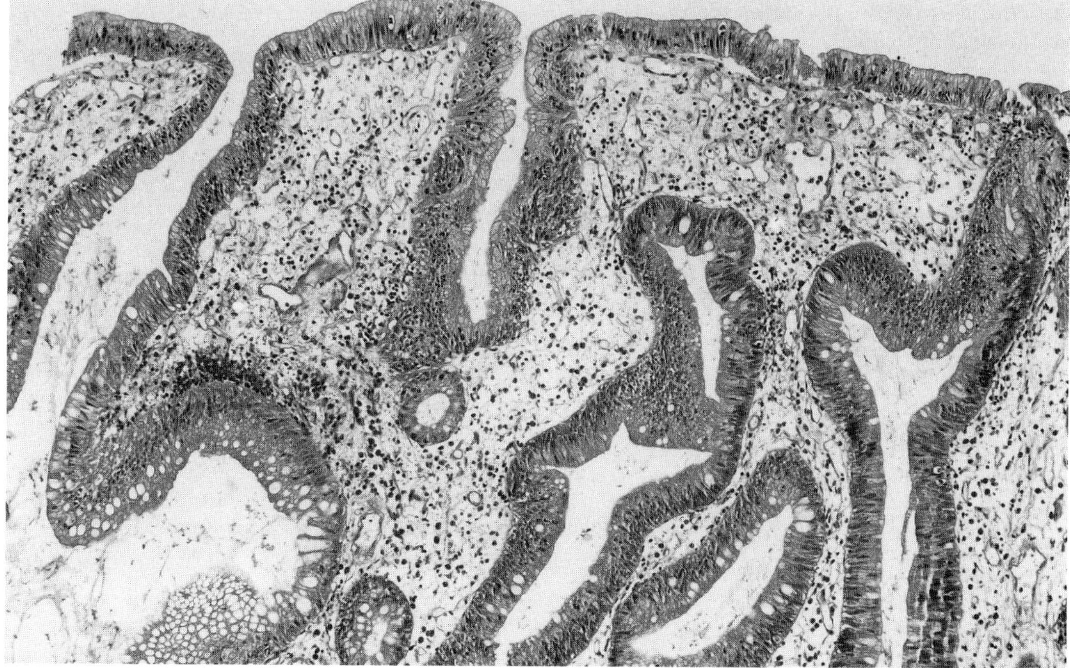

Fig. 10-16. Juvenile polyposis of the colon. **(A)** Section of slightly raised mucosa, showing an early polyp formation (right). Compared to the normal mucosa (left), there is elongation and cystic change of the crypts as well as increased inflammation near the surface (top) (× 42). **(B)** Focus of dysplastic (adenomatous) glands, seen in the three glands appearing at the right. They show elongation, palisading, and slight hyperchromatism of the epithelial cell nuclei. Compare with the non-dysplastic glands appearing at the left (× 105).

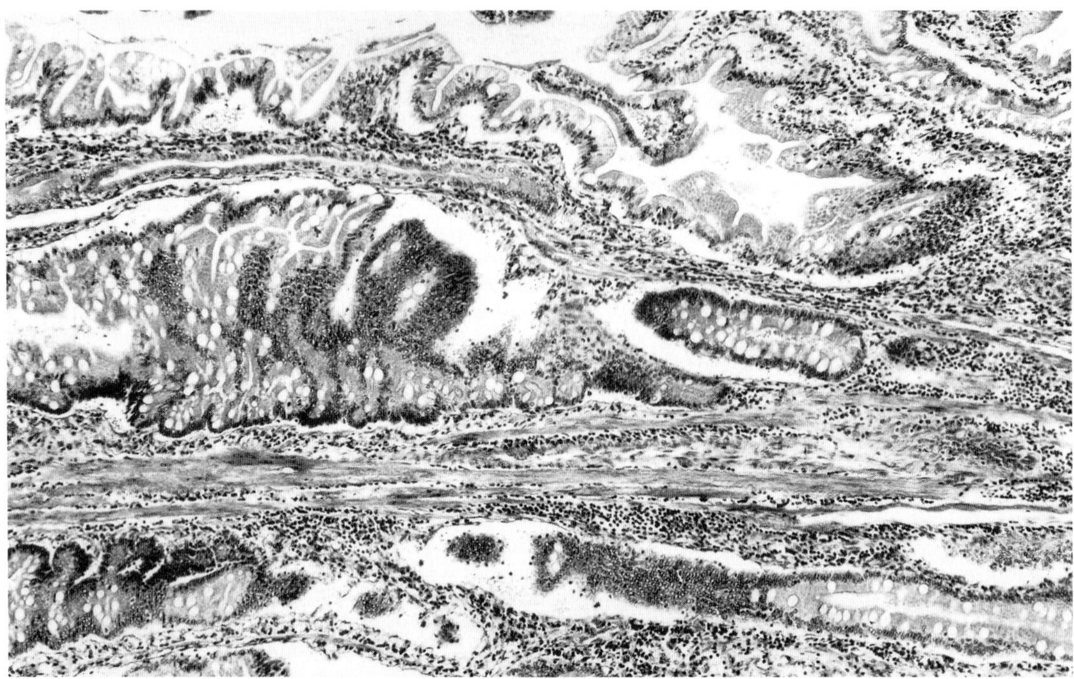

Fig. 10-17. Peutz-Jeghers polyp of the colon. The tumor reveals hyperplastic colonic glands and prominent smooth muscle strands in the lamina propria (× 105). See Figure 6-23 for another example in the small intestine.

hamartomatous polyps and also as separate lesions in the intestinal tract.[153, 154] Some of the larger polyps can be associated with extension of glands into the submucosa and muscularis propria, representing a localized form of enteritis or colitis cystica, and this must be distinguished from invasive carcinoma.[155] The malignant lesions reveal dysplastic epithelium together with tumor stroma, whereas the Peutz-Jeghers polyps show either normal or regenerative epithelium.

Cronkhite-Canada Syndrome

Cronkhite-Canada syndrome is an uncommon, acquired condition in which there are multiple small polyps throughout all portions of the gut, most pronounced in the stomach and in the colon.[156, 157] Compared to the polyps in the other syndromes, these tend to be flatter. Patients also develop an assortment of cutaneous, hair, and nail abnormalities. The symptomatology is largely related to the location of the major lesions, and patients may present with a protein-losing enteropathy, malabsorption, anemia, or simple diarrhea.

Biopsy of the polyps reveals inflammatory-type lesions with dilated crypts, prominent edema, and variable inflammation[158] (Fig. 10-18). The epithelial cells may be normal, atrophic, or show signs of degeneration. Samples of the non-polypoid areas frequently show similar changes. There is a small association with carcinoma both in the stomach and in the colon, and polyps in these cases frequently show adenomatous changes.[159, 160]

Other Syndromes

Other disorders may be associated with an increased likelihood of adenomas or a propensity of the mucosa to develop carci-

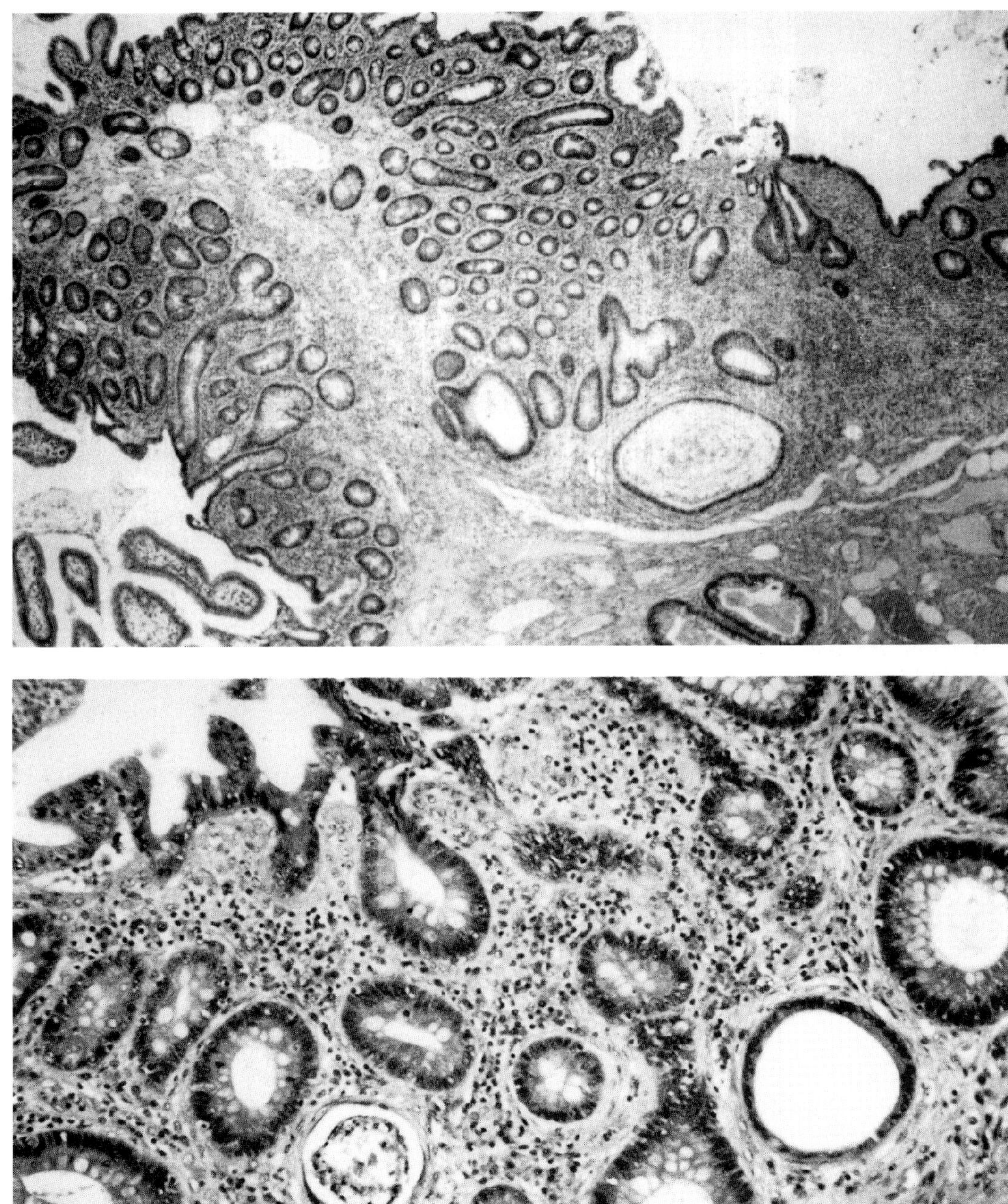

Fig. 10-18. Cronkhite-Canada syndrome. **(A)** Example of a polyp in the ileum. A small fragment of normal mucosa appears at the bottom left. The polyp shows increased glands with focal cystic change and localized extension into the submucosa (lower right). **(B)** Closer view of the polyp, revealing the bland nature of the epithelium and the slight cystic change.

noma. In Turcot syndrome the patients develop asytrocytomas as well as the adenomas.[161, 162] Since the brain tumors tend to be highly aggressive, these patients rarely survive to develop colonic carcinoma.

There are two major types of Lynch syndromes. Type I includes patients with an increased frequency of carcinoma in the absence of extensive adenomas.[163] Biopsies of grossly normal mucosa have revealed altered crypt kinetics, with enhanced mitoses and other growth parameters in the upper portion of the colonic crypts. The type II syndrome is associated with the appearance of flat adenomas in both the colon and the stomach.[164, 165] It is thought that these lesions may be more aggressive and lead to early malignant change.[111–113] (see above section on "Adenomas".)

Mucosal nodules can be seen in the Cowden syndrome and in the multiple endocrine neoplasia syndromes.[68, 166–168] In these lesions there is proliferation of nerves and excess ganglia within the mucosa, and these features can be readily appreciated in biopsy samples (Fig. 10-19). Some of these cases have been associated with other polyps and carcinoma of the colon.[169, 170]

TUMORS IN INFLAMMATORY BOWEL DISEASE

Types of Tumors

There is a considerable increase in neoplasms seen in patients with chronic inflammatory bowel disease, particularly ulcerative colitis and Crohn's disease[171–176] (Table 10-8). Most evident are adenocarcinomas that develop in the colon in both disorders and within the small intestine in Crohn's disease. These are typically associated with the prior formation of epithelial cell dysplasia.

A smaller but definite increase of other tumors has been seen in the colon in these patients, including the formation of carcinoid and composite tumors,[177–180] and of lymphomas and leukemias.[181–184] Microscopic foci of carcinoid tumors are also observed[185, 186] (Fig. 10-20). These are usually found in the region of the rectum at the time of a random biopsy. It is probable that they represent the earlier lesions of regular carcinoids and that they are detected at the time of sampling of the mucosa for some other reason. The lesions have no functional effect but can cause difficulty in decisions regarding their excision. There have been rare reports of adenosquamous cell carcinoma and of malignant melanoma occurring in patients with chronic colitis.[187, 188] All of these lesions are described in the section below on "Other Tumors."

Also noted is an increase in adenocarcinoma of the bile ducts in association with the sclerosing cholangitis that can develop in patients with chronic inflammatory bowel disease,[189] and there are reports of appendiceal adenocarcinoma occurring in cases of ulcerative colitis.[190]

Adenocarcinoma

Frequency and Risk Factors

Adenocarcinoma is the most common tumor seen as a complication of chronic inflammatory bowel disease. It is particularly frequent in patients with ulcerative colitis and is related largely to the extent of the disease and its duration.[171–173, 191] The complication becomes most important in patients with disease that lasts more than 8 to 10 years. Those with colitis involving one-half or more of the colon develop carcinoma in about 15 percent of cases, whereas patients with more limited left-sided colitis have a lesser frequency of 5 percent, but still much greater than in persons without chronic inflammatory bowel disease.[192]

Similarly, cases of Crohn's disease show an increased frequency of carcinoma development of about 3 percent; the lower incidence compared to UC cases probably re-

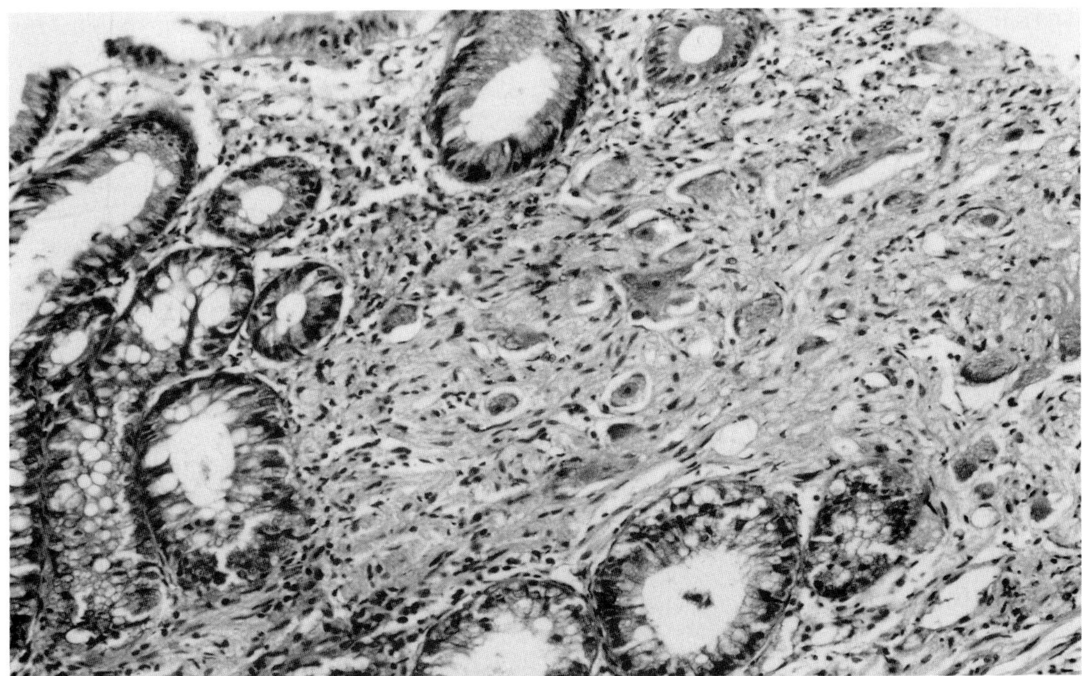

Fig. 10-19. Cowden syndrome, with an example of glanglioneuroma in the colonic mucosa appearing at the right. Noted is a nodule of edematous neural tissue with numerous ganglia (× 210).

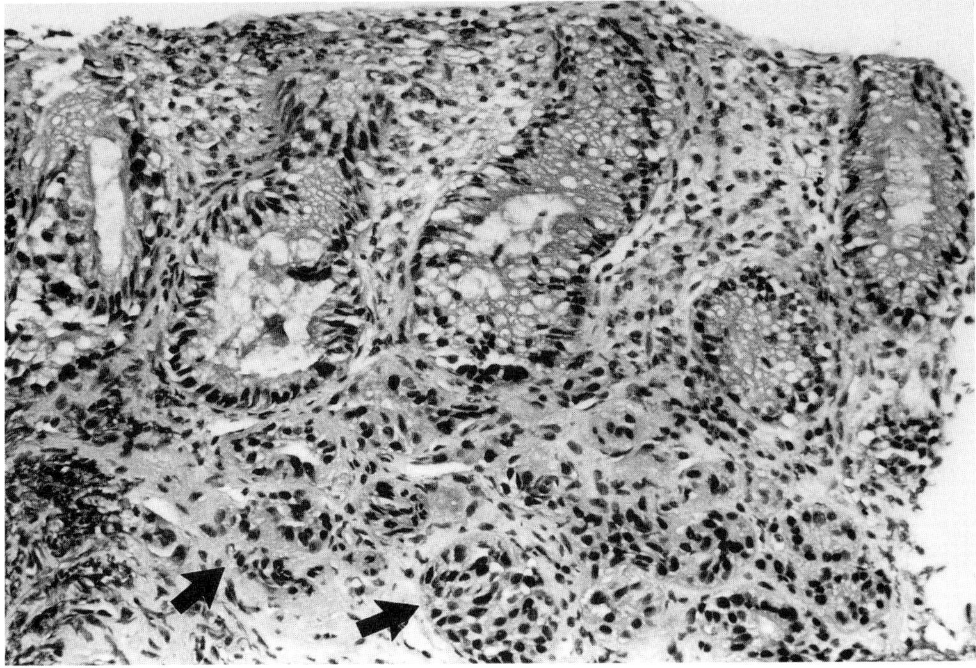

Fig. 10-20. Microcarcinoid tumor in a case of ulcerative colitis. Noted are the small nests of tumor cells (arrows) as well as the shortened crypts of the ulcerative colitis. The surface appears at the top (× 210).

Table 10-8. Malignant Tumors of the Colon in Inflammatory Bowel Disease

Adenocarcinoma
Carcinoid and adenocarcinoid tumors
Lymphoma and leukemia
Rare
Adenosquamous cell carcinoma
Malignant melanoma

flects the presence of more focal disease and of earlier surgery for other complications in patients with CD.[174–176, 193] The carcinomas in CD often affect the rectal and anal area, possibly related to long-standing perianal inflammation.[194, 195]

There also appears to be an increase in carcinoma frequency both in patients with ulcerative colitis and Crohn's disease who present with disease at an earlier age.[196, 197] In ulcerative colitis, this has tended to involve teenagers, whereas young adults have shown the increased incidence in Crohn's disease.

Clinical Features

Compared with patients without colitis, the carcinomas complicating IBD occur in patients about 1 decade younger and are commonly multiple (Table 10-9). It is often difficult to detect these carcinomas because of their gross and histologic aspects. Most of the carcinomas tend to be flat and to merge with the underlying inflammatory bowel disease rather than developing polyps as in noncolitic patients.[198] Also, about 40 percent of the carcinomas seen are relatively well differentiated, making it difficult to diagnose unless there is evident invasion. In this regard, superficial mucosal biopsies may appreciate that there is an epithelial neoplasm, but may not be capable of distinguishing benign dysplasia and carcinoma (Fig. 10-21).

Table 10-9. Characteristics of Carcinoma in Inflammatory Bowel Disease

Younger age of onset
Multiple tumors
Flat and infiltrative gross form
Mucinous histology is common
Frequent association with dysplasia

Given the considerable increase in carcinoma development, it was previously recommended that all patients with chronic colitis lasting for 10 years should be considered for a prophylactic colectomy. However, most patients and their physicians are unwilling to accept this recommendation since they are proceeding with otherwise controllable disease. Because of the macroscopic features, it has not been possible for gross examinations, either radiographic or endoscopic, to clearly identify early tumors. Accordingly, it is now most often urged that these patients at high risk have initial screening and subsequent surveillance to look for dysplasia that might be regarded as an even greater marker of existing or impending carcinoma, as described below.[199]

It was formerly thought that the carcinomas seen in patients with IBD had a worse prognosis, but it is now appreciated that this was probably due to delays in diagnosis.[200] Comparing patients with comparable stages, the responses to therapy are the same in both colitic and non-colitic patients. Indeed, surveillance programs have led recently to earlier detection and improved prognosis in cases of colitis-associated cancers.[201, 202]

Gross Features

Most of the advanced carcinomas complicating IBD are of the ulcerative and infiltrative type, and raised areas of dysplasia are commonly present in the adjacent mucosa.[198, 200, 201, 203–206] The carcinomas are often multiple and are almost always located in areas of prior inflammatory bowel disease. Carcinomas can also develop in strictures and in fistulous tracts[207–209]; making the diagnosis more difficult is the lack of dysplasia in the adjacent mucosa in many of these instances. Brushing and cytologic examination may be particularly useful in such cases when biopsies are not diagnostic.[8–11]

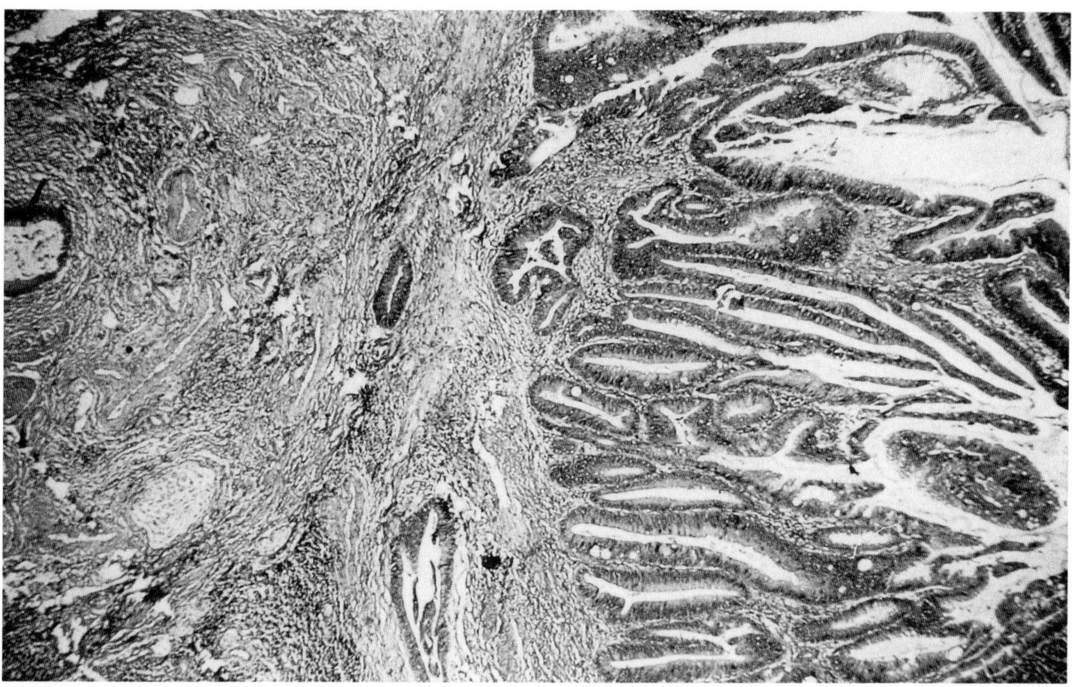

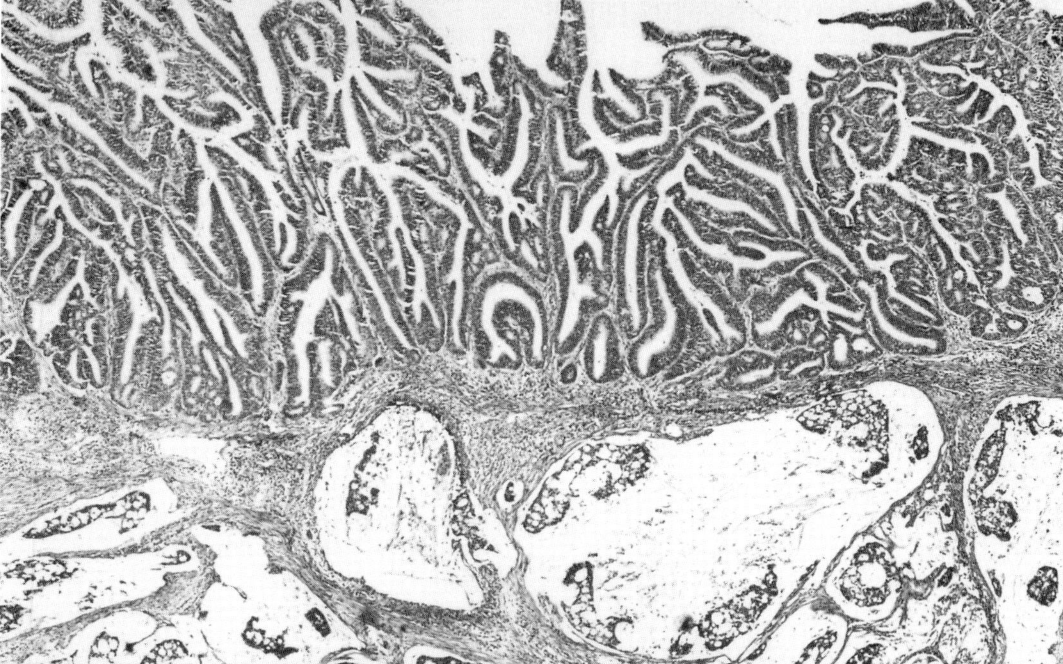

Fig. 10-21. Adenocarcinoma in ulcerative colitis. **(A)** The mucosa appearing at the right is diffusely replaced by neoplastic glands that are well differentiated. Biopsy of such areas may be diagnosed only as dysplasia, but the carcinomatous nature of the lesion is evidenced by the presence of the invasive glands into the submucosa (bottom center and left). **(B)** Example of adenocarcinoma with large mucinous pools containing tumor cells (bottom) (× 56).

Biopsy Features

Most carcinomas are detected in examination of mass, ulcerated, or stricture lesions. As previously noted, over 40 percent of the lesions are well differentiated or mucinous in character (Fig. 10-21B). This includes examples with signet ring cells; such lesions are more commonly seen in tumors of the stomach but can also be primary in the colon. It is particularly important to remember this at biopsy study and to look for sheets of mucus-filled malignant cells as well as for glands; otherwise, the tumors resemble the adenocarcinomas seen in patients without colitis. Noted are variable gland and mucin formation, highly irregular nuclei with hyperchromasia and loss of polarity, and both numerous and abnormal mitoses.

Currently, much more effort is undertaken in patients with long-standing chronic inflammatory bowel disease to look for the precursor lesion of dysplasia, either in random samples or as part of a mass lesion.[210, 211] In such instances, there is much less chance of finding carcinoma in the resected specimen. In patients with ulcerative colitis who have had less than a total colectomy, the residual stump mucosa remains at considerable risk for the development of neoplasia.[212, 213] Follow-up studies have demonstrated epithelial dysplasia and both adenocarcinoma and squamous cell carcinomas. Accordingly, if such rectal mucosa must remain, it is essential that it be routinely surveyed to look for dysplastic changes.

Epithelial Dysplasia

Nature and Significance

One of the common reasons for endoscopy and biopsy in patients with long-standing chronic IBD is to look for areas of epithelial dysplasia, which represents a neoplastic change.[201, 205, 210, 214] These lesions were seen next to carcinomas complicating UC in surgical specimens in many early studies, and it was later appreciated that they also could be found in mucosal biopsies adjacent to or away from the carcinomas at the time of endoscopy.[215–219] The dysplasia has also been noted in cases of CD, in both the small and large intestine.[204, 220–222] It is now well accepted that epithelial dysplasia is an excellent marker of existing or future development of carcinoma in high-risk patients.

It is suggested that patients with extensive UC have initial screening for dysplasia at about 8 to 10 years after the onset of the disease.[223–226] Given the lower frequency and possible later onset of tumors in patients with more limited UC and with Crohn's disease, it has been suggested that the surveillance procedure might be started at a slightly later time in those cases.

Gross Features

When prominent, the dysplasia is noted as a slightly raised, villiform or velvety lesion.[217, 227, 228] This is in contrast to the ordinary inflammatory pseudopolyps, which tend to have a smooth surface and to develop stalks when bigger. More often, there are no gross lesions suggestive of dysplasia, and random biopsies are taken from the flat, least inflamed mucosa. Areas of ulceration, inflammatory pseudopolyps, and other overt inflammation should be avoided, since this makes difficult the histologic diagnosis of dysplasia.

In evaluating a gross mass, it may be particularly difficult to distinguish a polypoid area of dysplasia from an incidental adenoma, since both are composed of the same benign neoplastic epithelium (Fig. 10-22). A separation based on patient age, with adenoma favored in older persons, is not entirely satisfactory. The isolated adenoma is more likely if the lesion occurs in an area of the bowel that is unaffected by the colitis or is associated with a stalk that is layered by normal mucosa; such polyps can be satisfactorily

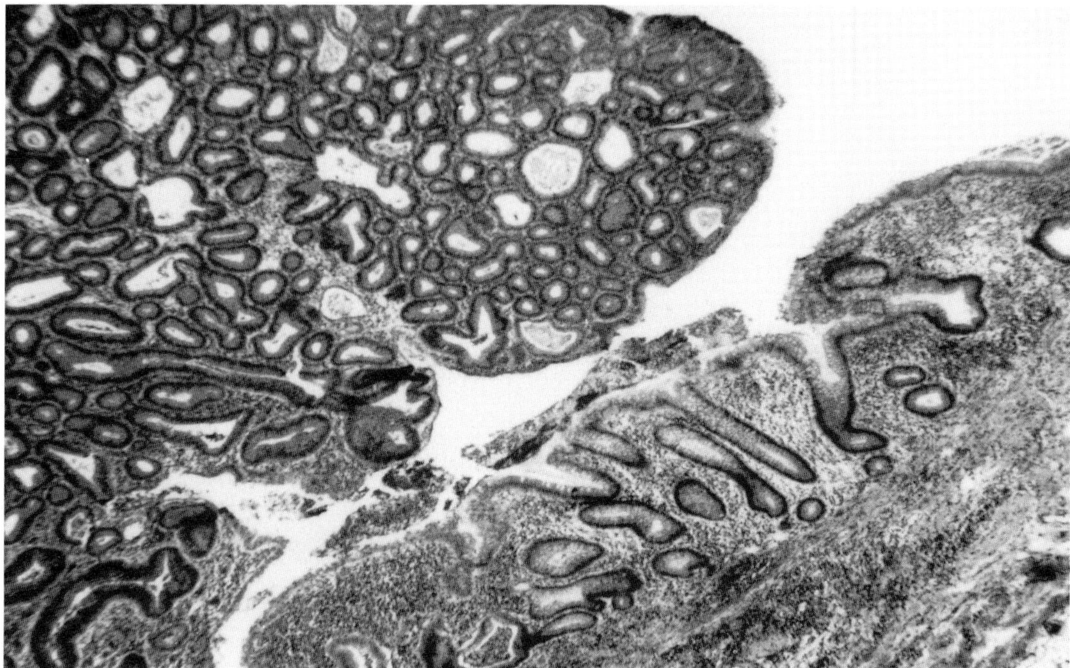

Fig. 10-22. Polypoid dysplasia in ulcerative colitis. At the left is a sessile mass of dysplastic tissue. The adjacent mucosa (right) shows the features of chronic colitis. There is no stalk.

treated by endoscopic excision. In contrast, a diagnosis of dysplasia is preferred in lesions that are sessile or located in regions of colitis. If there is doubt, more biopsies may be taken to look for additional foci of dysplasia in any stalk mucosa and in the adjacent colon to support the diagnosis.

Grades of Dysplasia

There have been numerous studies defining the features of dysplasia and its degrees. Considering the limited clinical responses, it is currently proposed that dysplasia be separated into only two categories, low-grade and high-grade dysplasia.[210] Low-grade dysplasia corresponds to most of the prevous cases called mild, revealing no change in architecture above that seen in chronic colitis but a cytologic alteration that cannot be explained (Fig. 10-23). Specifically, one sees an increase of elongated and palisaded nuclei involving the basal half of the cells, in the absence of any hyperchromasia or loss of cellular polarity. Such areas can also be seen as part of the regenerative response next to regions of ulceration and marked acute inflammation. Accordingly, the effects of active colitis must be excluded before a firm diagnosis of low-grade dysplasia is made.

High-grade dysplasia encompasses a much larger group, including the moderate to severe cases as well as carcinoma in-situ (Fig. 10-24). At the lower end of the spectrum are the lesions that show the palisading and elongated nuclei extending to involve more than one-half of the height of the cells, and architectural changes in excess of that ordinarily seen in chronic UC, usually in the form of beginning polyp formation. At the high end are samples with overt hyperchromasia, loss of cell polarity, and cribiform arrangement in the glands. Cases of high-grade dys-

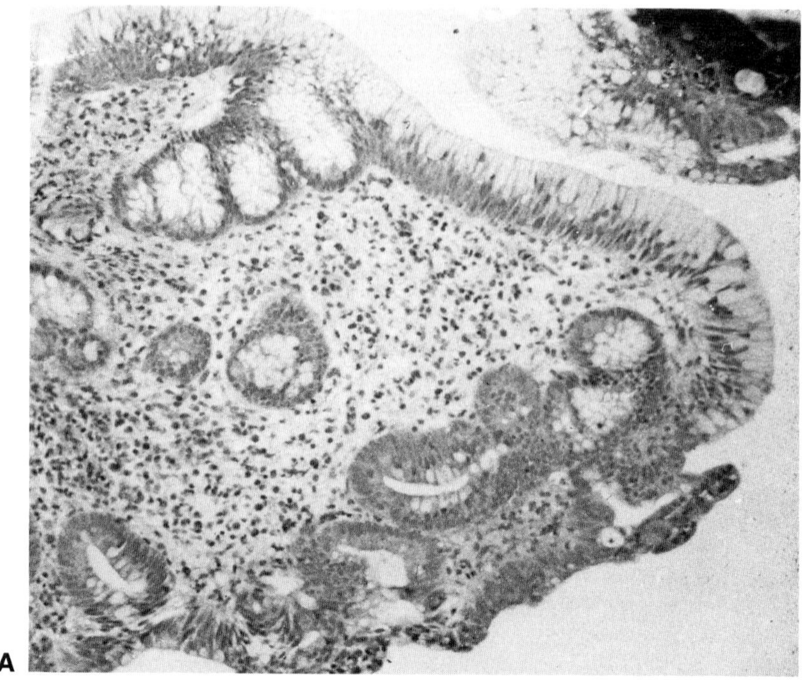

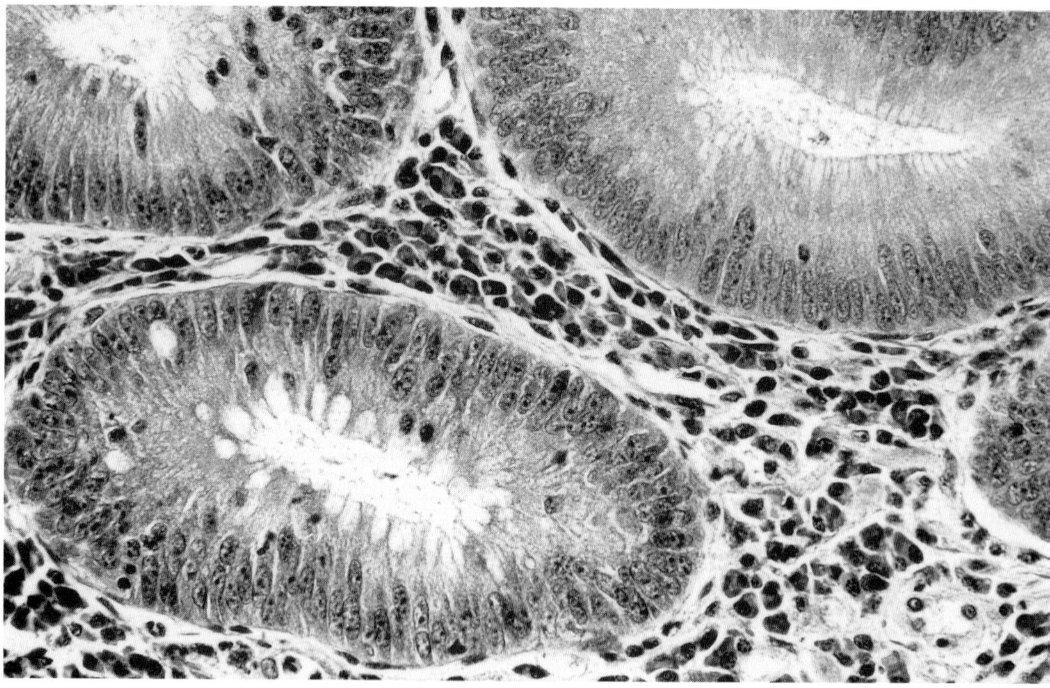

Fig. 10-23. Low-grade epithelial dysplasia in ulcerative colitis. **(A)** Biopsy showing irregular glands similar to that seen in ulcerative colitis. The surface epithelium reveals elongated nuclei that occupy the basal half of the cells. **(B)** Closer view of the glands to show the nuclear changes. They are elongated but otherwise regular in size and shape and lack hyperchromatism (× 425).

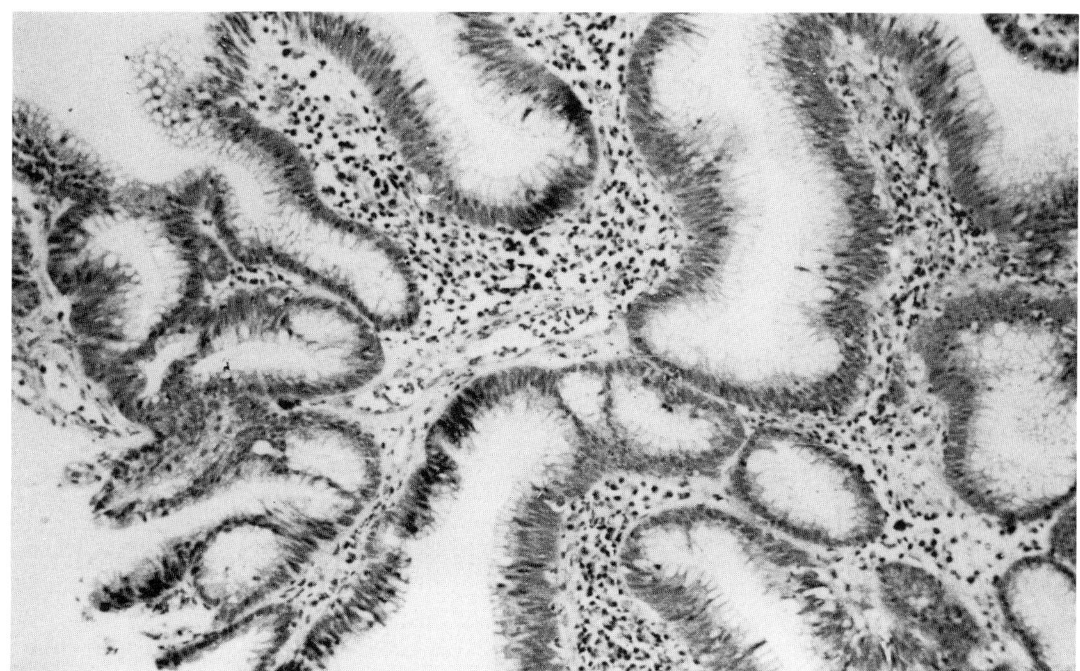

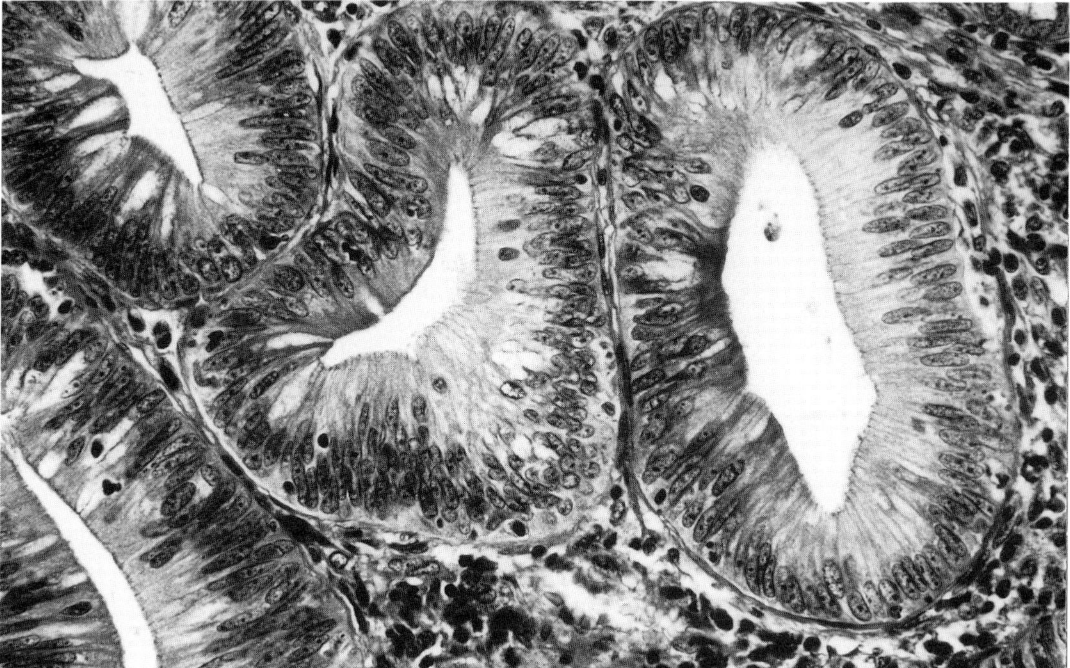

Fig. 10-24. High-grade epithelial dysplasia in ulcerative colitis. **(A)** Biopsy of gross polypoid lesion showing glandular proliferation and some epithelial cells with nuclei extending into the upper half of the cells. **(B)** Closer view of the glands, revealing nuclear palisading and variable hyperchromasia. Compared to the low-grade dysplasia in Figure 10-23B, there is greater variation in size and position of the nuclei within the cells (× 425).

plasia also may be associated with adjacent ulceration and acute inflammation, but the abnormal cytologic features are usually sufficient to permit the diagnosis of dysplasia in such cases.

Histologic Classification

The biopsies are categorized into three broad groups of *negative for dysplasia,* including the great majority of inactive and active samples; *indefinite for dysplasia,* representing those cases in which the diagnosis is not certain because of the presence of considerable confounding inflammation; and *positive for dysplasia,* separated into low-grade and high-grade degrees[210, 214] (Table 10-10). Most of the negative samples cause no difficulty since they are derived from areas of atrophic mucosa (see Fig. 9-10). Aside from the crypt irregularities, the individual epithelial cells show no atypism, and have basal nuclei. Problems can occur in the presence of active colitis because of the combination of irregular glands of the chronic colitis together with the effects of degeneration and regeneration (Fig. 10-25). In contrast, in a patient without colitis, the presence of an architectural abnormality might provide added support for a neoplasm. The cases with colitis show the active inflammation in the form of neutrophils or ulcers, and this should serve as an alarm for withholding a positive diagnosis except in the high-grade cases. This can be even more difficult when the active inflammation is gone and there persists a prominent regeneration. Such cases show, however, a great regularity of the nuclei. Although enlarged, they tend to be the same size and shape and to have the same position within the cell together with a lack of hyperchromasia, all supportive of their regenerative nature. There are many mitoses including rare abnormal forms, and this cannot be used as a distinguishing feature between regeneration and dysplasia.

Table 10-10. Classification of Epithelial Dysplasia

Negative for dysplasia
Normal
Inactive colitis
Active colitis
Indefinite for dysplasia
Probably inflammatory
Unknown
Probably dysplastic
Positive for dysplasia
Low-grade dysplasia
High-grade dysplasia

(Modified from Riddell et al.,[210] with permission.)

Clinical Response

There can be regular surveillance at an annual or biannual level in cases that are negative for dysplasia; the need for repeat biopsy in those that are indefinite or demonstrate just low-grade dysplasia; and serious consideration for a total colectomy in cases with confirmed high-grade dysplasia[201, 205, 223–226] (Table 10-11). Given the potential for observer variation and the importance of the diagnosis, it is always recommended that the diagnosis of dysplasia be confirmed by review with other morphologists or by additional biopsies.[210, 229] The above applies to samples taken from flat mucosa. If biopsies are derived from a grossly evident mass lesion, the finding of any degree of dysplasia, whether low grade or high grade, deserves consideration of colectomy, since such lesions more often have carcinoma.[227, 230]

Special Studies

Many other studies have been performed in an effort to refine the diagnosis of epithelial dysplasia in patients with chronic IBD. The demonstration of carcinoembryonic antigen proved to be nonspecific, elevated in most inflammatory and regenerative lesions as well as in the dysplastic areas.[231] Similar findings were noted in studies of epithelial mucins. Whereas the normal colon is espe-

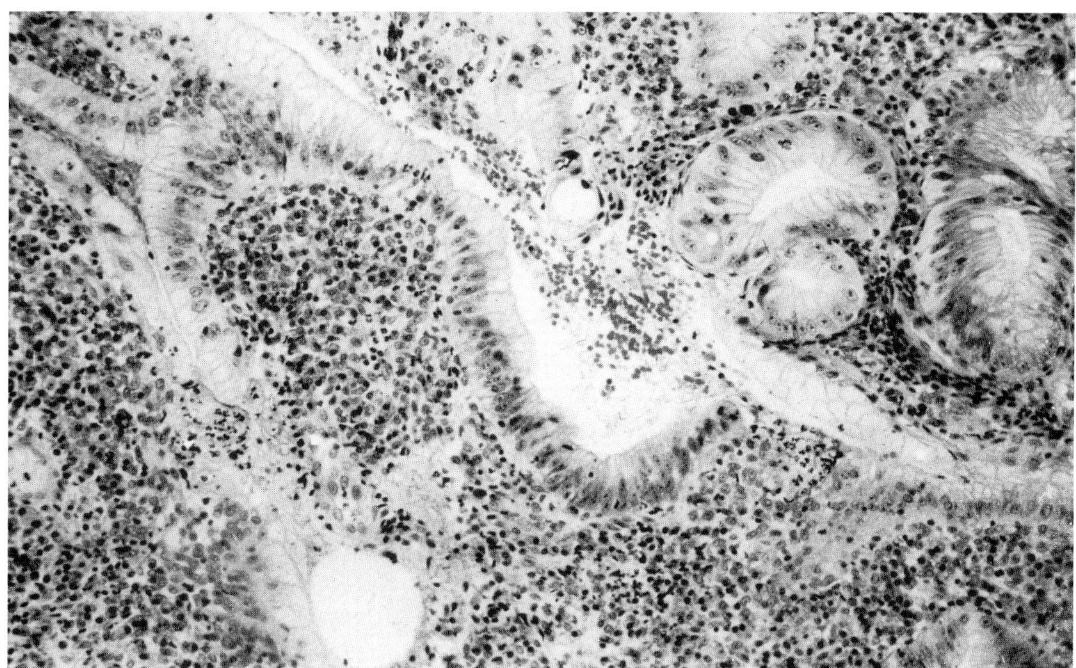

A

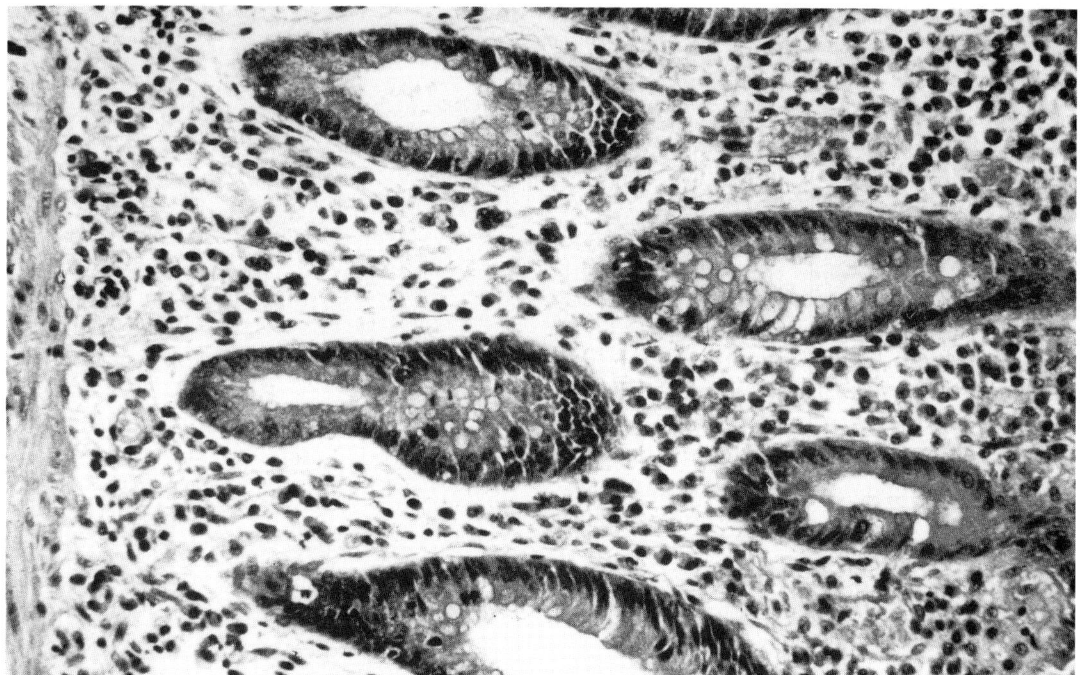

B

Fig. 10-25. Examples of biopsies that are negative or indefinite for dysplasia in ulcerative colitis. **(A)** Clump of glands with focal areas of epithelial nuclear crowding and elongation, similar to low-grade dysplasia. However, presence of prominent inflammation suggests that this is negative. **(B)** Biopsy revealing marked regeneration of the crypts. The epithelial cell nuclei are enlarged but regular in size, shape, and position in the cells. Muscularis mucosae appears at the left.

Table 10-11. Management of Epithelial Dysplasia

Classification	Flat Mucosa	Mass Lesion
Negative and probably negative	Regular surveillance	Regular surveillance
Other indefinite	Repeat biopsy	Repeat biopsy
Low grade	Repeat biopsy	Consider colectomy
High grade	Consider colectomy	Consider colectomy

(Modified from Riddell et al.,[210] with permission.)

cially rich in sulfomucins, an increase in sialomucins was seen in most dysplastic and carcinomatous areas but also in over one-half of the benign inflamed regions.[232] More recent stains include sucrase–isomaltase, with the finding of an aberrant cytoplasmic distribution of the enzyme in dysplastic and carcinomatous cells, whereas it was limited to the surface membrane in areas of inflammation and regeneration.[233]

Flow cytometry has revealed aneuploidal populations in most cancers and dysplastic areas and may serve as a tool for providing specificity.[234–238] Similar results have been noted with scanning electron microscopy, where abnormalities in number and size of the microvilli appear to be highly characteristic of the neoplastic epithelium.[239] Again, this technique might provide specificity in uncertain cases. Other studies have shown p53 mutation and aberrant overexpression in dysplastic and carcinomatous lesions.[240–242] Of interest, the p53 change appears to be a relatively early event in colitis-associated tumors, whereas it is a late finding in ordinary colonic cancers. There is a current boom in molecular and biochemical studies, resulting in the finding of many other alterations in the dysplasias and carcinomas.[243–248] Examples include K-*ras* and APC gene mutations, deletions of 8p chromosomes, and enhanced levels of the tyrosine kinases.

Summary

Initial screening should be considered in patients with long-standing colitis at 8 to 10 years. At endoscopy, the velvety or villiform lesions of gross dysplasia should be sought. In their absence, numerous samples should be taken from the flat and least inflamed mucosa. Up to three tissue levels should be provided for each biopsy site because of the potential for the existence of very tiny areas of dysplasia. The biopsies are classified as negative, indefinite, or positive for dysplasia, with an effort made to distinguish low-grade and high-grade degrees. With a positive finding for dysplasia, there should be confirmation, preferably by another morphologist, of this lesion. The clinical responses are as outlined above.

ADENOCARCINOMA

Adenocarcinoma is the most common malignant tumor of the colon and rectum and is seen with approximately equal frequency in men and women.[1, 2, 249, 250]

Epidemiology

There is an increased incidence of carcinoma related to a family history, both in polyposis and sporadic cases, and such tumors typically develop in younger patients.[251]

Dietary Aspects

Adenocarcinoma of the colon and rectum is most often observed in the developed countries and is thought to relate to the type of diet. It is considered that the extensive use of a low-fiber diet results in less frequent bowel activity and the potential for greater stasis and time for carcinogens to act on the mucosa. Diets rich in protein and fats are also subject to heavy bacterial action that might promote the tumors.

Genetic Aspects

Recent investigations have concentrated on the genetic features, revealing selective loss of tumor suppressor genes in polyposis syndromes and in other families with enhanced frequency of adenocarcinoma of the colon and rectum.[21–25] Such patients would be at an increased risk for tumor development by the subsequent action of any carcinogens and promoting agents. Mutations of K-*ras* appear as an early event, and of p53 as a later occurrence, in the develoment of the cancers.[29, 30] Furthermore, their overexpression tends to occur more often in aggressive tumors.[28] A variety of genetic deletions involving 17q, 18q, and 22q have also been noted in colonic carcinomas, and these tend to correlate with poor survival.[31, 32]

Premalignant Conditions and Lesions

The reader should refer to the earlier sections on "Adenomas" and on "Polyposis Syndromes" for further details.

Adenomas

By far the most common premalignant lesion is the adenoma, which is thought to be the starting point for over 90 percent of the adenocarcinomas[90, 104, 105] (Table 10-12).

Table 10-12. Premalignant Conditions and Lesions of Adenocarcinoma of the Colon

Adenoma
Polyposis syndromes
Chronic colitis
Ureterosigmoidostomy
Immunodeficiency disorders
Celiac disease
Duplication cyst

Studies of polypectomy specimens have greatly supported this notion, revealing the development of carcinoma in about 10 percent of lesions larger than 1 cm in diameter. All the stages, from tiny foci of in-situ carcinoma and early invasion of an adenoma, to almost complete loss of the adenoma by the overgrowth of the carcinoma, have been demonstrated.

It is most desirable to identify patients who have a familial history or other factors favoring the development of adenomas. Such patients should ideally have sigmoidoscopy or colonoscopy to look for and to remove any suspicious polyps. There does not appear to be any increased frequency of carcinoma related to isolated cases of the other types of polyps, including the inflammatory, juvenile, and hyperplastic types.

Polyposis Syndromes

The polyposis syndromes all are associated with an increased frequency of adenocarcinoma, especially the cases of adenomatous polyposis and its variant of the Gardner syndrome.[124–126] In this group, the risk of carcinoma is so great that prophylactic colectomy is routinely performed to prevent the development of malignant tumor.[138] A much smaller incidence is noted in the other polyposis syndromes, and these patients can probably be followed for the development of dysplastic lesions before considering the need for a colectomy.

Acquired Inflammatory Conditions

Any case of chronic colitis of long-standing duration has the potential for the development of carcinoma. It has been best documented in the patients with idiopathic inflammatory bowel disease, including both ulcerative colitis and Crohn's disease.[171–176, 192] It also occurs to a lesser extent in cases of chronic schistosomiasis of the colon and as a late effect of radiation in the large bowel.[252–256] In the case of IBD, it has proven helpful to look for the precursor lesion of epithelial dysplasia in surveillance biopsies and using this finding to select the patients who should have a colectomy.[201, 205, 210] (See above section on "Tumors in Inflammatory Bowel Disease" for details.)

Ureterosigmoidostomy

Patients with major urinary bladder defects, such as extrophy, formerly had their ureters diverted and implanted in the colon, usually in the sigmoid region. It was later appreciated that colonic adenomas and carcinomas developed in the stomal region at an early age, presumably due to the constant irritation from the urinary drainage.[257, 258] Endoscopy and biopsy are used to detect the masses and to identify the neoplastic lesions.[259, 260] Inflammatory and hyperplastic mucosal lesions also can occur and must be distinguished from the neoplasms.[261] The former tend to be small, sessile, and smooth surfaced, and biopsies reveal inflammation and no dysplasia. Colonic insertions of ureters is no longer employed and has been replaced by the formation of ileal bladders.

Other Conditions

An increase in tumors is seen in patients with AIDS, including more carcinomas and lymphomas involving the colon and rectum.[262–264] Patients with celiac disease develop tumors in the gut, principally lymphomas in the small intestine.[265] Noted, in addition, are a small increase of carcinomas involving the stomach and colon. Carcinomas are also seen in cases of duplication cysts involving the colon.[266, 267] Of interest, these frequently reveal a mixture of glandular and squamous differentiation. There are various systemic conditions that are thought to have a higher frequency of internal tumors, including colonic carcinoma. Examples include cases of scleroderma, dermatomyositis, and some skin disorders such as acantholysis nigricans.

Clinical Features

Most tumors develop in adults beyond the age of 50 but it can be seen in younger patients, especially if there is a positive family history.[251] There are two major modes of presentation: progressive constipation and bleeding from the colon and rectum. There is a tendency for the carcinomas involving the left side of the colon to be associated with early obstruction and greater symptoms related to change in bowel habit. In contrast, tumors developing in the right side of the colon, where the lumen is much larger, are more apt to reveal extensive bleeding before there are any obstructive signs.

Late findings relate to delays in diagnosis and include anemia from the bleeding and an obstructive form of colitis secondary to the tumor stenosis.

Pathologic Features

Gross Forms

The earliest and smallest carcinomas are typically found in polyps, and this subject is detailed above in the section on "Adenomas."[115–122] In the larger and more advanced tumors, there are three major forms of polypoid, ulcerative, and infiltrative carcinoma.[1, 2] The polypoid carcinomas represent about 10 percent of cases and are thought to be relatively early lesions in which preexisting adenomas have been overgrown by the malignant tissue. The large majority of the tumors are of the ulcerative type and are associated with markedly irregular edges. Least commonly noted are the diffusely infiltrative tumors of the linitis plastica form, similar to that noted in the stomach.[268–270] These tumors typically extend for several centimeters and are associated with marked stricture formation. They are usually comprised of a predominance of signet ring cell type carcinoma cells and tend to be more common in the cases complicating IBD.

Most of the lesions are easily accessed by endoscopy, permitting biopsy of the polypoid and ulcerated areas. Difficulties may occur with the stenotic lesions where finer scopes or brushes may be needed to acquire biopsy or cytologic material.

Histologic Features

The great majority of the adenocarcinomas reveal gland formation, and the tumors are roughly graded based on the quantity of well formed glands (Fig. 10-26). These are present in over 75 percent of the tumors in the well differentiated, 25 to 75 percent in the moderately differentiated, and less than 25 percent in the poorly differentiated lesions (see Fig. 10-14B). Clearly, this grading is best achieved in the examination of the entire tumor, but initial estimates can be provided in the biopsy. The potential importance is the rough correlation of lesser prognosis related to the poorly differentiated tumors.

Tumors with extensive mucin production are seen in about 10 to 15 percent of the cases overall and much more often in those complicating chronic IBD.[270,271] Such tumors reveal large mucus lakes that contain scattered epithelial cells and glandular tissue. They also may show foci of malignant signet ring cells, similar to tumors in the stomach (Fig. 10-27). The identification of mucinous carcinoma in biopsies can be particularly helpful, since it tends to predict the presence of more advanced cancers.[272] Least commonly observed are totally undifferentiated

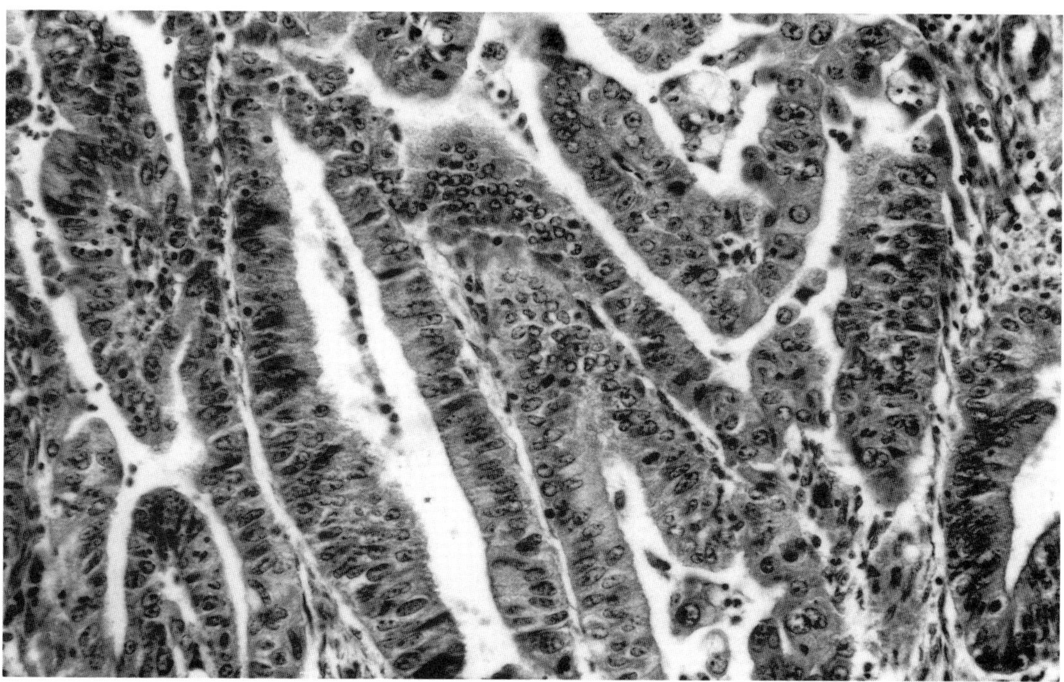

Fig. 10-26. Adenocarcinoma of the colon, with gland formation. Noted is a moderately differentiated tumor with large irregular glands (× 210). See Figure 10-14B for an example of poorly differentiated adenocarcinoma.

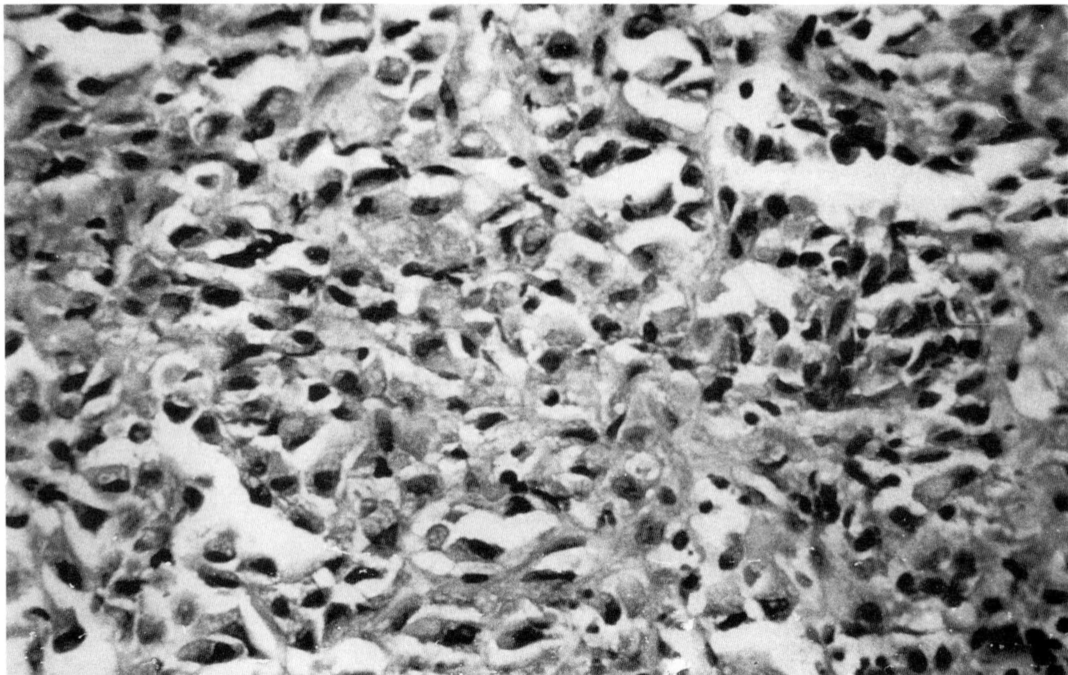

Fig. 10-27. Adenocarcinoma of the colon, signet ring cell type. Noted is a diffuse sheet of malignant cells with abundant cytoplasm, due to the presence of mucus, and nuclei at the edges.

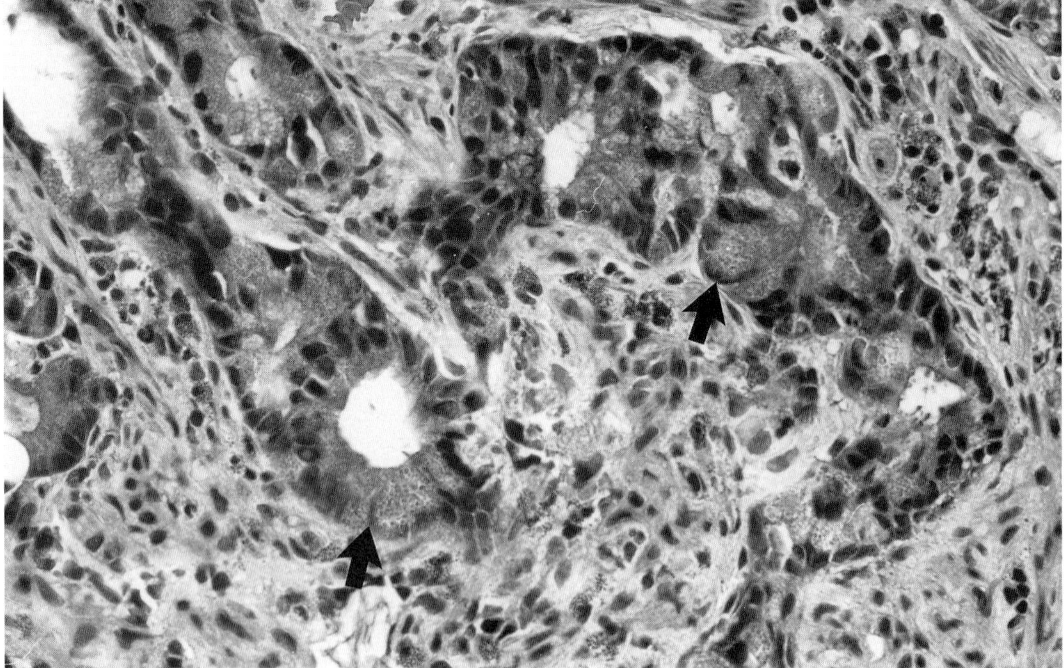

Fig. 10-28. Adenocarcinoma of the colon, with many Paneth cells. There are irregular tumor glands, and many of the epithelial cells contain Paneth granules (arrows) (× 425). See Figure 10-9C for Paneth cell differentiation in a colonic adenoma.

carcinomas, consisting of sheets of malignant cells with ample cytoplasm but with minimal mucus production. The epithelial nature of these tumors can be confirmed by immunocytochemical stains for cytokeratin and carcinoembryonic antigen as well as by electron microscopy[14] (see Fig. 10-1).

Commonly noted in adenocarcinomas are an increase in the amount of endocrine cells.[273, 274] Some studies have shown these to be present in almost one-half of the cases. The endocrine cells typically appear at the edges of glands and have either clear or granular pink cytoplasm; their nature can be readily confirmed by special stains. They have no special significance, as the tumors behave as other adenocarcinomas and depend strictly on the stage of tumor invasion. Other elements are much less commonly observed, including Paneth cells and squamous fragments[95, 96] (Fig. 10-28).

Special Studies

There have been numerous investigations involving flow cytometry of tumors in the colon and rectum.[15–20] Noted overall is the presence of aneuploidy in about 50 percent of adenomas and 75 to 80 percent of carcinomas. There appears to be a greater frequency in cancers that involve the left portion of the colon, in tumors that are highly mucinous, and in the more advanced lesions.

Recent studies of a tumor antigen designated as DF-3 show lack of immunocytochemical expression in normal colonic mucosa and in benign adenomatous tissue, but its appearance in adenocarcinoma cells.[38] This has been observed in extensive cancers and also in the carcinomatous foci arising within adenomas, raising the possibility that this may assist in the detection of malignancy in such lesions. The results of various molecular studies are discussed in the above section on "Epidemiology."

Biopsy Uses and Features

Detection of Carcinoma

Endoscopy and biopsy are performed for the detection of the tumors and to follow the patients after initial therapy (Table 10-13). The diagnosis is usually secured by taking multiple samples of any mass or ulcerated lesion, aiming for the most viable tissue. In the case of polypoid lesions, there is the potential that the biopsies will only demonstrate the preexisting benign adenomatous tissue. In such cases, one must consider the gross findings in conjunction with the biopsy results. For example, if there is a large ulcerated lesion revealing only adenoma in the small biopsy samples, there is the strong likelihood that the ulcerated area represents carcinoma and specific therapy can proceed.

The earlier carcinomas developing in the adenomas may reveal lesser degrees of cancer and its invasion. These include the findings of in-situ adenocarcinoma, which is probably best regarded as the extreme of high-grade dysplasia; the development of intramucosal carcinoma that is limited to the head of a polyp; and the appearance of invasive carcinoma into a stalk or submucosa.[103] (This subject is covered fully in the section above on "Adenomas.") It may be more difficult to acquire adequate biopsy material from lesions that are associated with marked strictures or that develop in fissure areas. In such cases, it may be necessary to obtain larger samples or cytologic brushings.

Table 10-13. Biopsy Uses in Malignant Tumors of the Colon

Diagnosis of malignant tumor
Determination of specific histologic type
Evaluation of differentiation and degree of invasion of tumor
Assessment of drug and radiation effects
Identification of opportunistic infections
Surveillance for coexisting and future tumors

Estimation of Grade and Stage

Because of the limited size of the biopsies, attempts at grading are not necessarily representative of the entire tumor. Nevertheless, efforts are made to indicate the degree of glandular formation, noting whether the tumor is of the well, moderate, or poorly differentiated type. Particularly helpful is the finding of the mucinous category including that with many signet ring cells, since this appears to correlate with more aggressive tumors.[272] Efforts are also made to determine the stage of the carcinoma, whether limited to the mucosa or extending into the adjacent underlying submucosal tissue. Unfortunately, the superficial endoscopic biopsies frequently contain only mucosal tissue. Again, one should consider the gross aspects of the tumor together with the mucosal findings in assessing the probable degree of invasion and what surgery is needed.

In summary, biopsies are used to detect the adenocarcinoma; to rate the degree of glandular formation, with particular note of the mucinous, signet ring cell, and undifferentiated forms; to assess the degree of invasion or note that the sample is limited to the mucosa; and to find any tumor extension into lymphatic or blood vascular spaces.

Other Uses of Endoscopy and Biopsy

Aside from the overt carcinomatous lesion, there is a strong likelihood that the patient has additional adenomas in other parts of the colon, and endoscopy is typically done to survey the entire area.[114, 275, 276] Furthermore, following surgical resection, there remains an increased chance for these patients to develop other adenomas and carcinomas. Accordingly, such patients are routinely surveyed by endoscopy to look for and to remove any polyps, and this clearly helps in preventing the development of future carcinomas of the colon and rectum.

Endoscopy may also be done to evaluate the effects or complications of therapy, such as any injury from radiation or chemotherapeutic agents or any erosions that develop in the anastomotic area.[277] In all such cases, biopsy helps to distinguish the inflammatory lesions from recurrent tumor.

Variant Forms

As indicated in the previous section, it is common to find neuroendocrine cells scattered throughout tumors that are otherwise adenocarcinomas, and this has no significance.

Paneth Cell Adenocarcinoma

Occasional adenocarcinomas have a few Paneth cells but this is rarely a conspicuous finding.[95, 96] An adenocarcinoma containing abundant Paneth cells has been described, with the suggestion that they might represent better-differentiated tumors with a favorable prognosis, but more studies are needed[278] (Table 10-14). Biopsies simply show adenocarcinoma together with the plentiful Paneth cells. The only potential problem would be to miss the diagnosis of malignancy because of the finding of the Paneth cells, since they

Table 10-14. Types of Malignant Colonic Tumors

Adenocarcinoma
Variants of adenocarcinoma
Paneth cell adenocarcinoma
Adenosquamous cell carcinoma
Carcinosarcoma
Endometrioid carcinoma
Endocrine tumors
Carcinoid and composite tumors
Neuroendocrine carcinoma
Malignant lymphoma
Sarcomas
Rare primary tumors
Squamous cell carcinoma
Choriocarcinoma
Cloacogenic carcinoma
Malignant melanoma
Secondary and metastatic tumors

are more commonly seen in benign adenomas and in inflammatory conditions.

Adenosquamous Cell Carcinoma

Adenosquamous cell carcinomas are rare tumors in which one can find foci of squamous differentiation in tumors that are otherwise of a glandular type[279–281] (see Fig. 3-17). The squamous cells can vary in differentiation, resembling benign or malignant tissue. The overall behavior is that of the adenocarcinoma. Biopsies show the combination and can cause problems if only the squamous element is seen in small samples.

Carcinosarcoma

Carcinosarcoma is a rare finding in which there is association of both glandular elements and spindle cell forms[282] (see Fig. 3-10). These are currently believed to be mainly of epithelial origin, with the spindle elements representing either undifferentiated tumor or reactive cells. Cytochemical stains and electron microscopy can help in confirming the predominant epithelial nature of the tumor. Again, small biopsies may underestimate the glandular component. Since sarcomas are generally rare in the colon, multiple sections or biopsies should be sought to determine the adenocarcinoma component.

Endometrioid Adenocarcinoma

Endometrioid adenocarcinomas are rare tumors, developing in foci of colonic endometriosis.[283] The lesion can be suspected by noting the tall columnar cells with ciliated border and without mucin granules. The diagnosis would be secured by finding the benign endometrial tissue in the adjacent tissue or in prior biopsies from that area.

OTHER TUMORS

Compared to adenocarcinoma, other tumors of the colon and rectum are all uncommon (Table 10-14).

Endocrine Tumors

Endocrine tumors are those that develop from the neuroendocrine cells that are scattered throughout the gut.[284] Although the number of cells in the intestine is plentiful, endocrine tumors in the large intestine are uncommon compared to the mid- and upper portions of the digestive tract.[285–287]

Carcinoid Tumors

Carcinoid tumors are uncommon and usually located in the distal colon and rectum.[288–290] The clinical presentation is variable, depending on the size and presumably the duration of the tumor. Earlier lesions are polypoid and tend to have an excellent prognosis following local resection. More advanced tumors reveal ulceration and are often more aggressive.

Biopsies are characteristic, revealing nests and sheets of extremely uniform cells with central peppered nuclei and finely granular cytoplasm (Fig. 10-29). The endocrine nature of the cells is readily provided by supportive stains such as those for chromagranin and synaptophysin.[291] The tumor cells also stain for argyrophylic reactions such as Grimelius' stain but are typically negative for the argentaffinic stains.[292] Accordingly, functional carcinoid tumors in this area are rare.[293] The nature of the cells can also be readily confirmed by electron microscopy, which shows the characteristic neuroendocrine granules in the cytoplasm.

Very tiny tumors, termed *microcarcinoids,* are seen in patients with ulcerative colitis (Fig. 10-20). These are not grossly evident and are typically detected in a rectal biopsy

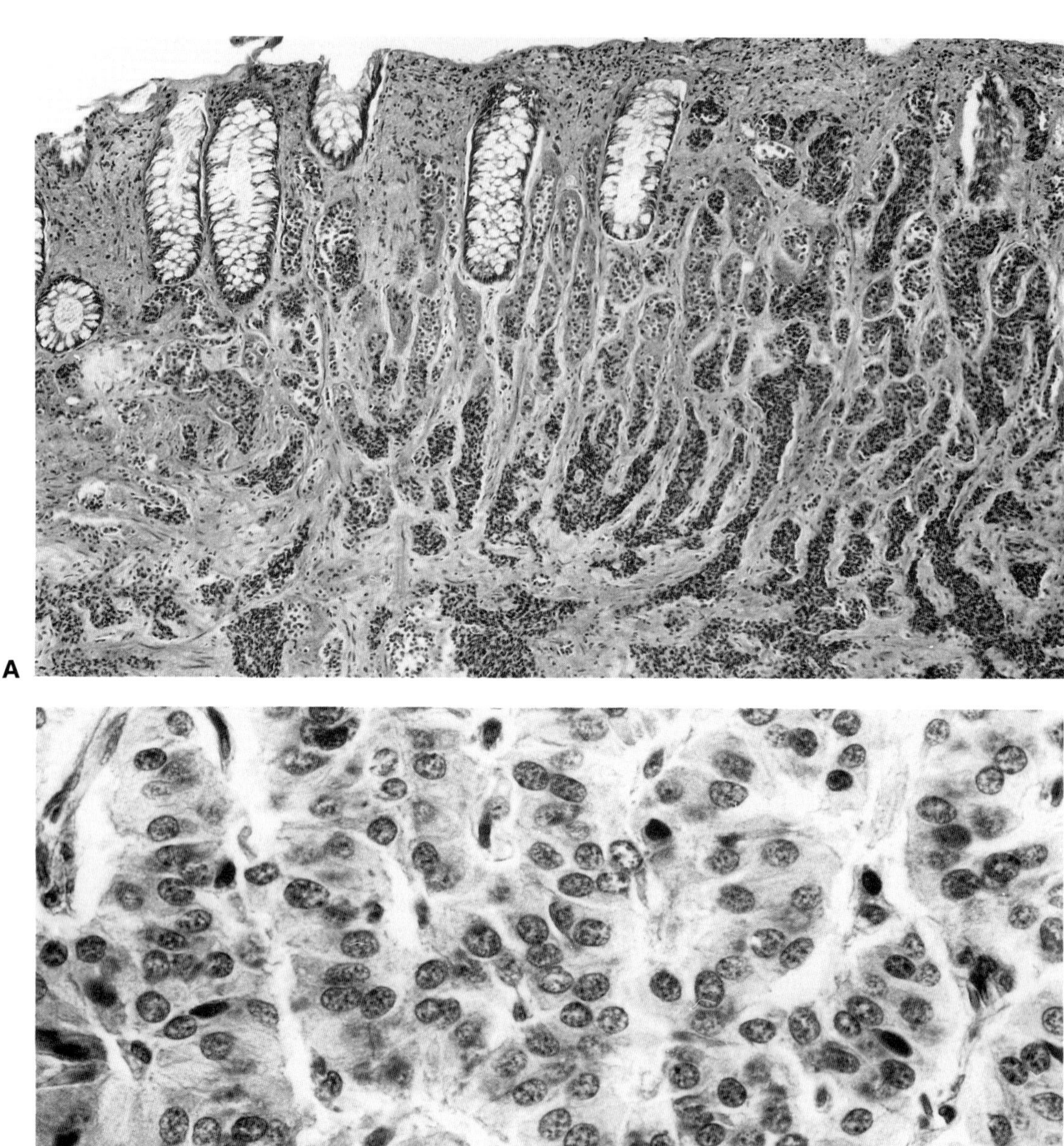

Fig. 10-29. Carcinoid tumor of the colon. **(A)** There are sheets and cords of monomorphic cells in the mucosa and the submucosa. Scattered crypts are present near the surface (top) (× 105). **(B)** Closer view of tumor, showing regularity of the cells and the finely stippled nuclei (× 635).

that is performed for other reasons.[185, 186] (See above section on "Tumors in Inflammatory Bowel Disease" for details.)

Composite Tumors

Composite tumors represent those that contain a considerable admixture of adenocarcinoma and carcinoid component.[294–296] As discussed in the section on Adenocarcinoma, it is common to find scattered endocrine cells within tumors that are otherwise adenocarcinomas, and these behave as such.[273, 292] The composite tumors are diagnosed only when there is a substantial component of both elements. They also have been referred to as adenocarcinoid tumors and as goblet cell carcinoids (Fig. 10-30). They are much more commonly seen in the appendix but can involve any part of the colon.[297] Their behavior seems to be more aggressive than that of pure carcinoid tumors and is probably similar to that of adenocarcinomas.

Biopsies reveal the mixture of glandular and endocrine cells, and these can be supported by the stains for mucin and for the endocrine granules. Also identified are individual tumor cells that contain both elements.

Neuroendocrine Carcinoma

Neuroendocrine carcinoma also has been referred to as small cell carcinoma and corresponds to the poorly differentiated and most aggressive form of neuroendocrine tumors in the gut.[298–300] Within the large intestine, the tumors are more often noted in the cecal and right colon region. They may occur alone or in combination with other areas revealing more mature glandular or endocrine elements.

Biopsies show poorly differentiated tumor, and immunocytochemical stains and electron microscopy are often needed to distinguish a highly undifferentiated carcinoma from the neuroendocrine tumor[301, 302] (see Fig. 3-19).

Lymphoid Tumors

Lymphoid Hyperplasia

Lymphoid hyperplasia presents as a nodular or, less commonly, as a diffuse area of proliferation of lymphoid tssue.[303, 304] It is most commonly seen in the rectum but can occur in any other part of the colon, and it usually appears as a polypoid lesion. Biopsies reveal very large lymphoid follicles with prominent centers showing a heterogeneity of the cells, surrounded by a large number of mature lymphocytes (Fig. 10-31). These have also been referred to as benign lymphoid polyps.[65, 66]

A lesser degree of lymphoid hyperplasia is more often noted and can be seen in any chronic inflammatory process involving the colon, either of a segmental or diffuse nature. These do not typically cause grossly large nodules or present as polyps, but may appear as areas of granularity.[305] Biopsy reveals the lymphoid hyperplasia and also the other features of active or chronic colitis. Biopsies of the colon may also show prominent lymphoid nodules but be otherwise normal. It has been suggested that this represents a healing phase, and the lymphoid tissue eventually disappears.

Malignant Lymphoma

The large intestine is the least common site for the development of primary malignant lymphoma of the gut.[306–309] The tumors are more often seen in the distal colon and rectal area and present as segmental, nodular, or ulcerated lesions.[310–312] An increase of lymphomas localized to the lower rectal and anal region has been noted in homosexual males, including those with AIDS, possibly

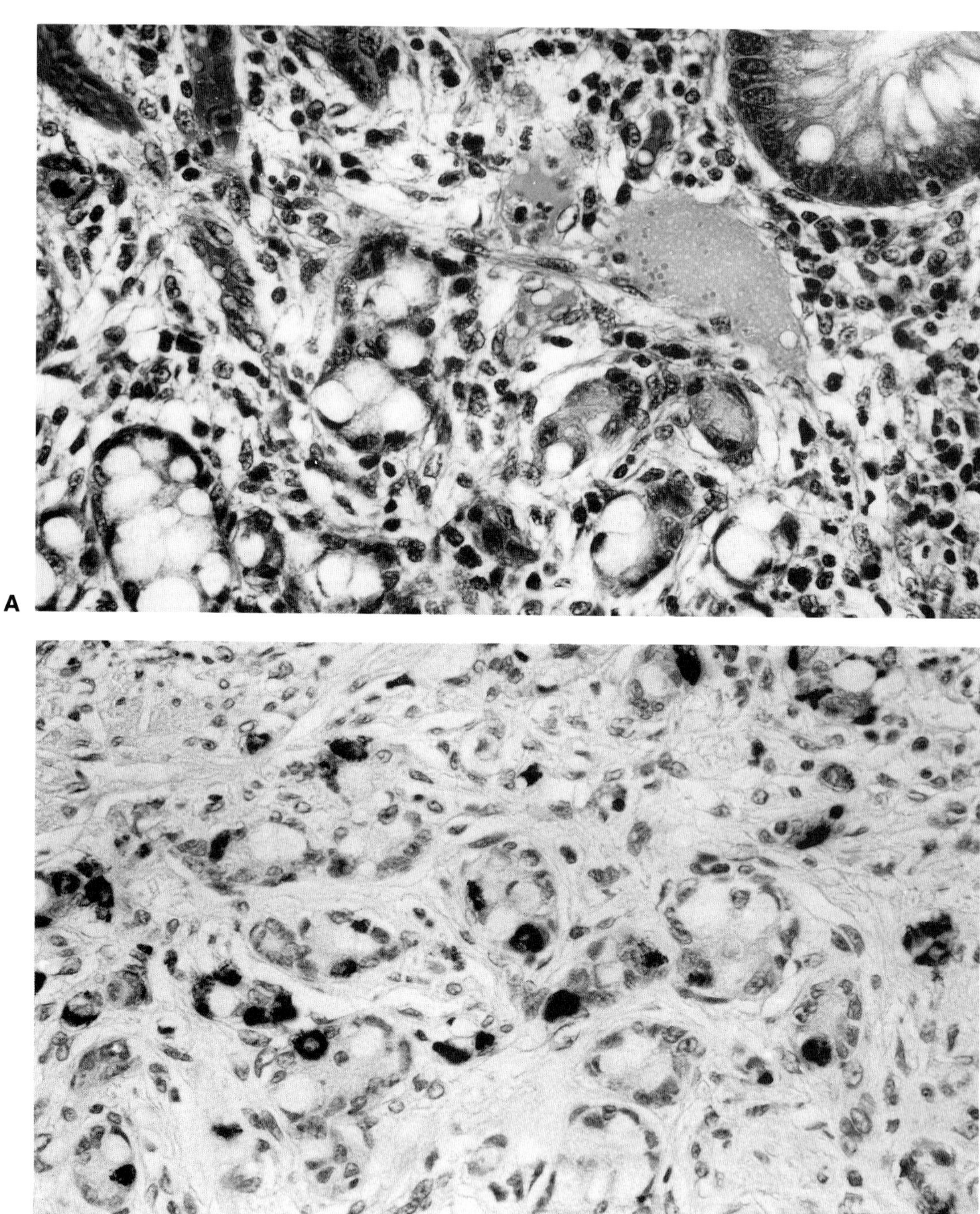

Fig. 10-30. Goblet cell carcinoid tumor. **(A)** Noted are small clumps of tumor cells with evident mucin in their cytoplasm. A part of a normal crypt appears at the upper right (× 425). **(B)** Chromogranin stain for endocrine cells, revealing positive cytoplasmic stain in many of the tumor cells (× 425).

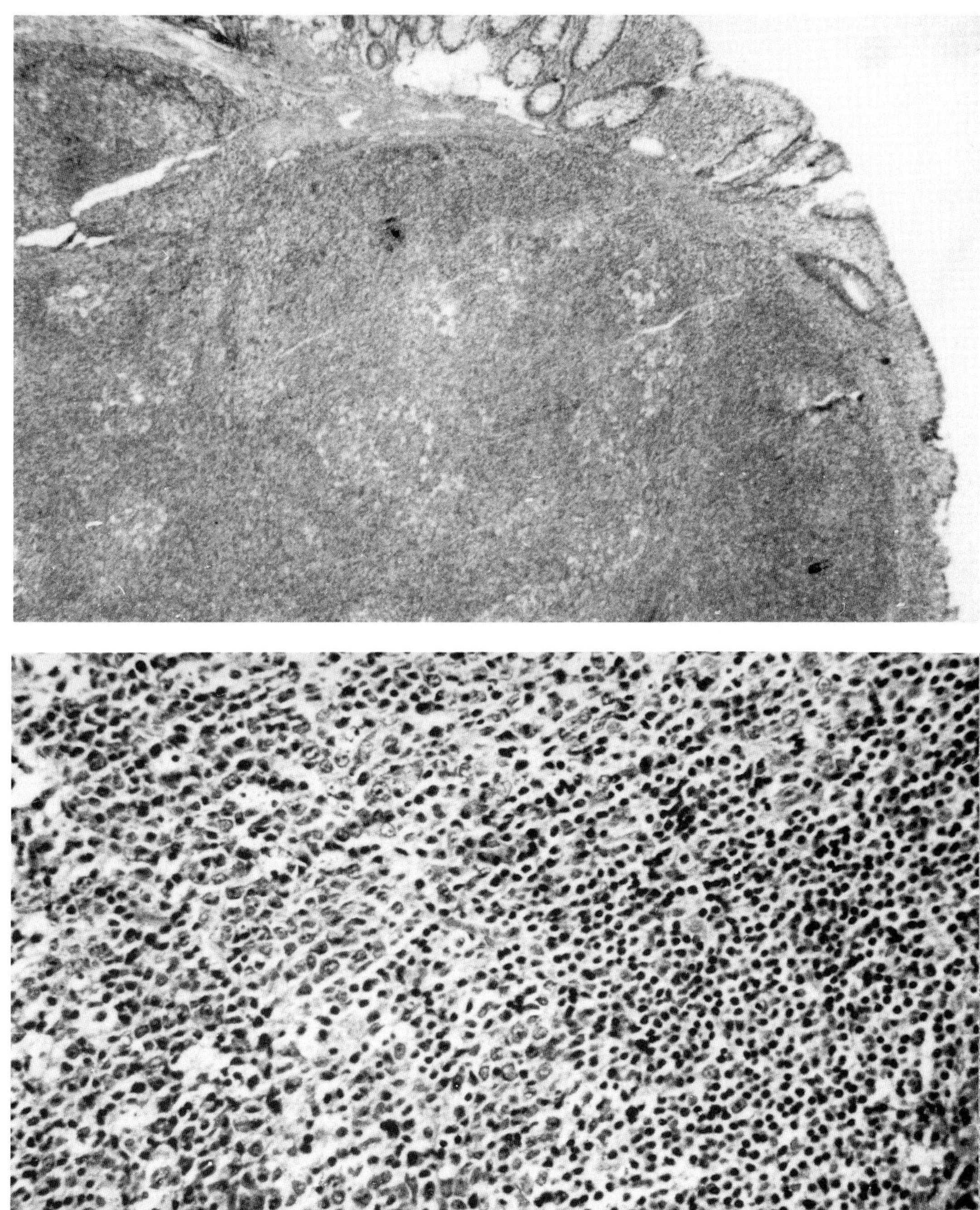

Fig. 10-31. Benign lymphoid polyp of the rectum. **(A)** The polyp is formed by a mass of lymphoid tissue in which there are several well formed follicles. The normal mucosa at the edge of the lesion is seen at the top. **(B)** Closer view of polyp, showing large follicular areas.

related to an increase of infections in this region.[313, 314] Lymphomas of the colon also have been seen in cases of long-standing colitis and as a late consequence of radiation.[181–183, 315]

As in other parts of the tract, most of the tumors are of the B-cell type and they can vary from highly differentiated nodular forms to the large cell types (Fig. 10-32). The former are differentiated from benign lymphoid hyperplasia by noting the greater homogeneity of the cells in the center of the nodules and the less mature lymphocytes in the surrounding tissue. In the more differentiated cases, marker studies may be required to look for monoclonality in securing the diagnosis.[316, 317]

The large cell type of lymphoma may resemble the undifferentiated forms of carcinoma, but these can readily be separated by immunocytochemical stains for leukocyte common antigen. More diffuse lymphoid tumors, such as lymphomatous polyposis and secondary tumor infiltrates, can also affect the colon, and there are rare reports of plasmacytoma.[318–320] In all of these cases, biopsy is done to provide the diagnosis.

Mesenchymal Tumors

Most of the mesenchymal tumors tumors are contained in the bowel wall and do not present at endoscopy.[321] As the lesions enlarge, however, they can project into the lumen or press on the mucosa, causing secondary ulceration. Some of the softer tumors residing mainly in the submucosa, such as lipomas, also can be causes of intussusception. Many of the diagnoses are suggested by radiographic and endoscopic studies, and biopsies indicate the specific type. In many instances, the superficial biopsies may reveal

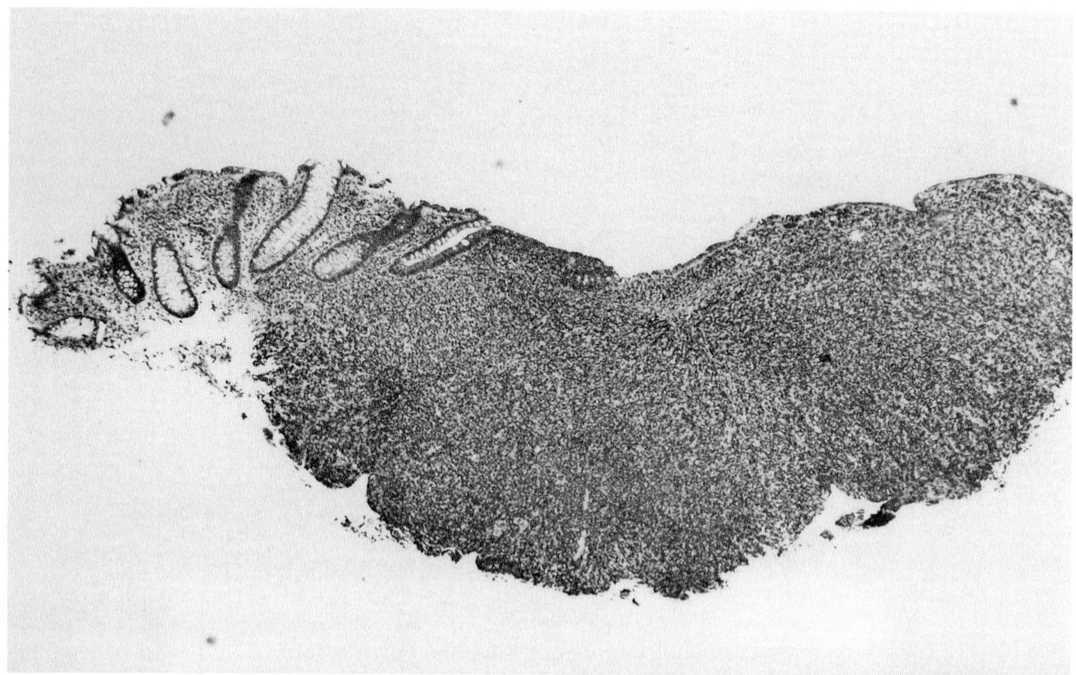

Fig. 10-32. Lymphomatous polyposis in the colon. The mass is compromised of a dense infiltrate of lymphoid cells without follicle formation. A small portion of the normal mucosa appears at the left (× 56).

only the overlying mucosa and serve to rule out an epithelial cause for the polyp or mass.

Smooth Muscle Tumors

Leiomyomas are most often found in the esophagus and stomach.[322, 323] A small mature leiomyoma can arise from the muscularis mucosae in the colon and present as a small polyp, usually in the distal portion. Biopsies reveal the nodule that is comprised of mature smooth muscle tissue and covered by a normal or slightly atrophic mucosa (Fig. 10-33). These are benign lesions and readily excised by the polypectomy.

The smooth muscle tumors located in the deeper portions of the wall, particularly in the muscularis propria, are more often malignant.[324–326] These can extend, as they enlarge, into the mucosal area causing compression, erosion, and rare polyp formation. Biopsies show a spindle cell tumor with elongated, irregular nuclei and numerous mitoses. It is important to distinguish this from a poorly differentiated spindle cell area in a carcinoma. Cytochemical stains for vimentin and muscle antigens as well as electron microscopy can be helpful.

Stromal Tumors

Some of the mesenchymal tumors lack complete differentiation and resemble the stromal tumors seen in the stomach and duodenum[321, 327] (see Figs. 5-24 and 5-25). These may stain for a variety of cytochemical markers of muscle and nervous substances, whereas electron microscopy typically fails to show complete differentiation.[328–330] In contrast to the tumors in the upper part of the gut, the stromal lesions in the colon tend to be more aggressive. The lesions are located in the wall and rarely extend into the mucosa to permit a biopsy.

Granular Cell Tumors

Granular cell tumors can occur in any part of the gut and present as single or multiple nodules extending from the submucosa into the mucosa.[331–333] They typically have a smooth surface, are sessile, and biopsies are characteristic, revealing large cells with small nuclei and a granular cytoplasm that stains moderately with the PAS reaction (see Figs. 3-21 and 5-29). The lesions need to be distinguished from nodules of macrophages that contain vacuolated or storage material. The granular cell tumors are typically benign and treated by local excision.

Neural Tumors

Mucosal neuromas consisting of a benign proliferation of the nerves, alone or together with increased ganglia, can be seen in some of the multiple endocrine neoplasia syndromes.[68, 168] These can also present as small polyps in Cowden syndrome[166, 167] (see above section on Polyps). Isolated benign schwannomas can occur and must be distinguished from leiomyomas and the less differentiated stromal tumors.[334]

A variety of soft tissue tumors can appear in the gut in patients with von Recklinghausen's disease.[335, 336] These include neurofibromas, schwannomas, ganglioneuromas, and various sarcomas. These are typically located in the wall and rarely reach the mucosa to allow for a diagnostic biopsy.

Adipose Tissue Tumors

Commonly noted in the region of the ileocecal valve is an increase in the adipose tissue that represents a simple hyperplastic process. This usually causes no problems; and biopsies show mature adipose tissue and serve to rule out other more significant lesions[337] (see Fig. 8-10).

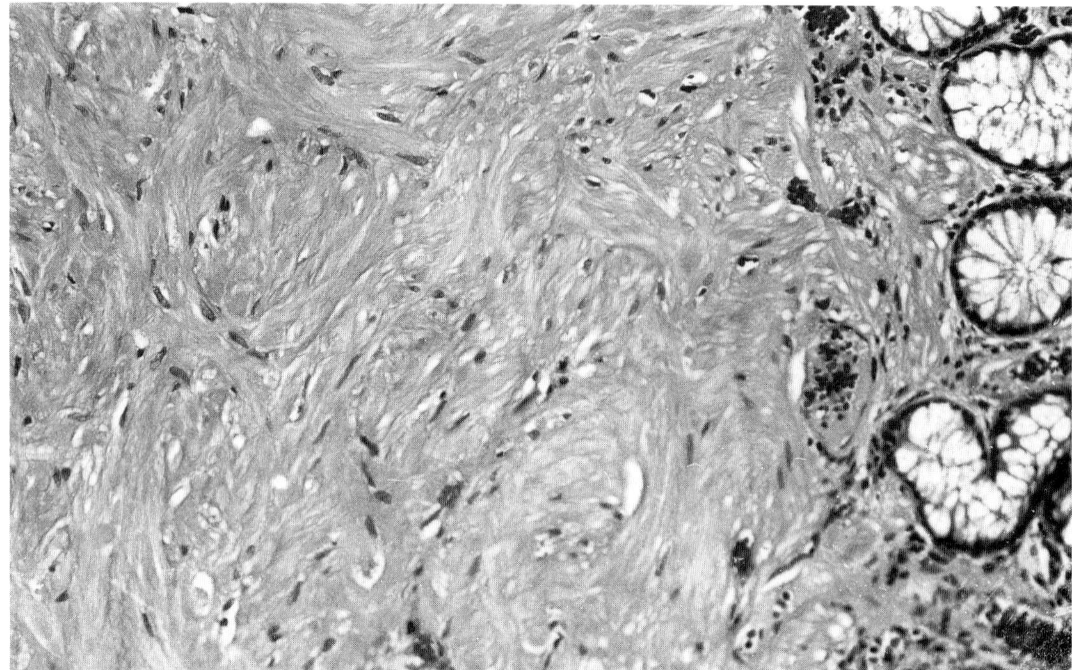

Fig. 10-33. Leiomyoma of the muscularis mucosae in the rectum. The lower part of the crypts appears at the right. The tumor is comprised of closely packed spindle cells and intercellular collagen, without cytologic atypism (× 210).

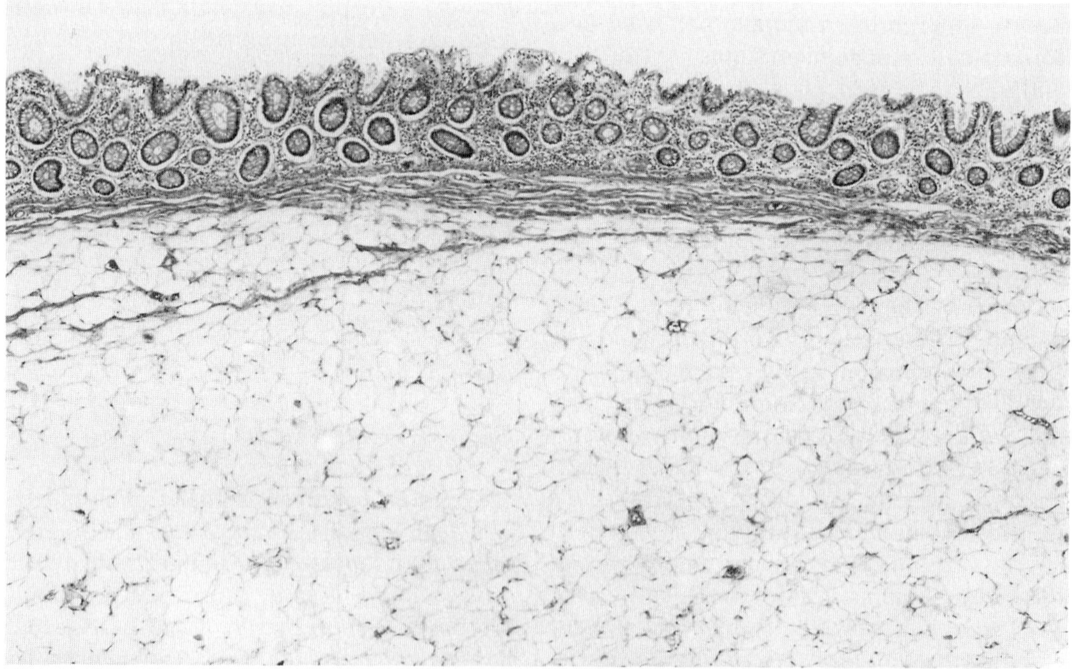

Fig. 10-34. Lipoma of the colon. The tumor is located in the submucosa and consists of mature adipose tissue. There is slight compression of the overlying mucosa (top) (× 42).

One of the more common submucosal tumors that extends into the bowel lumen of the large intestine is the lipoma, which consists of mature adipose tissue[338–340] (Fig. 10-34). These are usually grossly evident by their sessile and very soft nature. Rarely, these or other submucosal tumors that project into the lumen can serve as the lead point of an intussusception.

Fibrous Tissue Tumors

Inflammatory fibroid polyps are uncommon in the colon and must be distinguished from the mesenchymal neoplasms[62, 63] (see above section on "Polyps"). Ordinary fibromas are not seen. Occasional polyps are encountered that contain a core of mature collagen and an overlying normal or atrophic mucosa (Fig. 10-35). These probably represent nodules of old trauma or inflammation with excess scar production. They typically are single lesions and do not recur.

There are rare examples of undifferentiated sarcomas, sometimes termed *fibrosarcoma,* and of malignant fibrous histiocytoma within the bowel wall, and these do not ordinarily extend into the mucosa.[321, 341] It is possible that some of the poorly differentiated tumors are examples of the stromal tumors.

Vascular Tumors

Vascular tumors are generally uncommon and include benign hamartomas of vascular elements, represented as hemangiomas or lymphangiomas.[342–345] Some of these can get large and require excision. Biopsy is ordinarily not obtained but may help in removal of polypoid lesions.[346]

Kaposi's sarcoma can involve any part of the gut including the large intestine, and is most commonly noted in patients with AIDS.[347–349] It typically presents with ulcerations, resembling colitis or tumor, and biopsies may contain just a small amount of the diagnostic tissue[350, 351] (Fig. 10-36). Revealed are compact spindle cells with atypism and areas of fresh and old hemorrhage (see Fig. 6-28). There are other rare malignant vascular tumors that can occur in the large bowel, including angiosarcomas and malignant hemangiopericytoma that are ordinarily diagnosed by resection.[352, 353]

Other Primary Tumors

Squamous Cell Carcinomas

Squamous cell carcinomas are usually located in the anal region and are rare in the large intestinal mucosa.[354–357] They have been noted in all parts of the colon and appear to be more common in tumors that occur within duplication cysts.[267] It is thought that they arise from areas of ectopic or metaplastic squamous epithelium in the colonic mucosa.[354, 358] More often noted are foci of squamous tissue in ordinary adenocarcinomas, termed *adenosquamous cell carcinoma,* or *adenocanthoma.* Biopsies of the tumors reveal the squamous elements, and it is important to review sufficient sections to ensure that it is a pure squamous carcinoma (Fig. 10-37).

Choriocarcinomas

Choriocarcinomas are rarely noted in the large intestine and can occur either as pure lesions or mixed with adenocarcinoma[359, 360] (see Fig. 3-26). They are typically diagnosed in a resection specimen and not by biopsy.

Rectal Tumors

Inflammatory Lesions

Represented are a mixture of inflammatory lesions affecting the lower rectum and adjacent anal area. Anal skin tags can en-

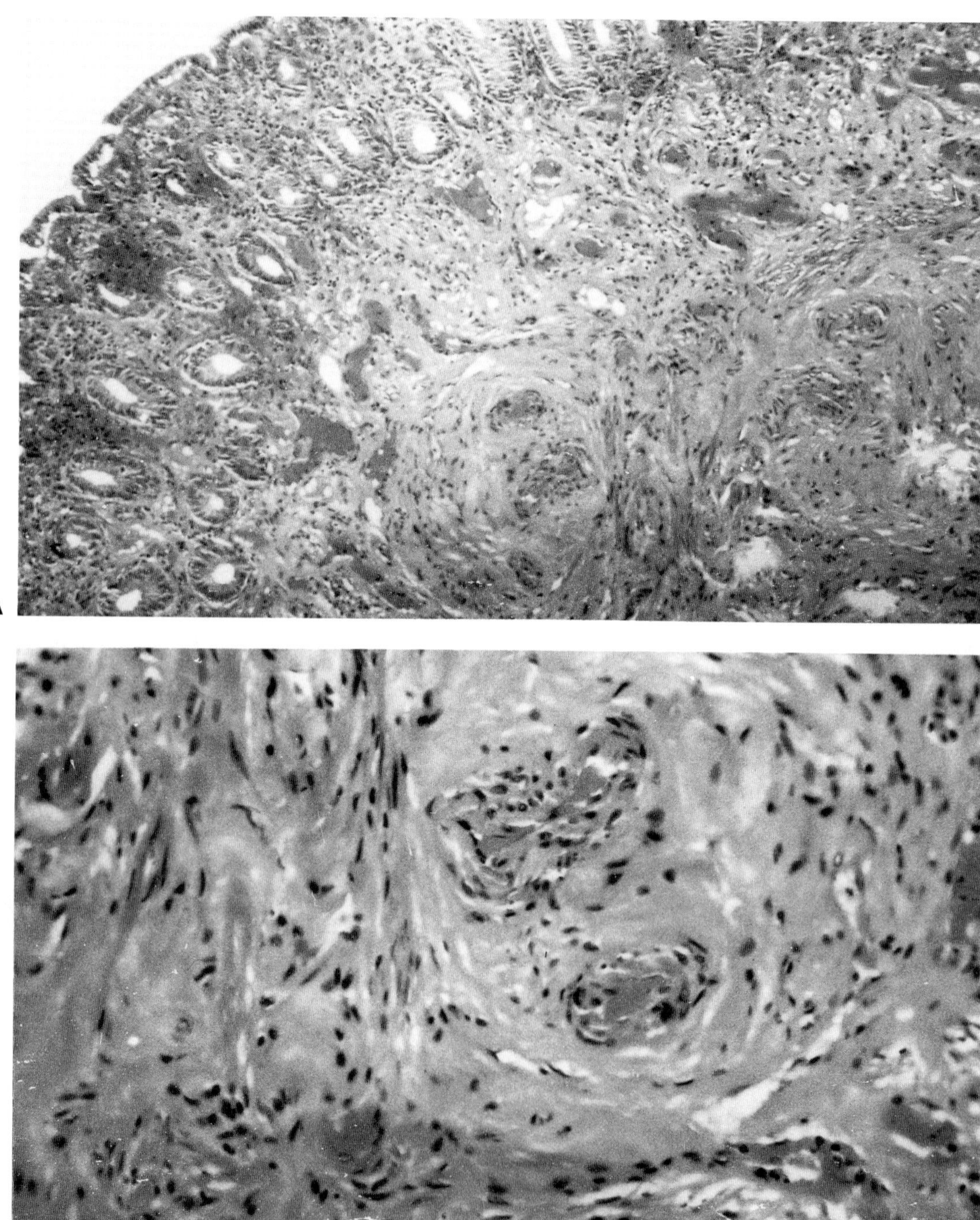

Fig. 10-35. Fibrous polyp of the colon. **(A)** The polyp is mainly formed of fibrovascular tissue with little inflammation. There is overlying mucosa appearing at the top and left. **(B)** Closer view of the core of polyp, showing the dense fibrous tissue and vessels.

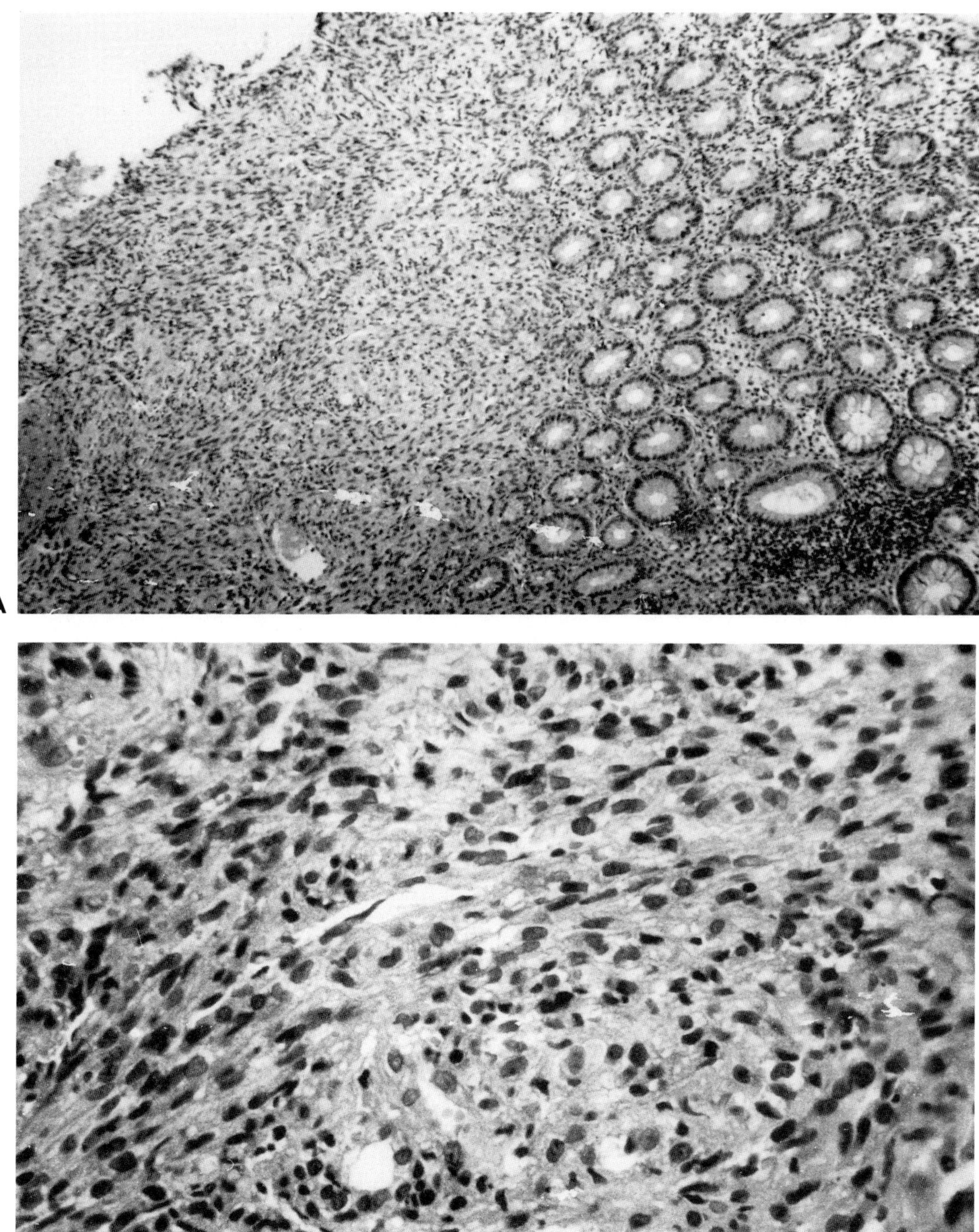

Fig. 10-36. Kaposi sarcoma of the colon. **(A)** Biopsy showing colonic mucosa (right) and a spindle cell lesion (left). **(B)** Closer view of tumor, revealing densely packed spindle cells. (See Fig. 6-28 of a Kaposi tumor in the small intestine.)

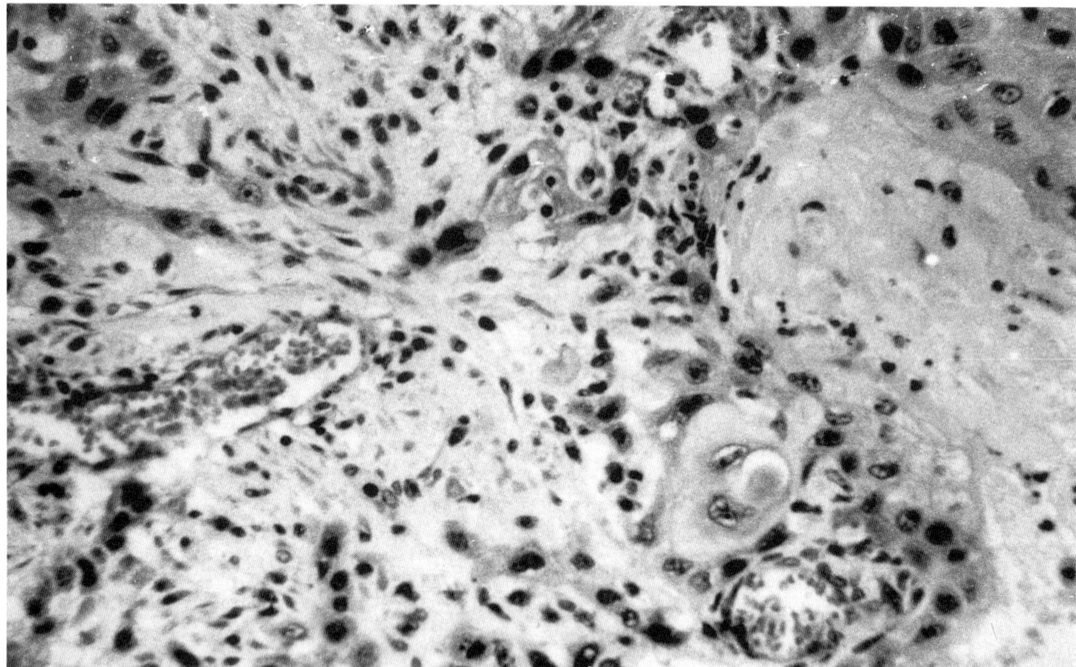

Fig. 10-37. Squamous cell carcinoma of the colon. Seen are sheets of squamous cells with focal keratin production. Multiple sections should be taken of such tumors to exclude a mixed adenosquamous cell carcinoma.

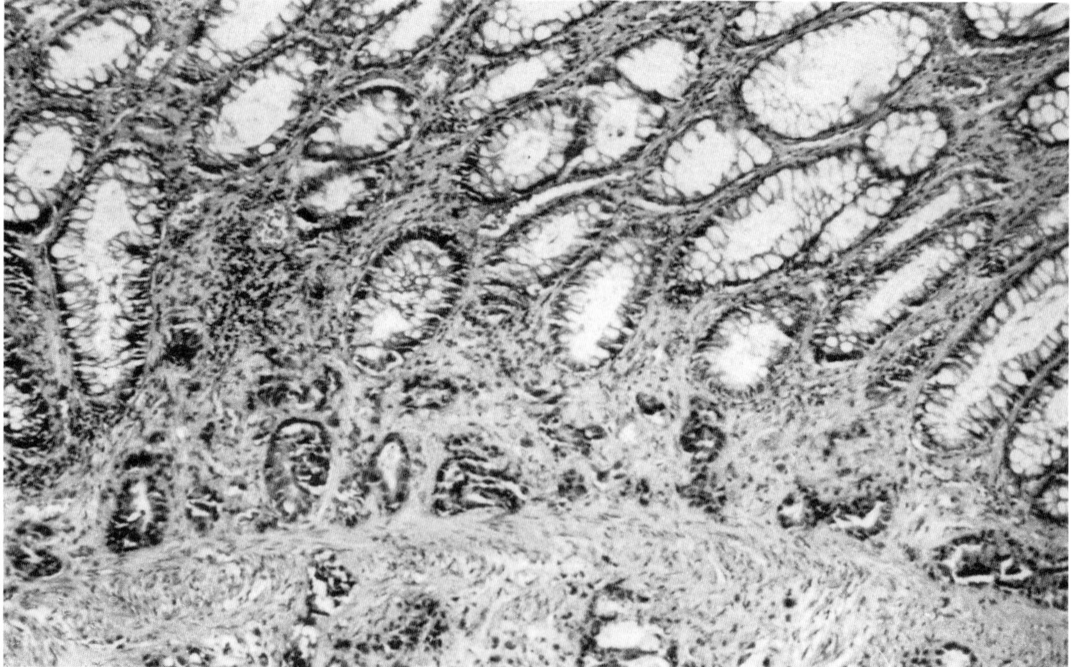

Fig. 10-38. Recurrent adenocarcinoma in the rectum. The malignant glands are present in the submucosa, muscularis, and basal part of the mucosa appearing at the bottom.

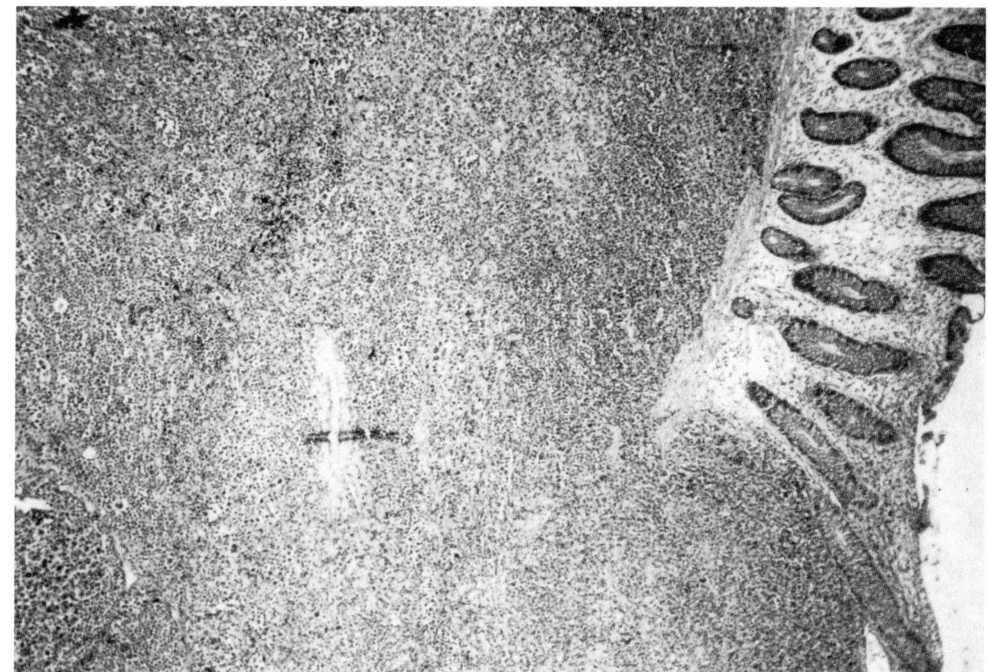

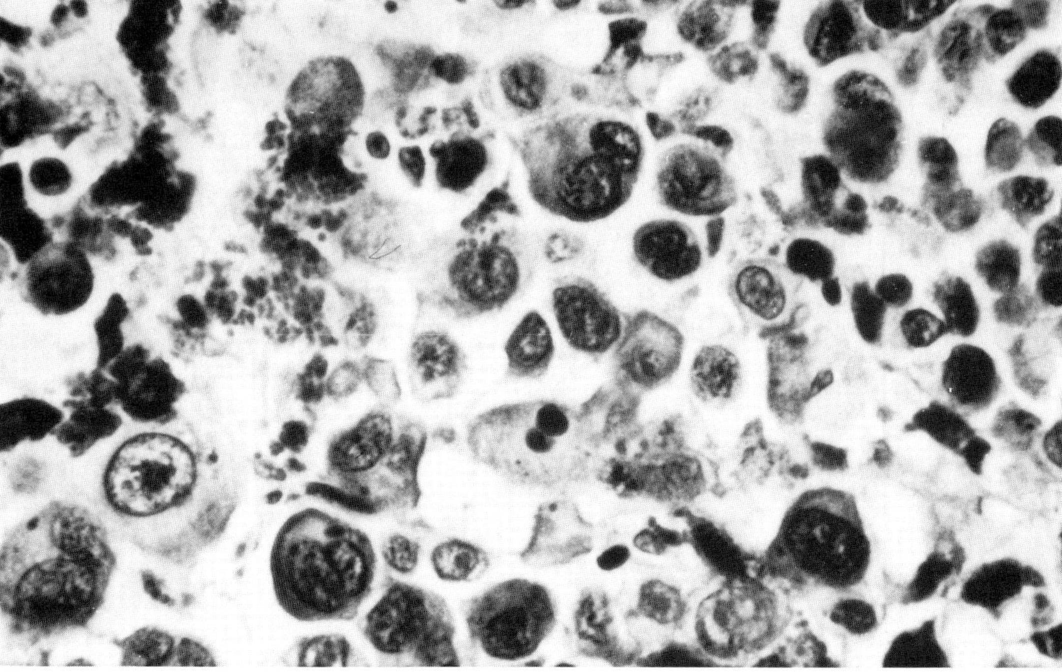

Fig. 10-39. Metastatic malignant melanoma in the colon, presenting as a polypoid lesion. **(A)** Mass of tumor in the bowel wall extends into the mucosa (lower right). A strip of normal mucosa appears at the upper right. **(B)** Closer view of tumor, showing diffuse sheet of malignant cells that contain abundant melanin pigment.

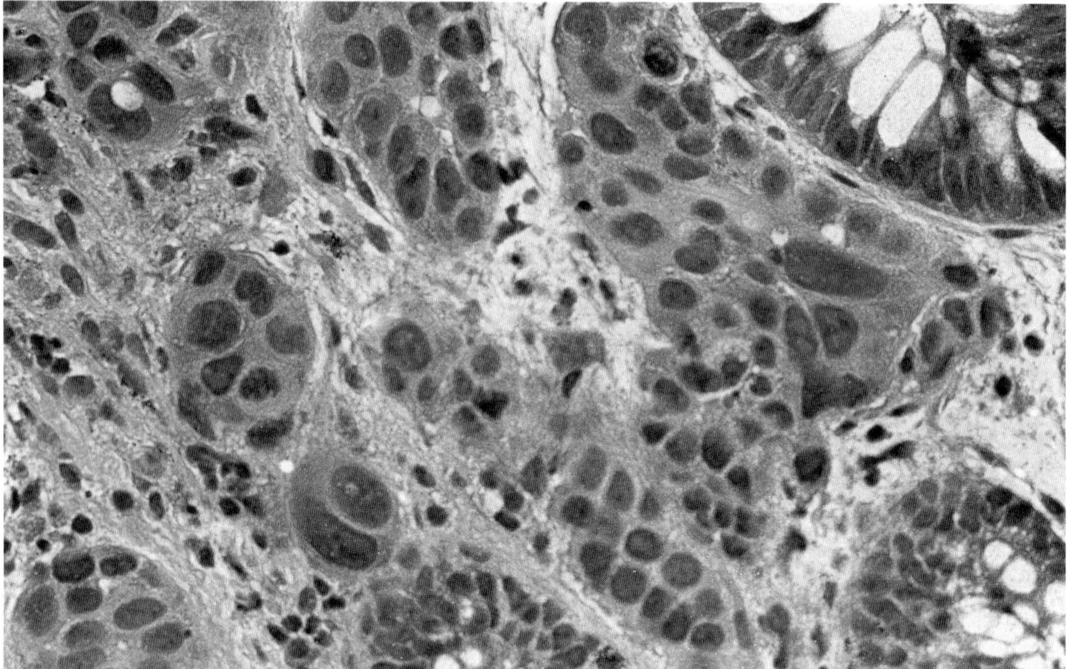

Fig. 10-40. Metastatic transitional cell carcinoma in the rectum. Colonic crypts are present in the upper and lower right. There are sheets of malignant cells with large and irregular nuclei (×425).

large and appear in the rectal area. They consist of a core of fibrovascular tissue covered by squamous epithelium. The solitary ulcer syndrome in its reparative phase can develop a prominent polyp, and this reveals a striking fibromuscular proliferation covered by serrated glands.[361, 362] This is discussed in Chapter 9.

Cloacogenic Carcinoma

Cloacogenic carcinoma typically occurs in the anal region and may extend into the lower rectum. There are rare instances of tumor development in higher sites within the rectum and the colon.[363, 364] Biopsies indicate the features of a poorly differentiated squamous or transitional tumor, usually associated with a predominance of basaloid cells (see Fig. 11-11).

Malignant Melanomas

Most of the melanomas seen in the rectum and colon are metastatic lesions. They can also develop in the anal region and rarely are primary in the rectum and lower colon[365–367] (see Fig. 3-23). They presumably arise from ectopic melanocytic tissue. Biopsies reveal the classical malignant cells with melanin pigment, and it is particularly important to exclude the much more common metastatic lesions that are frequently multiple, or a melanoma that has extended from the anal area.

Miscellaneous Tumors

There have been isolated reports of benign dermoid cyst and of cylindromatous carcinoma involving the rectum.[368, 369]

SECONDARY AND METASTATIC TUMORS

Secondary Tumors

There can be recurrence of adenocarcinoma that was previously treated and extension of tumors from adjacent tissues into the large intestine.[1, 2] The recurrent lesions show malignant glands concentrated in the submucosa (Fig. 10-38). Of the secondary tumors, most often noted is invasion of adenocarcinoma of the prostrate into the rectum, and this can appear as nodules in the submucosa or mucosa. Biopsies show the tumor cells that must be distinguished from a primary rectal carcinoma. Most of the prostratic carcinomas show more uniform cells with less nuclear atypism and uncommon mucus production. Of interest, they can sometimes resemble endocrine cell tumors. Immunocytochemical stains for acid phosphatase and for prostate specific antigen are particularly helpful in making the distinction. Other tumors that can locally invade include squamous cell carcinomas from the cervix and any other lesion that might be growing within the peritoneal cavity.

Metastatic Tumors

Metastases in the colon and rectum can derive from many types of malignant tumors. More commonly noted are nodules of Kaposi's sarcoma, of lymphomas and leukemias, and of malignant melanoma[349, 370–374] (Fig. 10-39). Less often seen are metastases of carcinomas from a large variety of tissues, including the stomach, pancreas, breast, lung, kidney, testis, and urinary bladder[2, 375–380] (Fig. 10-40). Most of the tumor nodules present as polyps that secondarily ulcerate.

Biopsy Uses

Biopsies serve to detect the tumor and occasionally reveal specific histologic features that help in determining its type. Clearly, the historical information is vital in such cases. Biopsies also are used to exclude other lesions that occur in tumor patients, including the effects of drugs and radiation as well as the appearance of opportunistic infections.

REFERENCES

1. Fenoglio-Preiser CM, Pascal RR, Perzin KH: Tumors of the intestines. Atlas of Tumor Pathology, second series, fascicle 27. Armed Forces Institute of Pathology, Washington, DC, 1990
2. Ming S-C: Adenocarcinoma and other malignant epithelial tumors of the intestines. pp. 816–857. In Ming S-C, Goldman H (eds): Pathology of the Gastrointestinal Tract. WB Saunders, Philadelphia, 1992
3. Jass JR, Sabin LH, Watanabe H: The World Health Organization's histologic classification in gastrointestinal tumors. A commentary on the second edition. Cancer 66:2162–2167, 1990
4. Reilly JC, Theuerkauf FJ Jr, Rusin LC: Colonoscopy: its role in cancer of the colon and rectum. Dis Colon Rectum 25:532–538, 1982
5. Hunt RH, Cotton PB, Crespi M et al: Role of endoscopy in the diagnosis of cancer. Cancer Res 49:6822–6827, 1989
6. Kline TS, Yum KK: Fiberoptic colonoscopy and cytology. Cancer 37:2553, 1976
7. Winawer SJ, Leidner SD, Hajdu SI, Sherlock P: Colonoscopic biopsy and cytology in the diagnosis of colon cancer. Cancer 42:2849, 1978
8. Jeevanandom V, Treat MR, Forde KA: A comparison of direct brush cytology and biopsy in the diagnosis of colorectal cancer. Gastrointest Endosc 33:370–371, 1987
9. Melville DM, Richman PI, Shepherd NA et al: Brush cytology of the colon and rectum in ulcerative colitis: an aid to cancer diagnosis. J Clin Pathol 41:1180–1186, 1988
10. Ehya H, O'Hara BJ: Brush cytology in the diagnosis of colonic neoplasms. Cancer 66:1563–1567, 1990
11. Marshall JB, Diaz-arias AA, Barthel JS et al: Prospective evaluation of optimal number of biopsy specimens and brush cytology in the

diagnosis of cancer of the colorectum. Am J Gastroenterol 88:1352–1354, 1993

12. Rosman AS, Federman Q, Feinman L: Diagnosis of colon cancer by lavage cytology with an orally administered balanced electrolyte solution. Am J Gastroenterol 89:51–56, 1994
13. Zargar SA, Khuroo MS, Mahajan R et al: Endoscopic fine needle aspiration cytology in the diagnosis of gastro-esophageal and colorectal malignancies. Gut 32:745–748, 1991
14. Hickey WF, Seiler MW: Ultrastructural markers of colonic adenocarcinoma. Cancer 47:140–145, 1981
15. Borkje B, Hostmark J, Shagen DN et al: Flow cytometry of biopsy specimens from ulcerative colitis, colorectal adenomas, and carcinomas. Scand J Gastroenterol 22:1231–1237, 1987
16. Banner BF, Chacho MS, Roseman DL, Coon JS: Multiparameter flow cytometric analysis of colon polyps. Am J Surg Pathol 87:313–318, 1987
17. Fischbach W, Zidianakis Z, Luke G et al: DNA mapping of colorectal neoplasms: a flow cytometric study of DNA abnormalities and proliferation. Gastroenterology 105: 1126–1133, 1993
18. Bosari S, Lee AKC, Wiley BD et al: Flow cytometric and image analyses of colorectal adenocarcinoma. A comparative study with clinical correlations. Am J Clin Pathol 99:187–194, 1993
19. Bottinger TC, Potratz D, Stockle M et al: Prognostic value of DNA analysis in colorectal carcinoma. Cancer 72:3579–3587, 1993
20. Lanza G, Maestri I, Ballotta MR: Relationship of nuclear DNA content to clinicopathologic features in colorectal cancer. Modern Pathol 7:161–165, 1994
21. Vogelstein B, Fearon ER, Nakamura Y et al: Genetic alterations during colorectal tumor development. N Engl J Med 319:525–532, 1988
22. Hamilton SR: The molecular genetics of colorectal neoplasia. Gastroenterology 105:3–7, 1993
23. Kinzler KW, Vogelstein B, Nakamura Y: Identification of FAP locus gene from chromosome 5q21. Science 253:661–665, 1991
24. Powell SM, Petersen GM, Krush AJ, et al: Molecular diagnosis of familial adenomatous polyposis. N Engl J Med 329:1982–1987, 1993
25. Tsao J-I, Shibata D: Short communication. Further evidence that one of the earliest alterations in colorectal carcinogenesis involves APC. Am J Pathol 145:531–534, 1994
26. Chang F, Syrjanen S, Kurinen K, Syrjanen K: The p53 tumor suppressor gene as a common cellular target in human carcinogenesis. Am J Gastroenterol 88:174–186, 1993
27. Kaklamanis L, Gatter KC, Mortensen N, et al: p53 expression in colorectal adenomas. Am J Pathol 142:87–93, 1993
28. Hamelin R, Laurent-Puig P, Olschwang S et al: Association of p53 mutations with short survival in colorectal cancer. Gastroenterology 106:42–48, 1993
29. Magrisso IJ, Richmond RE, Carter JH et al: Immunohistochemical detection of RAS, JUN, FOS, and p53 oncoprotein expression in human colorectal adenomas and carcinomas. Lab Invest 69:674–681, 1993
30. Benkattor J, Losi L, Chaubert P et al: Prognostic significance of K-ras mutations in colorectal carcinoma. Gastroenterology 104: 1044–1048, 1993
31. Jen J, Kim H, Piantadosi S et al: Allelic loss of chromosome 18q and prognosis in colorectal cancer. N Engl J Med 331:213–221, 1994
32. Iino H, Fukayama M, Maeda Y et al: Molecular genetics for clinical management of colorectal carcinoma. 17p, 18q, and 22q loss of heterozygosity and decreased DCC expression are correlated with the metastatic potential. Cancer 73:1324–1331, 1994
33. Kim H, Jen J, Vogelstein B et al: Clinical and pathological characteristics of sporadic colorectal carcinomas with DNA replication errors in microsatellite sequences. Am J Pathol 145:148–156, 1994
34. Kubben FJ, Peeters-Haesevoets A, Engels LG et al: Proliferating cell nuclear antigen (PCNA): a new marker to study human colonic cell proliferation. Gut 35:530–535, 1994
35. Linden MD, MA CK, Kubus J, Brown RD, Zarbo RJ: Ki-67 and proliferating cell nuclear antigen tumor proliferative indices in DNA diploid colorectal adenocarcinomas. Correlation with histopathologic characteristics and cell cycle analysis with two-color

DNA flow cytometry. Am J Clin Pathol 100:206–212, 1993

36. Al-Sheneber IF, Shibata HR, Sampalis J, Jothy S: Prognostic significance of proliferating cell nuclear antigen expression in colorectal cancer. Cancer 71:1954–1959, 1993
37. Teixeira CR, Tanaka S, Haruma K et al: Proliferating cell nuclear antigen expression at the invasive tumor margin predicts malignant potential of colorectal carcinomas. Cancer 73:575–579, 1994
38. Andrews Jr CW, Jessup JM, Goldman H et al: Localization of tumor-associated glycoprotein DF3 in normal, inflammatory, and neoplastic lesions of the colon. Cancer 72:3185–3190, 1993
39. Mulder JWR, Wielenga VJM, Polak MM et al: Expression of mutant p53 protein and CD44 variant proteins in colorectal tumorigenesis. Gut 36:76–80, 1995
40. Listron MB, Fenoglio-Preiser C: Short course. Gastrointestinal polyps. Modern Pathol 2:161–181, 1989
41. Cooper HS: Benign polyps of the intestines. pp. 786–815. In Ming S-C, Goldman H (eds): Pathology of the Gastrointestinal Tract. WB Saunders, Philadelphia, 1992
42. Teague RH, Read AE: Polyposis in ulcerative colitis. Gut 16:792, 1975
43. Kelly JK, Langevin JM, Price IM et al: Giant and symptomatic inflammatory polyps of the colon in idiopathic inflammatory bowel disease. Am J Surg Pathol 10:420–428, 1986
44. Hinrichs HR, Goldman H: Localized giant pseudopolyposis of the colon. JAMA 205:248, 1968
45. Goldenberg B, Mori K, Friedman IH et al: Fused inflammatory polyps simulating carcinoma in ulcerative colitis. Am J Gastroenterol 73:441, 1980
46. Bronza JP, Fisher RL, Barwick KW: Filiform polyposis: an unusual complication of inflammatory bowel disease. J Clin Gastroenterol 7:451–458, 1985
47. Jessurun J, Paplanus SH, Nagle RB et al: Pseudosarcomatous changes in inflammatory pseudopolyps of the colon. Arch Pathol Lab Med 110:883–886, 1986
48. Roth SI, Helwig EB: Juvenile polyps of the colon and rectum. Cancer 16:468–479, 1963
49. Nugent KB, Talbot IC, Hodgson SV, Phillips RKS: Solitary juvenile polyps: not a marker for subsequent malignancy. Gastroenterology 105:698–700, 1993
50. Arthur JF: Structure and significance of metaplastic nodules in the rectal mucosa. J Clin Pathol 21:735, 1968
51. Goldman H, Ming S-C, Hickok DF: Nature and significance of hyperplastic polyps of the human colon. Arch Pathol 89:349–354, 1970
52. Kaye GI, Fenoglio CM, Pascal RR, Lane N: Comparative electron microscopic features of normal, hyperplastic and adenomatous human colonic epithelium. Gastroenterology 64:926–945, 1973
53. Jass JR, Filipe MI, Abbas S et al: A morphologic and histochemical study of metaplastic polyps of the colorectum. Cancer 53:510–515, 1984
54. Williams GT, Arthur JF, Bussey HJR et al: Metaplastic polyps and polyposis of the colorectum. Histopathology 4:155, 1980
55. Hayashi T, Yatoni R, Apostol J et al: Pathogenesis of hyperplastic polyps of the colon: a hypothesis based on ultrastructure and in vitro cell kinetics. Gastroenterology 66:347, 1974
56. Sobin LH: Inverted hyperplastic polyps of the colon. Am J Surg Pathol 9:265–272, 1985
57. Shepherd NA: Inverted hyperplastic polyposis of the colon. J Clin Pathol 46:56–60, 1993
58. Longacre TA, Fenoglio-Preiser CM: Mixed hyperplastic adenomatous polyps/serrated adenomas. A distinct form of colorectal neoplasia. Am J Surg Pathol 14:524–537, 1990
59. Lillemoe T, Snover D: A clinicopathological analysis of mixed hyperplastic–neoplastic polyps of the large intestine. Modern Pathol 2:53A, 1989
60. Cooper HS, Patchefsky AS, Marks G: Adenomatous and carcinomatous changes within hyperplastic colonic epithelium. Dis Colon Rectum 22:152–156, 1979
61. Urbanski SJ, Kossakowsha AE, Marion N, Bruce WR: Mixed hyperplastic adenomatous polyps—an underdiagnosed entity. Report of a case of adenocarcinoma arising within a mixed hyperplastic adenomatous polyp. Am J Surg Pathol 8:551–556, 1984
62. Benjamin SP, Hawk WA, Turnbull RB: Fibrous inflammatory polyps of the ileum and cecum: review of five cases with emphasis on differentiation from mesenchymal neoplasms. Cancer 39:1300–1305, 1977

63. Kim YI, Kim WH: Inflammatory fibroid polyps of gastrointestinal tract. Am J Clin Pathol 89:721–727, 1988
64. Nakamura S-i, Kino I, Akagi T: Inflammatory myoglandular polyps of the colon and rectum. A clinicopathological study of 32 pedunculated polyps, distinct from other types of polyps. Am J Surg Pathol 16:772–779, 1992
65. Meissner WW: Benign lymphoma of the rectum: review of the literature and report of fifteen additional cases. J Int Coll Surg 26:739–749, 1956
66. Price AB: Benign lymphoid polyps and inflammatory polyps. pp. 33. In Morson BC (ed): Pathogenesis of Colorectal Cancer. WB Saunders, Philadelphia, 1978
67. Matsui K, Iwase T, Kitagawa M. Small, polypoid-appearing carcinoid tumors of the rectum: clinicopathologic study of 16 cases and effectiveness of endoscopic treatment. Am J Gastroenterol 88:1949–1953, 1993
68. d'Amore ESG, Manivel JC, Pettinato G et al: Intestinal ganglioneuromatosis. Hum Pathol 22:276–286, 1991
69. Gramlich TL, Hunter SB: Focal polypoid ischemia of the colon: atheroemboli presenting as a colonic polyp. Arch Pathol Lab Med 118:308–309, 1994
70. Cheville JC, Mitros FA, Vanderzalm G, Platz CE: Atheroemboli-associated polyps of the sigmoid colon. Am J Surg Pathol 17:1054–1057, 1993
71. Fellows IW, Clarke JMF, Roberts PF: Nonsteroidal anti-inflammatory drug-induced jejunal and colonic diaphragm disease: a report of two cases. Gut 33:1424–1426, 1992
72. Herman AH, Nabseth DC: Colitis cystica profunda: localized, segmental, and diffuse, Arch Surg 106:337, 1973
73. Caccese WJ, McKinley MJ, Bronzo RL, Bronson R: Endoscopic confirmation of colonic endometriosis. Gastrointest Endosc 30:191–193, 1984
74. Pemberton HW, Smith WG, Holman CB: Pneumatosis cystoides intestinalis diagnosed sigmoidoscopically. Am J Surg 94:472–477, 1957
75. Fazio RA, Wickremesinghe PC, Arsusa EL et al: Endoscopic removal of an intussuscepted appendix mimicking a polyp—an endoscopic hazard. Am J Gastroenterol 77: 556–558, 1982
76. Jevon GP, Daya D, Qizilbash AH: Intussusception of the appendix. A report of four cases and review of the literature. Arch Pathol Lab Med 116:960–964, 1992
77. Shah AN, Mazza BR: The detection of an inverted diverticulum by colonoscopy. Gastrointest Endosc 28:188–189, 1982
78. Kelly JK: Polypoid prolapsing mucosal folds in diverticular disease. Am J Surg Pathol 15:871–878, 1991
79. Franzin G, Fratton A, Manfrini C: Polypoid lesions associated with diverticular disease of the sigmoid colon. Gastrointest Endosc 31:196–199, 1985
80. Kelley JK, MacConnell KL, Hershfield NB: Residual stalks of pedunculated adenomas. An under-recognized type of colonic polyp. J Clin Gastroenterol 9:227–231, 1987
81. Dimmette RM, Sproat HF: Rectosigmoid polyps in schistosomiasis. Am J Trop Med Hyg 4:1057, 1067, 1955
82. Rutter K, Riddell RH: The solitary ulcer syndrome of the rectum. Clin Gastroenterol 4:505–530, 1975
83. Saul SH, Sollenberger LC: Solitary rectal ulcer syndrome. Its clinical and pathological underdiagnosis. Am J Surg Pathol 9:441–421, 1985
84. Chetty R, Bhathal PS, Slavin JL: Prolapse-induced inflammatory polyps of the colorectum and anal transition zone. Histopathology 23:63–67, 1993
85. Lobert PF, Appelman HD: Inflammatory cloacogenic polyp: a unique inflammatory lesion of the anal transitional zone. Am J Surg Pathol 5:761, 1981
86. Saul SH: Inflammatory cloacogenic polyp: relationship to solitary rectal ulcer syndrome/mucosal prolapse and other bowel disorders. Hum Pathol 18:1120, 1987
87. Levey JM, Banner B, Darrah J et al: Inflammatory cloacogenic polyp: three cases and literature review. Am J Gastroenterol 89:438–441, 1994
88. Rickert RR, Auerbach O, Garfinkel L et al: Adenomatous lesions of the large bowel: an autopsy study. Cancer 43:1847, 1979
89. Konishi F, Morson BC: Pathology of colorectal adenomas: a colonoscopic survey. J Clin Pathol 35:830–841, 1982

90. O'Brien MJ, Winawer SJ, Zauber AG et al: The national polyp study. Patient and polyp characteristics associated with high grade dysplasia in colorectal adenomas. Gastroenterology 98:371–379, 1990
91. Thompson JJ, Enterline HT: The macroscopic appearance of colorectal polyps. Cancer 48:151, 1981
92. Fung CHK, Goldman H: Incidence and significance of villous change in adenomatous polyps. Am J Clin Pathol 53:21–25, 1970
93. Lev R: Defects in the current histological classification of adenomatous polyps of the colon. Surg Pathol 5:199–210, 1994
94. Van den Ingh HF, Van den Broek L, Verkofstod AJ: Neuroendocrine cells in colorectal adenomas. J Pathol 148:231–237, 1986
95. Bansal M, O'Toole K, Smith SM, Fenoglio-Preiser CM: Endocrine antigenic profile of normal, hyperplastic, and neoplastic large intestinal tissues. Surg Pathol 1:93–112, 1988
96. Lewin KJ: Neoplastic Paneth cells. J Clin Pathol 21:476, 1968
97. Almagro UA, Pintar K, Zellmer RB: Squamous metaplasia in colorectal polyps. Cancer 53:2679–2682, 1984
98. Groisman GM, Benkov KJ, Adsay V, Dische MR: Osseous metaplasia in benign colorectal polyps. Arch Pathol Lab Med 118:64–65, 1993
99. Fulcheri E, Baracchini P, Lapertosa G, Bussolati G: Distribution and significance of the smooth muscle component in polyps of the large intestine. Hum Pathol 19:922–927, 1988
100. Dirschmid K, Kiesler J, Mathis G, et al: Epithelial misplacement after biopsy of colorectal adenomas. Am J Surg Pathol 17:1262–1265, 1993
101. Lundquest DE, Marcus JN, Thorson AG et al: Primary squamous cell carcinoma of the colon arising in a villous adenoma. Hum Pathol 19:362–364, 1988
102. Robert L, Lagace R, Delage C: Malakoplakia of the colon associated with a villous adenoma. Dis Colon Rectum 17:668–671, 1974
103. Goldman H, Antonioli DA: Mucosal biopsy of the rectum, colon and distal ileum. Human Pathol 13:981–1012, 1982
104. Muto T, Bussey HJR, Morson BC: The evolution of cancer of the colon and rectum. Cancer 36:2251–2270, 1975
105. Fenoglio CM, Pascal RR: Colorectal adenomas and cancer. Pathologic relationships. Cancer 50:2601–2608, 1982
106. Fenoglio CM, Kaye GI, Lane N: Distribution of human colonic lymphatics in normal, hyperplastic, and adenomatous tissue. Gastroenterology 64:51, 1973
107. Muto T, Bussey HJR, Morson BC: Pseudocarcinomatous invasion in adenomatous polyps of the colon and rectum. J Clin Pathol 26:25, 1973
108. Greene FL: Epithelial misplacement in adenomatous polyps of the colon and rectum. Cancer 33:206, 1974
109. Qizilbash AH, Meghju M, Castelli M: Pseudocarcinomatous invasion in adenomas of the colon and rectum. Dis Colon Rectum 23:529–535, 1980
110. Cheung DK, Attizeh FF: Pseudocarcinomatous invasion of colonic polyps. Dis Colon Rectum 24:399–401, 1981
111. Muto T, Kamiya J, Sawada T et al: Small "flat adenoma" of the large bowel with special reference to its clinicopathologic features. Dis Colon Rect 28:847–851, 1985
112. Wolber RA, Owen DA: Flat adenomas of the colon. Hum Pathol 22:70–74, 1991
113. Yao T, Tada S, Tsuneyoshi M: Colorectal counterpart of gastric depressed adenoma. A comparison with flat and polypoid adenomas with special reference to the development of pericryptal fibroblasts. Am J Surg Pathol 18:559–568, 1994
114. Winawer SJ, Zauber AG, Ho MN et al: Prevention of colorectal cancer by colonoscopic polypectomy. N Engl J Med 329:1977–1981, 1993
115. Lipper S, Kahn LB, Ackerman LV: The significance of microscopic invasive cancer in endoscopically removed polyps in the large bowel. A clinicopathologic study of 51 cases. Cancer 52:1691–1699, 1983
116. Cooper HS: Surgical pathology of endoscopically removed malignant polyps of the colon and rectum. Am J Surg Pathol 7:613–623, 1983
117. Morson BC, Whiteway JE, Jones EA et al: Histopatology and prognosis of malignant colorectal polyps treated by endoscopic polypectomy. Gut 25:437–444, 1984
118. Haggitt RC, Glotzbach RE, Soffer EE, Wruble LD: Prognostic factors in colorectal car-

cinomas arising in adenomas: implications for lesions removed by endoscopic polypectomy. Gastroenterology 89:328–336, 1985

119. Frei JV: Endoscopic large bowel polypectomy. Adequate treatment of some completely removed, minimally invasive lesions. Am J Surg Pathol 9:355–359, 1985
120. Gyorffy EJ, Amontree JS, Fenoglio-Preiser CM et al: Large colorectal polyps: colonoscopy, pathology, and management. Am J Gastroenterol 84:898–905, 1989
121. Muller S, Chesner IM, Igan MA et al: Significance of venous and lymphatic invasion in malignant polyps of the colon and rectum. Gut 30:1385–1391, 1990
122. Geraghty JM, Williams CB, Talbort IC: Malignant colorectal polyps: venous invasion and successful treatment by endoscopic polypectomy. Gut 32:774–778, 1991
123. Kazzer S, Begin LR, Gordon PH, Mitmaker B: The care of patients with colorectal polyps that contain invasive adenocarcinoma. Endoscopic polypectomy or colectomy? Cancer 70:2044–2050, 1992
124. Haggitt RC, Reid BJ: Hereditary gastrointestinal polyposis syndromes. Am J Surg Pathol 10:871–877, 1986
125. Rustgi AK: Hereditary gastrointestinal polyposis and non-polyposis syndromes. N Engl J Med 331:1694–1702, 1994
126. Bussey HJR: Familial Polyposis Coli. Johns Hopkins University Press, Baltimore, 1975
127. Gurbuz AK, Giardiello FM, Petersen GM et al: Desmoid tumours in familial adenomatous polyposis. Gut 35:377–381, 1994
128. Giardiello FM, Hamilton SR, Krush AJ et al: Nasopharyngeal angiofibroma in patients with familial adenomatous polyposis. Gastroenterology 105:1550–1552, 1993
129. Iida M, Yao T, Itoh H et al: Natural history of gastric adenomas in patients with familial adenomatosis coli/Gardner's syndrome. Cancer 61:605–611, 1988
130. Damizio P, Talbort IC, Spigelman AD et al: Upper gastrointestinal pathology in familial adenomatous polyposis—results from a prospective study of 102 patients. J Clin Pathol 43:738–743, 1990
131. Noda Y, Watanabe H, Iida M et al: Histologic follow-up of ampullary adenomas in patients with familial adenomatous coli. Cancer 70:1847–1856, 1992
132. Hamilton SR, Bussey HJR, Mendelsohn G et al: Ileal adenomas after colectomy in nine patients with adenomatous polyposis coli/Gardner's syndrome. Gastroenterology 77:1252, 1979
133. Suarez V, Alexander-Williams J, O'Connor HJ et al: Carcinoma developing in ileostomies after 25 or more years. Gastroenterology 95:205–208, 1988
134. Taylor BA, Wolff BG, Dozois RR et al: Ileal pouch–anal anastomosis for chronic ulcerative colitis and familial polyposis coli complicated by adenocarcinoma. Dis Colon Rectum 31:358–362, 1988
135. Stern H, Wolfisch S, Mullen B: Cancer in an ileoanal reservoir: a new late complication? Gut 31:473–475, 1990
136. Kubota O, Kino I: Depressed adenomas of the colon in familial adenomatous polyposis. Histology, immunohistochemical detection of proliferating cell nuclear antigen (PCNA), and analysis of the background mucosa. Am J Surg Pathol 19:318–327, 1995
137. Woda BA, Forde K, Lane N: A unicryptal colonic adenoma: the smallest colonic neoplasm yet observed in a non-polyposis individual. Am J Clin Pathol 68:631, 1977
138. Rhodes M, Bradburn DM: Overview of screening and management of familial adenomatous polyposis. Gut 33:125–131, 1992
139. Haggitt RC, Picock JA: Familial juvenile polyposis of the colon. Cancer 26:1232, 1970
140. Grotsky HW, Rickert RR, Smith WD, Newsome JF: Familial juvenile polyposis coli. A clinical and pathological study of a large kindred. Gastroenterology 82:494–501, 1982
141. Mestra JR: The changing pattern of juvenile polyps. Am J Gastroenterol 81:312–314, 1986
142. Goodman ZD, Yardley JH, Milligan FD: Pathogenesis of colonic polyps in multiple juvenile polyposis. Cancer 43:1906, 1979
143. Subramony C, Scott-Conner CEH, Skelton D, Hall TJ: Familial juvenile polyposis. Study of a kindred: evolution of polyps and relationship to gastrointestinal carcinoma. Am J Clin Pathol 102:91–97, 1994
144. Sandler RS, Lipper S: Multiple adenomas in juvenile polyposis. Am J Gastroenterol 75:361, 1981
145. Jarvinen H, Franssila KO: Familial juvenile polyposis coli: increased risk of colorectal cancer. Gut 25:792–800, 1984

146. Jass JR, Williams CB, Bussey HJR, Morson BC: Juvenile polyposis—a precancerous condition. Histopathology 13:619–630, 1988
147. O'Riordan DS, O'Dwyer RJ, Cullen AF et al· Familial juvenile polyposis coli and colorectal cancer. Cancer 68:889–892, 1991
148. Sachatello CR, Pickren JW, Grace JT: Generalized juvenile gastrointestinal polyposis. Gastroenterology 58:669, 1970
149. Williams GT, Bussey HJR, Morson BC: Hamartomatous polyps in Peutz-Jeghers syndrome. N Engl J Med 299:101, 1978
150. Estrada R, Spjut HJ: Hamartomatous polyps in Peutz-Jeghers syndrome. A light-, histochemical and electron-microscopist study. Am J Surg Pathol 7:747–754, 1983
151. Giardiello FM, Welsh SB, Hamilton SR et al: Increased risk of cancer in the Peutz-Jeghers syndrome. N Engl J Med 316:1511–1514, 1987
152. Hizawa K, Iida M, Matsumoto T et al: Cancer in Peutz-Jeghers syndrome. Cancer 72:2777–2781, 1993
153. Perzin KH, Bridge MF: Adenomatous and carcinomatous changes in hamartomatous polyps of the small intestine (Peutz-Jeghers syndrome). Cancer 49:971–983, 1982
154. Narita T, Eto T, Ito T: Peutz-Jeghers syndrome with adenomas and adenocarcinomas in colonic polyps. Am J Surg Pathol 11:76–81, 1987
155. Shepherd NA, Bussey HJR, Jass JR: Epithelial misplacement in Peutz-Jeghers polyps: a diagnostic pitfall. Am J Surg Pathol 11: 743–749, 1987
156. Ali M, Weinstein J, Biempica J et al: Cronkhite-Canada syndrome: report of a case with bacteriologic, immunologic, and electron microscopic studies. Gastroenterology 79:731, 1980
157. Daniel ES, Ludwig SL, Lewin KJ et al: The Cronkhite-Canada syndrome. An analysis of clinical and pathologic features and therapy in 55 patients. Medicine (Baltimore) 61: 293–309, 1982
158. Burke AP, Sobin LH: The pathology of Cronkhite-Canada polyps: A comparison to juvenile polyposis. Am J Surg Pathol 13: 940–946, 1989
159. Katayama Y, Kimura M, Konn M: Cronkhite-Canada syndrome associated with a rectal cancer and adenomatous changes in C-C polyps. Am J Surg Pathol 9:65–71, 1985
160. Malkotra R, Sheffield A: Cronkhite-Canada syndrome associated with colon carcinoma and adenomatous changes in C-C polyps. Am J Gastroenterol 83:772–776, 1988
161. Baughman FW Jr, List CF, Williams JR et al: The gliomapolyposis syndrome. N Engl J Med 281:1345, 1969
162. Schroder S, Moehrs D, Von Weltzien J et al: The Turcot syndrome. Report of an additional case and review of the literature. Dis Colon Rectum 26:533–538, 1983
163. Lynch HT, Smyrk TC, Watson P et al: Genetics, natural history, tumor spectrum, and pathology of hereditary non-polyposis colorectal cancer: an updated review. Gastroenterology 104:1535–1549, 1993
164. Lanspa SJ, Lynch HT, Smyrk TC et al: Colorectal adenomas in the Lynch syndromes. Results of a colonoscopy screening program. Gastroenterology 98:1117–1122, 1990
165. Lynch HT, Smyrk TC, Lanspa SJ, et al: Upper gastrointestinal manifestations in families with hereditary flat adenoma syndrome. Cancer 71:2709–2714, 1993
166. Carlson GJ, Nivatvongs S, Snover DC: Colorectal polyps in Cowden's disease (multiple hamartomatous syndrome). Am J Surg Pathol 8:763–770, 1984
167. Lashner BA, Riddell RH, Winans CS: Ganglioneuromatosis of the colon and extensive glycogenic acanthosis in Cowden's disease. Dig Dis Sci 31:213–216, 1986
168. Carney JA, Hayles AB: Alimentary tract manifestations of multiple endocrine neoplasia, type II B. Mayo Clin Proc 52: 543–548, 1977
169. Weidner N, Flanders DJ, Mitros FA: Mucosal ganglioneuromatosis associated with multiple colonic polyps. Am J Surg Pathol 8:779–786, 1984
170. Snover DC, Weigent CE, Sumner HW: Diffuse mucosal ganglioneuromatosis of the colon associated with adenocarcinoma. Am J Clin Pathol 75:225–229, 1981
171. Devroede GJ, Taylor WF, Sauer WG et al: Cancer risk and life expectancy of children with ulcerative colitis. N Engl J Med 285:17–21, 1971

172. Kewenter J, Ahlman H, Hulten L: Cancer risk in extensive ulcerative colitis. Ann Surg 188:824–828, 1987
173. Eklom A, Helmick C, Zack M, Adami H-O: Ulcerative colitis and colorectal cancer: a population-based study. N Engl J Med 323:1228–1233, 1990
174. Weedon DD, Shorter RG, Ilstrup DM et al: Crohn's disease and cancer. N Engl J Med 289:1099–1103, 1973
175. Lightdale CJ, Sternberg SS, Posner G et al: Carcinoma complicating Crohn's disease. Am J Med 59:262–268, 1975
176. Choi PM, Zelig MP: Similarity of colorectal cancer in Crohn's disease and ulcerative colitis: implications for carcinogenesis and prevention. Gut 35:950–954, 1994
177. Owen DA, Hwang WS, Thorlakson RH, Walli E: Malignant carcinoid tumor complicating chronic ulcerative colitis. Am J Clin Pathol 76:333–338, 1981
178. Miller RR, Sumner HW: Argyrophilic cell hyperplasia and an atypical carcinoid tumor in chronic ulcerative colitis. Cancer 50:2920–2925, 1982
179. Gledhill A, Hall PA, Cruse JP et al: Enteroendocrine cell hyperplasia, carcinoid tumours and adenocarcinoma in long-standing ulcerative colitis. Histopathology 10:501–508, 1986
180. Lyss AP, Thompson JJ, Glick JH: Adenocarcinoid tumor of the colon arising in preexisting ulcerative colitis. Cancer 48:833, 1981
181. Baker D, Chirput RO, Rimer D et al: Colonic lymphoma in ulcerative colitis. J Clin Gastroenterol 7:379–386, 1985
182. Shepherd NA, Hall PA, Williams GT et al: Primary malignant lymphoma of the large intestine complicating chronic inflammatory bowel disease. Histopathology 15:325–337, 1989
183. Greenstein AJ, Mullin GE, Strauchen JA et al: Lymphoma in inflammatory bowel disease. Cancer 69:1119–1123, 1992
184. Hanauer SB, Wong KK, Frank PH et al: Acute leukemia following inflammatory bowel disease. Dig Dis Sci 27:545–548, 1982
185. Haidor A, Dixon MF: Solitary microcarcinoid ulcerative colitis. Histopathology 21: 487–488, 1992
186. McNeely B, Owen DA, Pezim M: Multiple microcarcinoids arising in chronic ulcerative colitis. Am J Clin Pathol 98:112–116, 1992
187. Patterson FK: Adenocanthoma and ulcerative colitis. Case report and review of the literature. South Med J 66:681–690, 1973
188. Greenstein AJ, Sackar DB, Shafir M et al: Malignant melanoma in inflammatory bowel disease. Am J Gastroenterol 87:317–320, 1992
189. Mir-Madjlessi SH, Farmer RG, Easley KA, Beck GJ: Colorectal and extracolonic malignancy in ulcerative colitis. Cancer 58:1569–1574, 1986
190. Odze RD, Medline P, Cohen Z: Adenocarcinoma arising in an appendix involved with chronic ulcerative colitis. Am J Gastroenterol 89:1905–1907, 1994
191. Pinczowski D, Ekbom A, Baron J et al: Risk factors for colorectal cancer in patients with ulcerative colitis: a case-control study. Gastroenterology 107:117–120, 1994
192. Greenstein AJ, Sacher DB, Smith H et al: Cancer in universal and left-sided ulcerative colitis: factors determining risk. Gastroenterology 89:290–294, 1979
193. Gillen CD, Walmsley RS, Prior P et al: Ulcerative colitis and Crohn's disease: a comparison of the colorectal cancer risk in extensive colitis. Gut 35:1590–1592, 1994
194. Connell WR, Sheffield JP, Kamm MA et al: Lower gastrointestinal malignancy in Crohn's disease. Gut 35:347–352, 1994
195. Nikias G, Eisner T, Katz S et al: Crohn's disease and colorectal carcinoma: rectal cancer complicating longstanding active perianal disease. Am J Gastroenterol 90:216–219, 1995
196. Sugita A, Sackar DB, Ribeiro MB et al: Colorectal cancer in ulcerative colitis. Influence of anatomical extent and age at onset on colitis–cancer interval. Gut 32:167–169, 1991
197. Gillen CD, Andrews HA, Prior P, Allan RN: Crohn's disease and colorectal cancer. Gut 35:651–655, 1994
198. Goldgraber MB, Kirsner JB: Carcinoma of the colon in ulcerative colitis. Cancer 17:657, 1964
199. Bernstein CN, Shanahan F, Weinstein WM: Are we telling patients the truth about surveillance colonoscopy in ulcerative colitis? Lancet 343:71–74, 1994

200. Cook MG, Goligher JC: Carcinoma and epithelial dysplasia complicating ulcerative colitis. Gastroenterology 68:1127–1136, 1975
201. Nugent FW, Haggitt RC, Gilpin PA: Cancer surveillance in ulcerative colitis. Gastroenterology 100:1241–1248, 1991
202. Connell WR, Lennard-Jones JE, Williams CB et al: Factors affecting the outcome of endoscopic surveillance for cancer in ulcerative colitis. Gastroenterology 107:934–944, 1994
203. Hamilton SR: Colorectal carcinoma in patients with Crohn's disease. Gastroenterology 89:398–407, 1985
204. Petras RE, Mir-Madjlessi SH, Farmer RG: Crohn's disease and intestinal carcinoma. A report of 11 cases with emphasis on associated epithelial dysplasia. Gastroenterology 93:1307–1314, 1987
205. Lennard-Jones JE, Melville DM, Morson BC et al: Pre-cancer and cancer in extensive ulcerative colitis; findings among 401 patients over 22 years. Gut 31:800–806, 1990
206. Thompson EM, Clayden G, Price AB: Cancer in Crohn's disease—an "occult" malignancy. Histopathology 7:365–376, 1983
207. Yamazoki Y, Ribeiro MB, Sackar D et al: Malignant colroectal strictures in Crohn's disease. Am J Gastroenterol 86:882–885, 1991
208. Gumoste V, Sackar DB, Greenstein AJ: Benign and malignant colorectal strictures in ulcerative colitis. Gut 33:938–941, 1992
209. Reiser JR, Waye JD, Janowitz HD, Harpaz N: Adenocarcinoma in strictures of ulcerative colitis without antecedent dysplasia by colonoscopy. Am J Gastroenterol 89:119–122, 1994
210. Riddell RH, Goldman H, Ransohoff DF et al: Dysplasia in inflammatory bowel disease: Standardized classification with provisional clinical applications. Hum Pathol 14:931–968, 1983
211. Pascal RR: Dysplasia and early carcinoma in inflammatory bowel disease and colorectal adenomas. Hum Pathol 25:1160–1171, 1994
212. Johnson WR, McDermott FT, Hughes ESR: Mucosal dysplasia: a major predictor of cancer following ileorectal anastomosis. Dis Colon Rect 26:697–700, 1983
213. Thomas DM, Filipe MI, Smedley FH: Dysplasia and carcinoma in the rectal stump of total colitics who have undergone colectomy and ileo–rectal anastomosis. Histopathology 14:289–298, 1989
214. Goldman H: Ulcerative colitis and Crohn's disease. pp. 643–688. In Ming S-C, Goldman H (eds): Pathology of the Gastrointestinal Tract. WB Saunders, Philadelphia, 1992
215. Morson BC, Pang LSC: Rectal biopsy as an aid to cancer control in ulcerative colitis. Gut 8:423–434, 1967
216. Fenoglio CM, Pascal RR: Adenomatous epithelium, intraepithelial anaplasia, and invasive carcinoma in ulcerative colitis. Am J Dig Dis 18:556–562, 1973.
217. Yardley JH, Keren DF: Precancer lesions in ulcerative colitis: a retrospective study of rectal biopsy and colectomy specimens. Cancer 34:835–844, 1974
218. Gewertz BL, Dent TL, Appelman HD: Implications of precancerous rectal biopsy in patients with inflammatory bowel disease. Arch Surg 111:326–329, 1976
219. Vatn MH, Elgjo K, Bergan A: Distribution of dysplasia in ulcerative colitis. Scand J Gastroenterol 19:893–895, 1984
220. Craft CF, Mendelsohn G, Cooper HS et al: Colonic "pre-cancer" in Crohn's disease. Gastroenterology 80:578, 1981
221. Simpson S, Traube J, Riddell RH: The histological appearance of dysplasia (precarcinomatous change) in Crohn's disease of the small and large intestine. Gastroenterology 81:492–501, 1981
222. Cuvelier C, Bekaert E, De Potter C et al: Crohn's disease with adenocarcinoma and dysplasia. Macroscopical, histological, and immunohistochemical aspects of two cases. Am J Surg Pathol 13:187–196, 1989
223. Rosenstock E, Farmer RG, Petras R et al: Surveillance for colonic carcinoma in ulcerative colitis. Gastroenterology 89:1342–1346, 1985
224. Fozard JDJ, Dixon MF: Colonoscopic surveillance in ulcerative colitis—dysplasia through the looking glass. Gut 30:285–292, 1989
225. Lofberg R, Brostran O, Karlen P et al: Colonoscopic surveillance in longstanding total ulcerative colitis—a 15 year follow-up study. Gastroenterology 99:1021–1031, 1990
226. Choi PM, Nugent FW, Schoetz DJ et al: Colonoscopic surveillance reduces mortality

from colorectal cancer in ulcerative colitis. Gastroenterology 105:418–424, 1993

227. Blackstone MO, Riddell RH, Rogers RHG et al: Dysplasia-associated lesion or mass (DALM) detected by colonoscopy in longstanding ulcerative colitis: an indication for colectomy. Gastroenterology 80:366, 1981
228. Butt JH, Koniski F, Morson BC et al: Macroscopic lesions in dysplasia and carcinoma complicating ulcerative colitis. Dig Dis Sci 28:18–26, 1983
229. Dixon MF, Brown LJ, Gilmour HM et al: Observer variations in the assessment of dysplasia in ulcerative colitis. Histopathology 13:385–397, 1988
230. Woolrich AJ, DaSilva MD, Korelitz BI: Surveillance in the routine management of ulcerative colitis: the predictive value of low grade dysplasia. Gastroenterology 103:431–438, 1992
231. Fischbach W, Mossner J, Seyschab H, Hohn H: Tissue carcinoembryonic antigen and DNA aneuploidy in precancerous and cancerous colorectal lesions. Cancer 65:1820–1824, 1990
232. Ehsanullah M, Naunton-Morgan M, Filipe MI, Gazzard B: Sialomucins in the assessment of dysplasia and cancer-risk patients with ulcerative colitis treated with colectomy and ileo–rectal anastomosis. Histopathology 9:223–235, 1985
233. Andrews CW, O'Hara CJ, Goldman H et al: Sucrase–isomaltase expression in chronic ulcerative colitis and dysplasia. Hum Pathol 23:774–779, 1992
234. Cuvelier CA, Morson BC, Roels HJ: The DNA content in cancer and dysplasia in chronic ulcerative colitis. Histopathology 11:927–929, 1987
235. Melville DM, Jass JR, Shepherd NA et al: Dysplasia and deoxyribonucleic acid aneuploidy in the assessment of precancerous changes in chronic ulcerative colitis. Gastroenterology 95:668–675, 1988
236. Rutegard J, Ahsgren L, Stenling R, Roos G: DNA content and mucosal dysplasia in ulcerative colitis: flow cytometric analysis in patients with dysplastic or indefinite morphologic changes in the colorectal mucosa. Dis Colon Rectum 32:1055–1059, 1989
237. Lofberg R, Brostrom O, Karlen P et al: DNA aneuploidy in ulcerative colitis: reproducibility, topographic distribution, and relation to dysplasia. Gastroenterology 102:1149–1154, 1992
238. Rubin CE, Haggitt RC, Burner GC et al: DNA aneuploidy in colonic biopsies predicts future development of dysplasia in ulcerative colitis. Gastroenterology 103:1611–1620, 1992
239. Shields HM, Best CJ, Goldman H: Distinction of dysplasia from inflammatory changes in ulcerative colitis. A scanning electron microscopic study with quantitative analyses. Surg Pathol 1:183–192, 1988
240. Yin J, Harpaz N, Tong Y et al: p53 point mutations in dysplastic and cancerous ulcerative colitis lesions. Gastroenterology 104:1633–1639, 1993
241. Brentnall TA, Crispin DA, Rabinovitch PS et al: Mutations in the p53 gene: an early marker of neoplastic progression in ulcerative colitis. Gastroenterology 107:369–378, 1994
242. Harpaz N, Peck AL, Yin J et al: p53 protein expression in ulcerative colitis-associated colorectal dysplasia and carcinoma. Hum Pathol 25:1069–1074, 1994
243. Kern SE, Redston M, Seymour AB et al: Molecular genetic profiles of colitis-associated neoplasms. Gastroenterology 107:420–428, 1994
244. Chaubert P, Benhattar J, Saraga E, Costa J: K-ras mutations and p53 alterations in neoplastic and nonneoplastic lesions associated with longstanding ulcerative colitis. Am J Pathol 144:767–775, 1994
245. Redston MS, Papadopoulos N, Caldas C, et al: Common occurrence of APC and K-ras gene mutations in the spectrum of colitis-associated neoplasias. Gastroenterology 108:383–392, 1995
246. Chang M, Tsuchiya K, Batchelor RH et al: Deletion mapping of chromosome 8p in colorectal carcinoma and dysplasia arising in ulcerative colitis, prostatic carcinoma, and malignant fibrous histiocytomas. Am J Pathol 144:1–6, 1994
247. Cartwright CA, Coad CA, Egbert BM: Elevated c-src tyrosine kinase activity in premalignant epithelia of ulcerative colitis. J Clin Invest 93:509–515, 1994
248. Pena SV, Melhem MF, Meisler AI et al: Elevated c-Yes tyrosine kinase activity in pre-

malignant lesions of the colon. Gastroenterology 108:117–124, 1995
249. Thomas RM, Sobin LH: Gastrointestinal cancer. Cancer 75:154–170, 1995
250. Cooper GS, Yuan Z, Landefeld S et al: A national population-based study of incidence of colorectal cancer and age. Implications for screening in older Americans. Cancer 75:775–781, 1995
251. Fuchs CS, Giovannucci EL, Colditz GA et al: A prospective study of family history and the risk of colorectal cancer. N Engl J Med 331:1669–1674, 1994
252. Ming-Chai C, Chi-Yuan C, Pei-Yu C et al: Evolution of colorectal cancer in schistosomiasis: transitional mucosal changes adjacent to large intestinal carcinoma in colectomy specimens. Cancer 46:1661, 1980
253. Xu Z, Su DI: Schistosoma japonicum and colorectal cancer: an epidemiological study in the People's Republic of China. Int J Cancer 34:315–318, 1984
254. O'Connor TW, Rombeau JL, Levine HS et al: Late development of colorectal cancer subsequent to pelvic irradiation. Dis Colon Rectum 22:123–128, 1979
255. Sandler RS, Sandler DP: Radiation-induced cancers of the colon and rectum: assessing the risk. Gastroenterology 84:51–57, 1983
256. Jao SW, Beart RW Jr, Reiman HM et al: Colon and anorectal cancer after pelvic irradiation. Dis Colon Rectum 30:953–958, 1987
257. Ali MH, Satti MB, Al-Nafussi A: Multiple benign colonic polypi at the site of ureterosigmoidostomy. Cancer 53:1006–1010, 1984
258. Cipolla R, Garcia RL: Colonic polyps and adenocarcinoma complicating ureterosigmoidoscopy: report of a case. Am J Gastroenterol 79:453–457, 1984
259. Stewart M, Macrae FA, William CB: Neoplasia and ureterosigmoidostomy: a colonoscopy survey. Br J Surg 69:414–416, 1982
260. Sterling JR, Uehling DT, Gilchrist KW: Value of colonoscopy after ureterosigmoidostomy. Surgery 96:784–790, 1984
261. Williams JG, Williams LA, Colhoun E: Changes at ureteroenteric anastomosis masquerading as a neoplastic polyp. Dis Colon Rectum 31:313–314, 1988
262. Danzig JB, Brandt LJ, Reinus JF, Klein RS: Gastrointestinal malignancy in patients with AIDS. Am J Gastroentrol 86:715–718, 1991
263. Cappell MS, Yao F, Cho KC: Colonic adenocarcinoma associated with the acquired immune deficiency syndrome. Cancer 62:616–619, 1988
264. Klugman AD, Schaffner J: Colon adenocarcinoma in HIV infection: a case report and review. Am J Gastroenterol 89:254–256, 1994
265. Swinson CM, Slavin G, Coles EC, Booth CC: Coeliac disease and malignancy. Lancet 1:111–115, 1983
266. Orr MM, Edwards AJ: Neoplastic change in duplication of the alimentary tract. Br J Surg 62:269–274, 1975
267. Hickey WF, Corson JM: Squamous cell carcinoma arising in a duplication cyst: case report and literature review of squamous cell carcinoma of the colon and of malignancy complicating colonic duplication. Cancer 47:602, 1981
268. Giacchero A, Aste H, Baracchini P et al: Primary signet-ring carcinoma of the large bowel: report of nine cases. Cancer 56:2723–2726, 1985
269. Nakahara H, Ishikowa T, Haboshi M, Hirota T: Diffusely infiltrating primary colorectal carcinoma of linitis plastica and lymphangiosis types. Cancer 69:901–906, 1992
270. Symonds DA, Vickey AL: Mucinous carcinoma of the colon and rectum. Cancer 37:1891, 1976
271. Minsky BD, Mies C, Rich TA et al: Colloid carcinoma of the colon and rectum. Cancer 60:3103–3112, 1987
272. Younes M, Katikaneni PR, Lechago J: The value of the preoperative mucosal biopsy in the diagnosis of colorectal mucinous adenocarcinoma. Cancer 72:3588–3592, 1993
273. Iwashita A: Argyrophil and argentaffin cells in carcinoma of the colon and rectum. Fukuoka Acta Medica 70:370, 1979
274. Ulich RT, Cheng L, Glover H et al: A colonic adenocarcinoma with argentaffin cells. A immunoperoxidase study demonstrating the presence of numerous neuroendocrine products. Cancer 51:1483–1489, 1983
275. Lieberman D: Screening/early detection model for colorectal cancer. Cancer 74:2023–2027, 1994
276. Toribara NW, Sleisenger MH: Screening for colorectal cancer. N Engl J Med 332:861–867, 1995

277. Sunter JP, Higgs MJ, Cowan WK: Mucosal abnormalities at the anastomosis site in patients who have had intestinal resection for colonic cancer. J Clin Pathol 38:385–389, 1985
278. Shousha S: Paneth cell-rich papillary adenocarcinoma and a mucoid adenocarcinoma occurring synchronously in colon: a light and electron microscopic study. Histopathology 3:489–501, 1979
279. Comer TP, Beahrs OH, Docheertz MB: Primary squamous cell carcinoma and adenoacanthoma. Cancer 28:1111–1117, 1971
280. Crissman JD: Adenosquamous and squamous cell carcinoma of the colon. Am J Surg Pathol 2:47, 1978
281. Cerezo L, Alvarez M, Edwards O, Price G: Adenosquamous carcinoma of the colon. Dis Colon Rectum 28:597–603, 1985
282. Weidner N, Zekan P: Carcinosarcoma of the colon. Report of a unique case with light and immunohistochemical studies. Cancer 58: 1126–1130, 1986
283. Amano S, Yamada N: Endometrioid carcinoma arising from endometriosis of the sigmoid colon: a case report. Hum Pathol 12:845–849, 1981
284. Solcia E, Capella C, Fiocca R et al: Disorders of the endocrine system. pp. 240–263. In Ming S-C, Goldman H (eds): Pathology of the Gastrointestinal Tract. WB Saunders, Philadelphia, 1992
285. Sanders RJ, Axtell HK: Carcinoids of the gastrointestinal tract. Surg Gynecol Obstet 119:369–380, 1984
286. Ballantyne GH, Savoca PE, Flannery JT: Incidence and mortality of carcinoids of the colon. Data from the Connecticut Tumor Registry. Cancer 69:2400–2405, 1992
287. Lechago J: Gastrointestinal neuroendocrine cell proliferations. Hum Pathol 25:1114–1122, 1994
288. Taxy JB, Mendelsohn G, Gupta PK: Carcinoid tumors of the rectum: silver reactions, fluorescence and serotonin content of cytoplasmic granules. Am J Clin Pathol 74:791, 1980
289. O'Briain DS, Dayal Y, DeLellis RA et al: Rectal carcinoids as tumors of the hindgut endocrine cells: a morphological and immunohistochemical analysis. Am J Surg Pathol 6:131, 1982
290. Federspiel BH, Burke AP, Sobin LH, Shekitka KM: Rectal and colonic carcinoids. A clinicopathologic study of 84 cases. Cancer 65:135–140, 1990
291. Facer P, Bishop AE, Lloyd RV et al: Chromogranin: a newly recognized marker for endocrine cells of the human gastrointestinal tract. Gastroenterology 89:1366–73, 1985
292. Smith DM, Haggitt RC: A comparative study of generic stains for carcinoid secretory granules. Am J Surg Pathol 7:61, 1983
293. Yoshida A, Yano M, Fujinaga Y et al: Argentaffin carcinoid tumor of the rectum. Cancer 48:2103, 1981
294. Klappenbach RS, Kurman RJ, Sinclair CF, James LP: Composite carcinoma–carcinoid tumors of the gastrointestinal tract. A morphologic, histochemical and immunocytochemical study. Am J Clin Pathol 84:137–143, 1985
295. Lewin K: Carcinoid tumors and the mixed (composite) glandular-endocrine cell carcinomas. Am J Surg Pathol 11(suppl 1): 71–86, 1987
296. Moyana TN, Qizilbash AH, Murphy F: Composite glandular-carcinoid tumors of the colon and rectum: report of two cases. Am J Surg Pathol 12:607–611, 1988
297. Warner TF, Seo IS. Goblet cell carcinoid of the appendix: ultrastructural and histogenic aspects. Cancer 44:1700, 1979
298. Schwartz AM, Orenstein JM: Small cell undifferentiated carcinoma of the rectosigmoid colon. Arch Pathol Lab Med 109:629–632, 1985
299. Mills SE, Allen MS, Cohen AR: Small-cell undifferentiated carcinoma of the colon: a clinicopathological study of five cases and their association with colonic adenomas. Am J Surg Pathol 7:643–651, 1987
300. Burke AB, Shekita KM, Sobin LH: Small cell carcinomas of the large intestine. Am J Clin Pathol 95:315–321, 1991
301. Orenstein JM, Schwartz AM: Small-cell undifferentiated carcinoma of the colorectum. Ultrastruct Pathol 11:781–786, 1987
302. Wick MR, Weatherby RP, Weiland LH: Small cell neuroendocrine carcinoma of the colon and rectum: clinical, histologic, and ultrastructural study and immunohistochemical comparison with cloacogenic carcinoma. Hum Pathol 18:9–21, 1987

303. Ranchod M, Lewin KJ, Dorfman RF: Lymphoid hyperplasia of the gastrointestinal tract. Am J Surg Pathol 2:383, 1978
304. Capitanio MA, Kirkpatrick JA: Lymphoid hyperplasia of the colon in children. Radiology 94:323–327, 1970
305. Burbige EJ, Sobky RZF: Endoscopic appearance of colonic lymphoid nodules. Gastroenterology 72:524–526, 1977
306. Appelman HD, Hirsch SD, Schnitzer B, Coon WW: Clinicopathologic overview of gastrointestinal lymphomas. Am J Surg Pathol 9(3)(suppl):71–83, 1985
307. Filippa DA, Lieberman PH, Weingrad DN et al: Primary lymphoma of the gastrointestinal tract. Analysis of prognostic factors with emphasis on histological type. Am J Surg Pathol 7:363–372, 1983
308. Amer MH, El-Akkad S: Gastrointestinal lymphoma in adults: clinical features and management of 300 cases. Gastroenterology 106:846–858, 1994
309. Isaacson PG: Gastrointestinal lymphoma. Hum Pathol 25:1020–1029, 1994
310. Heule BV, Taylor CR, Terry R et al: Presentation of malignant lymphoma in the rectum. Cancer 49:2602–2607, 1982
311. Shepherd NA, Blackshaw AJ, Coates PJ et al: Primary malignant lymphoma of the colon. A histopathological and immunocytochemical study of 45 cases with clinicopathological correlation. Histopathology 12:235–252, 1988
312. Schmid C, Vazquez JJ, Diss TC, Isaacson PG: Primary B-cell mucosa-associated lymphoid tissue lymphoma presenting as a solitary colorectal polyp. Histopathology 24:357–362, 1994
313. Lee MH, Waxman M, Gillooley JF: Primary malignant lymphoma of the anorectum in homosexual men. Dis Colon Rectum 29: 413–416, 1986
314. Ioachim HL, Weinstein MA, Robbins RD et al: Primary anorectal lymphoma. A new manifestation of the acquired immune deficiency syndrome (AIDS). Cancer 60:1449–1453, 1987
315. Sibly TG, Keane RM, Lever JV et al: Rectal lymphoma in radiation injured bowel. Br J Surg 72:879–880, 1985
316. Yamanaha N, Ishil Y, Koshiba H et al: A study of surface markers in gastrointestinal lymphoma. Gastroenterology 79:673, 1980
317. Grody WW, Weiss LM, Warnke RA et al: Gastrointestinal lymphomas. Immunohistochemical studies on the cell of origin. Am J Surg Pathol 9:328–337, 1985
318. Fernandes BJ, Amato D, Goldfinger M: Diffuse lymphomatous polyposis of the gastrointestinal tract. A case report with immunohistochemical studies. Gastroenterology 88:1267–1270, 1985
319. Stessens L, Van Den Oord JJ, Geboes K et al: Gastrointestinal lymphomatous polyposis. Gastroenterology 90:2041–2042, 1986
320. Gleason TH, Hammar SP: Plasmacytoma of the colon. Cancer 50:130–133, 1982
321. Appelman HD: Mesenchymal tumors of the gastrointestinal tract. pp. 310–350. In Ming S-C, Goldman H (eds): Pathology of the Gastrointestinal Tract. WB Saunders, Philadelphia, 1992
322. Ranchod M, Kempson RL: Smooth muscle tumors of the gastrointestinal tract and retroperitoneum: a pathologic analysis of 100 cases. Cancer 39:255, 1977
323. Evans HL: Smooth muscle tumors of the gastrointestinal tract. A study of 56 cases followed for a minimum of 10 years. Cancer 56:2242–2250, 1985
324. Weiss RA, Mackay B: Malignant smooth muscle tumors of the gastrointestinal tract. Ultrastruct Pathol 2:231–240, 1981
325. Walsh TH, Mann CV: Smooth muscle neoplasms of the rectum and anal canal. Br J Surg 71:597–599, 1984
326. Khalifa AA, Bong WL, Rao VK et al: Leiomyosarcoma of the rectum—report of a case and review of the literature. Dis Colon Rectum 29:427–432, 1986
327. Hague S, Dean RJ: Stromal neoplasms of the rectum and anal canal. Hum Pathol 23:762–767, 1992
328. Saul SH, Rast ML, Brooks JJ: The immunohistochemistry of gastrointestinal stromal tumors. Am J Surg Pathol 11:464–473, 1987
329. Pike AM, Lloyd RV, Appelman HD: Cell markers in gastrointestinal stromal tumors. Hum Pathol 19:830–834, 1988
330. Franquemont DW: Differentiation and risk assessment of gastrointestinal stromal tumors. Am J Clin Pathol 103:41–47, 1995
331. Cohen RS, Cramm RE: Granular-cell myoblastoma. Dis Colon Rectum 12:120–124, 1969

332. Johnston J, Helwig EB: Granular cell tumors of the gastrointestinal tract and perianal region. A study of 74 cases. Dig Dis Sci 26:807–816, 1981
333. Yanai-Inbor I, Odes HS, Krugliak P et al: Granular cell myoblastoma of the sigmoid colon. Dig Dis Sci 26:852–854, 1981
334. Daimaru Y, Kido H, Hashimoto H, Enjoji M: Benign schwannoma of the gastrointestinal tract: a clinicopathologic and immunohistochemical study. Hum Pathol 19:257–264, 1988
335. Fuller CE, Williams GT: Gastrointestinal manifestations of type-1 neurofibromatosis (von Recklinghausen's disease). Histopathology 19:1–12, 1991
336. Shekitka KM, Sobin LH: Ganglioneurons of the gastrointestinal tract. Relation to Von Recklinghausen disease and other multiple tumor syndromes. Am J Surg Pathol 18: 250–257, 1994
337. Tawfik OW, McGregor DH: Lipohyperplasia of the ileocecal valve. Am J Gastroenterol 87:82–87, 1992
338. Castro EB, Stearns MW: Lipoma of the large intestine. Dis Colon Rectum 15:441–444, 1972
339. Michowitz M, Lazebnik N, Noy S et al: Lipoma of the colon: a report of 22 cases. Am Surg 51:449–454, 1985
340. Taylor BA, Wolff BG: Chronic lipomas: report of two unusual cases and review of the Mayo clinical experience, 1976–1985. Dis Colon Rectum 30:888–893, 1988
341. Wassman M, Faegenburg D, Waxman JS, Janelli PE: Malignant fibrous histiocytoma of the colon associated with diverticulitis. Dis Colon Rectum 26:339–343, 1983
342. Norris HT: Vascular disorders. pp. 214–239. In Ming S-C, Goldman H (eds): Pathology of the Gastrointestinal Tract. WB Saunders, Philadelphia, 1992
343. Pontecorvo C, Lombardi S, Mottola L et al: Hemangiomas of the large bowel. Report of a case. Dis Colon Rectum 26:818–820, 1983
344. Camilleri M, Satti MB, Wood CB: Cystic lymphangioma of the colon: endoscopic and histologic features. Dis Colon Rectum 25:813–816, 1982
345. Kuramoto S, Sakai S, Tsuda K et al: Lymphangioma of the large intestine. Dis Colon Rectum 31:900–905, 1988
346. Nakagawara G, Kojima Y, Mai M et al: Lymphangioma of the transverse colon treated by transendoscopic polypectomy: report of a case and review of the literature. Dis Colon Rectum 24:291–295, 1981
347. Rose HS, Balthazar EJ, Megibow AJ et al: Alimentary tract involvement in Kaposi's sarcoma: radiographic and endoscopic findings in 25 homosexual men. Am J Radiol 39:661–666, 1982
348. Saltz RK, Kurtz RC, Lightdale CJ et al: Kaposi's sarcoma. Gastrointestinal involvement and correlation with skin findings and immunologic function. Dig Dis Sci 29: 817–823, 1984
349. Freedman SL, Wright TL, Altman DF: Gastrointestinal Kaposi's sarcoma in patients with acquired immunodeficiency syndrome. Endoscopic and autopsy findings. Gastroenterology 89:102–108, 1985
350. Roth JA, Schell S, Panzarino S et al: Visceral Kaposi's sarcoma presenting as colitis. Am J Surg Pathol 2:209, 1978
351. Bianco J, Pratt-Bianco L: Kaposi's sarcoma of the rectum: a case report. Mt Sinai J Med 50:278–280, 1983
352. Taxy JB, Battifora H: Angiosarcoma of the gastrointestinal tract. A report of three cases. Cancer 62:210–216, 1988
353. Genter B, Mir K, Strauss R et al: Hemangiopericytoma of the colon: report of a case and review of the literature. Dis Colon Rectum 25:149–156, 1982
354. Williams GT, Blackshaw AJ, Morson BC: Squamous carcinoma of the colorectum and its genesis. J Pathol 29:139, 1979
355. Gould L, Shaw JM, Khedekor RR, Burns WA: Squamous cell carcinoma of the splenic flexure of the colon. Dig Dis Sci 28:918–922, 1983
356. Lafreniere R, Ketcham AS: Primary squamous carcinoma of the rectum: report of a case and review of the literature. Dis Colon Rectum 28:967–972, 1985
357. Michelassi F, Mishlove LA, Stipa F, Block GE: Squamous-cell carcinoma of the colon. Dis Colon Rectum 31:228–235, 1988
358. Cabera A, Pickren JW: Squamous metaplasia and squamous cell carcinoma of the rectosigmoid. Dis Colon Rectum 10:288, 1967
359. Ordonez NG, Luna MA: Choriocarcinoma of the colon. Am J Gastroenterol 79:39–42, 1984

360. Kubosawa H, Nagao K, Kondo Y et al: Coexistence of adenocarcinoma and choriocarcinoma in the sigmoid colon. Cancer 54:866–868, 1984
361. Rutter K, Riddell RH: The solitary ulcer syndrome of the rectum. Clin Gastroenterol 4:505–530, 1975
362. Saul SH, Sollenberger IC: Solitary rectal ulcer syndrome. Its clinical and pathological underdiagnosis. Am J Surg Pathol 9:411–421, 1985
363. Hall-Craggs M, Toker C: Basaloid tumor of the sigmoid colon. Hum Pathol 13:497–500, 1982
364. Strate RW, Richardson JD, Bannayan GA: Basosquamous (transitional cloacogenic) carcinoma of the sigmoid colon. Hum Pathol 13:497–500, 1982
365. Wanebo HJ, Woodruff JM, Farr GH, Quan SH: Anorectal melanoma. Cancer 47:1891–1900, 1981
366. Werdin C, Limas C, Knodell RG: Primary malignant melanoma of the rectum. Evidence for orgination from rectal mucosal melancytes. Cancer 61:1364–1371, 1988
367. Nicholson AG, Cox PM, Marks CG, Cook MG: Primary malignant melanoma of the rectum. Histopathology 22:261–264, 1993
368. Aldridge MC, Boylston AW, Sim AJW: Dermoid cyst of the rectum. Dis Colon Rectum 26:333–334, 1983
369. Johnston EV, Dockerty MB, Dixon CF: Cylindroma of rectum. Proc Mayo Clin 28:729–735, 1953
370. Barcos M, Lane W, Gomez GA et al: An autopsy study of 1206 acute and chronic leukemias (1958–1982). Cancer 60:827–837, 1987
371. Kothus R, Marsh F, Posner G et al: Endoscopic leukemic polyposis. Am J Gastroenterol 85:884–886, 1990
372. Sachs Ba, Joffe N, Antonioli DA: Metastatic melanoma presenting clinically as multiple colonic polyps. AJR 129:511, 1979
373. Geboes K, DeJaeger E, Rutgierts P, Vantrappen G: Symptomatic gastrointestinal metastases from malignant melanoma. A clinical study. J Clin Gastroenterol 10:64–70, 1988
374. Adair C, Ro, JY, Sahin AA et al: Malignant melanoma metastatic to gastrointestinal tract. Int J Surg Pathol 2:3–10, 1994
375. Katon RM, Brendler SJ, Ireland K: Gastric linitis plastica with metastases to the colon: a mimic of Crohn's disease. J Clin Gastroenterol 11:555–560, 1989
376. Rabau MY, Alon RJ, Werbin N, Yossipov Y: Colonic metastases from lobular carcinoma of the breast: report of a case. Dis Colon Rectum 31:401–402, 1988
377. Antler AS, Ough Y, Pitchumoni CS et al: Gastrointestinal metastases from malignant tumors of the lungs. Cancer 49:170–172, 1982
378. Wegener M, Borsch G, Reitemeyer E, Schafer K: Metastastis to the colon from primary bronchogenic carcinoma presenting as occult gastrointestinal bleeding: report of a case. Z Gastroenterol 26:358–362, 1988
379. Heymann AD, Vieta JO: Recurrent renal carcinoma causing intestinal hemorrhage. Am J Gastroenterol 69:582–585, 1978
380. Sweetenham JW, Whitehouse JM, Williams CJ, Mead GM: Involvement of the gastrointestinal tract by metastases from germ cell tumor of the testes. Cancer 61:2566–2570, 1988

11

Disorders of the Anal Region

GENERAL ASPECTS

A few disorders are often seen in the anal region, such as hemorrhoidal varices, anal fissures and fistulae.[1, 2] Tumors in the anal region occur much less frequently than in the large intestine. Many of the conditions have an increased prevalence in homosexual males, this presumably related to a greater number of chronic infections in this area.

Endoscopy and biopsy of the anal region are uncommonly performed, as compared to other parts of the alimentary tract. Most of the material used for evaluation is in the form of small mucosal and skin biopsies. The diagnoses are largely provided by examination of the routine H & E sections, and special stains including cytochemical reactions are helpful in delineating the various tumors.

NORMAL STRUCTURE

The anal region includes the lowest part of the rectum, the anal canal, and the adjacent anal skin.[3] The canal is separated from the rectum by a zone termed the *dentate,* or *pentinate, line.*[4] At the lower end of the anal canal, there is the junction with the anal skin, referred to as the *anal verge,* or *margin.*

At the dentate line there is an irregular interposition of the rectal mucosa and of the anal papillae extending for up to 1 cm. This has also been referred to as the *transitional zone,* and most of the ducts from the anal glands enter into this region.[5]

Lower Rectal Mucosa

As described in Chapter 9, the distal few centimeters of the rectum show a marked shortening of the crypts with irregularity, prominent lymphoid tissue, and a thickened muscularis mucosae, all features that also would be compatible with a chronic colitis in a more proximal location (see Fig. 9-7). Some of the disorders of the anal region, such as hemorrhoids, can extend into the lower rectum and are covered by this atrophic mucosa.

Transitional Zone

The transitional zone corresponds to the junction of the rectum and anal canal, and can extend for a few millimeters, up to

1 cm.[4] The epithelium in this region shows a stratified cuboidal and flattened type that has been called *transitional epithelium,* with an implication of similarity to that seen in the urinary tract (Fig. 11-1). However, there appear to be significant functional differences, and the epithelium in the anal area is probably more like a modified squamous tissue. The lack of complete squamous differentiation in this area might help to explain the histologic features seen in the tumors that arise from this area—the cloacogenic carcinomas.

Anal Glands

The openings of the anal glands and ducts are typically in this upper region of the anal canal, and their blockage is probably the key factor in the formation of anal fistulae and abscesses. There are scattered anal glands beneath the epithelium and extending part of the way down the anal canal; these most often have mucous-type cells.[5]

Anal Canal

The anal canal extends for about 4 to 5 cm and is covered by a non-keratinizing, stratified squamous epithelium (Fig. 11-2). Scattered in the basal region are endocrine and melanin-producing cells as well.[6] In the wall are the anal glands and a rich venous plexus that is subject to dilation.

Anal Skin

The anal skin is covered by a keratinized squamous epithelium and has all of the features of skin in other areas of the body, including the presence of hair as well as sebaceous, sweat, and apocrine glands. Accordingly, many of the inflammatory and tumor diseases affecting the skin can also develop in this area.

DEVELOPMENTAL DISORDERS

Most of these conditions are recognized by their gross characteristics, and biopsies are uncommonly employed to exclude complications such as infections and ischemic effects.

Anal Stenosis and Atresia

There are a large variety and combination of developmental defects in the anal canal, consisting of a mixture of agenesis, stenosis, and fistulae in this area.[7] A classification of these lesions is based on location, whether high, intermediate, or low in reference to the levator ani and other muscles. Imperforate anus is a separate condition due presumably to a failure of elimination of the outer anal membranes.[8] All of these conditions may be associated with an increase in sacrococcygeal teratomas.[1]

Exstrophy and Cysts

Failure of elimination of the developmental cloaca can result in persistent connections of the urinary and alimentary tracts with variable wide openings in the perineal region.[9] These are usually evident grossly and do not require biopsy studies. As mentioned in Chapter 10, the former technique of implanting the ureter into the colon of such patients was associated with the early development of adenomas and carcinomas in the colon. This technique has now been replaced by the creation of ileal bladders without this complication.

Duplication cysts are rare; they are typically located in the retrorectal region and

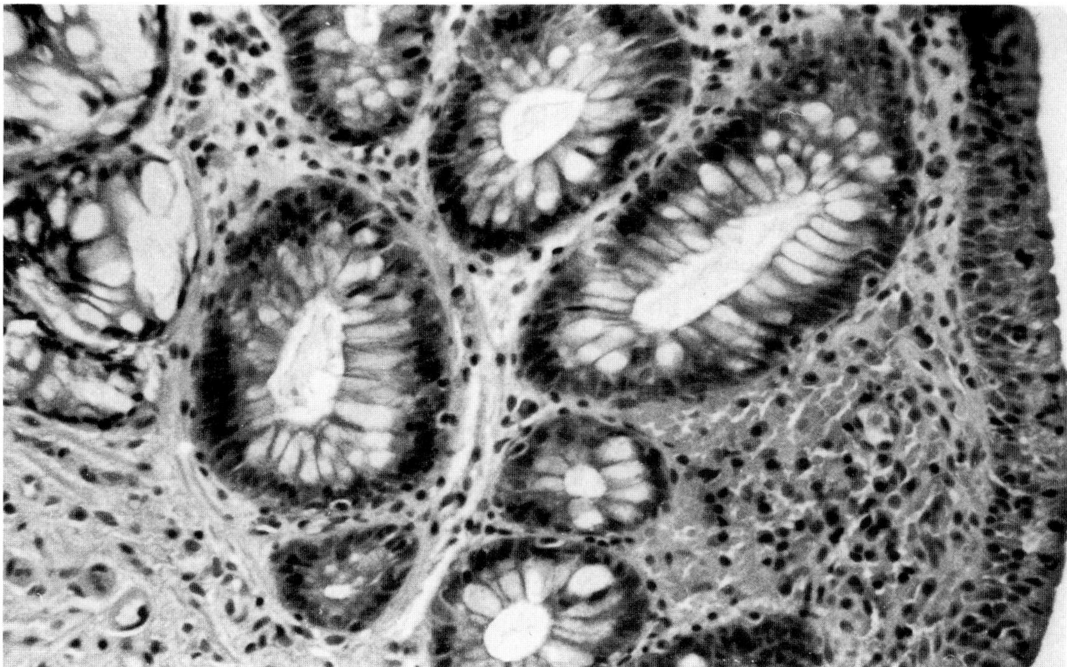

Fig. 11-1. Normal transitional zone at the anorectal junction. A relatively thin layer of squamous epithelium appears at the right, covering the rectal glands.

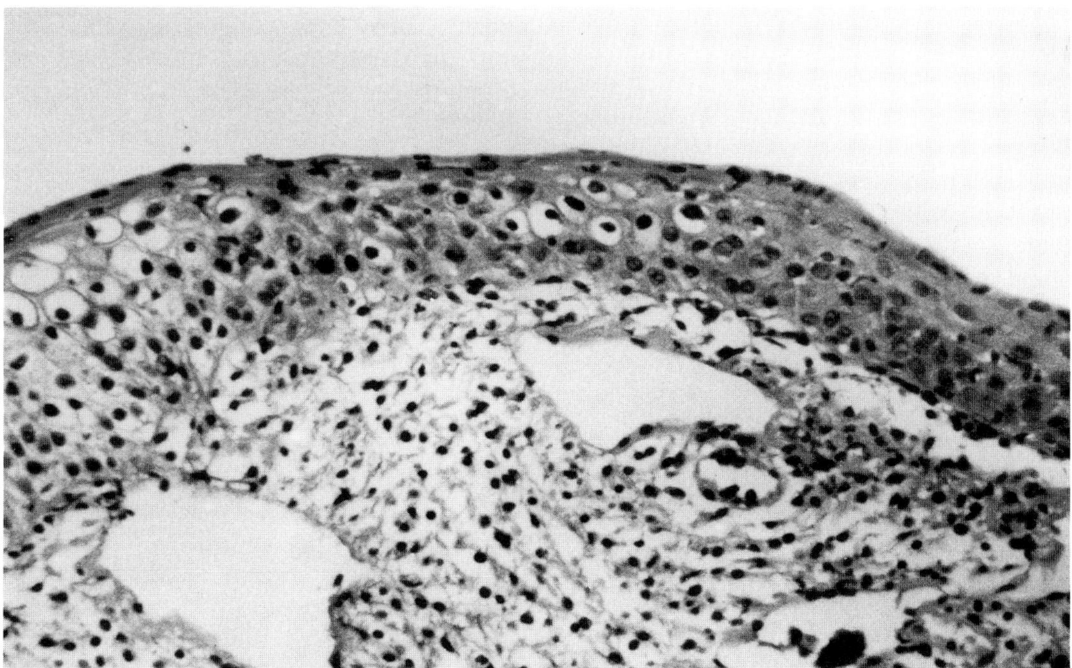

Fig. 11-2. Normal anal canal. The layer of stratified squamous epithelium appears at the top. This extends from the less mature tissue in the transitional zone (right) to the thicker layer of the anal canal (left). There is no keratin production.

may be associated with an increased chance of carcinoma development.

VASCULAR DISORDERS

Hemorrhoidal Varices

Hemorrhoidal varices is one of the most common conditions affecting both men and women and is due to a progressive dilation of the veins beneath the surface epithelium in the anal and lower rectal regions.[10–12] It is thought to be a consequence of prolonged and progressive stasis in this area, and can be accentuated in patients with portal hypertension, with various causes of increased intra-abdominal pressure, and probably with a general sedentary life-style. The varices are categorized as *internal* if located in the upper region and covered by atrophic rectal mucosa, and as *external* when in the anal area and surrounded by a squamous epithelium.

The patients present with acute or chronic bleeding, with prolapse of the varices, and with other complications. The dilated veins are prone to the development of secondary thrombi that can cause further expansion and increased pain. They also may ulcerate and result in prolonged bleeding. In healing, there is a tendency for the veins to undergo obliteration and to be associated with extensive fibrous tissue; these are covered by squamous epithelium and may present as anal skin tags.

Biopsy Features

Although there are currently many less surgical excisions than in former years, removal of hemorrhoidal varices is still a fairly common procedure. Examination reveals the subepithelial dilated veins, which typically show a thickened wall and thrombi of varying ages (Fig. 11-3). The healed lesions reveal a dense core of fibrous tissue. The overlying epithelium, whether atrophic rectal or squamous, is usually normal. Uncommonly, one may observe other conditions in the tissue samples that are submitted with the hemorrhoidal varices. These include the presence of infections, Crohn's disease, and dysplasia of the squamous epithelium.[13] Accordingly, histologic examination of hemorrhoidal tissue should be routinely performed.

Prolapse

Prolapse of the rectal and upper anal mucosa is a fairly common event. It is seen in younger patients in association with the solitary rectal ulcer syndrome. More commonly, it occurs in older patients, presumably as a result of acquired deficiencies in the anal sphincter area.[14, 15] Changes are most typically noted in the rectal mucosa and show the effects of ischemia in the form of marked edema, patchy hemorrhages, and focal erosions. In the solitary ulcer syndrome, the condition can be associated with a large polyp.[16, 17] (See Ch. 9 for further details.)

INFECTIONS

The infections may be limited to the anal region or involve both the anal canal and the adjacent rectum.

General Features

Anal infections are generally uncommon, but are decidedly increased in frequency in homosexual males with or without associated AIDS (Table 11-1). The biopsies help in identifying the ulcerative or other inflammatory lesions, and in acquiring material for the diagnosis of the specific infection.

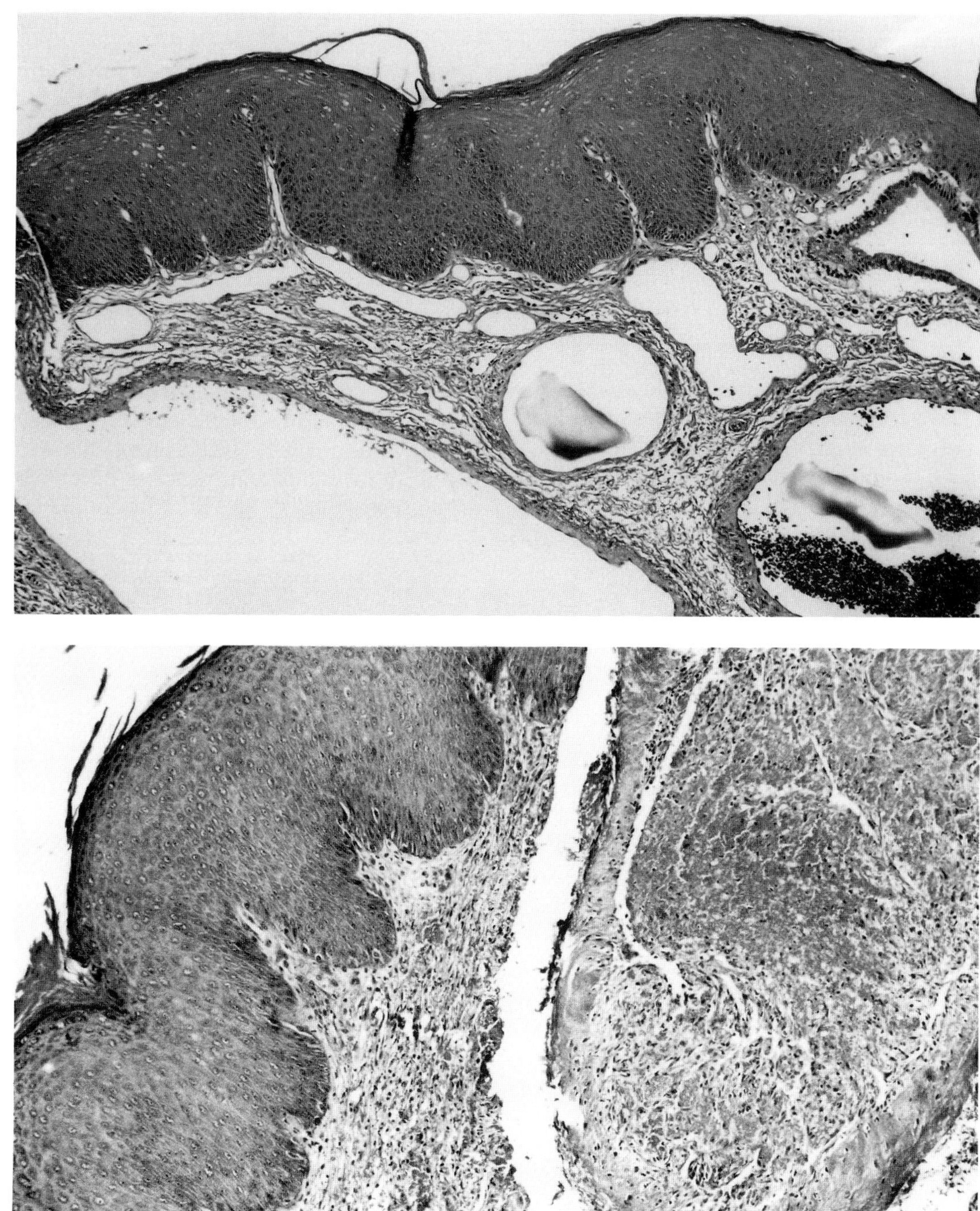

Fig. 11-3. Examples of hemorrhoidal varices. **(A)** Noted are several large dilated veins. The anal surface appears at the top (× 105). **(B)** A large dilated vein that contains an organizing thrombus appears at the right. The squamous epithelium appears at the left (× 105).

Table 11-1. Infections of the Anal Canal

Viral
Herpes simplex
HIV
Rare: CMV
Chlamydial
Bacterial
Gonorrhea
Syphilis
Granuloma inguinale
Tuberculosis
Rare: malakoplakia
Fungal
Parasitic
Enterobius

Most of the infections in the anal region are of the venereal type. They are more often seen in homosexual males and especially in patients with AIDS, showing a greater frequency of the usual infections and the appearance of opportunistic organisms.

VIRAL INFECTIONS

Herpes Simplex Infection

Herpes simplex is the most common viral infection seen in the anal area, related to the presence of the squamous epithelium as the target tissue.[18–20] Noted are multiple vesicles and small erosions. Biopsies show the typical features of multinucleated squamous cells together with intranuclear inclusions that have a prominent halo, and associated marked acute inflammation in the ulcerated areas (Plate 1A). The features can be readily diagnosed in brush cytologic material as well as in the biopsies.

Human Papillomaviruses

Human papillomaviruses are present in association with condylomas, with dysplasia, and squamous tumors. They are described in later sections.

Human Immunodeficiency Virus

Some of the ulcers noted in the anal and rectal mucosa are thought to be a direct infection by HIV.[21] Biopsies show nonspecific ulcer and inflammation, and the viral particles can be detected by electron microscopy (see Fig. 7-7).

Other Viral Infections

Cytomegalovirus infection is more commonly noted in the rectal and colonic mucosa but can complicate other ulcerating lesions in the anal area in patients with AIDS (see Ch. 9). There can be infection of the skin region from molluscum, which is described in the section below on "Skin Lesions".

CHLAMYDIAL INFECTIONS

The most important type of chlamydial infection is lymphogranuloma venereum, which can involve the anal mucosa but is much more commonly noted in the rectum.[22,23] It is associated with pronounced lymphoid hyperplasia and with sporadic granulomas.[24] The diagnosis is usually made by serologic study.

BACTERIAL INFECTIONS

Gonorrhea

Gonorrhea is a veneral infection associated with scattered ulcers and inflammation in the anal canal and rectal mucosa.[25,26] Biopsies show nonspecific erosions with marked acute inflammation, and smears may reveal the gram-negative diplococci. The diagnosis is dependent on culture.

Syphilis

Both primary and secondary syphilitic lesions can occur in the anal region.[27] In the primary chancre, there is pronounced proliferation of plasma cells and of endothelial cells. The spirochetes can be demonstrated by dark field examination of smears, and also in the tissue sections by the use of the Warthin-Starry silver stain.

The secondary form of syphilis presents as slightly raised papules referred to as *condyloma latum.* This shows less specific features in the form of acanthosis and scattered inflammatory cells in the underlying stroma.

Granuloma Inguinale

Granuloma inguinale usually presents as a perianal ulcer. Biopsies show the necrosis together with nonspecific inflammation, and there is often a marked pseudoepitheliomatous hyperplasia of the squamous tissue. The responsible bacteria can be found in the macrophages, termed *Donovan bodies,* and are best seen with Giemsa and silver stains.

Other Bacterial Infections

Tuberculosis can occur in the anal or perianal regions and is associated with ulceration or hypertrophic lesions.[28] An increase in the number of cases of tuberculosis is seen in AIDS patients.[29] Biopsies show the ulcers or hyperplasia together with granulomas (see Fig. 9-20). The diagnosis is dependent on finding the acid-fast organisms in the tissues and is made secure by culture. There are also rare reports of malakoplakia in the anal area[30, 31] (see Ch. 9 for a description).

Fungal and Parasitic Infections

These are rare and mostly restricted to patients with severe debilitation or immunodeficiency disorders. Reaction to the pinworm, *Enterobius vermicularis,* can occur in the anal area, resulting in localized abscess or granuloma formation, and these may be seen on biopsy.[32, 33]

OTHER INFLAMMATORY DISORDERS

Anal Fissure and Fistula

Anal fissure and fistula are relatively common and are often evaluated by endoscopy and biopsy for diagnosis and to follow the cases after therapy (Table 11-2).

Anal Fissure

The anal fissure presents as a longitudinal, narrow ulcer and is most often located on the posterior wall of the anal canal.[34] Biopsy features are variable, probably dependent on the age of the lesion, and initially show necrosis and acute inflammation (Fig. 11-4A). Later lesions reveal chronic inflammation, fibrosis, and the development of anal skin tags similar to those seen in hemorrhoidal varices. The differential diagnosis includes infections, which may show more specific features including the particular microorganisms; Crohn's disease, which may have granulomas; and tumors.

Fistula and Abscess

The fistula and abscess probably develop as a result of blockage of the anal ducts, particularly at their origin in the anal crypts.[35, 36] This can lead to a fistulous tract from that area into the underlying tissues,

Table 11-2. Other Inflammatory Disorders of the Anal Region

Anal fissure
Anal fistula and abscess
Crohn's disease
Foreign body reactions
Drug reactions
Skin diseases
Hidradenitis suppurativa
Molluscum contagiosum
Lichen sclerosis
Bowenoid papulosis

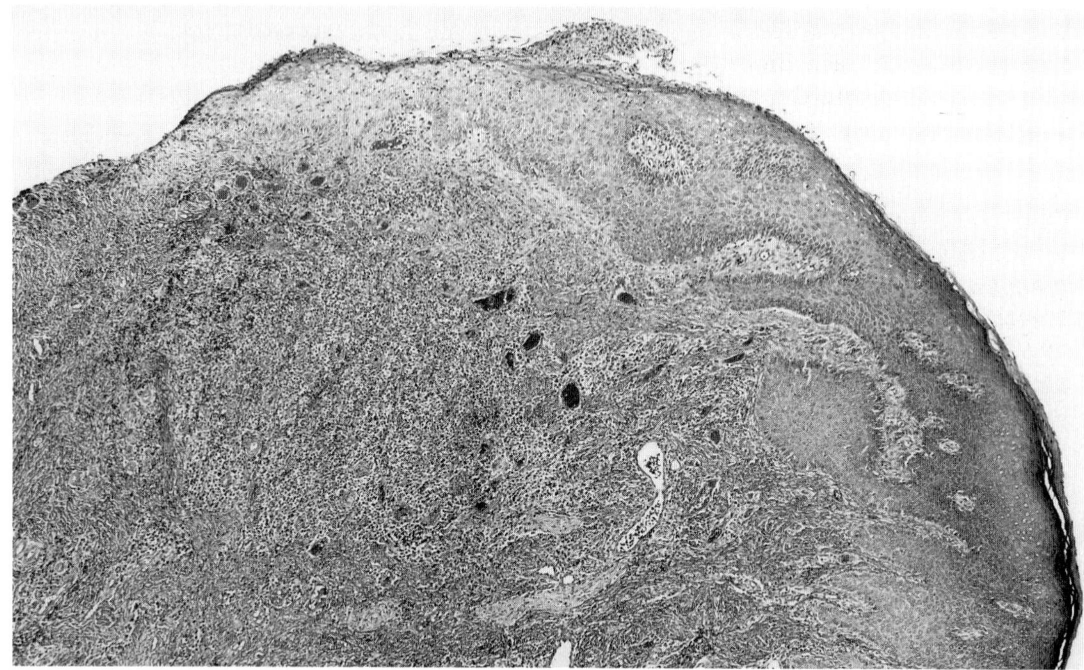

A

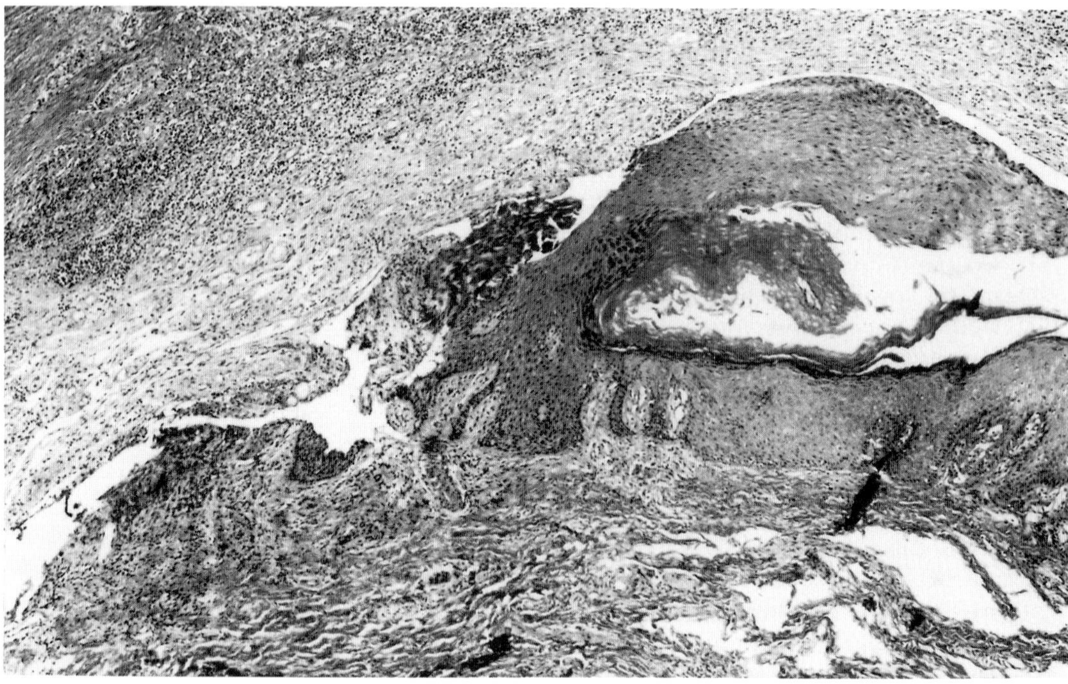

B

Fig. 11-4. (A) Anal fissure. Present are a superficial ulcer (top left) and marked inflammation in the underlying wall. The adjacent intact squamous epithelium (right) is thickened (× 42). **(B)** Anal fistula and abscess. Extending from the surface (right) is a tract that is partially lined by squamous epithelium. There is a rupture of the fistula (center left) with adjacent abscess and granulation tissue (× 56).

and it may extend to the perianal skin. There can be rupture with abscess formation anywhere along the tract. Biopsies are entirely nonspecific, showing the marked acute inflammation together with granulation tissue and variable fibrosis (Fig. 11-4B). The differential diagnosis includes Crohn's disease, which can be associated with multiple fistulae and abscesses but usually shows prominent granulomas and disease in other parts of the bowel; and tumors. Squamous cell carcinomas can occasionally present with an anal fistula or abscess, and adenocarcinomas can develop as a late complication of fistulae.[37–39]

Idiopathic Inflammatory Bowel Disease

Ulcerative Colitis

There are no special features of ulcerative colitis that affects the anal canal.[40] The patients can develop the common disorders, and it has been suggested that anal fissures may be slightly more frequent.

Crohn's Disease

The anal canal and perianal skin are frequently involved in patients with Crohn's disease.[41–44] It is estimated to occur in about 20 to 30 percent of cases with involvement of the small bowel, and from 50 to 80 percent of those with large intestinal disease. Indeed, the condition may primarily appear in the anal and perianal region in a small percentage of the cases, with a lag before there is evident gross intestinal disease. The patients present with marked ulcers, abscesses, and fistulae which usually do not respond to ordinary treatment regimens. The diagnosis should be grossly suspected by the finding of multiple fissures or fistulae.

Biopsy features are mostly nonspecific, showing the inflammation, granulation tissue, and fibrosis (Fig. 11-5). Granulomas are present in about one-half of the cases and may be well or poorly formed. They typically lack caseous necrosis, helping to distinguish Crohn's disease from tuberculosis. Unfortunately, granulomas responding to foreign material and to other bacteria are not rare in the perianal skin region, and it is important to link this finding with other features to support the diagnosis of Crohn's disease. It is helpful in these cases to recommend that endoscopy of the adjacent bowel be done, with the taking of biopsies from the rectal mucosa to look for associated granulomas. These may be present in this region even if there is no evidence of proctitis, and their finding can be used to support the diagnosis.[45–47.]

The cases of anal and perianal Crohn's disease can be associated with carcinoma.[48] Adenocarcinomas typically develop in the fistulous tracts and may be especially difficult to diagnose. A high index of suspicion and deep biopsies are often required. There is also an increased frequency of squamous cell carcinoma that involves the anal mucosa.[49, 50]

Foreign Body and Drug Reactions

Reactions can develop secondary to injected foreign materials such as oils.[51, 52] The lesions are usually more prominent in the rectum but can extend into the wall of the anal region. Biopsies show irregular spaces, corresponding to the oils dissolved in the preparation, together with chronic inflammation and prominent fibrosis (see Fig. 9-33).

Injury due to ergot drugs in suppositories has been noted in the anal and rectal regions, presumably due to the vascular effect.[53] Biopsies reveal mucosal erosions with inflammation.

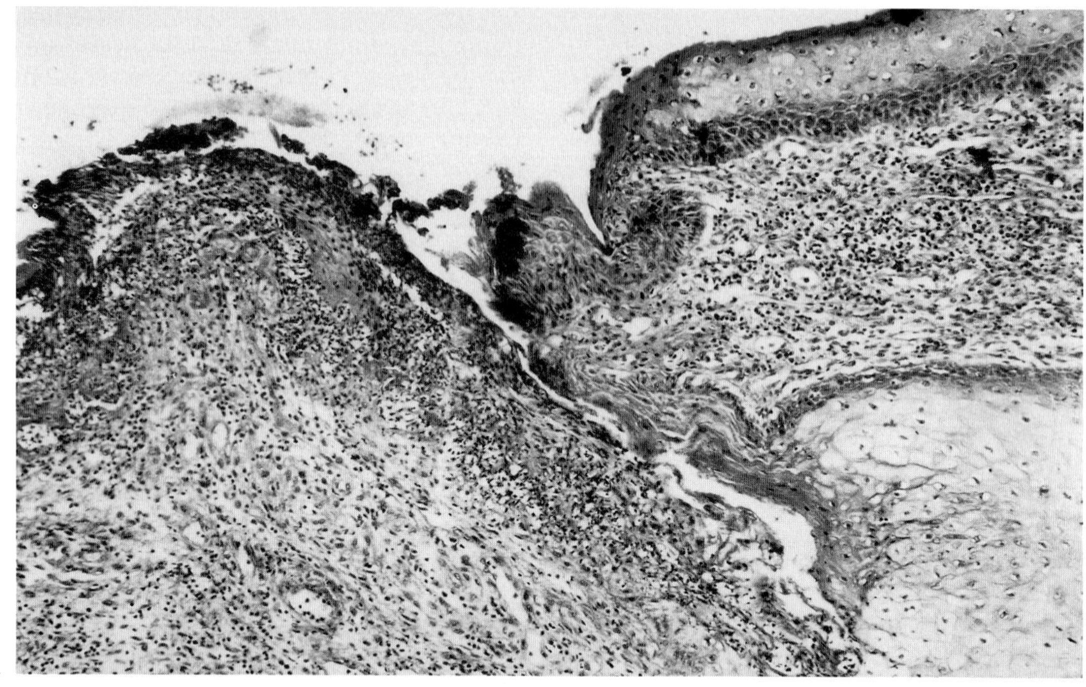

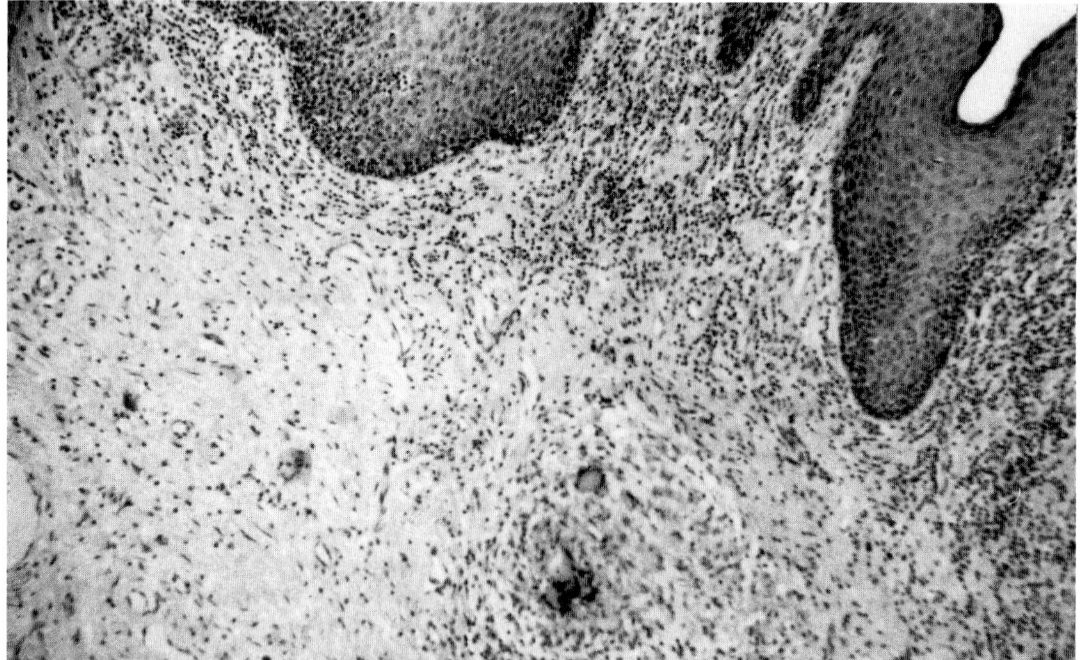

Fig. 11-5. Crohn's disease in the anal region. **(A)** Present are an ulcer with acute inflammation (left) and a sinus tract that extends into the underlying tissue (lower right) and is partly lined by squamous epithelium. The intact anal surface appears at the upper right (× 105). **(B)** Noted are poorly formed granulomas without central necrosis, together with inflammation and fibrosis. The squamous epithelium appears at the top.

Skin Lesions

Skin lesions occur in the adjacent anal skin.

Hidradenitis Suppurativa

Hidradenitis suppurativa results from rupture of apocrine glands in the area, typically presenting with a large abscess.[54] It mainly affects the skin but can extend into the wall of the lower anal canal. Biopsies show the marked acute inflammation, scattered giant cells, and rare fragments of the glands.

Molluscum Contagiosum

Molluscum contagiosum represents an infection by a pox virus. The lesion presents as a small umbilicated nodule, and excisional biopsy is highly characteristic, showing the squamous cells expanded by brightly eosinophilic inclusions.

Lichen Sclerosis et Atrophicus

The lesion of lichen sclerosis is more commonly seen in older and postmenopausal women but can develop in all ages. It presents as irregular thickenings or atrophy of the skin and often responds to applications of androgen ointments. Biopsies show the characteristic condensation of the collagen in the upper portion of the dermis, together with an irregular squamous epithelium. Biopsies are also done to exclude any dysplasia or carcinoma in the epithelium.

Bowenoid Papulosis

Bowenoid papulosis is an uncommon condition that must be distinguished from Bowen's disease. It presents as a pigmented papule, and biopsy shows acanthosis with some irregularity of the cells, but not as excessive as in dysplasia of the squamous epithelium.[55] The lesions typically regress rather than develop a carcinoma, in contrast to Bowen's disease.

BENIGN TUMORS

Inflammatory Polyps

Polyps can develop as a consequence of trauma, infection, or other inflammatory conditions (Table 11-3). They appear as nodules that are comprised of variable inflammation and granulation tissue, and are associated with a marked hyperplasia of the squamous epithelium together with prominent elongation of the rete pegs. In addition, polyps of an inflammatory nature can be seen as a consequence of the solitary rectal ulcer syndrome. These can extend into the anal region and are recognized by biopsies that show their glandular nature. They rarely may contain foci of squamous metaplasia, particularly in the very large lesions that are referred to as *inflammatory cloacogenic polyps*.[16, 17]

Lymphoid Polyps

There can be pronounced lymphoid hyperplasia resulting in plaques or polyps in the anal region.[56] Biopsies show the marked lymphoid tissue together with prominent follicles (see Fig. 10-31). They are differentiated from lymphoma by the heterogeneity of the follicle cells and the overall maturity of the surrounding lymphocytes. Marker studies

Table 11-3. Benign Tumors of the Anal Region

Inflammatory polyps
Lymphoid polyps
Anal skin tag
Condyloma acuminatum
Mesenchymal tumors
Adnexal tumors

used to look for monoclonal proliferation can be performed in uncertain cases.

Anal Skin Tags

Anal skin tags, which represent cores of fibrous tissue that are covered by squamous epithelium, with varying degrees of acanthosis and papillomatosis, can develop as a late consequence of inflammatory lesions (Fig. 11-6). They are most commonly seen in patients with external hemorrhoids, and as a consequence of anal fissures and of Crohn's disease in the area. It was previously suggested that the presence of anal skin tags was a sign of an increased frequency of colorectal adenomas, but this remains in dispute.[57, 58]

Condyloma Acuminatum

Condylomas present as single or multiple warty lesions, and are most often noted in the anal and genital regions. They are more common in women, and are thought to be principally due to infection from human papillomavirus (HPV), mainly of types 6, 11, 16, and 18.[59, 60] Studies indicate that the types 6 and 11 are typical of the totally benign lesions, whereas types 16 and 18 are more often noted in areas of squamous cell dysplasia.

Biopsy Features

The biopsy features are characteristic, revealing a papillary lesion covered by an acanthotic squamous epithelium (Fig. 11-7). There is a variable granular zone, together with patchy parakeratosis and hyperkeratosis. Most strikingly noted are the koilocytotic changes in the squamous epithelial cells, in the form of wrinkled nuclei together with adjacent vacuoles in the cytoplasm. These changes are most often seen in the squamous cells in the upper portion of the thickened epithelium, and are the typical cytopathic feature of HPV organisms.

The lesions can develop foci of dysplasia, and exceptionally be associated with large forms and with carcinoma formation, which are described below in the section on "Squamous Cell Carcinoma and Related Tumors."[61]

Mesenchymal Tumors

A variety of benign mesenchymal lesions are uncommonly seen in the anal and perianal region.

Granular Cell Tumors

Granular cell tumors can affect any part of the alimentary tract, including the anal region.[62, 63] They present as nodules, and biopsies show the distinctive features of large cells with very small nuclei and abundant cytoplasm of a granular nature, corresponding to a marked increase of lysosomes (see Fig. 3-21). The tumors can be single or multiple and involve other parts of the gut or skin.

Other Mesenchymal Tumors

There are rare examples of leiomyoma, schwannoma, lipoma, and hemangioma in this area as well.[64–68] The diagnosis is usually established by excision rather than by biopsy.

Adnexal Tumors

Adnexal tumors develop in the skin appendages, principally the sweat and apocrine glands.[1, 2] They are typically in the form of small nodules, and their excision reveals characteristic features. Noted are adenomas and fibroadenomas of the apocrine glands, and hidradenoma papilliferum derived from sweat glands.[69, 70] They are limited to the

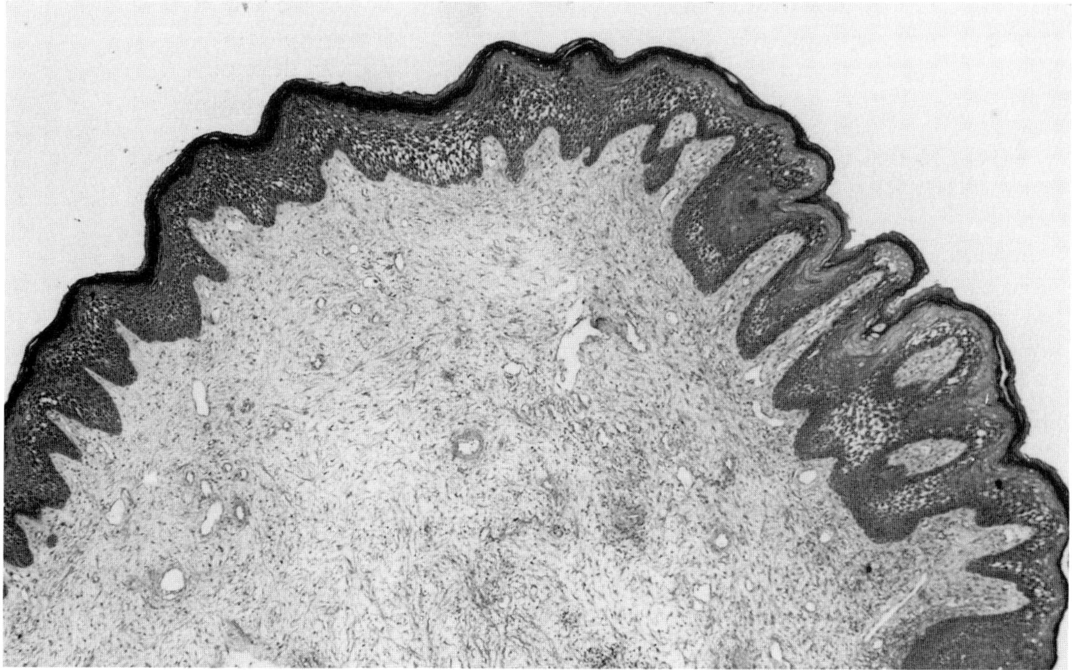

Fig. 11-6. Anal skin tag. There is a core of fibrovascular tissue covered by a slightly thickened squamous epithelial layer (× 42).

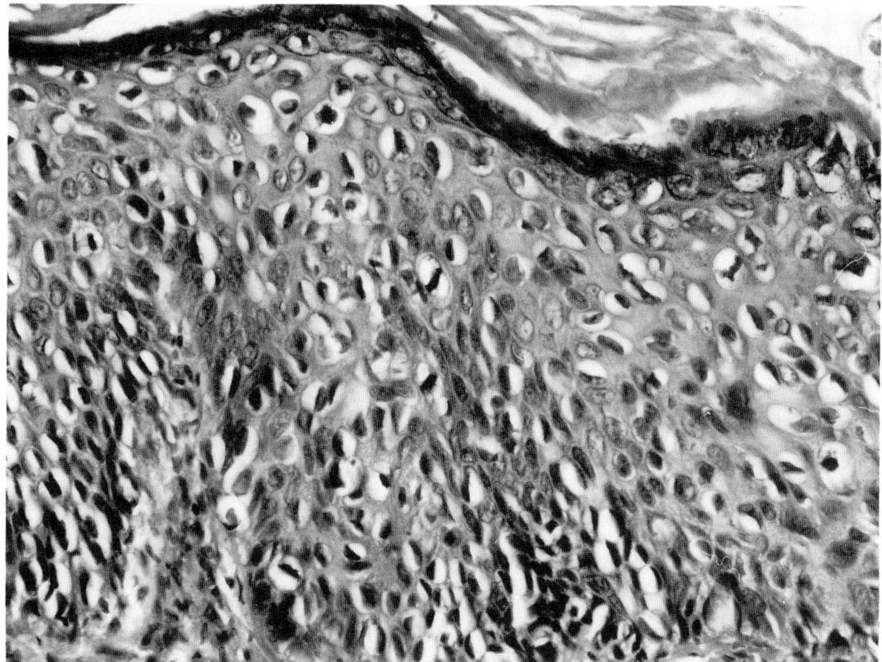

Fig. 11-7. Condyloma acuminatum. There are prominent acanthosis, hyperkeratosis, and squamous cells with dense wrinkled nuclei and cytoplasmic vacuoles, representing the cytopathic effects of human papillomavirus (× 280).

skin area and do not extend into the anal region.

SQUAMOUS CELL CARCINOMA AND RELATED TUMORS

Squamous cell carcinoma represents the most common form of malignant tumor in the anal region (Table 11-4). Biopsies are done to secure the diagnosis, to determine its extent, to follow the patients after therapy, and to exclude other lesions that can result from therapy, such as the effects of radiation and drugs as well as the appearance of opportunistic infections (Table 11-5).

Table 11-5. Biopsy Uses in Anal Tumors

Diagnosis
Extent of tumor
Evaluate after therapy
Exclude other diseases
Radiation effects
Chemotherapy effects
Opportunistic infections

General Features and Epidemiology

The majority of tumors develop in the anal canal, with less frequency of occurrence in the upper transitional area and at the lower anal margin.[71, 72] The carcinomas are more often seen in patients of lower socioeconomic status, and show a major increase of incidence in homosexual males, which is principally related to an increased number of infections in this area. It is thought that this is due to enhanced infection by human papillomavirus, which is important in the development of the dysplastic and carcinomatous lesions.[73, 74] Other factors that have been associated with an increase in squamous tumors include excess cigarette smoking, multiparity, and prior radiation exposure.

Table 11-4. Malignant Tumors of the Anal Region

Bowen's disease
Squamous cell carcinoma
Cloacogenic carcinoma
Adenocarcinomas
Anal ducts and glands
Fistulae
Paget's disease
Sarcomas
Malignant lymphoma
Malignant melanoma
Neuroendocrine carcinoma
Skin tumors
Secondary and metastatic tumors

Several types of tumors that involve the squamous epithelium have been noted, ranging from the pure squamous cell carcinomas to the cloacogenic carcinomas that develop in the transitional epithelium at the junction of the rectum and upper anal canal. The latter show less squamous features and more transitional or basaloid patterns, as discussed below. There are also verrucous and spindle cell types of squamous carcinoma, described below in the section on "Variant Forms of Squamous Carcinoma".

Premalignant Conditions and Lesions

Inflammatory Conditions

An increase of squamous cell carcinoma is noted in conditions associated with prolonged chronic inflammation, such as lymphogranuloma venereum and Crohn's disease,[49, 50] and in those lesions caused by HPV[59, 60] (Table 11-6). There is no enhanced frequency of squamous tumors related to the

Table 11-6. Premalignant Conditions in Anal Carcinoma

Chronic infections
Crohn's disease
Prolonged fistulas
Immunodeficiency
Human papillomavirus infection

common benign conditions, including varices, acute infections, and anal fissure.[75]

There appears to be a small increase of adenocarcinomas occurring in perianal fistulas of prolonged duration, including patients with Crohn's disease.[38, 39, 48] The tumors developing in these areas are often difficult to diagnose because of their location in the underlying tissue and the absence of associated dysplasia. The potential for carcinoma must be kept in mind, leading to deeper biopsies in such cases.

Human Papillomavirus

Human papillomavirus is noted in condylomas, in areas of dysplasia, and in the carcinomas.[59, 60, 76–79] In general, there is a tendency for types 6 and 11 to appear in the benign condylomas, whereas types 16 and 18 are seen more often in the dysplasia and better-differentiated carcinomas. Studies have linked the presence of HPV with alterations in the tumor suppressor gene p53. Mutations and overexpression of p53 have been seen in dysplastic and carcinomatous tissue as opposed to the benign conditions.[80] Patients with immunosuppression also show an increase of dysplasia and tumor, probably related to enhanced HPV infection.

Premalignant Lesions

Whatever the particular condition, the major premalignant lesion is dysplasia of the squamous epithelium, which can be categorized as of the low- or high-grade degree. The most severe form is called *squamous cell carcinoma in-situ,* or *Bowen's disease.* These lesions can be present in an isolated form or in conjunction with invasive carcinoma.

Squamous Dysplasia and Bowen's Disease

A full range of abnormal changes can be seen in the squamous epithelium, ranging from early dysplasia to carcinoma in-situ.[73, 81, 82] Collectively, these have been termed *intraepithelial neoplasia* and can be broadly divided into examples showing low-grade and high-grade dysplasia and Bowen's disease.

The lesions in Bowen's disease present as slightly raised plaques, and there is associated invasive cancer, usually superficial, in close to one-half of the cases.[83–85] As noted previously, all anal specimens removed from common lesions should be routinely examined, since areas of squamous dysplasia and Bowen's disease have been found.[13] Examples include the squamous epithelium overlying hemorrhoidal varices and that adjacent to anal fissures.

Biopsy Features

The lesions may show areas of dysplasia of a low- to high-grade degree as well as regions of more complete carcinoma in-situ (Bowen's disease) (Figs. 11-8 and 11-9). There is a lack of differentiation of the cells, resulting in the presence of immature and atypical squamous forms outside of the basal zone. Overall, there is a general uniformity of the cells but they show enlargement of the nuclei relative to the cytoplasm. There are also increased and irregular chromatin within the nuclei and mitoses above the basal layer. Keratin production is usually minimal or absent.

The determination of the lesion, whether squamous dysplasia of the low- or high-grade degree or Bowen's disease, is dependent on the extent of transformation of the squamous epithelium and the cytologic features. In general, low-grade dysplasia shows most abnormal cells limited to the lower third of the squamous epithelium; high-grade dysplasia reveals the cells in the mid and upper regions; and Bowen's disease has the atypical cells throughout the layer. The cytologic features also increase in abnormality from low-grade to high-grade dysplasia to Bowen's disease. Noted, in particular, are an increase in nu-

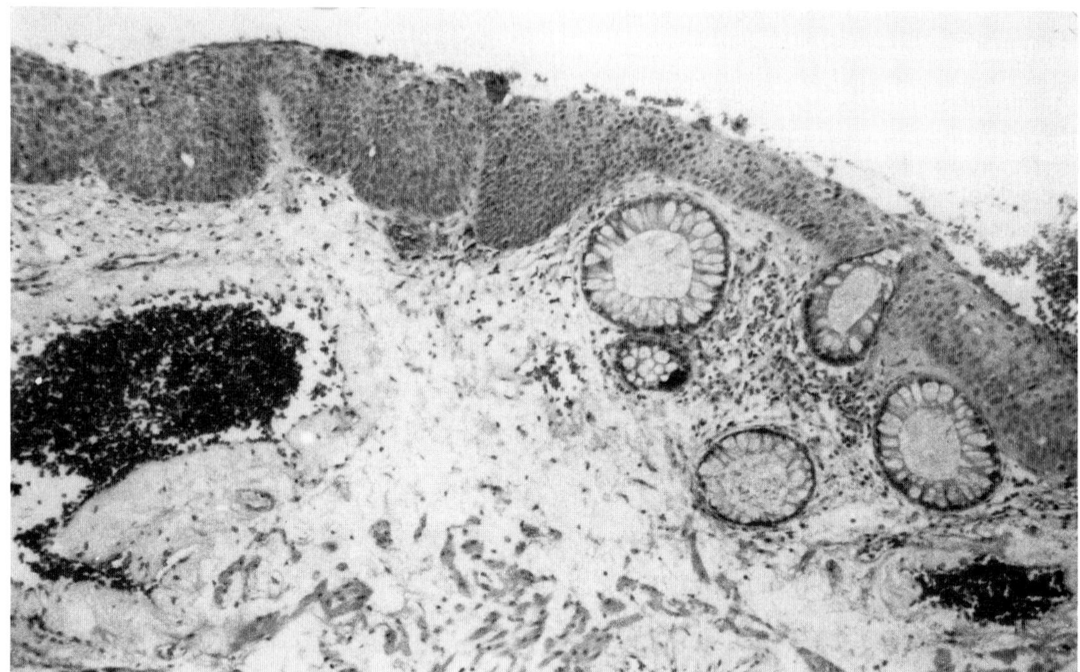

A

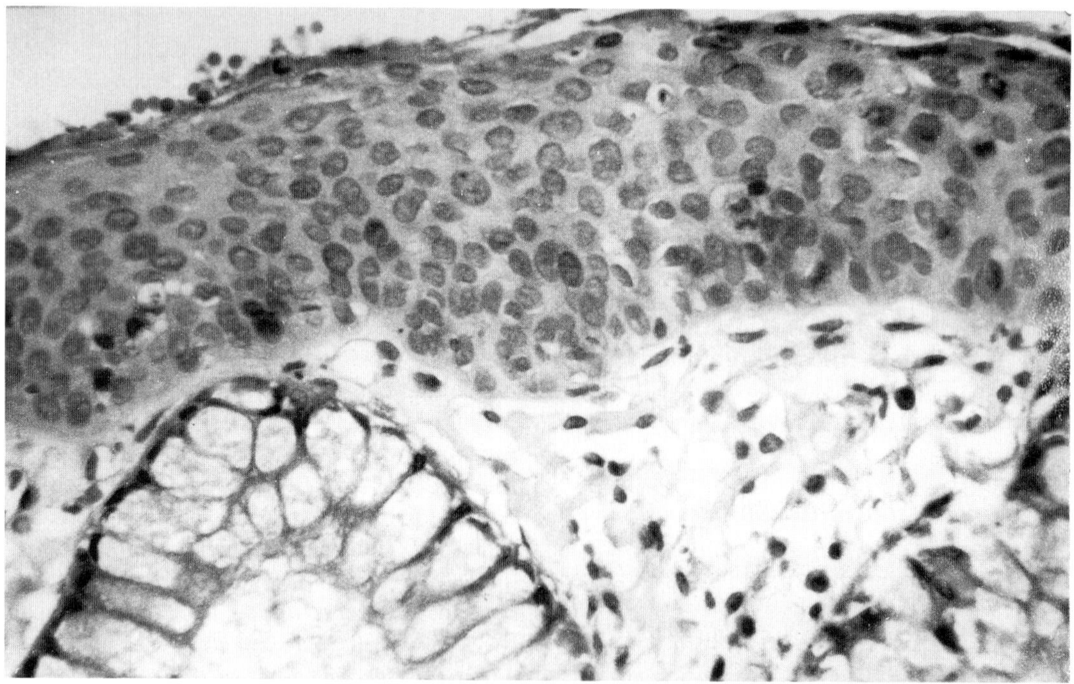

B

Fig. 11-8. Squamous cell dysplasia of the anal epithelium. **(A)** The thickened squamous layer of dysplasia appears at the upper left. **(B)** Closer view of squamous cell dysplasia of the high-grade degree, revealing immature and atypical squamous cells extending high into the layer.

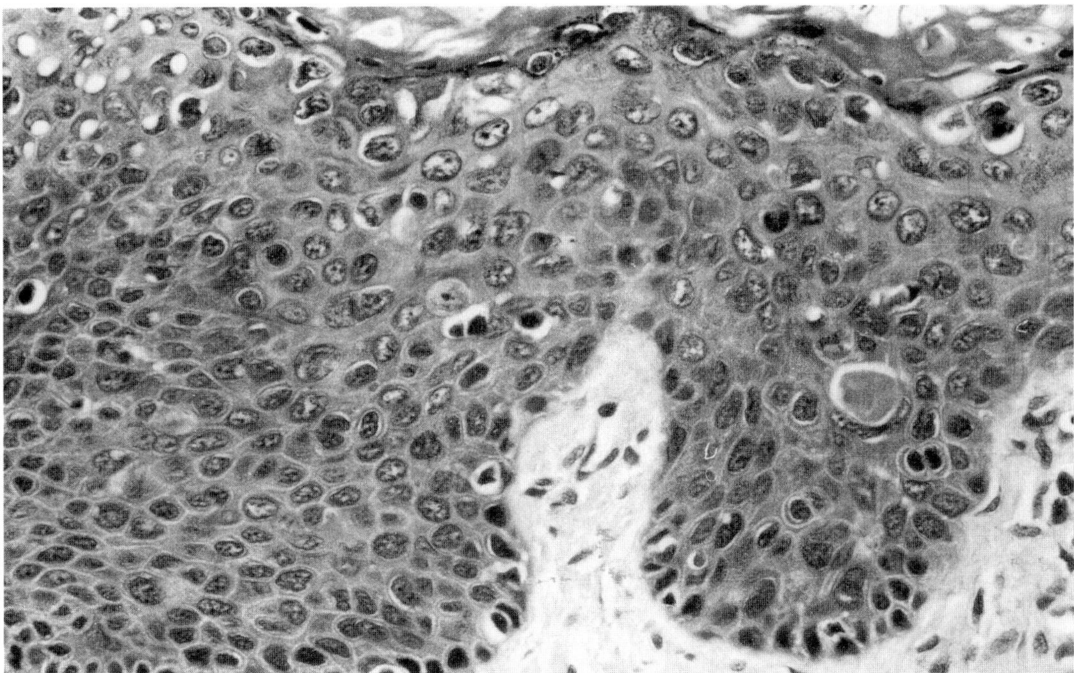

Fig. 11-9. Bowen's disease of the anal epithelium. There is a marked irregularity of the squamous cell nuclei, with several mitoses and extension of atypical cells to the surface (top) (× 425).

clear : cytoplasmic ratio and irregularity in nuclear chromatin.

In addition to the finding of dysplasia or Bowen's disease, the biopsies are scanned for the presence of early invasion into the subepithelial tissue. This is typically in the form of scattered individual cells or small cords.

Features of Squamous Cell Carcinoma

The diagnosis is usually secured by biopsies, and cytologic smears are uncommonly obtained from this area, although they could be helpful in cases with strictures. The carcinomas may be present alone or be associated with squamous cell dysplasia or Bowen's disease.[72, 86–90] The tumors appear as elevated polypoid lesions or more often as ulcerated masses.

Biopsy Features

The invasive areas reveal sheets of malignant cells with prominent pleomorphism and irregular edges, usually in conjunction with marked inflammatory cell infiltrate at the tumor margins (Fig. 11-10). Differentiation is variable, with most tumors showing good squamous cell and keratin production. The surrounding stroma consists of loose mesenchymal tissue together with marked inflammation, which helps in distinguishing the infiltrative tumor from areas of pseudoepitheliomatous hyperplasia. The tumors can be graded by the degree of squamous cell formation, with greater than 75 percent in the well, 25 to 75 percent in the moderately, and less than 25 percent in the poorly differentiated carcinomas. The overall behavior is largely more dependent on the extent of invasion and staging of the tumor. Most of the tumors present in an advanced stage and require extensive radiation therapy and surgery.

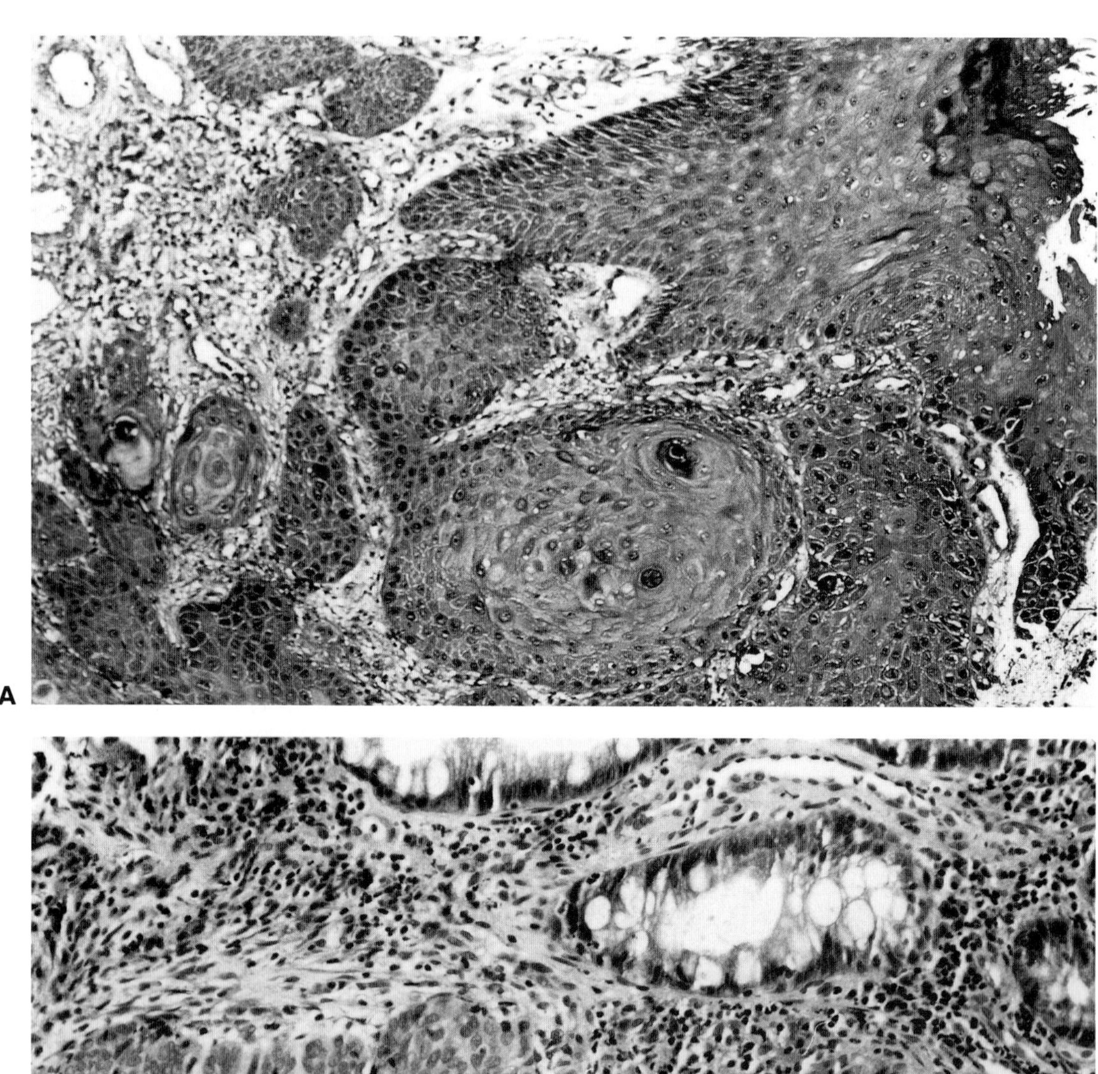

A

B

Fig. 11-10. Squamous cell carcinoma of the anal region. **(A)** Well differentiated squamous cell carcinoma. There are irregular nests of mature tumor cells with invasion into the stroma (left). The surface appears at the right (× 105). **(B)** Example of poorly differentiated squamous cell carcinoma (bottom) that extended into the rectal mucosa (top) (× 210).

The adjacent epithelium frequently shows areas of squamous cell dysplasia and of Bowen's disease. In the dysplastic areas there is the appearance of immature squamous cells that may extend to involve the mid or upper regions of the squamous epithelium, whereas Bowen's disease reveals almost no maturation.

Cytologic Features

The cytologic features of squamous cell carcinoma are similar to those noted in other squamous tissues, such as in the esophagus and cervix (Plates 3A–D). The squamous nature is determined by the central location of the nuclei. Dysplasia is associated with enlargement of the nuclei and total cell size together with the beginning of alteration of chromatin appearance within the nuclei. The carcinoma cells show further increase in nuclear : cytoplasmic ratio, denser chromatin, irregularites in the edge of the nuclei, and greater pleomorphism.

Cloacogenic Carcinoma

The term *cloacogenic carcinoma* is used for the tumors that arise preferentially from the transitional zone at the junction of the lower rectum and the anal canal.[91–93] Overall, they differ from the other squamous cell carcinomas of the anal canal by their location; by the greater histologic variation and types; and by the lack of a strong relation to HPV infection, which may relate to its higher position in the anal area (Table 11-7). Conversely, the behavior of the tumors is very similar to those of the other squamous carcinomas in the anal region, and some investigators have tended to consider the whole group in a similar way.

Biopsy Features

As indicated, these tumors reveal a greater variation in histologic forms, which probably relates to their origin from the transitional zone (Fig. 11-11). Most distinctive is the basaloid pattern in which the carcinoma shows broad sheets or bands of cells that are highly uniform, mainly consisting of nuclei and lacking in much cytologic differentiation. They, therefore, have a superficial resemblance to basal cell tumors but are much more aggressive.[94] Another form is the transitional, or intermediate, cell carcinoma that shows a larger amount of cytoplasm and greater pleomorphism; it may be difficult to distinguish such areas from poorly differentiated squamous tumors. Finally, squamous cell differentiation is seen in one-quarter to one-third of the cases, usually in the form of poorly differentiated squamous cell carcinoma. The more sections one takes of these tumors, the greater likelihood of seeing all forms. Otherwise, the features are typical of invasive carcinomas and show a tumor-type of stroma. Their ultimate behavior is dependent on the degree of invasion.

Commonly seen are regions of in-situ carcinoma involving the adjacent epithelium, as in ordinary squamous cell carcinomas.

Table 11-7. Distinction of Squamous and Cloacogenic Carcinomas

Feature	Squamous	Cloacogenic
Location of tumors	All parts of anal canal and skin	Transitional zone
Histologic types	Squamous	Basaloid, transitional, and squamous
Association with HPV	Yes	No

A
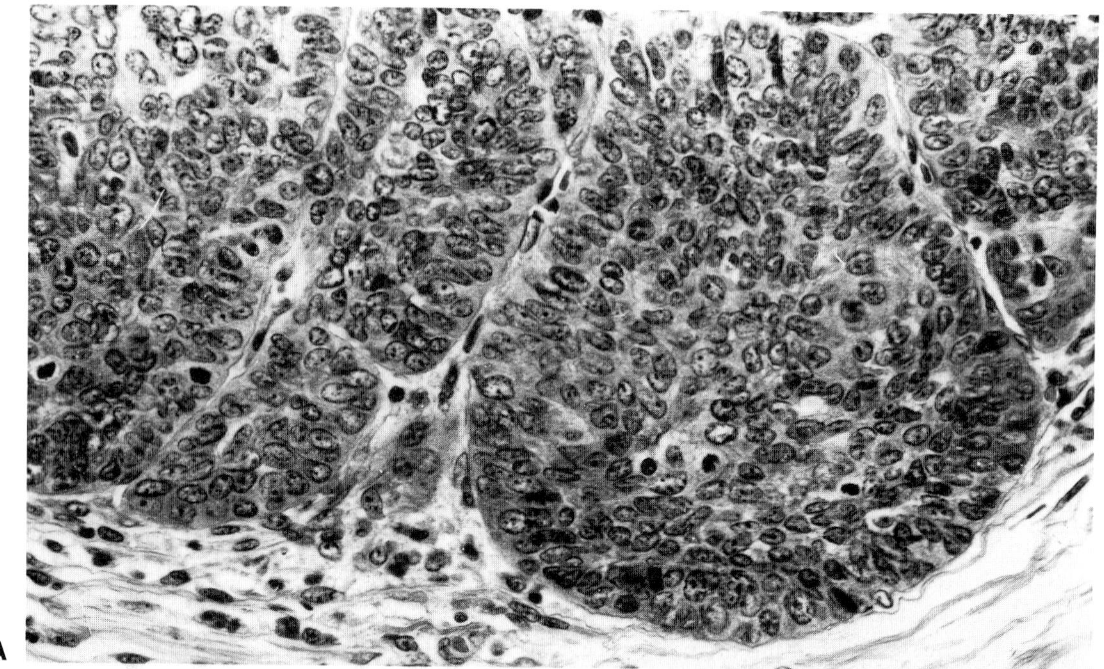

B
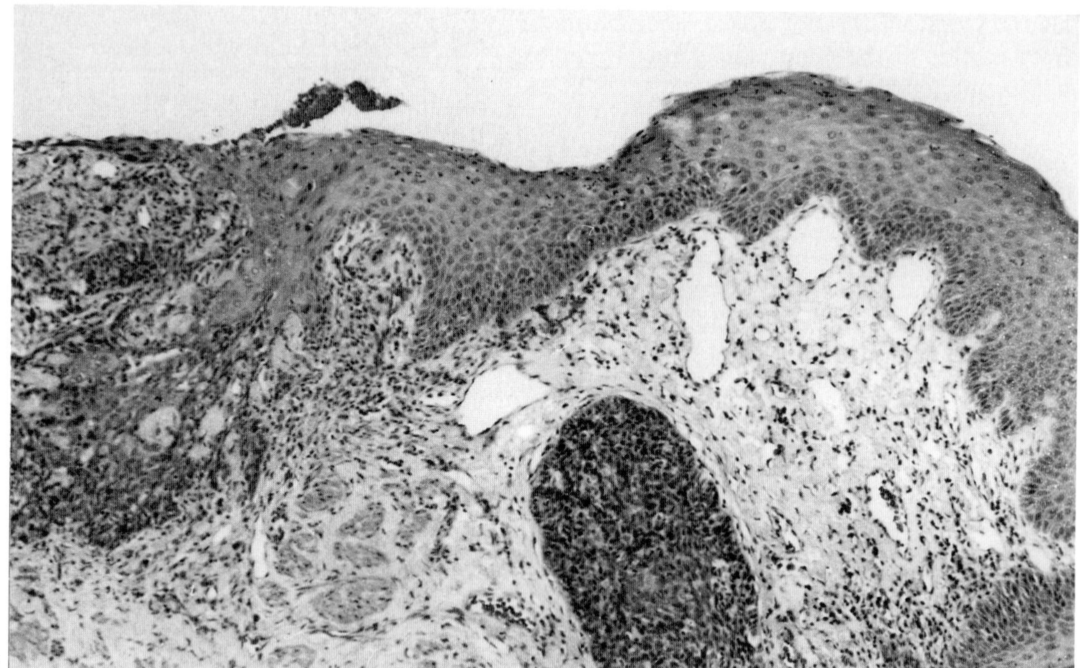

Fig. 11-11. Cloacogenic carcinoma of the anal region. The different histologic types are shown. **(A)** Baseloid pattern (× 425). **(B)** Intermediate (or transitional) type, appearing at the left. A portion of the baseloid form appears at the right (× 105). (*Figure continues.*)

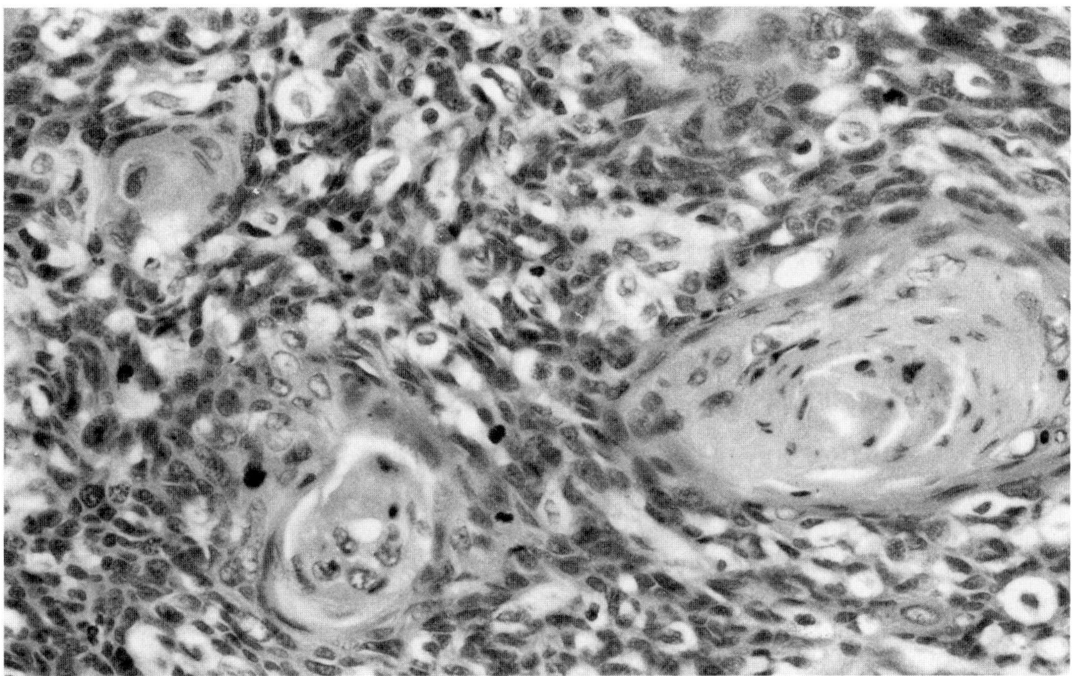

Fig. 11-11 (*Continued*). **(C)** Focus of squamous cell pattern (× 425).

Variant Forms of Squamous Carcinoma

Giant Condylomas

Uncommonly noted are very large condylomas, also referred to as Buschke-Löwenstein lesions.[95, 96] These show the typical features of the condyloma acuminatum with pronounced acanthosis and papillomatosis as well as the cytopathic features of HPV. Because of their very large size and extension of the squamous epithelium into the stroma, it is often difficult to distinguish them from well differentiated carcinoma. Indeed, these cases may develop small foci of carcinoma but still have an excellent prognosis because of the limited invasion. Biopsies generally show the features of a condyloma, and the entire diagnosis is based as well on the size of the lesion. It is best that they be removed because of the strong potential for the development of squamous cell carcinoma.

Verrucous Carcinoma

Verrucous carcinomas represent well differentiated squamous cell carcinomas that grow predominantly into the lumen and are associated with a great deal of mature squamous epithelium and keratin production[96, 97] (see Fig. 3-8). They are more commonly noted in the anal skin but also can occur in the canal region. Biopsies that are superficial may simply show the squamous epithelium without prominent atypism and fail to demonstrate the underlying invasive tumor. Again, one must consider the gross features and attempt to remove any large papillary lesion because of the possible presence of carcinoma.

Spindle Cell Tumor

As in other parts of the gut, the poorly differentiated squamous cell carcinomas can be associated with spindle cells, suggesting a sarcomatous element (see Fig. 3-9). However, these tumors reveal squamous epithelial features by virtue of cytochemical and electron microscopy studies.[98]

OTHER MALIGNANT TUMORS

The other malignant tumors of the anal region are all much less common than the squamous lesions (Table 11-4).

Glandular Tumors

Adenocarcinoma of the Anal Ducts and Glands

Carcinomas rarely develop in the anal ducts and glands.[99, 100] They are most often composed of mucous cells and must be distinguished from tumors that extend down from the rectum (Fig. 11-12). In general, the anal carcinomas contain cells that are more cuboidal, and the mucin tends to be more in the form of the neutral glycoproteins rather than the highly acidic types noted in the colon. The diagnosis is greatly dependent on the location and on the exclusion of an associated rectal tumor. Biopsies show sheets or glands composed of the mucous cells.

Adenocarcinoma in Fistulas

Mucinous adenocarcinomas have been observed in fistulas that involve the perianal region.[38, 39, 48] Some of these are associated with Crohn's disease, and others with longstanding localized anal fistulas. Deeper and larger biopsies are usually needed to detect the tumor because of its location in the wall.

Paget's Disease

Paget's disease is most commonly seen in the breast but can occur wherever apocrine glands are present. They are rarely found in the perianal skin region and are thought to arise in the apocrine glands in that area.[101, 102] Tumor cells extend into the overlying squamous epithelium, including that in the anal canal (Fig. 11-13). Such lesions are more often noted in the lower portion of the anal canal. Identical lesions can be seen in the upper part due to the extension of mucinous carcinoma from the lower rectum[103] (Fig. 11-14).

In either case, the histologic and biopsy features are the same, showing the presence of vacuolated cells scattered throughout the squamous layer. They are more concentrated in the lower region of the epithelium but can be found in the upper parts as well. Noted are enlarged and atypical nuclei indicative of their malignant nature, and the mucinous nature of the vacuoles can be confirmed by special stains, particularly the PAS reaction. The major differential is malignant melanoma, which can also have cells with clear cytoplasm; these stain for S-100 and other melanoma markers and not for mucins. The Paget cells can be in the single form or can appear as larger nodules. The particular origin of the lesion, whether from a rectal mucinous tumor or from an apocrine carcinoma, should be determined by a full examination of the area.

Mucoepidermoid Carcinoma

Mucoepidermoid tumors have rarely been noted in the anal canal and are thought to arise from the anal ducts.[104, 105] Biopsies show an admixture of squamous nests and mucus-producing cells (Fig. 11-15).

Sarcomas

Kaposi's sarcoma can occur in the anal region as well as in other parts of the gut. The lesions are recognized by the compact, atypical spindle cells in association with fresh or old hemorrhages (see Figs. 6-28 and

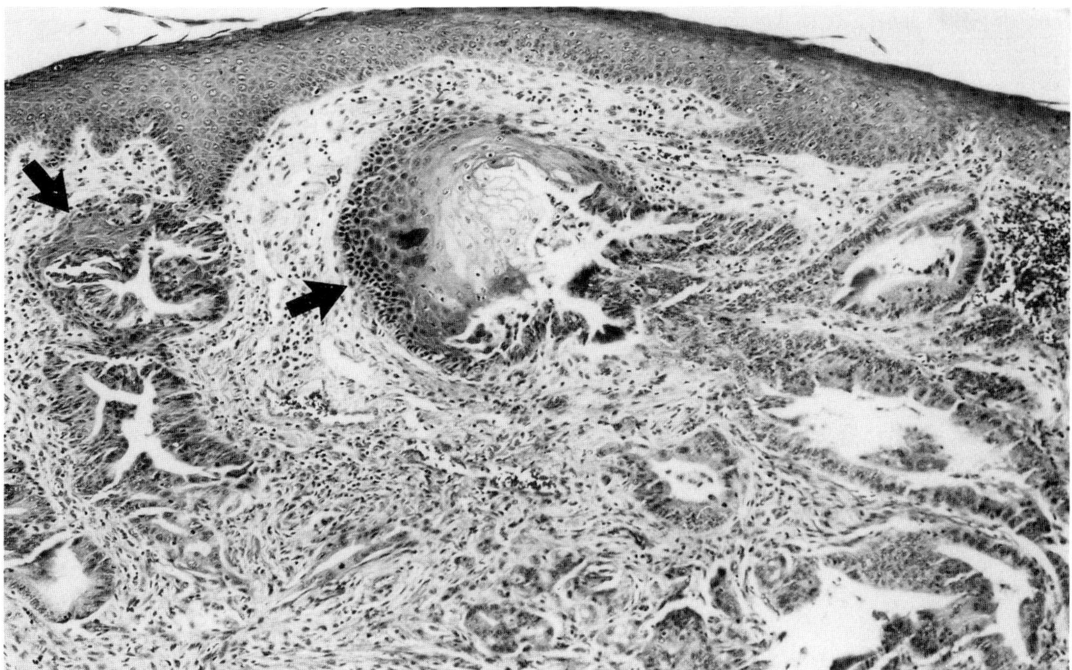

Fig. 11-12. Adenocarcinoma of the anal ducts. There are irregular malignant glands in the stroma, with focal squamous lining closer to the surface (arrows). The squamous epithelium of the anal canal appears at the top (× 105).

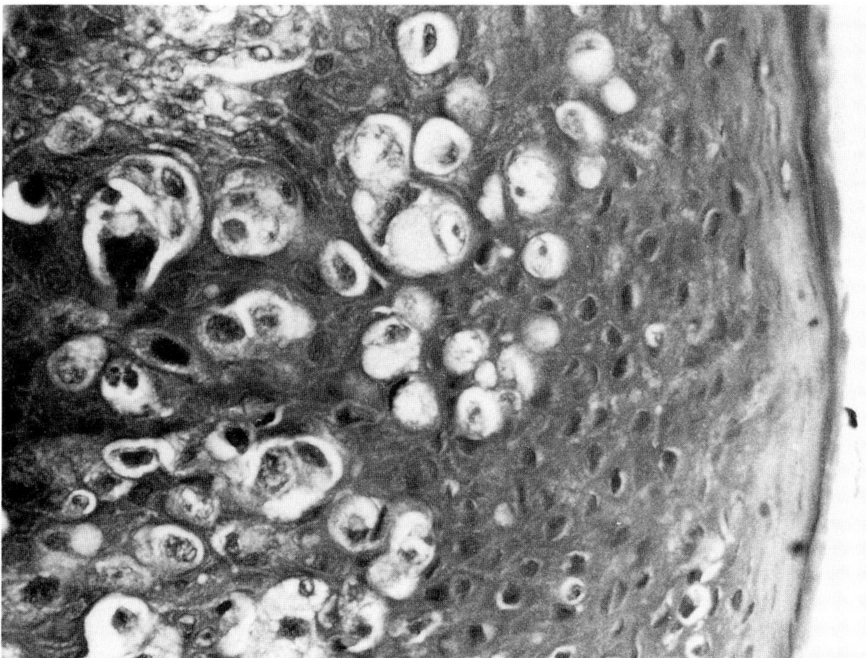

Fig. 11-13. Paget's disease of the anal epithelium. Many large vacuolated cells are noted in the basal and midzonal regions of the squamous layer. The surface appears at the right (× 425).

A

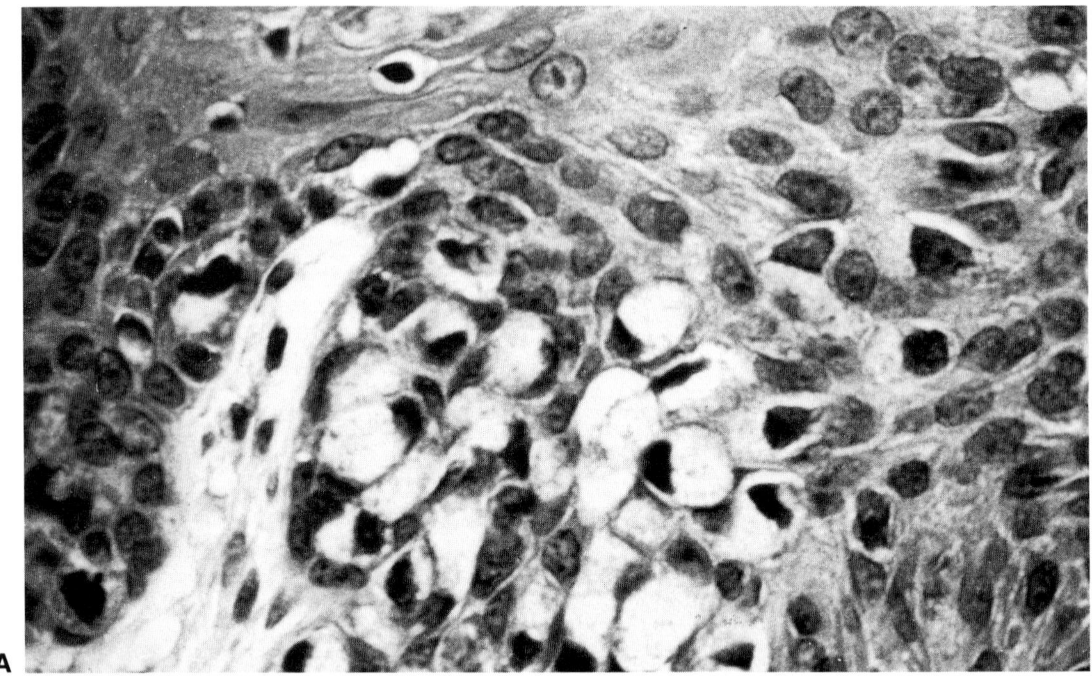

B

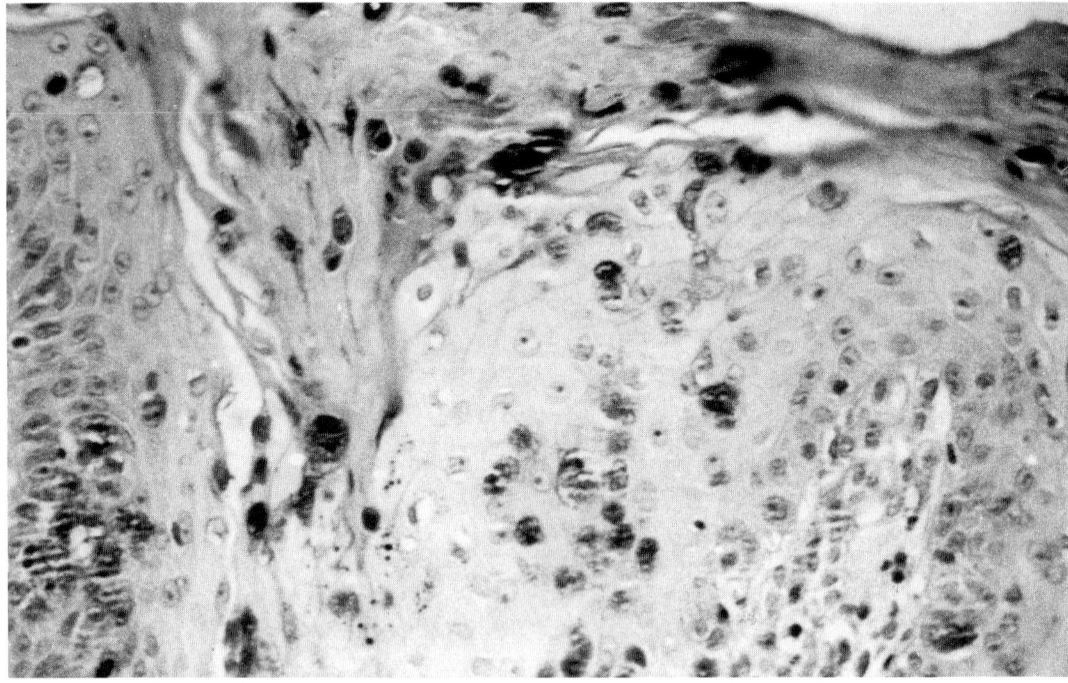

Fig. 11-14. Paget-type disease in the anal canal, secondary to invasion of a mucinous adenocarcinoma of the rectum. **(A)** Noted is a cluster of vacuolated tumor cells in the base of the epithelium (bottom center). **(B)** Mucin stain revealing the numerous tumor cells throughout the squamous layer (periodic acid–Schiff [PAS] reaction).

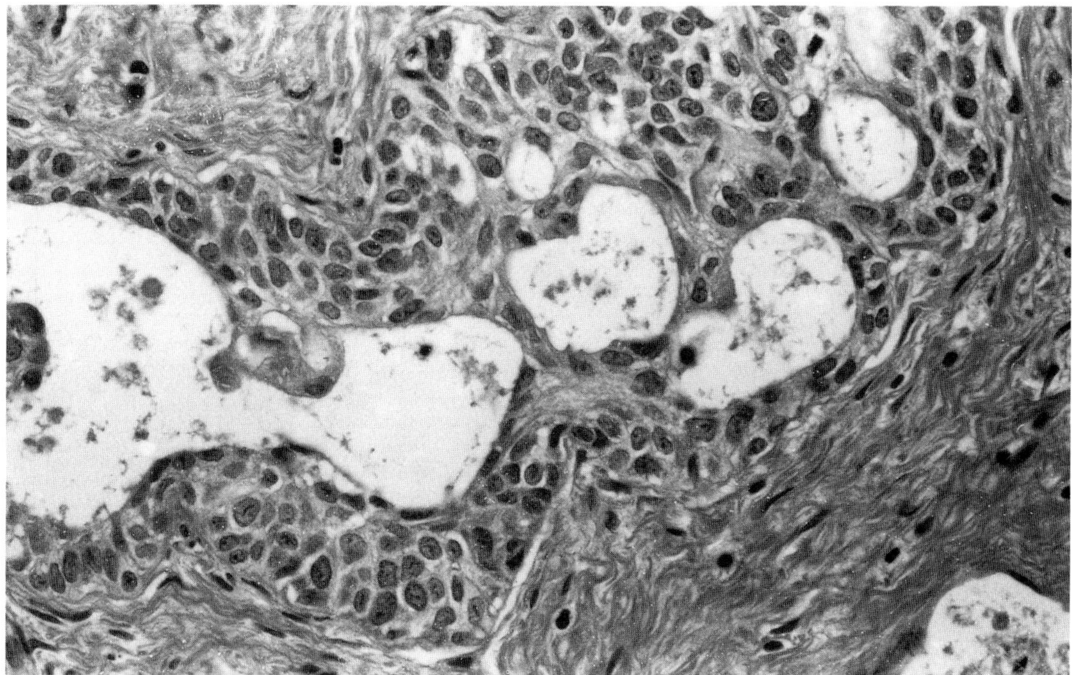

Fig. 11-15. Mucoepidermoid carcinoma of the anal region. The tumor is composed of sheets of immature squamous cells with central areas of mucin formation (× 425).

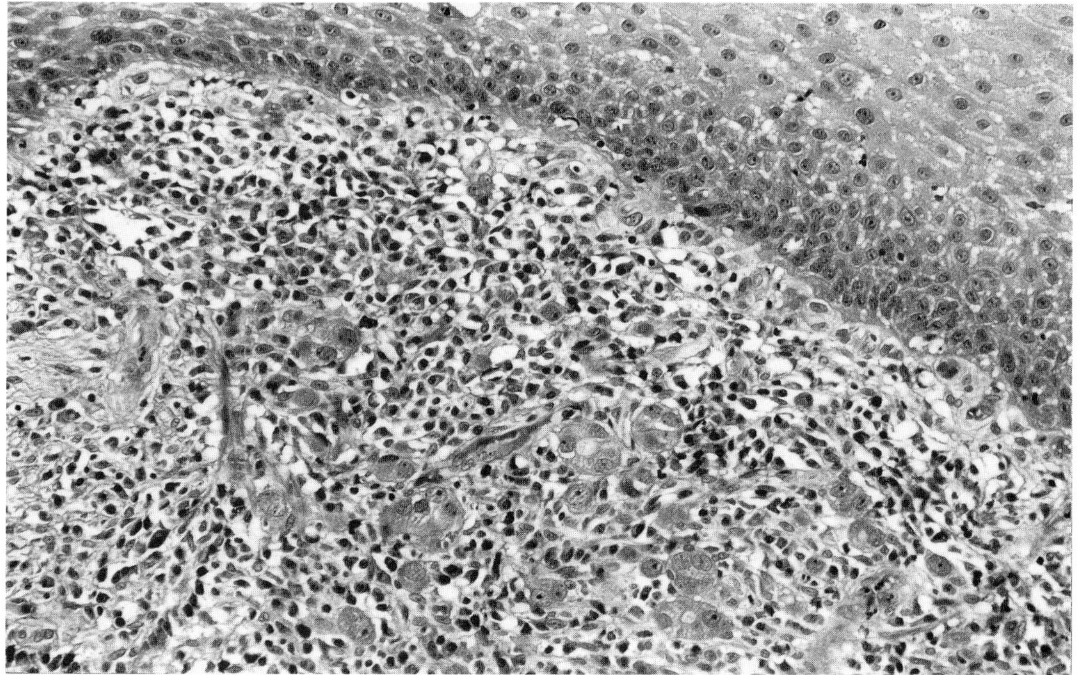

Fig. 11-16. Recurrent rectal carcinoma in the anal area. Noted are scattered, small tumor glands and cells in the subepithelial tissue. A portion of the squamous layer appears at the top (× 210).

10-36). Also noted are embryonal rhabdomyosarcoma or botryoides tumor, presenting as large, fleshy nodules and consisting of spindle cells with prominent stromal edema and focal striated muscle differentiation.[106] These are more common in young females and also can occur in the genital region. Rare instances of other malignant tumors include leiomyosarcoma and alveolar rhabdomyosarcoma.[2, 107]

Other Primary Tumors

Malignant Lymphomas

Malignant lymphomas are more often seen in patients with AIDS.[108, 109] Most tumors are composed of B cells and may be the small or large cell types (see Figs. 7-26 and 10-32). The biopsy diagnosis is usually evident, but it may be necessary to rule out florid lymphoid hyperplasia or other malignant tumors. The former requires cell markers and the latter cytochemical stains, as described in other chapters.

Malignant Melanomas

Malignant melanomas represent a few percent of all of the tumors that occur in the anal region, and arise from the melanocytes that are normally present in the anal canal epithelial tissue.[110–113] The melanomas present with masses or ulcers, and biopsies reveal the typical malignant cells that contain the melanin pigment. The adjacent epithelium frequently shows the junctional melanocytic lesions that are supportive of a primary tumor (see Figs. 3-23 and 3-25).

Small Cell Carinomas

Rarely noted in the anal area are neuroendocrine carcinomas that are derived from the endocrine cells in this area[1, 2] (see Fig. 3-19).

Epidermal Tumors

Epidermal tumors develop from the squamous epithelium in the adjacent perianal skin, and are similar to the tumors that arise in any other portions of the skin in the body. Examples include keratoacanthoma,[114] Bowen's disease,[84, 115] squamous cell carcinoma, and basal cell carcinoma.[94, 116]

Secondary and Metastatic Tumors

Most often noted are the extension of tumors from adjacent organs, particularly mucinous adenocarcinoma from the rectum, transitional cell carcinoma from the urinary bladder, and squamous cell carcinoma from the uterine cervix (Fig. 11-16). Biopsy can be used to detect the tumor and the particular cell type, but the historical information is often needed to define the original site. The anal region can also be rarely involved by systemic infiltrates of tumor, such as leukemia, and from metastases of remote tumors such as breast carcinoma.[1]

REFERENCES

1. Rickert RR: Disorders of the anal region. pp. 888–903. In Ming S-C, Goldman H (eds): Pathology of the Gastrointestinal Tract. WB Saunders, Philadelphia, 1992
2. Sommers SC: Anal canal. pp. 783–805. In Rotterdam H, Sheahan DG, Sommers SC: Biopsy Diagnosis of the Digestive Tract. 2nd Ed. Raven Press, New York, 1993
3. Fenger C: Histology of the anal canal. Am J Surg Pathol 12:41–55, 1988
4. Fenger C, Knoth M: The anal transitional zone: a scanning and transmission electron microscopic investigation of the mucosal surface. Ultrastruct Pathol 2:163–173, 1981
5. Fenger C, Filipe MI: Pathology of the anal glands with special reference to their mucin histochemistry. Acta Pathol Microbiol Scand, Sect A 85:273–285, 1977

6. Fenger C, Lyon H: Endocrine cells and melanin-containing cells in the anal canal epithelium. Histochem J 14:631–639, 1982
7. Santulli TV, Kiesewetter WB, Bill AH Jr: Anorectal anomalies: a suggested international classification. J Pediatr Surg 5:281–287, 1970
8. Bill AH Jr, Johnson RJ: Failure of migration of the rectal opening as the cause for most cases of imperforate anus. Surg Gynecol Obstet 106:643–651, 1958
9. Zarabi CM, Rupani M: Cloacal exstrophy: a hypothesis on the allantoic origin of the distal midgut. Pediatr Pathol 4:117–124, 1985
10. Norris HT: Vascular disorders. pp. 214–239. In Ming S-C, Goldman H (eds): Pathology of the Gastrointestinal Tract. WB Saunders, Philadelphia, 1992
11. Thomson WH: The nature of hemorrhoids. Br J Surg 62:542–552, 1975
12. Haas PA, Fox TA Jr, Haas GP: The pathogenesis of hemorrhoids. Dis Colon Rectum 27:442–450, 1984
13. Foust RL, Dean PJ, Stoler MH, Moinuddin SM: Intraepithelial neoplasia of the anal canal in hemorrhoidal tissue: a study of 19 cases. Hum Pathol 22:528–534, 1991
14. DuBoulay CE, Fairbrother J, Isaacson PG: Mucosal prolapse syndrome—a unifying concept for solitary ulcer syndrome and related disorders. J Clin Pathol 36:1264–1268, 1983
15. Chetty R, Bhathal PS, Slavin JL, Prolapse-induced inflammatory polyps of the colorectum and anal transition zone. Histopathology 23:63–67, 1993
16. Lobert PF, Appelman HD: Inflammatory colacogenic polyp: a unique inflammatory lesion of the anal transitional zone. Am J Surg Pathol 5:761, 1981
17. Saul SH: Inflammatory cloacogenic polyp: relationship to solitary rectal ulcer syndrome/mucosal prolapse and other bowel disorders. Hum Pathol 18:1120, 1987
18. Siegal FP, Lopez C, Hammer GS et al: Anal ulcerative herpes simplex in AIDS. N Engl J Med 305:1439–1444, 1981
19. Goodell SE, Quinn TC, Mertichinian E et al: Herpes simplex virus proctitis in homosexual men. Clinical, sigmoidoscopic and histopathological features. N Engl J Med 308:868–871, 1983
20. Kalb RE, Grossman ME: Chronic perianal herpes simplex in immunocompromised hosts. Am J Med 80:486–490, 1986
21. Wilcox CM, Schwartz DA: Idiopathic anorectal ulceration in patients with human immunodeficiency virus infection. Am J Gastroenterol 89:599–604, 1994
22. Geller SA, Zimmerman MJ, Cohen A: Rectal biopsy in early lymphogranuloma venereum proctitis. Am J Gastroenterol 74:433, 1980
23. Levine JS, Smith PD, Brugge WR: Chronic proctitis in male homosexuals due to lymphogranuloma venereum. Gastroenterology 79:563, 1980
24. Quinn TC, Goodell SE, Mkrtichian EE et al: Chlamydia trachomatis proctitis. N Engl J Med 305:195–200, 1981
25. Felman YM, Nikitas JA: Anorectal gonococcal infection. NY State J Med 80:231–233, 1980
26. Kilpatrick ZM: Gonorrheal proctitis. N Engl J Med 287:967, 1972
27. Samenius B: Primary syphilis of the anorectal region. Dis Colon Rectum 11:462–466, 1968
28. Nepomuceno OR, O'Grady JF, Eisenberg SW et al: Tuberculosis of the anal canal: report of a case. Dis Colon Rectum 14:313–316, 1971
29. Barnes PF, Bloch AB, Davidson PT, Snider DE: Tuberculosis in patients with human immunodeficiency virus infection. N Engl J Med 324:1644–1650, 1991
30. Colby TV: Malakoplakia: two unusual cases which presented diagnostic problems. Am J Surg Pathol 2:377–382, 1978
31. Damjanov I, Katz SM: Malakoplakia. Pathol Annu 16:103, 1981
32. Mortensen NJ, Thomson JP: Perianal abscess due to Enterobius vermicularis: report of a case. Dis Colon Rectum 27:677–678, 1984
33. Vafai M, Mohit P: Granuloma of the anal canal due to Enterobius vermicularis: report of a case. Dis Colon Rectum 26:349–350, 1983
34. Abcarian H, Alexander-Williams J, Christiansen J et al: Benign anorectal disease: definition, characterization and analysis of treatment. Am J Gastroenterol 89:S182–S193, 1994

35. Hanley PH: Anorectal abscess and fistula. Surg Clin North Am 58:487–503, 1978
36. Ramanujam PS, Prasad ML, Abcarian H et al: Perianal abscess and fistula. A study of 1023 patients. Dis Colon Rectum 23:593, 1984
37. Nelson RL, Prasad ML, Abcarian H: Anal carcinoma presenting as a perianal abscess or fistula. Arch Surg 120:632, 1983
38. Jones EA, Morson BC: Mucinous adenocarcinoma in anorectal fistulae. Histopathology 8:279–292, 1984
39. Onerkeun RM: A case of perianal mucinous adenocarcinoma arising in a fistula-in-ano. A clue to the early pathologic diagnosis. Am J Clin Pathol 89:809–812, 1988
40. Goldman H: Ulcerative colitis and Crohn's disease. pp. 643–688. In Ming S-C, Goldman H (eds): Pathology of the Gastrointestinal Tract. WB Saunders, Philadelphia, 1992
41. Rankin GB, Watts HD, Melnyk CS, Kelley MI Jr: National Cooperative Crohn's Disease Study: extraintestinal manifestations and perianal Crohn's. Gastroenterology 77:914–920, 1979
42. Alexander-Williams J, Bachman P: Perianal Crohn's. World J Surg 4:203, 1980
43. Williams DR, Coller JA, Corman ML et al: Anal complications in Crohn's disease. Dis Colon Rectum 24:22–24, 1981
44. Lockhart-Mummery HE: Anal lesions in Crohn's disease. Br J Surg 72:S95–S96, 1985
45. Price AB, Morson BC: Inflammatory bowel disease: the surgical pathology of Crohn's disease and ulcerative colitis. Hum Pathol 6:7, 1975
46. Surawicz CM, Meisel JL, Ylvisaker T et al: Rectal biopsy in the diagnosis of Crohn's disease: value of multiple biopsies and serial sectioning. Gastroenterology 81:66–71, 1981
47. Goldman H: Colonic mucosal biopsy in inflammatory bowel disease. Surg Pathol 4:3–24, 1991
48. Chaikhouni A, Requeyra FI, Stevens JR: Adenocarcinoma in perineal fistulas of Crohn's disease. Dis Colon Rectum 24:639–643, 1981
49. Slater G, Greenstein A, Aufses AH Jr: Anal carcinoma in patients with Crohn's disease. Ann Surg 199:348–350, 1984
50. Connell WR, Sheffield JP, Kamm MA et al: Lower gastrointestinal malignancy in Crohn's disease. Gut 35:347–352, 1994
51. Mazier WP, Sun KM, Robertson WG: Oil-induced granuloma (oleoma) of the rectum. Dis Colon Rectum 21:292–294, 1978
52. Goldman H: Systemic and miscellaneous disorders. pp. 351–380. In Ming S-C, Goldman H (eds): Pathology of the Gastrointestinal Tract. WB Saunders, Philadelphia, 1992
53. Eckardt VF, Kanzler G, Remmele W: Anorectal ergotism: another cause of solitary rectal ulcer. Gastroenterology 91:1123–1127, 1986
54. Culp CE: Chronic hidradenitis suppurativa of the anal canal: a surgical skin disease. Dis Colon Rectum 26:669–676, 1983
55. Patterson JW, Kao GF, Graham JH et al: Bowenoid papulosis. Cancer 57:823–836, 1986
56. Cornes JS, Wallace H, Morson BC: Benign lymphomas of the rectum and anal canal: a study of 100 cases. J Pathol Bacteriol 82:371–382, 1961
57. Leavitt J, Klein I, Kendricks F et al: Skin tags: a cutaneous marker of colonic polyps. Ann Intern Med 98:928–930, 1983
58. Dalton ADA, Coghill SB: No association between skin tags and colorectal adenomas. Lancet 1:1332–1333, 1985
59. Duggan MA, Boras VF, Inoue M et al: Human papillomavirus DNA determination of anal condylomata, dysplasias, and squamous carcinoma with in-situ hybridization. Am J Clin Pathol 92:16–21, 1989
60. Taxy JB, Gupta PK, Gupta JW, Shah KV: Anal cancer. Microscopic condyloma and tissue demonstration of human papillomavirus capsid antigen and viral DNA. Arch Pathol Lab Med 113:1127–1131, 1989
61. Kovi J, Tillman L, Lee SM: Malignant transformation of condyloma acuminatum: a light microscopic and ultrastructural study. Am J Clin Pathol 61:702–710, 1974
62. Rickert RR, Larkey IG, Kantor EB: Granular-cell tumors (myoblastomas) of the anal region. Dis Colon Rectum 21:413–417, 1978
63. Johnston J, Helwig EB: Granular cell tumors of the gastrointestinal tract and perianal region. A study of 74 cases. Dig Dis Sci 26: 807–816, 1981
64. Kalima TV, Peltokallio P: Leiomyoma of the ischioanal region: report of a case. Dis Colon Rectum 11:198–200, 1968

65. Walsh TH, Mann CV: Smooth muscle neoplasms of the rectum and anal canal. Br J Surg 71:597–599, 1984
66. Abel ME, Kingsley AEN, Abcarian H et al: Anorectal neurilemomas. Dis Colon Rectum 28:960–961, 1985
67. Sweeney K, Petrelli N, Herrera L et al: Cavernous hemangioma of the anus. J Surg Oncol 27:286–288, 1984
68. Appelman HD: Mesenchymal tumors of the gastrointestinal tract. pp. 310–350. In Ming S-C, Goldman H (eds): Pathology of the Gastrointestinal Tract. WB Saunders, Philadelphia, 1992
69. Weigand DA, Burgdorf WHC: Perianal apocrine gland adenoma. Arch Dermatol 116: 1051–1053, 1980
70. Assor D, Davis JB: Multiple apocrine fibroadenomas of the anal skin. Am J Clin Pathol 68:397–399, 1977
71. Fenger C: Anal tumors and their precursors. Pathol Annu 23(part 1):45–66, 1988
72. Williams GR, Talbot IC: Anal carcinoma—a histological review. Histopathology 25:507–516, 1994
73. Nash G, Allen W, Nash S: Atypical lesions of the anal mucosa in homosexual men. JAMA 256:873–876, 1986
74. Frazer IH, Crapper RM, Medley G et al: Association between anorectal dysplasia, human papillomavirus, and human immunodeficiency virus infection in homosexual men. Lancet 2:657–660, 1986
75. Frisch M, Olsen JH, Bautz A, Melbye M: Benign anal lesions and the risk of anal cancer. N Engl J Med 331:300–302, 1994
76. Gal AA, Saul SH, Stoler MH: In-situ hybridization analysis of human papillomavirus in anal squamous cell carcinoma. Modern Pathol 2:439–443, 1989
77. Scholefield JH, Shepherd NA, Miller KJ et al: Human papillomavirus type 16 DNA in anal cancers from six different countries. Gut 32:674–676, 1991
78. Duggan MA, Boras VF, Inoue M, McGregor SE: Human papillomavirus DNA in anal carcinomas. Comparison of in-situ and dot blot hybridization. Am J Clin Pathol 96:318–325, 1991
79. Zaki SR, Judd R, Coffield LM et al: Human papillomavirus infection and anal carcinoma. Retrospective analysis by in-situ hybridization and the polymerase chain reaction. Am J Pathol 140:1345–1355, 1992
80. Walts AE, Koeffler P, Said JW: Localization of p53 protein and human papillomavirus in anogenital squamous lesions. Immunohistochemical and in-situ hybridization studies in benign, dysplastic, and malignant epithelia. Hum Pathol 24:1238–1242, 1993
81. Fenger C, Nielsen VT: Precancerous changes in the anal canal epithelium in resection specimens. Acta Pathol Microbiol Immunol Scand 94:63–69, 1986
82. Surawicz CM, Kirby P, Critchlow C et al: Anal dysplasia in homosexual men: role of anoscopy and biopsy. Gastroenterology 105:658–666, 1993
83. Scoma JA, Levy EI: Bowen's disease of the anus: report of two cases. Dis Colon Rectum 18:137–140, 1975
84. Strauss RJ, Fazio VW: Bowen's disease of the anal and perianal area. A report and analysis of twelve cases. Am J Surg 137:231–234, 1979
85. Croxson T, Chabon AB, Rorat E, Barash IM: Intraepithelial carcinoma of the anus in homosexual men. Dis Colon Rectum 27: 325–330, 1984
86. Morson BC, Pang LSC: Pathology of anal cancer. Proc Roy Soc Med London 61:623–624, 1968
87. Boman BM, Moertel CG, O'Connell MJ et al: Carcioma of the anal canal: a clinical and pathologic study of 188 cases. Cancer 54: 114–125, 1984
88. Dougherty BG, Evans HL: Carcinoma of the anal canal: a study of 79 cases. Am J Clin Pathol 83:159–164, 1985
89. Greenall MJ, Quan SHQ, Stearns MW et al: Epidermoid cancer of the anal margin: pathologic features, treatment, and clinical results. Am J Surg 149:95–100, 1985
90. Papillon J, Montbaron JT: Epidermoid carcinoma of the anal canal: a series of 276 cases. Dis Colon Rectum 30:324–333, 1987
91. Serota AI, Weil M, Williams RA et al: Anal cloacogenic carcinoma. Classification and clinical behavior. Arch Surg 116:456–459, 1981
92. Wolber R, Dupuis B, Thiyagaratnam P, Owen D: Anal cloacogenic and squamous carcinomas: comparative histogenic analysis using in-situ hybridization for human papil-

lomavirus DNA. Am J Surg Pathol 14:176–182, 1990
93. Aparacio-Duque R, Mittal KR, Chan W, Schinella R: Cloacogenic carcinoma of the anal canal and associated viral lesions. An in-situ hybridization study for human papillomavirus. Cancer 68:2422–2425, 1991
94. White WB, Schneiderman H, Sayre JT: Basal cell carcinoma of the anus: clinical and pathological distinction from cloacogenic carcinoma. J Clin Gastroenterol 6:441–446, 1984
95. Alexander RM, Kaminsky DB: Giant condyloma acuminatum (Buschke-Löwenstein tumor) of the anus: case report and review of the literature. Dis Colon Rectum 22:561–565, 1979
96. Bogomoletz WV, Potet F, Molas G: Condylomata acuminata, giant condyloma acuminatum (Buschke-Loewenstein tumor) and verrucous squamous carcinoma of the perianal and anorectal region: a continuous precancerous spectrum? Histopathology 9: 1155–1169, 1985
97. Gingrass RJ, Burbrick MP, Hitchcock CR et al: Anorectal verrucose squamous carcinoma: report of two cases. Dis Colon Rectum 21:120–122, 1978
98. Kalogeropoulos NK, Antonakopoulos GN, Agapitos MB, Papacharalampoulos NX: Spindle cell carcinoma (pseudosarcoma) of the anus: a light, electron microscopic and immunocytochemical study of a case. Histopathology 9:987–994, 1985.
99. Lee SH, Zucker M, Sato T: Primary adenocarcinoma of an anal gland with secondary perianal fistulas. Hum Pathol 12:1034–1036, 1981
100. Jensen SL, Shokouli-Amiri MH, Hagen K et al: Adenocarcinoma of the anal ducts. Dis Colon Rectum 31:268–272, 1988
101. Helwig EB, Graham JH: Anogenital (extramammary) Paget's disease. Cancer 16:387–403, 1963
102. Merot Y, Mazoujian G, Pinkus G et al: Extramammary Paget's disease of the perianal and perineal regions: evidence of apocrine derivation. Arch Dermatol 121:750–752, 1985
103. Arminski TC, Pollard RJ: Paget's disease of the anus secondary to malignant papillary adenoma of the rectum. Dis Colon Rectum 16:46–55, 1973
104. Morson BC, Volkstadt H: Mucoepidermoid tumors of the anal canal. J Clin Pathol 16: 200–205, 1963
105. Seidenverg N, Kleinihenz RJ: Mucoepidermoid carcinoma of the anus. Am J Surg 117:413–415, 1969
106. Srouji MN, Donaldson MH, Chatten J, Koblenzer CS: Perianal rhabdomyosarcoma in childhood. Cancer 38:1008–1012, 1976
107. Ueyama T, Hashimoto H, Tsuneyoshi M: Leiomyosarcoma of the anus. A clinicopathologic and immunohistochemical study. Int J Surg Pathol 1:221–226, 1994
108. Lee MH, Waxman M, Gillooley JF: Primary malignant lymphoma of the anorectum in homosexual men. Dis Colon Rectum 29: 413–416, 1986
109. Ioachim HL, Weinstein MA, Robbins RD et al: Primary anorectal lymphoma. A new manifestation of the acquired immune deficiency syndrome (AIDS). Cancer 60:1449–1453, 1987
110. Morson BC, Volkstadt H: Malignant melanoma of the anal canal. J Clin Pathol 16: 126–132, 1963
111. Chiu YS, Unni KK, Beart RW Jr: Malignant melanoma of the anorectum. Dis Colon Rectum 23:122–124, 1980
112. Wanebo HJ, Woodruff JM, Farr GH, Quan SH: Anorectal melanoma. Cancer 47:1891–1900, 1981
113. Cooper PH, Miels SE, Allen MS Jr: Malignant melanoma of the anus. Report of 12 patients and analysis of 255 additional cases. Dis Colon Rectum 25:693–703, 1982
114. Jensen SL, Sjolin K-E: Keratocanthoma of the anus: report of three cases. Dis Colon Rectum 28:743–745, 1985
115. Beck DE, Fazio VW, Jagelman DG et al: Perianal Bowen's disease. Dis Colon Rectum 31:419–422, 1988
116. Nielsen OV, Jensen SL: Basal cell carcinoma of the anus: a clinical study of 34 cases. Br J Surg 68:856–857, 1981

Appendix

Electron Microscopic Illustrations

Index

Note: *Page numbers followed by an* f *denote figures; those followed by a* t *denote tables.*